CARDIOLOGY
1999

James T. Willerson, MD

William C. Roberts, MD

Charles E. Rackley, MD

Thomas P. Graham, Jr., MD

Dean T. Mason, MD

William W. Parmley, MD

Published by
Futura Publishing Company, Inc.
135 Bedford Road
Armonk, New York 10504

ISBN #: 0-87993-431-X
ISSN #: 0275-0066

Cardiology
1999

JAMES T. WILLERSON, MD
Edward Randall III Professor and Chairman
Department of Internal Medicine
The University of Texas—Houston Medical School
Chief of Medical Service
Hermann Hospital
Medical Director, Chief of Cardiology,
and Director of Cardiology Research
Texas Heart Institute
Chief of Cardiology, St. Luke's Episcopal Hospital
Houston, Texas
Editor in Chief, Circulation

William C. Roberts, MD
Executive Director
Baylor Cardiovascular Institute
Dean, A. Webb Roberts Center
for Continuing Education
Baylor University Medical Center
Dallas, Texas
Editor in Chief, The American Journal
of Cardiology
Editor in Chief, The Baylor University
Medical Center Proceedings

Charles E. Rackley, MD
Professor of Medicine
Division of Cardiology
Department of Medicine
Georgetown University Medical Center
Washington, D.C.

Thomas P. Graham, Jr., MD
Professor of Pediatrics
Ann & Monroe Carell Family
Professor of Pediatric Cardiology
Director of Pediatric Cardiology
Vanderbilt University Medical Center
Nashville, Tennessee

Dean T. Mason, MD
Physician in Chief, Western Heart Institute
Chairman, Department of
Cardiovascular Medicine
St. Mary's Medical Center
at Golden Gate Park, San Francisco
San Francisco, California

William W. Parmley, MD
Professor of Medicine
University of California
San Francisco, School of Medicine
San Francisco, California
Editor in Chief, Journal of the
American College of Cardiology

Futura Publishing
Company, Inc.
Armonk, NY

Preface

Cardiology 1999, the 19th volume to be published in this series, is a compilation of approximately 700 summaries highlighting the major developments in the cardiology literature from November 1997 to October 1998. The book is intended to serve as an overview of current trends and developments in clinical cardiovascular medicine.

Prominent topics in *Cardiology 1999* include interventional procedures used to treat coronary heart disease and peripheral atherosclerosis; infections and inflammation and their association with coronary heart disease; discussions concerning the importance of homocysteine and its role in promoting atherosclerosis; surgical bypass procedures; and developments in the treatment of congestive heart failure. Further emphasis has also been given to the antiplatelet therapies, especially the inhibitors of the platelet glycoprotein IIb/IIIa receptors.

Coronary stenting continues to increase in usage with and without associated radiotherapy. Local radiation therapy may be efficacious in reducing the risk of restenosis lesions and is relatively safe during short-term follow-up.

An attempt has been made to summarize the most important developments that have been presented in the major journals of cardiovascular medicine, including abstracts selected from *The New England Journal of Medicine; The Lancet; Circulation; Journal of the American College of Cardiology; Arteriosclerosis, Thrombosis, and Vascular Biology; American Heart Journal;* and *The American Journal of Cardiology.*

Cardiology 1999 also presents recent interviews of leaders of American cardiovascular medicine/surgery by Dr. William Roberts, editor of *The American Journal of Cardiology,* following *Cardiology 1998* in which similar interviews were made available. The editors of *Cardiology 1999* are pleased to be able to make these interviews of selected leaders of American cardiovascular medicine available in one volume.

We believe that *Cardiology 1999* will prove useful to all interested in clinical cardiovascular medicine. The summaries of major advances abstracted from leading journals of cardiovascular medicine should serve as a rich and permanent referral source for all who care for patients with these problems.

James T. Willerson, MD

Acknowledgments

The contributors to *Cardiology 1999* have attempted to identify and present recent developments from the literature to create this volume of important trends in the field of cardiology. Dr. Robert's articles were chosen from *The American Journal of Cardiology;* Dr. Rackley's were from *Arteriosclerosis, Thrombosis, and Vascular Biology;* Dr. Mason's from the *American Heart Journal*; and Dr. Parmley's were from the *Journal of the American College of Cardiology.* Dr. Graham's selections for the pediatric section were taken from a variety of medical journals. My summaries were from *Circulation, The New England Journal of Medicine,* and *The Lancet.*

In addition to the painstaking task of selection, several individuals also assisted in preparing these summaries for publication. We are grateful to Suzy Lanier for editorial assistance and to Barbara Capps, Joy Phillips, Linda Maddox, Dorothy Molero, and Angie Esquivel for typing the summaries in this volume. We also are grateful to Linda Shaw of Futura Publishing Company for editorial coordination of this project.

We continue to owe many thanks to Dr. William C. Roberts for having served as editor of this volume for 16 years. Additionally, I would like to thank Futura Publishing Company for continuing their tradition of excellence in bringing this book to the medical community.

James T. Willerson, MD

Contents

Conversion of Units

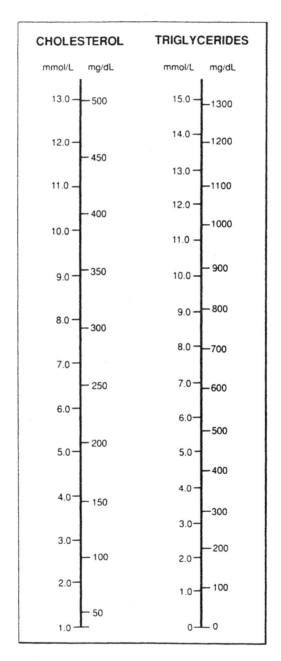

Cholesterol mg/dL = mmol/L x 38.6
Triglyceride mg/dL = mmol/L x 88.5

1
Atherothrombosclerosis

Biology of Atherosclerotic Plaques

Apoptosis and Related Proteins in Plaques

Kockx and colleagues[1] in Antwerp, Belgium, investigated the distribution of apoptotic cell death and apoptotic-related proteins in early and advanced atherosclerotic lesions. They used whole-mount carotid endarterectomy specimens (n = 18) to evaluate these variables in human atherosclerotic plaques. This approach allowed a comparison of adaptive intimal thickenings, fatty streak, and advanced atherosclerotic plaques in the same patient. The fatty streaks differed from adaptive intimal thickening by the presence of Bax, a proapoptotic protein of the BC1-2 family. Both regions were composed heavily of smooth muscle cells and macrophage infiltration was not at a high level. Apoptosis, as detected by DNA *in situ* end labeling and *in situ* nick translation was not present in these regions. Apoptosis of smooth muscle cells and macrophages, however, was present in advanced atherosclerotic plaques that were present mainly in the carotid sinus. A dense infiltration of macrophages was present in these advanced atherosclerotic plaques. Cytoplasmic remnants of apoptotic smooth muscle cells enclosed by a cage of thickened basal lamina were TUNEL negative and remained present in the plaques as matrix vesicles. The authors conclude that smooth muscle cells within human fatty streaks express Bax, which increases the susceptibility of these cells to undergo apoptosis. The localization of these susceptible smooth muscle cells in the deep layer of the fatty streaks might be important in the understanding of transition of fatty streaks into atherosclerotic plaques, which are characterized by regions of cell death (Figure 1-1).

Fas in Human Atherosclerotic Intima

The membrane protein Fas apolipoprotein-1 CD95 signals program cell death or apoptosis in activated T lymphocytes. Vascular smooth muscle cells bear markers for programmed cell death or apoptosis in advanced atherosclerotic plaques that contain immune cells, *e.g.*, macrophages and T lymphocytes. A study by Geng and coworkers[2] in Boston, Massachusetts, tested the hypothesis that the Fas death-signaling pathways contributed to apoptosis of smooth muscle cells exposed to pro-inflammatory cytokines produced by these immune cells during atherogenesis. All human carotid atherosclerotic plaques examined contain immunoreactive Fas. The majority of the Fas positive smooth muscle cells localized in the intima of the plaques, whereas the medial

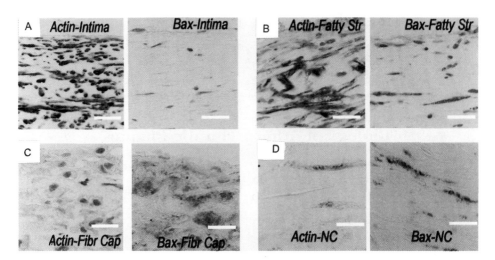

FIGURE 1-1. α-SMC actin expression and Bax expression in 4 different regions of a carotid endarterectomy specimen. **(A)** Adaptive intimal thickening. The SMCs show α-SMC actin but do not express Bax. **(B)** Fatty streak. Most SMCs express α-SMC actin and contain lipid vacuoles. These smooth muscle are immunoreactive for Bax. Scattered mononuclear cells, which are negative for Bax, are present. **(C)** Fibrous cap of an unstable atherosclerotic plaque. Residual smooth muscle can be detected between the foam cells. The foam cells are of macrophage origin, as detected by their expression for CD68 (not shown), and are immunoreactive for Bax. **(D)** Region within the necrotic core. Empty splitlike spaces or spaces filled with cytoplasmic remnants are present. These cytoplasmic remnants contain remnants that are immunoreactive for α-SMC actin and are often surrounded by a prominent cage of PAS, indicating their SMC origin. These cytoplasmic remnants are associated with matrix vesicles and are immunoreactive for Bax. Scale bar = 30 μm. Reproduced with permission from Kockx et al.[1]

smooth muscle cells expressed Fas antigen less prominently. Double staining for DNA fragments (TUNEL) and Fas or cell identification markers co-localized Fas with TUNEL positive smooth muscle cells in the areas that contain CD3 T cells and CD68 macrophages, suggesting a role for Fas in the induction of smooth muscle cell apoptosis by activated T cells during atherogenesis. In culture, stimulation with interferon-γ, tumor necrosis factor-α, and interleukin-1β increased expression of Fas in smooth muscle cells. Incubation with an activating anti-Fas antibody triggered apoptosis of the cytokine-primed, but not the untreated smooth muscle cells, as demonstrated by TUNEL and electrophoresis of oligonucleosomal DNA fragments. These data suggest that activation of the Fas death-signaling pathway contributes to the induction of smooth muscle cell apoptosis during atherogenesis and furnished a mechanism whereby immune cells and their cytokines promoted the cell death process related to vascular remodeling and plaque rupture.

Location of Phospholipase A₂ in Arterial Tissue

Romano and coinvestigators[3] in Gotenborg, Sweden, recently reported on the immunolocalization of type 2 secretory nonpancreatic phospholipase A_2

in human atherosclerotic lesions. In a subsequent study, the investigators presented data on the distribution and ultrastructural localization of phospholipase A_2 in adjacent nonatherosclerotic and atherosclerotic regions of human arteries. Electron microscopy of immunogold labeling techniques with a monoclonal antibody was used to analyze arterial tissue. The human specimens analyzed were obtained from autopsy and surgery cases. The results with electron microscopy showed a stronger phospholipase A_2 immunoreactivity in regions of arteries with atherosclerotic lesions than in regions without lesions in the same individuals. Phospholipase A_2 immunoreactivity was stronger in the arterial intima of atherosclerotic tissue than of nonatherosclerotic tissue. Electron microscopy–immunogold examination revealed that phospholipase A_2 was primarily localized along the extracellular matrix and was associated with collagen fibers and other extracellular matrix structures. Intracellular phospholipase A_2 was observed in electron-dense vesicals in intimal cells. Phospholipase A_2 was also found in contact with large, extracellular lipid droplets (Figure 1-2). These results support the hypotheses that extracellular phospholipase A_2 is localized at sites where it may hydrolyze phospholipids from lipoprotein and lipid aggregates retained in the extracellular matrix of the arterial wall. This may be a mechanism for *in situ* release of pro-inflammatory lipids, free fatty

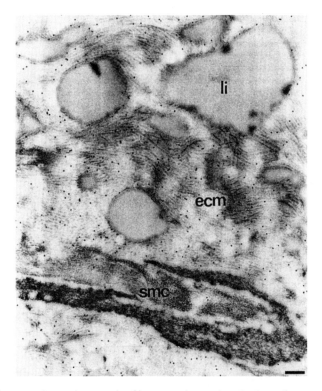

FIGURE 1-2. Electron photomicrograph of human atherosclerotic tissue from a coronary artery showing ultrastructural labeling pattern obtained with an mAb against snpPLA$_2$. Immunogold particles are found associated with the ECM (ecm) and in close proximity to lipid droplets (li). Original magnification, ×35,000; scale bar = 286 nm. Reproduced with permission from Romano et al.[3]

acids, and lysophosphatidylcholine in regions of apolipoprotein B accumulation, which are abundant in atherosclerotic lesions.

Macrophages Sustain Atheroma

Activated resident macrophages sustain atheroma, and a higher macrophage amount is associated with plaque vulnerability. Factors leading to differentiation and activation of these blood-derived cells remained largely uncharacterized. Wesley and colleagues[4] in Atlanta, Georgia, investigated the contribution of interaction with collagen type 1, the predominant component of atherosclerotic matrix, to differentiation and modulation of characteristic macrophage functions, including intracellular lipid accumulation and production of the typical matrix-degrading enzyme matrix metalloproteinase-9. When used as an adhesion substrate for human peripheral blood monocytes *in vitro*, collagen type 1 increased monocyte differentiation, assessed by analysis of CD71 expression and cell spreading. Culturing on collagen type 1 doubled the number of differentiated monocytes at 24 hours and was a stronger stimulus for differentiation than phorbol myristate acetate, a known inducer of monocyte differentiation. The effect of substrate on intracellular accumulation of modified lipoproteins was assessed by quantitative confocal microscopy of monocytes incubated with fluorescent acetylated LDL. The collagen type 1 substrate also doubled the number of macrophages containing intracellular lipid and significantly increased the individual intracellular loading. Monocytes cultured on collagen type 1 also released more matrix metalloproteinase-9 than did cells plated directly on plastic. The role of monocyte spreading was further assessed by treatment with colchicine, an inhibitor of cytoskeletal function or with genistein, a nonspecific inhibitor of tyrosine kinases, shown to participate in cell adhesion. Cell spreading was inhibited in 72% of colchicine-treated and in 62% of genistein-treated monocytes (Figure 1-3). The same conditions also decreased secretion of matrix metalloproteinase-9 and genistein reduced the number of acetylated LDL-containing cells. These data show a strong correlation between monocyte spreading on collagen type 1 and intracellular lipid accumulation. These results indicate that interaction with vascular matrix may play an important role in differentiation of peripheral blood monocytes into resident lipid-laden macrophages, which act as central simulators throughout the natural history of atheroma.

Oxidation of Lipids/Antioxidants

Restoration of Nitric Oxide Activity in Familial Hypercholesterolemia

Impaired NO activity is an early event in the pathogenesis of cardiovascular disease, resulting either from reduced formation or increased degradation.

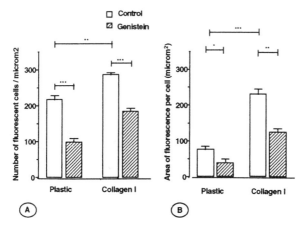

FIGURE 1-3. Inhibition of monocyte spreading abolishes the enhancing effect of collagen type 1 on intracellular lipid loading in cultured monocytes. Inhibition of protein phosphorylation reduced intracellular accumulation of fluorescently labeled (DiI)-acLDL in monocytes. Genistein treatment abolished increase in lipid accumulation caused by culturing monocytes on a collagen type 1 substrate. Treatment reduced total number of cells that accumulated fluorescent acLDL (A) and individual cell loading, as assessed by measurement of fluorescence area per labeled cell (B). Columns show mean values obtained from image analysis of confocal microscopy data ±SEM from a representative experiment. ***$p < .001$, **$p < .01$, * $p < .05$. Three independent experiments showed similar results. Reproduced with permission from Wesley et al.[4]

Tetrahydrobiopterin, an essential co-factor for NO production, can restore NO activity in familial hypercholesterolemia. Verhaar and colleagues[5] from Amsterdam, The Netherlands, hypothesized that administration of 5-methyltetrahydrofolate (5-MTHF), the active circulating form of folate, might improve NO formation in familial hypercholesterolemia. They studied the effects of 5-MTHF on NO bioavailability *in vivo* in 10 patients with familial hypocholesterolemia and 10 matched control subjects by venous occlusion plethysmography, using serotonin and nitroprusside as endothelium-dependent and -independent vasodilators. They investigated the effect of 5-MTHF on NO production by recombinant endothelial NO synthase by use of [³H]arginine to [³H]citrulline conversion. They also studied the effects of 5-MTHF on superoxide generation by endothelial NO synthase and xanthine oxidase by use of lucigenin chemiluminescence. The impaired endothelium-dependent vasodilation in familial hypocholesterolemia could be reversed by co-infusion of 5-MTHF, whereas 5-MTHF had no significant effect on the endothelium-dependent vasodilation in control subjects. 5-MTHF did not influence basal forearm vasomotion of endothelium-independent vasodilation. 5-MTHF had no direct effect on *in vitro* NO production by endothelial NO synthase. However, the authors did observe a dose-dependent reduction in both endothelium NO synthase and xanthine oxidase-induced superoxide generation. These data suggest that the active form of folic acid restores *in vivo* endothelial function in patients with familial hypocholesterolemia. The data also suggest that this effect is due to reduced catabolism of NO (Figure 1-4).

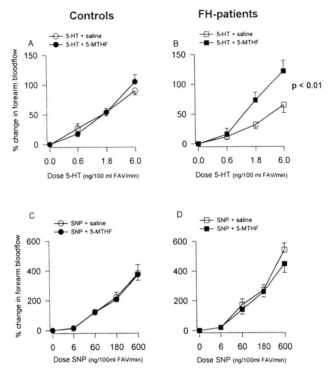

FIGURE 1-4. (A, C) Percentage change in forearm blood flow after stimulation of endothelium-dependent and endothelium-independent vasodilation with serotonin (5-HT) and sodium nitro-prusside (SNP), respectively, in control subjects. **(B, D)** Same parameters for patients with familial hypocholesterolemia. Reproduced with permission from Verhaar et al.[5]

Upregulation of Endothelial Nitric Oxide Synthase

Laufs and colleagues[6] determined whether HMG CoA reductase inhibitors restore endothelial function by directly upregulating endothelial NO synthase activity, as well as by reducing serum cholesterol levels. Human saphenous vein endothelial cells were treated with oxidized LDL (Ox-LDL) in the presence of HMG CoA reductase inhibitors, simvastatin and lovastatin. In a time-dependent manner, Ox-LDL decreased endothelial NO synthase activity and protein levels. Both simvastatin and lovastatin upregulated endothelial NO synthase expression by 3.8-fold and 3.6-fold, respectively, and prevented its downregulation by Ox-LDL. These effects of simvastatin on endothelial NO expression correlated with changes in endothelial NO activity. Although L-mevalonate alone did not cause endothelial NO synthase expression, co-treatment with L-mevalonate completely reversed endothelial NO synthase upregulation by simvastatin. Actinomycin D studies revealed that simvastatin stabilized endothelial NO synthase mRNA. Nuclear run-on assays and transient transfection studies with a -1.6 kb endothelial NO synthase promoter construct showed that simvastatin did not affect endothelial NO synthase gene transcription. Thus, inhibition of endothelial HMG CoA reductase upregulates endothelial NO synthase expression predominantly by post-transcriptional mechanisms.

Result of Oxidative Stress

Reactive oxygen species generated by treatment of smooth muscle cells (SMCs) with either phorbol 12-myristate 13-acetate or with the combination of H_2O_2 and vanadate strongly induce expression of the class A scavenger-receptive (SR-A) gene. In a study by Mietus-Snyder and colleagues[7] in San Francisco, California, cis-acting elements in the proximal 245 bp of the SR-A promotor were shown to direct luciferase report expression in response to oxidative stress in both human SMCs and macrophages. A composite (AP-1)/ets binding element located between -67 and -50 bp relative to the transcriptional start site is critical for the macrophage SR-A activity. Mutation of either the AP-1 or the ets component of this site also prevented promotor activity in SMCs. Mutation of a second site located between -44 and -21 bp, which the investigators identified as CCAAT/enhancer binding protein (C/EBP) element, reduced the inducible activity of the promotor in the SMCs by 50%, suggesting that a combinatorial interaction between these sites is necessary for optimal gene induction. Interaction between SMC nuclear extracts and the SR-A promotor were analyzed by electrophoretic mobility shift assay. c-Jun/activating protein-1 binding activity was induced in SMCs by the same conditions that increased scavenger receptor-A expression. Moreover, phorbol 12-myristate 13-acetate H_2O_2 or other combinations of H_2O_2 and vanadate activated c-Jun-activating kinase. The binding activity within SMC extracts specific for enhancer binding protein sites was shown to be C/EBPβ in SMCs. Taken together, these findings demonstrate that reactive oxygen species could regulate the interaction between c-Jun/AP-1 and C/EPBβ in the SR-A promotor. Furthermore, induction of oxidative stress in cells induced macrophage differentiation, adhesion, and scavenger receptor activity. These data suggest that vascular oxidative stress may contribute to the induction of SR-A gene expression and thereby promote the uptake of oxidatively modified LDL by both macrophage and SMCs to produce foam cells in the atherosclerotic lesions.

Exercise and Cardiovascular Disease

The oxidation of LDL has been suggested as a key event in atherogenesis. Paradoxically, exercise, which imposes an oxidative stress, is an important deterrent in cardiovascular disease. In study 1 by Shern-Brewer and colleagues[8] in Atlanta, Georgia, the oxidizability of LDL was enhanced in exercisers compared with sedentary controls. The lag time of isolated LDL subjected to copper-induced *in vitro* oxidation was significantly shortened in the exercises compared with sedentary subjects. This increased sensitivity was not due to a decreased presence of vitamin E. Instead, these findings suggested that the LDL of exercisers may contain increased amounts of preformed lipid peroxides, which account for the increased oxidizability. In study 2, a group gender analysis of variance (ANOVA) revealed that male exercisers had a significantly longer lag time than male sedentary subjects and that females had a similar lag time regardless of exercise group. This remained the case when statistical adjust-

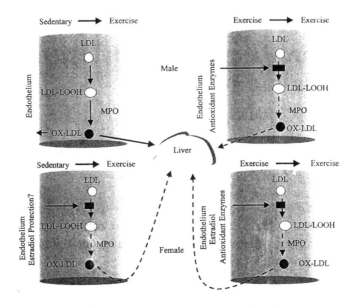

FIGURE 1-5. Top left: male subjects. Change from sedentary lifestyle to exercise induces oxidative stress, which results in "seeding" of LDL with peroxides. Exercise also induces neutrophil degranulation and increases plasma MPO. Seeded LDL and MPO are suggested to result in generation of oxidized (OX) LDL that is readily cleared by the liver. **Top right:** male subjects. Long-term exercisers have elevated cellular antioxidant enzymes that prevent generation of lipid hydroperoxides (LOOH) and seeding of LDL. Despite an increase in plasma MPO, LDL undergoes less oxidation due to lack of peroxides. **Bottom left:** female subjects. Change from sedentary lifestyle to exercise induces oxidative stress; however, female hormones or other factors prevent generation of LOOH and seeding of LDL. Despite an increase in plasma MPO, LDL undergoes less oxidation due to lack of peroxides. **Bottom right:** female subjects. Long-term exercise induces oxidative stress, which may also deplete estrogens. However, induction of antioxidant enzymes in the endothelium may prevent generation of LOOH and seeding of LDL. Despite an increase in plasma MPO, LDL undergoes less oxidation due to lack of peroxides. Reproduced with permission from Shern-Brewer.[8]

ment was made for age, body mass index, blood lipid levels, LDL, and plasma α-tocopherol levels. Study 1 exercisers had been in training for a shorter period of time (<1 year) than study 2 exercisers (>2 years). These findings suggest that truly chronic exercise (aerobic intensity over several months) decreases the susceptibility of male exercisers' LDL to undergo oxidation (Figure 1-5). Conversely, regular aerobic stress during an overall shorter time span creates a more oxidative environment in the body, thus increasing the susceptibility of LDL to undergo oxidation. The oxidative stress of aerobic exercise does not appear to adversely effect the oxidizability of LDL in women.

Oxidative Processes

Oxidative processes play an important role in atherogenesis. Because superoxide anion and NO are important mediators in vascular pathology, Luoma and coworkers[9] in Kuopio, Finland, studied the expression of extracellular superoxide dismutase and inducible NO synthase in human and rabbit athero-sclerotic lesions by using simultaneous *in situ* hybridization and immunocyto-chemistry and extracellular superoxide dismutase enzyme activity measure-ments. The investigators also analyzed the presence in the arterial wall of oxidized lipoprotein and peroxynitrate-modified proteins as indicators of oxi-dative damage and possible mediators in vascular pathology. Extracellular su-peroxide dismutase and inducible NO synthase mRNA and protein were ex-pressed in smooth muscle cells and macrophages in early advanced lesions. The expression of both enzymes was especially prominent in macrophages. As measured by enzyme activity, extracellular superoxide dismutase was the major superoxide dismutase isoenzyme in the arterial wall. Extracellular super-oxide dismutase activity was higher in highly cellular rabbit lesions, but lower in advanced, connective tissue-rich human lesions. Despite the abundant expression of extracellular superoxide dismutase, malondialdehyde-lysine, and hydroxynonenal-lysine epitopes characteristic of oxidized lipoproteins and ni-trotyrosine, residues characteristic of peroxynitrate-modified proteins were de-tected in inducible NO synthase-positive, macrophage-rich lesions, thus imply-ing that malondialdehyde, hydroxynonenal, and peroxynitrate are important mediators of oxidative damage. The investigators conclude that extracellular superoxide dismutase, inducible NO synthase, and the balance between NO and superoxide anion play important roles in atherogenesis. Extracellular su-peroxide dismutase and inducible NO synthase are highly expressed in lesion macrophages. High extracellular superoxide dismutase expression in the arte-rial wall may be required not only to prevent deleterious effects of superoxide anion, but also to preserve NO activities and prevent peroxynitrate formation. Modulation of arterial extracellular superoxide dismutase and inducible NO synthase activities could provide means to protect arteries against atheroscle-rotic vascular disease.

Low-Density Lipoprotein Oxidation

Accumulated evidence indicates that oxidative modification of LDL plays an important role in the atherogenic process. Therefore, van de Vijver and investigators[10] in Leiden, The Netherlands, investigated the relation between coronary atherosclerosis and susceptibility of LDL to oxidation in a case con-trol study in men between 45 and 80 years of age. Case subjects and hospital control subjects were selected from subjects undergoing a first coronary angi-ography. Subjects with severe coronary stenoses (>85% stenosis in 1 and greater than 50% stenosis in a second major coronary vessel) were classified as case subjects. Hospital control subjects with no or minor stenosis (<50% stenosis in no more than 2 of the 3 major coronary vessels) and population control subjects free of plaques in the carotid artery were pooled for the statisti-cal analysis into one control category. Enrollment procedures allowed for simi-lar distributions in age and smoking habits. Case subjects had higher levels of total and LDL cholesterol and triglycerides and lower levels of HDL cholesterol. Resistance time, maximum rate of oxidation, and maximum diene production were measured *ex vivo* using copper-induced LDL oxidation. A borderline significant inverse trend was observed for coronary atherosclerosis risks at increasing resistance time. No relation with maximum rate of oxidation was found, and higher maximum diene levels were found in control subjects. The main determinate of oxidation was the fatty acid composition of LDL. No effect of smoking or use of medication was observed. The investigators conclude that although LDL resistance to oxidation may be a factor in atherogenesis, the *ex vivo* measure is not a strong predictor of the severity of coronary atherosclerosis.

Inhibition of Nitric Oxide Release

Recent studies have demonstrated that, unlike cholesterol, cholesterol oxidized in position 7 can reduce the maximal endothelium-dependent relaxation of isolated rabbit aortas (Circulation 1997; 95:723–731). The aim of a study by Deckert and colleagues[11] in Paris, France, was to determine whether cholesterol oxide reduced the release of NO from human umbilical vein endothelial cells. The amount of NO released by histamine-stimulated human umbilical vein endothelial cells was determined by differential pulse amperometry using a nickel porphyrin- and Nafion-coated carbon microfiber electrode. The effects of cholesterol (preserved from oxidation by butylated hydroxytoluene), 7-ketocholesterol, 7β-hydroxycholesterol, 5α, 6α-epoxycholesterol, 19-hydroxycholesterol, and α-lysophosphatidylcholine were compared. Pretreatment of human umbilical vein endothelial cells with cholesterol, 5α, 6α-epoxycholesterol, or 19-hydroxycholesterol did not alter histamine-activated NO production. In contrast, pretreatment with 7-ketocholesterol or 7β-hydroxycholesterol significantly decreased NO release. The inhibitory effect of 7-ketocholesterol was time- and dose-dependent when maintained in the presence of L-arginine. In the absence of serum, lysophosphatidylcholine also reduced NO production. In ionomycin-stimulated cells, pretreatment with 7-ketocholesterol did not inhibit NO release. These results demonstrate that cholesterol derivatives oxidized at the 7 position, the main products of LDL oxidation, reduce histamine-activated NO release in human umbilical vein endothelial cells. Such an inhibitory effect of cholesterol oxides may account, at least in part, for the ability of oxidized LDL to reduce endothelium-dependent relaxation of arteries.

Antigenicity Oxidized Low-Density Lipoprotein

Lysophosphatidylcholine is formed by the hydrolysis of phosphatidylcholine in LDL and cell membranes by phospholipase A_2 or by oxidation. Oxidized LDL activates endothelial cells, an effect mimicked by lysophosphatidylcholine. Oxidized LDL also has the capacity to activate T and B cells, and antibody titers to oxidized LDL are related to the degree of atherosclerosis. The antigen in oxidized LDL responsible for its immune stimulatory capacities is not well characterized, and Wu and coinvestigators[12] in Stockholm, Sweden, hypothesized that lysophosphatidylcholine was involved. The investigators demonstrated the presence of antibodies against lysophosphatidylcholine, both of the

TABLE 1-1
Antibody Titers Against LPC, Ox-LDL, LDL, and CL in 210 Healthy Individuals

Antibody	Type	OD₄₀₅ Range	Mean ± SD
Anti-LPC	IgG	0–1.027	0.25 ± 0.119
	IgM	0.017–0.707	0.203 ± 0.097
Anti-oxLDL	IgG	0.017–0.777	0.149 ± 0.11
	IgM	0–1.663	0.324 ± 0.23
Anti-LDL	IgG	0–1.235	0.093 ± 0.105
	IgM	0–0.764	0.177 ± 0.091
Anti-CL	IgG	0–0.873	0.242 ± 0.132
	IgM	0–0.765	0.134 ± 0.074

OD_{405} indicates optical density lv 405 nm.
Reproduced with permission from Wu et al.[12]

IgG and IgM isotopes in 210 healthy individuals (Table 1-1). This antibody activity was not specifically related to oxidation of the fatty acid moiety in lysophosphatidylcholine since lysophosphatidylcholine, containing only palmitic acid, showed antibody titers equivalent to those of lysophosphatidylcholine-containing unsaturated fatty acids. Antibody titers to phosphatidylcholine were low compared with lysophosphatidylcholine, and hydrolysis of phosphatidylcholine at the sn-2 position was thus essential for immune activity. There was a close correlation between antioxidized LDL and anti-lysophosphatidylcholine antibodies. Furthermore, lysophosphatidylcholine competitively inhibited antioxidized LDL reactivity, which indicated that lysophosphatidylcholine may explain a significant part of the immune stimulatory properties of oxidized LDL. Lysophosphatidylcholine, being a lipid, is not likely to be an antigen itself. Instead, lysophosphatidylcholine could form immunogenetic complexes with peptides, which may induce and potentiate immune reactions in the vessel wall. This study adds to the evidence that lysophosphatidylcholine is an important component of oxidized LDL and emphasizes the potential role of phospholipase A_2 in atherosclerosis.

Macrophages and Oxidized Low-Density Lipoprotein

The interaction between macrophages and oxidatively modified LDL appears to play a central role in the development of atherosclerosis, not only through foam cell formation, but also via the induction of numerous cytokines and growth factors. A study by Ramos and colleagues[13] in Nagoya, Japan, demonstrated that oxidized LDL upregulated vascular endothelial growth factor mRNA expression in RAW 264 cells, a monocyte cell line, in a time- and concentration-dependent manner, and that oxidized LDL stimulated vascular endothelial growth factor protein secretion from the cells. Lysophosphatidylcholine, a component of oxidized LDL, also enhanced vascular endothelial growth factor mRNA expression in RAW 264 cells and vascular endothelial growth factor secretion from RAW 264 cells with a maximal effect at a concentration of 10 mmol/L lysophosphatidylcholine. Immunohistochemical studies showed that early atherosclerotic lesions in humans exhibited intense vascular endothelial growth factor immunoreactivity in subendothelial macrophage-rich regions of the thickened intima. In atherosclerotic plaques, vascular endothelial growth factor staining was also observed in foam cell-rich regions adjacent to the lipid core or the neovascularized basal regions of plaque consisting predominantly of smooth muscle cells. High-power–field observation revealed that vascular endothelial growth factor was localized in the extracellular space, as well as at the macrophage cell surface. These observations suggest the possible involvement of oxidized LDL in the development of human atherosclerosis through vascular endothelial growth factor induction in macrophages.

Oxidized Low-Density Lipoprotein and Cytokines

CD36 is a glycoprotein with an M_r of 88 kDa that is expressed on platelets, monocytes, macrophages, capillary endothelial cells, and adipocytes. Nakagawa and coinvestigators[14] in Osaka, Japan, previously demonstrated that CD36 is involved in the uptake of oxidized LDL by using CD36-deficient macrophages (Journal of Clinical Investigation 1995; 96:1859). However, the regulation of CD36 expression in human monocyte-derived macrophages has not been fully elucidated. The current study attempts to clarify the effect of oxidized LDL and cytokines, both of which are present in atherosclerotic lesions and may play an important role in atherogenesis and on the expression of CD36. A cell enzyme link immunosorbent assay and flow cytometry were used to detect CD36 protein. Ribonuclease protection system was used to measure CD36 and mRNR in human monocyte-derived macrophages. The expression of CD36 was increased during the differentiation of monocytes to macrophages. Incubation of macrophages with oxidized LDL for 24 hours increased the level of CD36 protein by 56% and that of CD36 mRNA by 58% (Figure 1-6). Lysophosphatidylcholine did not affect the expression of CD36. The effects of oxidized LDL were demonstrated in macrophages that had already differentiated to the point where CD36 expression was almost maximal. Interferon-γ reduced the expression of CD36 in a dose-dependent manner. A concentration of 1,000 U/mL interferon-γ significantly reduced the expression of CD36 protein by 57% and that of CD36 mRNA by 30%. In conclusion, CD36 may be important in the formation of foam cells by induction through its ligand oxidized LDL. Moreover, some local factors, such as interferon-γ, may suppress CD36 expression on macrophages in human atherosclerotic lesions.

Cytokine Modulation

There is considerable evidence to suggest that cytokines modulate pathological cellular events that occur in human atherosclerosis. Folcik and coworkers[15] in Cleveland, Ohio, sought to determine the effects of T-helper lymphocyte-1 and lymphocyte type 2 cytokines on the ability of human monocytes to oxidize LDL, one of the pathological processes believed to occur in atheroscle-

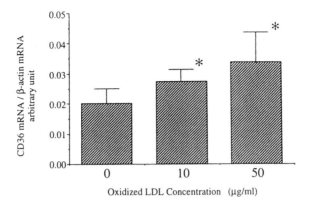

FIGURE 1-6. Induction of CD36 mRNA expression by Ox-LDL in macrophages. Bar graph shows expression of CD36 mRNA in macrophages, as detected by ribonuclease protection assay. Total RNA (2.0 μg) from human monocyte-derived macrophages incubated with and without Ox-LDL (0, 10, and 50 μg/mL) for 24 hours was hybridized with ^{32}P-labeled human CD36 cRNA. Annealed materials were digested with RNase A and T1. Protected fragments were analyzed by electrophoresis on 6% polyacrylamide/urea gel. Data were normalized to the β-actin signal and presented as arbitrary units. Data represent mean ±SD of triplicate experiments. *p < 0.05 compared with control values (without addition of Ox-LDL). Reproduced with permission from Nakagawa et al.[14]

rosis. The ability of opsonized zymosan-activated human monocytes to oxidize LDL in a 24-hour period was significantly enhanced by pretreatment of the monocytes with the lymphocyte type 2 cytokine, interleukin-4 or interleukin-13, compared with untreated monocytes. In contrast, interferon-γ, a T-helper lymphocyte-1 cytokine, inhibited LDL oxidation by activated monocytes. Treatment with interferon-γ also prevented the interleukin-4 and interleukin-13 mediated enhancement of LDL oxidation by zymosan-activated monocytes. Untreated or cytokine-treated inactivated monocytes did not oxidize LDL. The enhancement of LDL oxidation mediated by interleukin-4 or interleukin-13 treatment was not due to a mitogenic effect of the cytokines on the monocytes or to modulation of superoxide anion production. The cytokine regulation of 15-lipoxygenase in the monocytes was also examined. Interleukin-4 and interleukin-13 induction of 15-lipoxygenase-mRNA and 15-lipoxygenase activity in the monocytes was confirmed, as was the previously reported inhibition of induction by interferon-γ. In summary, interleukin-4 and interleukin-13 enhance the ability of activated human monocytes to oxidize LDL, whereas interferon-γ inhibits the cell-mediated oxidation. The up- and downregulation of activated monocyte-mediated LDL oxidation by these cytokines correlates with the expression of 15-lipoxygenase activity. Considerable evidence suggests that the progression of atherosclerosis includes events that are immunologically mediated, lending potential physiological relevance to these *in vitro* observations.

Inhibition of Low-Density Lipoprotein Expression

The regulation of macrophage lipoprotein lipase and mRNA expression by atherogenic lipoproteins is of critical relevance to foam cell formation. Lipoprotein lipase is present in arterial lesions and constitutes a bridging ligand between lipoproteins, proteoglycans, and cell receptors, thus favoring macrophage lipoprotein uptake and lipid accumulation. Stengel and coinvestigators[16] in Paris, France, investigated the effects of native and of oxidized lipoproteins on the expression of lipoprotein lipase in an *in vitro* human monocyte-macrophage system. Exposure of mature macrophages to highly copper-oxidized human LDL led to marked reduction in the regression of lipoprotein lipase activity and mRNA level; native LDL, acetylated LDL, and LDL oxidized for less than 6 hours were without effect. Reduction in lipoprotein lipase activity became significant at a threshold of 6 hours of LDL oxidation. Among the biologically active sterols formed during LDL oxidation, only 7β-hydroxycholesterol induced a minor reduction in macrophage lipoprotein lipase activity, whereas 25-hydroxycholesterol was without effect. In contrast, lysophosphatidylcholine whose LDL content increased parallel with the degree of oxidation induced significant reductions in lipoprotein lipase activity and mRNA levels at concentrations of 2 to 20 mmol/L. The results demonstrated that highly oxidized LDL by greater than 6 hours of oxidation exerted negative feedback on lipoprotein lipase secretion in human monocytes-macrophages via a reduction in mRNA levels. By contrast, negative LDL and mildly oxidized LDL with less than 6 hours of oxidation did not exert a feedback effect on lipoprotein lipase expression. The investigators speculate that the content of lysophosphatidylcholine and, to a lesser degree, of 7β-hydroxycholesterol in oxidized LDLs is responsible for the downregulation of lipoprotein lipase activity and mRNA abundance in human monocyte-derived macrophages and may, therefore, modulate lipoprotein lipase-mediated pathways of lipoprotein uptake during conversion of macrophages to foam cells.

Lysophosphatidylcholine

Lysophosphatidylcholine, which is generated in oxidized LDL and abundantly exists in atherosclerotic arterial walls, has been shown to alter various endothelial functions and induces several endothelial genes expressed in atherosclerotic arterial walls. Nuclear factor-κB, a pleiotropic transcription factor, plays an important role in regulation of expression of various genes implicated in atherosclerosis. Sugiyama and colleagues[17] in Kumamoto, Japan, had previously reported that lysophosphatidylcholine transferred from oxidized LDL to endothelial surface membrane activates endothelial protein kinase C, leading to modulated endothelial function. A subsequent study was aimed at determining whether lysophosphatidylcholine could modulate activity of transcription factors in cultured human umbilical vein endothelial cells by using electrophoretic mobility shift assay. Lysophosphatidylcholine was found to increase DNA binding activity of nuclear factor-κB in human umbilical vein endothelial cells within 15 minutes, which peaked at 1 to 2 hours and subsequently could climb to the baseline level at 6 hours. Lower concentrations of lysophosphatidylcholine markedly increased nuclear factor-κB activity, but higher concentrations of lysophosphatidylcholine inhibited the activity. Phorbol 12-myristate 13-acetate, a potent activator of protein kinase C, also augmented nuclear factor-κB activity in human umbilical vein endothelial cells, mimicking the effects of lysophosphatidylcholine; furthermore, calphostin C and chelerythrine chloride, specific phosphokinase C inhibitors and α-tocopherol, a clinically potent phosphokinase C inhibitor, suppress the lysophosphatidylcholine-induced nuclear factor-B activation. These results indicate that lysophosphatidylcholine regulated nuclear factor-κ B activity in a biphasic manner dependent on its concentrations and incubation time in human endothelial cells and the endothelial phosphokinase C activation may in part be involved in the lysophosphatidylcholine-induced nuclear factor-κ B activation. Thus, the time course in the positive and negative biphasic regulatory actions of lysophosphatidylcholine on nuclear factor-κ C activities and endothelial cells might exhibit a unique effect of lysophosphatidylcholine in arterial walls on the different stages of atherosclerosis.

Antibodies Against Oxidatively Modified Low-Density Lipoprotein

Autoantibodies against oxidatively modified LDL and cardiolipin occur in patients with vascular disease, including atherosclerosis. The ability of such antibodies to predict AMI was investigated by Wu[18] and colleagues in Uppsala, Sweden, in a prospective nested case-control study in which healthy 50-year-old men were followed-up for 20 years. Raised levels of autoantibodies against oxidized LDL and cardiolipin at age 50 correlated positively with the incidence of AMI and mortality related to AMI 10–20 years later. IgG and IgA antibodies against cardiolipin were associated with AMI between 50 and 60 years of age and IgG and IgA antibodies against oxidized LDL with AMI at 60–70 years of age. Moreover, higher antibody levels were noted in those who died from acute AMI in comparison to those who survived. The predictive power of IgA and IgG antibodies was strong and largely independent of that of other strong risk factors. In conclusion, raised levels of antibodies against oxidized LDL and cardiolipin may predict AMI and AMI-related death.

Low-Density Lipoprotein Oxidation

Much data have accrued in support of the concept that oxidation of LDL is a key early step in atherogenesis. The most consistent data with respect to micronutrient antioxidants and atherosclerosis appear to relate to α-tocopherol, the predominant lipid-soluble antioxidant in LDL. There are scant data on the direct comparison of RRR-α-tocopherol and all-racemic α-tocopherol on LDL oxidizability. Hence the aim of a study by Devaraj and colleagues[19] in Dallas, Texas, was to examine the relative effects of RRR-α-tocopherol and all-racemic α-tocopherol on plasma antioxidant levels and LDL oxidation in healthy persons in a dose-response study. The effects of RRR-α-tocopherol and all-racemic α-tocopherol at doses of 100, 200, 300, and 800 IU/day on plasma and LDL α-tocopherol levels and LDL oxidation were tested in a randomized, placebo-controlled study of 79 healthy subjects. Copper-catalyzed oxidation of LDL was monitored by measuring the formation of conjugated dienes and lipid peroxides over an 8-hour time course at baseline and again at 8 weeks. Plasma α-tocopherol, lipid-standardized α-tocopherol, and LDL α-tocopherol levels rose in a dose-dependent fashion in both the RRR-α-tocopherol and all-racemic α-tocopherol groups at baseline. There were no significant differences in plasma, lipid-standardized, and LDL α-tocopherol levels between RRR-α-tocopherol and all-racemic α-tocopherol supplementation at any dose comparison. The lag phases of oxidation were significantly prolonged with doses greater than 400 IU/day of RRR-α-tocopherol and all-racemic α-tocopherol, as measured by the conjugated dienes assay and at 400 IU/day of RRR-α-tocopherol and 800 IU/day of both forms of α-tocopherol by lipid peroxide assay. Again, there were no significant differences in the lag phase of oxidation at each dose for the RRR-α-tocopherol when compared with all-racemic α-tocopherol. Also, there were no significant differences in LDL oxidation after *in vitro* enrichment of LDL with RRR-α-tocopherol and all-racemic α-tocopherol. Thus, supplementation with either RRR-α-tocopherol or all-racemic α-tocopherol results in similar increases in plasma and LDL α-tocopherol levels at equivalent international unit doses, and the degree of protection against cooper-catalyzed LDL oxidation is evident only at doses greater than 400 IU/day for both forms.

Antioxidants and Atherosclerosis

Increased antioxidant intake is associated with decreased coronary risk. Vita and colleagues[20] from Boston, Massachusetts, and Nashville, Tennessee, sought to investigate the relation between plasma antioxidant status, extent of atherosclerosis, and activity of coronary artery disease. Plasma samples were obtained from 149 patients undergoing cardiac catheterization (65 with stable angina, 84 with unstable angina or acute myocardial infarction within 2 weeks). Twelve plasma antioxidant markers were measured and correlated with the extent of atherosclerosis in the presence of an unstable coronary syndrome. By multiple linear regression analysis, age, diabetes mellitus, male gender, and hypercholesterolemia were independent predictors of the extent of atherosclerosis. No antioxidant/oxidant marker correlated with the extent of atherosclerosis. However, lower plasma ascorbic acid concentrations predicted the presence of an unstable coronary syndrome by multiple logistic regression (odds ratio .59). The severity of atherosclerosis also predicted the presence of an unstable coronary syndrome (odds ratio 1.7) when all patients were considered. These authors conclude that their data are consistent with the hypothesis that the beneficial effects of antioxidants in coronary artery disease may result, in part, by an influence on lesion activity rather than a reduction in the overall extent of fixed disease.

Peroxidation of Low-Density Lipoprotein

The effects of marine omega-3 polyunsaturated fatty acids and antioxidants on the oxidative modification of LDL were studied by Brude and coworkers[21] in Oslo, Norway, in a randomized, double-blind placebo-controlled trial. Male smokers (n = 41) with combined hyperlipidemia were allocated to 1 of 4 groups receiving supplementation with omega-3 fatty acids (5 gm eicosapentaenoic acid and docosahexaenoic acid/day), antioxidants (75 mg of vitamin E, 150 mg of vitamin C, 15 mg β-carotene, and 30 mg co-enzyme Q_{10}/day), both omega-3 fatty acids and antioxidants or controlled oils. LDL and human mononuclear cells were isolated from the patients at baseline and after 6 weeks of supplementation. LDL was subjected to cell-mediated oxidation by the patient's own mononuclear cells, as well as to CU^{2+} catalyzed and 2,2' AZOBIS-initiated oxidation. The extent of LDL modification was measured as lag time, the formation rate of conjugated dienes, the maximum amount of conjugated dienes formed, formation of liquid peroxides, and the relative electrophoretic mobility of LDL on agarose gels. Dietary supplementation with omega-3 fatty acids increased the concentration of total omega-3 fatty acids in LDL and reduced the concentration of vitamin E in serum. The omega-3 fatty acid enriched LDL particles were not more susceptible to CU^{2+} catalyzed, AZOBIS-initiated, or autologous cell-mediated oxidation than control LDL. In fact, enrichment with omega-3 fatty acids significantly reduced the formation rate of conjugated dienes when LDL was subjected to AZOBIS-induced oxidation. Supplementation with moderate amounts of antioxidants significantly increased the concentration of vitamin E in serum and increased the resistance of LDL to undergo cooper-catalyzed oxidation, measured as increased lag time, reduced formation of liquid peroxides, and reduced relative electrophoretic mobility compared with control LDL. Supplementation with omega-3 fatty acid antioxidants showed oxidizability of LDL similar to that of control LDL and omega-3 fatty acid-enriched LDL. In conclusion, omega-3 fatty acids neither render the LDL particles more susceptible to undergo *in vitro* oxidation nor influence the ability of mononuclear cells to oxidize autologous LDL, whereas moderate amounts of antioxidants protect LDL against oxidative modification.

Genistein Prevents Low-Density Lipoprotein Oxidation

There is now growing evidence that the oxidative modification of LDL plays a potential role in atherosclerosis. In a study by Kapiotis and coworkers[22] in Vienna, Austria, genistein, a compound derived from a soy dye with flavonoid chemical structure, which was found to inhibit angiogenesis, was evaluated for its ability to act as an LDL antioxidant and a vascular cell protective agent against oxidized LDL. The results showed that genistein was able to inhibit the oxidation of LDL in the presence of copper ions or superoxide/nitric oxide radicals as measured by thiobarbituric acid-reactive substance formation, alteration in electrophoretic mobility, and lipid hydroperoxides. Bovine aortic endothelial cell- and human endothelial cell-mediated LDL oxidation was also inhibited in the presence of genistein (Figure 1-7). The 7-0 glucoside of genistein, genistin, was much less effective in inhibiting LDL oxidation in the cell-free and cell-mediated lipoprotein-oxidating system. Incubating human endothelial cells in the presence or absence of genistein and challenging the cells with already oxidized lipoprotein revealed that in addition to its antioxi-

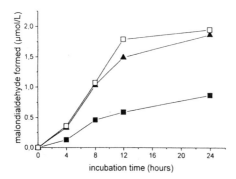

FIGURE 1-7. LDL oxidation by genistein-pretreated cells. HUVECs were preincubated with or without genistein (100 μmol/L) for 24 hours in RPMI-1640. Subsequently the cells were washed, RPMI-1640 containing 50 μg/mL LDL was added, and cell-mediated LDL oxidation was monitored by TBARS formation in the media. □ = no genistein; ▲ = pregenistein. In cultures designated co-genistein ■ = genistein (100 μmol/L) was present during LDL oxidation. Reproduced with permission from Kapiotis et al.[22]

dant potential during LDL oxidating processes, genistein effectively protected the vascular cells from damage by oxidized lipoproteins. The tyrosine kinase inhibitor genistein was found to block upregulation of 2 tyrosine-phosphory-lated proteins of 132 and 69 kDa in endothelial cells induced by oxidized LDL. Parallel experiments with the inactive analog daidzein, however, showed that the cytoprotective effect of the isoflavones seemed not to be dependent on tyrosine phosphorylation. The findings of the investigators support the suggested and documented beneficial action of a soy diet in preventing chronic vascular diseases and early atherogenic events.

Oxidized Low-Density Lipoprotein

Oxidized LDL may play a key role in the initiation and progression of atherosclerosis. Risk factors for elevated levels of oxidized LDL are not well established. Mosca and associates[23] from Ann Arbor, Michigan, and Rochester, New York, evaluated the relation between clinical parameters and oxidized LDL in 45 nonsmoking, nondiabetic patients (39 men and 6 women) with CAD. Oxidized LDL was assessed by measurement of conjugated dienes, lipid peroxides, and thiobarbituric reactive substances (TBARS) at 0 hours to evaluate baseline oxidant stress and postincubation with an oxidizing agent to assess the capacity of LDL for peroxidation. Results were lipid standardized and were not materially altered by multivariate adjustment. Significant predictors of increased oxidized LDL included female gender, family history of premature cardiovascular disease, increased percent body fat, increased body mass index, increased heart rate at rest, history of smoking, exercise less than 4 times per week, and no regular wine consumption. These data suggest that clinical parameters correlate with levels of oxidized LDL and may be useful in identifying patients at risk for increased oxidant stress.

Vitamin C Protects Human Arterial Smooth Muscle Cells

Glutathione (GSH) plays a key role in cellular antioxidant defenses by scavenging reactive oxygen species and reducing lipid peroxides. Intracellular

GSH levels are regulated by transport of this precursor L-cystine via system X_c^- which can be induced by oxidant stress. As oxidase-modified LDLs contribute to impaired vascular reactivity and the formation of atherosclerotic lesions, Siow and coinvestigators[24] in London, England, examined the effects of oxidized LDL and the antioxidant vitamins C and E on the L-cystine GSH pathway in human umbilical artery smooth muscle cells (HUASMCs). Oxidized LDL, but not native LDL, elevated intracellular GSH levels and L-cystine transport via system X_c^- in a time-dependent and dose-dependent manner. These increases were dependent on protein synthesis and the extent of LDL oxidation, but the induction of L-cystine transport activity was independent of GSH synthesis. Pretreatment of HUASMCs for 24 hours with vitamin E (100 μmol/L) attenuated oxidized LDL-mediated increases in GSH, whereas pretreatment with vitamin C depressed basal levels and abolished oxidized LDL-induced increases in GSH and L-cystine transport in a time-dependent and dose-dependent manner. Pretreatment of cells with dehydroscorbate had no effect on oxidized LDL-mediated increases in L-cystine transport and only marginally attenuated increases in GSH. These investigators' findings provide the first evidence that vitamin C spares endogenous adaptive antioxidant responses in human vascular smooth muscle cells exposed to atherogenic oxidized LDL.

Altered Low-Density Lipoprotein

The mechanisms underlying the selective accumulation of macrophages in early atherosclerotic lesions are poorly understood, but they are likely to be related to specific properties of altered LDL deposited in the subendothelium. Enzymatic, nonoxidative degradation of LDL converts the lipoprotein to a potentially atherogenic moiety, enzymatically altered LDL, (E-LDL), which activates complement and is taken up by human macrophages via a scavenger receptor-dependent pathway. Immunohistological evidence indicates that E-LDL is present in an extracellular location in the early lesion. Klouche and associates[25] in Mainz, Germany, reported that E-LDL causes massive release of monocyte chemotactic protein-1 (MCP-1) from human macrophages and that expression of interleukin A or RANTES remains unchanged. Release of MCP-1 was preceded by a rapid expression of MCP-1 mRNA that was detectable after 15 minutes, reached maximum levels after 1 hour, and remained detectable for 12 hours after exposure to concentrations as low as 10 μ/mL E-LDL. MCP-1 mRNA induction and protein release by E-LDL exceeded that evoked by oxidized LDL. Release of MCP-1 was dependent on *de novo* protein synthesis and on the activity of tyrosine kinase. At higher concentrations, E-LDL, but not oxidized LDL, exerted toxic effects on macrophages that in part appear to be due to apoptosis. These results show that E-LDL possesses major properties of an atherogenic lipoprotein.

Thyroid Function

In a study by Costantini and coinvestigators[26] in Chieti, Italy, the effect of different levels of thyroid hormone and metabolic activity on LDL oxidation

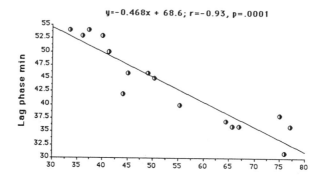

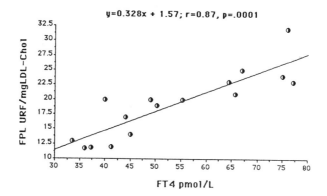

FT4 pmol/L

FIGURE 1-8. In hyperthyroid patients, the lag phase and LDL content in lipid peroxides (FPLPs) are significantly related to serum FT$_4$ levels. Reproduced with permission from Costantini et al.[26]

was investigated. Thus, in 16 patients with hyperthyroidism, 16 with hypothyroidism, and 16 age- and sex-matched healthy normolipidemic control subjects, the native LDL content in lipid peroxides, vitamin E, β-carotene and lycopene, as well as the susceptibility of these particles to undergo lipid peroxidation was assessed. Hyperthyroidism was associated with significantly higher lipid peroxidation, characterized by a higher native LDL content in lipid peroxide, a lower lag phase, and a higher oxidation rate than in the other 2 groups (Figure 1-8). This elevated lipid peroxidation was associated with a lower LDL antioxidant concentration. Interestingly, hypothyroid patients showed an intermediate behavior. In fact, in hypothyroidism, LDL oxidation was significantly lower than in hyperthyroidism, but higher than in the control group. Hypothyroidism was also characterized by the higher β-carotene LDL content, whereas vitamin E was significantly lower than in control subjects. In hyperthyroidism, but not in the other 2 groups, LDL oxidation was strongly influenced by free thyroxine blood content. In fact, in this group, the native LDL lipid peroxide content in the lag phase was directly and indirectly, respectively, related to free thyroxine blood levels. On the contrary, in hypothyroidism, LDL oxidation was strongly and significantly related to serum lipids. In conclusion, both hypothyroidism and hyperthyroidism are characterized by higher levels of LDL oxidation when compared with normolipidemic control subjects. In hyperthyroid patients, the increased lipid peroxidation is strictly related to free thyroxine levels, whereas in hypothyroidism, it is strongly influenced by serum lipids.

Smooth Muscle Cell Cytotoxicity

Oxidation of LDL is associated with degradation of phosphatidylcholine into platelet-activating factor-like phospholipids and lysophosphatidylcholine. Exposure of cultured human smooth muscle cells to platelet activating factor and lysophosphatidylcholine in a concentration of 25 μmol/L was found by Nillson and coinvestigators[27] in Stockholm, Sweden, to result in complete cell death as assessed by MTT cytotoxicity assay and cell counting. Addition of 50 gm/mL apolipoprotein A-I and apolipoprotein A-I$_{Milano}$ containing phospholipid particles completely inhibited this cytotoxicity (Figure 1-9). Phospholipid complexes alone were almost as effective, whereas free apolipoprotein A-I$_{Milano}$ and albumin were without effect, suggesting that the effect was phospholipid dependent. Experiments using [^{14}C] lysophosphatidylcholine demonstrated that apolipoprotein A-I and apolipoprotein A-I$_{Milano}$-containing phospholipid

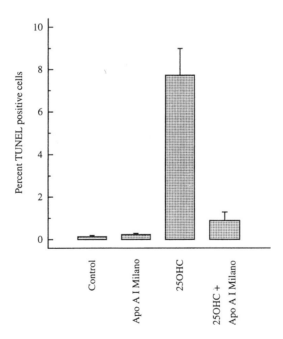

FIGURE 1-9. Effect of apo A-I$_{Milano}$-containing phospholipid particles on 25-hydroxycholesterol-induced apoptosis. Subconfluent cultures of SMCs were exposed to 5 μmol/L 25-hydroxycholesterol (25OHC) with or without addition of 50 μg/mL apo A-I$_{Milano}$-containing phospholipid particles for 24 hours. Apoptotic cells were identified by the TUNEL technique. Values are expressed as mean ±SD of at least triplicate experiments. Reproduced with permission from Nielson et al.[27]

particles effectively bind lysophosphatidylcholine. The results show that HDL-like phospholipid particles effectively inhibit the toxic effect of phospholipids and other lipid soluble factors. The ability of HDL to inhibit the proinflammatory and toxic effects of phospholipids generated during oxidation of LDL may be responsible for part of the antiatherogenic properties of HDL.

Reactive Oxygen Species

Vascular endothelial cells are constantly subjected to flow-induced shear stress. Although the effects of shear stress on endothelial cells are well known, the intracellular signal mechanisms remain unclear. Reactive oxygen species have recently been suggested to act as intracellular second messengers. The potential role of reactive oxygen species in shear-induced gene expression was examined by Chiu and colleagues[28] in Taipei, Taiwan, in a study by subjecting endothelial cells to a shear force using a parallel plate-flow chamber system. Endothelial cells under shear-flow increased the intracellular reactive oxygen species as indicated by superoxide production. This superoxide production was maintained at an elevated level as increased shear flow remained. Sheared endothelial cells, similar to tumor necrosis factor-α, PMA, or H_2O_2-treated cells, increased their intracellular adhesion molecule-1 mRNA levels in a time-dependent manner. Pretreatment of endothelial cells with an antioxidant, N-acetylcysteine or catalase, inhibited the shear-induced or oxidant-induced intracellular adhesion molecule-1 expression. Reactive oxygen species that were involved in the shear-induced adhesion molecule-1 gene expression were further substantiated by functional analysis using a chimera containing the adhesion molecule-1 promoter region and the reporter gene luciferase. Shear-induced promoter activities were attenuated by pretreating sheared endothelial cells with N-acetylcysteine and catalase. Flow cytometric analysis and monocyte adhesion assay confirmed the inhibitor effect of N-acetylcysteine and catalase on the shear-induced adhesion molecule-1 expression on endothelial cells. These results clearly demonstrated that shear-flow to endothelial cells can induce intracellular reactive oxygen species generation that may result in an increase in intracellular adhesion molecule-1 mRNA levels via transcriptional events. The investigators' findings thus support the importance of intracellular reactive oxygen species in modulating hemodynamically induced endothelial responses.

Hypercholesterolemia and Dietary L-Arginine

Hypercholesterolemia reduces vascular NO activity. This dysfunction may promote endothelial monocyte interaction, as NO is a potent inhibitor of cell adhesion. Theilmeier and coinvestigators[29] in Stanford, California, have previously shown that in hypercholesterolemic rabbits, chronic oral supplementations of L-arginine restored NO activity and inhibited monocyte-endothelial cell interaction, in association with a reduction in atherogenesis. The investigators hypothesized that enhancement of endothelial NO activity in hypercholesterolemic humans would reduce monocyte adhesiveness. The investigators used a functional binding assay to assess the adhesiveness of human mononuclear cells *ex vivo* to determine the effects of hypercholesterolemia and L-arginine administration. Mononuclear cells from hypercholesterolemic subjects adhered in greater numbers than in cells derived from subjects with normal cholesterol values. To determine whether enhancement of endogenous NO activity could inhibit mononuclear cell adhesiveness, in a double-blind placebo-controlled study, oral arginine hydrochloride (8.4 g/d) was administered to hypercholesterolemic subjects. Over a course of 2 weeks, this treatment abolished the increased adhesiveness of hypercholesterolemic mononuclear cells (160 vs. 104%: before and after 2 weeks of L-arginine treatment; results expressed as a percentage of the binding values obtained using cells derived from paired normal cholesterolemic subjects). In contrast, mononuclear cell adhesion remained significantly elevated in the placebo-treated hypercholesterolemic subjects (Figure 1-10). To examine whether endothelium-derived NO could act as a paracrine modulator of monocyte behavior, monocytes were exposed to NO donors or co-cultured in the presence of endothelial cells exposed to antagonists of NO synthase in the presence or absence of L-arginine. NO donors inhibited monocyte adhesiveness. Furthermore, the adhesiveness of monocytes cocultured with endothelial cells was increased by antagonists of NO synthase; this effect was reversed by L-arginine. This study shows that the adhesiveness of mononuclear cells was increased by hypercholesterolemia. The increase in adhesiveness was reversed *in vivo* by administration of the NO precursor L-arginine. NO donors or endothelium-derived NO inhibited the adhesiveness of monocytes *in vitro*, supporting the hypothesis that the effects of L-arginine are mediated by NO.

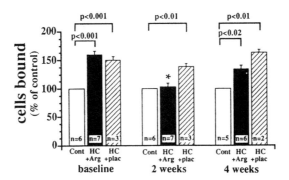

FIGURE 1-10. Reduction of mononuclear cell (MNC) adhesiveness by dietary arginine supplementation. Hydroxycholesterolemic (HC) individuals were randomized to arginine supplementation or placebo. At baseline (before the initiation of study drug), MNCs from both HC groups exhibited greater adhesiveness than monocytes derived from NC individuals. After 2 weeks of arginine supplementation, monocytes derived from these HC individuals demonstrated a significant reduction in adhesiveness. At the 4-week time point (after discontinuing the study drugs for 2 weeks), the adhesiveness of MNCs derived from HC individuals previously treated with dietary arginine had returned to levels significantly greater than that of NC individuals. The number in the bars refers to the number of individuals participating at each time point. Cont = control (NC) subjects; Arg = arginine; plac = placebo. *Significantly different from baseline value. Reproduced with permission from Theilmeier et al.[29]

Endothelial Function, Vasodilation, Vascular Remodeling, and Inflammation

Reversal of Abnormal Coronary Vasomotion

Kaufmann and colleagues[30] evaluated the effects of calcium channel blockers on coronary vasomotion of angiographically normal smooth coronary arteries in 57 patients with hypercholesterolemia. Vasomotion of angiographically normal coronary arteries was evaluated in 37 control subjects (group 1) without and 20 patients (group 2) with calcium channel blocker administration before physical exercise. Both groups were subdivided into subgroup A (normal cholesterol values of 212 mg% or lower) and subgroup B (elevated cholesterol values >212 mg%). Coronary luminal area at rest and during exercise was assessed by biplane quantitative coronary arteriography. The normal vessels showed a significant increase in coronary luminal area during exercise in subgroup A with normal cholesterol values but not in subgroup B. In contrast, all patients in group 2 showed similar vasodilation during exercise in subgroups A and B. Independent of the actual cholesterol value, the stenotic lesions showed coronary vasoconstriction during exercise in group 1 but vasodilation in group 2 after pretreatment with a calcium antagonist. Thus, coronary vasomotor response to exercise is inversely related to actual serum cholesterol level in angiographically normal vessels. Administration of calcium antagonists normalizes exercise-induced vasodilatation and eliminates cholesterol-induced abnormal vasomotion, probably by direct effect on the smooth muscles of the vasculature (Figures 1-11, 1-12).

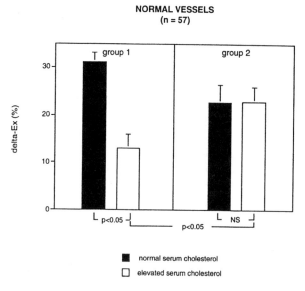

FIGURE 1-11. Coronary vasomotion of the normal vessel segments in control subjects (group 1) and in patients pretreated with calcium antagonists (group 2). delta-Ex indicates percent change of luminal cross-sectional area during exercise. Reproduced with permission from Kaufmann et al.[30]

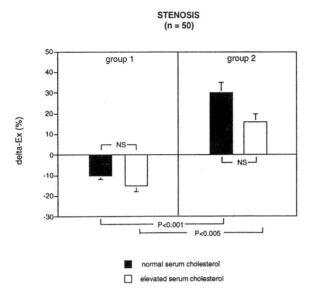

STENOSIS
(n = 50)

FIGURE 1-12. Coronary vasomotion of the stenotic vessel segments in control subjects (group 1) and in patients pretreated with calcium antagonists (group 2). Note that there was stenosis constriction in control subjects that was prevented by calcium antagonists in group 2. delta-Ex indicates percent change of stenosis cross-sectional area and during exercise. Reproduced with permission from Kaufmann et al.[30]

Atherosclerosis Risk in Communities Study

Hwang and colleagues[31] in Houston, Texas, determined the ability of circulating vascular cell adhesion molecule-1 (VCAM-1), endothelial leukocyte adhesion molecule-1 (E-selectin), and intercellular adhesion molecule-1 (ICAM-1) to serve as molecular markers of atherosclerosis and predictors of incident CAD. They studied 204 patients with incident CAD, 272 patients with carotid artery atherosclerosis, and 316 control subjects from the large, biracial Atherosclerosis Risk In Communities (ARIC) study. Levels of VCAM-1 were not significantly different among the patients with incident CAD, those with carotid artery atherosclerosis, and control subjects. Higher levels of E-selectin and ICAM-1 were observed for patients with CAD and those with carotid artery atherosclerosis. Logistic regression analysis indicated that the relationship of ICAM-1 and E-selectin with CAD and carotid artery atherosclerosis was independent of other known CAD risk factors and was most pronounced in the highest quartile. The odds of CAD and carotid artery atherosclerosis were 5.53 and 2.64, respectively, for those with serum levels of ICAM-1 in the highest quartile compared with those in the lowest quartile. Odds of carotid artery atherosclerosis were 2.03 for those with levels of E-selectin in the highest quartile compared with those in the lowest quartile (Table 1-2). Thus, these data indicate that plasma levels of ICAM-1 and E-selectin may serve as molecular markers for atherosclerosis and the risk of developing CAD.

TABLE 1-2
Odds Ratios and 95% CIs of Incident CHD and CAA Occurrence for Those with E-Selectin or ICAM-1 in the Second, Third, and Fourth Quartiles

Adhesion Molecules	Quartile	Model 1	Model 2	Model 3
CHD				
E-selectin	Second	1.91 (1.15–3.16)	1.62 (0.87–3.04)	1.52 (0.80–2.89)
	Third	2.23 (1.34–3.72)	1.67 (0.88–3.16)	1.53 (0.79–2.95)
	Fourth	2.98 (1.74–5.10)	1.78 (0.88–3.60)	1.60 (0.78–3.30)
ICAM-1	Second	1.62 (0.95–2.75)	1.41 (0.72–2.77)	1.37 (0.69–2.73)
	Third	1.78 (1.05–3.01)	1.53 (0.79–2.94)	1.46 (0.75–2.84)
	Fourth	7.93 (4.48–14.04)	5.85 (2.81–12.19)	5.53 (2.51–12.21)
CAA				
E-selectin	Second	1.19 (0.73–1.92)	0.93 (0.53–1.63)	0.86 (0.48–1.53)
	Third	1.76 (1.10–2.82)	1.35 (0.78–2.34)	1.16 (0.65–2.07)
	Fourth	3.45 (2.14–5.59)	2.25 (1.28–3.95)	2.03 (1.14–3.62)
ICAM-1	Second	1.62 (1.01–2.58)	1.25 (0.73–2.16)	1.17 (0.67–2.03)
	Third	1.70 (1.07–2.72)	1.10 (0.64–1.92)	1.02 (0.58–1.79)
	Fourth	4.95 (2.93–8.34)	2.86 (1.54–5.30)	2.64 (1.40–5.01)

Reference groups are those with measurements in the lowest quartile.

Model 1 adjusted for race, age, and sex.

Model 2 adjusted for race, age, sex, body mass index, hypertension, diabetes, total cholesterol, HDL cholesterol, and cigarette-years for smokers.

Model 3 adjusted for race, age, sex, body mass index, hypertension, diabetes, total cholesterol, HDL cholesterol, cigarette-years for smokers, triglyceride, fibrinogen, von Willebrand factor, and white blood cell count.

Reproduced with permission from Hwang et al.[31]

Effect of Glutathione on Endothelial Vasomotor Function

Kugiyama and colleagues[32] in Kumamoto, Japan, examined the effect of reduced glutathione, an antioxidant, on human coronary circulation, believing that inhibition of the accumulation of oxygen free radicals would improve endothelial vasomotor function. Responses of epicardial diameter and blood flow of the LAD to intracoronary infusion of acetylcholine was determined by quantitative coronary arteriography and Doppler flow-wire techniques, before and during combined intracoronary infusion of glutathione or saline in 26 subjects with no significant coronary stenoses. Glutathione infusion decreased the constrictor response of epicardial diameter to acetylcholine and enhanced the increase in blood flow response to acetylcholine (Figure 1-13). Glutathione administration also potentiated the coronary vasodilator effect of nitroglycerin. A beneficial effect of glutathione on the epicardial diameter response to acetylcholine was observed in a subgroup of subjects with 1 or greater coronary risk factor, but not in the subgroup without risk factors. Saline infusion had no physiologic effects. These data indicate that glutathione improves coronary endothelial vasomotor function, especially in patients with coronary risk factors, and it potentiated the vasodilator effect of nitroglycerin in human coronary arteries.

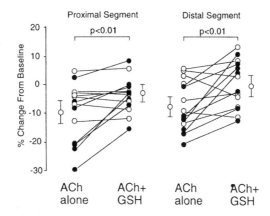

FIGURE 1-13. Percent changes in lumen diameter from baseline in response to acetylcholine (Ach) alone and in combination with glutathione (GSH) in proximal and distal segments of epicardial coronary arteries. ● = Subjects with coronary risk factors; ○ = subjects without risk factors. Mean ± SEM was calculated from subjects with and without risk factors. Reproduced with permission from Kugiyama et al.[32]

Aspirin Improves Endothelial Dysfunction

Husain and colleagues[33] in Bethesda, Maryland, hypothesized that a cyclooxygenase-dependent constricting factor contributes to the endothelial dysfunction in atherosclerosis and that its action can be reversed by aspirin. They evaluated 14 patients with coronary atherosclerosis and 5 with risk factors in whom they tested femoral vascular endothelial function with acetylcholine and substance P and endothelium-independent function with sodium nitroprusside before and after intravenous aspirin. Drugs were infused into the femoral artery and Doppler flow velocity was measured. Acetylcholine-induced but not substance P- or sodium nitroprusside-induced vasodilation was lower in patients with atherosclerosis than in those with only risk factors. Aspirin had no effect at baseline, but it improved acetylcholine-mediated vasodilation in patients with atherosclerosis. At peak dose, acetylcholine-mediated femoral vascular resistance index was 19% ± 5%, p = .002 (Figure 1-14). There was

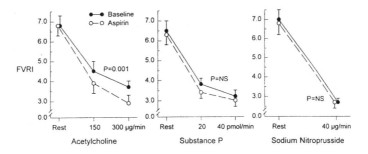

FIGURE 1-14. Effect of aspirin on response to acetylcholine (left), substance P (middle), and sodium nitroprusside (right) in 14 patients with atherosclerosis. FVRI = femoral vascular resistance index (mm Hg·cm^{-1}·s^{-1}). Reproduced with permission from Husain et al.[33]

a correlation between the baseline response to acetylcholine and the magnitude of improvement with aspirin. Patients with a depressed response to acetylcholine had greater improvement with aspirin and vice versa. Atherosclerosis was an independent determinant of improvement with aspirin. Aspirin had no effect on the responses to either substance P or sodium nitroprusside. Thus, these data suggest that cyclooxygenase-dependent, endothelium-derived vasoconstrictor release modulates acetylcholine-induced peripheral vasodilation in patients with atherosclerosis. Improvement of endothelial dysfunction with aspirin may involve vasodilation, reduction in thrombosis, and inhibit progression of atherosclerosis.

Physiological Function of ET_A and ET_B Receptor Subtypes

Verhaar and colleagues[34] evaluated the physiological function of ET_A and ET_B receptor subtypes in human blood vessels by studying human forearm resistance vessels *in vivo* and determined the mechanism underlying the vasodilatation to ET_A-selective receptor antagonist BQ-123. Two studies were performed, both in groups of 8 healthy subjects. Brachial artery infusion of BQ-123 caused significant forearm vasodilatation in both studies. This vasodilatation was reduced by 95% with inhibition of the endogenous generation of nitric oxide and by 38% with coinfusion of the ET_B receptor antagonist, BQ-788 (Figure 1-15). Inhibition of prostanoid generation did not affect the response to BQ-123. Infusion of BQ-788 alone produced a 20% reduction in forearm blood flow. Thus, selective ET_A receptor antagonism causes vasodilation of human forearm resistance vessels *in vivo*. The response appears to result in major part from an increase in nitric oxide generation. ET_B receptor antago-

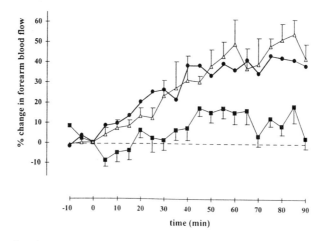

FIGURE 1-15. Eight subjects received brachial artery infusion of BQ-123 (100 nmol/min) during co-infusion of saline (●), BQ-123 (100 nmol/min) during inhibition of prostanoid generation (△), or BQ-123 (100 nmol/min) during inhibition of NO generation (■). Slow-onset vasodilation occurred in response to BQ-123; this response was attenuated during NO clamp but not during inhibition of prostanoid generation. Reproduced with permission from Verhaar et al.[34]

nism either alone or on a background of ET_A antagonism causes local vasoconstriction, indicating that ET_B receptors in blood vessels respond to endothelin-1 predominantly by causing vasodilatation.

Study of Endothelial Function in Families with Premature Coronary Artery Disease

Clarkson and colleagues[35] in London, England, studied endothelial function in 50 first-degree relatives of patients with proven CAD. There were 31 men and 19 women among the 50 first-degree relatives. The patients with premature CAD included men 45 years of age or younger and women 55 years of age or younger. The patients were well, lifelong nonsmokers, nondiabetic and nonhypertensive, and they took no medications. High-resolution external vascular ultrasound was used to measure brachial artery diameter at rest and in response to reactive hyperemia using endothelium-dependent and endothelium-independent vasodilators. Vascular responses were compared with those of 50 healthy control subjects matched for age and sex. Flow-mediated dilatation was impaired in the first-degree relatives from the patients with premature CAD. However, the endothelium-independent vasodilator caused dilatation in all subjects to a similar degree. When the family history subjects were subdivided, those with a serum cholesterol higher than 4.2 mmol/L had mildly impaired flow compared with control subjects. However, even in subjects with no risk factors and whose affected relatives had a normal cardiovascular risk factor profile, there was a markedly impaired flow-mediated dilatation among the first-degree relatives. Thus, healthy young adults with a family history of premature CAD may have impaired endothelium-dependent vasodilatation even in the absence of other cardiovascular risk factors (Figure 1-16).

Effect of Hyperglycemia on Endothelium-Dependent Vasodilation

Williams and colleagues[36] in Boston, Massachusetts, examined the effects of acute hyperglycemia on endothelium-dependent vasodilation in nondiabetic humans *in vivo*. Endothelium-dependent vasodilation was assessed through brachial artery infusion of methacholine chloride both before and during 6 hours of local hyperglycemia with blood sugars of 300 mg/dL achieved by intra-arterial infusion of 50% dextrose. Forearm blood flow was determined by plethysmography. In a group of 10 subjects, there was a trend toward attenuated methacholine-mediated vasodilation during hyperglycemia compared with euglycemia. The systemic serum insulin levels increased significantly during the dextrose infusion. In order to eliminate the confounding vasoactive effects of insulin, the protocol was repeated during systemic infusion of octreotide to inhibit pancreatic secretion of insulin. In these subjects, hyperglycemia significantly attenuated forearm blood flow response to methacholine during hyperglycemia. Methacholine-mediated vasodilation was not attenuated by an equi-

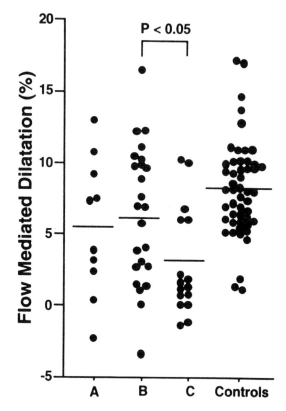

FIGURE 1-16. Flow-mediated dilation in subjects with a history of premature CAD divided into 3 cohorts: group A, subjects who had an elevated serum LDL cholesterol (>4.2 mmol/L); group B, subjects whose first-degree relative had identifiable cardiovascular risk factors (cigarette smoker >1 pack-year, LDL cholesterol >4.2 mmol/L or total cholesterol >5.5 mmol/L, BP >140/90 mm Hg); and group C, subjects with no identifiable cardiovascular risk factors and whose affected relative also had no identifiable cardiovascular risk factors. Group C subjects had the most markedly impaired flow-mediated dilation. Reproduced with permission from Clarkson et al.[35]

molar infusion of mannitol, nor did hyperglycemia reduce endothelium-independent vasodilation to verapamil. Thus, these data strongly indicate that acute hyperglycemia impairs endothelium-dependent vasodilation in healthy humans *in vivo* (Figure 1-17).

Hyperlipidemia Treatment Effect on Vasodilator Function

Huggins and colleagues[37] tested the hypothesis that correction of hyperlipidemia improves coronary vasodilator response and maximal perfusion in myocardial regions having substantial impairment of pretreatment vasodilator capacity. Measurements of myocardial blood flow were made with PET[^{13}N]ammonia in 12 patients with CAD at rest and during adenosine administration for 5 minutes at different doses before and again 4 months after

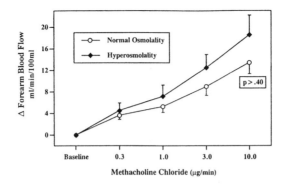

Figure 1-17. Absolute increase in forearm blood flow from baseline during graded intra-arterial infusion of methacholine chloride before and during hyperosmolar clamping. There was no significant effect of osmolality on the response to methacholine chloride as analyzed by repeated-measures ANOVA ($p > .40$). Reproduced with permission from Williams et al.[36]

simvastatin treatment (40 mg daily). Simvastatin reduced LDL from a mean value of 171 ± 13 before to 99 ± 18 mg/dL after therapy and increased HDL from 39 ± 8 to 45 ± 9 mg/dL. Myocardial segments were classified on the basis of pretreatment blood flow response to adenosine as normal or abnormal flow. In normal segments, baseline myocardial blood flow increased at both low- and high-dose adenosine and was unchanged both at rest and with adenosine after simvastatin. However, in abnormal segments, myocardial blood flow at rest increased at low- and high-dose adenosine. After simvastatin, myocardial blood flow increased more compared with pretreatment at both low- and high-dose adenosine (Figure 1-18). Thus, short-term lipid-lowering therapy increases stenotic segment maximal myocardial blood flow by about 45%. The

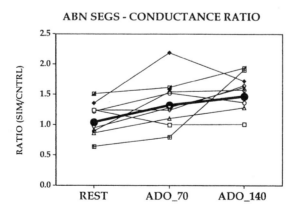

Figure 1-18. Group mean ($\pm$ SEM) values of myocardial conductance (G) of abnormal segments (ABN SEGS) at each stage of study before (solid line) and after (dashed line) simvastatin. Data conform to a linear model ($r^2 = 1.0$ for each) and demonstrate a clear-cut left shift of the adenosine (Ado) dose-response relationship with near doubling of the regression slope after simvastatin. Before simvastatin, the equation for the line is $G = 0.04 \times$ (Ado dose) $+ 6.9$. After simvastatin, the equation is $G = 0.07 \times$ (Ado dose) $+ 6.9$. Reproduced with permission from Huggins et al.[37]

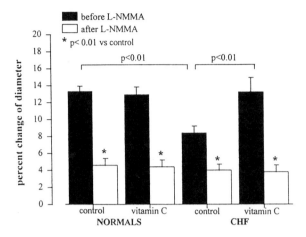

FIGURE 1-19. Change in radial artery diameter (%) during reactive hyperemia (flow-dependent dilation) after wrist occlusion in normal individuals (n = 8) and patients with congestive heart failure (n = 10) before (black bars) and after L-NMMA (open bars); effect of intra-arterial infusion of vitamin C. Reproduced with permission from Hornig et al.[38]

mechanism involves enhanced, flow-mediated dilation of stenotic epicardial conduit arteries and may account at least in part for the efficacy of lipid lowering in secondary prevention trials and in reducing CAD episodes in ambulatory patients.

Vitamin C Improves Endothelial Function of Conduit Arteries

Hornig and colleagues[38] tested the hypothesis that increased radical formation in patients with CHF impairs endothelial function using the antioxidant vitamin C to evaluate high-resolution ultrasound and Doppler measurements of radial artery diameter and blood flow. Fifteen patients with congestive heart failure (CHF) and 8 healthy volunteers were studied. Vascular effects of vitamin C given as 25 mg/min intra-arterially and placebo were determined at rest and during reactive hyperemia before and after intra-arterial infusion of N-monomethyl-L-arginine (L-NMMA) to inhibit endothelial synthesis of NO. Vitamin C restored flow-dependent dilation in patients with CHF after acute intra-arterial administration of vitamin C and after 4 weeks of oral therapy (Figure 1-19). The portion of flow-dependent dilation mediated by NO was increased after acute as well as chronic treatment with vitamin C. Thus, vitamin C improves flow-dependent dilation in patients with CHF as a result of increasing availability of NO. These observations support the hypothesis that endothelial dysfunction in patients with CHF is at least partly due to the relative inhibition of NO effects probably by oxygen-derived free radicals.

Lipid-Lowering Therapy Improves Endothelial Function

John and colleagues[39] in Nürnberg, Germany, hypothesized that lipid-lowering therapy improves endothelial function and that this effect is mediated

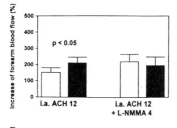

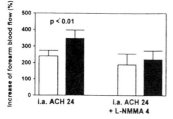

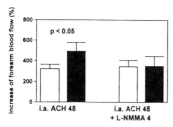

FIGURE 1-20. Comparison of increases in forearm blood flow before (open bars) and after (solid bars) therapy between intra-arterial (i.a.) acetylcholine (ACH) and i.a. acetylcholine plus co-infusion with i.a. L-NMMA 4 μmol/min. **Top:** i.a. acetylcholine 12 μg/min. **Middle:** i.a. acetylcholine 24 μg/min. **Bottom:** i.a. acetylcholine 48 μg/min. Reproduced with permission from John et al.[39]

mainly by increased bioavailability of NO. In a randomized, double-blind, placebo-controlled trial, they studied 29 patients with a mean age of 50 years with hypercholesterolemia and an LDL cholesterol of 160 mg/dL or higher, who were randomly assigned to receive either fluvastatin (40 mg twice daily in 17 patients) or placebo (12 patients). Forearm blood flow was measured by plethysmography before and after 24 weeks of treatment. Endothelium-dependent vasodilation was determined by intra-arterial infusion of acetylcholine and basal NO synthesis rate by intra-arterial infusion of N^G-monomethyl-L-arginine (L-NMMA). Intra-arterial infusion of L-NMMA and acetylcholine was used to test whether any increase in endothelium-dependent vasodilation after lipid-lowering therapy could be blocked by the NO synthase inhibitor. Endothelium-dependent vasodilation improved significantly after 24 weeks of lipid-lowering therapy compared with before therapy and placebo. This improvement in endothelium-dependent vasodilation was blocked by simultaneous administration of L-NMMA. Thus, lipid-lowering therapy with fluvastatin can improve disturbed endothelial function in hypercholesterolemic patients, and this improvement is mediated by increased bioavailability of NO (Figure 1-20).

Cocaine Increases Endothelin Release

Wilbert-Lampen and colleagues[40] in Munich, Germany, investigated whether vasoconstrictive endothelin-1 is released by cocaine in the supernatant

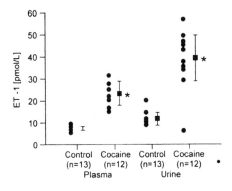

FIGURE 1-21. Deterioration of immunoreactive endothelin-1 (ET-1) in plasma and urine of patients intoxicated with cocaine (n = 12) compared with a control group (n = 13). Data and mean $\pm$ SD are in pmol/L. Statistical comparisons were made by t test; *p < 0.05 vs. control. Reproduced with permission from Wilbert-Lampen et al.[40]

of porcine aortic endothelial cells after treatment with cocaine and an δ-receptor antagonist, haloperidol or ditolylguanidine and in plasma and urine of 12 cocaine-intoxicated subjects and 13 healthy control individuals. Radioligand binding assays were performed on endothelial membrane preparations. In the cell culture, cocaine significantly increased endothelin accumulation above baseline at 3 to 24 hours. Endothelin release rates per hour increased dose-dependently, reaching a plateau of 175% $\pm$ 23% of control at hour 4 to 5. Coincubation of cocaine with haloperidol or ditolylguanidine abolished or reduced cocaine-induced endothelin release. Endothelial membrane preparations specifically and displaceably bound the highly selective δ-adrenergic ligand. Endothelin-1 levels in plasma and urine of cocaine-intoxicated patients were significantly increased compared with control values (Figure 1-21). These data suggest that cocaine increases the endothelin release *in vitro* and *in vivo* and the cocaine-induced vasoconstriction may be facilitated by the release of endothelin-1.

Effect of Hormone Therapy on Endothelium-Dependent Vasolilation

Gerhard and colleagues[41] in Boston, Massachusetts, studied 17 postmenopausal women with mild hypercholesterolemia who were enrolled in a placebo-controlled, crossover trial to evaluate the effect of transdermal estradiol, with and without vaginal micronized progesterone, on endothelium-dependent vasodilation in a peripheral artery. Brachial artery diameter was measured with high-resolution B-mode ultrasonography. In order to assess endothelium-dependent vasodilation, brachial artery diameter was determined at baseline and after a flow stimulus induced by reactive hyperemia. In order to assess endothelium-independent vasodilation, brachial artery diameter was measured after administration of sublingual nitroglycerin. During estradiol therapy, reactive hyperemia caused an 11% change in brachial artery diameter compared with a 4% change during placebo therapy. Progesterone did not significantly attenuate this improvement. During combined estrogen and progesterone therapy, flow-mediated vasodilation of the brachial artery was 9.6%. Endothelium-independent vasodilation was not altered by estradiol therapy, either with or with-

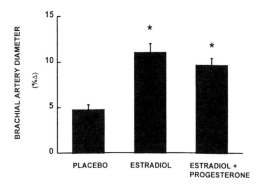

FIGURE 1-22. Flow-mediated, endothelium-dependent vasodilation of brachial artery during placebo therapy, estradiol therapy, and estradiol plus progesterone therapy. Values are mean ± SEM. *p < 0.001 vs. placebo. Reproduced with permission from Gerhard et al.[41]

out progesterone compared with placebo. There was a moderate decrease in total and LDL cholesterol during treatment both with estradiol alone and when estradiol was combined with progesterone. In a multivariate analysis that included serum estradiol, progesterone, total and LDL cholesterol concentrations, blood pressure, and heart rate, only the estradiol level was a significant predictor of endothelium-dependent vasodilation. Thus, the addition of micronized progesterone does not attenuate the favorable effect of estradiol on endothelium-dependent vasodilation (Figure 1-22).

Effect of Vitamin C on Endothelium-Dependent Vasodilation

Endothelium-dependent vasodilation is impaired with diabetes mellitus. Oxidatively mediated degradation of endothelium-derived nitric oxide may contribute to this abnormal function. Timimi and colleagues[42] from Boston, Massachusetts, evaluated the effects of the antioxidant vitamin C on endothelium-dependent vasodilation of forearm resistance vessels in patients with insulin-dependent diabetes mellitus. The study group included 10 patients with diabetes and 10 age-matched control subjects. Forearm blood flow was determined by venous occlusion plethysmography. Endothelium-dependent vasodilation was assessed by intra-arterial infusion of methacholine 0.3-10 μg/min. Endothelium-independent vasodilation was assessed by intra-arterial infusion of nitroprusside. In diabetic subjects, endothelium-dependent vasodilation was augmented by the concomitant infusion of vitamin C (24 mg/min). Endothelium-independent vasodilation was not affected by the concomitant infusion of vitamin C. Similarly, in control subjects, vitamin C infusion did not affect endothelium-dependent vasodilation. These authors conclude that vitamin C selectively restores the impaired endothelium-dependent vasodilation in the forearm resistance vessels of patients with insulin-dependent diabetes mellitus. These data suggest that nitric oxide degradation by oxygen-derived free radicals contributes to the abnormal vascular reactivity seen in humans with insulin-dependent diabetes mellitus.

Human Monocyte Gene Expression

Human monocyte chemoattractant protein-1 is expressed by a variety of cell types in response to various stimuli. Monocyte chemoattractant protein-1 expressed by the endothelium plays an important role in cell migration activation. Monocyte chemoattractant protein-1 is a major chemoattractant for monocytes, T lymphocytes, and basophils. Parry and coinvestigators[43] in La Jolla, California, presented evidence that the proteasome complex is involved in mediating the interleukin-1β induction of monocyte chemoattractant protein-1 in endothelial cells. The investigators presented evidence that a proteasome inhibitor, N-acetyl-leucinyl-leucinyl-norleucinal, and the protease inhibitor, tosyl-Phe-chloromethylketone, block interleukin-1β induction of monocyte chemoattractant protein-1 protein expression. norLeu and tosyl-Phe-chloromethylketone also blocked interleukin-1β-induced monocyte chemoattractant protein-1 promotor driven reporter gene expression as well as nuclear factor kB-mediated reporter gene expression. The effects of norLeu were due to its inhibition of the proteasome rather than calpain, because other calpain inhibitors had no effect on monocyte chemoattractant protein-1 expression. In contrast to the tosyl-Phe-chloromethylketone, which blocked nuclear factor kB translocation to the nucleus, norLeu had no effect on nuclear factor kB nuclear translocation or interleukin-1β-induced phosphorylation of p65. This study demonstrates that the proteasome pathway is involved in interleukin-1β-induced monocyte chemoattractant protein-1 gene expression in human endothelial cells.

Calcification of Human Vascular Cells

The cellular and molecular events leading to calcification in atherosclerotic lesions are unknown. Proudfoot and associates[44] in Cambridge, United Kingdom, have shown that bone-associated proteins, particularly matrix Gla and osteopontin, can be detected in atherosclerotic lesions, thus suggesting an active calcification process. In this study, the investigators aimed to determine whether human vascular smooth muscle cells could calcify *in vitro* and to determine whether matrix Gla protein and osteopontin have a role in vascular calcification. The investigators established that human aortic vascular smooth muscle cells and placental microvascular pericytes spontaneously formed nodules in cell culture and induced calcification, as detected by von Kossa's method, alizarin red S staining and electron microscopy. The cells in calcifying nodules differed from those in monolayer cultures by expressing higher levels of the smooth muscle cell markers α-smooth muscle actin, smooth muscle 22 α, and calponin. In addition, Northern blot analysis revealed that in human vascular smooth muscle cells, calcification was associated with increased levels of matrix Gla protein mRNA. In contrast, osteopontin mRNA was barely detectible in calcified human vascular smooth muscle cells and pericyte nodules, and osteopontin protein was not detected, suggesting that osteopontin was not necessary for calcification to occur. These studies reveal that human vascular smooth muscle cells are capable of inducing calcification and that matrix Gla protein may have a role in human vascular calcification.

Endothelial Dysfunction in the Pathogenesis of Atherosclerosis

Endothelial dysfunction, or activation, elicited by oxidized low-density lipoprotein (OX-LDL) and its lipid constituents has been shown to play a key role in the pathogenesis of atherosclerosis. Moriwaki and associates[45] in Kyoto, Japan, recently identified a novel receptor OX-LDL-designated lectin-like OX-LDL receptor (LOX-I) in vascular endothelial cells. To examine ligand specificity of LOX-I, the investigators established CHO cell line stably expressing both human and bovine LOX-I (LOX-I-CHO). LOX-I-CHO bound and degraded I^{125}-labeled OX-LDL but did not significantly degrade I^{125}-labeled acetylated LDL (Ac-LDL). Fucoidin and maleylated BSA (M-BSA), which inhibit I^{125}-OX-LDL binding to class A scavenger receptors, did not inhibit I^{125}-OX-LDL binding or degradation in LOX-I-CHO. Polyinosinic acid and carrageenan, in contrast, significantly reduced I^{125}-OX-LDL binding to LOX-I-CHO by 62% and 60%, respectively. Delipidated and untreated I^{125}-OX-LDL were bound and degraded equally and LOX-I-CHO; furthermore, excessive amounts of unlabeled, delipidated OX-LDL inhibited binding and degradation of untreated I^{125}-OX-LDL. Taken together, LOX-I is a receptor for OX-LDL but not for Ac-LDL. LOX-I recognizes protein moiety of OX-LDL, and its ligand specificity is distinct from other receptors for OX-LDL, including class A and B scavenger receptors.

Role of Adhesion Molecules in Serine Proteases

Polymorphonuclear leukocytes (PMNs) and endothelial cells interact at sites of vascular injury during inflammatory response and during the development of atherosclerotic lesions. Such close proximity leads to the modulation of several of the biological functions of the 2 cell types. Because Totani and colleagues[46] in Santa Maria Imbaro, Italy, had shown previously that PMNs enhance release of growth factors from resting endothelial cells, the investigators decided to evaluate whether co-incubation of PMNs with interleukin-Iβ (IL-Iβ) stimulated human umbilical vein endothelial cells (HUVEC) could further modulate mitogen release from HUVEC. The investigators found that PMN-HUVEC co-incubation resulted in a 10-fold increase in mitogen release, compared with HUVEC alone. When PMNs were incubated with IL-Iβ-treated HUVEC, a further increase in mitogen release up to 35-fold was observed (Figure 1-23). The mitogenic activity was immunologically related to platelet-derived growth factor (PDGF) because the activity was abolished by an anti-PDGF antibody. PDGF-AB antigen, detected in low concentrations in conditioned media from HUVEC alone, was increased 4-fold when IL-Iβ or PMNs were incubated with HUVEC and dramatically upgraded up to 40-fold when PMNs were co-cultured with IL-Iβ-treated HUVEC. The presence of the protease inhibitor eglin C abolished mitogenic activity generation, suggesting a role of PMN-derived elastase and cathepsin G. Indeed, purified elastase and cathepsin G mimicked PMN-induced mitogen release from HUVEC. Because PMNs firmly adhered to IL-Iβ-treated HUVEC, the investigators examined the role of cell-cell adhesion in mitogen release. Adhesion and PDGF release were inhibited by 60% in the presence of anti-CD11a/CD18 and anti-intercellular adhesion molecule-1 monoclonal antibodies. This study suggests a new role for PMNs and their interaction with endothelium and pathological conditions in which intimal hyperplasia is a common feature.

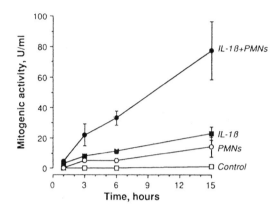

FIGURE 1-23. Line plots showing the effect of PMNs on mitogen release from untreated or IL-1β-treated HUVEC: kinetics. HUVEC (2.5 × 10⁵/well) were incubated in the absence or presence of PMNs (10⁶/mL), for 1, 3, 6, and 15 hours. Conditioned medium was collected, sedimented by centrifugation, and tested for [³H]-TdR incorporation into BALB/c 3T3. Each point represents mean ± SEM of 3 experiments. Reproduced with permission from Totani et al.[46]

Expression of Adhesion Molecules in Endothelial Cells

Ashby and colleagues[47] in Adelaide, Australia, had previously reported that HDLs inhibit the cytokine-induced expression of adhesion molecules in endothelial cells. The investigators further examined whether different preparations of HDLs vary in their ability to inhibit the expression of vascular cell adhesion molecule-1 (VCAM-1) in human umbilical vein endothelial cells (HUVECs) activated by tumor necrosis factor-α (TNF-α). HDLs selected from a number of different human subjects all inhibited VCAM-1 expression in a concentration-dependent manner, although the extent of the inhibition varied widely among subjects. The inhibitory activities of HDL_2 and HDL_3 subfractions isolated from individual subjects also differed. Whether equated for concentrations of apolipoprotein A-I or cholesterol, inhibitory activity of HDL_3 was superior to that of HDL_2. The difference remained apparent even when the HDL subfractions were present only during preincubations with the human HUVECs and were removed before activation by TNF-α. To determine whether the inhibitory effect of HDL_3 was influenced by apolipoprotein composition, preparations of HDL_3 were modified by replacing all of their apolipoprotein A-I with apolipoprotein A-II. This change in apolipoprotein composition had no effect on the ability of the HDL_3 to inhibit endothelial VCAM-1 expression. Thus, the investigators show that different preparations of HDL differ markedly in their abilities to inhibit VCAM-1 expression in cytokine-activated HUVECs. The mechanism underlying the differences remains to be determined.

Role of Endogenous Prostanoids

Two isoforms of cyclooxygenase (COX) have been identified: a constitutive isoform (COX-1) found in abundance in platelets and the vascular endothelium, and an inflammatory cytokine-inducible isoform (COX-2). Because COX metabolites regulate vascular smooth muscle cell (SMC) function and the interaction between the vessel and circulating components, Bishop-Bailey and associates[48] in London, United Kingdom, investigated the possibility that COX-2 can be induced in human arterial or venous SMC. Untreated venous or arterial cells contained undetectable levels of COX-1 or COX-2 and released low levels of metabolites. After stimulation with interleukin-1β, tumor necrosis factor-α, interferon-γ, and bacterial lipopolysaccharide, both venous and arterial SMC expressed COX-2 protein and released increased amounts of prostaglandins. In addition, the induced release of PGE_2 was inhibited by the COX-2-selective inhibitor, L-745, 337. When cells were treated with a mixture of cytokines, venous SMCs expressed greater amounts of COX-2 protein and released more prostaglandin than arterial SMC. Furthermore, when COX-2 activity was blocked by L-745,337, COX-2 expression in arterial SMC, but not in venous SMC, increased. Thus, the investigation described, for the first time, that COX-2 is expressed in greater amounts in venous SMC than in arterial SMC. Moreover, the investigators showed that this "differential induction" is due to a negative feedback pathway for COX-2 expression in arterial SMC but not in venous SMC. The ability of COX-2 activity to limit COX-2 expression in some cells but not others may contribute to the highly developed mechanisms involved in prostanoid release.

Effect of Gemfibrozil on Endothelial Function

Andrews and associates[49] from San Antonio, Texas, studied endothelial function using the brachial artery ultrasound model in 100 subjects from the Armed Forces Regression Study, a placebo-controlled, angiographic regression trial in subjects with normal or moderately elevated LDL cholesterol and low levels of HDL cholesterol. These subjects were treated for 30 months with gemfibrozil and (if necessary) niacin and/or cholestyramine to raise HDL by 25% and lower LDL to less than 110 mg/dL. Although the treatment group had highly significant improvements in LDL and HDL cholesterol, there was no difference between the 2 groups in flow-mediated dilation (treatment vs. control subjects 6.9% ± 6.5% vs. 6.3% ± 7.3%) or nitroglycerin-induced dilation (12.4% ± 9.6% vs. 11.9% ± 7.4%). Treatment and control subjects without a history of systemic hypertension had flow-mediated dilation similar to that of a normal reference population (10.6% ± 8.3% vs. 8.4% ± 4.5%), whereas subjects with a history of systemic hypertension had markedly impaired flow-mediated dilation that was not significantly improved with treatment (treatment vs. control subjects 6.0% ± 5.5% vs. 4.3% ± 5.9%). Thus, nonhypertensive subjects with angiographic CAD and low HDL cholesterol had normal endothelial function in the brachial artery model. Patients with a history of hypertension had marked endothelial dysfunction despite blood pressure treated to normal levels, and this dysfunction is not attenuated by pharmacologic therapy for dyslipidemia.

Shear Stress-Mediated Inhibition of Apoptosis

Physiological levels of shear stress reduce endothelial cell turnover and exert a potent anti-arteriosclerotic effect. Hermann and coworkers[50] in Frankfurt, Germany, demonstrated that oxidative stress-induced apoptosis of human endothelial cells was inhibited by shear stress exposure. Incubation with H_2O_2 (200 μmol/L) for 18 hours induced apoptosis of human umbilical venous endothelial cells as demonstrated by an enzyme-linked immunosorbent assay specific for histone-associated DNA fragments and visual analysis of fluorescence-stained nuclei. Shear stress-mediated inhibition of apoptosis was partially prevented by pharmacological inhibition of glutathione biosynthesis with buthionine sulfoximine or NO synthase with N^G-monomethyl-L-arginine, where inhibition of catalase by aminotriazol did not affect the inhibitor action of shear stress. Combined inhibition of NO synthase and glutathione biosynthesis completely reversed the protective effect of shear stress suggesting that both NO synthase and the glutathione redox cycle system are involved in the apoptosis of suppressing effect of shear stress. Similar results were obtained when apoptosis was stimulated by tumor necrosis factor-α. To gain further insights into the interference of shear stress with apoptosis signal transduction, the investigators measured caspase-3-like activity, a cysteine protease that has been shown to play a predominant role in the cell death effector pathway. Indeed, shear stress prevented the activation of caspase-3-like activity induced by H_2O_2 or tumor necrosis factor-α. The inhibitory effect of shear stress was prevented by N-monomethyl-L-arginine and buthionine sulfoximine, suggesting that the reduction of oxidative flux by shear stress prevents the activation of caspase-3-like proteases and thereby inhibits apoptotic cell death in human endothelial cells.

Use of Vitamin C to Prevent Development of Nitrate Tolerance

Decreased intracellular production of cyclic guanosine monophosphate (GMP) is a mechanism of nitrate tolerance. Increased supraoxide levels and reduced activation of guanylate cyclase have been observed *in vitro*. Watanabe and colleagues[51] from Ibaraki, Japan, evaluated the potential preventive effects of vitamin C, an antioxidant, on the development of nitrate tolerance. In a double-blind, placebo-controlled study, 24 normal volunteers and 24 patients with CAD were randomized to receive either vitamin C (2 g 3 times daily) or placebo. The vasodilator response to nitroglycerin was assessed with forearm plethysmography before and 5 minutes after sublingual administration of 0.3 mg of nitroglycerin. Blood samples were simultaneously obtained to measure platelet cyclic GMP levels. There were no differences between the vitamin C and placebo groups in the percent increase in forearm blood flow or platelet cyclic GMP levels after administration of sublingual nitroglycerin on day 0. The percent forearm blood flow and percent cyclic GMP in the placebo group were significantly lower on day 6 than in the vitamin C group. These results indicate that therapy with vitamin C is potentially useful for preventing the development of nitrate tolerance.

Platelet Aggregation

Chronolog Whole-Body Aggregometer

Mascelli and colleagues[52] in Malvern, Pennsylvania, adapted the chronolog whole-body aggregometer to test platelet function at the bedside with the hope of allowing an improved assessment of platelet glycoprotein llb/llla receptor blockade. They used this device to measure GP llb/llla receptor blockade, which measures platelet aggregation by electrical impedance. Platelet aggregation to collagen, and turbidimetric aggregation to 5 and 20 μmol/L adenosine diphosphate (ADF)-induced platelet aggregation was measured in 14 patients undergoing PTCA who received the standard bolus plus a 12-hour infusion of the platelet glycoprotein llb/llla receptor antagonist, abciximab. During abciximab administration, a mean GP llb/llla receptor blockade was greater than 91%, and both impedance and turbidimetric aggregation were inhibited by 90% or more. At 12 hours after abciximab treatment, the mean inhibition of turbidimetric platelet aggregation to 5 and 20 μmol/L ADP was 65% $\pm$ 20% and 49% $\pm$ 14%, respectively, and inhibition of impedance aggregation was 69% $\pm$ 12%. GP llb/llla receptor blockade was 67% $\pm$ 8%. After 36 hours following abciximab treatment in 8 patients, the mean inhibition of turbidimetric platelet aggregation to 5 and 20 μmol/L ADP was 44% $\pm$ 21% and 30% $\pm$ 14%, respectively. Thus, during and at 12 hours after abciximab therapy, impedance and turbidimetric platelet aggregation to ADP were comparable and closely correlated with GP llb/llla receptor blockade. However, 36 hours after treatment, the impedance platelet aggregation more closely paralleled GP llb/llla receptor blockade and indicates a slower recovery of platelet function than turbidimetric aggregometry (Figure 1-24).

Cell Adhesion Molecules

Hypertriglyceridemia may contribute to the development of atherosclerosis by increasing expression of cell adhesion molecules. Although the cellular expression of cell adhesion molecules is difficult to assess clinically, soluble forms of cell adhesion molecules are present in the circulation and may serve as markers for cellular adhesion molecules. Abe and coworkers[53] in Houston, Texas, examined the association between soluble forms of cell adhesion molecules and other risk factors occurring with hypertriglyceridemia, the effect of triglyceride reduction on soluble cell adhesion molecule levels and the role of soluble vascular cell adhesion molecule-1 in monocyte adhesion *in vitro*. Compared with normal control subjects (n = 20), subjects with hypertriglyceridemia and low HDL (n = 39) had significantly increased levels of soluble intercellular adhesion molecule-1, soluble vascular cell adhesion molecule-1, and soluble E-selectin. Analysis of covariance (ANCOVA) showed that the higher soluble forms of cell adhesion molecule levels in patients occurred independently of diabetes mellitus and other risk factors. In 27 patients who received purified n-3 fatty acids (OMACOR) 4 g/day for 7 months, triglyceride level was

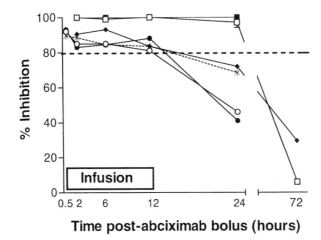

Time post-abciximab bolus (hours)

FIGURE 1-24. Inhibition of electrical impedance (20 μmol/L ADP [-□-], 6 μmol/L TRAP [-■-], and 5 μg/mL collagen [♦]) and turbidimetric (5 μmol/L [-○-] and 20 μmol/L [-●-] ADP), platelet aggregation, as well as GP IIb/IIIa receptor blockade [-*-] in two subjects who received the 0.25-mg/kg bolus and a 12-hour infusion of abciximab. One individual received a 0.125-μg·kg^{-1}·min^{-1} infusion, and the other subject received a 10-μg/min infusion of abciximab. Degree of GP IIb/IIIa receptors that are blocked by abciximab. Levels of inhibition of electrical impedance and light transmission aggregation are expressed as the percent inhibition of aggregation present after abciximab administration. Results represent the mean values at each time point. Reproduced with permission from Mascelli et al.[52]

reduced by 47%, soluble intercellular adhesion molecule-1 level was reduced by 9%, and soluble E-selectin level was reduced by 16%, with the greatest reduction in diabetic patients (Figure 1-25). These results support previous *in vitro* data showing that disorders in triglyceride and HDL metabolism influenced cell adhesion molecule expression and treatment with fish oils might

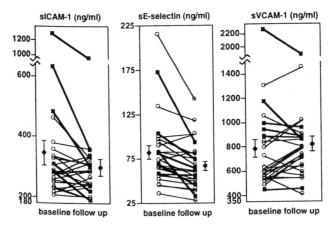

FIGURE 1-25. Levels of sICAM-1, sE-selectin, and sVCAM-1 in the serum of 27 hypertriglyceridemic patients before and after long-term treatment with Omacor. ■ and ○ indicate hypertriglyceridemic patients with and without NIDDM, respectively. ♦ = arithmetic mean; error bars = SE. Reproduced with permission from Abe et al.[53]

alter vascular cell activation. In a parallel-plate growth chamber, recombinant soluble vascular cell adhesion molecule-1 at the concentration seen in patients significantly inhibited adhesion of monocytes to interleukin-1-stimulated cultured endothelial cells under conditions of flow by 28%. Thus, elevated soluble forms of cell adhesion molecules may negatively regulate monocyte adhesion.

Inhibition of Thrombin-Induced Platelet Aggregation

Nofer and coinvestigators[54] in Munster, Germany, demonstrated that physiologic concentrations of HDL_3 from human volunteers inhibit the thrombin-induced platelet fibrinogen binding and aggregation in a time- and concentration-dependent fashion. The underlying mechanism included HDL_3-mediated inhibition of phosphatidylinositol 4,5-bis-phosphate turnover, 1,2-diacylglycerol, and inositol 1,4,5-tris-phosphate formation, and intracellular calcium mobilization. The inhibitory effects of HDL_3 on inositol 1,4,5-tris-phosphate formation and intracellular calcium mobilization were abolished after covalent modification of HDL_3 with dimethylsuberimidate. Furthermore, they could be blocked by calphostin C and bis-indolymaleimide, 2 highly selective and structurally unrelated protein kinase C inhibitors. However, the inhibitory effects of HDL_3 were not blocked by H89, a protein kinase A inhibitor. In addition, HDL_3 failed to induce cAMP formation but stimulated the phosphorylation of the protein kinase C 40 to 47 kD major protein substrate. The investigators observed a close temporal relationship between the HDL_3-mediated inhibition of thrombin-induced inositol 1,4,5-tris-phosphate formation, intracellular calcium mobilization, and fibrinogen binding and the phosphorylation of the protein kinase C 40 to 47 kD major protein substrate (Figure 1-26). Taken together, these findings indicate that the HDL_3-mediated inhibition of thrombin-induced fibrinogen binding and aggregation occur via inhibition of phosphatidylinositol 4,5-bis-phosphate turnover and formation of 1,2-diacylglycerol and inositol 1,4,5-tris-phosphate. Protein kinase C may be involved in this process.

Human Platelet Activation

The mechanisms that underlie reocclusion during thrombolytic therapy have not yet been clarified. The purpose of this study by Kawano and associates[55] from Tokyo, Japan, was to investigate the activating effects of tissue-type plasminogen activator and urokinase and the inhibitory effects of acetylsalicylic acid by measuring platelet surface P-selectin as a marker of platelet activation. After addition of urokinase (final concentration 192 U/mL, 1920 U/mL, or 19,200 U/mL) or tissue-type plasminogen activator (final concentration 120 U/mL, 1200 U/mL, or 12,000 U/mL) to platelet-rich plasma from 12 healthy persons, platelet surface P-selectin expression was measured by means of flow cytometry with an anti-CD62 monoclonal antibody. The presence of urokinase and tissue-type plasminogen activator increased platelet surface P-selectin expression in a concentration-dependent manner. In the next step,

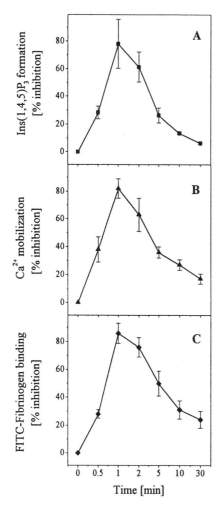

FIGURE 1-26. Influence of the incubation time on the HDL_3-induced inhibition of $Ins(1,4,5)P_3$ formation, $[Ca^{2+}]_i$ mobilization, and fibrinogen binding. Washed platelets (1×10^9/mL) were preincubated for the indicated times with 1.0 g/L HDL_3 and then stimulated with 0.1 U/mL thrombin. $Ins(1,4,5)P_3$ formation (A), Ca^{2+} mobilization (B), and fibrinogen binding (C) were determined. The results are given as mean ±SD of the relative inhibition and are representative of at least 3 independent experiments. Reproduced with permission from Nofer et al.[54]

either 160 mg/day (n = 6) or 660 mg/day (n = 6) acetylsalicylic acid was administered to the 12 healthy persons, and venous blood samples were collected after 7 days of treatment. Platelet surface P-selectin expression was measured with the method used earlier and after addition of tissue-type plasminogen activator or urokinase. Although the effect of acetylsalicylic acid at 160 mg/day on P-selectin expression was minimal, a dose of 660 mg/day suppressed platelet P-selectin expression and inhibited the platelet-activating effects of tissue-type plasminogen activator and urokinase in a statistically significant way. Platelets were activated by tissue-type plasminogen activator or urokinase, and this platelet activation was suppressed with administration of acetylsalicylic acid at 660 mg/day.

Role of Enhanced Responses of Platelets in Atherosclerosis

Elevated levels of lipoprotein(a) [Lp(a)] are correlated with an increased risk of atherosclerotic disease. Rand and colleagues[56] in Ontario, Canada, ex-

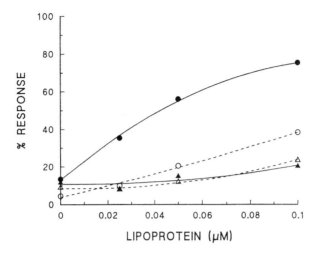

FIGURE 1-27. Effects of purified Lp(a) (O, ●) and LDL (△, ▲) on aggregation (●, ▲) and secretion of [^{14}C]serotonin (O, △) when platelets were stimulated by 7.5 μmol/L SFLLRN. Data, expressed as percentages, are representative of 2 experiments with similar results. Reproduced with permission from Rand et al.[56]

amined the effect of recombinant apolipoprotein(a) [r-apo(a)] and Lp(a) on responses of washed human platelets, pre-labeled with C^{14} serotonin and suspended in Tyrode's solution, to ADP and the thrombin receptor-activated peptide SFLLRN. No effect of the 17-kringle, 12-kringle, or 6-kringle r-apo(a) derivatives or Lp(a) on primary ADP-induced platelet aggregation was observed. In contrast, weak platelet responses stimulated by SFLLRN were significantly enhanced by the r-apo(a) derivatives. Significant enhancement of aggregation and release of granule contents was observed at low concentrations of 17-kringle r-apo(a). Purified lipoprotein(a) also enhanced SFLLRN-induced aggregation and release in a dose-dependent manner. Although plasminogen and LDL both exhibited potentiating effects on SFLLRN-mediated platelet aggregation, the magnitude of the responses was less than that observed with either the r-apo(a) derivatives or Lp(a) (Figure 1-27). The enhanced responses of platelets via the protease-activated receptor-1 thrombin receptor in the presence of Lp(a) may contribute to the increased risk of thromboembolic complications of atherosclerosis associated with this lipoprotein.

Effect of Estrogen on Platelet Function

The low prevalence of CAD in premenopausal women and its increase after menopause are well established. Although estrogen is thought to play a role in protecting the vasculature, the mechanism has not been fully clarified. The contribution of platelets to atherosclerotic cardiovascular diseases is well recognized. A study by Nakano and coworkers[57] in Hiroshima, Japan, focused on the still-controversial effect of estrogen on platelet function. The investigators examined the *in vitro* effects of estrogen on human platelets, including the aggregation, Ca^{2+} metabolism, the synthesis of cyclic nucleotides and NO synthesis after stimulation with thrombin or ADP. Pretreatment of platelets with 17β-estradiol reduced the platelet aggregation induced by thrombin or ADP, whereas 17α-estradiol had no effect. 17β-Estradiol accelerated the recovery of Ca^{2+} after the agonist-induced peak and reduced the area under the curve of accumulated platelet Ca^{2+}, but did not alter the baseline value Ca^{2+} influx induced by thrombin or ADP, the release of Ca^{2+} from internal stores, or the size of internal Ca^{2+} stores. Pretreatment of platelets of 17β-estradiol had no effect on the intracellular concentration of cAMP, but increased that of cGMP in agonist-stimulated platelets. Additionally, 17β-estradiol increased the platelet concentration of NO in a dose-dependent manner. These effects of 17β-estradiol on platelet aggregation, Ca^{2+} metabolism, and NO synthesis were abolished by exposure to N^{G}-monomethyl-L-arginine, an NO synthesis inhibitor. These results suggest that 17β-estradiol plays an important role in inhibiting platelet aggregation by promoting Ca^{2+} extrusion or reuptake activity that is dependent on the production of cGMP by increasing NO synthesis.

Atherogenesis/Thrombosis/Fibrosis

Relationship Between Tissue Factor Pathway Inhibitor and Tissue Factor Activity Within Plaques

Caplice and colleagues[58] in Rochester, Minnesota, measured the level of tissue factor pathway inhibitor (TFPI) antigen in human carotid plaques and determined the relationship between TFPI and tissue factor activity within the plaque. TFPI is an endogenous inhibitor of tissue factor-induced coagulation that binds to factor Xa and the TF-FVIIa catalytic complex. TFPI was detectable in 22 of 34 specimens (Figure 1-28). In the plaques without detectable TFPI, normalized tissue factor activity was greater than in those plaques with detecta-

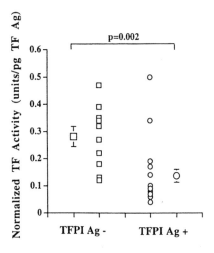

FIGURE 1-28. Scatterplot of normalized TF activity in homogenized carotid plaque specimens with undetectable TFPI antigen (□ = TFPI Ag−) and detectable TFPI antigen (○ = TFPI Ag+). Mean ±SEM values are presented adjacent to the individual data points. Reproduced with permission from Caplice et al.[58]

ble TFPI activity. Neutralization of TFPI activity using a polyclonal antibody resulted in an 8-fold increase in tissue factor activity in the TFPI positive group, but had no effect in the TFPI negative group. Immunostaining for TFPI showed localization to endothelial cells, vascular smooth muscle cells within the fibrous cap region of the plaque, and macrophages within the shoulder region of the plaque. These data suggest that biologically active TFPI is present within human atherosclerotic plaque and is associated with an attenuation of tissue factor activity.

Vascular Smooth Muscle Cell Proliferation

Vascular smooth muscle cell proliferation still remains a poorly understood process, although it is believed to play a critical role in pathological states including atherosclerosis and hypertension. Several reports have suggested that proteases might be directly involved in this process; however, it was still unclear which protease is responsible for vascular smooth muscle cell proliferation. In a study by Ariyoshi and colleagues[59] in Osaka, Japan, by use of a cell-permeable calpain inhibitor, its analog, the cell-impermeable semine protease inhibitor, leupetin, and antisense oligonucleotide against m-calpain to inhibit proliferation of primarily cultured smooth muscle cells, the investigators examined whether calcium-activated neutral protease (calpain) was involved in vascular smooth muscle cell proliferation. Calpeptin and its analog, more specific for m-calpain, equally inhibited the proliferation of vascular smooth muscle cells in a dose-related manner, whereas a more limited antiproliferative effect was observed in lupeptin-treated vascular smooth muscle cells. Antisense oligonucleotide against m-calpain, but not scrambled antisense, dose-dependently inhibited m-calpain expression and proliferation of vascular smooth muscle cells. Maximal inhibition was a 50% reduction of cell number and m-calpain antigen observed at 50 mol/L of antisense oligonucleotide. Calpeptin or antisense oligonucleotide against m-calpain increased the expression of the endogenous calpain substrate pp 125 focal adhesion kinase, whereas the expression of the endogenous calpain inhibitor, calpastatin was not affected. These results suggest that the proliferation of vascular smooth muscle cells requires protease activity, some of which was due to m-calpain.

Plasma Fibrinogen Levels

Increased plasma fibrinogen levels have been identified as a risk indicator for myocardial infarction, stroke, and thrombosis. Both environmental and genetic factors make an important contribution to plasma fibrinogen levels in humans. deMaat and coinvestigators[60] in Leiden, The Netherlands, evaluated in patients with serum cholesterol levels between 4 and 8 mmol/L, the relation of plasma levels and polymorphisms of fibrinogen with CAD, cross-sectionally at baseline and after a 2-year follow-up period, in which they received either a placebo or pravastatin. Higher plasma fibrinogen levels were observed at baseline in patients with the − 455 AA genotype than in patients with the − 455

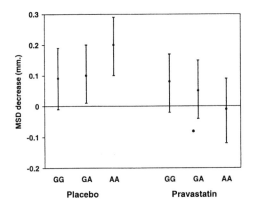

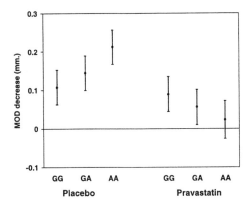

FIGURE 1-29. Mean (SE) decrease of MSD and MOD in patients according to genotypes of the −455G/A polymorphism and to treatment (placebo or pravastatin), after adjustment for baseline values. Reproduced with permission from deMaat et al.[60]

GA and −455 GG genotypes of the −455 G/A fibrinogen β-gene polymorphism. Plasma levels of fibrinogen were not related to the baseline angiographic variables (mean segment diameter and minimum obstruction diameter), or to the quantitative changes in these angiographic variables. However, in the placebo group, patients with the −455 AA genotype had more progression of CAD, expressed by the significantly greater decrease of the mean segment diameter and minimum obstruction diameter after the 2-year follow-up than patients with the other genotypes. The −455 G/A polymorphism was related to the progression of CAD, and pravastatin therapy seems to offset this deleterious effect (Figure 1-29). The investigators hypothesize that the −455 A allele may promote a stronger acute phase response in fibrinogen and that the resulting higher fibrinogen levels may form the pathogenic basis for the stronger progression of coronary atherosclerosis. Experiments to verify this hypothesis are being proposed and advocated, in view of the possibility of identifying a genetic marker that can recognize a subgroup of patients with an increased risk who may benefit from early treatment with lipid-lowering or anticoagulant drugs.

Plasma Viscosity

Plasma viscosity is determined by various macromolecules, e.g., fibrinogen, immunoglobulins, and lipoproteins. It may, therefore, reflect several aspects involved in cardiovascular disease, including the effects of classic risk factors, hemostatic disturbances, and inflammation. Koenig and colleagues[61] in Ulm, Germany, examined the association of plasma viscosity with the instance of a first major coronary heart disease event (fatal and nonfatal myocardial infarction and cardiac death, n = 50) in 933 men, age 45–64 years, of the MONICA project of Augsburg, Germany. The incidence rate was 7.23/1,000 person-years and the subjects were followed-up for 8 years. All suspected cases of an incident coronary heart disease event were classified according to the MONICA protocol. There was a positive and statistically significant unadjusted relationship between plasma viscosity and the incidence of coronary heart disease events. Relative risk of coronary heart disease events associated with a 1 SD increase in plasma viscosity was 1.6. After adjustments for age, total cholesterol, HDL cholesterol, smoking, blood pressure, and body mass index, the relative risk was reduced only moderately (1.42). The relative risk of coronary heart disease events for the men in the highest quintile of the plasma viscosity distribution in comparison with the lowest quintile was 3.31, after adjustment for the aforementioned variables. A large proportion of events (40%) occurred among men in the highest quintile. These findings suggest that plasma viscosity may have considerable potential to identify subjects at risk for coronary heart disease events.

Intracellular Receptors

Peroxisome proliferator-activated receptors and retinoid X receptors are members of the intracellular receptor superfamily. Peroxisome receptors bind to peroxisome proliferator response elements as heterodimers with retinoid X receptors and as such activate gene transcription in response to activators. Fibrates like gemfibrozil are well-known peroxisome α-activators and are used in the treatment of hyperlipidemia. Mukherjee and associates[62] in San Diego, California, showed that the retinoid X receptors ligand LGD1069 (targretin), like gemfibrozil, can activate the peroxisome α/retinoid X receptor signal transduction pathway including transactivation of the bifunctional enzyme or acyl-CoA oxidase response elements in a cotransfection assay. The activation also occurs *in vivo*, whereby in rats treated with LGD1069 or gemfibrozil, bifunctional enzyme and acyl-CoA oxidase RNA are induced, and the combination of LGD1069 and gemfibrozil leads to a greater induction. Importantly, in hypertriglyceridemic mice treated with retinoid X receptors or peroxisome α agonists, triglyceride levels are lowered and the combination again had significantly greater efficacy. Retinoid X receptor agonists also raised HDL levels without changing Apo-I RNA expression. This observation suggests the use of retinoid X receptor-selective agonist "rexinoids" either alone or in combination with a fibrate as a new therapeutic approach to treating patients with high triglyceride and low HDL levels.

Role of Complement Activation in Atherogenesis

There is increasing evidence that complement activation may play a role in atherogenesis. Complement proteins have been demonstrated to be present in early atherosclerotic lesions in animals and in humans. Cholesterol-induced atherosclerotic lesion formation is reduced in complement-deficient animals. Potential complement activators in atherosclerotic lesions are now a subject matter of debate. C-reactive protein (CRP) is an acute phase protein that is involved in inflammatory processes in numerous ways and binds to lipoproteins and activates the complement system via the classic pathway. Torzewski and coinvestigators[63] in Dusseldorf, Germany, investigated early atherosclerotic lesions of human coronary arteries by means of immunohistological staining. The investigators demonstrated that CRP deposited in the arterial wall in early atherosclerotic lesions with 2 predominant manifestations. First, there was a diffuse rather than a focal deposition in the deep fibroblastic layer and in the fibromuscular layer of the intima. In this location, CRP frequently co-localized with the terminal complement complex. Second, the majority of cells below the endothelium showed positive staining for CRP. In this location, no co-localization with the terminal complement protein was observed. The data suggest that CRP may promote atherosclerotic lesion formation by activating the complement system and being involved in foam cell formation.

Analysis of Plasma Fibrinogen Concentration

Elevated plasminogen-activated inhibitor-1 (PAI-1) and fibrinogen concentrations are risk factors for CAD. Pankow and coinvestigators[64] in Chapel Hill, North Carolina, investigated environmental, familial, and genetic influences on PAI-1 antigen and fibrinogen concentrations in 2,029 adults from 512 randomly ascertained families in 4 US communities. The investigators used maximum likelihood segregation analysis to fit several genetic and nongenetic modes of inheritance to the data to determine whether mendelian inheritance of a major gene could best explain the familial distributions of these 2 hemostatic factors. Age- and gender-adjusted familial correlations for PAI-1 antigen averaged 0.16 in first-degree relatives; the spouse correlation was positive but not statistically significant. Complex segregation analysis indicated a major gene associated with high PAI-1 concentration in 65% of individuals from these families. Demographic, anthropometric lifestyle, and metabolic characteristics together explained 37% to 47% of the variation in PAI-1 antigen levels, and the inferred major gene explained an additional 17% of the variance. Positive and statistically significant age- and gender-adjusted familial correlations in first-degree relatives indicated a possible heritable component influencing plasma fibrinogen concentration; however, segregation analysis did not provide statistical evidence of a major gene controlling fibrinogen level. These family data suggest that there are modest familial and genetic effects on the concentration of PAI-1.

Role of Chemokines in Atherosclerosis

Arteriosclerotic lesions are characterized by accumulation of T lymphocytes and monocytes and the proliferation of intimal smooth muscle cells. Expression of the chemokine monocyte chemoattractant protein-1 has been observed in arteriosclerotic plaques and has been proposed to mediate the transendothelial migration of mononuclear cells. More recently, monocyte chemoattractant protein-1 has been proposed to affect the proliferation migration of smooth muscle cells. Hayes and coinvestigators[65] in Essex, United Kingdom, have used reverse transcription polymerase chain reaction to investigate chemokine mRNA expression in human arteriosclerotic lesions obtained from surgical biopsy of diseased vascular tissue and have shown, in addition to monocyte chemoattractant protein-1, expression of the chemokine macrophage inflammatory protein-1 α at higher levels than in normal aortic tissue. The investigators also used polymerase chain reaction to characterize the expression of known chemokine receptors by primary human vascular smooth muscle cells. mRNA for the macrophage inflammatory protein/receptor and the chemokine monocyte attractant protein receptor was expressed by unstimulated vascular smooth muscle cells grown under serum-free culture conditions for 24 hours. The receptors were not expressed by vascular smooth muscle cells. The presence of functionally coupled receptors for the macrophage inflammatory protein-1 α on smooth muscle vascular cells was demonstrated by specific binding by biotinylated macrophage inflammatory protein-1 and increases in intracellular CA^{2+} levels after exposure to this chemokine. Taken together, these results suggest that chemokines are likely to be involved in arteriosclerosis and may play a role in modulating the function of vascular smooth muscle cells *in vivo*.

Predictive Value of Lipid Profiles and Fibrinolytic Parameters

There is as yet no definite consensus on the predictive value of the various lipid profiles and fibrinolytic parameters that became available in clinical use recently for CAD. Levels of lipoprotein(a), HDL cholesterol, remnant-like particles cholesterol (RLP-C), tissue plasminogen activator (t-PA), t-PA inhibitor, antithrombin III, and protein C were measured in 124 patients who underwent diagnostic coronary angiograms in this study by Masuoka and associates[66] from Owase and Tsu, Japan. Of these patients, 37 had no significant stenoses (group N) and 87 had significant stenoses (group S). There were no significant differences in patient characteristics between the 2 groups. HDL cholesterol was significantly lower and RLP-C was significantly higher in group S. When a product and a ratio of each of 2 factors were calculated, RLP-C/HDL was demonstrated to be a highly significant predictor for coronary artery stenoses. There were also significant increases in RLP-C/HDL levels with increasing number of vessels involved. This study discloses the predictive value of RLP-C/HDL ratio as a new indicator of CAD.

Concentrations of Tissue Plasminogen Activator

Tissue plasminogen activator (t-PA) is a major plasminogen activator responsible for dissolving blood clots found in blood vessels. However, elevated concentrations of t-PA antigens were found to be related to adverse events in patients with CAD. Considerable controversy about the significance of these results exists. The goal of a cross-sectional study by Geppart and colleagues[67] in Vienna, Austria, was to study independent determinates for t-PA antigen concentrations in patients with CAD to possibly identify the above paradoxical relationship. The baseline t-PA antigen concentrations of 366 patients with angiographic evidence of coronary sclerosis were determined. Univariate analysis showed that age, angiographic extent of disease, presence of angina at rest, diabetes mellitus, hypercholesterolemia, hypertriglyceridemia, and chronic intake of nitrates were significantly and positively related to t-PA antigen concentration, while the chronic intake of aspirin was inversely related to t-PA antigen (Figure 1-30). In addition, plasminogen activator inhibitor type 1 (PAI-1) activity was found to be significantly and positively associated with t-PA antigen concentration. A multivariate analysis identified chronic low-dose aspirin therapy, PAI-1 activity, hypertriglyceridemia, the type of angina, multivessel disease, and hypercholesterolemia as significant and independent determinates of t-PA antigen. While both hypertriglyceridemia and hypercholesterolemia were related to the underlying disease, the type of angina and the number of involved vessels were linked to the severity and extent of disease,

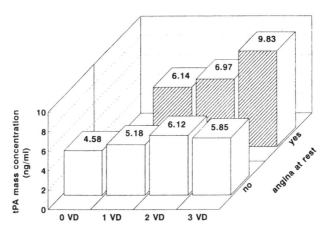

FIGURE 1-30. Mean t-PA antigen concentrations (geometric means) of patients with CAD in relation to the angiographic extent of disease (0-, 1-, 2- or 3-vessel disease) according to the presence or absence (bars in front) of angina at rest. Because there were no patients with angina at rest presenting with 0-vessel disease at time of angiography, only the mean t-PA antigen concentrations of patients with 0-vessel disease and angina on exertion can be shown. The number on top of each bar is the mean t-PA antigen concentration of the respective group. Reproduced with permission from Geppart et al.[67]

and all of them were indicators of a prothrombotic state found during the progression of CAD. In contrast, low-dose aspirin decreased the likelihood of thrombotic events. The relation of t-PA antigen to PAI-1 activity furthermore underlined the relationship between t-PA antigen concentration and a prothrombotic state. Therefore, the positive or—in the case of aspirin therapy—negative correlation of these parameters with t-PA antigen concentration indicates that thrombus formation and simultaneous endothelial cell activation might be major determinates for t-PA antigen concentration in CAD.

Effect of Controlled Alcohol Consumption on Lipoproteins

McConnell and associates[68] from 3 US medical centers (Boston, Massachusetts; Salt Lake City, Utah; and Nashville, Tennessee) studied 20 healthy nonsmoking volunteers (11 men and 9 women, age 23–54 years), free of hyperlipidemia, coronary or vascular disease, systemic hypertension, and diabetes mellitus. Each completed a 10-week program of controlled alcohol consumption. The subjects abstained from all alcohol for 2 weeks, then consumed 13.5 g of ethyl alcohol every evening for 6 weeks (one 12 oz Samuel Adams Boston Lager), and then abstained from all alcohol for an additional 2 weeks. Phlebotomy was performed after the first abstention, after the 6 weeks of daily beer consumption, and again after the second abstention. The findings are summarized in Table 1-3. There was a significant increase in HDL and HDL_2, but not HDL_3 cholesterol, associated with alcohol consumption. HDL increased 4.4%, HDL_2 increased 8%, and HDL_3 increased 1.6%. No significant changes were observed with alcohol consumption for t-PA antigen and activity, PAI-I antigen and activity, von Willebrand factor, thrombin, antithrombin III complex, prothrombin fragment F 1 + 2, and lipoprotein (a).

TABLE 1-3
Changes in Lipoproteins with Consumption of One Daily Alcoholic Beverage

Lipoprotein (mg/dL)	Alcohol Abstention	Alcohol Consumption	p Value
HDL	52 ± 2	54 ± 3	0.03
HDL_2	19 ± 1	21 ± 1	0.04
HDL_3	32 ± 2	32 ± 2	0.4
Apo A-I	146 ± 4	150 ± 5	0.09
Apo B	89 ± 4	92 ± 4	0.08
Apo E	5.6 ± 0.2	5.5 ± 0.2	0.3
LDL	94 ± 5	95 ± 5	0.7
VLDL	12 ± 1	11 ± 2	0.8
Triglycerides	79 ± 5	80 ± 8	0.9

Values are expressed as mean ± SEM. Apo = apolipoprotein; HDL = high-density lipoprotein cholesterol; LDL = low-density lipoprotein cholesterol; VLDL = very low-density lipoprotein cholesterol.
Reproduced with permission from McConnell et al.[68]

Impaired Fibrinolysis of Hypertriglyceridemia

Hypertriglyceridemia and impaired fibrinolytic function are linked to CAD and other atherothrombotic disorders. Triglyceride-rich lipoproteins may attenuate fibrinolysis by increasing the plasma levels of plasminogen activator inhibitor-1. Furthermore, a common 4/5 guanosine polymorphism in the promoter region of the platelet activator inhibitor-1 gene has been indicated to influence plasma platelet-activating inhibitor-1 activity and to be involved in an allele-specific response to triglycerides. Eriksson and coworkers[69] in Stockholm, Sweden, showed by transfection assays that VLDLs induce transcription of a human plasminogen activator inhibitor-1 promoter in endothelial cells. A VLDL response element was located to residues -672 to -657 in the promoter region by the electromobility shift assay, methylation interference, deoxyribonuclease (DNase) I footprinting, and if activity was shown to be influenced by the common 4/5 guanosine polymorphism located adjacent to and upstream of the binding site of a VLDL-inducible transcription factor. These findings may provide a molecular explanation for the link between VLDL and platelet activator inhibitor-1 activity elevation in plasma and for the interaction between the 4/5 guanosine polymorphism and plasma triglycerides.

Tissue Factor Pathway Inhibitor-2

Tissue factor pathway inhibitor-2, also known as placental protein 5, is a serine protease inhibitor consisting of 3 tandemly arranged Kunitz-type protease inhibitor domains. While tissue factor pathway inhibitor-2 is a potent inhibitor of trypsin, plasmin, kallikrein, and factor XIa in the test tube, the function of this inhibitor *in vivo* remains unclear. Iino and colleagues[70] in Seattle, Washington, investigated the synthesis and secretion of tissue factor pathway inhibitor-2 by cultured endothelial cells derived from human umbilical vein, aorta, saphenous vein, and dermal microvessels to gain insight into its biological function. While all endothelial cells examined synthesized and secreted tissue factor pathway inhibitor-2, dermal microvascular endothelial cells synthesized 3-fold to 7-fold higher levels of tissue factor pathway inhibitor-2. Approximately 60% to 90% of the tissue factor inhibitor-2 secreted by endothelial cells was directed to the subendothelial cell extracellular matrix. When cultured human umbilical vein endothelial cells were stimulated with inflammatory mediators, such as phorbol 12-myristate, 13-acetate, endotoxin, and tumor necrosis factor-α, tissue factor pathway inhibitor-2 synthesis by these cells increased 2-fold to 14-fold. Recombinant tissue factor pathway inhibitor-2 bound to dermal microvascular endothelial cell monolayers and its extracellular matrix in a specific, dose-dependent, and saturable manner with Kd values of 21 and 24 nmol/L, respectively. Tissue factor pathway inhibitor-2 interacted with endothelial cells and extracellular matrix, respectively. In the presence of rabbit anti-tissue factor pathway inhibitor-2 IgG, but no pre-immune IgG, endothelial cells disassociated from the culture flask in a time- and IgG concentration-dependant manner. These findings provide evidence that endothelial cell-derived tissue factor pathway inhibitor-2 is primarily secreted into the abluminal space and presumably plays an important role in maintaining the integrity of the extracellular matrix essential for cell attachment.

Preferential Cholesteryl Ester Acceptors

Triglyceride-rich lipoproteins, namely chylomicorns, VLDL, and their remnants, are implicated in the atherogenic features of postprandial lipemia. In human plasma, cholesteryl ester transfer protein mediates the heteroexchange of neutral lipids, *i.e.*, triglycerides and cholesteryl esters, between distinct subpopulations of apo B- and apo AI-containing proteins. In fasting normolipidemic plasma, cholesterol ester transfer protein plays an anti-atherogenic role by promoting preferential cholesteryl ester redistribution from HDL to LDL particles of intermediate subclass with optimal binding affinity for the cellular LDL receptor. While the relative proportions and chemical compositions of donor and acceptor lipoproteins are known to influence cholesteryl ester transfer protein activity, elevated levels of triglyceride-rich lipoproteins during alimentary lipemia have been proposed to be associated with enhanced cholesteryl ester to transfer protein activity. To identify the preferential cholesteryl ester acceptor particles among postprandial triglyceride-rich lipoprotein subfractions, Lassel and colleagues[71] in Paris, France, investigated the effects of a typical Western meal (1,200 kcal, 14% protein; 38% carbohydrates; and 48% fat, monounsaturated/polyunsaturated ratio 4:1) on the rates of postprandial cholesteryl ester transfer from HDL to apo B-containing lipoprotein in normolipidemic subjects (n = 13). Two hours postprandially, plasma levels of triglyceride-rich lipoproteins were significantly elevated. Total rates of cholesteryl ester transferred from HDL to apo B-containing protein were not significantly modified by alimentary lipemia over a period of 8 hours. Quantitatively, VLDL-1 was the major cholesteryl ester acceptor among triglyceride-rich lipoproteins; thus, VLDL-1, but not chylomicrons, represented the major cholesteryl ester acceptor among triglyceride-rich lipoproteins. Quantitatively, however, VLDL-2 and IDL displayed a high capacity to accept cholesteryl ester from HDL/hour/mg lipoprotein, respectively, compared with chylomicrons, VLDL-1 and LDL. In conclusion, elevated postprandial triglyceride-rich lipoprotein levels were not associated with enhanced cholesteryl ester transfer to these particles. Furthermore, the qualitative features of postprandial cholesteryl ester transfer from HDL to chylomicrons and VLDL-1 were not related to the relative triglyceride content of these particles. The cholesterol ester transfer protein-facilitated enrichment of VLDL-1 in cholesterol esters, therefore, identifies them as potentially atherogenic particles during the postprandial phase.

Stimulation of Cholesterol Production

Kwiterovich and Motevalli[72] in Baltimore, Maryland, studied further the basis for the abnormal effect of human serum basic protein-2 on cholesterol production in hyperapobetalipoproteinemia fibroblasts and whether this effect involved protein tyrosine kinase phosphorylation. Genistein, a specific inhibitor of protein tyrosine kinase phosphorylation was used as a probe. Compared with normal cells, basic protein-2 stimulated significantly the cellular mass of total cholesterol, unesterified cholesterol, and esterified cholesterol in hyperapo B fibroblasts. The addition of genistein to basic protein-2 in hyperapo B cells markedly inhibited these abnormal stimulatory effects of basic protein-2 on cell sterol mass. In normal cells, the addition of genistein to basic protein-2 produced an opposite effect: a marked stimulation in the mass of total and esterified cholesterol and a decrease in unesterified cholesterol. These effects of genistein on the formation of cellular cholesterol by basic protein-2 were both time- and concentration-dependent. Inhibition of the stimulatory effect of basic protein-2 on cholesterol production by genistein and hyperapo B cells may be mediated through 3-hydroxy 3-methylglutaryl co-enzyme A reductase, the rate-limiting enzyme of cholesterol biosynthesis, since the rate of incorporation of acetate, but not mevalonate, into unesterified cholesterol was decreased by genistein in the hyperapo B cells. When the mass of total cholesterol in cells treated with basic protein-2 was subtracted from those treated with basic protein-2 plus genistein, a negative number was produced in each of the 6 hyperapo B cell lines, while each of the normal cell lines retained a positive number. The mean difference for the mass of total cholesterol between the hyperapo B and normal fibroblasts under these conditions was 128 nmol/mg cell protein, a difference that was separated by greater than 3 SD. This study supports further the tenet that there is a defect in the response of hyperapo B cells to basic protein-2 and this defect results in an abnormality in cholesterol metabolism that appears to be mediated through a protein tyrosine kinase phosphorylation-mediated process.

Effects of Alcohol Withdrawal on Low-Density Lipoproprotein Particle Size

LDL subclass pattern B, reported to have a higher prevalence in hypertriglyceridemics, is considered to be associated with an increased risk for CAD, and the small dense LDL characteristic of this pattern is susceptible to oxidative modification. Alcohol is considered one of the most frequent causes of increases in plasma and triglyceride levels. Ayaori and coinvestigators[73] in Saitama, Japan, investigated the effects of alcohol withdrawal on LDL subclass distribution and oxidizability in drinkers with different plasma triglyceride levels. Thirty-seven male subjects with relatively heavy alcohol consumption habits were divided into 4 groups: normotriglyceridemic-withdrawal, normotriglyceridemic-control, hypertriglyceridemic-withdrawal, and hypertriglyceridemic-control. Both withdrawal groups abstained from alcohol for 4 weeks, while the control subjects maintained their usual intake of alcohol. Peak LDL particle diameter was smaller in the combined hypertriglyceridemic groups than in the combined normotriglyceridemic groups before abstinence, although particle diameter increased significantly in the hypertriglyceridemic group/withdrawal group. Before abstinence, lag times preceding LDL oxidation in the combined hypertriglyceridemic groups were shorter than in the combined normotriglyceridemic groups. After withdrawal, lag time was prolonged significantly in the hypertriglyceridemic-withdrawal group. No significant changes in particle diameter and lag time were observed in the other 3 groups. Significant correlations were observed between the change in lag time and change in triglycerides and between change in lag time and change in particle diameter. The investigators conclude that in alcohol-induced hypertriglyceridemic group subjects, alcohol withdrawal has beneficial effects on the LDL profile by shifting the particle size from smaller to larger and decreasing its susceptibility of oxidation.

Effect of Alcohol Withdrawal

Lipoprotein(a) is an important risk factor for cardiovascular disease. Alcohol is one of the few nongenetic factors that lowers lipoprotein(a) levels, but the metabolic mechanisms of this action are unknown. Alcohol inhibits the growth hormone/insulin-like growth factor I axis. Alcohol might also affect insulin-like growth factor-binding protein-I (IGFBP-I), which is an acute inhibitor of insulin-like growth factor I. Paassilta and colleagues[74] in Oulu, Finland, studied how alcohol withdrawal affected lipoprotein(a) levels and the GH/IGF-I/IGFBP-I axis. Male alcohol abusers (n = 27; 20-64 years old) were monitored immediately after alcohol withdrawal for 4 days. Twenty-six healthy men, mainly moderate drinkers, served as control subjects. Fasting blood samples were drawn to determine lipoprotein(a), insulin-growth factor I, and IGFBP-I. Nocturnal urine collection was performed in 9 alcoholics and in 11 control subjects for growth hormone analyses. The groups were similar in age and body mass. Lipoprotein(a), growth hormone, and insulin growth factor I tended to be lower and IGFBP-I higher in the alcoholics immediately after alcohol withdrawal than in the control subjects. During the 4-day observation of alcoholics, lipoprotein(a) levels increased by 64% and insulin growth factor I levels by 41%, whereas IGFBP-I levels decreased by 59%. Urinary growth hormone levels tended to decline. The increase in lipoprotein(a) correlated inversely with the changes in IGFBP-I and growth hormone, but not with insulin-like growth factor I. In multiple regression analysis, the main predictors for the increase in lipoprotein(a) were IGFBP-I and urinary growth hormone. In conclusion, alcohol withdrawal induces interrelated and potentially atherogenic changes in lipoprotein(a) predictors and IGFBP-I levels.

Tissue Factor Expression on Macrophages

Tissue factor is a membrane-bound glycoprotein that functions in the extrinsic pathway of blood coagulation by acting as a co-factor for factor VII and the resulting complex leads to thrombin production *in vivo*. The purpose of a study by Kaikita and coworkers[75] in Kumanoto, Japan, was to determine whether macrophages expressed tissue factor in human coronary atherosclerotic plaques. The investigators examined directional coronary atherectomy specimens from 24 patients with unstable angina and 23 with stable exertional angina. In these specimens, macrophages were detected in 22 (92%) of 24 patients with unstable angina versus 12 (52%) of 23 with stable exertional angina. The percentage of macrophage infiltration was significantly larger in patients with unstable angina than in those with stable exertional angina. The immunohistochemical double staining revealed the expression of tissue factor on macrophages in 18 (75%) of 24 patients with unstable angina versus 3 (13%) of 23 with stable exertional angina. Thrombus was identified in 20 (83%) of 24 patients with unstable angina versus 12 (52%) of 23 with stable exertional angina. Fibrin deposition was observed mainly around macrophages expressing tissue factor in the patients with unstable angina. These investigators show that tissue factor expression on macrophages is more frequent in coronary atherosclerotic plaques in patients with unstable angina. Tissue factor expressed on macrophages may play an important role in the thrombogenicity in coronary atherosclerotic plaques in these patients.

Lipid Metabolism/Genetics

Evaluation of the Aortic Root by Magnetic Resonance Imaging

Summers and colleagues[76] evaluated the aortic root by using MRI in 17 patients with homozygous familial hypercholesterolemia and 12 normal control subjects in a prospective blinded, control study. Morphologic assessment of the aortic root was done with spin-echo and gradient-echo MRI scanning. Comparisons were made with a number of measures of disease severity, including cholesterol-year score, calcium score on electron-beam CT, and size of Achilles tendon xanthomas. Atherosclerotic plaque, visible on fat-suppressed images but never on water-suppressed images, was present in 9 homozygous familial hypercholesterolemia patients. Supravalvular aortic stenosis was present in 7 patients with the familial hypercholesterolemia. Maximum supravalvular aortic wall thickness was greater and lumen cross-sectional areas were smaller in patients than in control subjects. Maximum wall thickness was associated with a greater calcium score on electron-beam CT. Thus, this study demonstrates the utility of MRI for detecting and characterizing aortic root atherosclerotic plaques and supravalvular aortic stenosis in patients with homozygous familial hypercholesterolemia (Figure 1-31).

Molecular Defect in High-Density Lipoprotein Cholesterol Deficiency

Miller and colleagues[77] in Baltimore, Maryland, investigated the molecular defect causing HDL cholesterol deficiency in a male proband and his family members. Amplification and sequencing of genomic DNA disclosed a novel based-pair substitution at residue 159 of the apolipoprotein A-I gene. This substitution resulted in the loss of AviII restriction site and a predicted substitution of leucine with prolene at residue 159. Restriction enzyme analysis demon-

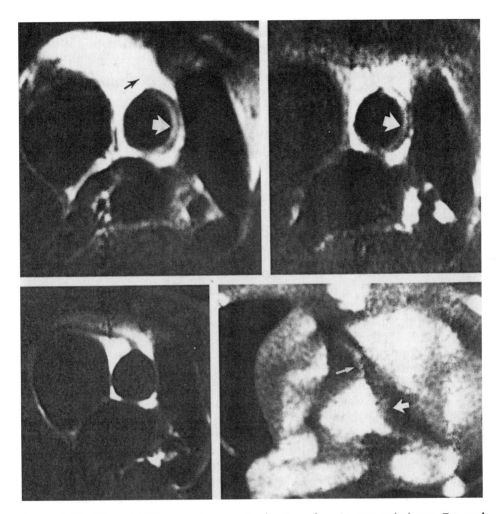

FIGURE 1-31. Effect of MRI parameters on visualization of aortic root and plaque. **Top and bottom left:** Transverse spin-echo MRI of supravalvular aortic root in a 4-year-old female homozygous familial hypercholesterolemia patient. Nonsuppressed **(top left)**, fat-suppressed **(top right)**, and water-suppressed **(bottom left)** images are shown. Right main coronary artery is visible (small arrow). Aortic wall is asymmetrically thickened on patient's left side (large arrow). Thickened wall, presumably due to plaque, is invisible on water-suppressed images. **Bottom right:** electron-beam CT at same level also shows right main coronary artery (small arrow) and thickened wall of aorta (large arrow). Reproduced with permission from Summers et al.[76]

strated absence of the AviII site in 19 of 40 biological family members. Compared with familial controls, subjects with the apolipoprotein A-I$_{Zavalla}$ had reduced HDL cholesterol and apolipoprotein A-I and A-II levels. Two subjects who have developed CAD to date possessed additional cardiovascular risk factors. Other heterozygotes with apolipoprotein-I$_{Zavalla}$ were without symptomatic CAD. This study identifies a monogenic cause of hypoalphalipoproteinemia with a single base pair substitution having a dominant effect on the low HDL phenotype. In addition, it extends recent observations that HDL cholesterol deficiency states may be more prone to the development of premature CAD when accompanied by additional cardiovascular risk factors.

European Atherosclerosis Research Study

The H-allele of the intron 8 Hind III polymorphism in the lipoprotein lipase gene has been associated with a lower risk of AMI and plasma levels of triglycerides. To test whether the Hind III site was in linkage disequilibrium with the functional variant lipoprotein lipase serine 447 stop, subjects from the European Atherosclerosis Research Study[78] were genotyped for both polymorphic sites. This study included 515 offspring of fathers with a premature (<55 years old) AMI, who were designated cases, and 930 age and sex match of control subjects from 5 different regions of Europe. The linkage disequilibrium between the 2 sites was very strong, with only 3 of the 4 possible haplotypes identified: H + S 447, H − S 447 and H − X 447. The frequency of H − X 447, but not of the H − S 447 haplotype, was significantly lower in patients than in control subjects, suggesting a protective effect for AMI with this difference being consistent in all 5 regions of Europe. Compared with individual homozygotes for the H + S 447 haplotype, the odds ratio of having a paternal history of premature AMI for H − X 447 heterozygotes was 0.71. In addition, there was an increase of the H − X 447 haplotype frequency from north to south in control subjects. Compared with the H + S 447 haplotype, the H − X 447 haplotype was associated with significantly lower concentrations of plasma triglycerides, with this effect being consistent over the regions of Europe. There was no significant evidence for a heterogeneity effect between males and females or between cases and control subjects, although the effect on triglyceride levels appeared to be the greatest in male patients. In a second study of the European Atherosclerosis Research Study of 332 cases and 342 control subjects, postprandial clearance of triglycerides after a standard fat meal was examined. H − X 447 haplotype was associated with significantly lower postprandial triglyceride levels than was the H + S 447 haplotype. Thus, the effects on AMI risks and plasma lipids associated with the H-allele appear to be mediated mainly by the X 447 mutation, and although the lowering effects associated with H − X 447 haplotype on fasting and postprandial triglycerides are not large, they are consistent with the lowering effect observed on AMI risk throughout Europe.

Analysis of Postprandial Lipemia

Polymorphism of the fatty acid-binding protein-2 (FABP-2) gene has been shown to affect the affinity of intestinal FABP for fatty acids. This could cause changes in postprandial triglyceride metabolism. Agren and coinvestigators[79] from Kuopio, Finland, studied postprandial lipemia in normotriglyceridemic subjects with genetic variation in the FABP-2 gene. Oral fat-loading tests were performed in 8 subjects homozygous for the Thr-encoding allele at codon 54 of the FABP-2 gene and in 7 subjects homozygous for the Ala-encoding allele (wild type). There were no significant differences between these 2 groups in age, body mass index, fasting plasma triglyceride and cholesterol levels, or fasting glucose and insulin levels. The increase of plasma triglyceride concentration after the fat test meal was significantly greater in subjects who were homozygous for the Thr-54 allele. The difference was seen in both chylomicron and VLDL triglycerides. Postprandial triglyceride response correlated with fasting triglycerides in the Ala-54 homozygotes but not in the Thr-54 homozygotes, and showed a strong correlation between triglyceride and insulin responses. With reservations related to a small number of subjects studied, these results indicate that the Thr-encoded allele of the FABP-2 gene is associated with increased postprandial lipemia. The lipemic response is associated with postprandial insulin response, suggesting that in the Thr-54 homozygotes, altered postprandial lipemia may also modify insulin action or vice versa.

Serum Paroxonase

Serum paroxonase (PON) is an HDL-bound enzyme protecting LDL from oxidation. A common polymorphism of the paroxonase gene (PON1) involving a Gln-to-Arg interchange at position 192 has been demonstrated to modulate PON activity toward paroxon, a nonphysiological substrate; Arg 192 (allele B) is associated with higher activity than Gln 192 (allele A). This polymorphism has been proposed as a genetic marker of risk for CAD. However, the relationships between codon 192 PON1 genotypes, coronary atherosclerosis, and the occurrence of AMI are still controversial. PON1 genotypes were determined by Ombres and coinvestigators[80] in Rome, Italy, in 472 consecutive subjects over 40 years old who underwent coronary angiography. CAD (>50% stenosis) was detected in 310 patients; 162 patients with less than 10% stenosis served as controls (CAD−). The investigators evaluated 204 randomly selected individuals as population controls. PON1 genotypes were determined by PCR and AlwI restriction enzyme digestion. Frequencies of alleles A and B were 0.70 and 0.30 in angiographically assessed subjects and 0.73 and 0.27 in population controls, respectively. Distribution of PON1 genotypes in CAD+ was not significantly different from those in CAD−. Similarly, no differences were observed in the subgroup of CAD+ with AMI or in those at higher oxidative risk (smokers and/or diabetics). After controlling for other coronary risk factors, no association was found between PON1 alleles and the presence of CAD. PON1 AA genotype was associated with reduced concentration of apolipoprotein B triglyceride-rich lipoprotein. This study does not provide evidence of a significant association between codon 192 PON1 genotypes and CAD in Italian patients. However, it does confirm that the PON1 low-activity allele is associated with a less atherogenic profile.

Effect of Cyclic Mechanical Stretch

In vivo, vascular walls are exposed to mechanical stretch, which may promote atherogenesis. A study by Okada and colleagues[81] in Tokyo, Japan, was designed to investigate the effect of mechanical stretch on the production and gene expression of cytokines in endothelial cells of human umbilical veins. Endothelial cells were cultured on flexible silicon membranes and exposed to cyclic mechanical stretch. Although the secretion levels of interleukin-1β, tumor necrosis factor-α, and interleukin-6, granulocyte colony stimulating factor G and macrophage granulocyte stimulating factor and macrophage colony stimulating factor were not effected by cyclic stretch over 24 hours, the levels of interleukin-8 and monocyte chemotactic and activating factor/monocyte chemoattractant protein-1 were significantly increased by cyclic stretch. Northern blot analysis indicated that mRNA levels of interleukin-8 and monocyte chemoattractant factor/monocyte chemoattractant protein-1 were upregulated by cyclic stretch as a function of its intensity. Cytochalasin D, which disrupts the actin cytoskeleton, abolished stretch-induced gene expression of interleukin-8 and monocyte chemoattractant factor/monocyte chemoattractant protein-1. In contrast, neither inhibition of stretch-activated ion channels nor distribution of microtubules affected the induction of these cytokines by cyclic stretch. Northern blot analysis using enzyme inhibitors show that phospholipase C, protein kinase C, and tyrosine kinase are involved in the stretch-induced gene expression of interleukin-8 and monocyte chemoattractant factor/monocyte chemoattractant protein-1, whereas cAMP- or gGMP-dependent protein kinase is not. In conclusion, cyclic stretch enhances the secretion in gene expression of interleukin-8 and monocyte chemoattractant factor/monocyte chemoattractant protein-1 in a stretch-dependent fashion, and the integrity of the actin cytoskeleton and activities of phospholipase C, protein kinase C, and tyrosine kinase may be essential in the process of stretch-induced gene induction of interleukin-8 and monocyte chemoattractant factor/monocyte chemoattractant protein-1.

Effect of Low-Density Lipoprotein Apheresis

The short-term effectiveness of LDL apheresis using a dextran sulfate cellulose adsorption technique was previously examined in a 9-center, 22-week control trial in 64 patients with familial hypercholesterolemia who did not adequately respond to diet and drug therapy. Forty-nine patients (40 treatment, 9 controls) subsequently received LDL apheresis procedures as part of an optional follow-up phase. Gordon and associates for the Liposorber Study Group[82] reported on the long-term safety, lipid lowering, and clinical efficacy of LDL apheresis for the 5-year period that includes both the initial control study and the follow-up phase. During this time, patients received a total of 3,902 treatments of which 3,314 treatments were given during the follow-up phase. Adverse events were infrequent, occurring in 142 procedures (3.6%). Immediate reduction in LDL cholesterol was 76% both in homozygotes and in heterozygotes. Patients with homozygous familial hypertension had a progressive decrease in pretreatment LDL cholesterol level along with an increase in HDL cholesterol level. There was no appreciable change in pretreatment lipoprotein level over time in heterozygotes. The rate of cardiovascular events during therapy with LDL apheresis and lipid-lowering drugs was 3.5

events/1,000 patient-months of treatment compared with 6.3 events/1,000 patient-months for the 5 years before LDL apheresis therapy. These findings support the long-term safety and clinical efficacy of LDL apheresis in patients with heterozygous and homozygous familial hypertension who are inadequately controlled with drug therapy.

Familial Hypercholesterolemia

Familial hypercholesterolemia is caused by mutations in the LDL receptor gene and is usually associated with hypercholesterolemia, lipid deposition in tissues, and premature CAD. However, individuals with heterozygous familial hypercholesterolemia in China exhibit a milder phenotype despite having deleterious mutations in the LDL receptor gene. Nineteen Chinese familial hypercholesterolemic heterozygotes living in Canada were screened by Pimstone and colleagues[83] in Vancouver, Canada, for the 11 mutations that had been described in familial hypercholesterol patients living in China. One Chinese Canadian carried 1 of these mutations, 2 carried a previously unreported single base mutation substitution, and 1 carried a mutation observed in French Canadian patients. Twelve additional carriers of these mutations were identified in the families of the index patients. Significantly higher LDL cholesterol concentrations were observed in familial hypercholesterolemic heterozygotes with defined mutations living in Canada than in those living in China. Six of the 16 familial hypercholesterolemic heterozygotes residing in Canada had evidence of tendon xanthomata and 4 had a history of premature CAD, whereas none of those in China had tendon xanthomata or CAD. Complete segregation between hypercholesterolemia and inheritance of a mutant allele was observed in 3 Canadian Chinese familial hypercholesterolemic families. Thus, Chinese familial hypercholesteremic heterozygotes living in Canada exhibited a phenotype similar to that of other familial hypercholesterolemic patients in Western societies. The differences between patients living in Canada and those living in China could be ascribed to differences in dietary fat consumption, showing that environmental factors, such as diet, play a significant role in modulating the phenotype of heterozygous familial hypercholesterolemia.

Genetic Relationships Between High-Density Lipoprotein Phenotypes and Insulin Concentrations

Rainwater and coworkers[84] in San Antonio, Texas, used data from the San Antonio Family Heart Study to determine the HDL correlates of the insulin-resistant syndrome, as reflected by insulin concentrations in nondiabetic subjects. The investigators measured insulin concentration both in the fasting state and 2 hours after a glucose challenge (2-hour insulin) and assessed 7 aspects of HDL phenotype, including size and concentration of both lipid and protein components. Measurements were obtained from 1,202 nondiabetic members of 42 families. Initial quantitative genetic analyses reveal that a substantial portion of phenotypic variation in the 9 variables was due to genes (inheritabilities h^2 ranged from 0.32 to 0.47). Investigators then conducted a series of bivariate genetic analyses, which indicated that there were significant additive genetic correlations (pleiotropy) between the 2 measures of insulin and 5 of the 7 HDL measures tested, including concentrations of HDL cholesterol (fasting insulin only) and triglyceride, and HDL size distributions of apo A-I, apo A-II and cholesterol; concentrations of apo A-I and apo A-II were not genetically related to either insulin measure. Increased insulin levels were associated with relatively small HDL phenotypes, and considering a similar association with small, dense LDLs, this finding suggested a common effect of insulin resistance on particle size distribution for these lipoproteins. Thus, these results suggest the existence of genes that pleiotropically influence variation in both HDLs and insulin levels and therefore contribute to the clustering of proatherogenic traits in the insulin-resistant syndrome.

Genetic Variation in Familial Hypercholesterolemia

Plasma lipid response to dietary fat and cholesterol is, in part, genetically controlled. The apolipoprotein A-IV has been shown to influence the response to dietary changes in normolipidemic individuals. The response to diet in subjects with familial hypercholesterolemia is also variable, and no studies are available on the influence of apolipoprotein A-IV mutations on dietary response in these subjects. Carmena-Ramon and colleagues[85] in Boston, Massachusetts, studied the effect of 2 common apolipoprotein A-IV genetic variants ($Gln_{360} \rightarrow$ His and $Thr_{347} \rightarrow$ SER) on the lipid response to the National Cholesterol Education Program type 1 diet in 67 familial hypercholesterolemia heterozygotes (43 women, 24 men). Subjects were studied at baseline (after consuming a 1-month diet with 35% fat [10% saturated] and 300 mg/dL cholesterol) and after 3 months of consuming a low-fat diet. No gender-related differences were found, and results were combined for men and women. The apolipoprotein A-IV-360 mutation was assessed in 67 subjects; 51 were genotype 1/1 and 16 were genotyped 1/2. The apolipoprotein A-IV-2 allele was associated with marginally significant lower LDL cholesterol levels and significantly lower apo B levels independent of diet. After consuming a National Cholesterol Education Program type 1 diet, carriers of the apolipoprotein A-IV-2 allele showed a significantly lower reduction in apoB concentration than 1/1 subjects; however, no significant differences in response were noted for LDL cholesterol. The apolipoprotein A-IV-347 mutation was assessed in 63 individuals, 44 with the A/A allele and 19 with A/T and T/T alleles. No significant differences were observed at baseline or post-diet values of these 2 groups in total LDL and HDL cholesterol and plasma apoB levels. After dietary intervention, A/A individuals showed significant reductions in plasma triglycerides and VLDL cholesterol levels; no changes were found in carriers of the T allele. Haplotype analysis suggested that in these familial hypercholesterolemic subjects, the apolipoprotein A-IV-360-2 allele was associated with lower plasma lipid levels during the National Cholesterol Panel 1 diet period, whereas no significant effects were observed for the apolipoprotein A-IV-347-T allele.

Influence of Antibodies on Familial Hypercholesterolemia

Antibodies against oxidized LDL have been proposed to be independent predictors of atherosclerosis development. The main aim of a study by Hulthe and colleagues[86] in Stockholm, Sweden, was to compare antibody titers to oxidized LDL in patients with heterozygous familial hypercholesterolemia (n = 51) with those in matched controls (n = 45) and to analyze whether the antibody titers were related to the extent of atherosclerosis as assessed cross-sectionally and prospectively by ultrasonography in the 2 study groups. Antibody titers were determined with a solid phase ELISA, and plates were coated with the antigen oxidized LDL or malondialdehyde-treated LDL as well as with the postcoat only. Antibody titers were expressed as absorbance [(value in patient's serum minus that in postcoat) divided by (Internal Standard Serum minus postcoat)]. There were no significant differences in antibody titers against oxidized LDL or malondialdehyde LDL between the group of patients with familial hypercholesterolemia and the controls. In cross-sectional comparison, no significant associations were observed between the intima-media thickness of the carotid or femoral arteries and antibody titers against oxidized LDL or between plaque occurrence and these titers. Patients with a history of AMI had significantly lower IgM titers against oxidized LDL compared with patients without a history of AMI and with controls (Figure 1-32). In conclusion, mean values for antibody titers against oxidized LDL were not increased in the patient group compared with a healthy control group, and no positive significant relationship was observed between antibody titers and the extent of atherosclerosis, as measured by ultrasound, in the carotid or femoral arteries. Taken together, these findings indicate that the relationship between the autoimmune response to oxidized LDL and the extent of atherosclerosis is more complex than previously anticipated.

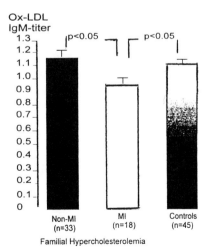

FIGURE 1-32. Bar graph showing mean values with SEs for IgM titer against Ox-LDL in patients with familial hypercholesterolemia and a history of MI compared with patients without such a history and compared with controls. Reproduced with permission from Hulthe et al.[86]

Hypertriglyceridemia

Reduced myocardial vasodilatation in hypercholesterolemics without overt coronary stenosis has been reported. However, the status of myocardial vasodilation in hypertriglyceridemics has not been clarified. The aim of a study by Yokoyama and coinvestigators[87] in Tokyo, Japan, was to investigate whether myocardial vasodilatation is impaired in patients with hypertriglyceridemia without overt coronary stenosis. Twenty-three hypertriglyceridemics (10 normal cholesterolemic hypertriglyceridemics and 13 mixed combined hyperlipidemics) and 13 age-matched controls were studied. All patients were proven to have more than 1 normal coronary artery, as diagnosed by coronary angiography, and those segments that were perfused by anatomically normal coronary arteries were used in the study. Myocardial blood flow during dipyridamole loading and baseline myocardial blood flow were measured by using positron emission tomography and N^{13} ammonia, after which myocardial vasodilatation was calculated. Baseline myocardial blood flow was comparable among hypertriglyceridemics, mixed combined hyperlipidemics, and controls. However, myocardial blood flow during dipyridamole loading was significantly lower in mixed combined hyperlipidemics than in control subjects, while it was comparable in normal cholesterolemic hypertriglyercidemics and controls. Myocardial vasodilatation was significantly reduced in both hypertriglyceridemics and mixed combined hyperlipidemics compared with controls (Figure 1-33). Myocardial vasodilatation in mixed combined hyperlipidemics tended to be reduced compared with that in hypertriglyceridemics, but the difference was statistically insignificant. There was a significant relationship

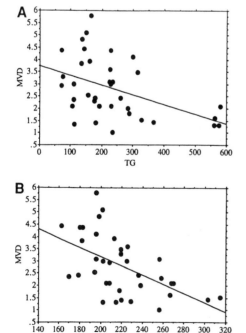

FIGURE 1-33. Relationship between myocardial vasodilation (MVD) and plasma TG level (top) or total TC level (bottom) in the three groups. There was a significant negative correlation between MVD and plasma TG (r = −.47, p < .01) and also between MVD and total TC (r = −.55, p < .01). Reproduced with permission from Yokoyama et al.[87]

between myocardial vasodilatation and both plasma triglycerides (TG) and plasma total cholesterol (TC). When controls and hypertriglyceridemics were combined, the relationship between myocardial vasodilatation and plasma total triglycerides became more prominent, and the significant relationship between cholesterol levels and myocardial vasodilatation disappeared. Multivariate regression analysis reveals that the triglyceride level is independently related to myocardial vasodilatation. In conclusion, myocardial vasodilatation is reduced in hypertriglyceridemics in anatomically normal coronary arteries. Hypertriglyceridemia is an independent factor for this abnormality.

Use of Niaspan for Hypercholesterolemia

Guyton and associates[88] from 5 different US medical centers performed a multicenter, open label study to determine the long-term safety and efficacy of a new extended-release once-a-night niacin preparation, Niaspan, in the treatment of hypercholesterolemia. Niaspan, 0.5 to 3.0 g once a night at bedtime, was used alone or in combination with a statin (inhibitor of hydroxymethylglutaryl co-enzyme A reductase), a bile acid sequestrant, or both. Patients included 269 hypercholesterolemic male and female adults enrolled in a 96-week study, and 230 additional adults for whom short-term safety data were available. The dosages of Niaspan attained by 269 patients were 1,000 mg (95% of patients), 1,500 mg (86%), and 2,000 mg (65%). After 48 weeks of treatment, Niaspan alone (median dose 2,000 mg) reduced LDL cholesterol (18%), apolipoprotein B (15%), total cholesterol (11%), triglycerides (24%), and lipoprotein(a) (36%), and increased HDL cholesterol (29%). Niaspan plus a statin lowered LDL cholesterol (32%), apolipoprotein B (26%), total cholesterol (23%), triglycerides (30%), and lipoprotein(a) (19%), and increased HDL cholesterol (26%). Reversible elevations of aspartate aminotransferase or alanine aminotransferase more than twice the normal range occurred in 2.6% of patients. One patient discontinued Niaspan because of transaminase elevations. Intolerance to flushing, leading to discontinuation of Niaspan, occurred in 4.8% of patients. The overall rate of discontinuance due to flushing in this study combined with 2 previous randomized trials was 7.3%. In the long-term treatment of hypercholesterolemia, Niaspan produced favorable changes in LDL and HDL cholesterol, triglycerides, and lipoprotein(a). Adverse hepatic effects were minor and occurred at rates similar to those reported for statin therapy (Table 1-4).

Use of the Hyperinsulinemic Euglycemic Clamp Technique

Familial combined hyperlipidemia (FCHL) is characterized by hyperlipidemia and insulin resistance, but intracellular defect in insulin action is unknown. Therefore, Karjalainen and associates[89] in Kuopio, Finland, investigated insulin action by applying the hyperinsulinemic euglycemic clamp technique with direct telemetry in 58 FCHL family members (28 with FCHL; 30 without dyslipidemia; average age 49 years; body mass index 25 kg/m^2) and

TABLE 1-4
Percent Change (SE) from Baseline in Mean Lipid, Lipoprotein, and Apolipoprotein Results at 48 and 96 Weeks

	Week 48			Week 96		
	Niaspan Only (n = 101)	Niaspan + Statin (n = 45)	Niaspan + BAS (n = 15)	Niaspan Only (n = 73)	Niaspan + Statin (n = 37)	Niaspan + BAS (n = 7)
LDL cholesterol	−17.7*	−31.7*	−19.5*	−17.5*	−32.2*	−27.8*
(mg/dL)	(1.3)	(2.6)	(3.7)	(1.6)	(2.3)	(4.2)
Apolipoprotein B	−15.4*	−26.2*	−19.2*	—	—	—
(mg/dL)†	(1.3)	(2.6)	(3.1)			
Total cholesterol	−10.5*	−23.1*	−11.3*	−10.0*	−23.8*	−15.1*
(mg/dL)	(0.9)	(1.8)	(1.8)	(1.2)	(2.1)	(2.6)
Triglycerides	−23.5*	−30.4*	−12.7	−26.4*	−32.2*	+5.1
(mg/dL)	(2.9)	(6.0)	(9.8)	(3.8)	(4.1)	(21.4)
HDL cholesterol	+29.0*	+25.8*	+36.2*	+32.1*	+24.7*	+31.2*
(mg/dL)	(2.0)	(3.1)	(5.2)	(2.5)	(2.4)	(9.4)
Lipoprotein(a)	−36.3*	−19.2	−24.0*	—	—	—
(mg/dL)‡	(2.7)	(17.6)	(5.8)			
Total cholesterol/HDL	−29.1*	−37.5*	−33.0*	−30.1*	−38.4*	−33.5*
cholesterol ratio	(1.3)	(2.4)	(4.2)	(1.6)	(1.8)	(3.9)

* p <0.01 by matched pair t test.

† Apolipoprotein B was analyzed in a subset of patients (n = 70, 30, and 11 for the respective columns at 48 weeks).

‡ Lipoprotein(a) was analyzed in a subset of patients (n = 74, 32, and 12 for the respective columns at 48 weeks).

BAS = bile acid sequestrant, either colestipol or cholestyramine; LDL = low-density lipoprotein; HDL = high-density lipoprotein; Statin = either lovastatin, pravastatin, or simvastatin; — = no information available.

Reproduced with permission from Guyton et al.[88]

in 72 healthy control subjects. In the fasting state, FCHL patients had higher levels of total cholesterol, total triglycerides, and apolipoprotein B than control subjects. During the euglycemia clamp, FCHL patients had lower rates of glucose oxidation and higher rates of lipid oxidation as well as higher levels of serum-free fatty acids (FFA) compared with those of control subjects (Figure 1-34). Relatives without dyslipidemia differed similarly from control subjects with respect to rates of glucose and lipid oxidation and FFA suppression during

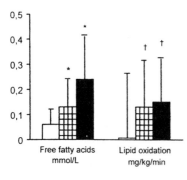

FIGURE 1-34. Free fatty acids (mmol/L) and the rates of lipid oxygenation (mg/kg/min) during the hyperinsulinemic clamp in control subjects (open bars), relatives without FCHL (hatched bars), and FCHL patients (filled bars). *p < 0.001 (control subjects vs. other groups); †p < 0.05 (control subjects vs. other groups). Reproduced with permission from Karjalainen et al.[89]

the hyperinsulinemic clamp. In FCHL family members, during the euglycemic clamp, FFAs correlated negatively with the rates of glucose oxidation but not with the rates of glucose nonoxidation. In FCHL family members without dys-lipidemia and in control subjects, FFAs during the clamp correlated positively with levels of total triglycerides and VLDL cholesterol. The investigators con-clude that in patients with FCHL and also in their first-degree relatives, insulin-suppressive effect on FFA levels is impaired which might precede dyslipidemia in FCHL.

Lipids/Prognosis

C-Reactive Protein Levels as Predictor

Ridker and colleagues[90] determined the prognostic utility of measure-ments of C-reactive protein (CRP) in 14,916 apparently healthy men participat-ing in the Physicians' Health Study. Baseline values of CRP, total cholesterol, and HDL cholesterol were measured among 245 study subjects who subse-quently developed a first AMI among 372 subjects who remained free of cardio-vascular disease during an average follow-up period of 9 years. In univariate analyses, high baseline values of CRP, total cholesterol, and total cholesterol: HDL cholesterol ratio were each associated with significantly increased risks of future AMI. In multivariate analyses, models incorporating CRP and lipid value variables provided a significantly better method to predict risk than did models using lipid alone. Relative risk of future AMI among those with high levels of CRP and total cholesterol were greater than the product of the individ-ual risks associated with isolated elevations of either CRP or total cholesterol. In stratified analyses, baseline CRP level was predictive of risk for those with low as well as high levels of total cholesterol and total cholesterol:HDL ratio (Figure 1-35). These findings were essentially identical when they were applied

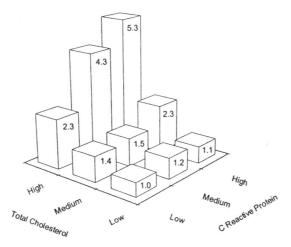

FIGURE 1-35. Relative risks of first MI among among apparently healthy men associated with high (>223 mg/dL), middle (191 to 223 mg/dL), and low (<191 mg/dL) tertiles of total choles-terol and high (>1.69 mg/L), middle (0.72 to 1.69 mg/L), and low (<0.72 mg/L) tertiles of CRP. Reproduced with permission from Ridker et al.[90]

to nonsmokers and after control of other cardiovascular risk factors. Thus, in prospective data from a large cohort of apparently healthy men, baseline CRP values add to the predictive value of lipid variables in determining risk of first MI.

Effect of Dyslipidemias

Several large scale trials have shown that lipid-lowering interventions are associated with reduced coronary events and mortality. Whether dyslipidemias have a detrimental effect on the evolution of AMI is still unknown. To examine whether dyslipidemias can aggravate myocardial vulnerability following AMI, Tsung-Dau Wang and colleagues[91] from Taipei, Taiwan, Republic of China, studied 165 patients with a first AMI. All patients underwent measurements of serum lipid profiles 1 week and 3 months after AMI, a radionuclide ventriculographic study, and a coronary angiographic study. The patients were divided into 3 groups according to their 3-month serum cholesterol levels (group 1, <200 mg/dL; group 2, 200-240 mg/dL, group 3, >240 mg/dL). Groups 1, 2, and 3 consisted of 66, 59, and 40 patients, respectively. Group 3 had a higher Gensini score than groups 1 and 2, although this was not statistically significant. The postinfarct LVEF was highest in group 1 (53% ± 13%), at mid-level in group 2 (43% ± 14%), and lowest in group 3 (35% ± 11%). A significant negative correlation between 3-month LDL cholesterol ($r = -0.55$) and the postinfarct LVEF was found. The product of peak creatine kinase (CK_{max}) and time to CK_{max}, and patency of the infarct-related artery, rather than variables of coronary atherosclerosis, were also independent predictors of the postinfarct LVEF. Increases in 1-week LDL cholesterol and decreases in 1-week HDL cholesterol were associated with a higher CK_{max} and a lower patency rate of the infarct-related artery, respectively. This study reveals that dyslipidemias *per se*, especially LDL cholesterol, have detrimental effects on the postinfarct LVEF; this effect might be independent of the atherogenic properties of dyslipidemias.

Cholesterol Reduction

Encouraging intervention trials drive our expectations toward more aggressive cholesterol-lowering therapies, lower target levels, and less severe hypercholesterolemia. Available studies may predict which patients, degrees of total cholesterol reduction, baseline and target level of total cholesterol provide the most clinical benefit. Data were pooled by Fager and Wiklund,[92] in Gotenborg, Sweden, from 7 primary and 9 secondary controlled trials with major CAD as primary endpoints. Analyses showed that we can expect large reductions in CAD from total cholesterol reduction in primary and secondary prevention. However, the reduction is much larger in subjects with high total cholesterol and/or previous CAD events. The percent reduction in CAD increased exponentially with increasing percent in total cholesterol reductions, which predicted greater than 70% of the change in CAD. Consequently, we cannot expect cost-effective clinical benefits from mean reductions in total cholesterol greater than 15% (LDL >20%). The total cholesterol level at the study endpoint correlated with CAD incidence irrespective of the study group and explained almost 45% of the CAD incidence. The relationship was progressive and leveled off at a total cholesterol level below about 150 mg/dL. Little extra clinical benefit can be expected from further reductions. We can expect an average 2% reduction in CAD events per percent reduction in total cholesterol. We can also expect a 2-fold greater clinical benefit among subjects with high initial total cholesterol level than among those with low levels. Finally, we can expect that the cholesterol-attributable risk is reset to that predicted by the total cholesterol level achieved within 4 to 6 years.

Lipid Regression Trials and Prognosis

West of Scotland Coronary Prevention Study

The West of Scotland Coronary Prevention Study (WOSCOPS)[93] was a primary prevention trial that demonstrated the effectiveness of pravastatin (40 mg/day) in reducing morbidity and mortality from CAD in moderately hypercholesterolemic men. In this study, the investigators examined the extent to which differences in LDL and other plasma lipids, both at baseline and on treatment, influenced CAD risk reduction. Relationships between baseline lipid concentrations and future incidence for cardiovascular events and between on-treatment lipid concentrations and risk reduction in patients taking pravastatin were examined by Cox regression models and by division of the cohort into quintiles. Variation in plasma lipids at baseline did not influence the relative risk reduction generated by pravastatin therapy. Fall in LDL levels in the pravastatin-treated group did not correlate with CAD risk reduction in multivariate regression. Furthermore, maximum benefit of an about 45% risk reduction was observed in the middle quintile of LDL reduction, *i.e.*, a mean of 24% reduction. Further reductions in LDL concentrations (up to 39%) were not associated with greater decreases in CAD risk. Comparison of event rates between placebo- and pravastatin-treated subjects with the same LDL cholesterol level provided evidence for an apparent treatment effect that was independent of LDL concentrations. The authors conclude that a treatment effect of 40 mg/day of pravastatin is the same regardless of baseline lipid phenotype. There is no CAD risk reduction unless LDL levels are reduced, but a fall in the range of 24% is sufficient to see the full benefit in patients taking this dose of pravastatin.

Scandinavian Simvastatin Survival Study

Pedersen and colleagues[94] for the Scandinavian Simvastatin Survival Study (4S) randomized 4,444 patients with CAD and serum cholesterol values of 213 to 310 mg/dL with triglycerides of less than 220 mg/dL to simvastatin 20 to 40 mg or placebo once daily. During the median follow-up period of 5.4 years, one or more major coronary events occurred in 622 (28%) of the 2,223

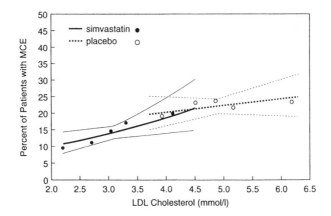

FIGURE 1-36. Relationship between LDL cholesterol levels at year 1 and subsequent risk of major coronary events in the placebo and simvastatin groups, with 95% confidence intervals. Points represent the mean value for each quintile. To convert mmol/L to mg/dL, multiply by 38.7. Reproduced with permission from Pedersen et al.[94]

patients in the placebo group and in 431 (19%) of the 2,221 patients in the simvastatin group for a 34% risk reduction. The Cox proportional hazards model was used to assess the relationship between lipid values at baseline, at year 1, and the percentage changed from baseline to year 1, and major coronary events. The reduction in major coronary events within the simvastatin group was highly correlated with on-treatment levels and changes from baseline in total and LDL cholesterol, apolipoprotein B, and less so with HDL cholesterol, but there was no clear relationship with triglycerides. The authors estimated that each additional 1% reduction in LDL cholesterol reduces major coronary events by 1.7%. These data suggest that the beneficial effect of simvastatin in individual patients in the 4S was determined mainly by the magnitude of the change in LDL cholesterol (Figure 1-36).

Results of the Long-Term Intervention with Pravastatin in Ischemic Disease Atherosclerosis Substudy

MacMahon and associates[95] randomized 522 patients with a history of AMI or unstable angina and with baseline levels of total cholesterol between 4 and 7 mmol/L to treatment with a low-fat diet plus pravastatin (40 mg daily) or a low-fat diet plus placebo. Pravastatin treatment reduced the levels of total cholesterol by 19%, LDL cholesterol by 27%, apolipoprotein B by 19%, and triglycerides by 13%, and increased apolipoprotein A-I and HDL cholesterol levels by 4% in comparison with placebo. Carotid atherosclerosis was estimated from B-mode ultrasound measurements of the common carotid artery. After 4 years, mean carotid wall thickness had increased by 0.048 mm in the placebo group and declined by 0.014 mm in the pravastatin-treated group (p < 0.0001)

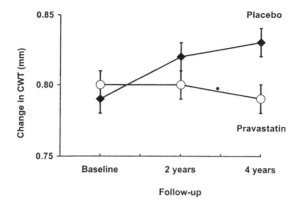

FIGURE 1-37. Carotid artery wall thickness in pravastatin and placebo groups at baseline, year 2 and year 4. Reproduced with permission from MacMahon et al.[95]

(Figure 1-37). The effect of treatment on wall thickness was similar in 3 groups classified by tertiles of total cholesterol at baseline with mean levels of 4.8, 5.7, and 6.6 mmol/L, respectively. Thus, these data suggest that treatment with pravastatin reduces the development of carotid atherosclerosis among patients with CAD and a wide range of pretreatment cholesterol levels.

Scandinavian Simvastatin Survival Study

Miettinen and colleagues[96] in Helsinki, Finland, studied the influence of simvastatin therapy in patients randomized in the Scandinavian Simvastatin Survival Study (4S) among those 65 years of age or older and those under 65 years of age, and women and men. The 4S cohort of 4,444 CAD patients included 827 women and 1021 patients 65 years of age or older. Total cholesterol at baseline was 5.5 to 8.0 mmol/L with triglycerides 2.5 mmol/L or less. Patients were randomized to therapy with simvastatin 20 to 40 mg/day or placebo for a mean follow-up period of 5.4 years. Endpoints consisted of all-cause and CAD mortality, major coronary events, including CAD death and nonfatal AMI, other acute CAD and atherosclerotic events, hospitalizations for CAD and cardiovascular events, and coronary revascularization procedures. Major changes in serum lipids were similar in the different subgroups. In patients 65 years of age or older in the simvastatin-treated group, relative risks for clinical events were as follows: all-cause mortality, 0.66; CAD mortality, 0.57; major coronary events, 0.66; any atherosclerosis-related event, 0.67; and revascularization procedures, 0.59. In women, the corresponding figures were 1.16, 0.86, 0.66, 0.71, and 0.51. Thus, these data indicate that cholesterol lowering with simvastatin produces similar reductions in relative risk for major coronary events in women compared with men and in those 65 years of age or older compared with younger patients (Figure 1-38).

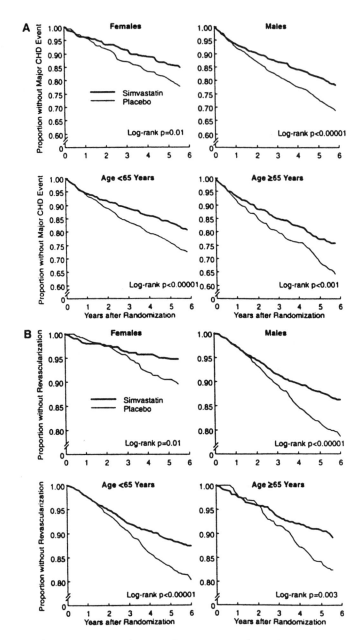

FIGURE 1-38. Kaplan-Meier survival curves for women, men, patients age 65 years of age or older for the proportion of patients remaining free of any major coronary event (A) and the proportion of patients not requiring coronary revascularization surgery (B). Reproduced with permission from Miettinen et al.[96]

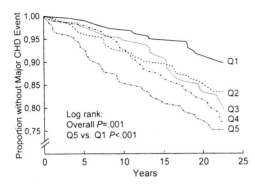

FIGURE 1-39. Kaplan-Meier survival curves for remaining free of major CAD events during 22-year follow-up by quintiles of AUC insulin. The risk of having a major CAD event was significantly higher in men in the highest quintile than in those in the lowest quintile (p < 0.001; age-adjusted p < 0.001). The overall trend for the risk of a major CHD event tested over all AUC insulin quintiles was also statistically significant (p = 0.001; age-adjusted p = 0.006). Reproduced with permission from Pyörälä et al.[97]

Follow-Up of Helsinki Policemen Study

Pyörälä and colleagues[97] in Kuopio, Finland, investigated the predictive value of hyperinsulinemia with regard to the development of CAD during a 22-year follow-up of the Helsinki Policemen Study population. This study was based on a cohort of 970 men who were 34 to 64 years of age and free of CAD, other cardiovascular disease, and diabetes. Risk factor measurements at baseline examination included an oral glucose tolerance test with blood glucose and plasma insulin measurements at 0, 1, and 2 hours. Area under the plasma insulin response curve during the oral glucose tolerance test was used as a composite variable reflecting plasma insulin levels. During the 22-year follow-up, 164 men had a major CAD event, including death or nonfatal AMI. Age-adjusted hazard ratio for major CAD events comparing men in the highest insulin response curve quintile with those in the combined 4 lower quintiles during 5, 10, 15, and 22 year follow-up periods were 3.29, 2.72, 2.14, and 1.61, respectively (Figure 1-39). Further adjustment for other risk factors attenuated these hazard ratios to 2.36, 2.29, 1.76, and 1.32, respectively. These data suggest that hyperinsulinemia predicts CAD risk in Helsinki policemen over a 22-year follow-up and to a large extent independently of other CAD risk factors, but its predictive value diminishes with lengthening follow-up time.

Bezafibrate Treatment

A subgroup analysis of the Bezafibrate Coronary Atherosclerosis Intervention Trial (BECAIT) data was undertaken by Ericsson and colleagues[98] from Danderyd, Sweden, to determine the effects of bezafibrate in relation to baseline coronary narrowing. BECAIT included 92 male post-AMI patients 45 years old or younger. Each received double-blind treatment with bezafibrate (200 mg 3 times daily) or placebo for 5 years, together with a low-fat diet. Coronary angiography was performed at baseline and after 2 and 5 years. The mean minimum lumen diameter of lesions causing 20% to less than 50% diameter stenosis at baseline did not narrow over 5 years in the bezafibrate group and decreased by 0.15 mm in the placebo group. In segments with 50% or greater diameter stenosis at baseline, no change was seen in either of the 2 groups. In the analysis including only segments with 20% to less than 50% stenosis at baseline, coronary events were seen in 7 of 40 patients with a progression in minimum lumen diameter of more than the median value and in 3 of 41 patients with a change less than the median value. Thus, bezafibrate had a preferential effect in slowing the progression of narrowings causing less than 50% diameter stenosis at baseline in young men followed up for a 5-year period after AMI.

Insulin Research/Diabetes Mellitus

Hyperinsulinemia

Hyperinsulinemia has been associated with cardiovascular disease, but whether this relation is independent of other coronary artery disease risk factors is uncertain. Most studies have focused on CAD, but few have included peripheral vascular disease and stroke. Moreover, evidence in elderly and minority populations is limited. Between 1991 and 1993, 3,562 elderly (71–93 years) Japanese-American men from the Honolulu Heart Program were examined by Burchfiel and coworkers[99] in Bethesda, Maryland, and had fasting insulin levels measured. Hyperinsulinemia defined as a fasting insulin greater than the 95th percentile among nonobese men with normal glucose tolerance and no dietary history of medication was observed in 22% of the population. Subjects with hyperinsulinemia had a more adverse CAD risk factor profile and had higher age-adjusted prevalences of CAD, angina, peripheral vascular disease, and thromboembolic and hemorrhagic strokes compared to with those without hyperinsulinemia. Age-adjusted fasting insulin levels, but not 2-hour levels, were also significantly elevated in those with prevalent CAD compared with those without. In logistic regression analyses, adjustment for multiple CAD risk factors attenuated the relations of hyperinsulinemia with CAD, angina, and peripheral vascular disease to nonsignificant levels, whereas those involving thromboembolic and hemorrhagic strokes were strengthened and remained significant (Table 1-5). When multivariate analyses were restricted

TABLE 1-5
Age-Adjusted Odds Ratios for Association of Hyperinsulinemia with Prevalent CVD by Cholesterol Level*

	<240 mg/dL (n = 3,317)	≥240 mg/dL (n = 244)	<200 mg/dL (n = 2,213)	≥200 mg/dL (n = 1,348)
CHD	1.54 (1.25–1.90)	1.66 (0.74–3.75)	1.56 (1.21–2.00)	1.54 (1.10–2.14)
Angina	1.38 (1.08–1.76)	0.92 (0.33–2.57)	1.24 (0.91–1.69)	1.53 (1.06–2.22)
ABI<0.9	1.36 (1.06–1.74)	2.56 (1.24–5.29)	1.53 (1.14–2.07)	1.34 (0.93–1.94)
Thromboembolic stroke	1.71 (1.12–2.60)	7.45 (0.65–85.20)	1.49 (0.92–2.43)	2.75 (1.26–6.00)
Hemorrhagic stroke	2.81 (1.32–5.98)	. . .	2.15 (0.93–4.96)	11.87 (1.23–114.7)

Values in parentheses are 95% CIs.
* Cholesterol levels were measured in 3,561 subjects.
Reproduced with permission from Burchfiel et al.[99]

to nondiabetic subjects, associations were slightly weaker and in general non-significant. Nondiabetic men with thromboembolic stroke were twice as likely to have hyperinsulinemia as those who were stroke free, although this association was of borderline significance. In subjects with elevated total cholesterol levels, somewhat stronger associations were observed for peripheral vascular disease and stroke, but not for CAD. Although further prospective studies are indicated, particularly for peripheral vascular disease and stroke, these cross-sectional results are consistent with an indirect role for insulin in CAD, wherein hyperinsulinemia or an underlying insulin-resistant state may adversely affect other CAD risk factors or serve as a marker for an atherogenic or thrombogenic state.

Insulin Resistance as an Independent Risk Factor

Studies have shown the presence of insulin resistance together with compensatory hyperinsulinemia and vasospastic angina, as well as obstructive CAD. There is growing evidence that the development of coronary atherosclerosis may be closely related to systemic atherosclerosis as well as coronary spasm. However, no information is available about the possible relationship between insulin resistance and the existence of carotid atherosclerosis and vasospastic angina without segmental stenosis or luminal irregularities of the coronary angiogram. To evaluate the independent effect of insulin resistance on carotid intima medial thickening, Shinozaki and colleagues[100] in Osaka, Japan, performed insulin sensitivity tests on 40 patients with vasospastic angina and 24 control subjects with angiographically intact coronary arteries. Both oral glucose tolerance tests and lipid analyses were performed. Using B-mode ultrasonography, the investigators assessed intima media thickness and plaque formation of common carotid arteries in these subjects. Steady-state plasma glucose levels in the vasospastic angina group were about 2-fold higher than those of the control group, confirming the presence of insulin resistance in patients with vasospastic angina. The patients with vasospastic angina showed a significant increase in the average intima media thickness of the carotid wall and frequency of plaque formation, although they were comparable to the control subjects in risk factors other than insulin resistance. The intima medial thickness was correlated with age, 2-hour insulin area, and steady-state plasma glucose level in patients with vasospastic angina. Similar correlations were observed in the control subjects. Multiple regression analyses of data indicate that 67% of the variation in the intima media thickness could be accounted for by age, steady-state plasma glucose level, and cigarette years in vasospastic angina. In addition, differences in intima media thickness were independently related to vasospastic angina. These results suggest that insulin resistance in association with compensatory hyperinsulinemia may be an important pathogenic factor for the development of coronary artery spasm and early atherosclerosis.

Insulin and Glucose Levels

Rainwater and Haffner[101] in San Antonio, Texas, assessed the relationship of lipoprotein(a) with diabetes status and with measures of glucose and insulin in a population of Mexican-Americans having a large prevalence for non-insulin-dependent diabetes mellitus. Because of enormous allelic diversity at the locus encoding the apo(a) protein that directly influences lipoprotein(a) concentration, it was first necessary to adjust for the large effects of variation of the locus encoding protein. The investigators calculated residual lipoprotein(a) concentration as the difference between observed and expected; expected lipoprotein(a) concentration was based on information from all family members sharing each identical by-descent allele. The investigators found significant effects of gender and age on residual lipoprotein(a) concentration that increased with age and in females. Although diabetes status *per se* was not related to residual lipoprotein(a) concentrations, investigators found that residual lipoprotein(a) concentrations were inversely correlated with fasting insulin and glucose concentrations measured 2 hours after glucose challenge. Furthermore, significant inverse correlations with the 2 insulin measures were observed for a subgroup of nondiabetic patients. Inclusion of 2 lipid measures (plasma concentrations of cholesterol and triglycerides) in the models showed that the correlation with insulin and glucose were independent of the relationship between lipoprotein(a) concentrations and the lipid measures. Also, the investigators determined the residual size for each apolipoprotein(a) isoform by adjusting for the identical by-descent allele isoform group average. Although not related to diabetes status, residual apolipoprotein(a) isoform size was positively correlated with fasting insulin and with 2-hour glucose and 2-hour insulin concentration. In addition, significant correlations for all 4 measures were found for the subgroup of nondiabetic individuals. Thus, the results demonstrate that glucose-intolerant individuals have significantly lower residual lipoprotein(a) concentrations and a significant increase of residual apolipoprotein(a) size.

Plasminogen Activator Inhibitor-1

Increased levels of plasminogen activator inhibitor-1 have been discussed as a part of the insulin resistance syndrome. However, it is not clear whether the relationship between plasminogen activator inhibitor-1 and insulin resistance is independent of or mediated by increased triglyceride levels. The aim of a study by Byberg and colleagues[102] in Uppsala, Sweden, was to investigate whether plasminogen activator inhibitor-1 activity is associated with insulin sensitivity independently of serum triglycerides and of other potential confounders. Seventy-year-old men participating in a cohort study undergoing extensive metabolic investigations had blood samples taken for determination of plasminogen activator inhibitor-1 activity. Insulin sensitivity was determined by the euglycemic hyperinsulinemic clamp. In multivariate and regression analyses, insulin sensitivity was a statistically significant determinant of plasminogen activator inhibitor-1 activity, independent of total triglycerides, body mass index, waist-hip ratio, and other potential confounders. The levels of triglycerides were also independently related to plasminogen activator inhibitor-1 activity. The relationship between the plasminogen activator inhibitor-1 and insulin sensitivity and triglycerides were independent of fasting glucose levels. Aggregation of risk factors of the insulin resistance syndrome was associated with increased activity of plasminogen activator inhibitor-1 in men with normal glucose tolerance. The investigators conclude that plasminogen activator inhibitor-1 activity was related to insulin sensitivity and triglycerides independent of each other and of other potential confounders, and that increased levels of plasminogen activator inhibitor-1 should be regarded as a component of the insulin resistance syndrome.

Leptin and Insulin Sensitivity

In humans, production of the adiposity-derived peptide leptin has been linked to adiposity, insulin, and insulin sensitivity. Leyva and coinvestigators[103] in London, United Kingdom, therefore, considered that alterations in plasma leptin concentrations could constitute an additional component of a metabolic syndrome of cardiovascular risk. To explore this hypothesis, the investigators used factor analysis, a multivariate statistical technique that allows reduction of large numbers of highly intercorrelated variables to composite, biological meaningful factors. Seventy-four men, average age 48 years, body mass index (BMI) 26 kg/m^2, who were free of CAD and diabetes, underwent anthropometric measurements (subscapular-to-triceps) [S:T] and subscapular-to-biceps [S:B], skinfold thickness ratios, measurement of fasting plasma leptin, and an intravenous glucose tolerance test (IVGTT) for assessment of insulin sensitivity. Plasma leptin concentrations were correlated with BMI, S:B, systolic and diastolic blood pressures, fasting triglycerides, uric acid, fasting glucose and insulin, and IVGTT insulin. A negative correlation was observed between leptin and insulin sensitivity. No significant correlations emerged between plasma leptin concentrations and age, HDL, or IVGTT glucose. In multivariate regression analyses, BMI, fasting insulin, and IVGTT insulin emerged as independent predictors of plasma leptin concentrations. After adjustment for BMI, only IVGTT insulin emerged as a significant predictor of plasma leptin concentrations. Factor analysis of plasma leptin concentration and the variables that are considered relevant to the insulin resistant syndrome revealed a clustering of plasma leptin concentrations with a factor dominated by insulin resistance and high IVGTT insulin, separate from a high IVGTT glucose/central obesity factor and a high triglyceride/LDL cholesterol factor. Together, these factors accounted for 56% of the total variants in the data set. In conclusion, interindividual variations in plasma leptin concentrations are strongly related to the principle components of the insulin resistant syndrome. Further studies are needed to determine whether the insulin–leptin axis plays a coordinating role in this syndrome and whether plasma leptin concentrations could provide an additional measure of cardiovascular risk.

Atherosclerosis in Insulin-Treated Diabetics

Kornowski and colleagues[104] from Washington, DC, assessed the impact of diabetes mellitus on atherosclerotic mass formation. Seventy insulin-treated diabetics, 150 non-insulin-treated diabetics, and 607 nondiabetics with chronic anginal syndrome and *de novo* native coronary stenoses were studied using (1) angiography, and (2) intravascular ultrasound (reference and lesion arterial, lumen, and plaque areas; area stenosis [reference-lesion/reference lumen area]; remodeling index [reference-lesion lumen area/lesion-reference plaque area]; and slope of the regression line relating lumen area to plaque burden [plaque/arterial area]). Despite being diabetic for a longer time and having similar lumen compromise, insulin-treated patients had (1) less reference plaque (8.3 ± 3.4 mm^2 vs. 10.5 ± 4.5 mm^2), (2) less stenosis plaque (13.0 ± 4.9 mm^2 vs. 16.9 mm^2), (3) smaller reference arterial areas (17.1 ± 5.4 mm^2 vs. 19.7 ± 6.2 mm^2), and (4) smaller stenosis arterial areas (15.3 ± 4.9 mm^2 vs. 19.5 ± 6.5 mm^2) than non-insulin-treated diabetics. With use of multivariate linear regression analysis, insulin use was an independent (and *negative*) predictor of reference plaque and arterial areas and stenosis plaque and arterial areas. This was also true when normalized for body surface area. The remodeling index showed that insulin treatment resulted in an exaggerated impact of plaque accumulation on lumen compromise. This was confirmed by the slope of the regression line relating lumen area to plaque burden. Patients with a longer duration of diabetes who were treated with insulin for 1 year or more had (paradoxically) less reference segment and stenosis plaque accumulation. Possible explanations include impaired adaptive remodeling and/or arterial (and plaque) shrinkage.

Insulin Resistance and Its Metabolic Consequences

A study was performed by Carantoni and coworkers[105] in San Francisco, California, in 36 healthy volunteers to define the relationship between plasma concentrations of partially oxidized LDL, plasma glucose, and insulin responses to oral glucose and steady-state plasma glucose concentration after a 180-minute infusion of somatostatin, insulin, and glucose. The concentration of partially oxidized LDL was estimated by determining the amount of conjugated dienes formed during *in vitro* LDL oxidation in the presence or absence of alanine. Under these conditions, the greater the *in vitro* antioxidant effect of alanine, the lower the amount of partially oxidized LDL that was present in the plasma. The results demonstrated that plasma partially oxidized LDL concentration was significantly correlated with plasma glucose and insulin responses, steady-state plasma glucose concentrations, and plasma triglycerides and HDL cholesterol concentrations (Figure 1-40). Furthermore, these relationships persisted when the data were corrected for differences in age, sex, body mass index, and the ratio of waist to hip girth. Of note, there was no correlation between partially oxidized LDL and LDL cholesterol concentrations. When steady-state plasma glucose was entered along with age, sex, body mass index, and waist to hip ratio in a multiple regression model, steady-state plasma glucose alone was a significant prediction of partially oxidized LDL. The addition of plasma glucose and insulin responses and triglyceride and HDL cholesterol concentrations increased the r^2 to only 0.47. These results show that the amount of partially oxidized LDL in plasma is significantly correlated with insulin resistance and its metabolic consequences.

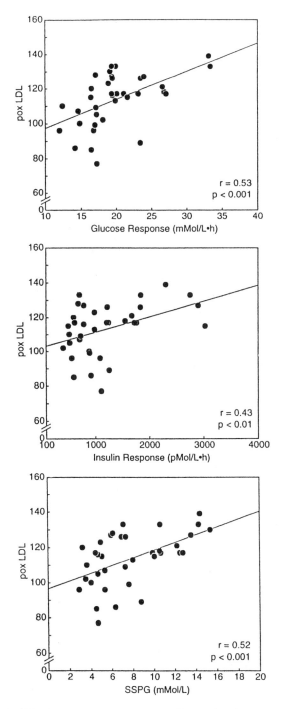

FIGURE 1-40. Relationship between pox LDL (partially oxidized LDL) and plasma glucose response (top), plasma insulin response (middle), and SSPG (steady-state plasma glucose) concentration (bottom). Reproduced with permission from Carantoni et al.[105]

Insulin Sensitivity

Human obesity is associated with an increased tumor necrosis factor-α mRNA expression in adipose tissue. Tumor necrosis factor-α decreases insulin-dependent glucose uptake by inhibiting autophosphorylation of the insulin receptor, suggesting that tumor necrosis factor-α may play a role in insulin resistance. Nilsson and coinvestigators[106] in Stockholm, Sweden, analyzed plasma levels of tumor necrosis factor-α in 40 70-year-old men with newly detected, non-insulin-dependent diabetes mellitus and in 20 age-matched controls. Twenty of the patients had a moderate level of insulin resistance and 20 were severely insulin resistant. The plasma levels of tumor necrosis factor-α were higher in patients moderately insulin resistant and in severely insulin-resistant subjects than in control subjects. Tumor necrosis factor-α was significantly related to body mass index, fasting glucose levels, and serum triglyceride levels and inversely related to the HDL cholesterol level. The finding of an association between high plasma levels of tumor necrosis factor-α and several metabolic abnormalities characteristic for the insulin-resistant syndrome suggests that tumor necrosis factor-α may be involved in the pathogenesis of non-insulin-dependent diabetes mellitus.

Diabetes/Lipids

Deferoxamine Versus L-Arginine to Improve Blood Flow

Nitenberg and colleagues[107] in Colombes, France, examined the mechanism by which acetylcholine produces coronary artery constriction in diabetic patients, itself suggesting an impairment of endothelium-dependent dilation. Two physiological tests were used: (1) a cold pressor test with coronary flow increases induced by an injection of 10 mg of papaverine in the distal LAD before and after either intravenous L-arginine or intravenous deferoxamine in 22 normotensive nonsmoking diabetics with angiographically normal coronary arteries and normal cholesterols. Coronary surface area was measured by quantitative angiography. Before the administration of L-arginine or deferoxamine, cold pressor test-induced coronary artery constriction in both groups and papaverine injection in the distal LAD did not modify significantly proximal LAD dimensions. In the 10 diabetic patients receiving L-arginine, responses to cold pressor test and papaverine were not modified. In the 12 patients receiving deferoxamine, the LAD dilated in response to the two tests (Figure 1-41). Intracoronary isosorbide dinitrate, an endothelium-independent dilator, produced similar dilation in the two groups. Thus, these data indicate that responses of angiographically normal coronary arteries to cold pressor test and to flow increases are impaired in diabetic patients; these abnormal responses are not improved by L-arginine, but they are improved by deferoxamine, suggesting that inactivation of nitric oxide by free radicals may be partly responsible for the coronary artery flow impairment in diabetic patients.

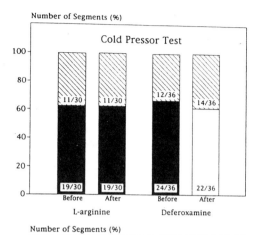

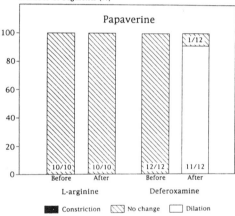

FIGURE 1-41. Prevalence among the two groups of patients of dilation, no change, and constriction in coronary segment responses to CPT and to injection of papaverine in the distal LAD. Numbers at the bottom of each column indicate the number of segments for each type of response divided by the number of segments analyzed. All of the segments were analyzed for the CPT; only dimensions of the proximal LAD were analyzed after papaverine injection. Reproduced with permission from Nitenberg et al.[107]

Coronary Atherosclerosis

The presence or absence of CAD in diabetic patients has been related to the level of circulating plasma lipoproteins. A study by Tkac and colleagues[108] in Toronto, Canada, examined whether there is a relationship between the actual severity of CAD and the plasma concentrations of major classes of plasma lipoprotein (HDL, LDL, triglyceride-rich lipoproteins and their subfractions) particularly the numbers of lipoprotein particles, in men and women with type 2 diabetes. One hundred seventy four diabetic patients (136 men, 38 women) who underwent angiography were studied. Nine specific coronary segments were scored. The population was divided into tertiles, according to the angiographic severity of their coronary disease: mild CAD: coronary score 1–10; moderate CAD: coronary score 11–13; or severe CAD: coronary score 14–22. The main findings were that the numbers of particles (as reflected by the apo B levels) of the triglyceride-rich lipoproteins were greater in those with moderate and severe disease than in those with mild disease. There was a significant correlation between the coronary score and the apo B in triglyceride-rich lipoproteins. There were parallel but not significant changes in triglyceride levels. Apo A-I was lower in patients with moderate and severe disease. These differences were more striking in women than in men. There were no differences in plasma LDL or HDL cholesterol or in LDL apo B or Lp(a). Multiple linear regression analysis, when adjusted for sex, age, and body mass index, showed that 3 lipid variables (triglyceride-rich lipoprotein apo B, LDL cholesterol, plasma apo A-I) significantly and independently predicted the coronary score. This study demonstrates that in type 2 diabetes, the severity of the angiographically evaluated CAD is possibly related to the numbers of triglyceride-rich lipoprotein particles in the plasma. This relationship is stronger in women than in men and is independent of HDL and LDL.

The Strong Heart Study

Small, dense LDLs have been shown to be associated with the insulin resistance syndrome and CAD. Gray and coworkers[109] in Washington, DC, examined the distribution of LDL size and phenotype within a population-based sample of American Indians to determine the relationships with prevalent CAD and to examine associations with hyperinsulinemia and other components of the insulin resistance syndrome. Data were available for 4,505 men and women between 45 and 74 years of age who are members of 13 American Indian communities in 3 geographic areas. Diabetes, CAD, and CAD risk factors were assessed by standardized techniques and LDL size was measured by gradient gel electrophoresis. LDL size was smaller in men than in women and in individuals with diabetes than in those without diabetes. In multivariate analysis, LDL size was significantly related to several components of the insulin resistance syndrome, including triglycerides (inversely) and HDL cholesterol (positively). Although univariate relations were positive, LDL size was not significantly related to fasting insulin concentration or body mass in the multivariant model. LDL size also showed no relationship to apolipoprotein E phenotype. When LDL size was compared in individuals with and without CAD, no significant differences were observed in either nondiabetic or diabetic patients. The investigators conclude that LDL size is most strongly related to lipoprotein components of the insulin resistance syndrome, especially plasma triglycerides. However, in this population with low LDL, it is not related to cardiovascular disease.

Body Mass Index, Smoking, and Other Risk Factors

Effect of Passive Smoking on Atherogenic Changes

Valkonen and Kuusi[110] in Helsinki, Finland, obtained blood samples during 2 ordinary working days from healthy, nonsmoking subjects (n = 10) before and after (up to 5.5 hours) spending half an hour in a smoke-free area (day 1) or in a room for smokers (day 2). Passive smoking caused an acute decrease in serum ascorbic acid and in serum antioxidant defense, a decreased capacity of LDL to resist oxidation, and the appearance of increased amounts of lipid

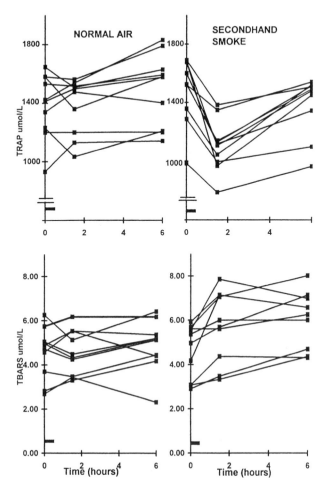

FIGURE 1-42. Effect of passive smoking on serum antioxidant defense (measured TRAP) and on serum lipid peroxidation end products (TBARS). Individual changes were noted after the subjects spent half an hour in a smoke-free area or in a smoking room. Exposure period was 30 minutes. Reproduced with permission from Valkonen and Kuusi.[110]

peroxidation end products in serum (Figures 1-42, 1-43). LDL isolated from subjects after passive smoking was taken up by cultured macrophages at an increased rate. Thus, exposure of nonsmoking subjects to second-hand smoke breaks down the serum antioxidant defense, leading to accelerated lipid peroxidation.

Coronary Artery Disease in Women

The association between plasma apolipoprotein B concentrations and angiographically determined CAD was investigated by Westerveld and colleagues[111] in Utrecht, The Netherlands, in women in a cross-sectional study.

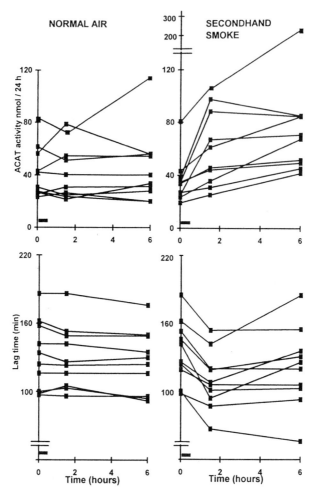

FIGURE 1-43. Effect of passive smoking on the capacity of LDL to resist peroxidation (lag time) and on the accumulation of LDL cholesterol in cultured human macrophages (ACAT activity). Individual changes were noted after subjects spent half an hour in a smoke-free area or in a smoking room. Exposure period was 30 minutes (■). Reproduced with permission from Valkonen and Kuusi.[110]

Stenosis of greater than 60% in 1 or more coronary arteries was classified as positive coronary artery disease. Negative CAD was defined as a maximum stenosis of 10% in any coronary artery. Fasting plasma concentrations of apolipoprotein B, apolipoprotein A-I, cholesterol, LDL, HDL, and triglycerides were determined. Information on nonlipid risk factors was obtained from questionnaires. Positive CAD women (n = 160) were older than negative CAD women. Positive CAD compared with negative CAD women had higher frequencies of diabetes, hypertension, and smoking. CAD positive women had higher plasma concentrations of apolipoprotein B, cholesterol, LDL cholesterol, and triglycerides and lower levels of HDL cholesterol (Table 1-6). After correction for nonlipid risk factors, apolipoprotein B, cholesterol, LDL, HDL, and triglycerides were independently related to CAD. In the lowest quartiles of cholesterol, LDL,

TABLE 1-6
Fasting Plasma Lipids and Lipoproteins in CAD − and CAD + Women as Assessed by
Angiography

	CAD −	CAD +	p*	p* (Age as Covariate)
Chol, mmol/L	6.38 ± 1.22 (n=129)	7.01 ± 1.19 (n=160)	<0.001	0.0011
TGS, mmol/L†	1.71 ± 0.93 (n=113)	1.98 ± 0.84 (n=145)	0.001*	0.0065
HDL-chol, mmol/L	1.37 ± 0.38 (n=111)	1.28 ± 0.28 (n=146)	0.028	0.019
LDL-chol, mmol/L	4.13 ± 1.13 (n=111)	4.74 ± 1.09 (n=146)	<0.001	0.0008
Apo A-I, g/L	1.53 ± 0.34 (n=96)	1.49 ± 0.24 (n=131)	NS	NS
Apo B, g/L	1.25 ± 0.34 (n=96)	1.48 ± 0.32 (n=131)	<0.001	<0.0001
Age, y	58.74 ± 11.09	64.19 ± 8.2	<0.001	

* By logistic regression.
† Logarithmically transformed.
Reproduced with permission from Westerveld et al.[111]

and triglycerides, CAD positive women had higher apolipoprotein B concentrations than CAD negative women. In contrast, cholesterol, LDL, triglycerides, or HDL levels were not different in any quartile of apolipoprotein B. Apolipoprotein B showed the most significant relation with the number of stenotic vessels, and apolipoprotein B was associated with CAD in the normolipidemic subgroup. In conclusion, apolipoprotein B is superior to cholesterol, LDL, HDL, triglycerides, and apo A-I in discriminating between positive and negative angiographic CAD.

Risk Factors for Atherosclerosis

In a cooperative multicenter study, the Pathobiological Determinants of Atherosclerosis in Youth, McGill and coworkers[112] in San Antonio, Texas, measured atherosclerosis of the aorta and right coronary artery in 2,403 black and white men and women 15–34 years of age who died of external causes and were autopsied in forensic laboratories. The investigators measured the diameter of the open, flattened, and fixed right coronary artery and the diameter, intimal thickness, intimal cross-sectional area, medial thickness, and medial cross-sectional area of the pressure-perfused, fixed left anterior descending coronary artery. Using the ratio of intimal thickness to outer diameter of the small renal arteries to predict mean arterial pressure during life, the investigators classified the cases as normotensive (mean arterial pressure <110 mm Hg) or hypertensive (mean arterial pressure >110 mm Hg). The prevalence of hypertension by age, sex, and race corresponded closely with that measured in a survey of the living population. Hypertension had little or no effect on fatty streaks. Hypertension was associated with more extensive raised lesions in the abdominal aorta and right coronary arteries of blacks older than 20 years of age and in the right coronary arteries of whites older than 25 years of age. At all ages, women had less extensive raised lesions in the right coronary arteries than did men, but the effect of hypertension on raised lesions was similar to that in men. Adjustment for serum lipoprotein cholesterol levels and smoking in a subset of cases yielded results similar to those obtained without adjustment. Hypertension was associated with large diameters of the right coronary artery and left anterior descending coronary artery and with larger cross-sectional intimal and medial areas of the left anterior descending coronary artery. In conclusion, hypertension augments atherosclerosis in both men and women primarily by accelerating the conversion of fatty streaks to raised lesions beginning in the third decade of life, and the effect of hypertension increases with age.

Arterial Stiffness in Pre- and Postmenopausal Women

Increased arterial stiffness is thought to contribute to the increased incidence of cardiovascular disease with age. Little, however, is known about the influence of aging on central and peripheral arterial stiffness in women. Moreover, it is unknown whether physical activity status influences age-related increases in arterial stiffness in women. Arterial pulse wave velocity and augmentation index were measured by Tanaka and colleagues[113] in Denver, Colorado, in 53 healthy women, including 10 premenopausal and 18 postmenopausal sedentary women, and 9 menopausal and 16 postmenopausal physically active women. In the sedentary women, there were no age-related differences in arterial blood pressure, but aortic pulse wave velocity and carotid augmentation index were higher in postmenopausal sedentary versus premenopausal sedentary women; however, there were no significant differences in leg and arm pulse wave velocity. Systolic and mean arterial blood pressures were higher in postmenopausal physically active women versus premenopausal physically active women. Despite this and in contrast to the sedentary women, aortic pulse wave velocity and augmentation index were not different in postmenopausal physically active versus premenopausal physically active women. Stepwise, multiple regression analysis indicated that maximal oxygen consumption, plasma total cholesterol, and plasma LDL cholesterol were significant independent predictors and together explained up to 50% of the variability in central arterial stiffness. The investigators conclude that (1) central, but not peripheral, arterial stiffness increased with age in sedentary healthy women in the absence of age-related increases in arterial blood pressure; (2) significant age-related increases in central arterial stiffness are not observed in highly physically active women; and (3) aerobic fitness and plasma total cholesterol and LDL cholesterol level are significant independent physiological correlates of central arterial stiffness in this population.

Patterns of Change in Lipids as Persons Age

Limited data are available on patterns of change in lipids and lipoproteins as persons age. Abbott and associates[114] from several US medical centers described a 10-year change in total and HDL cholesterol according to suspected determinants in 898 Japanese-American men enrolled the Honolulu Heart Pro-

TABLE 1-7
Average Baseline Levels of Total and HDL Cholesterol (mg/dL) and Average Changes Between Adjacent Examinations by Baseline Age in the Honolulu Heart Program

	Age Group	Sample Size	Baseline (mg/dl) 1970–1972	Average Change (mg/dL) from	
				Baseline to 1980–1982	1980–1982 to 1991–1993
Total cholesterol	51–54	346	221 ± 35	−7 ± 30‡	−24 ± 33‡
	55–59	331	222 ± 36	−11 ± 30‡	−22 ± 30‡
	60–72	221	219 ± 38	−10 ± 28‡	−26 ± 31‡
	Total	898	221 ± 36	−9 ± 29‡	−24 ± 32‡
HDL cholesterol§	51–54	345	44.0 ± 11.5	3.0 ± 10.0‡	1.2 ± 9.2†
	55–59	329	45.1 ± 12.1	2.1 ± 9.8‡	2.1 ± 9.3‡
	60–72	221	45.9 ± 11.9	1.5 ± 10.8*	2.7 ± 11.0‡
	Total	895	44.9 ± 11.9	2.3 ± 10.1‡	1.9 ± 9.7‡

Significant change in 10 years: *$p < 0.05$; †$p < 0.01$; ‡$p < 0.001$.

Values are expressed as mean ± SD.

§ Baseline values (1970 to 1972) increased significantly with age ($p < 0.05$).

Reproduced with permission from Abbott et al.[114]

gram. Data were based on examinations that occurred from 1970 to 1972 and at repeat examinations received 10 and 20 years later. At the last examination, men were aged 71 to 93 years. Mean reductions in total cholesterol in the second 10 years of follow-up (24 mg/dL) were more than double the reductions observed in the first 10 years (9 mg/dL). Levels of total cholesterol declined and levels of HDL cholesterol increased regardless of beginning levels of systolic blood pressure, body mass index, physical activity, cigarette smoking status, or the use of treatment for hypertension or elevated total cholesterol. Men with prevalent CAD experienced greater reductions in total cholesterol during the second 10 years of follow-up (32 mg/dL) versus men with CAD (22 mg/dL). Adjustment for baseline covariates failed to alter these findings appreciably. The authors conclude that alterations in total and HDL cholesterol with advancing age may be expected to occur regardless of risk factor status, disease prevalence, or pharmacological intervention. In the presence of such effects, evaluation of treatment programs to alter levels of total and HDL cholesterol in older persons should take into account the possibility that even in the absence of intervention, changes could also occur due to aging alone (Table 1-7).

Estradiol Therapy May Reduce Cardiovascular Risk

Estrogen therapy increases plasma HDL levels, which may reduce cardiovascular risk in postmenopausal women. The mechanism of action of estrogen in influencing various steps in hepatic HDL and apolipoprotein A-I synthesis and secretion are not fully understood. Jin and colleagues[115] in Long Beach, California, used the human hepatoblastoma cell line as an *in vitro* model system to delineate the effect of estradiol on multiple regulatory steps involved in hepatic HDL metabolism. Incubation of hepatoblastoma G2 cells with estradiol resulted in the following statistically significant findings: (1) increased accumulation of apolipoprotein A-I in the medium without affecting uptake/removal of radiolabeled HDL protein; (2) accelerated incorporation of [H^3] of leucine into apolipoprotein A-I; (3) selective increase of [H^3] leucine incorporation into apolipoprotein A-I, but not apolipoprotein A-I plus apolipoprotein A-II HDL particles without and with apolipoprotein A-II, respectively; (4) increased ability of apolipoprotein A-I-containing particles to efflux cholesterol from fibroblast; (5) stimulated steady-state apolipoprotein A-I but not apolipoprotein A-II mRNA expression; and (6) increased newly transcribed apolipoprotein A-I mRNA message without effect on apolipoprotein A-I mRNA half-life. The data indicate that estradiol stimulates newly transcribed hepatic apolipoprotein A-I mRNA, resulting in a selective increase in lipoprotein A-I, a subfraction of HDL that is associated with decreased atherosclerotic cardiovascular disease, especially in postmenopausal women.

Soy Isoflavones

The possibility that the heightened cardiovascular risk associated with menopause, which is said to be ameliorated by soybeans, can be reduced with soy isoflavones was tested in 21 women by Nestel and colleagues[116] in Adelaide, Australia. Although several were perimenopausal, all were included in this study. A placebo-control crossover trial tested the effects of 80 mg/day of isoflavones (45 mg genistein) over 5- to 10-week periods. Systemic arterial compliance (arterial elasticity), which declined with age in this group, improved 26% compared with placebo. Arterial pressure and plasma lipids were unaffected. The vasodilatory capacity of the microcirculation was measured in 9 women; high acetylcholine-mediated dilation in the forearm vasculature was similar with active and placebo treatment. LDL oxidizability measured *in vitro* was unchanged. Thus, one important measure of arterial health, systemic arterial compliance, was significantly improved in perimenopausal and in menopausal women taking soy isoflavones to approximately the same extent as is achieved with conventional hormone replacement therapy.

Chlamydia Pneumoniae: Risk Factor for Atherosclerosis

Chlamydia pneumoniae infection has been associated with CAD. To evaluate the mechanisms of this association, Laurila and coworkers[117] in Oulu, Finland, studied whether chronic *Chlamydia pneumoniae* infection affected serum lipid values similarly to acute infection. Triglycerides, total and HDL cholesterol concentrations, and *Chlamydia pneumoniae* antibodies were measured from paired serum samples of 415 Finnish males taken 3 years apart. Chronic infection, defined as persistent IgG and IgA antibodies, was found in 20% and the antibodies were negative in 15% of the cases studied. The serum triglyceride and total cholesterol concentrations were higher in the subjects with a chronic *Chlamydia pneumoniae* infection than in the subjects with no antibodies. The

HDL cholesterol concentrations and the ratios of HDL cholesterol to total cholesterol were significantly decreased in the subjects with chronic infection. Chronic *Chlamydia pneumoniae* infection seemed to be associated with a serum lipid profile considered to increase the risk of atherosclerosis. This finding supports the hypothesis that infections play a role in the pathogenesis of atherosclerosis.

Homocysteine

Hyperhomocysteinemia as a Risk Factor in End-Stage Renal Disease

Moustapha and colleagues[118] studied the association between total homocysteine and cardiovascular outcomes in 167 patients with end-stage renal disease. Included were 93 men and 74 women with a mean age of 56 years who were followed for a mean duration of 17 months. Cardiovascular events and causes of mortality were related to total homocysteine values and other cardiovascular risk factors. Cox regression analysis was used to identify the independent predictors for cardiovascular events and mortality. Fifty-five patients (33%) developed cardiovascular events and 31 (19%) died, 12 (8%) of cardiovascular causes. Total plasma homocysteine values ranged between 7.9 and 315 μmol/L. Levels were higher in patients who had cardiovascular events or died of cardiovascular causes (Figure 1-44). The relative risk for cardiovascular events, including death, increased 1% per μmol/L in total homocysteine concentration. These data suggest that hyperhomocysteinemia is an independent risk factor for cardiovascular morbidity and mortality in end-stage renal disease.

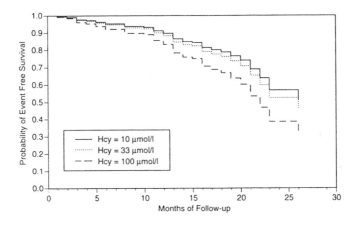

FIGURE 1-44. Probability for event-free survival during the follow-up period for patients with mean homocysteine (Hcy) values of 10, 33, and 100 μmol/L. Reproduced with permission from Moustapha et al.[118]

Hyperhomocysteinemia as a Risk Factor

A high serum total homocysteine level is an independent risk factor for cardiovascular disease. Because it is not known whether the strength of the association between hyperhomocysteinemia and cardiovascular disease is similar for peripheral arterial, coronary artery, and cerebral vascular disease, Hoogeveen and coworkers[119] in Amsterdam, The Netherlands, compared 3 separate risk estimates in an age-, sex-, and glucose tolerance-stratified random sample (n = 631) from a 50- to 75-year-old general white population. Furthermore, the investigators examined the combined effect of homocysteinemia and diabetes mellitus with regard to cardiovascular disease. The prevalence of fasting hyperhomocysteinemia (>14.0 μmol/L) was 26%. After adjustment for age, sex, hypertension, hypercholesterolemia, diabetes, and smoking, the odds ratios per 5-μmol/L increment in homocysteine were 1.44 for peripheral arterial, 1.25 for coronary artery, 1.24 for cerebral vascular, and 1.39 for any cardiovascular disease (Figure 1-45). After stratification by glucose tolerance category and adjustment for the classic risk factors and serum creatinine, the odds ratios per 5-μmol/L increment in homocysteine for any cardiovascular disease were 1.38 in normal glucose tolerance, 1.55 in impaired glucose tolerance, and 2.33 in non-insulin-dependent diabetes mellitus. The investigators conclude that the magnitude of the association between hyperhomocysteinemia and cardiovascular disease is similar for peripheral arterial, coronary artery, and cerebral vascular disease in a 50- to 75-year-old general population. High serum homo-

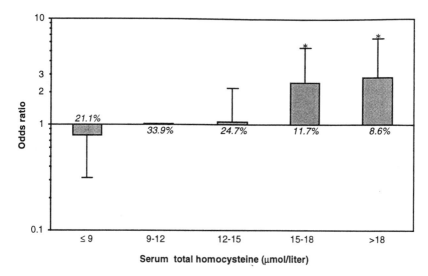

FIGURE 1-45. OR for cardiovascular disease according to serum total plasma homocysteine (tHcy) level adjusted for age and sex. The reference category was serum tHcy values of 9 to 12 μmol/L. Percentages of the subsample for each serum tHcy range are presented. The error bars represent the lower or upper half of the 95% CI. *p < .05, significantly different from the reference category (A logarithmic scale was used because the OR is a multiplicative measure of association; equal differences on the logarithmic scale correspond to equal ratios between OR). Reproduced with permission from Hoogeveen et al.[119]

cysteine may be a stronger (1.6-fold) risk factor for cardiovascular disease in subjects with non-insulin-dependent diabetes mellitus than in nondiabetic patients.

Vitamin Supplementation and Homocysteine Levels

Hyperhomocysteinemia is a risk factor for atherosclerosis and thrombosis and is inversely related to plasma folate and vitamin B_{12} levels. den Heijer and coworkers[120] in Nijmegen, The Netherlands, assessed the effects of vitamin supplementation on plasma homocysteine levels in 89 patients with a history of recurrent venous thrombosis and in 227 healthy volunteers. Patients and hyperhomocysteinemic (homocysteine level >16 μmol/L) volunteers were randomized to placebo or high-dose multivitamin supplements containing 5 mg folic acid, 0.4 mg hydroxy cobalamin, and 50 mg of pyridoxine. A subgroup of volunteers without hyperhomocysteinemia was also randomized into 3 additional regimens of 5 mg folic acid, 0.5 mg folic acid, or 0.4 mg hydroxy cobalamin. Before and after the intervention period, blood samples were taken for measurements of homocysteine, folate, cobalamin, and pyridoxal-5'-phosphate levels. Supplementation with high-dose multivitamin preparation normalized plasma homocysteine levels (<16 μmol/L) in 26 of 30 individuals compared with 7 of 30 in the placebo group. Also, in normohomocysteinemic subjects, multivitamin supplementation strongly reduced homocysteine levels (Figure 1-46). In this subgroup, the effect of folic acid alone was similar to that of multivitamins: median reduction, 26% for 5 mg folic acid and 25% for 0.5 mg folic acid. Cobalamine supplementation had only a slight effect on homocysteine lowering. This study shows that combined vitamin supplementation reduces homocysteine levels effectively in patients with venous thrombosis and in healthy volunteers either with or without hyperhomocysteinemia. Even supplementation with 0.5 mg of folic acid led to a substantial reduction of blood homocysteine levels.

Plasma Homocysteine Levels

The proteolytic enzyme-activated protein C (APC) is a normal plasma component, indicating that protein C (PC) is continuously activated *in vivo*. High concentrations of homocysteine inhibit activation of PC *in vitro*; this effect may account for the high risk of thrombosis in patients with hyperhomocysteinemia. Cattaneo and associates[121] in Milan, Italy, measured the plasma levels of APC in 128 patients with previous venous thromboembolism and in 98 age- and sex-matched healthy controls, and correlated them with the plasma levels of total homocysteine measured before and after oral methionine loading. Forty-eight patients had hyperhomocysteinemia and 80 had normal levels of homocysteine. No subject was known to have any of the congenital or acquired thrombolytic states at the time of the study. Because the plasma levels of APC and PC were correlated in healthy controls, the APC/PC ratios were also analyzed. Plasma APC levels and APC/PC ratios were significantly higher

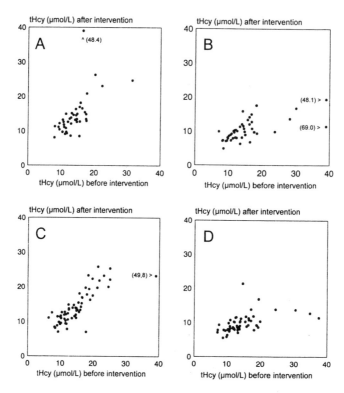

FIGURE 1-46. Total plasma homocysteine (tHcy) levels before (x axis) and after (y axis) 8 weeks of daily multivitamin or placebo supplementation in patients with a history of recurrent venous thrombosis (A = placebo group; B = multivitamin group) and in healthy volunteers (C = placebo group; D = multivitamin group). The multivitamin tablets contained 5 mg folic acid, 0.4 mg hydroxycobalamin, and 50 mg pyridoxine. Reproduced with permission from Cattaneo et al.[121]

in venous thromboembolism patients than in controls. Most of the increase in APC levels and APC/PC ratios were attributable to patients with hyperhomocysteinemia. Patients with normal homocysteine had intermediate values, which did not differ significantly from those of healthy controls. There was no correlation between the plasma levels of homocysteine or its plasma level increments and APC or APC/PC ratios in controls (Figure 1-47). Fasting plasma levels of

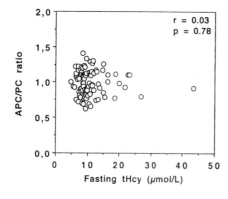

FIGURE 1-47. Correlation between the fasting plasma levels of total homocysteine (tHcy) and APC/PC ratios of 98 healthy volunteers. Reproduced with permission from Cattaneo et al.[121]

APC and APC/PC ratios of 10 controls did not increase 4 hours after oral methionine, despite a 2-fold increase in homocysteine. This study indicates that APC plasma levels are sensitive markers of activation of the hemostatic system *in vivo* and that homocysteine does not interfere with the activation of PC *in vivo*.

Diet

The Coronary Artery Risk Development in Young Adults Study

Hemostatic factors play an important role in the complications of ischemic heart and vessel disease. Dietary fats, such as n-3 fatty acids, have been shown to possibly influence hemostatic factors. However, most studies reporting an inverse association between cardiovascular disease and fish and n-3 fatty acid consumption used supplemental doses of fish oil or intakes exceeding the typical amount consumed by the US population. A report by Archer and coworkers[122] in Chicago, Illinois, examined the associations of usual intakes of fish, linolenic acid, and eicosapentaenoic acid and docosahexaenoic acid with fibrinogen, factor VII, factor VIII and von Willebrand factor in the Coronary Artery Risk Development in Young Adults (CARDIA) study. The analyses reported included 1,672 black and white men and women age 24 to 42 years from 1992 to 1993. After adjustment for age, body mass index, diabetes, number of cigarettes smoked per day, race, energy, and alcohol consumption, no significant associations were observed between those who consumed no fish versus those who consumed the highest level of dietary fish with respect to fibrinogen, factor VIII, or von Willebrand factor for any race–gender group. Comparisons of tertile I versus tertile III for dietary linolenic acid, eicosapentaenoic acid and docosahexaenoic acid were also not significantly associated with fibrinogen, factor VII, factor VIII, or von Willebrand factor for any race–gender group. These data suggest that customary intakes of fish and n-3 fatty acids in populations that generally do not consume large amounts of these food items are not associated with these hemostatic factors.

Modification of Dietary Fat

Modification of dietary fat composition may influence hemostatic variables, which are associated with increased risk of CAD. To address this question, Sanders and coinvestigators[123] in London, United Kingdom, performed a control feeding study on 26 healthy male, nonsmoking subjects with diets of differing fat composition. For the first 3 weeks, the subjects were given a diet calculated to supply 30% energy as total fat: 8% as monounsaturated, 4% as polyunsaturated, and 16% energy as saturated fatty acids, respectively (saturated diet). This was followed immediately by 2 diets taken in random order, each of 3-week duration and separated by an 8-week washout on the subject's usual diet. Both diets were calculated to supply 30% of energy as fat: 14% monounsaturated, 6% as polyunsaturated, and 8% energy as saturated fatty acids. They both provided 5 gm more of polyunsaturated fatty acids than the saturated fat diet—in 1 diet as long-chain n-3 fatty acids and in the other as linoleic acid (n-6 diet). Fasting plasma lipids, lipoproteins, and hemostatic factors were measured on the final 3 days of each dietary period. In a subset of 9 subjects, the postprandial responses to a test meal were studied on the penultimate day of each period, each meal having the fat composition of its parent diet. On the n-3 diet compared with the n-6 diet, plasma triglyceride, HDL_3 cholesterol, apoprotein AII, and fibrinogen concentrations were lower and HDL_2 cholesterol concentration was higher. On both the n-3 and n-6 diets compared with the saturated diet, fasting plasma total and LDL cholesterol, apoprotein B, β-thromboglobulin concentrations, and platelet counts were lower and the plasma Lp(a) and von Willebrand factor concentrations were higher. Fasting factor VII coagulant activity was increased and apo A-I protein concentration reduced following the n-3 diet, compared with the saturated diet. Plasma fibrinogen concentration was significantly greater following the n-6 diet than on the saturated diet. Postprandially, plasma triglyceridemia was greater on the n-6 diet and lowest on the n-3 diet with the saturated diet being in the median. Plasma VIIc was increased at 4 hours following the standardized test meals on the n-3 and n-6 diets but not on the saturated diet. An increased intake of long-chain n-3 fatty acids decreased fasting plasma triglycerides in apoprotein A-II concentrations and increased HDL_2 cholesterol concentrations and resulted in less postprandial lipemia, but led to an increase in VIIc. Thus, an increased intake of linoleic acid may raise plasma fibrinogen concentration. Decreasing the intake of saturated fatty acids reduces plasma LDL cholesterol and apoprotein B without affecting HDL cholesterol concentration independent of the type of polyunsaturated fatty acids in the diet. When advice is given to reduce saturated fat intake, it is important to ensure an appropriate ratio of n-3/n-6 fatty acids in the diet.

Reducing Dietary Saturated Fatty Acids

Few well-controlled diet studies have investigated the effects of reducing dietary saturated fatty acid intake in premenopausal and postmenopausal women or in blacks. Ginsberg and coworkers[124] in New York, New York, conducted a multicenter, randomized, crossover design trial of the effects of reducing dietary saturated fatty acid on plasma lipids and lipoproteins in 103 healthy adults 22–67 years old. There were 46 men, 57 women of whom 26 were black; 18 were postmenopausal women and 60 were men over 40 years old. All meals and snacks, except Saturday dinner, were prepared and served by the research centers. The study was designed to compare 3 diets: an average American diet, a step 1 diet, and a low saturated fatty acid diet. Dietary cholesterol was constant. Diet composition was validated and monitored by a central laboratory. Each diet was consumed for 8 weeks. Blood samples were obtained during weeks 5 through 8. The compositions of the 3 diets were as follows: the average American diet was 34% kcal fat and 15% kcal saturated fatty acid; the step 1 diet was 29% kcal fat and 9% kcal saturated fatty acid; the low saturated fatty acid diet was 25% kcal fat and 6% kcal saturated fatty acid. Each diet provided

275 mg cholesterol/day. Compared with the average American diet, plasma total cholesterol in the whole group fell 5% on the step 1 diet and 9% on the low saturated fatty acid diet. LDL cholesterol was 7% lower on the step 1 diet and 11% lower on the low saturated fatty acid diet than on the average American diet. Similar responses were seen in each subgroup. HDL cholesterol fell 7% on the step 1 diet and 11% on the low saturated fatty acid diet. Reductions in HDL cholesterol were seen in all subgroups, except in blacks and in older men. Plasma triglyceride levels increased 9% between the average American diet and the step 1 diet, but did not increase further from the step 1 diet to the low saturated fatty acid diet. Changes in triglyceride levels were not significant in most subgroups. Surprisingly, plasma Lp(a) concentrations increased in a stepwise fashion as saturated fatty acid was reduced. In a well-controlled feeding study, stepwise reductions in saturated fatty acids resulted in parallel reductions in plasma total and LDL cholesterol. Dietary effects were remarkably similar in several subgroups of men and women and in blacks. The reductions in total and LDL cholesterol achieved in these different subgroups indicate that diet can have a significant impact on risk for atherosclerotic cardiac disease in the total population.

Consumption of Green and Black Tea

Intake of flavonoids is associated with a reduced cardiovascular risk. Oxidation of LDL is a major step in atherogenesis, and antioxidants may protect LDL from oxidation. Because tea is an important source of flavonoids, which are strong antioxidants, Princen and coinvestigators[125] in Leiden, The Netherlands, assessed in a randomized, placebo-controlled study, the effect of consumption of black and green tea and of intake of isolated green tea polyphenols on LDL oxidation *ex vivo*, and on plasma levels of antioxidants and lipids. During a 4-week period, healthy male and female smokers (aged 34 years) consumed 6 cups of black or green tea or water/day, or they received as a supplement 3.6 gm of green tea polyphenol/day (equivalent to the consumption of 18 cups of green tea/day). Consumption of black or green tea had no effect on plasma cholesterol or triglycerides, HDL and LDL cholesterol, plasma vitamins C and E, β-carotene, and uric acid. No differences were found in parameters of LDL oxidation. Intake of green tea polyphenols decreased plasma vitamin E significantly in that group compared with the control group, but had no effect on LDL oxidation *ex vivo*. The investigators conclude that consumption of black or green tea up to 6 cups/day had no effect on plasma lipids and no sparing effect on plasma antioxidant vitamins, and that intake of a higher dose of isolated green tea polyphenols decreased plasma and vitamin E. Although tea polyphenols had a potent antioxidant activity on LDL oxidation *in vitro*, no effect was found on LDL oxidation *ex vivo* after consumption of green or black tea or intake of a green tea polyphenol isolate.

Effects of Diet on Metabolic Parameters

There is little information comparing the effects of a high-monounsaturated fat versus a high-carbohydrate diet in patients with type I diabetes mellitus. In a study by Georgopoulos and colleagues[126] in Minneapolis, Minnesota, the effects of these diets on a number of metabolic parameters were compared. Seventeen normolipidemic, nonobese patients with type I diabetes were provided with the diets for 4 weeks each in a randomized, crossover design study. The percentages of monounsaturated fat in the 2 diets were 25% monounsaturated fat versus 9% carbohydrates, with the corresponding total fat of 40% versus 24%, and a total carbohydrate content of 45% versus 61%. At the end of each dietary period, parameters of glycemic control, coagulation factors, and fasting and postprandial lipoproteins were assessed. There were no differences in weight, glycemia, insulin dose, fasting lipid profile, or coagulation factors between the 2 diets. However, the metabolism of postprandial lipoproteins after a fat load differed; after the monounsaturated fat diet was compared with the carbohydrate diet, mean plasma triglyceride levels over 10 hours were higher. The levels of triglycerides and retinyl esters and the total particle number (apolipoprotein B levels) in chylomicron remnants and small VLDLs were also higher. These data suggest that in patients with type I diabetes, a carbohydrate diet might be preferable to a monounsaturated fat diet, since adherence to the former results in a lower number of circulating postprandial lipoprotein particles that are potentially atherogenic.

Imaging Modalities

Lipoprotein Subclasses

Although each of the major lipoprotein fractions is composed of various subclasses that may differ in atherogenicity, the importance of this heterogeneity has been difficult to ascertain due to the labor-intensive nature of subclass measurement methods. Freedman and coinvestigators[127] in Atlanta, Georgia, recently developed a procedure, using proton nuclear magnetic resonance spectroscopy, to simultaneously quantify levels of subclasses of VLDL, LDL, and HDL lipoproteins; subclass distributions determined with this method agreed well with those derived by gradient gel electrophoresis. The objective of the current study of 158 men was to examine whether nuclear magnetic resonance-derived lipoprotein subclass levels improved the predictions of angiographically documented CAD when levels of lipids and lipoproteins were known. The investigators found that a global measure of CAD severity was possibly associated with levels of large VLDL and small HDL particles and inversely associated with intermediate size HDL particles; these associations were independent of age and standard lipid measurements. At comparable lipid and lipoprotein levels, for example, men with relatively high levels of either small HDL or large VLDL particles were 3 to 4 times more likely to have extensive CAD than were the other men; 27 men with high levels of both large VLDL and small HDL particles were 15 times more likely to have extensive CAD than were men with low levels. In contrast, adjustment for levels of triglycerides or HDL cholesterol greatly reduced the relation of small LDL particles to CAD. These findings suggest that large VLDL and small HDL particles may play important roles in the development of occlusive disease and that their measurement, which is not possible with routine lipid testing, may lead to more accurate risk assessment.

Lipid-Lowering Medication

Postmenopausal Hormone Therapy Reduces Lipoprotein Concentration

Espeland and colleagues[128] in Winston-Salem, North Carolina, report findings from a large, prospective, placebo-controlled clinical trial that allowed a determination of the influence of postmenopausal hormonal therapy to decrease levels of lipoprotein (Lp)(a) in cross-sectional studies and short or short-term longitudinal evaluations. The Postmenopausal Estrogen/Progestin Interventions Study was a 3-year, placebo-controlled, randomized clinical trial to assess the effects of hormone regimens on cardiovascular disease risk factors in postmenopausal women 45 to 65 years of age. Active regimens were conjugated equine estrogen therapy at 0.625 mg daily, alone or in combination with each of 3 regimens of progestational agents: medroxyprogesterone acetate 2.5 mg/day, medroxyprogesterone acetate at 10 mg/day, and micronized progesterone at 200 mg/day. Plasma levels of Lp(a) were measured at baseline, 12 months, and 36 months of treatment. Assignment to hormone therapy resulted in a 17% to 23% average drop in Lp(a) concentrations relative to placebo, which was maintained across 3 years of follow-up (Figure 1-48). No significant differences

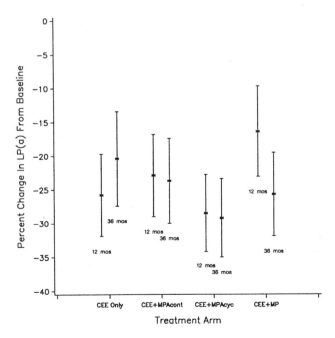

FIGURE 1-48. Mean changes in Lp(a) concentrations from baseline among adherers to active hormone regimens (relative to adherers to placebo) at 12 and 36 months after randomization. Reproduced with permission from Espeland et al.[128]

were observed among the 4 active arms. Changes in Lp(a) associated with hormone therapy were positively correlated with changes in LDL cholesterol, total cholesterol, apolipoprotein B, and fibrinogen levels and they were similar across subgroups defined by age, weight, ethnicity, and prior hormone use. Thus, postmenopausal estrogen therapy, with or without concomitant progestin, produces consistent and sustained reductions in Lp(a) concentrations.

Efficacy of Simvastatin in Familial Hypercholesterolemia

In familial hypercholesterolemia, the efficacy of the inhibitors of 3-hydroxy-3-methylglutaryl co-enzyme A reductase has shown considerable interindividual variation, and several genetic and environmental factors can contribute to explaining this variability. Couture and associates[129] conducted a randomized, double-blind, placebo-controlled clinical trial with simvastatin, a 3-hydroxy-3-methyglutaryl co-enzyme A reductase inhibitor, was conducted in 63 children and adolescents with heterozygous familial hypercholesterolemia. The patients were grouped according to known LDL receptor genotype. After 6 weeks of treatment with 20 mg/day of simvastatin, the mean reduction in plasma LDL cholesterol in patients with the W66G mutation (n = 14) was 31%, whereas in the deletion greater than 15 kb (n = 23) and the C646Y mutation group (n = 10), it was 38% and 42%, respectively. After treatment with simvastatin, HDL cholesterol levels were increased in all groups and triglyceride concentrations were significantly reduced. Multiple regression analyses suggested that 42% of the variation of the HDL cholesterol response to simvastatin can be attributed to variation in the mutant LDL receptor locus, apolipoprotein E genotype, and body mass index, while 35% of the variation to HDL cholesterol response was explained by gender and baseline HDL cholesterol. These results show that simvastatin was an effective and well-tolerated therapy for familial hypercholesterolemia in the pediatric population for all LDL receptor gene mutations. Moreover, the nature of LDL receptor gene mutations and other genetic and constitutional factors play a significant role in predicting the efficacy of simvastatin in the treatment of familial hypercholesterolemia in children and in adolescents.

Comparative Dose Efficacy Study of Reductase Inhibitors

Jones and associates[130] for the CURVES Investigators from multiple US medical centers reported results of a multicenter, randomized, open label parallel-group, 8-week study to evaluate the comparative dose efficacy of the 3-hydroxy-3-methylglutaryl co-enzyme A (HMG CoA) reductase inhibitor atorvastatin 10, 20, 40, and 80 mg compared with simvastatin 10, 20, and 40 mg, pravastatin 10, 20, and 40 mg, lovastatin 20, 40, and 80 mg, and fluvastatin 20 and 40 mg. Investigators enrolled 534 hypercholesterolemic patients (LDL cholesterol ≥160 mg/dL and triglycerides ≤400 mg/dL). The efficacy and points were mean percent change in plasma LDL cholesterol (primary), total cholesterol, triglycerides, and HDL cholesterol concentrations from baseline to the

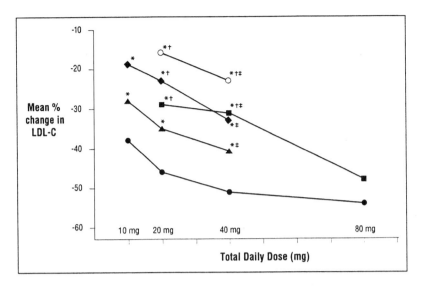

Figure 1-49. Percent reduction in low-density lipoprotein cholesterol (LDL-C) after 8 weeks of treatment with atorvastatin (●), simvastatin (▲), pravastatin (♦), lovastatin (■) and fluvastatin (○). *p ≤ 0.01 versus atorvastatin at mg equivalent doses; †p ≤ 0.02 versus atorvastatin 10 mg; ‡p ≤ versus atorvastatin 20 mg. Reproduced with permission from Jones et al.[130]

end of treatment (week 8). Atorvastatin 10, 20, and 40 mg produced greater reductions in LDL cholesterol, − 38%, − 46%, and − 51%, respectively, than the milligram equivalent doses of simvastatin, pravastatin, lovastatin, and fluvastatin. Atorvastatin 10 mg produced LDL cholesterol reductions comparable to or greater than simvastatin 10, 20, and 40 mg, pravastatin 10, 20, and 40 mg, lovastatin 20 and 40 mg, and fluvastatin 20 and 40 mg. Atorvastatin 10, 20, and 40 mg produced greater reductions in total cholesterol than the milligram equivalent doses of simvastatin, pravastatin, lovastatin, and fluvastatin. All reductase inhibitors studied had similar tolerability. There were no incidences of persistent elevations in serum transaminases or myositis (Figure 1-49; Tables 1-8, 1-9).

Efficacy and Safety of Simvastatin

Stein and associates[131] for the Expanded Dose Simvastatin US Study Group performed a randomized multicenter, double-blind, parallel-group study to evaluate the lipid-altering efficacy and safety of simvastatin 80 mg/day, a dose twice the current maximum recommended dose. At 20 centers in the US, 521 male and female hypercholesterolemic patients were randomly assigned in a ratio of 2:3 to receive simvastatin 40 or 80 mg once daily, respectively, for 24 weeks in conjunction with a lipid-lowering diet. Patients met National Cholesterol Education Program (NCEP) LDL cholesterol criteria for pharmacological treatment. The mean percentage reductions from baseline in LDL cholesterol averaged at weeks 18 and 24 were 38% (−4 to −36) and 46% (−47 to

Table 1-8
Mean Percent Change (±SD) in Lipoprotein Concentrations

Treatment	Dose (mg)	Number of Patients	Total Cholesterol	Triglycerides	HDL Cholesterol	LDL Cholesterol
Atorvastatin	10	73	−28 (9)	−13 (25)	5.5 (12)	−38 (10)
Pravastatin	10	14	−13 (12)†	3 (46)	9.9 (13)	−19 (14)†
Simvastatin	10	70	−21 (9)†	−12 (30)	6.8 (9)	−28 (12)†
Atorvastatin	20	51	−35 (6)	−20 (25)	5.1 (11)	−46 (8)
Pravastatin	20	41	−18 (7)†	−15 (17)	3.0 (8)	−24 (9)**,†
Simvastatin	20	49	−26 (8)†	−17 (22)	5.2 (10)	−35 (11)**
Fluvastatin	20	12	−13 (6)†	−5 (32)	0.9 (8)	−17 (8)**,†
Lovastatin	20	16	−21 (9)†	−12 (23)	7.3 (12)	−29 (13)**,†
Atorvastatin	40	61	−40 (8)	−32 (19)	4.8 (12)	−51 (10)
Pravastatin	40	25	−24 (7)†	−10 (22)†	6.2 (11)	−34 (9)**,‡
Simvastatin	40	61	−30 (10)†	−15 (29)†	9.6 (13)*	−41 (13)**,‡
Fluvastatin	40	12	−19 (9)†	−13 (34)*	−3.0 (10)	−23 (10)**,†‡
Lovastatin	40	16	−23 (6)†	−2 (27)†	4.6 (13)	−31 (7)**,†‡
Atorvastatin	80	10	−42 (7)	−25 (22)	−0.1 (9)	−54 (9)
Lovastatin	80	11	−36 (6)	−13 (28)	8.0 (13)	−48 (8)

* p ≤0.05; †p ≤0.01, Dunnett's test of significance compared with atorvastatin at milligram-equivalent doses.

† Atorvastatin 10 mg statistically significantly better (p≤0.02).

‡ Atorvastatin 20 mg statistically significantly better (p≤0.01).

Values are expressed as mean percent change from baseline.

Reproduced with permission from Jones et al.[130]

Table 1-9
Comparison of Percent Change in Low-Density Lipoprotein (LDL) Cholesterol:
Atorvastatin 10 and 20 mg Versus All Treatments

Treatment Group	Dose (mg)	Number of Patients	Mean* Percent Change from Baseline LDL Cholesterol	p Value vs Atorvastatin 10 mg	p Value vs Atorvastatin 20 mg
Atorvastatin	10	73	−38	Referent	—
Atorvastatin	20	51	−46	—	Referent
Fluvastatin	20	12	−17	0.0001	0.0001
Fluvastatin	40	12	−23	0.0001	0.0001
Lovastatin	20	16	−29	0.0019	0.0001
Lovastatin	40	16	−31	0.0197	0.0001
Lovastatin	80	11	−48	NS	NS
Pravastatin	10	14	−19	0.0001	0.0001
Pravastatin	20	41	−24	0.0001	0.0001
Pravastatin	40	25	−34	NS	0.0001
Simvastatin	10	70	−28	0.0001	0.0001
Simvastatin	20	49	−35	NS	0.0001
Simvastatin	40	61	−41	NS	0.0083

* Least-squares mean.

NS = atorvastatin not statistically significantly better.

Reproduced with permission from Jones et al.[130]

TABLE 1-10
Effect of Simvastatin 40 and 80 mg on Fasting Lipid and Lipoprotein Levels

Parameter	No.	Baseline Value (mg/dl)*	% Change†	95% CI‡	Between-Group p Value
Total cholesterol					
40 mg	206	291 (52)	−29	−30.1 to −27.3	<0.001
80 mg	311	289 (44)	−35	−36.2 to −34.0	
LDL cholesterol					
40 mg	205	209 (50)	−38	−40.1 to −36.2	<0.001
80 mg	310	205 (41)	−46	−47.3 to −44.6	
Apolipoprotein B					
40 mg	72	201 (42)	−31	−34.0 to −28.7	<0.001
80 mg	112	194 (31)	−38	−40.2 to −35.6	
HDL cholesterol					
40 mg	206	48 (11)	6.0	4.3 to 7.8	0.849
80 mg	311	48 (11)	6.1	4.8 to 7.5	
Apolipoprotein A-1					
40 mg	72	144 (27)	8.6	5.3 to 11.8	0.009
80 mg	112	151 (25)	3.5	1.2 to 5.7	
VLDL cholesterol					
40 mg	66	37 (22)	−31	−40.8 to −20.5	0.676
80 mg	103	36 (18)	−36	−42.7 to −28.7	
Triglycerides					
40 mg	206	162 (71)	−17	−21.4 to −12.6	0.002
80 mg	311	165 (76)	−25	−27.7 to −21.7	

Baseline values for triglycerides and VLDL cholesterol are median (SD); baseline values for all other parameters are mean (SD).

* To convert to SI units, divide by 38.7 for cholesterol and 88.6 for triglycerides.

† Percent change from baseline at week 24 (VLDL cholesterol and apolipoproteins A-I and B) or for the average at weeks 18 and 24 (all other parameters). The percent change represents the median for triglycerides and VLDL cholesterol and the mean for all other parameters.

‡ 95% confidence interval for the mean or median reported.

Reproduced with permission from Stein et al.[131]

−45) for the 40- and 80-mg groups, respectively. One third of patients on the 40- and 80-mg doses achieved an LDL cholesterol reduction of 46% and ≥53%, respectively. Decreases in apolipoprotein B, total cholesterol, and triglycerides were also significantly greater among patients receiving 80 mg/day. Simvastatin was well tolerated in both groups. Two patients (0.6%) in the 80-mg group developed myopathy. Consecutive, clinically significant hepatic transaminase elevations occurred in 3 (1.0%) and 6 (1.9%) patients in the 40- and 80-mg groups, respectively. In conclusion, simvastatin 80 mg/day provided substantial reduction in LDL cholesterol, allowing most patients to reach their NCEP target levels; it also had an excellent safety and tolerability profile (Table 1-10; Figure 1-50).

Lovastatin

Cuchel and coinvestigators[132] in Milan, Italy, investigated the effect of lovastatin, an inhibitor of 3-hydroxy-3-methylglutaryl co-enzyme, a reductase

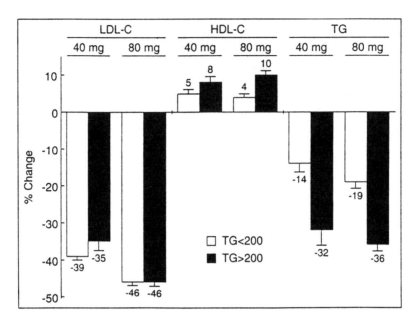

FIGURE 1-50. Percent change in lipids and lipoproteins with simvastatin 40 and 80 mg/day by baseline triglyceride level (triglyceride levels ≤200 mg/dL or > 200 mg/dL). Values represent average of 18- and 24-week data. For patients in the 40-mg group, n = 154 and 52 for triglyceride levels ≤200 mg/dL and >200 mg/dL, respectively. For patients in the 80-mg group, n = 205 and 105 for triglyceride levels ≤200 mg/dL and >200 mg/dL, respectively. HDL-C = high-density lipoprotein cholesterol; LDL-C = low-density lipoprotein cholesterol; TG = triglycerides. Reproduced with permission from Stein et al.[131]

activity on the kinetics of *de novo* cholesterol synthesis and apolipoprotein B in VLDL, IDL, and LDL in 5 male patients with combined hyperlipidemia. Subjects were counseled to follow a step 2 diet and were treated with lovastatin and placebo in a randomly assigned order for 6-week periods. At the end of each experimental period, subjects were given deuterium oxide orally and *de novo* cholesterol synthesis was assessed from deuterium incorporation into cholesterol and expressed as fractional synthesis rate and production rate. Simultaneously, the kinetics of VLDL, IDL, LDL, and apolipoprotein B-100 were studied in the fed state using a primed-constant infusion of deuterated leucine to measure fractional catabolic rates and production rates. Drug treatment resulted in significant decreases in total cholesterol (− 29%), VLDL (− 40%), LDL (− 27%) and apolipoprotein B (− 16%) levels and increases in HDL cholesterol (+ 13%) and apolipoprotein A-I (+ 11%) levels. Associated with these plasma lipoprotein increases was a significant reduction in both fractional synthesis rate and reduction rate. Treatment with lovastatin in these patients had no significant effect on the fractional catabolic rate of apolipoprotein B-100, VLDL, IDL, or LDL, but resulted in a significant decrease in the production rates of the apolipoprotein B-100 in IDL and LDL. Comparing the kinetic data of these patients with 10 normolipidemic control subjects indicated that lovastatin treatment normalized apolipoprotein B-100, IDL, and LDL density rates. The results of these studies suggest that the declines in plasma lipid levels observed after treatment of hyperlipidemic patients with lovastatin were attributable to reductions in the fractional synthesis rate and production rate of *de novo* cholesterol synthesis and the production rate of apolipoprotein B-100-containing lipoprotein. The decline in *de novo* cholesterol synthesis, rather than an increase in direct uptake of VLDL and IDL, may have contributed to the decline in the production rates observed.

Treatment Patterns to Lower Cholesterol Levels

To estimate the fraction of US adults who are eligible for treatment to reduce elevated LDL cholesterol levels based on Adult Treatment Panel II (ATP II) guidelines, and the percent reduction in LDL cholesterol required by those who qualify for treatment, Hoerger and associates[133] from New Orleans, Louisiana, analyzed data on 7,423 respondents to phase 2 of the third National Health and Nutrition Examination Survey (NHANES III) administered between 1991 and 1994. Approximately 28% of the US adult population aged 20 years or older is eligible for treatment based on ATP II guidelines. Eighty-two percent of adults with CAD are not at their target LDL cholesterol level of 100 mg/dL. Of those eligible for treatment, 65% report that they receive no treatment. Overall, 40% of people who qualify for drug therapy require an LDL cholesterol reduction of more than 30% to meet their ATP II treatment goal. Approximately 75% of those with CAD who qualify for drug therapy require an LDL cholesterol reduction of more than 30%. Although elevated LDL cholesterol levels can be treated, prevalence rates in the US adult population remain high. Several recent studies indicate that a considerable percentage of people treated with drug therapy do not reach their treatment goals; they require a larger reduction in LDL cholesterol than many therapies can provide (Tables 1-11, 1-12).

Simvastatin Therapy

Some patients with CAD experience continued progression of more coronary lesions despite treatment with drugs that inhibit 3-hydroxy-3-methylglutaryl co-enzyme A reductase activity and markedly lower plasma cholesterol levels. Sutherland and coworkers[134] in Dunedin, New Zealand, examined relationships between the progression of coronary artery lesions and plasma lipoproteins, in particular, IDL and its composition, in 38 patients with CAD who had been treated with simvastatin for 2 years. Patients were given lipid-lowering dietary advice; 3 months later they were started on simvastatin therapy (10 mg/day) for 1 month and, after review of the plasma cholesterol levels, the dose was increased to 20 mg/day and later to 40 mg/day if the target level of plasma cholesterol had not been attained. Progression of lesions was determined by serial quantitative coronary angiography and was defined as an increase in percent diameter stenosis greater than 10%; nonprogression was defined as a decrease in percent stenosis of greater than 10%. The proportions of cholesteryl esters and free cholesterol decreased significantly, and proportions of protein and triglycerides increased significantly in IDL during simvas-

TABLE 1-11
Percentage of U.S. Adults* Who Qualify for Treatment Under
Adult Treatment Panel II Guidelines

	Qualify for Treatment		
	Dietary Therapy Alone (%)	Drug Therapy† (%)	Total (%)
All	16.4	11.8	28.2
Race			
White	17.2	11.8	29.0
Black	12.4	12.1	24.5
Race/ethnicity			
Mexican-American	10.8	7.4	18.2
Non-Hispanic black	12.5	12.2	24.7
Non-Hispanic white	17.7	11.8	29.5
Men (age)	17.6	12.8	30.3
20–44	11.5	7.2	18.7
45–54	26.9	22.1	48.9
55–64	26.3	21.1	47.4
65–74	26.0	19.7	45.7
75+	25.1	18.5	43.6
Women (age)	15.3	10.8	26.1
20–44	9.3	2.8	12.2
45–54	17.9	10.2	28.1
55–64	26.4	24.3	50.7
65–74	26.5	27.3	53.8
75+	23.7	29.1	52.8

* ≥20 years.
† Subjects who qualify for drug therapy also qualify for dietary therapy.
Reproduced with permission from Hoerger et al.[133]

tatin therapy. The cholesteryl content of IDL decreased significantly in non-progressors and did not change significantly in progressors. This decrease in IDL cholesteryl ester content in nonprogressors was significantly different compared with the corresponding change in patients classified as progressors. Mean plasma cholesterol concentration tended to increase in progressors and tended to decrease in nonprogressors during the initial 3-month diet period, and these changes were significantly different (Figure 1-51). Furthermore, this change in plasma cholesterol level during the initial diet period was correlated significantly with the change in IDL cholesteryl ester content during the entire study. These data suggest that IDL cholesteryl ester content may be a determinant of progression of coronary lesions and may be influenced by compliance with a metabolic response to lipid-lowering dietary advice in patients with CAD during simvastatin treatment.

Effect of Simvastatin

Pedersen and associates[135] from Oslo, Norway, Kuopio, Finland, Linköping, Sweden, Odense, Denmark, and Rahway, New Jersey, reported the effect

TABLE 1-12
U.S. Population by Coronary Heart Disease Risk Group: Number and Percentage Not Meeting Goals

	Coronary Heart Disease Risk Group		
	Without Coronary Heart Disease		**With Coronary Heart Disease (treatment goal ≤100 mg/dL)**
	<2 Risk Factors (treatment goal <160 mg/dL)	**≥2 Risk Factors (treatment goal <130 mg/dL)**	
Estimated number in risk group (millions)	121.1	48.7	10.2
Not meeting treatment goals			
Estimated number (millions)	15.7	26.6	8.4
Percentage of risk group	12.9%	54.6%	82.5%
Qualify for dietary therapy alone			
Estimated number (millions)	11.0	15.6	2.9
Percentage of risk group	9.1%	32.1%	28.3%
Qualify for drug therapy*			
Estimated number (millions)	4.7	11.0	5.5
Percentage of risk group	3.8%	22.6%	54.2%
Not meeting desirable level of 130 mg/dL			
Estimated number (millions)	44.6	26.6	NA
Percentage of risk group	36.8%	54.6%	NA

* People who qualify for drug therapy also qualify for dietary therapy.
NA = not applicable.
Reproduced with permission from Hoerger et al.[133]

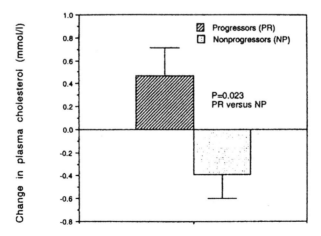

FIGURE 1-51. Bar graph shows mean ± SEM change in plasma cholesterol concentration between baseline and the end of the initial 3-month lipid-lowering diet period in patients treated with simvastatin who were classified as progressors (n = 14) or nonprogressors (n = 20). Progressors showed progression (increase percent lesion stenosis ≥10%) of 1 or more lesions without regression (decrease in percent lesion stenosis ≥10%) of any lesion. Nonprogressors did not show progression of any lesion. The changes in plasma cholesterol during the diet period were marginally significant in the progressors (p = .06) and nonprogressors (p = .08). Reproduced with permission from Sutherland et al.[134]

TABLE 1-13
Patients with New or Worsening Angina Pectoris, Intermittent Claudication, or Bruits

	Placebo (n = 2,223)	Simvastatin (n = 2,221)	RR (95% CI)	p Value
Angina pectoris	725 (32.6)	568 (25.5)	0.74 (0.67–0.83)	<0.0001
Intermittent claudication	81 (3.6)	52 (2.3)	0.62 (0.44–0.88)	0.008
≥1 bruit	92 (4.1)	66 (3.0)	0.70 (0.51–0.96)	0.025
Carotid bruit	45 (2.0)	24 (1.1)	0.52 (0.32–0.85)	0.009
Femoral bruit	43 (1.9)	39 (1.8)	0.89 (0.58–1.37)	0.59

Relative risk was obtained using the Cox regression method, and p values by the log rank test.
Values are expressed as number of patients (%).
CI = confidence intervals; RR = relative risk.
Reproduced with permission from Pedersen et al.[135]

of lipid intervention with simvastatin (20–40 mg/day) on noncoronary ischemic symptoms and signs during a median follow-up of 5.4 years. In addition, the authors provided new information on the effect of simvastatin on angina pectoris. There were 4,444 men and women aged 45 to 70 years with prior AMI or angina pectoris. All adverse experiences likely to be caused by atherosclerotic disease for which there was a significant difference between the treatments are listed in Table 1-13. The risk of new or worsening intermittent claudication, bruits, and angina pectoris was reduced by simvastatin. Over 90% of the bruits were carotid or femoral. There was no statistically significant effect on femoral bruits, but the risk of a new or worsening carotid bruit was substantially reduced. Transient ischemic attacks accounted for 19 patients with events in the simvastatin group and 29 in the placebo group. The risk of new or worsening intermittent claudication was reduced by 38% in the simvastatin group. The risk of developing new or worsening angina was reduced by 26% as would be expected given the 37% reduction in the risk of undergoing a coronary revascularization procedure. The effect of simvastatin on carotid bruits is consistent with reductions in cerebrovascular events with simvastatin in the Scandinavian Simvastatin Survival Study and with the provastatin in the cholesterol and recurrent events study. Thus, this analysis provides evidence that effective cholesterol lowering with simvastatin 20–40 mg/day will retard progression of atherosclerosis in the arterial vasculature, not limited to the coronary circulation, resulting in fewer ischemic signs and symptoms (Figure 1-52).

Miscellaneous

Kuopio Ischemic Heart Disease Study Results

Kamarck and colleagues[136] from Pittsburgh, Pennsylvania, examined the hypothesis that exaggerated cardiovascular reactivity to mental stress is associated with increased atherosclerotic risk. They used the cross-sectional data from the Kuopio Ischemic Heart Disease (KIHD) Study, a population-based

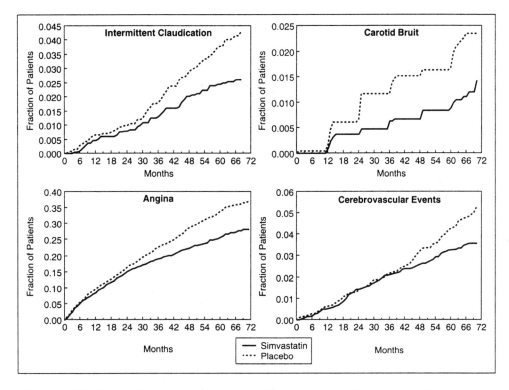

Figure 1-52. Kaplan-Meier curves for patients with new or worsening angina pectoris or intermittent claudication, carotid bruits, or cerebrovascular events. Reproduced with permission from Pedersen et al.[135]

epidemiological study in Eastern Finnish men to test the hypothesis. In this evaluation, 901 Eastern Finnish men from 4 age cohorts, including ages 42 to 60 years, were administered a standard testing battery to assess cardiovascular reactivity to mental stress. Ultrasound measures of intimal medial thickness and plaque height from the common carotid arteries were used as noninvasive markers of atherosclerosis. Diastolic BP responses to mental stress were significantly associated with intimal medial thickness, maximal intimal medial thickness, and mean plaque height (Figure 1-53). Significant associations were also found between stress-related systolic BP reactivity and mean intimal medial thickness. When examined separately by age, associations with intimal medial thickness were significant only in the youngest half of the sample, those patients aged 46 to 52 years. For mean intimal medial thickness, diastolic BP and maximum intimal medial thickness diastolic BP were also significant variables. The results remain significant in the younger subjects after adjustment for smoking, lipid profiles, fasting glucose, and resting BP. Thus, these data indicate that exaggerated pressor responses to mental stress are significant independent risk factors for atherosclerosis in Eastern Finnish men in the age groups studied.

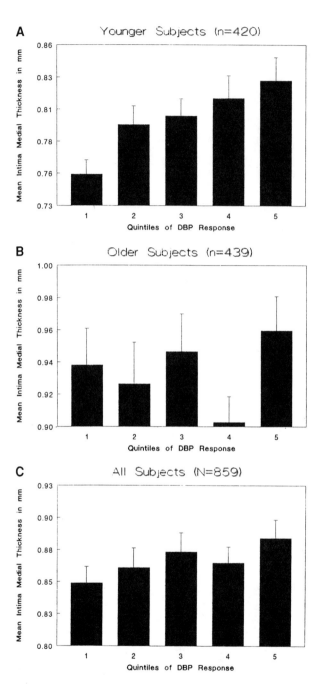

FIGURE 1-53. Covariate-adjusted common carotid mean IMT (in mm) by quintiles diastolic BP reactivity in the KIHD study. A = younger subjects (n = 420); B = older subjects (n = 439); C = all subjects (n = 859). Reproduced with permission from Kamarck et al.[136]

1. Kockx MM, De Meyer GRY, Muhring J, Jacob W, Bult H, Herman AG: Apoptosis and related proteins in different stages of human atherosclerotic plaques. Circulation 1998 (June 16);97:2307–2315.
2. Geng Y-J, Henderson LE, Levesque EB, Muszynski M, Libby P: FAS is expressed in human atherosclerotic intima and promotes apoptosis of cytokine-primed human vascular smooth muscle cells. Arterioscler Thromb Vasc Biol 1997 (October);17: 2200–2208.
3. Romano M, Romano E, Bjorkerud S, Hurt-Camejo E: Ultrastructural localization of secretory type II phospholipase A_2 in atherosclerotic and non-atherosclerotic regions of human arteries. Arterioscler Thromb Vasc Biol 1998 (April);18:519–525.
4. Wesley RB II, Meng X, Godin D, Galis ZS: Extracellular matrix modulates macrophage functions characteristic to atheroma: Collagen type I enhances acquisition of resident macrophage traits by human peripheral blood monocytes *in vitro.* Arterioscler Thromb Vasc Biol 1998 (March);18:432–440.
5. Verhaar MC, Wever RMF, Kastelein JJP, van Dam T, Koomans HA, Rabelink TJ: 5-methyltetrahydrofolate, the active form of folic acid, restores endothelial function in familial hypercholesterolemia. Circulation 1998 (January 27);97: 237–241.
6. Laufs U, La Fata V, Plutzky J, Liao JK: Upregulation of endothelial nitric oxide synthase by HMG CoA reductase inhibitors. Circulation 1998 (March 31);97: 1129–1135.
7. Mietus-Snyder M, Glass CK, Pitas RE: Transcriptional activation of scavenger receptor expression in human smooth muscle cells requires AP-1/c-Jun and C/EBPβ: Both AP-1 binding and JNK activation are induced by phorbol esters and oxidative stress. Arterioscler Thromb Vasc Biol 1998 (September);18:1440–1449.
8. Shern-Brewer R, Santanam N, Wetzstein C, White-Welkley J, Parthasarathy S: Exercise and cardiovascular disease: A new perspective. Arterioscler Thromb Vasc Biol 1998 (July);18:1181–1187.
9. Luoma JS, Stralin P, Marklund SL, Hiltunen TP, Sarkioja T, Yla-Herttuala S: Expression of extracellular SOD and iNOS in macrophages and smooth muscle cells in human and rabbit atherosclerotic lesions: Colocalization with epitopes characteristic of oxidized LDL and peroxynitrite-modified proteins. Arterioscler Thromb Vasc Biol 1998 (February);18:157–167.
10. van de Vijver LPL, Kardinaal FM, van Duyvenvoorde W, Kruijssen DACM, Grobbee DE, van Poppel G, Princen HMG: LDL oxidation and extent of coronary atherosclerosis. Arterioscler Thromb Vasc Biol 1998 (February);18:193–199.
11. Deckert V, Brunet A, Lantoine F, Lizard G, Millanvoye-van Brussel E, Monier S, Lagrost L, David-Dufilho M, Gambert P, Devynck M-A: Inhibition by cholesterol oxides of NO release from human vascular endothelial cells. Arterioscler Thromb Vasc Biol 1998 (July);18:1054–1060.
12. Wu R, Huang YH, Elinder LS, Frostegard J: Lysophosphatidylcholine is involved in the antigenicity of oxidized LDL. Arterioscler Thromb Vasc Biol 1998 (April); 18:626–630.
13. Ramos MA, Kuzuya M, Esaki T, Miura S, Satake S, Asai T, Kanda S, Hayashi T, Iguchi A: Induction of macrophage VEGF in response to oxidized LDL and VEGF accumulation in human atherosclerotic lesions. Arterioscler Thromb Vasc Biol 1998 (July);18:1188–1196.
14. Nakagawa T, Nozaki S, Nishida M, Yakub JM, Tomiyama Y, Nakata A, Matsumoto K, Funahashi T, Kameda-Takemura K, Kurata Y, Ymashita S, Matsuzawa Y: Oxidized LDL increases and interferon-gamma decreases expression of CD36 in human monocyte-derived macrophages. Arterioscler Thromb Vasc Biol 1998 (August);18:1350–1357.
15. Folcik VA, Aamir R, Cathcart MK: Cytokine modulation of LDL oxidation by an activated human monocyte. Arterioscler Thromb Vasc Biol 1997 (October);17: 1954–1961.
16. Stengel D, Antonucci M, Gaoua W, Dachet C, Lesnik P, Hourton D, Ninio E, Chapman MJ, Griglio S: Inhibition of LPL expression in human monocyte-derived macrophages is dependent on LDL oxidation state: A key role of lysophosphatidylcholine. Arterioscler Thromb Vasc Biol 1998 (July);18:1172–1180.

17. Sugiyama S, Kugiyama K, Ogata N, Doi H, Ota Y, Ohgushi M, Matsumura T, Oka H, Yasue H: Biphasic regulation of transcription factor nuclear factor-kB activity in human endothelial cells by lysophosphatidylcholine through protein kinase C-mediated pathway. Arterioscler Thromb Vasc Biol 1998 (April);18:568–576.
18. Wu R, Nityanand S, Berglund L, Lithell H, Holm G, Lefvert AK: Antibodies against cardiolipin and oxidatively modified LDL in 50-year-old men predict myocardial infarction. Arterioscler Thromb Vasc Biol 1997 (November);17:3159–3163.
19. Devaraj S, Adams-Huet B, Fuller CJ, Jialal I: Dose-response comparison of RRR-alpha-tocopherol and all-racemic alpha-tocopherol of LDL oxidation. Arterioscler Thromb Vasc Biol 1997 (October);17:2273–2279.
20. Vita JA, Keaney FJ, Jr., Raby KE, Morrow JD, Freedman JE, Lynch S, Koulouris SN, Kankin BR, Frei B: Low plasma ascorbic acid independently predicts the presence of an unstable coronary syndrome. JACC 1998 (April);31:980–986.
21. Brude IR, Drevon CA, Hjermann I, Seljeflot I, Lund-Katz S, Saarem K, Sandstad B, Sovoll K, Halvorsen B, Arnesen H, Nenseter MS: Peroxidation of LDL from combined hyperlipidemic male smokers supplied with Omega-3 fatty acids and antioxidants. Arterioscler Thromb Vasc Biol 1997 (November);17:2576–2588.
22. Kapiotis S, Hermann M, Held I, Seelos C, Ehringer H, Gmeiner BMK: Genistein, the dietary-derived angiogenesis inhibitor, prevents LDL oxidation and protects endothelial cells from damage by atherogenic LDL. Arterioscler Thromb Vasc Biol 1997 (November);17:2868–2874.
23. Mosca L, Rubenfire M, Tarshis T, Tsai A, Pearson T: Clinical predictors of oxidized low-density lipoprotein in patients with coronary artery disease. Am J Cardiol 1997 (October 1);80:825–830.
24. Siow RCM, Sato H, Leake DS, Pearson JD, Bannai S, Mann GE: Vitamin C protects human arterial smooth muscle cells against atherogenic lipoproteins: Effects of antioxidant vitamins C and E on oxidized LDL-induced adaptive increases in cystine transport and glutathione. Arterioscler Thromb Vasc Biol 1998 (October);18: 1662–1670.
25. Klouche M, Gottschling S, Gerl V, Hell W, Husmann M, Dorweiler B, Messner M, Bhakdi S: Atherogenic properties of enzymatically degraded LDL: Selective induction of MCP-1 and cytotoxic effects on human macrophages. Arterioscler Thromb Vasc Biol 1998 (September);18:1376–1385.
26. Costantini F, Pierdomenico SD, De Cesare D, De Remigis P, Bucciarelli T, Bittolo-Bon G, Cazzolato G, Nubile G, Guagnano MT, Sensi S, Cuccurullo F, Mezzetti A: Effect of thyroid function on LDL oxidation. Arterioscler Thromb Vasc Biol 1998 (May);18:732–737.
27. Nilsson J, Dahlgren B, Ares M, Westman J, Nilsson AH, Cercek B, Shah PK: Lipo-protein-like phospholipid particles inhibit the smooth muscle cell cytotoxicity of lysophosphatidylcholine and platelet-activating factor. Arterioscler Thromb Vasc Biol 1998 (January);18:13–19.
28. Chiu JJ, Wung BS, Shyy JYJ, Hsieh HJ, Wang DL: Reactive oxygen species are involved in shear stress-induced intercellular adhesion molecule-1 expression in endothelial cells. Arterioscler Thromb Vasc Biol 1997 (December);17:3570–3577.
29. Theilmeier G, Chan JR, Zalpour C, Anderson B, Wang B, Wolf A, Tsao PS, Cooke JP: Adhesiveness of mononuclear cells in hypercholesterolemic humans is normalized by dietary L-arginine. Arterioscler Thromb Vasc Biol 1997 (December);17: 3557–3564.
30. Kaufmann PA, Frielingsdorf J, Mandinov L, Seiler C, Hug R, Hess OM: Reversal of abnormal coronary vasomotion by calcium antagonists in patients with hypercholesterolemia. Circulation 1998 (April 14);97:1348–1354.
31. Hwang S-J, Ballantyne CM, Sharrett AR, Smith LC, Davis CE, Gotto AM, Jr., Boerwinkle E: Circulating adhesion molecules VCAM-1, ICAM-1, and E-selectin in carotid atherosclerosis and incident coronary heart disease cases: The Atherosclerotic Risk in Communities (ARIC) Study. Circulation 1997 (December 16);96: 4219–4225.
32. Kugiyama K, Ohgushi M, Motoyama T, Hirashima O, Soejima H, Misumi K, Yoshimura M, Ogawa H, Sugiyama S, Yasue H: Intracoronary infusion of reduced gluta-

thione improves endothelial vasomotor response to acetylcholine in human coronary circulation. Circulation 1998 (June 16);97:2299–2301.

33. Husain S, Andrews NP, Mulcahy D, Panza JA, Quyyumi AA: Aspirin improves endothelial dysfunction in atherosclerosis. Circulation 1998 (March 3);97: 716–720.

34. Verhaar MC, Strachan FE, Newby DE, Cruden NL, Koomans HA, Rabelink TJ, Webb DJ: Endothelin-A receptor antagonist-mediated vasodilatation is attenuated by inhibition of nitric oxide synthesis and by endothelin-B receptor blockade. Circulation 1998 (March 3);97:752–756.

35. Clarkson P, Celermajer DS, Powe AJ, Donald AE, Henry RMA, Deanfield JE: Endothelium-dependent dilatation is impaired in young healthy subjects with a family history of premature coronary disease. Circulation 1997 (November 18);96: 3378–3383.

36. Williams SB, Goldfine AB, Timimi FK, Ting HH, Roddy M-A, Simonson DC, Creager MA: Acute hyperglycemia attenuates endothelium-dependent vasodilation in humans *in vivo*. Circulation 1998 (May 5);97:1695–1701.

37. Huggins GS, Pasternak RC, Alpert NM, Fischman AJ, Gewirtz H: Effects of short-term treatment of hyperlipidemia on coronary vasodilator function and myocardial perfusion in regions having substantial impairment of baseline dilator reserve. Circulation 1998 (September 29);98:1291–1296.

38. Hornig B, Arakawa N, Kohler C, Drexler H: Vitamin C improves endothelial function of conduit arteries in patients with chronic heart failure. Circulation 1998 (February 3);97:363–368.

39. John S, Schlaich M, Langenfeld M, Weihprecht H, Schmitz G, Weidinger G, Schmieder RE: Increased bioavailability of nitric oxide after lipid-lowering therapy in hypercholesterolemic patients: A randomized, placebo-controlled, double-blind study. Circulation 1998 (July 21);98:211–216.

40. Wilbert-Lampen U, Seliger C, Zilker T, Arendt RM: Cocaine increases the endothelial release of immunoreactive endothelin and its concentrations in human plasma and urine: Reversal by coincubation with δ-receptor antagonists. Circulation 1998 (August 4);98:385–390.

41. Gerhard M, Walsh BW, Tawakol A, Haley EA, Creager SJ, Seely EW, Ganz P, Creager MA: Estradiol therapy combined with progesterone and endothelium-dependent vasodilation in postmenopausal women. Circulation 1998 (September 22);98:1158–1163.

42. Timimi FJ, Ting MH, Haley EA, Roddy M-A, Ganz P, Creager MA: Vitamin C improves endothelium-dependent vasodilation in patients with insulin-dependent diabetes mellitus. JACC (March 1);31:552–557, 1998.

43. Parry GCN, Martin T, Felts KA, Cobb RR: IL-1 beta-induced monocyte chemoattractant protein-1 gene expression in endothelial cells is blocked by proteasome inhibitors. Arterioscler Thromb Vasc Biol 1998 (June);18:934–940.

44. Proudfoot D, Skepper JN, Shanahan CM, Weissberg PL: Calcification of human vascular cells *in vitro* is correlated with high levels of matrix Gla protein and low levels of osteopontin expression. Arterioscler Thromb Vasc Biol 1998 (March);18: 379–388.

45. Moriwaki H, Kume N, Sawamura T, Aoyama T, Hoshikawa H, Ochi H, Nishi E, Masaki T, Kita T: Ligand specificity of LOX-1, a novel endothelial receptor for oxidized low density lipoprotein. Arterioscler Thromb Vasc Biol 1998 (October); 18:1541–1547.

46. Totani L, Cumashi A, Piccoli A, Lorenzet R: Polymorphonuclear leukocytes induce PDGF release from IL-1β-treated endothelial cells: Role of adhesion molecules in serine proteases. Arterioscler Thromb Vasc Biol 1998 (October);18:1534–1540.

47. Ashby DT, Rye K-A, Clay MA, Vadas MA, Gamble JR, Barter PJ: Factors influencing the ability of HDL to inhibit expression of vascular cell adhesion molecule-1 in endothelial cells. Arterioscler Thromb Vasc Biol 1998 (September);18:1450–1455.

48. Bishop-Bailey D, Pepper JR, Larkin SW, Mitchell JA: Differential induction of cyclooxygenase-2 in human arterial and venous smooth muscle: Role of endogenous prostanoids. Arterioscler Thromb Vasc Biol 1998 (October);18:1655–1661.

49. Andrews TC, Whitney EJ, Green G, Kalenian R, Personius BE: Effect of gemfibrozil ± niacin ± cholestyramine on endothelial function in patients with serum low-density lipoprotein cholesterol levels <160 mg/dl and high-density lipoprotein cholesterol levels <40 mg/dl. Am J Cardiol 1997 (October 1);80:831–835.

50. Hermann C, Zeiher AM, Dimmeler S: Shear stress inhibits H_2O-induced apoptosis of human endothelial cells by the modulation of the glutathione redox cycle in nitric oxide synthase. Arterioscler Thromb Vasc Biol 1997 (December);17: 3588–3592.

51. Watanabe H, Kakihana M, Ohtsuka S, Sugishita Y: Randomized, double-blind, placebo-controlled study of the preventive effect of supplemental oral vitamin C on attenuation of development of nitrate tolerance. JACC 1998 (May);31:1323–1329.

52. Mascelli MA, Worley S, Veriabo NJ, Lance ET, Mack S, Schaible T, Weisman HF, Jordan RE: Rapid assessment of platelet function with a modified whole-blood aggregometer in percutaneous transluminal coronary angioplasty patients receiving anti-GP IIb/IIIa therapy. Circulation 1997 (December 2);96:3860–3866.

53. Abe Y, El-Masri B, Kimball KT, Pownall H, Reilly CF, Osmundsen K, Smith CW, Balltyne CM: Soluble cell adhesion molecules in hypertriglyceridemia and potential significance on monocyte adhesion. Arterioscler Thromb Vasc Biol 1998 (May);18:723–731.

54. Nofer J-R, Walter M, Kehrel B, Wierwille S, Tepel M, Seedorf U, Assmann G: HDL_3-mediated inhibition of thrombin-induced platelet aggregation and fibrinogen binding occurs via decreased production of phosphoinositide-derived second messengers 1,2-diacylglycerol and inositol 1,4,5-tris-phosphate. Arterioscler Thromb Vasc Biol 1998 (June);18:861–869.

55. Kawano K, Aoki I, Aoki N, Homori M, Maki A, Hioki Y, Hasu Terano A, Arai T, Mizuno H, Ishikawa K: Human platelet activation by thrombolytic agents: Effects of tissue-type plasminogen activator and urokinase on platelet surface P-selectin expression. Am Heart J 1998 (February);135:268–671.

56. Rand ML, Sangrar W, Hancock MA, Taylor DM, Marcovina SM, Packham M, Koschinsky ML: Apolipoprotein (a) enhances platelet responses to the thrombin receptor-activating peptide SFLLRN. Arterioscler Thromb Vasc Biol 1998 (September);18:1393–1399.

57. Nakano Y, Oshima T, Matsuura H, Kajiwama G, Kambe M: Effect of 17 beta-estradiol on inhibition of platelet aggregation in vitro is mediated by an increase in NO synthesis. Arterioscler Thromb Vasc Biol 1998 (June);18:961–967.

58. Caplice NM, Mueske CS, Kleppe LS, Simari RD: Presence of tissue factor pathway inhibitor in human atherosclerotic plaques is associated with reduced tissue factor activity. Circulation 1998 (September 15);98:1051–1057.

59. Ariyoshi H, Okahara K, Sakon M, Kambayashi J, Kawashima S, Kawasaki T, Monden M: Possible involvement of M-calpain in vascular smooth muscle cell proliferation. Arterioscler Thromb Vasc Biol 1998(March);18:493–498.

60. deMaat MPM, Kastelein JJP, Jukema JW, Zwinderman AH, Jansen H, Groenemeir B, Bruschke AVG, Kluft C on behalf of the REGRESS Group: −455 G/A polymorphism of the beta-fibrinogen gene is associated with the progression of coronary atherosclerosis in symptomatic men: Proposed role for an acute phase reaction pattern of fibrinogen. Arterioscler Thromb Vasc Biol 1998 (February);18:265–271.

61. Koenig W, Sund M, Filipiak B, Doring A, Lowel H, Ernest E: Plasma viscosity and the risks of coronary heart disease: Results from the MONICAR-Augsburg Cohort Study, 1984–1992. Arterioscler Thromb Vasc Biol 1998 (May);18:768–772.

62. Mukherjee R, Strasser J, Jow L, Hoener P, Paterniti JR, Jr., Heyman RA: RXR agonists activate PPAR alpha-inducible genes, lower triglycerides, and raise HDL levels in vivo. Arterioscler Thromb Vasc Biol 1998 (February);18:272–276.

63. Torzewski J, Torzewski M, Bowyer DE, Fröhlich M, Koenig W, Waltenberger J, Fitzsimmons C, Hombach V: C-reactive protein frequently colocalizes with the terminal complement complex in the intima of early atherosclerotic lesions of human coronary arteries. Arterioscler Thromb Vasc Biol 1998 (September);18: 1386–1392.

64. Pankow JS, Folsom AR, Province MA, Rao DC, Williams RR, Eckfeldt J, Sellers

TA: Segregation analysis of plasminogen activator inhibitor-1 and fibrinogen levels in the NHLBI family heart study. Arterioscler Thromb Vasc Biol 1998 (October); 18:1559–1567.

65. Hayes IM, Jordan MJ, Towers S, Smith G, Paterson JR, Earnshaw JJ, Roach AG, Westwick J, Williams RJ: Human vascular smooth muscle cells express receptors for CC chemokines. Arterioscler Thromb Vasc Biol 1998 (March);18:397–403.

66. Masuoka H, Ishikura K, Kamel S, Obe T, Seko T, Okuda K, Koyabu S, Tsuneoka K, Tamai T, Sugawa M, Nakano T: Predictive value of remnant-like particles cholesterol/cholesterol ratio as a new indicator of CAD. Am Heart J 1998 (August); 136:226–230.

67. Geppert A, Graf S, Beckmann R, Hornykewycz S, Schuster E, Binder BR, Huber K: Concentration of endogenous tPA antigen in coronary artery disease: Relation to thrombotic events, aspirin treatment, hyperlipidemia and multivessel disease. Arterioscler Thromb Vasc Biol 1998 (October);18:1634–1642.

68. McConnell MV, Vavouranakis I, Wu LL, Vaughan DE, Ridker PM: Effects of a single, daily alcoholic beverage on lipid and hemostatic markers of cardiovascular risk. Am J Cardiol 1997 (November 1);80:1226–1228.

69. Eriksson P, Nilsson L, Karpe F, Hamsten A: Very low-density lipoprotein response element in the promoter region in the human plasminogen activator inhibitor-1 gene implicated in the impaired fibrinolysis of hypertriglyceridemia. Arterioscler Thromb Vasc Biol 1998 (January);18:20–26.

70. Iino M, Foster DC, Kisiel W: Quantification and characterization of human endothelial cell-derived tissue factor pathway inhibitor-2. Arterioscler Thromb Vasc Biol 1998 (January);18:40–46.

71. Lassel TS, Guerin M, Auboiron S, Chapman MJ, Guy-Grand B: Preferential cholesteryl ester acceptors among triglyceride-rich lipoproteins during alimentary lipemia in normolipidemic subjects. Arterioscler Thromb Vasc Biol 1998 (January);18:65–74.

72. Kwiterovich PO, Jr., Motevalli M: Differential effect of Genistein on the stimulation of cholesterol production by basic protein II in normal and hyperapo B fibroblasts. Arterioscler Thromb Vasc Biol 1998 (January);18:57–64.

73. Ayaori M, Ishikawa T, Yoshida H, Suzukawa M, Nishiwaki M, Shige H, Ito T, Nakajima K, Higashi K, Yonemura A, Nakamura H: Beneficial effects of alcohol withdrawal on LDL particle size distribution and oxidative susceptibility in subjects with alcohol-induced hypertriglyceridemia. Arterioscler Thromb Vasc Biol 1997 (November);17:2540–2547.

74. Paassilta M, Kervinen K, Linnaluoto M, Kesaniemi YA: Alcohol withdrawal-induced change in lipoprotein(a): Association with the growth hormone/insulin like growth factor-I (IGF-I)/IGF-binding protein-1 (IGFBP-1) axis. Arterioscler Thromb Vasc Biol 1998 (April);18:650–654.

75. Kaikita K, Ogawa H, Yasue H, Takeya M, Takahashi K, Saito T, Hayasaki K, Horiuchi K, Takizawa A, Kamikubo Y, Nakamura S: Tissue factor expression on macrophages in coronary plaques in patients with unstable angina. Arterioscler Thromb Vasc Biol 1997 (October);17:2232–2237.

76. Summers RM, Andrasko-Bourgeois J, Feuerstein IM, Hill SC, Jones EC, Busse MK, Wise B, Bove KE, Rishforth BA, Tucker E, Spray TL, Hoeg JM: Evaluation of the aortic root by MRI: Insights from patients with homozygous familial hypercholesterolemia. Circulation 1998 (August 11);98:509–518.

77. Miller M, Aiello D, Pritchard H, Friel G, Zeller K: Apolipoprotein A-I:$_{Zavalla}$ (Leu$_{15}$ → Pro) HDL cholesterol deficiency in a kindred associated with premature coronary artery disease. Arterioscler Thromb Vasc Biol 1998 (August);18:1242–1247.

78. Humphries SE, Nicaud V, Margalef J, Tiret L, Talmud PJ for the EARS: Lipoprotein lipase gene variation is associated with a paternal history of premature coronary artery disease and fasting and postprandial plasma triglycerides: The European Atherosclerosis Research Study (EARS). Arterioscler Thromb Vasc Biol 1998 (April);18:526–534.

79. Agren JJ, Valve R, Vidgren H, Laakso M, Uusitupa M: Postprandial lipemic response is modified by the polymorphism at codon 54 of the fatty acid-binding protein 2 gene. Arterioscler Thromb Vasc Biol 1998 (October);18:1606–1610.

80. Ombres D, Pannittrei G, Montali A, Candeloro A, Seccareccia F, Campagna F, Cantini R, Campa PP, Ricci G, Arca M: The Gln-Arg 192 polymorphism of human paroxonase gene is not associated with coronary artery disease in Italian patients. Arterioscler Thromb Vasc Biol 1998 (October);18:1611–1616.

81. Okada M, Matsumori A, Ono K, Furukawa Y, Shioi T, Iwasaki A, Matsushima K, Sasayama S: Cyclic stretch upregulates production of interleukin-8 and monocyte chemotactic and activating factor/monocyte chemoattractant protein-1 in human endothelial cells. Arterioscler Thromb Vasc Biol 1998 (June);18:894–901.

82. Gordon BR, Kelsey SF, Dau PC, Gotto AM, Jr., Graham K, Illingworth R, Isaacsohn J, Jones PH, Leitman SF, Saal SD, Stein EA, Stern TN, Troendle A, Zwiener RJ, for the Liposorber Study Group: Long-term effects of low-density lipoprotein apheresis using an automated dextran sulfate cellulose adsorption system. Am J Cardiol 1998 (February 15);81:407–411.

83. Pimstone SN, Sun X-M, duSouich C, Frohlich JJ, Hayden MR, Soutar AK: Phenotypic variation in heterozygous familial hypercholesterolemia: A comparison of Chinese patients with the same or similar mutations in the LDL receptor gene in China or Canada. Arterioscler Thromb Vasc Biol 1998 (February);18:309–315.

84. Rainwater DL, Mitchell BD, Mahaney C, Haffner SM: Genetic relationships between measures of HDL phenotypes and insulin concentrations. Arterioscler Thromb Vasc Biol 1997 (December);17:3414–3419.

85. Carmena-Ramon R, Ascaso JF, Real JT, Ordovas JM, Carmena R: Genetic variation at the apo A-IV gene locus and response to diet in familial hypercholesterolemia. Arterioscler Thromb Vasc Biol 1998 (August);18:1266–1274.

86. Hulthe J, Wikstrand J, Lidell A, Wendelhag I, Hansson GK, Wiklund O: Antibody titers against oxidized LDL are not elevated in patients with familial hypercholesterolemia. Arterioscler Thromb Vasc Biol 1998 (August);18:1203–1211.

87. Yokoyama I, Ohtake T, Momomura S, Yonekura K, Kobayakawa N, Aoyagi T, Sugiura S, Sasaki Y, Omata M: Altered myocardial vasodilatation in patients with hypertriglyceridemia in anatomically normal coronary arteries. Arterioscler Thromb Vasc Biol 1998 (February);18:294–299.

88. Guyton JR, Goldberg AC, Kreisberg RA, Sprecher DL, Superko HR, O'Connor CM: Effectiveness of once-nightly dosing of extended-release niacin alone and in combination for hypercholesterolemia. Am J Cardiol 1998 (September 15);82: 737–743.

89. Karjalainen L, Pihlajamaki J, Karhapaa P, Laakso M: Impaired insulin-stimulated glucose oxidation and free fatty acid suppression in patients with familial combined hyperlipidemia: A precursor defect for dyslipidemia? Arterioscler Thromb Vasc Biol 1998 (October);18:1548–1553.

90. Ridker PM, Glynn RJ, Hennekens CH: C-reactive protein adds to the predictive value of total and HDL cholesterol in determining risk of first myocardial infarction. Circulation 1998 (May 26);97:2007–2011.

91. Wang T-D, Wu C-C, Chen W-J, Lee C-M, Chen M-F, Liau C-S, Sung F-C, Lee Y-T: Dyslipidemias have a detrimental effect on left ventricular systolic function in patients with a first acute myocardial infarction. Am J Cardiol 1998 (March 1); 81:531–537.

92. Fager G, Wiklund O: Cholesterol reduction and clinical benefit: Are there limits to our expectations? Arterioscler Thromb Vasc Biol 1997 (December);17:3527–3533.

93. West of Scotland Coronary Prevention Study Group: Influence of pravastatin and plasma lipids on clinical events in the West of Scotland Coronary Prevention Study (WOSCOPS). Circulation 1998 (April 21);97:1440–1445.

94. Pedersen TR, Olsson AG, Fægeman O, Kjekshus J, Wedel H, Berg K, Wilhelmsen L, Haghfelt T, Thorgeirsson G, Pyörälä K, Miettinen T, Christophersen B, Tobert JA, Musliner TA, Cook TJ, for the Scandinavian Simvastatin Survival Study Group: Lipoprotein changes and reduction in the incidence of major coronary heart disease events in the Scandinavian Simvastatin Survival Study (4S). Circulation 1998 (April 21);97:1453–1460.

95. MacMahon S, Sharpe N, Gamble G, Hart H, Scott J, Simes J, White H, on behalf of the LIPID Trial Research Group: Effects of lowering average or below-average

cholesterol levels on the progression of carotid atherosclerosis: Results of the LIPID Atherosclerosis Substudy. Circulation 1998 (May 12);97:1784–1790.

96. Miettinen TA, Pyörälä K, Olsson AG, Musliner TA, Cook TJ, Faergeman O, Berg K, Pedersen T, Kjekshus J, for the Scandinavian Simvastatin Study Group: Cholesterol-lowering therapy in women and elderly patients with myocardial infarction or angina pectoris: Findings from the Scandinavian Simvastatin Survival Study (4S). Circulation 1997 (December 16);96:4211–4218.

97. Pyörälä M, Miettinen H, Laakso M, Pyörälä K: Hyperinsulinemia predicts coronary heart disease risk in healthy middle-aged men: The 22-year follow-up results of the Helsinki policemen study. Circulation 1998 (August 4);98:398–404.

98. Ericsson C-G, Nilsson J, Grip L, Svane B, Hamsten A: Effect of bizafibrate treatment over five years on coronary plaques causing 20% to 50% diameter narrowing (The Bezafibrate Coronary Atherosclerosis Intervention Trial [BECAIT]). Am J Cardiol 1997 (November 1);80:1125–1129.

99. Burchfiel CM, Sharp DS, Curb JD, Rodriguez BL, Abbott RD, Arakaki R, Yano K: Hyperinsulinemia and cardiovascular disease in elderly men: The Honolulu Heart Program. Arterioscler Thromb Vasc Biol 1998 (March);18:450–457.

100. Shinozaki K, Hattori Y, Suzuki M, Hara Y, Kanazawa A, Takaki H, Tsushima M, Harano Y: Insulin resistance as an independent risk factor for carotid artery wall intima media thickening in vasospastic angina. Arterioscler Thromb Vasc Biol 1997 (November);17:3302–3310.

101. Rainwater DL, Haffner SM: Insulin and 2-hour glucose levels are inversely related to lipoprotein(a) concentrations controlled for LPA genotype. Arterioscler Thromb Vasc Biol 1998 (August);18:1335–1341.

102. Byberg L, Siegbahn A, Berglund L, McKeigue P, Reneland R, Lithell H: Plasminogen activator inhibitor-1 activity is independantly related to both insulin sensitivity and serum triglycerides in 70-year-old men. Arterioscler Thromb Vasc Biol 1998 (February);18:258–264.

103. Leyva F, Godsland IF, Ghatei M, Proudler HA, Aldis S, Walton C, Bloom S, Stevenson JC: Hyperleptinemia as a component of a metabolic syndrome of cardiovascular risk. Arterioscler Thromb Vasc Biol 1998 (June);18:928–933.

104. Kornowski R, Mintz GS, Lansky AJ, Hong MK, Kent KM, Pichard AD, Satler LF, Popma JJ, Bucher TA, Leon MB: Paradoxic decreases in atherosclerotic plaque mass in insulin-treated diabetic patients. Am J Cardiol 1998 (June 1);81:1298–1304.

105. Carantoni M, Abbasi F, Warmerdam F, Klebanov M, Wang P-W, Chen Y-D I, Azhar S, Reaven GM: Relationship between insulin resistant and partially oxidized LDL particles in healthy nondiabetic volunteers. Arterioscler Thromb Vasc Biol 1998 (May);18:762–767.

106. Nilsson J, Jovinge S, Niemann A, Reneland R, Lithell H: Relation between plasma tumor necrosis factor-alpha and insulin sensitivity in elderly men with non-insulin dependent diabetes mellitus. Arterioscler Thromb Vasc Biol 1998 (August);18:1199–1202.

107. Nitenberg A, Paycha F, Ledoux S, Sachs R, Attali J-R, Valensi P: Coronary artery responses to physiological stimuli are improved by deferoxamine but not by L-arginine in non-insulin-dependent diabetic patients with angiographically normal coronary arteries and no other risk factors. Circulation 1998 (March 3);97:736–743.

108. Tkac I, Kimball BP, Lewis G, Uffelman K, Steiner G: The severity of coronary atherosclerosis in type 2 diabetes mellitus is related to the number of circulating triglyceride-rich lipoprotein particles. Arterioscler Thromb Vasc Biol 1997 (December);17:3633–3638.

109. Gray RS, Robbins DC, Wang W, Yeh JL, Fabsitz RR, Cowan LD, Welty TK, Lee ET, Krauss RM, Howard BV: Regulation of LDL size to the insulin resistent syndrome in coronary heart disease in American Indians: The Strong Heart Study. Arterioscler Thromb Vasc Biol 1997 (November);17:2713–2720.

110. Valkonen M, Kuusi T: Passive smoking induces atherogenic changes in low-density lipoprotein. Circulation 1998 (May 26);97:2012–2016.

111. Westerveld HT, Roeters van Lennep JE, Roeters van Lennep HWO, Liem A-H, de Boo JAJ, van der Schouw YT, Erkelens DW: Apolipoprotein B and coronary artery disease in women: A cross-sectional study in women undergoing their first coronary angiography. Arterioscler Thromb Vasc Biol 1998 (July);18:1101–1107.
112. McGill HC, Jr., McMahan CA, Tracy RE, Oalmann MC, Cornhill JF, Herderick EE, Strong JP: for the Pathobiological Determinants of Atherosclerosis in Youth (PDAY) Research Group: Relation of a postmortem renal index of hypertension to atherosclerosis and coronary artery size in young men and women. Arterioscler Thromb Vasc Biol 1998 (July);18:1108–1118.
113. Tanaka H, DeSouza CA, Seals DR: Absence of age-related increase in central arterial stiffness in physically active women. Arterioscler Thromb Vasc Biol 1998 (January);18:127–132.
114. Abbott RD, Yano K, Hakim AA, Burchfiel CM, Sharp DS, Rodriguez BL, Curb JD: Changes in total and high-density lipoprotein cholesterol over 10- and 20-year periods (the Honolulu Heart Program). Am J Cardiol 1998 (July 15);82:172–178.
115. Jin F-Y, Kamanna VS, Kashyap ML: Estradiol stimulates apolipoprotein A-I- but not A-II-containing particle synthesis and secretion by stimulating mRNA transcription rate in Hep G2 cells. Arterioscler Thromb Vasc Biol 1998 (June);18:999–1006.
116. Nestel PJ, Yamashita T, Sasahara T, Pomeroy S, Dart A, Komesaroff P, Owen A, Abbey M: Soy isoflavones improve systemic arterial compliance but not plasma lipids in menopausal and perimenopausal women. Arterioscler Thromb Vasc Biol 1997 (December);17:3392–3398.
117. Laurila A, Bloigu A, Nayha S, Hassi J, Leinonen M, Saikku P: Chronic Chlamydia pneumoniae infection is associated with a serum lipid profile known to be a risk factor for atherosclerosis. Arterioscler Thromb Vasc Biol 1997 (November);17:2910–2913.
118. Moustapha A, Naso A, Nahlawi M, Gupta A, Arheart KL, Jacobsen DW, Robinson K, Dennis VW: Prospective study of hyperhomocysteinemia as an adverse cardiovascular risk factor in end-stage renal disease. Circulation 1998 (January 20);97:138–141.
119. Hoogeveen EK, Kostense PJ, Beks PJ, Mackaay AJC, Jakobs C, Bouter LM, Heine RJ, Stehouwer CDA: Hyperhomocysteinemia is associated with an increased risk of cardiovascular disease, especially in non-insulin-dependent diabetes mellitus: A population-based study. Arterioscler Thromb Vasc Biol 1998 (January);18:133–138.
120. den Heijer M, Brouwer IA, Bos GMJ, Blom HJ, vander Put NMJ, Spaans AP, Rosendaal FR, Thomas CMG, Haak HL, Wijermans PW, Gerrits WBJ: Vitamin supplementation reduces blood homocysteine levels: A controlled trial in patients with venous thrombosis and healthy patients. Arterioscler Thromb Vasc Biol 1998 (March);18:356–361.
121. Cattaneo M, Franchi F, Zighetti ML, Martinelli I, Asti D, Mannucci M: Plasma levels of activated protein C in healthy subjects and patients with previous venous thromboembolism: Relationships with plasma homocysteine levels. Arterioscler Thromb Vasc Biol 1998 (September);18:1371–1375.
122. Archer SL, Green D, Chamberlain M, Dyer AR, Liu K: Association of dietary fish and n-3 fatty acid intake with hemostatic factors in the coronary artery risk development in young adults (CARDIA) study. Arterioscler Thromb Vasc Biol 1998 (July);18:1119–1123.
123. Sanders TAB, Oakley FR, Miller GJ, Mitropoulos KA, Crook D, Oliver MF: Influence of n-6 versus n-3 polyunsaturated fatty acids in diets low in saturated fatty acids on plasma lipoproteins and hemostatic factors. Arterioscler Thromb Vasc Biol 1997 (December);17:3449–3460.
124. Ginsberg HN, Kris-Etherton P, Dennis B, Elmer PJ, Ershow A, LeFevre M, Pearson T, Roheim P, Ramakrishnan R, Reed R, Stewart K, Stewart P, Phillips K, Anderson N, for the DELTA Research Group: Effects of reducing dietary saturated fatty acids on plasma lipids and lipoproteins in healthy subjects: The DELTA Study, Protocol I. Arterioscler Thromb Vasc Biol 1998 (March);18:441–449.

125. Princen HMG, van Duyvenvoorde W, Buytenhek R, Blonk C, Tijburg LBM, Langius JAE, Meinders AE, Pijl H: No effect of consumption of green and black tea on plasma lipid and antioxidant levels and on LDL oxidation in smokers. Arterioscler Thromb Vasc Biol 1998 (May);18:833–841.

126. Georgopoulos A, Bantle JP, Noutsou M, Swaim WR, Parker SJ: Differences in the metabolism of post prandial lipoproteins after a high monosaturated-fat versus a high-carbohydrate diet in patients with type I diabetes mellitus. Arterioscler Thromb and Vasc Biol 1998 (May);18:773–782.

127. Freedman DS, Otvos JD, Jeyarajah EJ, Barboriak JJ, Anderson AJ, Walker JA: Reduction of lipoprotein subclasses as measured by proton nuclear magnetic resonance spectroscopy to coronary artery disease. Arterioscler Thromb Vasc Biol 1998 (July);18:1046–1053.

128. Espeland MA, Marcovina SM, Miller V, Wood PD, Wasilauskas C, Sherwin R, Schrott H, Bush TL, for the PEPI Investigators: Effect of postmenopausal hormone therapy on lipoprotein(a) concentration. Circulation 1998 (March 17);97:979–986.

129. Couture P, Brun LD, Szots F, Lelievre M, Gaudet D, Despres J-P, Simard J, Lupien PJ, Gagne C: Association of specific LDL receptor gene mutations with differential plasma lipoprotein response to simvastatin in young French Canadians with heterozygous familial hypercholesterolemia. Arterioscler Thromb Vasc Biol 1998 (June);18:1007–1012.

130. Jones P, Kafonek S, Laurora I, Hunninghake D, for the CURVES Investigators: Comparative dose efficacy study of atorvastatin versus simvastatin, pravastatin, lovastatin, and fluvastatin in patients with hypercholesterolemia (The CURVES Study). Am J Cardiol 1998 (March 1);81:582–587.

131. Stein EA, Davidson MH, Dobs AS, Schrott H, Dujovne CA, Bays H, Weiss SR, Melino MR, Stepanavage ME, Mitchel YB, for the Expanded Dose Simvastatin US Study Group: Efficacy and safety of simvastatin 80 mg/day in hypercholesterolemic patients. Am J Cardiol 1998 (August 1);82:311–316.

132. Cuchel M, Schafer EJ, Millar JS, Jones PJH, Dolnikowski GG, Vergani C, Lichtenstein AH: Lovastatin decreases *de novo* cholesterol synthesis and LDL apo B-100 production rates in combined-hyperlipidemic males. Arterioscler Thromb Vasc Biol 1997 (October);17:1910–1917.

133. Hoerger TJ, Bala MV, Bray JW, Wilcosky TC, LaRosa J: Treatment patterns and distribution of low-density lipoprotein cholesterol levels in treatment-eligible United States adults. Am J Cardiol 1998 (July 1);82:61–65.

134. Sutherland WHF, Restieaux NJ, Nye ER, Williams MJA, de Jong SA, Robertson MC, Walker HL: IDL composition and angiographically determined progression of atherosclerotic lesions during Simvastatin therapy. Arterioscler Thromb Vasc Biol 1998 (April);18:577–583.

135. Pedersen TR, Kjekshus J, Pyörälä K, Olsson AG, Cook TJ, Musliner TA, Tobert JA, Haghfelt T: Effect of simvastatin on ischemic signs and symptoms in the Scandinavian Simvastatin Survival Study (4S). Am J Cardiol 1998 (February 1);81: 333–335.

136. Kamarck TW, Everson SA, Kaplan GA, Manuck SB, Jennings JR, Salonen R, Salonen JT: Exaggerated blood pressure responses during mental stress are associated with enhanced carotid atherosclerosis in middle-aged Finnish men: Findings from the Kuopio Ischemic Heart Disease study. Circulation 1997 (December 2);96: 3842–3848.

2

Coronary Artery Disease

Coronary Artery Disease

Induction of Neoangiogenesis in Ischemic Myocardium by Human Growth Factors

Schumacher and colleagues[1] in Freiburg, Germany, have presented some of the first clinical trials using the human growth factor FGF-I (basic fibroblast growth factor) to induce neoangiogenesis in the ischemic myocardium in humans. FGF-I (0.01 mg/kg body weight) was injected close to the vessels after the completion of an internal mammary artery/LAD coronary artery anastomosis in 20 patients with 3-vessel disease. All of the patients had additional peripheral stenoses of the LAD or 1 of its diagonal branches. Twelve weeks later, the internal mammary artery bypasses were selectively imaged by intra-arterial digital subtraction angiography and were quantitatively evaluated. The development of new vessels in the ischemic myocardium could be demonstrated angiographically (Figure 2-1). Formation of capillaries could also be demonstrated in humans and was found in all cases around the site of injection. These data suggest that FGF-I may be used for myocardial revascularization in patients undergoing coronary bypass surgery.

The Effect Walking Has on Mortality

Hakim and colleagues[2] studied 707 nonsmoking retired men, 61 to 81 years of age, who were enrolled in the Honolulu Heart Program. They hypothesized that walking would reduce mortality in this cohort of retired men who were nonsmokers and physically capable of participating in low-intensity exercise on a daily basis. The distance walked was recorded at baseline examination. Data on overall mortality were collected over a 12-year period of follow-up. During the follow-up period, there were 208 deaths. After adjustment for age, the mortality rate among the men who walked less than 1 mile per day was nearly twice that among those who walked more than 2 miles per day. The cumulative incidence of death after 12 years for the most active walkers was reached in less than 7 years among the men who were least active. The distance walked remained inversely related to mortality after adjustment for overall measures of activity and other risk factors. Thus, these data indicate that regu-

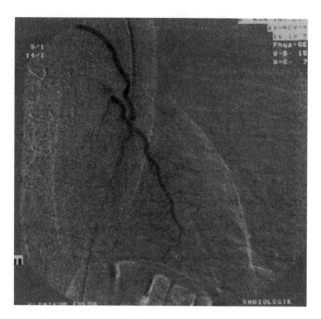

FIGURE 2-1. Angiography after injection of the growth factor into the human heart. Angiography in the control group does not show any increased accumulation of contrast medium around the inferior mesenteric artery/LAD anastomosis. HBGF-I indicates human FGF-I. Reproduced with permission from Schumacher et al.[1]

lar walking is associated with a lower overall mortality rate. Encouraging elderly people to walk may prolong their lives.

Influence of Estrogen on Cellular Adhesion Molecules

Atherosclerotic plaque demonstrates features similar to inflammation. Endothelial cell activation by inflammatory cytokines induces expression of cellular adhesion molecules, thereby perhaps augmenting leukocyte adhesion and recruitment, and subsequent development of atherosclerosis. Caulin-Glaser and colleagues[3] from New Haven and West Haven, Connecticut, evaluated whether the cardioprotective effects of estrogen might be due to an influence on cellular adhesion molecules. They evaluated consecutive eligible subjects with CAD admitted for cardiac catheterization. The groups included men, postmenopausal women receiving estrogen, postmenopausal women not receiving estrogen, and premenopausal women. Control groups included men and women without CAD. They observed a statistically significant increase in circulating adhesion molecules in men with CAD and in postmenopausal women with CAD not receiving estrogen, compared with postmenopausal women with CAD receiving estrogen. Premenopausal women with CAD and postmenopausal women with CAD receiving estrogen had a significant increase in circulating adhesion molecules alone compared to the female control group. This group concludes that a possible mechanism by which estrogen exerts one of its cardioprotective effects is by limiting the inflammatory response to injury by modulating the expression of circulating adhesion molecules from the endothelium.

Endothelial Dysfunction in Patients with Myocarditis

Recent reports indicate that myocarditis can be associated with acute myocardial ischemia and even myocardial infarction in patients with normal arteriograms. Klein and associates[4] from Dusseldorf, Germany, therefore tested the hypothesis that patients with biopsy-proven myocarditis have endothelial dysfunction despite angiographically smooth epicardial coronary arteries. Graded concentrations of the endothelium-dependent vasodilator acetylcholine (10^{-6} to 10^{-4} mol/L) and for comparison, the non-endothelium-dependent vasodilator nitroglycerin (0.3 mg intracoronary), were infused into the left coronary arteries of 18 patients (mean age 47 $\pm$ 9 years; 8 women and 10 men) with biopsy-proven myocarditis but without angiographically demonstrable CAD. Vascular responses were analyzed by quantitative coronary angiography. Three patients had an intact vasodilator response to acetylcholine concentrations of up to 10^{-4} mol/L in all segments of the left coronary artery, with a mean dilatation of $+9.9\% \pm 2\%$. In contrast, paradoxical constriction by acetylcholine occurred in 9 patients, who showed a mean change in coronary artery diameter of $-11\% \pm 3\%$. Six patients had no significant change in any segments in response to acetylcholine ($-2.5\% \pm 4\%$). There was a significant inverse correlation between the number of T lymphocytes in the myocardium and the response of the epicardial coronary arteries to acetylcholine. It can be assumed that the process of myocarditis is associated with impairment of endothelium-dependent vasodilation in response to acetylcholine in most patients. Vasoconstriction in the presence of acetylcholine in myocarditis is likely to reflect an abnormality of endothelial function. Endothelial dysfunction of coronary arteries may explain the occurrence of myocardial ischemia in patients with myocarditis.

Edinburgh Artery Study

Plasma fibrinogen is a consistent predictor of CAD in prospective studies, but there are fewer data relating other hemostatic variables to CAD and also to stroke. Smith and coworkers[5] in Glasgow, Scotland, therefore, studied the relationships of plasma fibrinogen, von Willebrand factor antigen, tissue plasminogen activator antigen, factor VII, and fibrin d-dimer to incidence of CAD and stroke and determined whether any associations could be explained by conventional risk factors and baseline heart disease. In the Edinburgh Artery Study, 1,592 men and women age 55–74 years, randomly sampled from the general population were followed prospectively over 5 years to detect fatal and nonfatal CAD and stroke events. During the 5 years, 268 new vascular events were identified. Baseline plasma fibrinogen was independently related to risk of stroke in multivariate analysis that adjusted for cigarette smoking, LDL cholesterol, systolic blood pressure, and pre-existing CAD. Tissue plasminogen activator antigen and fibrin d-dimer were also independently associated with risk of stroke. Significant relationships were found between tissue plasminogen activator antigen and acute myocardial infarction. In older men and women, increased coagulation activity and disturbed fibrinolysis appeared to be predictors of future vascular events (both CAD and stroke).

Coronary Endothelial Dysfunction

Coronary artery endothelial dysfunction has been proposed as a cause of myocardial ischemia and symptoms in patients with angina-like chest pain despite normal coronary angiograms, especially in those with ischemic-appearing ST-segment depression during exercise (syndrome X). Cannon and associates[6] from Bethesda, Maryland, measured coronary vasomotor responses to acetylcholine (3–300 μg/min) in 42 patients (27 women and 15 men) with effort angina and normal coronary angiograms who also had normal electrocardiograms and echocardiograms at rest. All patients underwent treadmill exercise testing and measurement of systolic wall thickening responses to dobutamine (40 μg/kg/min) during transesophageal echocardiography. There were no differences in the acetylcholine-stimulated epicardial coronary diameter (+5% ± 13% vs. +1% ± 13%) and flow (+179% ± 90% vs. +169% ± 96%), or in the systolic wall thickening responses (+134% ± 65% vs. +118% ± 57%) from baseline values in the 12 syndrome X patients compared with the 30 patients with negative exercise test results. In patients in the lowest quartile of coronary flow responses to acetylcholine, dobutamine increased systolic wall thickening by 121% ± 73%; 3 had ischemic-appearing ST-segment depression during this stress. This contractile response to dobutamine was no different than the increase in systolic wall thickening (129% ± 48%) in patients in the highest quartile of coronary flow responses, 3 of whom also had ischemic-appearing ST-segment depression during this stress. Thus, coronary endothelial dysfunction in the absence of CAD does not account for ischemic-appearing ST-segment depression in patients with chest pain despite normal coronary angiograms. Further, coronary endothelial dysfunction is not associated with myocardial contractile responses to stress consistent with myocardial ischemia (Figure 2-2).

Strategies to Predict Myocardial Ischemia

Myocardial ischemia identified by ambulatory electrocardiography, exercising treadmill testing (ETT), or 12-lead electrocardiogram at rest is associated with an adverse prognosis, but the effect of improving these myocardial ischemic manifestations by treatment on outcome is unknown. The Asymptomatic Cardiac Ischemic Pilot (ACIP) Study was a National Heart, Blood, and Lung Institute funded study to determine the feasibility of conducting a large-scale prognosis study and to assess the effect of 3 treatment strategies (angina-guided strategy, ambulatory electrocardiography ischemia-guided strategy, and revascularization strategy) in reducing the manifestations of myocardial

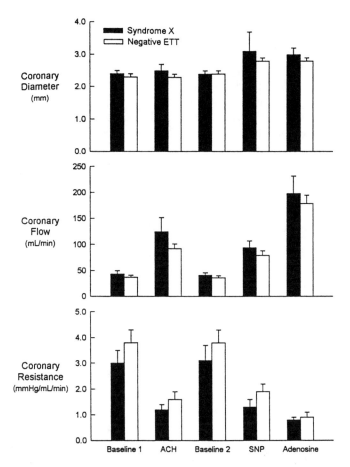

FIGURE 2-2. Epicardial coronary diameter, coronary flow, and calculated coronary resistance values are provided for the 5 measurement periods during the study, with values in 12 syndrome X patients compared with 30 patients with negative treadmill exercise tests. The acetylcholine (ACH) dose producing the maximum coronary flow response to this agonist was 100 μg/min for 2 minutes. Sodium nitroprusside (SNP) was infused at 40 μg/min for 3 minutes to 41 patients and adenosine was infused at 2.2 mg/min for 2 minutes to 40 patients. Data are expressed as mean ± SEM (p value >0.180 for all comparisons between values for syndrome X patients and patients with negative exercise tests). ETT = exercise treadmill test. Reproduced with permission from Cannon et al.[6]

ischemia as indicated by ambulatory electrocardiography and ETT. The study was reported by Stone and associates[7] from multiple US medical centers. The study cohort for this database consisted of 496 randomized patients who performed the ambulatory electrocardiography, ETT, and 12-lead electrocardiogram at rest of both the qualifying and week 12 visits. The effect of modifying ischemia by treatment on the incidence of cardiac events (death, MI, coronary revascularization procedure, or hospitalization for an ischemic event) at 1 year was examined. In the 2 medical treatment groups (n = 328), there was an association between the number of ambulatory electrocardiographic ischemic episodes of the qualifying visit and combined cardiac events at 1 year. In the ambulatory electrocardiography ischemia-guided patients, there was a trend associating greater reduction in the number of ambulatory electrocardiographic ischemia episodes with a reduced incidence of combined cardiac events. In the revascularization strategy patients, this association was absent. In the medical treatment patients, the exercise duration on the baseline ETT was inversely associated with an adverse prognosis. The medical treatment strategies only slightly improved the exercise time and the exercise duration remained of prognostic significance. In the revascularization group strategy patients, this association was absent. Thus, myocardial ischemia detected by ambulatory electrocardiography and an abnormal ETT are each independently associated with an adverse cardiac outcome in patients subsequently treated medically.

Myocardial Ischemia in Master Athletes

Physical activity levels are associated with reduced risk of symptomatic CAD. There are a number of reports of exercise-related sudden death and AMI in aerobically trained athletes. Katzel and associates[8] from Baltimore, Maryland, compared the prevalence of exercised-induced myocardial ischemia on maximum graded exercise tests with tomographic thallium scintigraphy in 70 master male athletes (63 ± 6 years, mean $\pm$ SD) (maximum aerobic capacity, VO_2 max > 40 mL/kg/min) and in 85 healthy untrained men (61 ± 7 years) with no history of CAD. The prevalence of silent ischemia (exercise-induced ST-segment depression on electrocardiogram and perfusion abnormalities on thallium scintigraphy) was similar in athletes and untrained men; 16% of the athletes (11 of 70) had silent ischemia compared with 21% of the untrained men (chi square = 81). No athletes had hyperlipidemia, systemic hypertension, or diabetes mellitus. However, the apolipoprotein E4 allele was present in 9 of the 11 athletes with silent ischemia compared with 2 of 32 athletes with normal exercise tests (chi square = 24). These results suggest that older male athletes with the apolipoprotein E4 allele are at increased risk for the development of exercise-induced silent ischemia.

Silent Myocardial Ischemia

β-Endorphin has been reported to play a role in the mechanism of silent myocardial ischemia. Plasma β-endorphin levels during coronary angioplasty-induced silent and symptomatic myocardial ischemia were compared with those during exercise-induced silent ischemia in this study by Hikita and associates[9] from Saitama, Japan. The study population consisted to 40 nondiabetic patients with angioplasty-indicated CAD. All patients underwent exercise treadmill testing 2 to 4 days before angioplasty. Patients were divided into 3 groups: group 1, 10 patients with silent ischemia during exercise and angioplasty; group 2, 15 patients with silent ischemia during exercise and symptomatic ischemia during angioplasty; and group 3, 15 patients with symptomatic ischemia during both exercise and angioplasty. In group 1, plasma β-endorphin levels during balloon inflation were significantly higher than in groups 2 and 3 and also significantly higher than during exercise. In group 2, plasma β-endorphin levels were significantly elevated at exercise-induced silent myocardial ischemia and balloon-induced symptomatic myocardial ischemia, but the levels between exercise and balloon inflation were not significantly different. For silent myocardial ischemia, it may be necessary for β-endorphin levels to increase to sufficiently high levels to suppress anginal symptoms in response to the degree of ischemic stimuli.

Depressed Heart Rate Variability

Little is known about the value of heart rate variability in patients with symptomatic CAD preserved LV function. Van Boven and associates[10] from Groningen, Utrecht, and Leiden, The Netherlands, hypothesized that in these patients, heart rate variability might be a helpful adjunct to conventional parameters to predict clinical events. In a prospective 2-year follow-up study, ambulatory electrocardiographic recordings were performed in 263 consecutive male patients (mean age 56 ± 8 years) with stable angina pectoris and a mean LVEF of 71% ± 12%. Clinical events consisted mainly of coronary events such as PTCA or CABG. Low measures of standard deviation of normal R-R intervals, standard deviation of the mean R-R intervals of 5 minutes, and 2 spectral components of heart rate variability were found in patients who had had an event compared with patients with no event. Adjusted for severity of angina, the presence of a previous myocardial infarction, and the use of β-blockers in a logistic regression model, this relation remained statistically significant. Healthy volunteers appeared to have the highest measures of heart rate variability. In patients with ischemic heart disease and normal or near normal ventricular function, decreased heart rate variability is associated with adverse clinical events.

Risk Stratification and Detection of Coronary Artery Disease

Role of Dobutamine Stress Echocardiography in Predicting Cardiac Events

Chuah and colleagues[11] in Rochester, Minnesota, obtained follow-up information from 860 patients who underwent dobutamine stress echocardiography over a 2-year period. They wished to determine the value of this test in predicting future cardiac events, including cardiac death and AMI. Clinical and rest and stress echocardiographic data were considered in a stepwise Cox multivariate regression model. During follow-up of up to 52 months, 72 patients underwent coronary revascularization before any cardiac event and were censored. Eighty-six patients had cardiac events, including nonfatal MI in 36 and cardiac death in 50. In a multivariate model, a history of CHF, the percentage of abnormal segments at peak stress, and an abnormal LV end-systolic volume response

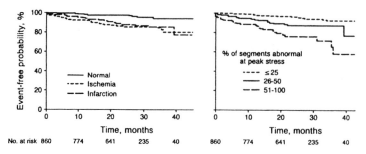

FIGURE 2-3. **Left:** Effects of ischemia and fixed wall motion abnormalities (infarction) by dobu-tamine stress echocardiography on cumulative cardiac event-free probability. Cardiac event-free probabilities were significantly worse in patients with ischemia than in normal subjects ($\chi^2 = 20$; p < .0001) and worse in patients with fixed wall motion abnormalities than in normal subjects ($\chi^2 = 15$; p = .0001). **Right:** Effect of percentage of segments that were abnormal at peak stress on cumulative cardiac event-free probability. Reproduced with permission from Chuah et al.[11]

to stress were independent predictors of cardiac events. The model that best predicted subsequent cardiac events included clinical and stress echocardio-graphic data (Figure 2-3).

Role of a Common Deoxyribonucleic Acid Variant to Predict Progression of Coronary Artery Disease

Kuivenhoven and colleagues[12] emphasized the role of the cholesteryl ester transfer protein and the metabolism of HDL and speculated that the cholesteryl ester transfer protein may alter susceptibility to atherosclerosis. The DNA of 807 men with angiographically documented CAD was analyzed for the presence of a polymorphism in the gene encoding for cholesteryl ester transfer protein. The presence in this DNA variation was referred to as *B1,* and its absence as *B2.* All patients participated in a cholesterol-lowering trial designed to induce the regression of CAD and were randomly assigned to treatment with either pravastatin or placebo for 2 years. The *B1* variant of the cholesteryl ester trans-fer protein gene was associated with both higher plasma cholesteryl ester trans-fer protein concentrations and lower HDL cholesterol concentrations. The in-vestigators observed a significant dose-dependent association between this marker and the progression of CAD in the placebo group. This association was abolished by pravastatin. Pravastatin therapy slowed the progression of CAD in *B1B1* carriers, but not in *B2B2* carriers. Thus, there is a significant relationship between variation at the cholesteryl ester transfer protein gene locus and the progression of CAD that is independent of plasma HDL cholesterol levels and the activities of lipolytic plasma enzymes. This common DNA variant appears to predict whether men with CAD will benefit from treatment with pravastatin to delay the progression of CAD (Figure 2-4).

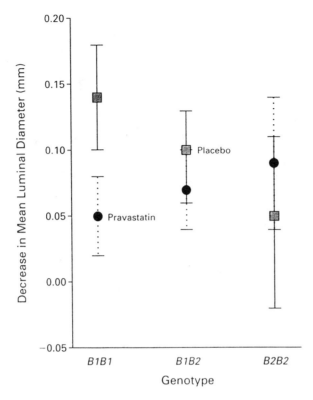

FIGURE 2-4. Changes in mean luminal diameter (and 95% confidence intervals) according to the *CETP* TaqIB genotype in patients with established coronary atherosclerosis treated with either placebo or pravastatin. Higher values reflect increased diffuse progression of coronary atherosclerosis. Reproduced with permission from Kuivenhoven et al.[12]

Use of Electron-Beam Computed Tomography in Detection of Stenoses and Occlusions

Achenbach and colleagues[13] in Erlangen, Germany, investigated the accuracy of contrast-enhanced electron-beam computed tomography for the detection of high-grade coronary artery stenoses and occlusions in 125 patients. Following intravenous injection of a contrast agent, 40 cross-sectional images of the heart were acquired during inspiration, triggered by the electrocardiogram in diastole. Three-dimensional reconstructions of the heart and coronary arteries were obtained to facilitate evaluation of the images; the proximal and middle segments of the major coronary arteries were evaluated for the presence or absence of high-grade stenoses and occlusions. The results were compared with those of invasive coronary angiography in a blinded fashion. In 124 (25%) of the 500 coronary arteries studied, technical problems that impaired the quality of the images required their exclusion from further evaluation. No vessels could be evaluated in 19 patients (15%), and another 28 patients (22%) had 1, 2, or 3 vessels that could not be evaluated. In the remaining coronary arteries with adequate image quality, electron-beam CT permitted

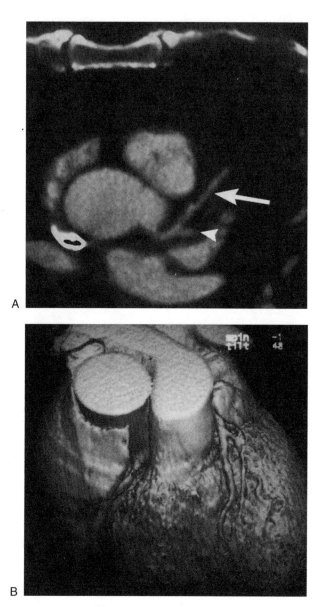

FIGURE 2-5. Electron-beam CT images of the heart. Panel **A** shows a cross-section of the heart at the level of the aortic root. The origin of the left main coronary artery from the aortic root as well as the proximal left anterior descending coronary artery (arrow) and left circumflex coronary artery (arrowhead) can be seen. Panels **B** and **C** show a 3-dimensional reconstruction (shaded-surface display) of the heart and coronary arteries. The reconstruction is designed to show only contrast-enhanced structures. Panel **B** shows a reconstruction of the complete heart. In panel **C,** the main stem of the pulmonary artery and the atrial appendages have been removed to show the left main coronary artery (LM), the left anterior descending coronary artery (LAD), and the right coronary artery (RCA). Reproduced with permission from Achenbach et al.[13]

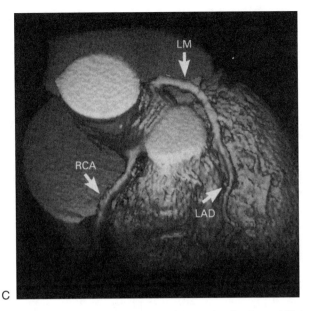

C

FIGURE 2-5. Reproduced with permission from Achenbach et al.[13] *(continued)*

visualization of 69 of 75 high-grade stenoses and occlusions with a sensitivity of 92%, whereas in 282 of 301 arteries, the absence of high-grade stenoses and occlusions was correctly detected (specificity 94%). Thus, when image quality is adequate, electron-beam CT may be useful to detect or rule out high-grade coronary-artery stenoses and occlusions (Figure 2-5).

Use of Electron-Beam Computed Tomography to Predict Atherosclerosis

Electron-beam CT scanning is correlated with the severity of atherosclerosis. Guerci and colleagues[14] from Roslyn, New York, evaluated whether this information adds to conventional risk factor assessment in the prediction of angiographic CAD. Electron-beam CT scans and conventional risk factors were measured in 290 men and women undergoing coronary arteriography for clinical reasons. Age, the ratio of total cholesterol to HDL, and the coronary calcium score were significantly and independently associated with the presence of any CAD and obstructive CAD. For obstructive CAD, highest quartile versus lower quartile, the respective odds ratio for age, the ratio of total cholesterol to HDL, and calcium score were 3.86, 4.11, and 34.12. Male gender was also significantly associated with any CAD as was cigarette smoking. After adjustment for the coronary calcium score and other risk factors, it appeared that triglycerides, family history, and hypertension were not significantly associated with any disease state. A coronary calcium score greater than 80 (Agatston method) was associated with an increased likelihood of any CAD regardless of the number of risk factors. A coronary calcium score greater than 170 was associated with an increased likelihood of obstructive CAD regardless of the number of risk factors. These authors conclude that electron-beam CT scanning offers improved discrimination over conventional risk factors in the identification of persons with any angiographic CAD or angiographic obstructive CAD.

Value of Early Acute Rest Sestamibi Perfusion Imaging

Evaluation of patients presenting to the emergency department with possible acute coronary syndromes and nondiagnostic electrocardiograms is problematic. Kontos and colleagues[15] from Richmond, Virginia, evaluated 532 such consecutive patients who underwent serial myocardial marker analysis and rest perfusion images. Perfusion imaging with technetium-99m sestamibi was positive in 32%. Positive perfusion imaging was the only multivariate predictor of AMI and was the most important independent predictor of AMI or revascularization, followed by diabetes, typical angina, and male gender. The sensitivity of positive perfusion for AMI was 93%, and AMI or revascularization, 81%. These authors conclude that positive rest perfusion imaging accurately identified patients at high risk for adverse cardiac outcomes whereas negative perfusion imaging identified a low-risk patient group. Thus, early perfusion imaging has the potential for rapid and accurate risk stratification of emergency department patients with possible cardiac ischemia and nondiagnostic electrocardiograms.

Prognostic Value of Stress Echocardiography

Patients with atypical chest pain frequently lack significant CAD and are, therefore, at low risk for future adverse cardiovascular events. Colon and colleagues[16] from New Orleans, Louisiana, hypothesized that in this group of patients, stress echocardiography could identify those at risk for cardiac events. The authors retrospectively reviewed (mean follow-up 23 ± 7 months) the prognostic value of stress echocardiography for major (cardiac death, AMI, CHF, and unstable angina) and total (major events plus coronary revascularization) cardiac events in 661 patients with atypical chest pain, normal global LV systolic function, and no history of myocardial ischemia. A positive stress echocardiogram was defined as the development of new or worsening wall motion abnormalities with exercise stress (80%) or dobutamine (20%). A total of 41 cardiac and 16 major events were noted. The event-free survival for total cardiac events was 97% for a normal stress echocardiogram and 93% for a normal stress electrocardiogram at 30 months. A positive stress electrocardiogram predicted an event-free rate of 86% compared with 74% for stress-induced wall motion abnormalities and 42% if stress-induced LV dysfunction accompanied the wall motion abnormalities. A strategy recommending invasive studies based on positive stress echocardiogram results increased the per-patient cost, but led to greater savings per cardiac event predicted, and provided incremental prognostic value for future cardiac events beyond clinical and

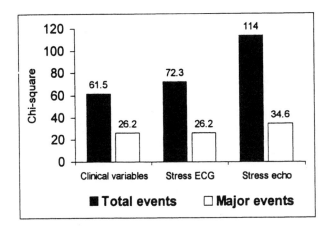

FIGURE 2-6. Comparison of cumulative chi square for stepwise analysis of clinical, stress electrocardiographic, and stress echocardiography variables for the prediction of total and major cardiac events. Reproduced with permission from Colon et al.[16]

stress electrocardiogram data. Thus, stress echocardiography in low-risk patients for CAD appears to be more cost-effective than a stress electrocardiogram (Figure 2-6).

Electrocardiographic and Clinical Predictors of Risk

Among patients with unstable angina pectoris (UAP), those who have non-ST elevation AMI are at higher risk for subsequent adverse events. To determine predictors of AMI in patients with UAP, Lloyd-Jones and associates[17] from Boston and Framingham, Massachusetts, and Los Angeles, California, studied consecutive nonreferral patients with UAP or AMI admitted from the emergency department to the intensive care or telemetry units of an urban teaching hospital over 1 year. There were 280 study patients (mean age 66 years; 1/3 women); 24% had AMI at presentation, whereas 76% had UAP without evidence of AMI. Thresholds of 3 or more involved leads (odds ratio [OR] 3.3) and 0.2 mV or more (OR 5.1) of ST depression on the presenting electrocardiogram were strongly associated with AMI. The multivariate predictors of AMI were reported duration of symptoms of 4 hours or more (OR 3.8), absence of prior revascularization (OR 3.5), absence of β-blocker use before presentation (OR 2.8), and presence of new ST depression (OR 2.8). Using the 4 multivariate predictors, a prediction rule was developed. The percentages of patients with AMI when 0, 1, 2, 3, or 4 characteristics were present, respectively, were 7%, 6%, 24%, 46%, and 83%. A similar prediction rule developed from the Thrombolysis in Myocardial Ischemia III trial was validated in this cohort. Among patients with UAP, electrocardiographic and clinical variables can help immediately identify those at high risk for AMI at presentation.

Incremental Prognostic Value of Single Photon Emission Computed Tomography

Hachamovitch and colleagues[18] in Los Angeles, California; New York City, New York; Durham, North Carolina; and Atlanta, Georgia, determined the incremental prognostic value of stress single photon emission computed tomography (SPECT) for the prediction of cardiac death as an individual endpoint, and the implications for risk stratification in 5,183 consecutive patients who underwent stress/rest SPECT and were followed for the occurrence of cardiac death or AMI. Over a mean follow-up of 642 ± 226 days, 119 cardiac deaths and 158 MIs occurred, i.e., 3% cardiac death rate, 2.3% AMI rate. Patients with normal scans were at low risk, i.e., ≤0.5%/year and rates of both outcomes increased significantly with worsening scan abnormalities (Figure 2-7). Patients who underwent exercise stress and had mildly abnormal scans had low rates of cardiac death, but higher rates of AMI (0.7%/year vs. 2.6%/year). After adjustment for pre-scan information, scan results provided incremental prognostic value toward the prediction of cardiac death. The identification of patients at intermediate risk of nonfatal MI and low risk for cardiac death by

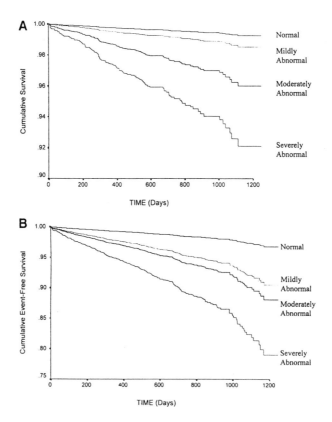

FIGURE 2-7. Risk-adjusted survival as a function of scan result using (A) cardiac death and (B) hard events as an endpoint. p < .00001 across scan results for both endpoints. Reproduced with permission from Hachamovitch et al.[18]

SPECT may result in significant cost savings when applied in a clinical testing strategy in the future.

Value of Tomographic Myocardial Perfusion Imaging for Left Bundle Branch Block

Wagdy and colleagues[19] from Rochester, Minnesota, determined the prognostic value of tomographic myocardial perfusion imaging with dipyridamole or adenosine in patients with left bundle branch block (LBBB). The study group consisted of 245 patients with LBBB who underwent tomographic myocardial perfusion imaging with thallium-201 or technetium-99m sestamibi and either dipyridamole or adenosine stress. Patients were classified into 2 groups. They were classified as "high risk" if they had (1) a large severe fixed defect (n=28); (2) a large reversible defect (n=36); or (3) cardiac enlargement and either increased pulmonary uptake with thallium or a decreased resting LVEF with sestamibi. The remaining 161 patients were at "low risk." Follow-up was 99% complete at 3 ± 1.4 years. Three-year overall survival was 57% in the high-risk group compared to 87% in the low-risk group. Survival free of cardiac death/nonfatal AMI/cardiac transplantation was 55% in the high-risk group and 93% in the low-risk group. The presence of a high-risk scan had significant incremental prognostic value after adjustment for age, gender, diabetes, and previous AMI. Patients with a low-risk scan had an overall survival rate that was not significantly different from that of a US age-matched population. Thus, tomographic myocardial perfusion imaging with adenosine or dipyridamole stress provides important prognostic information in patients with LBBB that is incremental to clinical assessment (Figure 2-8).

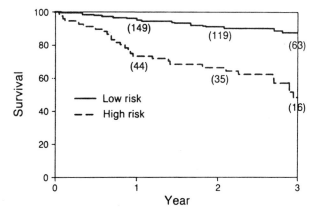

FIGURE 2-8. Survival free of hard and soft events (cardiac death, nonfatal myocardial infarction, cardiac transplantation, late revascularization) in low- (solid line) and high- (dotted line) risk groups. Three-year survival free of hard and soft events was 49% in the high-risk group compared to 87% in the low-risk group (p < .001). Reproduced with permission from Wagdy et al.[19]

Detection of Plaques

Schmermund and associates[20] from Herdecke and Mülheim an der Ruhr, Germany, compared intracoronary ultrasound (ICUS) and electron-beam computed tomography (EBCT) on a coronary segmental basis in 40 consecutive patients with acute coronary syndromes and no or minimal to moderate angiographic coronary artery narrowing. The patients were aged 53 ± 10 years; 34 were men and 6 were women. ICUS was used to define plaques, and EBCT was used to quantify coronary calcium (using a threshold of a CT density greater than 130 Hounsfield units in an area larger than 1.03 mm^2). In a site-by-site analysis, coronary segments were defined as normal if both methods were negative, as containing noncalcified plaques if only ICUS were positive, and as containing calcified plaques if both methods were positive. A total of 222 coronary segments were analyzed (5.6 ± 1.9 segments per patient). In 36 patients (90%), a total of 95 segments with plaques were identified, whereas in 4 patients (10%), only normal segments were seen. Of the 95 segments with plaques, 61 (64%) were calcified and 34 (36%) were noncalcified. There was a linear relationship between the number of segments with calcified and with noncalcified plaques (r = 0.86), but the mean relative frequency of segments with calcified plaques (55 ± 38%) was highly variable. Calcium was found in 15 of 16 patients (93%) with 3 or more segments with plaques, while it was found in only 12 of 20 patients (60%) with 1 or 2 segments with plaques. Younger age, high LDL levels, diabetes, and active smoking predicted a higher relative frequency of segments with noncalcified plaques. Thus, in patients with acute coronary syndromes but no angiographically critical stenoses, there is a linear relationship between segments with calcified plaques versus segments with noncalcified plaques. However, while the mean ratio of these segments is close to 1:1, it is highly variable among individual patients.

Detection of Multivessel Coronary Artery Disease

Dobutamine stress echocardiography has been shown to accurately detect CAD, but it is not clear whether it has the ability to detect multivessel CAD relative to clinical and exercise electrocardiography. Senior and colleagues[21] from Harrow, United Kingdom, evaluated the ability of dobutamine stress echocardiography to detect multivessel CAD and ascertain its incremental value when combined with clinical and exercise test variables. One hundred twenty-one consecutive patients referred for coronary arteriography on the basis of symptoms and exercise electrocardiography underwent dobutamine stress echocardiography. Significant multivessel CAD was defined as the presence of 70% or greater diameter stenosis in 2 or more major epicardial arteries. Stepwise logistic regression analysis was performed using the clinical exercise test and echocardiographic variables. The strongest independent variables predicting the presence of multivessel CAD were systolic wall thickening index at peak stress, presence of wall thickening abnormalities in multiple vascular territories, and a history of AMI. Furthermore, dobutamine echocardiography significantly enhanced the prediction of multivessel disease when combined with clinical and exercise test variables. Dobutamine stress echocardiography adds independent and incremental information to clinical and exercise test variables for identifying multivessel CAD.

Angioscopic Evaluation

Coronary angioscopy provides direct visualization of the endoluminal surface of coronary vessels. The usefulness of coronary angioscopy during coronary angioplasty of angiographically complex lesions remains to be established. This study by Alfonso and associates[22] from Madrid, Spain, was designed to determine the value of coronary angioscopy to elucidate the underlying substrate of angiographically complex lesions. Forty-seven consecutive patients with angiographically complex lesions were studied with coronary angioscopy before coronary intervention. Mean age of the group was 59 ± 9 years; 6 patients were women. Forty (85%) patients had unstable angina. Complex angiographic lesions included coronary occlusions (n=23) (14 with Thrombolysis in Myocardial Infarction [TIMI] coronary flow grade 0 and 9 with flow grade 1), lesions with intraluminal filling defects suggestive of thrombus or ulceration (n=8), and lesions that were highly eccentric (n=16). Items analyzed with coronary angioscopy included red thrombus (lining or protruding) and plaque color (yellow, white, or mixed). In all patients, coronary angioscopy visualized the protruding material causing the angiographic appearance. At this site coronary angioscopy detected red thrombus in 34 (72%) patients (14 protruding, 20 lining) and atherosclerotic plaque in 45 (96%) patients. At the site of the angiographically complex lesion, plaque was classified as predominantly yellow in 24 patients, mixed in 12, and white in 9. The incidence of thrombus on coronary angioscopy was higher for occluded vessels (91%) or lesions with intraluminal filling defects or ulceration (87%) than in eccentric lesions (37%). However, plaque coloration was not significantly different among these 3 angiographic subgroups. Initial procedural success (without stent requirement) was lower in lesions showing protruding thrombus on coronary angioscopy (64% vs. 91%). Thus most angiographically complex lesions contain thrombus. On coronary angioscopy, red thrombus was more frequently identified on occluded vessels and lesions with filling defects or ulceration than in eccentric lesions. Yellow or mixed plaques are common in these patients, suggesting lipid-laden plaques as the underlying pathologic substrate of angiographically complex lesions.

Isometric Hand Grip Exercise in Detecting Coronary Artery Disease

Dobutamine atropine stress echocardiography (DASE) detects CAD by increasing myocardial oxygen demand causing myocardial ischemia. The sensitivity of the test for detection of CAD is reduced in patients with submaximal stress. Afridi and associates[23] from Dallas, Texas, hypothesized that increasing workload by adding isometric exercise would improve the detection of myocardial ischemia during DASE. The authors studied 31 patients, mean age 57 ± 11 years, with angiographically documented CAD. Patients underwent DASE using incremental dobutamine doses from 5 to 40 μg/kg/min, followed by atropine if peak heart rate was higher than 85% of predicted maximal. Hand grip was then performed for 2 minutes of 33% of maximal voluntary contraction, while dobutamine infusion was maintained at the peak dose. The addition of hand grip during dobutamine stress was associated with a significant increase in systolic BP (143 ± 21 vs. 164 ± 24 mm Hg) and LV end-systolic circumferential wall stress ($72 ± 30 × 10^3$ dynes/cm^2 vs. $132 ± 34 × 10^3$ dynes/cm^2). Wall motion score index increased from 1.0 at rest to 1.15 ± 0.18 with dobutamine and increased further to 1.29 ± 0.22 with the addition of hand grip. Ischemia was detected in 19 patients (62%) with dobutamine-atropine stress alone and in 25 (83%) after the addition of hand grip. The addition of hand grip during DASE is feasible, and improves the detection of myocardial ischemia.

Repeat Coronary Angiography

Of the 1 million Americans who undergo coronary angiography each year, about one-third have angiographically normal or only minimally narrowed coronary arteries. Although subjects with angiographically normal coronary arteries have excellent long-term survival, many continue to have chest pain and some are disabled by their symptoms. In subjects with known epicardial CAD, repeat coronary angiography demonstrates clinically significant progression of narrowing in 25% to 33% of patients each year, but it is unknown if such progression is likely to occur in subjects in whom a previous angiogram showed normal coronary arteries. Pitts and associates[24] from Dallas, Texas, reviewed the records of all 10,366 cardiac catheterizations performed at Parkland Memorial Hospital from July 1970 to March 1997. During this period, 17 patients with a previously normal coronary angiogram had repeat angiography for the evaluation of continued chest pain. The group consisted of 15 women and 2 men aged 43 to 73 years (mean 55) at initial angiography. All had coronary angiography for evaluation of chest pain. No patient had an AMI before the first angiogram. The initial angiogram demonstrated normal epicardial coronary arteries in all 17 patients. The elapsed time between angiograms was 8.9 ± 3 years during which 2 patients developed single-vessel CAD, one of whom had an AMI. Thus, 15 of the 17 patients had no angiographically demonstrable CAD. It is recommended that repeat coronary angiography in a patient with a previously normal coronary angiogram should be reserved for those patients with objective evidence of spontaneous or provocable myocardial ischemia.

Detection of Coronary Artery Disease in Women

The detection of CAD by noninvasive methods has been hindered in women by the high rate of false positive results. To determine the feasibility and accuracy of transesophageal dobutamine and stress echocardiography for identification of CAD in women, Laurienzo and associates[25] from Bethesda, Maryland, studied 84 patients (age 51 ± 11 years) who underwent symptom-limited exercise treadmill testing, exercise thallium-201 scintigraphy, and coronary angiography for the evaluation of anginal-type chest pain. Of the 84 patients, 62 had normal coronary arteries or nonsignificant coronary lesions, and 22 had significant stenosis of 1 or more major coronary arteries. During treadmill exercise, repolorization changes were observed in 16 of 21 patients with CAD and in 19 of 60 patients with normal coronary arteries. With thallium scintigraphy, a reversible defect was observed in 19 of 22 patients with CAD and in 12 of 60 patients with normal coronary arteries. Regional wall motion abnormalities during dobutamine infusion developed in 18 of 22 patients with CAD and in none of the 62 patients with normal coronary arteries. All 3 tests had similar sensitivity for detection of CAD (76% for exercise treadmill test, 86% for thallium scintigraphy, and 82% for transesophageal dobutamine stress echocardiography). However, transesophageal dobutamine stress echocardiography had significantly higher specificity than the other 2 tests (100% vs. 68% for exercise treadmill test and 80% for thallium scintigraphy). Thus, transesophageal dobutamine stress echocardiography is accurate for evaluation of CAD among women presenting with chest pain; its use should be considered when more conventional tests are equivocal or technically suboptimal.

Coronary Flow Velocity

The intracoronary Doppler tipped guidewire has been shown to be highly accurate in the measurement of coronary flow velocity. Recent studies have indicated that blood flow velocity in the LAD coronary artery can be determined by transesophageal echocardiography (TEE). The purpose of this study by Gadallah and associates[26] from Los Angeles, California, was to compare flow velocity recordings and coronary flow reserve measurements in the LAD by TEE with those obtained by Doppler guidewire. The study population consisted of 14 patients with chest pain and normal coronary arteriograms. After routine coronary arteriography was performed, a 0.014-inch Doppler guidewire was advanced into the proximal part of the LAD. After baseline measurement of coronary flow velocity was obtained, 140 μg/kg/min adenosine was administered intravenously for 3 minutes, and the flow velocity was recorded. TEE was performed within 24 hours of the cardiac catheterization. After baseline measurements of coronary flow velocity in the LAD, heart rate, and BP were obtained, 140 μg/kg/min adenosine was administered intravenously, and the coronary flow velocity was recorded. Coronary flow reserve was calculated as the ratio of the peak diastolic coronary flow velocity during adenosine infusion to the peak diastolic coronary flow velocity at baseline. A good correlation was also found between the coronary flow reserve assessed by Doppler guidewire and that determined by TEE. These data indicate that the coronary flow velocity and coronary flow reserve in the LAD can be accurately estimated by transesophageal echocardiography.

Electron-Beam Computed Tomography Versus Conventional Risk Factor Assessment

Electron-beam CT scanning is correlated with the severity of atherosclerosis. Guerci and colleagues[27] from Roslyn, New York, evaluated whether this information adds to conventional risk factor assessment in the prediction of angiographic CAD. Electron-beam CT scans and conventional risk factors were measured in 290 men and women undergoing coronary arteriography for clinical reasons. Age, the ratio of total cholesterol to HDL, and the coronary calcium score were significantly and independently associated with the presence of any CAD and obstructive CAD. For obstructive CAD, highest quartile versus lower quartile, the respective odds ratio for age, the ratio of total cholesterol to HDL, and calcium score were 3.86, 4.11, and 34.12. Male gender was also significantly associated with any CAD as was cigarette smoking. After adjustment for the coronary calcium score and other risk factors, it appeared that triglycerides, family history, and hypertension were not significantly associated with any disease state. A coronary calcium score of 80 or more (Agatston method) was associated with an increased likelihood of any CAD regardless of the number of risk factors. A coronary calcium score of 170 or more was associated with an increased likelihood of obstructive CAD regardless of the number of risk factors. These authors conclude that electron-beam CT scanning offers improved discrimination over conventional risk factors in the identification of persons with any angiographic CAD or angiographic obstructive CAD.

Risk Factors Associated with Coronary Artery Disease

Increased Plasminogen Activator Inhibitor Type 1 in Diabetics Versus Nondiabetics

Sobel and colleagues[28] hypothesized that increased plasminogen activator inhibitor type 1 (PAI-1) would be present in excess in atheroma from patients with type 2 diabetes. They had previously shown that insulin stimulates PAI-1 synthesis *in vivo*, and it is well documented that increases in PAI-1 in blood are associated with insulin resistance, hyperinsulinemia, and type 2 diabetes mellitus. Samples were acquired by directional coronary atherectomy from 25 patients with type 2 diabetes and 18 patients without diabetes and were characterized qualitatively histologically for cellularity and immunohistochemistry and by quantitative image analysis for assessment of urokinase-type plasminogen activator and PAI-1. Patients with and without diabetes were similar with respect to their demographic features and the distribution and severity of CAD. However, substantially more PAI-1 and less urokinase-type plasminogen activator were present in the atherectomy samples from subjects with dia-

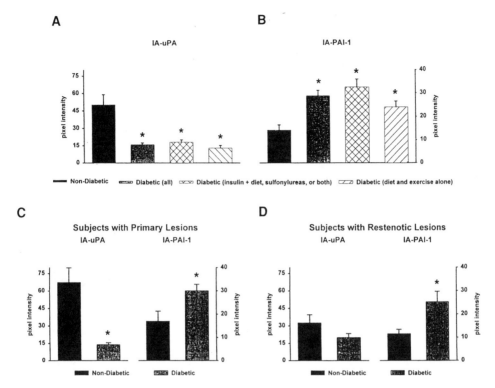

FIGURE 2-9. Results of quantitative image analysis (IA) for detection of u-PA and PAI-1 in nondiabetic versus diabetic subjects **(A),** nondiabetic versus all diabetic subjects and only diabetic subjects treated with insulin, sulfonylureas, or both **(B),** diabetic and nondiabetic subjects with primary lesions **(C),** and diabetic versus nondiabetic subjects with restenotic lesions **(D).** *p < 0.05 for comparisons between diabetic and nondiabetic subjects in each case. Reproduced with permission from Sobel et al.[28]

betes (Figure 2-9). The disproportionate elevation of PAI-1 compared with the urokinase-type plasminogen activator observed in atheromatous material extracted from vessels of diabetic patients is consistent with increased gene expression of PAI-1 in vessels as well as the known increase of PAI-1 in blood, presumably reflecting increased synthesis. The authors speculate that the increased PAI-1 detected in the atheroma may contribute *in vivo* to accelerated or persistent thrombosis and to vasculopathy in patients with type 2 diabetes.

Family History as a Risk Factor for Cardiac Arrest

Friedlander and associates[29] from Jerusalem, Israel, examined the hypothesis that a family history of MI or primary cardiac arrest is an independent risk factor for primary cardiac arrest in a population-based case-control study. They investigated whether recognized risk factors account for the familial aggregation of these cardiovascular events. Primary cardiac arrest cases attended by paramedics during the period 1988 to 1994 in individuals 25 to 74 years old and population-based control subjects matched for age and gender were identified from the community by random digit dialing. All subjects were free of recognized clinical heart disease and major comorbidity. A detailed history of MI and primary cardiac arrest in first-degree relatives was collected in interviews with the spouses of case and control subjects by trained interviewers using a standardized questionnaire. For each familial relationship, there was a higher rate of MI or primary cardiac arrest in relatives of cases compared with relatives of control subjects. Overall, the rate of MI and primary cardiac arrest among first-degree relatives of cardiac arrest patients was almost 50% higher than in first-degree relatives of control subjects. In a multivariate logistic model, family history of MI and primary cardiac arrest was associated with primary cardiac arrest even after adjustment for other common risk factors. Thus, family history of MI or primary cardiac arrest is associated with the risk of primary cardiac arrest. This association is largely independent of familial aggregation of other common risk factors.

Cigarette Smoking Increases Sympathetic Outflow

Narkiewicz and colleagues[30] in Iowa City, Iowa, examined the effects of sham smoking, cigarette smoking, and cigarette smoking in combination with nitroprusside on muscle sympathetic nerve activity in 10 healthy habitual smokers. The 3 sessions were performed in random order, each study on a separate day. In an additional study, they also investigated the effects of sham and cigarette smoking on skin sympathetic nerve activity in 9 subjects. Compared with sham smoking, cigarette smoking alone increased blood pressure and decreased muscle sympathetic nerve activity. When the blood pressure increase in response to smoking was blunted by nitroprusside, there was a striking increase in muscle sympathetic nerve activity. Muscle sympathetic nerve activity increased up to 3-fold the levels seen before smoking, accompanied by an increase in heart rate of up to 37 ± 4 beats/minute. Cigarette smoking also induced a $102\% \pm 22\%$ increase in skin sympathetic nerve activity. These data provide the first direct evidence that cigarette smoking increases sympathetic outflow (Figure 2-10).

Cardiac Sympathetic Dysinnervation in Diabetes

Stevens and colleagues[31] proposed in this study that in diabetes, regional cardiac denervation may elsewhere induce regional sympathetic hyperactivity, which may in turn act as a focus for chemical and electrical instability. In this study, they wished to explore whether regional changes in sympathetic neuronal density and tone exist in diabetic patients with and without diabetic autonomic neuropathy. They used positron-emission tomography and the sympathetic neurotransmitter analog ^{11}C-labeled hydroxyephedrine to characterize LV sympathetic innervation in diabetic patients by assessing regional disturbances in myocardial tracer retention and washout. The subject groups comprised 10 diabetic subjects without diabetic autonomic neuropathy, 10

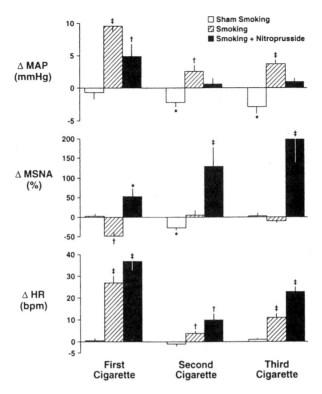

FIGURE 2-10. Group data showing changes in MAP, muscle SNA (MSNA), and heart rate (HR) during sham smoking, smoking, and smoking with infusion of nitroprusside (n=10). *p < 0.05, †p < 0.01, ‡p < 0.001 versus pre-smoking period. Both MSNA and HR increases were particularly striking when the blood pressure increase with smoking was attenuated with nitroprusside. Data are mean ±SEM. Reproduced with permission from Narkiewicz et al.[30]

diabetic subjects with mild diabetic autonomic neuropathy, 9 subjects with severe diabetic autonomic neuropathy, and 10 healthy subjects. Abnormalities of cardiac ^{11}C-labeled hydroxyephedrine retention were found in 40% of diabetic autonomic neuropathy-free diabetics. In subjects with mild neuropathy, tracer defects were observed only in the distal inferior wall of the left ventricle, whereas with more severe neuropathy, defects extended to involve the distal and proximal anterolateral and inferior walls. Absolute ^{11}C-labeled hydroxyephedrine retention was found to be increased by 33% in the proximal region of the severe diabetic autonomic neuropathy subjects compared with the same regions in the diabetic autonomic neuropathy-free subjects. No appreciable amount of tracer was observed in the proximal segments, consistent with normal regional tone but increased sympathetic innervation. Distally, ^{11}C-labeled hydroxyephedrine retention was decreased in severe diabetic autonomic neuropathy by 33% compared with diabetic autonomic neuropathy-free patients with diabetes. Thus, diabetes results in LV sympathetic dysinnervation with proximal hyperinnervation complicating distal denervation. This combination could play a role in electrical instability and explain the enhanced cardioprotection from β-blockers in these patients.

Evaluation of Lipoprotein(a) Concentrations in Cardiovascular Events

Several but not all studies have shown that elevated lipoprotein(a) (Lp(a)) concentrations may be associated with CAD. To further investigate this association, Cantin and associates[32] from Ste-Foy and Montreal, Quebec, Canada, conducted a 5-year prospective follow-up study in 2,156 French Canadian men age 47 to 36 years, who did not have any clinical evidence of CAD. During the follow-up period, 116 first events (AMI, angina, death) occurred. Lp(a) was not an independent risk factor for CAD but seemed to increase the deleterious effects of mildly elevated LDL cholesterol and elevated total cholesterol and apoprotein B levels. It also seemed to counteract the beneficial effects associated with elevated HDL cholesterol levels. These authors conclude that Lp(a) is not an independent risk factor for ischemic heart disease but appears to increase the risk associated with other lipid risk factors.

Abdominal Obesity and Hyperinsulinemia in Men with Mutated Low-Density Lipoprotein Receptor Gene

Gaudet and colleagues[33] in Quebec, Canada, determined whether the hyperinsulinemic-insulin-resistant state of abdominal obesity affects coronary atherosclerosis among familial hypercholesterol (FH) patients. The relationship between abdominal obesity and hyperinsulinemia and angiographically assessed CAD was evaluated in a sample of 120 French Canadian men 60 years old or younger who were heterozygous for FH and in a group of 280 men without FH. The risk of CAD associated with abdominal obesity, as estimated by waist circumference, was largely dependent on the concomitant variation in plasma lipoprotein and insulin concentrations. The association between fasting insulin and CAD was independent of variations in waist girth and triglyceride, HDL, and apolipoprotein B concentrations. However, the most substantial increase in the risk of CAD was observed among abdominally obese (waist circumference >90 cm) and hyperinsulinemic FH patients who had an odds ratio of 12.9 (Figure 2-11). The increase in risk remained significant even after adjustment for LDL cholesterol and apolipoprotein B concentrations. Thus, these data support the concept that the hyperinsulinemic-insulin-resistant state of abdominal obesity is a powerful predictor of CAD in men, even among patients with raised LDL cholesterol concentrations due to FH.

Oxidized Low-Density Lipoprotein and Malondialdehyde-Modified Low-Density Lipoprotein

Holvoet and colleagues[34] evaluated 63 patients with acute coronary syndromes, including 45 with AMI and 18 with unstable angina, 35 patients with stable angina, 28 heart transplant patients with post-transplant CAD, 79 heart transplant patients without CAD, and 65 control individuals to determine the

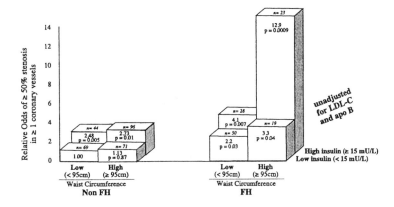

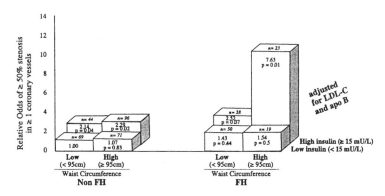

FIGURE 2-11. Relative odds of CAD among men with (FH) or without (non-FH) mutations in the LDL receptor gene according to the 50th percentiles of waist circumference and of fasting insulin concentration, before **(top)** and after **(bottom)** adjustment for plasma LDL-C and apo B concentrations. Odds ratios are from a logistic regression model. Low-waist circumference <50th percentile (95 cm); High-waist circumference >50th percentile (95 cm). Reproduced with permission from Gaudet et al.[33]

association between plasma levels of oxidized LDL and malondialdehyde (MDA)-modified LDL and the development of acute coronary syndromes. After correction for age, gender, and LDL and HDL cholesterol, plasma levels of oxidized LDL and MDA-modified LDL were higher in patients with CAD than in individuals without CAD. Plasma levels in MDA-modified LDL were significantly higher in patients with acute coronary syndromes than in individuals with stable CAD and were associated with increased levels of troponin I and C-reactive protein (Figure 2-12). Plasma levels of oxidized LDL were not associated with increased levels of troponin I and C-reactive protein. Thus, these data suggest that elevated plasma levels of oxidized LDL are associated with CAD. Elevated plasma levels of malondialdehyde-modified LDL suggest plaque

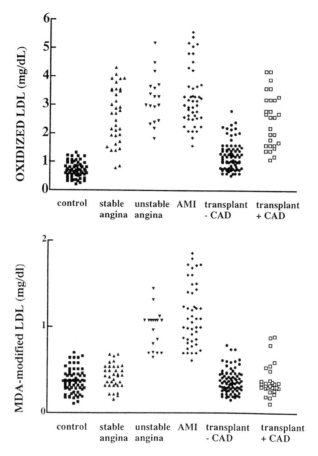

FIGURE 2-12. Individual values of oxidized LDL and MDA-modified LDL in control subjects; nontransplanted patients with stable angina and unstable angina and AMI; and heart transplant patients without and with post-transplant CAD. Reproduced with permission from Holvoet et al.[34]

instability and may be useful for the identification of patients with acute coronary syndromes.

Early Familial Coronary Artery Disease

An interaction between high plasma lipoprotein(a), unfavorable plasma lipids, and other risk factors may lead to very high risk for premature CAD. Plasma lipoprotein(a), lipids, and other CAD risk factors were examined by Hopkins and coworkers[35] in Salt Lake City, Utah, in 170 cases with early familial CAD and 165 control subjects to test this hypothesis. In univariate analysis, relative odds for CAD were 2.95 for plasma lipoprotein(a) above 40 mg/dL. Nearly all of the risk associated with elevated lipoprotein(a) was found to be restricted to persons with historically elevated plasma total cholesterol or with a total/HDL cholesterol ratio greater than 5.8. Nonlipid risk factors were also

TABLE 2-1
**Risks Associated with High Lipoprotein(a) in the Presence and Absence
of Nonlipid Risk Factors**

	Risk Factor Absent		Risk Factor Present	
	Lp(a) ≤40	Lp(a) >40	Lp(a) ≤40	Lp(a) >40
Hypertension				
Relative odds	1.0	3.0	3.6	16.6
95% CI	. . .	1.6–6.7	3.0–8.9	4.8–56
p	. . .	.0008	2.4×10^{-9}	8.6×10^{-6}
Hypertension and/or diabetes				
Relative odds	1.0	3.4	6.1	20.5
95% CI	. . .	1.6–6.9	3.6–10.3	6.3–67
p	. . .	.0009	3.0×10^{-11}	5.1×10^{-7}
Cigarette smoking (ever)				
Relative odds	1.0	3.3	3.7	7.2
95% CI	. . .	1.5–7.2	2.2–6.4	2.9–17.8
p	. . .	.003	.000001	.00002
H(e) >90th percentile				
Relative odds	1.0	2.4	3.4	31.7
95% CI	. . .	1.2–4.7	1.8–6.6	6.5–155
p	. . .	.01	.0003	.00002
Bilirubin <40th percentile				
Relative odds	1.0	2.9	4.5	11.4
95% CI	. . .	1.1–7.7	2.7–7.6	5.0–26.0
p	. . .	.03	1.4×10^{-8}	5.7×10^{-9}

Lp(a) = lipoprotein(a); CI = confidence interval; H(e) = homocyst(e)ine. Odds ratios were determined for each gender separately and then pooled by the Mantel-Haenszel method. There were too few control subjects with diabetes for separate evaluation. Sex-specific 90th percentile cut points for [H(e)] were 12 μmol/L for women and 15 μmol/L for men. For bilirubin, 40th percentile cut points were 12 μmol/L for women and 13.6 μmol/L for men.
Reproduced with permission from Hopkins et al.[35]

found to at least multiply the risks with lipoprotein(a) (Table 2-1). When lipoprotein(a) was over 40 mg/dL and plasma total/HDL cholesterol was greater than 5.8, relative odds for CAD were 25 in multiple logistic regression. If 2 or more nonlipid risk factors were also present (including hypertension, diabetes, cigarette smoking, high total homocysteine, or low serum bilirubin) relative odds were 122. The ability of nonlipid risk factors to increase risks associated with lipoprotein(a) was dependent on at least a mild elevated total/HDL cholesterol ratio. In conclusion, high lipoprotein(a) is found to greatly increase risks only if the total/HDL cholesterol ratio is at least mildly elevated, an effect exaggerated by other risk factors. Aggressive lipid lowering in those with elevated lipoprotein(a) therefore appears indicated.

Multiple Risk Factor Intervention Trial

A nested case-control study was undertaken involving men participating in the Multiple Risk Factor Intervention Trial, and Evans and coworkers[36] in Pittsburgh, Pennsylvania, analyzed serum samples from 712 men stored for

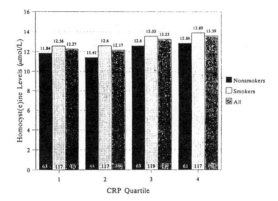

FIGURE 2-13. Average levels of homocyst(e)ine within quartiles of C-reactive protein (CRP) for MRFIT cases and matched controls (combined) by smoking status at entry to trial. Reproduced with permission from Evans et al.[36]

up to 20 years for homocyst(e)ine. Cases involved fatal AMIs, identified through the active phase of the study that ended on February 28, 1982, and deaths due to CAD, monitored through 1990. The nonfatal AMIs occurred within 7 years of sample collection, whereas the majority of CAD deaths occurred more than 11 years after sample collection. Mean homocyst(e)ine concentrations were in the expected range and did not differ significantly between case patients and control subjects: AMI cases, 12.6 mmols/L; AMI controls, 13.1 mmols/L; CAD death cases, 12.8 mmols/L; and CAD controls, 12.7 mmols/L. The odds ratios versus quartile 1 for CAD deaths and AMIs combined were as follows: quartile 2, 1.03; quartile 3, 0.84; quartile 4, 0.92. Thus, in this prospective study, no association of homocyst(e)ine concentration with heart disease was detected. Homocyst(e)ine levels were weakly associated with the acute phase protein (C-reactive protein) (Figure 2-13). These results suggest that homocyst(e)ine is an independent risk factor for heart disease.

Subclinical Vascular Disease

A composite measure of subclinical vascular disease has been developed in the Cardiovascular Health Study. In previous reports Kuller and associates[37] in Pittsburgh, Pennsylvania, measured the prevalence of subclinical disease among the original 5,201 participants in the Cardiovascular Health Study, the relationship of risk factors of subclinical disease, and the association of subclinical disease to clinically evident CAD. In 1992–1993 (year 4 of the study), a larger cohort of 424 black women and 248 black men was added to the study. In this study, the investigators compared the prevalence of subclinical disease among blacks and whites in the Cardiovascular Health Study and the association with cardiovascular risk factors. The prevalence of subclinical disease for all participants was 41% for white women, 40% for black women, 42% for white men, and 44% for black men. The prevalence increased with age (Figure

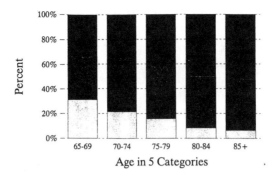

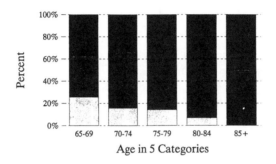

FIGURE 2-14. **Top:** Distribution of prevalent disease by age in white males. **Bottom:** Distribution of prevalent disease by age in black males. Solid portion of bars represents clinical disease; dark shaded portion, subclinical disease; and light shaded portion, no disease. Reproduced with permission from Kuller et al.[37]

2-14). The risk factor associations of subclinical disease were similar among blacks and whites. In multivariate analysis, age, systolic blood pressure, LDL cholesterol, smoking, and family history of AMI were independently associated with subclinical disease among both black and white women, while for white men systolic blood pressure, use of antihypertensive medication, smoking, body mass index, and diastolic blood pressure (inverse) were related to subclinical disease. In black men, blood triglyceride level, use of antihypertensive medications, and family history of myocardial infarction (inverse) were associated with subclinical disease.

Relationship of Helicobacter Pylori Infection to Heart Disease

Strachan and colleagues[38] collected plasma samples during 1979 to 1983 from 1,796 men in Caerphilly, South Wales, and they were analyzed for IgG antibodies to *Helicobacter pylori*. Causes of death and occurrence of incident CAD events were ascertained over an average of 13.7 years from death certificates, hospital records, and electrocardiogram changes at 5-year follow-up examinations. Seventy percent of men were seropositive. The prevalence of CAD at entry was similar in men with and without *H. pylori* antibodies. Seropositivity was significantly associated with poorer socioeconomic status currently and in childhood, shorter stature, and poorer ventilatory function at entry, but not with age, smoking, body mass index, blood pressure, total cholesterol, HDL cholesterol, LDL cholesterol, fibrinogen, plasma viscosity, or heat shock protein antibodies. Thirteen-year incidence of CAD was not significantly associated with *H. pylori*, but there was a strong relationship with all-cause mortality. After adjustment for cardiovascular risk factors and both adult and childhood socioeconomic status, odds ratios were slightly reduced and lost statistical significance for all-cause mortality (odds ratio = 1.52). Thus, these data suggest that *H. pylori* infection is unlikely to be a strong risk factor for CAD, but its relationship to mortality, including fatal CAD, deserves further investigation.

Association of Helicobacter Pylori *with Ischemia*

Pasceri and colleagues[39] in Rome, Italy, determined the prevalence of infection by *Helicobacter pylori* and by strains bearing the cytotoxin-associated gene-A, a strong virulence factor, in 88 patients with CAD with a mean age of 57 ± 8 years with 74 men and in 88 age- and gender-matched controls with a mean age of 57 ± 8 years and 74 men with similar social backgrounds. Prevalence of *H. pylori* infection was significantly higher in patients than in controls (62% vs. 40%) with an odds ratio of 2.8 adjusted for age, gender, main cardiovascular risk factors, and social class. Patients with CAD also had a higher prevalence of cytotoxin-associated gene-A positive strains (43% vs. 17%) with an adjusted odds ratio of 3.8. Conversely, prevalence of the cytotoxic-associated gene-A negative strains were similar in patients and controls. Thus, the association between *H. pylori* and CAD appears to be due to a higher prevalence of more virulent *H. pylori* strains in patients. The data are consistent with a hypothesis that *H. pylori* may influence atherogenesis through low-grade, persistent inflammatory infection (Figure 2-15).

Helicobacter Pylori *Seropositivity and Coronary Artery Disease*

Folsom and colleagues[40] in Minneapolis, Minnesota, used a prospective, case-cohort design to determine *Helicobacter pylori* seropositivity in relation to CAD incidence over a median follow-up period of 3.3 years among middle-

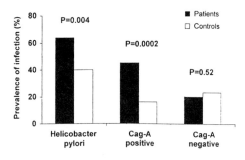

FIGURE 2-15. Prevalence of *Helicobacter pylori* infection and of cytotoxin-associated gene-A (CagA)-positive or CagA-negative strains in patients and controls. Reproduced with permission from Pasceri et al.[39]

aged men and women. There were 217 incident CAD cases and a cohort sample of 498. They determined *H. pylori* antibody status by measuring IgG antibody to the high molecular weight cell associated proteins of *H. pylori* using a sensitive and specific ELISA. The prevalence of *H. pylori* seropositivity was higher in blacks than in whites, in those with less than high school education, and in those with lower plasma pyridoxal 5'-phosphate and higher homocyst(e)ine concentrations, in those who did not use vitamin supplements, in those with higher fibrinogen levels, and in individuals seropositive for cytomegalovirus and herpes simplex type 1. The age-, gender-, race-, and field center-adjusted hazard ratio CAD for *H. pylori* seropositivity was 1.03. After adjustment for other risk factors, including fibrinogen, cytomegalovirus seropositivity, and herpes simplex type 1 seropositivity, the hazard ratio was 0.85. *H. pylori* seropositivity was not associated with increased mean intima-media thickness of the carotid artery, a measure of subclinical atherosclerosis. These data cast doubt on the likelihood that *H. pylori* infection is an important contributor to clinical CAD events.

Role of Chronic Infection in Development of Coronary Artery Disease

Davidson and colleagues[41] performed a retrospective investigation to evaluate premortem serum specimens and autopsy tissue from 60 indigenous Alaska Natives at low risk for CAD, selected by the potential availability of their stored specimens. Serum specimens were drawn a mean of 8.8 years prior to death, which occurred at a mean age of 34 years, primarily from noncardiovascular causes (97%). Coronary artery tissues were independently examined histologically and, for *C. pneumoniae* organism and DNA, by immunocytochemistry and polymerase chain reaction with species-specific monoclonal antibody in primers. Microimmunofluorescence detected species-specific IgG, IgA, and IgM antibody in stored serum. *C. pneumoniae*, frequently within macrophage foam cells, was identified in coronary fibrolipid atheroma (raised lesions) in 15 subjects (25%) and in early flat lesions in 7 (11%) either by polymerase chain reaction or by immunocytochemistry. The odds ratio for *C. pneumoniae* in raised atheroma after a level of IgG antibody 1:256 or more at least 8 years earlier was 6.1 and for all coronary tissues after adjustment for multiple potential confounding variables, including tobacco exposure, was 9.4. Thus, serological evidence for *C. pneumoniae* infection frequently precedes both the earliest and the most advanced lesions of coronary atherosclerosis that contain this intracellular pathogen, suggesting a chronic infection and developmental role in CAD.

Human Paraoxonase Gene Polymorphism

Recent reports have suggested that polymorphism in the human paraoxonase gene may be a genetic risk factor for CAD in a white population. However, this association has not yet been confirmed in other ethnic populations. Zama and coworkers[42] in Tokyo, Japan, studied 75 Japanese patients with CAD whose coronary lesions were confirmed by angiography and 115 Japanese control subjects with no history of CAD and a normal resting electrocardiogram. The assays for genotyping the polymorphisms in the human paraoxonase gene were based on changes in restriction enzyme digestion patterns. For codon 192, the frequencies of the Arg-coding allele in both patients and control subjects were much higher than those in published results of whites and the difference between patients and control subjects was statistically significant. The patient group had a high proportion of Arg/Arg (B/B) homozygotes. For codon 55, the frequencies of Leu-coding allele control subjects and patients were much higher than published results for whites, but there was no difference between Japanese control subjects and Japanese patients. When subjects with the [55]Leu/Leu genotype only were analyzed, [192]Arg/Arg homozygotes were still significantly more frequent in the patients than in the control subjects, and the frequency of [192]Arg and allele was also higher in patients than in control subjects. Logistic regression analysis including conventional coronary risks factors revealed that [192]Arg is an independent risk factor for CAD. Thus, in the Japanese population, the association of CAD with the [192]Arg variant of the human paraoxonase gene is similar to that reported for whites, although the allele frequency for [192]Arg and [55]Leu is much higher in the former than the latter population.

Depression in the Elderly

The role of duration of depressed mood in the prediction of CVD is unclear. Penninx and colleagues[43] from multiple US medical centers and also from Padua, Italy, studied prospectively 3,701 men and women over 70 years of age using 3 measurement occasions of depressive symptomatology (Center for Epidemiological Studies—Depression Scale) during a 6-year period to distinguish persons who were newly (depressed at baseline but not at 3 and 6 years before baseline) and chronically (depressed at baseline and at 3 or 6 years before baseline) depressed. Their risk of subsequent CVD events and all-cause mortality was compared with that of subjects who were never depressed during the 6-year period. Outcome events were based on death certificates and Medicare hospitalization records. During a median follow-up of 4.0 years, there were 732 deaths (46.2/1,000 person-years) and 933 new CVD events (64.7/1,000 person-years). In men, but not in women, newly depressed mood was associated with an increased risk of CVD mortality (relative risk 1.75), new CVD events (relative risk 2.07), and new coronary heart disease events (relative risk 2.03) after adjustment for traditional CVD risk factors. The association between newly depressed mood and all-cause mortality was smaller (relative risk 1.40). Chronic depressed mood was not associated with new CVD events or all-cause mortality. These findings suggest that newly depressed older men, but not women, were approximately twice as likely to have a CVD event than those who were never depressed. In men, recent onset of depressed mood is a better predictor of CVD than long-term depressed mood.

Relationship of Plasma Viscosity and Cardiovascular Disease

Several studies have indicated that plasma viscosity contributes to cardiovascular risk in men. Thus far, a significant relationship between plasma viscos-

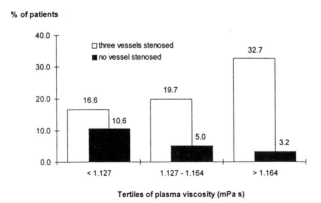

% of patients

FIGURE 2-16. Percentages of MI patients without any and with 3 stenosed vessels referring to the total number of MI patients within tertiles of plasma viscosity. Reproduced with permission from Junker et al.[44]

ity and the severity of CAD has not been found. Thus, a study by Junker and colleagues[44] in Munster, Germany, was the first to report on the relationship of plasma viscosity and the severity of CAD. In a collective study of 1,142 male AMI patients, plasma viscosity and additional laboratory parameters were determined. Atherosclerotic changes were quantified by coronary angiography. The patients were divided into groups without any, and with 1, 2, 3 stenosed vessels. The investigators found a positive relationship between plasma viscosity and the severity of CAD, even after adjusting groups for age, fibrinogen, and use of diuretics. Mean plasma viscosity ranged from 1.141 mPa s in patients without stenosed vessels to 1.162 mPa s in patients who had 3 coronary vessels with stenoses greater than 50% (Figure 2-16). Differences between the groups were significant with 2 exceptions: differences between patients without any and with 1 stenosed vessel, as well as between patients with 1 and 2 stenosed vessels, did not reach the significance level. On the whole, the investigators gave further support to the hypothesis that cardiovascular risk factors and CAD may be linked by plasma viscosity.

Offspring of Women with Premature Coronary Artery Disease

Some studies suggest that the first-degree relatives of female patients with premature CAD are at greater risk for early disease than if the proband is a male patient. To examine coronary risk factors, related knowledge, attitudes, and beliefs concerning CAD risk, Allen and Blumenthal[45] from Baltimore, Maryland, screened a sample of 87 apparently healthy offspring (56 female subjects and 31 male subjects) of women with documented premature CAD. More than half of the offspring had total and LDL cholesterol levels above the recommended levels for primary prevention, 31% were current smokers, and 56% exercised fewer than 3 times a week. A high proportion were overweight with a high prevalence of central obesity. A total of 13% had only 1 major risk factor, a family history of premature CAD, 10% had 2 risk factors, 23% had 3, and 54% had 4 or more CAD risk factors. When compared with the Framingham cohort, 29% of sons and 30% of daughters exceeded their age- and gender-specific average risk for having CAD in 10 years. Only 28% identified heredity as a major cause of CAD, and 47% perceived their risk for future myocardial infarction as less than or equal to that of others their age. These findings suggest that adult children of women with premature CAD have a high prevalence of modifiable risk factors and do not perceive themselves to be at risk for CAD.

Effect of Smoking on C-Reactive Protein

Blood levels of C-reactive protein, a marker of inflammation, are related to cardiovascular disease risks. To determine cross-sectional correlates in the elderly, Tracy and coinvestigators[46] in Colchester, Vermont, measured C-reactive protein in 400 men and women older than 65 years and free of clinical cardiovascular disease at baseline as part of the Cardiovascular Health Study. Only 2% of the values were greater than 10 mg/L, the cut point usually used to identify inflammation. C-reactive protein levels appeared tightly regulated, since there were strong bivariate correlations between C-reactive protein and the following: inflammation – sensitive proteins such as fibrinogen; measures of fibrinolysis such as plasmin – antiplasmin complex; pack – years of smoking; and body mass index. The association with pack years was independent on the length of time since cessation of smoking. C-reactive protein levels were also associated with coagulation factors VIIc, IXc, Xc; HDL (negative) and triglyceride; diabetes status; diuretic use; electrocardiogram abnormalities; and level of exercise. Because of effect modification, 2 multiple linear regression prediction models were developed for C-reactive protein, 1 each for never smokers and ever smokers. An *a priori* physiological model was used to guide these analyses, which disallowed the use of other inflammation-sensitive variables such as fibrinogen. In never smokers, the independent predictors were body mass index, diabetes status, plasmin-antiplasmin complex, and presence of electrocardiogram abnormalities; this model predicted 15% of the C-reactive protein and population variance. In ever smokers, the predictors were body mass index, plasmin-antiplasmin complex, pack years of smoking, HDL cholesterol (negative), and ankle/arm blood pressure index (negative); this model predicted 42% of the population variance. The investigators conclude that levels of C-reactive protein in the healthy elderly population are tightly regulated and reflect lifetime exposure to smoking, as well as level of obesity, ongoing level of fibrinolysis, diabetes status, and level of subclinical atherothrombotic disease. Moreover, exposure to smoking affects the relation of C-reactive proteins to these other factors.

Role of Infectious Agents in Coronary Artery Disease

Chlamydia pneumoniae, cytomegalovirus and *Helicobacter pylori* have been linked to the risk of myocardial infarction or coronary artery disease. Anderson and colleagues[47] from Salt Lake City, Utah, tested whether C-reactive protein and seropositivity to any of these 3 infectious agents were associated with angiographic CAD and clinical AMI. Blood samples were collected from 363 patients undergoing coronary arteriography and tested for C-reactive protein and IgG titers to the infectious agents. C-reactive protein was higher in patients with CAD (1.32 mg/dL vs. 0.5 mg/dL) than in those with AMI (2.05 mg/dL vs. 0.4 mg/dL) than in respective control subjects. Seropositivity for each agent was present in a high proportion of patients with CAD (58% to 77%) or AMI (54% to 75%) as well as in control subjects (no CAD 46% to 74%, no AMI 50% to 77%). However, subjects seropositive to both *C. pneumoniae* and *H. pylori* had an increased prevalence of CAD (odds ratio = 2.6) and tended to have higher C-reactive protein levels than those seronegative to both infectious agents. These authors concluded that C-reactive protein is elevated more than 2-fold in patients with CAD and 4-fold in patients with AMI. Infectious serology is highly prevalent in both patients and control subjects. These data provide additional support for the potential role of infectious agents in patients with CAD.

Coronary Disease-Prone Behavior in Japanese Men

In Japan, the type A behavior pattern, particularly its component of hostility, is known to have less value as a risk for CAD than in the United States. Hayano and associates[48] from Nagoya, Warabi, Isehara, Tokyo, Naruto, and Iwaki, Japan, developed a questionnaire (Japanese Coronary-Prone Behavior Scale) to investigate the behavioral correlates with CAD among contemporary Japanese persons. The Japanese Coronary-Prone Behavior Scale was administered to 419 Japanese men undergoing coronary angiography; 310 of them had angiographic or clinical evidence or both of CAD, and 109 had no evidence of CAD. The group with CAD had more coronary risk factors than the group without CAD, but the 2 groups did not differ in type A behavior pattern as assessed with the Jenkins-Activity Survey. Stepwise discriminant analysis, in which standard coronary risk factors were forced into the model, revealed that inclusion of 9 Japanese Coronary-Prone Behavior Scale items (scale C) in the model resulted in the best discrimination between the 2 groups. Cross-validation results showed that the error-rate estimates for the discriminant models that consisted only of standard coronary risk factors, only of scale C items, and of their combination were 35%, 32%, and 27%, respectively. The scale C items represented a job-centered lifestyle, social dominance, and suppressed overt type A behaviors. These results indicate that an independent behavior pattern prone to CAD is discernible among Japanese men and suggest that the behavior pattern may contain characteristics that can be differentiated from those that constitute the type A behavior pattern.

Insulin Resistance in Nondiabetic Men

Variants of the angiotensinogen gene may increase the risk of having arterial hypertension and CAD, but their effect on insulin resistance remains unknown. Sheu and associates[49] from Taiwan, Republic of China, determined M235 and T174 allele status and fasting plasma glucose, insulin, and lipid values in nondiabetic men with CAD documented on angiography (n = 102) and in a control group (n = 145). Plasma glucose and insulin responses to 75 gm oral glucose tolerant test and insulin resistance as measured by an insulin suppression test were also carried out in 46 (45%) patients with CAD and in 73 (50%) members of a control group. There was no association between M235T status and BP, fasting plasma glucose, insulin, most of the lipids values, and insulin resistance in patients with CAD and normal subjects. Nevertheless, compared with individuals with homozygotes T174, subjects with heterozygotes T174M were associated with greater glucose and insulin response to the oral glucose tolerance test and insulin resistance indicated by higher steady-state plasma glucose concentrations in patients with CAD. Similar findings were found in the control group, with higher steady-state plasma glucose values in individuals with heterozygotes T174M than in those with homozygotes T174. These data suggest that the angiotensinogen T174M allele might be associated with insulin resistance in nondiabetic men with and without CAD.

Vascular Stress Response in Postmenopausal Women

This study by Merz and associates[50] from Los Angeles, California; Bethesda, Maryland; Toronto, Canada; and New York, New York, tested the hypothesis that postmenopausal women demonstrate greater vascular instability, measured by enhanced cardiovascular stress responses during mental stress, compared with men and premenopausal women. Recent data suggest that estrogen plays a role in regulating vascular tone. The possible consequences of estrogen deficiency during menopause on systemic vascular reactivity is largely unexplored. One hundred subjects (84 men and 16 women) underwent mental stress testing with radionuclide ventriculography. Study subjects included 19 normal volunteers, 23 control subjects with chest pain syndromes or hypertension but without CAD, and 58 CAD subjects. The subjects performed a series of 3 mental stress tasks, during which hemodynamic data and radionuclide ventriculograms were obtained. Overall, women demonstrated greater hemodynamic responses during mental stress measured by changes in heart rate, systolic and diastolic BP, and double product stress responses compared with those of men. Women with CAD demonstrated greater heart rate, diastolic BP, and double product stress responses than their male counterparts. Women of postmenopausal age demonstrated significantly greater systolic BP reactivity than men or premenopausal women. Women of postmenopausal age have greater cardiovascular responses to stress than men or premenopausal women. These findings suggest an additional mechanism by which estrogen deficiency conveys a poor prognosis in female patients with CAD.

Coronary Side Effects Potential of Antimigraine Drugs

VanDenBrink and colleagues[51] in Rotterdam, The Netherlands, compared the coronary vasoconstrictor potential of a number of current and prospective antimigraine drugs, including ergotamine, dihydroergotamine, methysergide

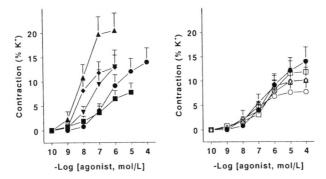

FIGURE 2-17. Concentration-response (expressed as % of response to 100 mmol/L K⁺) curves in human isolated coronary arteries (n = 9) obtained with current **Left:** ergotamine, ▲; dihydroergotamine, ◆; methysergide, ■; and its metabolite methylergometrine ▼, and potential. **Right:** zolmitriptan, □; rizatriptan, ◇; naratriptan, △; and avitriptan, ○, antimigraine drugs compared with sumatriptan (●). Data are mean ± SEM. Reproduced with permission from VanDenBrink et al.[51]

and its metabolite methylergometrine, sumatriptan, naratriptan, zolmitriptan, rizatriptan, and avitriptan. Concentration-response curves to the antimigraine drugs were constructed in human isolated coronary artery segments to obtain the maximal contractile response and the concentration eliciting 50% of E_{max}. The EC_{50} values were related to maximal plasma concentrations (C_{max}) reported in patients, obtaining C_{max}/EC_{50} ratios as an index of coronary vasoconstriction occurring in the clinical setting. They studied the duration of contractile responses after washout of the acutely acting antimigraine drugs to assess their disappearance from the receptor biophase. Compared with sumatriptan, all drugs were more potent in contracting the coronary artery but had similar efficacies. The C_{max} of avitriptan was 7- to 11-fold higher than its EC_{50} value, whereas those of the other drugs were <40% of their respective EC_{50} values. The contractile responses to ergotamine and dihydroergotamine persisted even after repeated washings, but those to other drugs declined rapidly after washing. Thus, all current and prospective antimigraine drugs contract the human coronary artery *in vitro,* but these drugs are unlikely to cause myocardial ischemia at therapeutic plasma concentrations in healthy subjects. In patients with coronary heart disease, however, these drugs should remain contraindicated. The sustained contraction by ergotamine and dihydroergotamine seems to be an important disadvantage compared with sumatriptan-like drugs (Figure 2-17).

Detection and Prognostic Implications for Coronary Artery Disease in Exercise Testing

Prognostic Significance of Ischemic ST-Segment Response

Rywik and colleagues[52] in Baltimore, Maryland, analyzed the treadmill exercise tests of 825 healthy volunteers between 22 and 89 years of age in the Baltimore Longitudinal Study of Aging. All subjects were without clinical evidence of CAD as indicated by history, physical exam, and resting electrocardiogram. Among 825 participants, 611 had no ischemic ST-segment changes during or after treadmill exercise, but 214 subjects developed 1 mm or more flat or downsloping ST-segment depression. Among these 214 subjects, 151 (group 1) had ST-segment changes starting during exercise, and 63 (group 2) had changes limited to recovery. Groups 1 and 2 were similar in age, gender, smoking status, hypertension prevalence, fasting plasma glucose, and serum cholesterol. However, both groups were older and had higher serum cholesterol values and prevalence of hypertension than the patients who had no ischemic ST-segment changes during or after treadmill exercise. Treadmill exercise duration, peak oxygen consumption, and maximal heart rate were similar between groups 1 and 2, but they were lower than in the group without ischemic changes with exercise stress. During a mean follow-up time of 9 years, 55 subjects developed coronary events, including angina, AMI, or coronary death: 21 of 611 (3%) in the group without ischemic ST-segment changes during or after treadmill exercise, 22 of 151 (15%) in the group with ST-segment changes starting during exercise, and 12 of 63 (19%) in the group with ST-segment changes limited to the recovery period. By survival analysis, the risk of coronary events was similar in the patients who had ST-segment changes at the beginning of exercise and only during the recovery period, but they were significantly higher than in those patients who had no ischemic ST-segment changes during or following exercise stress. Multiple logistic regression showed that age, total serum cholesterol, and presence of ST-segment depression were independent predictors of events (Figure 2-18). Therefore, ischemic ST-segment changes developing during recovery from treadmill exercise in apparently healthy individuals have the same adverse prognostic significance as those patients in whom ST-segment changes occurred during exercise.

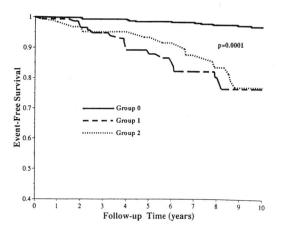

FIGURE 2-18. Event-free survival for groups 0 (normal exercise tests), 1 (ischemic ST response during exercise), and 2 (ischemic ST response limited to recovery). Survival curves for groups 1 and 2 are similar but lie significantly below that of group 0. Reproduced with permission from Rywik et al.[52]

Use of Exercise Training to Improve Thallium Uptake and Contractile Response

Belardinelli and colleagues[53] in Los Angeles, California, investigated whether exercise training can improve thallium uptake and contractile response of low-dose dobutamine of dysfunctional myocardium in 46 patients with chronic CAD and impaired LV systolic function with LVEFs less than 40% and were randomly assigned to 2 groups. The exercise group (n = 26) underwent exercise training at 60% of peak oxygen uptake for 8 weeks. The control group (n = 20) was not exercised. At baseline and after 8 weeks, all patients underwent an exercise test with gas exchange analysis and stress echocardiography using low-dose dobutamine (5 to 10 μg/kg/min) followed by thallium myocardial scintigraphy. Coronary arteriography was performed in 23 patients at baseline and after 8 weeks. After 8 weeks, peak oxygen uptake increased significantly only in trained patients. Significant improvements in contractile performance to dobutamine and thallium activity were observed in training patients versus controls (Figure 2-19). In a subgroup of trained patients, both improvements were correlated with an increase in coronary collateral score. Thus, moderate exercise training improves both thallium-201 uptake and the contractile response of dysfunctional myocardium to low-dose dobutamine in patients with ischemic cardiomyopathy.

Clinical Value of Exercise Treadmill Testing

Exercise treadmill testing is frequently performed to screen for CAD in asymptomatic individuals. Its clinical value, however, is unclear. Pilote and associates[54] from Cleveland, Ohio, examined a consecutive cohort of asymptomatic adults undergoing exercise treadmill testing at the Cleveland Clinic Foundation between September 1990 and December 1993. Endpoints included

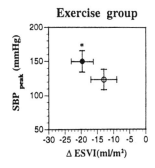
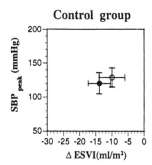

Figure 2-19. Effect of exercise training on systolic blood pressure–end-systolic volume index (SBP-ESVI) relationship. In the exercise group, an increase in SBP was accompanied by a reduction in ESVI from rest to peak dobutamine. The pressure-volume relationship was shifted upward and to the left (p < 0.001). No significant changes in the pressure-volume relationship were observed in the control group. ○ = Baseline; ● = 8 weeks. Reproduced with permission from Belardinelli et al.[53]

(1) identification of subjects with severe CAD and (2) performance of any second diagnostic study within 90 days of the index exercise treadmill test. Screening exercise treadmill testing was performed in 4,334 adults (median age 51, 89% men); only 34% had 1 or more cardiac risk factors and 15% exhibited an abnormal response to exercise. A second test after treadmill testing was performed in 215 patients (in 110, coronary angiography; in 105, stress thallium scintigraphy, followed by coronary angiography in 16). The strongest predictor of referral for a second test was an ischemic ST-segment response (adjusted odds ratio [OR] 34). The only clinical variable independently associated with referral for a second test was female gender (adjusted OR 0.35). Of the 126 patients who underwent coronary angiography, severe CAD was identified in only 19 individuals (0.44% of the original cohort); CABG was performed in 14 of these patients. The estimated cost of exercise treadmill testing to identify 1 case of severe CAD for which surgical revascularization may provide a survival benefit was $39,623. The estimated cost per year of lives saved was at least $55,274. Thus, as used in actual practice in 1 center, screening exercise treadmill testing has a low yield and is costly. This is perhaps in part because of the low-risk population that was selected and the failure to incorporate pre-test variables, increasing probability of disease into post-test clinical decision making.

Comparison of Indicators of Myocardial Ischemia

Sheps and associates[55] from multiple US medical centers compared and contrasted indicators of myocardial ischemia in a well-characterized group of 196 patients with CAD documented angiographically or by verified history of AMI and a positive exercise test result. Myocardial ischemia occurs frequently in response to every day stressors in patients with CAD. The Psychophysiological Interventions in Myocardial Ischemia Study provides a unique opportunity to study neuroendocrine and psychological manifestations of myocardial ischemia. Patients with exercise-induced ischemia underwent exercise radionuclide ventriculography and electrocardiographic monitoring and 2 laboratory mental stressors (Speech and Stroop) after being withdrawn from cardiac medications. In addition, 48-hour ambulatory electrocardiograms were recorded during routine daily activities. Patients with a history of angina within the past 3 months reported angina during the bicycle or treadmill test with a much higher frequency than patients without such an anginal history (77% vs. 26%). Ejection fraction (EF) responses to the Stroop test were abnormal in 48% of patients with an abnormal EF response to the Speech task, versus 17% in patients with a normal EF response. Seventy-six percent of patients had an abnormal EF response to bicycle exercise. Three indicators of ischemia (ST-segment depression, wall motion abnormality, and EF response) were compared during the same laboratory stressor and across different types of stress tests. Presence of the 3 indicators was only moderately associated during exercise, and only weak or nonsignificant associations occurred among the presence of the 3 ischemic markers during mental stress. Occurrence of the same ischemic markers was moderately associated between the 2 mental stress tasks, but few associations were found between the occurrence of the same ischemic marker during exercise and mental stress. There is a marked heterogeneity of responses to psychological and exercise stress testing using electrocardiography, ambulatory electrocardiography, or radionuclide criteria for ischemia during stress. The heterogeneity may be related to differences in the magnitude or types of physiologic responses provoked and to differences in the sensitivity and specificity of the different tests used to identify ischemia.

Evaluation of Exercise Thallium Scintigraphy Versus Exercise Electrocardiography

Studies have demonstrated the value of stress nuclear cardiac scintigraphy in the prognosis of patients with CAD. Parisi and colleagues[56] from Providence, Rhode Island; West Haven, Connecticut; and Worcester, Massachusetts, focused a study on patients with proven angiographic low-risk profile (single- and double-vessel CAD). Three hundred twenty-eight patients with documented single- and double-vessel disease were treated by random assignment to PTCA or medical therapy in the Angioplasty Compared to Medicine (ACME) trial. Six months after randomization, maximal symptom limited exercise tests were performed with electrocardiography (n = 300) and thallium scintigraphy (n = 270). Patients were followed for a minimum of 5 years thereafter. A reversible thallium perfusion deficit documented after 6 months of either therapy was associated with an adverse mortality outcome (18% mortality vs. 8% with no reversible defect). Moreover, an important mortality gradient was demonstrated in relation to the number of reperfusing defects (0 = 7%, 1–2 = 5%, >3 = 20%). Exercise electrocardiogram did not predict this mortality outcome. These authors conclude that a reversible thallium perfusion deficit demonstrated 6 months after medical therapy or PTCA is a valuable prognostic marker in patients with angiographically documented single- and double-vessel disease and is superior to exercise electrocardiography.

Effect of Gender on Diagnostic Evaluation with Treadmill Testing

Controversy exists as to whether a gender bias exists that affects the diagnostic approach to suspected CAD: previous studies have used coronary angiography, but not other noninvasive testing, as a primary endpoint. This investigation by Lauer and associates[57] from Cleveland, Ohio, examined post-test gender differences in diagnostic evaluation after exercise treadmill testing according to a broader endpoint than just coronary angiography alone. The design was a cohort analytic study with a 90-day follow-up. The study was done at the Cleveland Clinic Foundation, an academic group practice. Patients included consecutive adults (1,023 men and 579 women) with chest pain but no documented CAD who were referred for symptom-limited exercise treadmill testing without adjunctive imaging; none had undergone prior invasive cardiac procedures. Main outcomes measures included (1) performance of any subsequent diagnostic study (invasive or noninvasive) and (2) performance of coronary angiography as the next diagnostic study. During follow-up, 89 (8.7%) men and 48 (8.3%) women underwent a second diagnostic study, whereas 64 (6.3%) men and 21 (3.6%) women went straight to coronary angiography. In multivariable logistic regression analyses, which considered baseline clinical characteristics, the ST-segment response, and other prognostically important exercise responses, women tended to be less likely than men to be referred to any second test but were markedly and significantly less likely to be referred straight to coronary angiography. After exercise treadmill testing, women are only slightly less likely than men to be referred for subsequent diagnostic testing; they are, however, much less likely to be referred straight to coronary angiography as opposed to another noninvasive study.

Hibernation and Stunning

Effects of Altered Patterns of Expression of Connexin43

In this study, Kaprielian and colleagues[58] in London, United Kingdom, investigated the hypothesis that altered patterns of expression of connexin43, the principal gap junctional protein responsible for passive conduction of the cardiac action potential, contributes to the pathogenesis of hibernation. Patients with reduced LVEFs and severe CAD underwent thallium-201 scanning and magnetic resonance imaging to predict regions of normally perfused, reversibly ischemic, or hibernating myocardium. Twenty-one patients went on to CABG during which biopsies representative of each of the above classes were taken. Hibernation was confirmed by improvement in segmental wall motion at reassessment 6 months after CABG. Connexin43 was measured by quantitative immunoconfocal laser scanning microscopy and using image software. Analyses revealed a significant reduction in relative connexin43 content per unit area in reversibly ischemic and hibernating tissue compared with normal tissue (Figure 2-20). The hibernating region was further characterized by loss of the larger gap junctions normally seen at the disk periphery, reflected by a significant reduction in mean junctional plaque size in the hibernating tissues compared with reversibly ischemic and normal segments. These data suggest progressive reduction and disruption of connexin43 gap junctions in reversibly ischemic and hibernating myocardial tissue.

Predicting Recovery of Left Ventricular Function After Revascularization

Kitsiou and colleagues[59] in Bethesda, Maryland, hypothesized that stress-induced reversible thallium-201 defects may better differentiate reversible from irreversible regional LV dysfunction after revascularization. Twenty-four patients with chronic CAD underwent pre-revascularization and post-revascu-

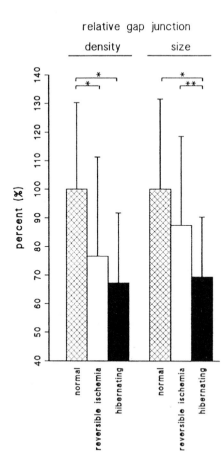

FIGURE **2-20.** Histograms showing results of quantification of disk gap junction density and gap junction size expressed relative to values obtained from control segments. Reversibly ischemic and hibernating tissues show significant reductions in gap junctional density in individual disks (ANOVA p < 0.001). Hibernating tissue contains significantly smaller gap junctions than other groups (ANOVA p < 0.001). Bars = SD; *p′ < 0.001; **p′ = 0.012. Reproduced with permission from Kaprielian et al.[58]

larization exercise-redistribution-reinjection thallium single photon emission CT, gated MRI, and radionuclide ventriculography. After revascularization, mean LVEF increased from 30% ± 9% to 37% ± 13% at rest. In this study, revascularization included the use of CABG and PTCA. Before revascularization, abnormal contraction at rest was observed in 56 of 110 reversible and 20 of 37 mild-to-moderate irreversible thallium defects. After revascularization, regional contraction improved in 44 of 56 reversible compared with 6 of 20 mild-to-moderate irreversible thallium defects (79% and 30%, respectively, p<0.001) (Figure 2-21). The final thallium content was significantly higher in regions with reversible defects that improved than in those that did not improve after revascularization. Final thallium-201 content was similar in regions with mild-to-moderate irreversible defects that improved and in those that did not improve after revascularization. When asynergic regions were grouped according to the final thallium content, functional recovery was observed in 83% of regions with reversible defects compared with 33% of regions with mild-to-moderate irreversible defects. Thus, these data suggest that although both reversible and mild-to-moderate irreversible thallium defects after stress contain viable myocardium, the identification of reversible thallium defect on stress in an asynergic region accurately predicts recovery of function after revascularization.

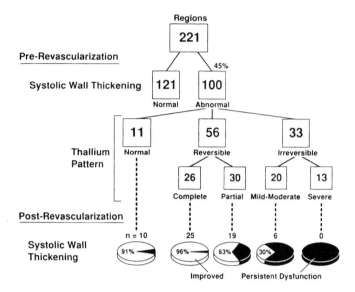

FIGURE 2-21. Flow diagram of pre-revascularization systolic wall thickening and thallium pattern and post-revascularization functional outcome of the 221 revascularized regions. Reproduced with permission from Kitsiou et al.[59]

Ultrasonic Tissue Characterization Predicts Myocardial Viability

Takiuchi and colleagues[60] in Osaka, Japan, characterized temporal changes in cyclic variation of ultrasonic integrated backscatter, which reflects intrinsic contractile performance in patients with reperfused AMI and determined clinical value of tissue characterization in predicting myocardial viability. They recorded short-axis ultrasonic integrated backscatter images before and 3, 7, and 21 days after reperfusion in 26 patients with AMI and obtained the cyclic variation for these images in the normal and infarct zones. When cyclic variation showed synchrony and asynchrony, they expressed its magnitude as positive and negative values, respectively, called the phase-corrected magnitude. They also measured average wall motion score of the infarct segments. The phase-corrected magnitude was lower in the infarct zone than in the normal zone before reperfusion. At day 3, the phase-corrected magnitude increased despite no improvement in wall motion. Improvement in wall motion was observed only at day 21. The patients with the phase-corrected magnitude of 2.0 dB or higher at day 3 showed significantly lower wall motion score at day 21 than did the other patients. Thus, in patients with AMI, cyclic variation of ultrasonic integrated backscatter is blunted during ischemia, but recovers much faster after reperfusion than improvement in wall motion. The greater phase-corrected magnitude at day 3 may be a predictor of better functional improvement.

Assessment of Myocardial Viability with Magnetic Resonance Tagging

Geskin and colleagues[61] in Pittsburgh, Pennsylvania, hypothesized that magnetic resonance tagging could be used to quantify the intramyocardial response to low-dose dobutamine in patients with first AMI. Twenty patients with a first reperfused AMI, including 11 with inferior AMIs were evaluated. Patients underwent breath-hold magnetic resonance tagged short-axis imaging on day 4 after MI and during dobutamine infusions at 5 and 10 μg/kg/min. At 8 weeks after AMI, patients returned for a follow-up magnetic resonance tagging study without dobutamine. Quantification of recent intramyocardial circumferential segment shortening was performed. Low-dose dobutamine magnetic resonance imaging was well tolerated. Overall, mean percent circumferential segment shortening was 15% ± 11% at baseline, increased to 16% ± 10% at 5 μg/kg/min dobutamine and 18% ± 10% at 8 weeks. The increase in percent segmental shortening with peak dobutamine was greater in dysfunctional myocardium. In dysfunctional regions, the percent segmental shortening also increased from 6% ± 7% at baseline to 14% ± 10% at 8 weeks after MI. In dysfunctional segments that responded normally to peak dobutamine, i.e., a 5% or greater increase in segmental shortening, the increase in percent segmental shortening from baseline to 8 weeks after MI was greater than in those regions that did not respond normally. Mid-myocardial and subepicardial responses to dobutamine were predictive of functional recovery, but the subendocardial response was not. The response of intramyocardial function to low-dose dobutamine after reperfused AMI can be quantified with magnetic resonance tagging. Dysfunctional tissue after MI demonstrates a larger contractile response to dobutamine than normal myocardium. A normal increase in shortening elicited by dobutamine within dysfunctional midwall and subepicardium predicts greater functional recovery at 8 weeks after MI, but the response within the subendocardium is not predictive.

Assessment of Myocardial Viability

Srinivasan and colleagues[62] determined whether single photon emission computed tomography (SPECT) cameras allow imaging of positron-emitting tracers, such as [18F]fluorodeoxyglucose (18FDG) to be accomplished. They examined differences between SPECT and PET technologies and between 18FDG and thallium tracers to determine whether 18FDG SPECT could be adopted for assessment of myocardial viability. Twenty-eight patients with chronic CAD and with mean LVEF of 33% ± 15% underwent 18FDG SPECT, 18FDG PET, and thallium SPECT studies. Receiver operating characteristic curves showed overall good agreement between SPECT and PET technologies and thallium and 18FDG tracers for assessing viability regardless of the level of 18FDG PET cutoff (ranging from 40% to 60%). However, in the subgroup with LVEF 25% or greater at 60% 18FDG PET threshold, thallium-201 underestimated myocardial viability. In a subgroup of patients with LV regions with severe asynergy, there was considerably more thallium/[18]FDG discordance in the inferior wall than elsewhere indicating attenuation of thallium-201 as a possible explanation. When uptake of [18]FDG by SPECT and PET was compared in 137 segments exhibiting severely irreversible thallium defects, i.e., scars as detected by thallium-201, 59 (43%) were viable by [18]FDG PET, of which 52 (88%) were also viable by [18]FDG SPECT. However, among 78 segments confirmed to be nonviable by [18]FDG PET, 57 (73%) were nonviable by [18]FDG SPECT (p<.001). Therefore, although [18]FDG SPECT increases the sensitivity for detection of viable myocardium in tissue declared nonviable by thallium, it sometimes falsely identifies as viable tissue nonviable tissue identified by both PET and thallium-201 scans.

Echo Dobutamine International Cooperative Study

Picano and colleagues[63] in Pisa, Italy, assessed the impact on survival of echocardiographically detected viability in medically treated patients with global LV dysfunction after AMI that was uncomplicated. The data bank of a large-scale, prospective, multicenter, observational Echo Dobutamine International Cooperative (EDIC) study was used to select 314 medically treated patients who were administered low-dose dobutamine for the detection of myocardial viability and high-dose dobutamine for the detection of myocardial ischemia performed 12 ± 6 days after AMI and showing a moderate to severe resting LV dysfunction. Patients were followed for 9 ± 7 months. Low-dose dobutamine stress echocardiography identified myocardial viability in 130 patients (52%). Dobutamine-atropine stress echocardiography was positive for ischemia in 148 patients (47%) and negative in 166 patients (53%). During the follow-up, there were 12 cardiac deaths. With the use of the Cox proportional hazards model, the delta low-dose wall motion score index was shown to exert a protective effect by reducing cardiac death by 0.8 for each decrease in wall motion score index at low-dose dobutamine. Wall motion score index at peak stress was the best predictor of cardiac death in these patients (Figure 2-22). Thus, in medically treated patients with severe global LV dysfunction early after AMI that is uncomplicated, the presence of myocardial viability identified as inotropic reserve after low-dose dobutamine is associated with a higher probability of survival.

Viable Myocardium After Acute Myocardial Infarction

Viable myocardium after AMI may be characterized by magnetic resonance imaging (MRI) either by demonstration of recovery of wall motion under dobutamine stress or by perfusion patterns after contrast medium administration. This study by Dendale and associates[64] from Brussels, Belgium, and Leiden, The Netherlands, examines the relation between the 2 techniques. Gradient-echo MRI at rest and under low-dose dobutamine stress was performed in 28 patients within the first 2 weeks after AMI. In addition, spin-echo MRI

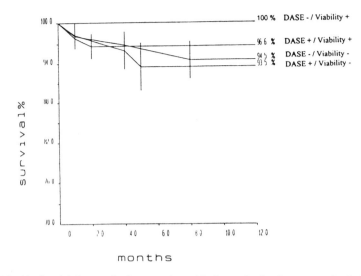

FIGURE 2-22. Kaplan-Meier survival curves (considering only death as an endpoint) in patients stratified according to presence or absence of echocardiographically assessed viability and ischemia at low and high doses of dobutamine, respectively. Best survival is observed in patients with low-dose viability and no inducible ischemia; worst survival is observed in patients without viability and with inducible ischemia. Viability + and viability − indicate presence or absence of myocardial viability at low-dose dobutamine, respectively; DASE + and DASE − indicate presence or absence of myocardial ischemia at high-dose dobutamine, respectively. Reproduced with permission from Picano et al.[63]

was performed after gadolinium-DOTA administration. Wall motion at rest and under stress was scored to assess the contractile reserve of the infarct regions. Infarct enhancement patterns were classified as subendocardial, transmural, or as a doughnut pattern. Subendocardial or absent infarct enhancement was related to functional recovery under stress in 31 of 37 infarct segments. Transmural infarct enhancement was correlated with the absence of functional recovery in 10 of 17 infarct segments, indicating nonviability. The doughnut pattern was exclusively associated with the absence of viability. Contrast enhancement patterns are related to residual myocardial viability.

Histologic Changes in Hibernating Myocardium

The objective of this study by Hennessey and associates[65] from Dublin, Ireland, was to correlate histologic change in hibernating myocardium with dobutamine stress echocardiography (DSE). Patients (n = 8) with anterior regional wall motion abnormalities in the 7 echocardiographic segments representing the territory supplied by a significantly stenosed LAD coronary artery had preoperative DSE performed (yielding 56 segments for analysis). Two transmural biopsy specimens were taken from the anterior wall of the left ventricle during CAGB. Morphometric histologic analysis of biopsy specimens showed significantly less fibrosis in segments demonstrating inotropic reserve and significantly less fibrosis in segments demonstrating improvement in wall motion on echocardiography 3 months after revascularization. DSE had a sensitivity of 100% and a specificity of 62% for detection of hibernating myocardial segments. Percent fibrosis was inversely correlated with percent nucleated cells and directly correlated with cytoplasmic clearance. Inotropic response during DSE correlates with histologic evidence of hibernating myocardium.

Assessment of Myocardial Viability

The aim of this study by Vernon and associates[66] from Charlottesville, Virginia, was to compare perfusion patterns on myocardial contrast echocardiography with those on myocardial perfusion scintigraphy for the assessment of myocardial viability in patients with previous myocardial infarction. Accordingly, perfusion scores with the 2 techniques were compared in 91 ventricular regions in 21 patients with previous (>6 weeks old) myocardial infarction. Complete concordance between the 2 techniques was found in 63 (69%) regions; 25 (27%) regions were discordant by only 1 grade, and complete discordance (2 grades) was found in only 3 (3%) regions. A kappa statistic of 0.65 indicated good concordance between the 2 techniques. Although the scores on both techniques demonstrated a relation with the wall motion score, the correlation between the myocardial contrast echocardiography and wall motion scores was closer. It is concluded that myocardial contrast echocardiography provides similar information regarding myocardial viability as myocardial perfusion scintigraphy in patients with CAD and previous myocardial infarction.

Viable Myocardium

The recognition of dysfunctional but viable myocardium after AMI may be of importance for both patient prognostication and the decision for revascularization. Low-dose dobutamine echocardiography has been shown to be a reliable technique in detecting reversibility of dysfunctional myocardium. The aim of the present study by Knudsen and associates[67] from Aarbus, Denmark, was to assess by low-dose dobutamine echocardiography possible time-dependent changes in myocardial viability and to evaluate the utility of low-dose dobutamine echocardiography in the postinfarction period. Twenty-seven patients with AMI underwent low-dose dobutamine echocardiography on days 6, 30, and 90. At low-dose dobutamine day 6, 41% of the affected segments showed a positive response to low-dose dobutamine echocardiography. At later examination on days 30 and 90, only 32% and 18%, respectively, of the dysfunctioning segments responded to dobutamine stimulation with a significant decline in response, indicating loss of viability. Spontaneous segmental outcome was significantly better for low-dose dobutamine echocardiography-responding segments than for nonresponding segments. This study indicates that myocardial viability may be temporary and that a time-dependent loss of viability may take place during the first months after AMI.

Coronary Blood Flow

Regional Myocardial Blood Flow Redistribution

Baliga and colleagues[68] in London, United Kingdom, determined whether redistribution of myocardial blood flow, from a region supplied by a severely stenotic artery to those supplied by less diseased or normal vessels, is a mechanism responsible for postprandial angina. They determined the effects of a standard liquid meal on whole heart and regional myocardial blood flow measured by dynamic positron emission tomography (PET) with ^{15}O-labeled water in 14 patients with a reproducible history of postprandial angina and 7 matched control subjects. The standard liquid meal precipitated angina in all patients. Baseline whole heart blood flow was similar and increased normally after the meal in patients as in control subjects. However, the coefficient of variation of blood flow increased significantly after the standard liquid meal in patients, but not in control subjects. In these patients, regional myocardial blood flow decreased in territories supplied by stenotic arteries, but there was an increase in blood flow in territories supplied by normal arteries after the meal (Figure 2-23). Thus, a standard liquid meal inducing angina pectoris in patients with CAD is associated with the redistribution of regional blood flow from territories supplied by severely stenotic coronary arteries to those supplied by less diseased or normal arteries.

Radionuclide Measures of Blood Flow

In a previous study from a single center, radionuclide measures of collateral flow with technetium 99m (^{99m}Tc) sestamibi have been shown to be signifi-

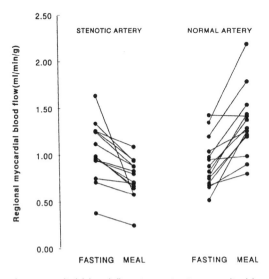

FIGURE 2-23. Regional myocardial blood flow in territories supplied by stenotic and normal arteries, in the fasting state, and after the standard liquid meal in patients with postprandial angina. Reproduced with permission from Baliga et al.[68]

cantly associated with angiographic residual (antegrade and collateral) flow and independent predictors of final infarct size in AMI. This study by Chareon-thaitawee and associates[69] from Rochester, Minnesota; Royal Oak, Michigan; Kansas City, Missouri; and Tulsa, Oklahoma, examined whether the previously described radionuclide measures of blood flow to the infarct zone were reproducible with different laboratories and imaging systems. Residual flow to the infarct zone was assessed by both invasive and noninvasive methods in 77 patients with first-time myocardial infarction (32 anterior, 45 nonanterior). All patients underwent acute coronary angiography before any intervention within 8 hours of the onset of chest pain (4.0 $\pm$ 1.5 hours; range 1.2 to 7.9 hours). ^{99m}Tc sestamibi was injected intravenously before reperfusion therapy, and tomographic imaging was performed 1 to 6 hours after injection. A central core laboratory processed the acquired images from 3 centers, each with a unique camera and computer system. Three previously published methods based on the severity of the acute perfusion defect were used to measure residual flow to the infarct zone (nadir, severity index, area). Antegrade (Thrombolysis in Myocardial Infarction [TIMI] flow) and collateral flow before direct angioplasty were blindly graded on a 4-point scale (0 to 3) from the acute angiogram. The simple sum of the 2 grades was defined as the angiographic flow index, representing residual flow to the jeopardized zone. All 3 noninvasive measures of residual flow were highly associated with the angiographic flow index in a linear fashion: severity index, area, and nadir. This association was independent of the laboratory where the data were acquired. Despite different laboratories and camera systems, radionuclide measures of residual flow were highly associated with the angiographic flow index before reperfusion therapy. These results suggest that these measures are applicable on a broader scale for the noninvasive determination of collateral and antegrade flow in AMI.

Use of Long-Term L-Arginine Supplementation

Lerman and colleagues[70] at the Mayo Clinic conducted a double-blind, randomized study to test the hypothesis that long-term, 6-month supplementation of L-arginine, the precursor of the endothelium-derived vasodilator NO, reverses coronary endothelial dysfunction to acetylcholine in patients with nonobstructive CAD. Twenty-six patients without significant CAD on coronary angiography and intravascular ultrasound were randomized to receive either oral L-arginine or placebo 3 g 3 times a day. Endothelium-dependent coronary blood flow reserve to acetylcholine was assessed at baseline and after 6 months of therapy. There were no differences between the 2 study groups in clinical characteristics or in the coronary blood flow in the response to acetylcholine at baseline. After 6 months, the coronary blood flow in response to acetylcholine increased in the subjects taking L-arginine compared with the placebo group (Figure 2-24). There was a decrease in plasma endothelin concentrations and an improvement in patients' symptom scores in the L-arginine treatment group compared with the placebo group. Thus, long-term oral L-arginine supplementation for 6 months in humans improves coronary small vessel endothelial function in association with a significant improvement in symptoms and a

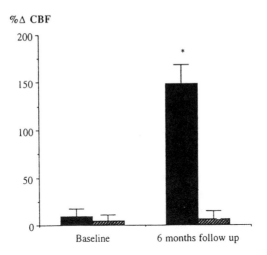

%Δ CBF

FIGURE 2-24. Percent changes in CBF in response to 10^{-4} mol/L of acetylcholine at baseline and at 6-month follow-up in 2 study groups (solid bars = group 1, L-arginine; hatched bars = group 2, placebo; *p<0.05 between groups and compared with baseline). Reproduced with permission from Lerman et al.[70]

decrease in plasma endothelin concentrations. These data suggest a role for L-arginine as a therapeutic option for patients with coronary endothelial dysfunction and nonobstructive CAD.

Stable Angina

Differences in Plasma Endothelin Levels

Raised plasma endothelin concentrations have previously been reported in patients with cardiac syndrome X, but it is not known whether these levels vary between clinically distinct subgroups in this heterogeneous condition. Kaski and associates[71] from London, United Kingdom, compared plasma immunoreactive endothelin levels in 54 patients with angina pectoris and normal coronary angiograms and in 21 healthy control subjects. The patient group was divided into 4 clinically distinct subgroups: 7 with left BBB (group A); 7 with previous myocardial infarction (group B); 24 with positive exercise electrocardiography (group C); and 16 with negative exercise electrocardiography (group D). The plasma endothelin concentration was significantly higher in patients compared with control subjects (3.7 [2.9 to 4.3] vs. 3.0 [2.4 to 3.4] pg/mL, respectively). Endothelin concentrations were most significantly elevated in group A and group B (4.5 [3.6 to 5.2] pg/mL; and 4.1 [3.9 to 4.5] pg/mL, respectively). Plasma endothelin concentrations were also significantly elevated in group C (3.7 [2.8 to 4.1] pg/mL) but not in group D (3.0 [2.5 to 3.8] pg/mL). Plasma endothelin concentration is elevated in patients with angina pectoris and angiographically normal coronary arteries, particularly in those with left BBB or previous myocardial infarction.

Evaluation of Coronary Calcium Patterns

Although coronary calcium is invariably associated with atherosclerosis, its role in the pathogenesis of acute and chronic coronary syndromes remains unclear. Utilizing double helical computerized tomography, Shemesh and associates[72] from Tel-Aviv, Israel, evaluated the coronary calcium patterns in 149 patients: 47 with chronic stable angina, compared with 102 patients surviving a first AMI. Prevalence of coronary calcium was 81% among the AMI patients and 100% in the stable angina patients. The 547 calcific lesions identified in the AMI patients and the 1,242 lesions in the stable angina patients were categorized into 3 groups according to their extent: mild, intermediate, and extensive. The age-adjusted percentages of the highest level of calcification among AMI versus stable angina patients were: mild 18% versus 3%, intermediate 49% versus 18%, and extensive lesions 33% versus 79%, respectively. In the AMI group, 73 culprit arteries were identified: 16 (22%) had no calcium detected, whereas 30 (41%) had mild lesions, 20 (27%) had intermediate forms, and only 7 (10%) had extensive lesions. The age-adjusted mean of the natural logarithm transformation of total calcium scores + 1 was significantly lower in patients with AMI than in those with stable angina (4.1 vs. 5.3). Thus, double helical computerized tomography demonstrates that extensive calcium characterizes the coronary arteries of patients with chronic stable angina, whereas a first AMI most often occurs in mildly calcified or noncalcified culprit arteries (Figure 2-25; Table 2-2).

Evaluation of the "Warm-Up" Phenomenon

Most patients with chronic stable angina show improvement in ischemic threshold when a second exercise test is performed a few minutes after a first

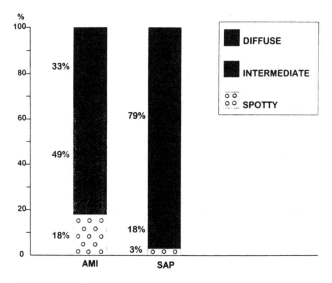

FIGURE 2-25. Distribution of different coronary calcium patterns among AMI and stable angina groups. The age-adjusted percentage of the highest level of calcification is shown. Only patients with detected calcium deposits were included. Reproduced with permission from Shemesh et al.[72]

TABLE 2-2
Extent of Coronary Calcium in Patients with Calcium

	AMI (n = 83)*	Stable Angina (n = 47)	p Value
Number of calcified coronary arteries			0.001
1	34 (41%)	5 (11%)	
2	24 (29%)	16 (34%)	
3	25 (30%)	26 (55%)	
Number of calcific lesions			
Total	547	1,242	
Median (range)	7 (1–67)	12 (1–72)	0.005
Total calcium score			
Median (range)	41.3 (1–1,851)	311 (1–3,727)	0.0001
Log transformed (total calcium score + 1) (mean ± SD)			
All patients	3.9 ± 1.8	5.5 ± 1.8	<0.0001
Age ≤55 years	3.2 ± 1.5	4.7 ± 2.2	0.03
Age >55 years	4.8 ± 1.8	5.9 ± 1.5	0.01
Age-adjusted mean (95% CI)	4.1 (3.7–4.4)	5.3 (4.8–5.8)	<0.05

* The 19 patients without coronary calcium in the AMI group were not included.
Reproduced with permission from Shemesh et al.[72]

positive test. Lupi and associates[73] from Rome, Italy, evaluated whether this "warm-up" phenomenon also occurs in patients with syndrome X. They performed 2 consecutive exercise tests in 14 patients with chronic stable angina and in 11 patients with syndrome X. The second exercise test was performed after 10 minutes from the end of the first one, always after complete recovery to baseline of ST segment. In patients with stable angina, heart rate (108 ± 18 vs. 99 ± 16 beats/min), rate-pressure product (17,020 ± 4,541 vs. 15,215 ± 3,734 beats/min × mm Hg), and exercise time (587 ± 297 vs. 444 ± 244 seconds) at 1-mm ST depression were higher in the second test than in the first one and a significant improvement in these parameters during the second test was also observed at peak exercise. Conversely, in patients with syndrome X, there were no significant differences between the 2 tests in heart rate (128 ± 18 vs. 131 ± 23 beats/min), rate-pressure product (19,922 ± 5,153 vs. 19,390 ± 5,654 beats/min × mm Hg), and exercise time (592 ± 243 vs. 566 ± 228 seconds) at 1-mm ST-segment depression. Similarly, in this group of patients, no significant differences in exercise variables between the 2 tests were observed at peak exercise. Thus, unlike patients with chronic stable angina, patients with syndrome X have no evidence of warm-up in response to repeated exercise testing.

Treatment

Calcium Channel Blocking Agents and Risk of Cancer

Some recent reports have raised the possibility that short-acting calcium channel blockers may increase the risk of cancer. Braun and colleagues[74] from

Tel-Aviv and Tel Hashomer, Israel, evaluated 11,575 patients screened for the Bezfibrate Infarction Prevention study, one-half of whom were treated at the time of screening with calcium channel blockers. Patients were followed over a mean of 2.8 years and cause-specific mortality was analyzed. Of 246 incident cancer cases, 129 occurred among the users and 117 among nonusers of calcium channel blockers. After adjustment for age, gender, and smoking, the odds ratio estimate for all cancers combined was 1.07. This was not statistically significant. These authors conclude that in patients treated with short-acting calcium channel blockers, there is a similar risk of cancer incidence and total cancer-related mortality compared with nonusers of calcium channel blockers.

Direct Costs of Coronary Artery Disease

To generate current incidence-based estimates of the direct costs of CAD in the US, Russell and associates[75] from Morris Plains, New Jersey, and New York, New York, developed a Markov model of the economic costs of CAD-related medical care. Risk of initial and subsequent CAD events (sudden CAD death, fatal/nonfatal AMI, unstable angina, and stable angina) were estimated using new Framingham Heart Study risk equations and population risk profiles derived from national survey data. Costs were assumed to be those related to treatment of initial and subsequent CAD events ("event-related") and follow-up care ("nonevent-related"), respectively. Cost estimates were derived primarily from national public-use databases. First-year direct medical costs of treating CAD events are estimated to be $17,532 for fatal AMI, $15,540 for nonfatal AMI, $2,569 for stable angina, $12,058 for unstable angina, and $713 for sudden CAD death. Nonevent-related direct costs of CAD treatment are estimated to be $1,051 annually. The annual incidence of CAD in the US is estimated at 616,900 cases, with first-year costs of treatment totaling $5.54 billion. Five- and 10-year cumulative costs in 1995 dollars for patients who are initially free of CAD are estimated at $9.2 billion and $16.5 billion, respectively; for all patients with CAD, these costs are estimated to be $71.5 billion and $126.6 billion, respectively. The direct medical costs of CAD create a large economic burden for the US health care system.

Vitamin E Therapy

Epidemiologic studies have suggested that vitamin E (α-tocopheral) may play a preventive role in reducing the frequency of atherosclerosis. Davey and associates[76] from Harrow, United Kingdom, conducted a cost-effectiveness analysis of vitamin E supplementation in patients with CAD using data from the Cambridge Heart Antioxidant Study (CHAOS). The study compared cost-effectiveness in the context of Australian and US health care utilization. The main clinical outcome used in the economic evaluation was the incidence of AMI that was nonfatal. Utilization of health care resources was estimated by conducting a survey of Australian clinicians and published Australian and US cost data. Cost savings of $127 (A$181) and $578/patient randomized to vitamin

E therapy compared with patients receiving placebo was found for Australian and US settings, respectively. Savings in the vitamin E group were due primarily to reduction in hospital admissions for AMI. This occurred because the vitamin E group had a 4.4% lower absolute risk of AMI than did the placebo group. Less than 10% of health care costs in the Australian evaluation was due to vitamin E ($150 [A$214/patient]). The authors' evaluation indicates that vitamin E therapy in patients with angiographically proven coronary atherosclerosis is cost-effective in the Australian and US settings.

Impact of Hormonal Replacement Therapy

Epidemiological evidence suggests that hormonal replacement therapy reduces morbidity and mortality from cardiovascular diseases in postmenopausal women. In a study by McGrath and coinvestigators[77] in Victoria, Australia, indices of arterial function (total systemic arterial compliance and carotid arterial distensibility coefficient), structure (carotid intimal medial thickness), and lipid profiles were compared in postmenopausal women on long-term hormonal replacement therapy and age-matched controls. One hundred nine women aged 44 to 77 years taking hormone replacement therapy and an age-matched group of 108 female controls were entered into the study. The 2 groups were similar for body mass index, smoking status, exercise level, alcohol intake, and BP. Fasting cholesterol, LDL, and lipoprotein(a) were reduced and HDL increased in the hormonal replacement therapy group. Intimal medial thickness increased with age; systemic arterial compliance and distensibility coefficient were reduced with age in both groups. The hormonal replacement therapy group had a higher mean systemic arterial compliance and a lower mean intimal medial thickness than did controls (Figure 2-26). Subgroup analysis for

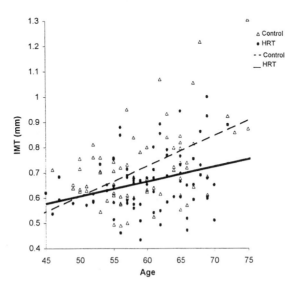

FIGURE 2-26. Intimal medial thickness (IMT)-age relationship in women on HRT and controls. HRT IMT-age regression is represented by $y = 0.006 \times + 0.31$, $r = 0.32$. Control IMT-age regression is represented by $y = 0.012 \times - 0.003$, $r = 0.51$. Reproduced with permission from McGrath et al.[77]

estrogen versus estrogen plus progestin revealed no differences for systemic arterial compliance and intimal medial thickness; distensibility coefficient, however, was greater in estrogen-only users. Smokers on hormonal replacement therapy had higher mean systemic arterial compliance and a lower intimal medial thickness than did smokers not on such therapy. A protective effect of long-term estrogen therapy on age-related changes in arterial structure and function in postmenopausal women was evident in smokers and nonsmokers alike. Progestin appeared to counteract the effects of estrogen on carotid compliance only. The investigators conclude that long-term control trials are needed to determine the significance of these findings.

Protection of Estrogen Replacement Therapy

Estrogen replacement therapy (ERT) in women after menopause is associated with prevention of clinical evidence of myocardial ischemia. Few studies, however, have investigated possible benefits from ERT in postmenopausal women undergoing treatment for established CAD. Abu-Halawa and colleagues[78] from Houston, Texas, retrospectively reviewed the clinical outcomes of 428 postmenopausal women undergoing PTCA to test the hypothesis that ERT has a beneficial effect in this setting. The women were divided into 2 groups based on ERT status at the time of the procedure. Estrogen users were younger (60 ± 10 vs. 68 ± 9 years), more commonly had family histories of CAD (54% vs. 41%), had less incidence of systemic hypertension (63% vs. 76%), and had slightly fewer diseased narrowed coronary arteries per patient (1.3 ± 0.5 vs. 1.5 ± 0.7) compared with nonusers. No in-hospital deaths occurred in estrogen users compared with 5% hospital mortality in nonusers. The combined outcome of death or AMI was also lower in estrogen users (4% vs. 12%). Of 348 women discharged after successful PTCA, 336 (97%) were able to be contacted at an average follow-up interval of 22 ± 17 months (range 5 to 82). Estrogen users had superior event-free survival both for death as well as for death or nonfatal AMI. Repeat revascularization was similar in both groups (32% vs. 24%). In a Cox proportional hazards model, nonusers had 4 times the likelihood of death after coronary angioplasty compared with estrogen users (odds ratio = 4.025). The authors conclude that estrogen replacement may offer protection against coronary events in postmenopausal women who already have established CAD and are undergoing coronary angioplasty. The benefit is independent of age, smoking, presence of diabetes mellitus, or the number of narrowed coronary arteries. It did not include a reduction in repeat revascularization procedures, suggesting no reduction in restenosis (Figure 2-27).

Hormone Replacement Therapy and Coronary Artery Disease

Many studies have suggested that hormone replacement therapy reduces the risk of coronary heart disease. Electron-beam tomography is a highly sensitive noninvasive method by which to detect CAD disease. The objective of

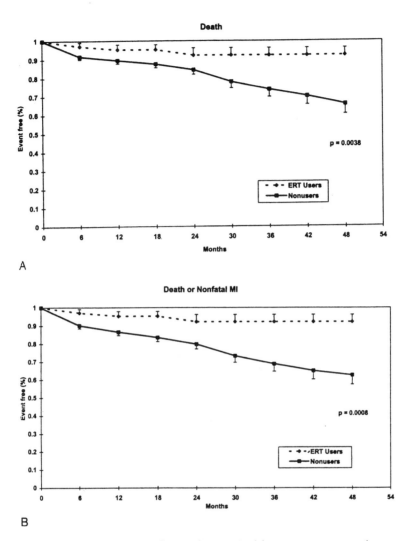

FIGURE 2-27. Kaplan-Meier estimated event-free survival for estrogen users and nonusers. **(A))** death. **(B)** Death or nonfatal myocardial infarction. Reproduced with permission from Abu-Halawa et al.[78]

McLaughlin and associates[79] from Chicago, Illinois, was to investigate whether hormone replacement therapy had an effect on CAD as determined by electron-beam tomography in postmenopausal women. Nine hundred fourteen self-referred postmenopausal women older than 50 years underwent electron-beam tomography. Each woman completed a questionnaire regarding age, risk factors, menopausal status, and hormone replacement therapy. Women taking hormone replacement therapy were slightly younger (58 years) than those not (61 years). A significantly higher frequency of a family history of myocardial infarction and smoking history was found in the group taking hormone replacement therapy, whereas more diabetics were in the group not taking hormone replacement therapy. The mean total coronary artery scores for women receiving hormone replacement therapy and not receiving hormone replacement therapy were 54 and 86, respectively. Independent predictive variables of a positive coronary artery calcium score with multiple logistic regression analysis were age, hypercholesterolemia, diabetes, and estrogen use. These results suggest that hormone replacement therapy is associated with less CAD in postmenopausal women as determined by electron-beam tomography.

Nosocomial Infections

To describe the epidemiology of nosocomial infections in coronary care units in the US, Richards and associates[80] from Atlanta, Georgia, analyzed data collected between 1992 and 1997 using the standard protocols of the National Nosocomial Infectious Surveillance (NNIS) Intensive Care Unit (ICU) surveillance component. Data on 227,451 patients with 6,698 nosocomial infections were analyzed. Urinary tract infections (35%), pneumonia (24%), and primary bloodstream infections (17%) were almost always associated with use of an invasive device (93% with a urinary catheter, 82% with a ventilator, 82% with a central line, respectively). The distribution of pathogens differed from that reported from other types of ICUs. *Staphylococcus aureus* (21%) was the most common species reported from pneumonia and *Escherichia coli* (27%) from urine. Only 10% of reported urine isolates were *Candida albicans*. *S. aureus* (24%) was the more common bloodstream isolate than enterococci (10%). The mean overall patient infection rate was 2.7 infections per 100 patients. Device-associated infection rates from bloodstream infections, pneumonia, and urinary tract infections did not correlate with length of stay, number of hospital

TABLE 2-3
Specific Infection Site Distribution in Coronary Care Unit Patients (NNIS 1992 to 1997)

Infection	Number	Percentage of Selected Major Sites
BSI	1,159	
Laboratory-confirmed BSI	1,085	94
Clinical sepsis	74	6
Pneumonia	1,635	100
UTI	2,321	
Symptomatic UTI	1,282	55
Asymptomatic UTI	1,024	44
Other	15	1
Cardiovascular infection	309	
Vascular	300	97
Endocarditis	8	3
Eye, ear, nose, and throat infection	147	
Sinusitis	79	54
Oral	30	20
Conjunctivitis	27	18
Other	11	8

BSI = bloodstream infection; UTI = urinary tract infection.
Reproduced with permission from Richards et al.[80]

TABLE 2-4

Commonly Reported Pathogens from Patients in Coronary Care Units (NNIS 1992 to 1997)

Pathogen	Bloodstream Infection % (n=1,159)	Pneumonia % (n=1,635)	Urinary Tract Infection % (n=2,321)	Cardiovascular % (n=300)	Eye, Ear, Nose, and Throat Infection % (n=147)
Coagulase-negative staphylococci	37	2	3	46	18
S. aureus	24	21	3	20	17
Enterococcus	10	2	14	11	5
E. coli	3	4	28	2	3
Enterobacter	3	9	4	2	6
C. albicans	3	6	10	4	5
Klebsiella pneumoniae	2	8	6	2	3
Serratia marcescens	2	4	1	1	2
P. aeruginosa	2	14	7	2	8
Other candida	2	1	4	2	12
C. glabrata	2	0.2	3	0.3	
Acinetobacter	1	3	0.2	1	
Other fungi	1	3	5	1	3
Proteus mirabilis	0.6	2	4	1	1
Streptococcus pneumoniae	0.4	2			
Haemophilus influenzae	0.1	3			
Other	7	16	8	5	17

Reproduced with permission from Richards et al.[80]

beds, number of CCU beds, or the hospital teaching affiliation, and were the best rates for comparisons between units. Use of invasive devices was lower than in other types of ICUs. Overall patient infection rates were lower than in other types of ICUs, which is largely explained by lower rates of invasive device usage (Tables 2-3, 2-4).

Erythrocyte Promotion of Platelet Reactivity Decreases Aspirin Effectiveness

Valles and colleagues[81] from Valencia, Spain, had previously shown that platelet reactivity is enhanced by a prothrombotic effect of erythrocytes in a thromboxane-independent manner. This diminishes the antithrombotic therapeutic potential of aspirin. In the present study, the effects of platelet erythrocyte interactions were evaluated *ex vivo* in 82 patients with vascular disease, 62 patients with CAD treated with 200 mg of aspirin/day and 20 patients with ischemic stroke treated with 300 mg ASA/day. Platelet activation (release reaction) and platelet recruitment were assessed after collagen stimulation of platelets, platelet-erythrocyte mixtures, or whole blood. Platelet thromboxane A_2 synthesis was inhibited by more than 94% by aspirin in all patients. Platelet recruitment followed 1 of 3 distinct patterns. In group A (n = 32, 39%), platelet recruitment was blocked by aspirin both in the presence and absence of erythrocytes. In group B (n = 37, 45%), recruitment was abolished when platelets were evaluated alone but continued in the presence of erythrocytes, indicating a suboptimal effect of aspirin on erythrocytes in this patient group. In group C (n = 13, 16%), detectable recruitment in stimulated platelets alone persisted and was markedly enhanced by the presence of erythrocytes. Thus, in two-thirds of the patients with vascular disease, 200 to 300 mg of aspirin was insufficient to block platelet reactivity in the presence of erythrocytes despite abolishing thromboxane A_2 synthesis. Platelet activation in the presence of erythrocytes can induce the release reaction and generate biologically active products that recruit additional platelets into a developing thrombus.

Effect of β-Blocker Therapy

Haim and associates[82] for the Bezafibrate Infarction Prevention (BIP) Study Group investigated the effect of bezafibrate on a large cohort of patients with CAD in functional classes II and III according to the New York Heart Association (NYHA) Classification. Among 11,575 patients with CAD screened for participation, but not included in the BIP study, 3,225 (28%) were in NYHA classes II and III. In the latter group of patients, the prognosis of 1,109 patients (34%) treated with β-blockers was compared with 2,116 counterparts not receiving β-blocker therapy. After a mean follow-up of 4 years, all-cause and cardiac mortality rates were significantly lower among β-blocker therapy patients. After a mean follow-up of 4 years, all-cause and cardiac mortality rates were significantly lower among β-blocker users, 9% and 5%, respectively, than among β-blocker nonusers, 17% and 11%, respectively. After multivariate adjustment, treatment with β-blockers was associated with a lower all-cause mortality risk (hazards ratio [HR] 0.62), and a lower cardiac mortality risk (HR = 0.61) than was no treatment with a β-blocker. Lower total mortality risk was noted among patients in NYHA class II (HR = 0.63) and in NYHA class III (HR = 0.57) as well as in patients with (HR = 0.62) or without (HR = 0.70) a previous AMI. The authors conclude that β-blocker therapy in coronary patients in NYHA classes II or III is safe and associated with a lower risk for all-cause and cardiac mortality.

The Second Transdermal Intermittent Dosing Evaluation (TIDES II) Study

Transdermal nitroglycerin given continuously may cause nitrate tolerance. There are some data, however, to suggest that intermittent transdermal nitrate use may be associated with rebound ischemia. Pepine and colleagues[83] from Gainesville, Florida, and Morgantown, West Virginia, conducted a multicenter, randomized, double-blind, placebo-controlled, crossover trial. Transdermal nitroglycerin (0.2–0.4 mg/hour) significantly reduced the magnitude of ST-segment depression at angina onset during exercise testing compared with placebo. Total angina frequency was not significantly different between transdermal nitroglycerin and placebo (3.2 vs. 3.3). During patch-off hours (10 PM to 8 AM) angina frequency increased with nitroglycerin (1.1 compared with placebo 0.7). Similar trends were noted for silent ischemia during ambulatory electrocardiogram monitoring. These authors conclude that an increase in ischemia frequency during patch-off hours after the use of intermittent transdermal nitroglycerin was perceived by patients, and this subjective finding was supported by a corresponding trend for ambulatory electrocardiogram ischemia to increase during these same hours.

Treatment for Symptomatic Anginal Patients

Anginal patients who remain symptomatic despite optimally dosed β-blockade also may be given dihydropyridine calcium antagonists. Dunselman and associates[84] from several centers in The Netherlands examined this treatment regimen in a double-blind parallel, randomized, controlled study in 147 patients with angina and positive bicycle exercise tests despite optimal β-blockade with atenolol (heart rate at rest <60 beats/min). Patients were randomized to atenolol and/or placebo (control), and atenolol and/or amlodipine. The main outcome measurement was exercise tolerance after 8 weeks compared with baseline. After 8 weeks, no significant differences in time to 0.1-mV ST-segment depression, time to chest pain, and time to end of exercise were observed. The number of patients with chest pain during exercise decreased significantly in the amlodipine group. The subgroup of patients with an early (<6 minutes) onset of chest pain at baseline showed a significant increase in time to chest pain after amlodipine. In the amlodipine group, ST depression and rate-pressure product at submaximum comparable workload decreased to 0.4 mm (0.56) and 1.223 (2.652) beats/min × mm Hg. The number of patients in each group with adverse events was not different. The addition of amlodipine to the treatment of patients with myocardial ischemia, despite optimal β-blockade, is well tolerated and may lead to improvement in symptomatic anginal patients who have a rapid onset of exercise-induced ischemia.

Concomitant Treatment with Captopril

The anti-ischemic efficacy of organic nitrates is rapidly blunted by the development of nitrate tolerance. The underlying mechanisms may be multifactorial and may involve increased vasoconstrictor responsiveness. In 40 male patients with stable CAD, Heitzer and associates[85] from Frieburg and Hamburg, Germany, evaluated vascular reactivity responses to intra-arterial angiotensin II and phenylephrine. The patients were randomized into 4 groups receiving 48 hours of treatment with nitroglycerin or placebo, with or without the ACE-inhibitor captopril. In patients treated with nitroglycerin alone, the maximal reduction in forearm blood flow response to angiotensin II and phenylephrine were markedly greater than in patients receiving placebo. Captopril treatment completely prevented the nitroglycerin-induced hypersensitivity to angiotensin and phenylephrine, but had no significant effect on blood flow responses in patients with nitroglycerin treatment. These authors conclude that continuous administration of nitroglycerin is associated with increased sensitivity to phenylephrine and angiotensin II that is prevented by concomitant treatment with captopril. The prevention of nitroglycerin-induced hypersensitivity to vasoconstrictors by ACE inhibition suggests an involvement of the renin-angiotensin system in mediating this phenomenon.

Comparison of Antianginal Treatments

The antianginal efficacy and tolerability of amlodipine and diltiazem were compared in a double-blind randomized trial of 97 patients with angina resistant to atenolol alone by Knight and Fox on behalf of the Centralized European Studies in Angina Research (CESAR) Investigators.[86] Both amlodipine and diltiazem significantly reduced the frequency of anginal attacks and glycerol trinitrate consumption. During Holter monitoring, both treatments reduced the overall frequency of ambulatory myocardial ischemia, although changes did not reach statistical significance. Exercise test parameters (total exercise time, time to angina, time to ST depression, and maximum ST depression) tended to improve with both treatments, but changes did not achieve statistical significance relative to baseline or to each other. Both drugs were generally well tolerated. Adverse events occurred in 15 patients in the amlodipine group (30%) and in 17 patients in the diltiazem group (36%), but patients taking diltiazem reported almost twice as many adverse events (30) as patients taking amlodipine (18). Quality of life, as assessed by total Nottingham Health Profile Scores, was not significantly different between treatments. The addition of either once-daily amlodipine or twice-daily sustained release diltiazem improved symptoms in patients with angina resistant to atenolol alone, but diltiazem was associated with more frequent and more serious adverse events.

Unstable Angina Pectoris

Inflammatory Profile in Unstable Versus Stable Angina

Inflammatory markers have been shown to be elevated in acute coronary syndromes. Recently, interleukin-6 was demonstrated to be elevated in unstable angina compared with stable angina. However, the effect of percutaneous coronary interventions on the levels of inflammatory markers is less well known. In this study, Yazdani and associates[87] from New York and Roslyn, New York, measured the levels of interleukin-6 and interleukin-1 by using enzyme-linked immunosorbent assays in patients with angina pectoris undergoing coronary interventions and in healthy control subjects. Interleukin-6 was significantly elevated in patients with unstable angina compared with patients with stable angina. There were no significant differences between the levels of interleukin-1 in patients with unstable angina versus patients with stable angina and healthy control subjects. Furthermore, at 1-month follow-up after percutaneous coronary interventions, there were no longer any significant differences between the levels of interleukin-6 in patients with unstable angina versus patients with stable angina and healthy control subjects. These data suggest that interleukin-6 levels may correlate with instability of atheromatous plaques and that the decrease of interleukin-6 levels after percutaneous coronary interventions may represent plaque re-endothelialization and stabilization.

Functional Testing for Risk Stratification in Unstable Angina

Functional testing is recommended for risk stratification of medically treated patients with unstable angina. Exercise echocardiography is used in this situation, but its safety and prognostic value are not well defined. Lin and associates[88] from Cleveland, Ohio, assessed the incremental prognostic value of exercise echocardiography in 226 consecutive patients (128 men, aged 59 ± 13 years) with medically treated unstable angina who underwent exercise echocardiography from 1991 to 1996. Clinical risk was designated as low in 108 patients, intermediate in 116, and high in 2 patients according to the unstable angina practice guidelines. There were no major complications from the stress tests. The exercise electrocardiogram was nondiagnostic in 57 patients (25%). Ischemia was identified by exercise electrocardiography in 33 patients and exercise echocardiography in 55 patients. Patients were followed for 29 ± 18 months. After exclusion of 38 patients who underwent early revascularization, 28 patients had cardiac death, nonfatal infarction, and late (>3 months) revascularization. Ischemia at exercise echocardiography was associated with a 24-month event-free survival of 81%, compared to 95% with negative exercise echocardiography. A positive exercise electrocardiogram was associated with a 24-month event-free survival of 84%, compared to 93% with negative exercise electrocardiograms. In a Cox regression model, event-free survival was predicted by ischemia at exercise echocardiography (relative risk 2.8), but not at exercise electrocardiography (relative risk 2.1) (Figures 2-28, 2-29).

Prognostic Role of Troponin T Versus Troponin I

Controversy exists as to the clinical roles and relative specificities of cardiac troponin T and I in patients with unstable angina pectoris (UAP). Olatidoye and colleagues[89] from Hartford and Framingham, Connecticut, measured troponin T and I levels on admission in 123 patients with UAP. Of the 107 patients with normal creatine kinase during the first 24 hours, troponin T and I were elevated in 14 and 13 patients, respectively. At 30 days, 5 of 14 patients (36%) with elevated troponin T and 3 of 93 patients (3.2%) with normal troponin T had AMI (odds ratio [OR], 16.7). Of 13 patients with elevated troponin I, 5

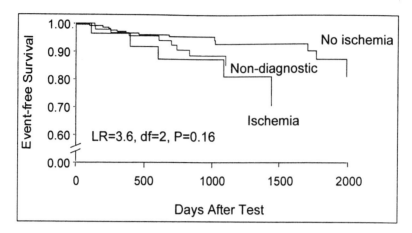

FIGURE 2-28. Event-free survival of patients with nondiagnostic studies, and with and without ischemia on exercise ECG. DF = degrees of freedom; LR = log-rank. Reproduced with permission from Lin et al.[88]

patients (39%) and 3 of 94 patients (3.2%) with normal troponin I had AMI (odds ratio, 21.7). No deaths occurred within 30 days. Both markers demonstrated equivalent sensitivity (63%) and specificities (troponin T: 91%; troponin I: 92%) for AMI. Meta-analysis of 12 published troponin T and 9 troponin I studies in patients with UAP produced risk ratios of 4.2 for troponin I compared with 2.7 for troponin T. Comparison of the sensitivities and specificities of both markers using summary receiver operating characteristic curves showed no significant difference in their abilities to predict AMI and cardiac death. Troponin T and I show similar prognostic significance for AMI or death in the same patients with UAP. The 2 markers are equally sensitive and specific, as confirmed by meta-analysis, and this supports a role in risk stratification.

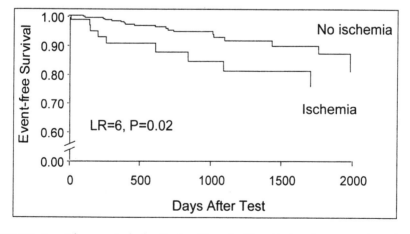

FIGURE 2-29. Event-free survival of patients with and without ischemia on exercise echocardiography. LR = log-rank. Reproduced with permission from Lin et al.[88]

Nuclear Factor κB in Unstable Angina Pectoris

Ritchie[90] in Cincinnati, Ohio, determined whether nuclear factor κB (NF-κB) is activated in patients with unstable angina pectoris. NF-κB resides inactive in the cytoplasm of lymphocytes, monocytes, endothelial cells, and smooth muscle cells, and after stimulation, it transcriptionally activates interleukins, interferon, tumor necrosis factor α, and adhesion molecules. Since acute inflammation appears to play a role in coronary artery plaque rupture, the author hypothesized that NF-κB activation correlated with CAD activity. Evidence of NF-κB activation in the circulation of 102 consecutive patients without an AMI who were undergoing a cardiac catheterization was determined. Among these, 19 had unstable angina and were within 24 hours of the last episode of chest pain. The remaining 83 were being evaluated for stable angina, valvular heart disease, atypical chest pain, or CHF. Evidence of NF-κB activation was determined by electromobility shift assays. Analyses showed that 17 of 19 patients with unstable angina had marked activation of NF-κB. Only 2 of the 83 patients without unstable angina showed marked NF-κB activation. There was no relationship between drugs used, hemodynamic status, or other clinical characteristics and state of NF-κB activation. Thus, these data suggest that NF-κB is specifically and significantly activated in unstable angina and this occurs independent of other clinical characteristics.

Enhanced Coagulation Activation

Intracoronary thrombus formation and systemic activation of coagulation have been demonstrated in unstable angina pectoris. Circulating troponin T as a marker of minor myocardial cell injury is associated with adverse outcome in this condition. Little information exists about the interrelation of coagulation activation and myocardial cell injury in unstable angina. Terres and associates[91] from Hamburg, Germany, quantitatively assessed systemic activation of coagulation and myocardial cell injury in serial blood samples obtained up to 10 days from 22 patients with angiographically documented coronary heart disease and unstable angina pectoris at rest. In the 9 patients with increased maximal levels of serum troponin T, maximal concentrations of fibrin monomers during the first 48 hours were higher than those in patients with persistently normal troponin T concentrations (6.3 ± 4.8 vs. 2.9 ± 2.3 mg/L). The proportion of patients with at least 1 blood sample showing an increased concentration of plasma fibrin monomer was also higher in the group with increased troponin T (67% vs. 15%). Plasma prothrombin fragment F1 + 2 levels showed a nonsignificant trend toward higher values in troponin T-positive patients. Enhanced activation of coagulation in patients with troponin T-positive unstable angina may contribute to the adverse outcome associated with this condition.

Treatment of Unstable Angina

Studies of Left Ventricular Dysfunction (SOLVD) Trial

Antiplatelet agents play an important role in the prevention and treatment of coronary disease. Their effect in patients with LV systolic dysfunction are less well known. Al-Kadra and associates[92] from Boston, Massachusetts, reviewed data on antiplatelet agent use in 6,800 patients enrolled in the Studies of Left Ventricular Dysfunction (SOLVD) trial and analyzed their use and all-cause mortality. Antiplatelet agent use (46% of patients) was associated with significantly reduced mortality from all causes, hazard ratio .82, and reduced risk of death or hospital admission for heart failure, adjusted risk .81. There was no influence of trial assignment, gender, LVEF, New York Heart Association class, or etiology. The association between antiplatelet agent use and survival was not observed in the enalapril group, nor was an enalapril benefit on survival detectable in patients receiving antiplatelet agents at baseline. However, randomization to enalapril therapy significantly reduced the combined endpoint of death or hospital admission for heart failure in antiplatelet agent users. These authors conclude that in patients with LV systolic dysfunction, use of antiplatelet agents is associated with improved survival and reduced morbidity. Antiplatelet agent use is associated with retained but reduced benefit from enalapril (Figure 2-30).

Drug Therapy for Patients with Unstable Angina

Both aspirin and β-adrenergic blocking drugs have been shown to reduce the risk of death or AMI in patients with unstable angina, but their effect during

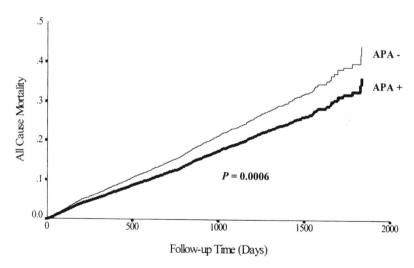

FIGURE 2-30. Antiplatelets and survival. Reproduced with permission from Al-Kadra et al.[92]

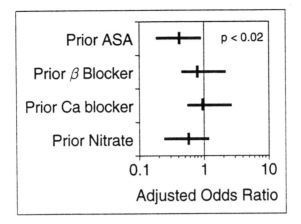

FIGURE 2-31. Effect of prior medical therapy on presentation as myocardial infarction or unstable angina. Adjusted odds ratios (vertical tick) and 95% confidence intervals (horizontal line) are shown. ASA = acetylsalicylic acid; Ca = calcium. Reproduced with permission from Borzak et al.[93]

chronic use on the presentation of acute coronary syndromes is less well defined. Calcium antagonists and oral nitrates also are widely prescribed for patients with CAD, but their effect on presentation of acute myocardial ischemia is unknown. Borzak and associates[93] for the Thrombin Inhibition in Myocardial Ischemia (TIMI) 7 investigators retrospectively examined the effects of prior aspirin and anti-ischemic medical therapy on clinical events in 410 patients hospitalized for unstable angina. Ischemic pain occurred at rest for a duration of 5 to 60 minutes. During hospitalization, 97% of patients received aspirin and all received the direct thrombin inhibitor bivalirudin for at least 72 hours. Despite being older and more likely to have risk factors for CAD and poor outcome, patients receiving aspirin before admission were less likely to present with non-Q-wave AMI (5% vs. 14% in patients not on aspirin). Prior β-blocker, calcium antagonist, or nitrate administration did not appear to modify presentation as unstable angina or non-Q-wave AMI. In a multivariate model, the combined incidence of death, AMI not present at enrollment, or recurrent angina was best predicted by age (adjusted odds ratio 2.38) and presence of electrocardiogram changes with pain on presentation (adjusted odds ratio 2.83 [1.50 to 5.35]) but was not related to prior or in-hospital medical therapy. Thus, aspirin, but not anti-ischemic therapy before hospitalization of patients with unstable angina, is associated with a decreased incidence of non-Q-wave AMI on admission (Figures 2-31, 2-32).

Heparin Versus Inogatran

Thrombin has been suggested as one of the main pharmacological targets in unstable coronary syndromes. Electrocardiographic signs of myocardial ischemia during continuous monitoring convey prognostic information in these patients. Andersen and associates[94] from Göteborg, Sweden, assessed the anti-

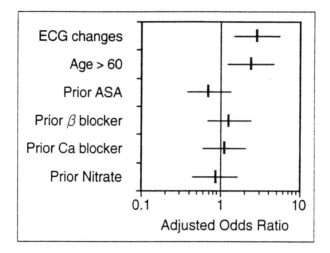

FIGURE 2-32. Effect of prior medical therapy on death, myocardial infarction, or recurrent ischemia: multivariate analysis. Adjusted odds ratios and 95% confidence intervals are shown. ECG = electrocardiographic; other abbreviations as in Figure 31. Reproduced with permission from Borzak et al.[93]

ischemic and clinical effects of the novel low-molecular-weight thrombin inhibitor inogatran in patients with unstable angina pectoris and non-Q-wave AMI without persistent ST-segment elevation on hospital admission. Within 24 hours of the last episode of chest pain, 324 patients were randomized to 72 hours of treatment with inogatran or heparin. Continuous ST-segment analysis with computerized vectorcardiography was used to monitor ischemia for 24 hours. The occurrence of cardiac events during the first 7 days were studied and compared with ischemic episodes during the initial 24 hours. The heparin-treated patients had less episodes of ischemia (ST vector magnitude [ST-VM]: 1 ± 2.6 vs. 2 ± 4.5, and ST change vector magnitude [STC-VM]: 3 ± 4.7 vs. 6 ± 7.6) than the patients receiving inogatran. This was paralleled by a lower incidence of the combined endpoint of death, nonfatal infarction, refractory or recurrent angina during the first 7 days for the heparin-treated patients (35%) compared with the inogatran-treated patients (50%). Patients who had episodes of ischemia in spite of anti-ischemic therapy were at increased risk of all events studied. Heparin is more effective than inogatran in suppressing myocardial ischemia and clinical events at short-term follow-up. Continuous ST-segment monitoring with vectorcardiography identifies nonresponders who are at an increased level of risk.

PARAGON Trial of Lamifiban

The PARAGON investigators[95] tested the benefit of different doses of a platelet IIb/IIIa antagonist, lamifiban, a small molecule member of the new class of IIb/IIIa inhibitors developed for intravenous administration alone and

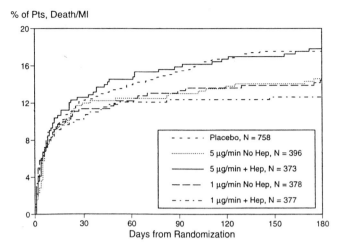

% of Pts, Death/MI

Placebo, N = 758
5 µg/min No Hep, N = 396
5 µg/min + Hep, N = 373
1 µg/min No Hep, N = 378
1 µg/min + Hep, N = 377

Days from Randomization

FIGURE 2-33. Kaplan-Meier estimates of the probability of death or nonfatal myocardial (re)infarction (MI) during 6-month follow-up separated according to treatment assignment. At 30 days, all groups had similar outcomes, whereas at 6 months the group receiving low-dose lamifiban with heparin had the fewest endpoint events compared with controls (p=0.025). Pts = patients; Hep = heparin. Reproduced with permission from the PARAGON Investigators.[95]

in combination with heparin in patients with unstable angina and non-Q-wave AMI at 273 hospitals in 20 countries and in 2,282 patients. These patients were randomly assigned to receive lamifiban with and without heparin at 2 different doses of lamifiban (1 µg/min and 5 µg/min) or to receive standard therapy with placebo and heparin. All patients received aspirin. The composite primary endpoint of death or nonfatal AMI at 30 days occurred in 11.7% of those receiving standard therapy, 10.6% of those receiving the lower dose of lamifiban, and 12% receiving the higher dose of lamifiban. At 6 months, this composite was lowest for those assigned to low-dose lamifiban and intermediate for those assigned to high-dose lamifiban (Figure 2-33). The combination of high-dose lamifiban and heparin resulted in more intermediate or major bleeding and a similar rate of ischemic events. Thus, in patients with unstable angina and non-Q-wave AMI, the use of a small molecule inhibitor of the platelet IIb/IIIa receptors with lamifiban reduces adverse ischemic events at 6 months beyond that of aspirin and heparin therapy. The role of heparin appears most favorable when given with low-dose IIb/IIIa antagonism.

Organization to Assess Strategies for Ischemic Syndromes (OASIS) Pilot Study

Anand and colleagues[96] in Hamilton, Canada, studied the effects of long-term warfarin at two intensities in patients with acute ischemic syndromes without ST-segment elevation in 2 consecutive randomized controlled studies.

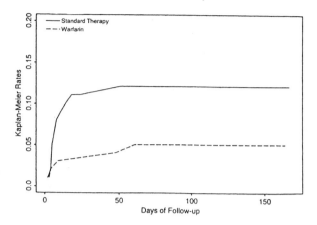

FIGURE 2-34. Cumulative rates of CV death, MI, and refractory angina: phase 2. Reproduced with permission from Anand et al.[96]

In phase 1, after the cessation of 3 days of intravenous antithrombotic therapy, 309 patients were randomized to receive fixed low-dose (3 mg/day) warfarin for 6 months that produced a mean international normalized ratio (INR) of 1.5 ± 0.6 or to standard therapy. Eighty-seven percent of patients received aspirin in both groups. The rates of cardiovascular death, new AMI, and refractory angina at 6 months were 6.5% in the warfarin group and 3.9% in the standard therapy group. The rates of death, new AMI, and stroke were 6.5% in the warfarin group and 2.6% in the standard therapy group. The overall rate of rehospitalization for unstable angina was 21% and it did not differ significantly between the groups. Four patients in the warfarin group and none in the control group experienced a major bleed, and there was an excess of minor bleeds in the warfarin group. In phase 2, the protocol was modified and 197 patients were randomized <48 hours from the onset of symptoms to receive warfarin at an adjusted dose that produced a mean INR of 2.3 ± 0.6 or standard therapy for 3 months. Eight-five percent of patients received aspirin in both groups. The rates of cardiovascular death, new AMI, and refractory angina at 3 months were 5.1% in the warfarin group and 12.1% in the standard group (RR 0.42; p=0.08). The rates of all death, new AMI, and stroke were 5.1% in the warfarin group and 13% in the standard therapy group (RR 0.39; p=0.05). There were significantly fewer patients rehospitalized for unstable angina in the warfarin group than in the control group (7% vs. 17%, p=0.03). Two patients in the warfarin group and 1 in the control group experienced a major bleed and there was an excess of minor bleeds in the warfarin group. Thus, long-term treatment with moderate-intensity warfarin (INR 2.0 to 2.5) plus aspirin but not low-intensity warfarin (INR 1.5) plus aspirin appears to reduce the rate of acute ischemic events in patients with previous acute coronary syndromes without ST-segment elevation (Figure 2-34).

c7E3 Fab Antiplatelet Therapy in Unstable Refractory Angina (CAPTURE) Study

Klootwijk and colleagues[97] have used the c7E3 Fab Antiplatelet Therapy in Unstable Angina (CAPTURE) database to investigate the incidence of recurrent

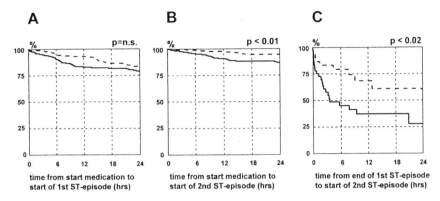

A p=n.s.

B p < 0.01

C p < 0.02

time from start medication to
start of 1st ST-episode (hrs)

time from start medication to
start of 2nd ST-episode (hrs)

time from end of 1st ST-episode
to start of 2nd ST-episode (hrs)

FIGURE 2-35. Kaplan-Meier estimate of the probability to remain free of an ST episode during the course of the monitoring period. **(A)** Probability to remain free from a recurrent ST episode from the start of medication. The continuous curve represents the patients treated with placebo (163) and the dashed curve represents the patients treated with abciximab (169). **(B)** Probability to remain free from a second ST episode from the start of medication. **(C)** Probability to remain free from a second ST episode after the first one has ended. The continuous curve represents the patients with at least 1 ST episode treated with placebo (37) and the dashed curve represents the patients with at least 1 ST episode treated with abciximab (31). Both the probability to remain free from a second ischemic episode after the start of medication and the probability to remain free from a second ischemic episode after the first one appear significantly better for patients treated with abciximab. Reproduced with permission from Klootwijk et al.[97]

ischemia and the ischemic burden in a subset of 332 patients who underwent continuous vector-derived 12-lead ECG ischemia monitoring. In the CAPTURE trial, patients with refractory unstable angina were treated with abciximab or placebo in addition to standard treatment from 16 to 24 hours preceding coronary intervention through 1 hour after intervention. Patients were monitored from start of treatment through 6 hours after coronary intervention in this substudy. Ischemic episodes were detected in 31 (18%) of 169 abciximab and in 37 (23%) of the placebo-treated patients. Only 9 (5%) of abciximab compared to 22 (14%) of placebo patients had 2 or more episodes of ST depression (Figure 2-35). In patients with ischemia, abciximab significantly reduced total ischemic burden, which was calculated as the total duration of ST-segment episodes per patient, the area under the curve of the ST vector magnitude during episodes, or the sum of the areas under the curves of 12 leads during episodes. Twenty-one patients (6%) suffered an AMI (18) or died (3) within 5 days of treatment. The presence of asymptomatic and symptomatic ST episodes during this monitoring period preceding coronary intervention was associated with an increased relative risk of these events (3.2 and 4.1, respectively). Thus, recurrent ischemia predicts MI or death within 5 days of follow-up. Treatment with abciximab is associated with a reduction of frequent ischemia and a reduction of total ischemic burden in patients with refractory unstable angina.

Management of Unstable Angina

Management of unstable angina is largely determined by symptoms, yet some symptomatic patients stabilize, whereas others develop AMI after waning

TABLE 2-5
Outcome at 3 Months After Discharge in Relation to Risk Factors

	Overall (102 pts.)	Pain		ECG		Troponin T		CRP		Holter	
		No (42 pts.)	Yes (60 pts.)	Normal (63 pts.)	Abnormal (39 pts.)	<0.2 μg/L (88 pts.)	>0.2 μg/L (14 pts.)	<3 mg/L (49 pts.)	>3 mg/L (53 pts.)	Neg. (69 pts.)	Pos. (33 pts.)
Myocardial infarction	15 (15%)	3 (7%)	12 (20%)	9 (14%)	6 (15%)	8 (9%)§	7 (50%)	2 (4%)†	13 (24%)	3 (4%)§	2 (36%)
Myocardial revascularization	28 (27%)	5 (12%)‡	23 (38%)	15 (24%)	13 (33%)	26 (30%)	2 (14%)	10 (20%)*	18 (34%)	16 (23%)	12 (36%)

* p = 0.04; † p < 0.01; ‡ p = 0.006; § p < 0.001.
Pos. = positive; Neg. = negative.
Reproduced with permission from Rebuzzi et al.[98]

of symptoms. Therefore, markers of short-term risk, available on admission, are needed. The value of 4 prognostic indicators available on admission (pain in the last 24 hours, electrocardiogram, troponin T, and C-reactive protein [CRP]), and of Holter monitoring available during the subsequent 24 hours was analyzed in 102 patients with Braunwald class IIIB unstable angina hospitalized in 4 centers by Rebuzzi and associates[98] from Rome, Italy, and London, United Kingdom. The patients were divided into 3 groups: group 1, 27 with pain during the last 24 hours and ischemic electrocardiographic changes; group 2, 45 with pain or electrocardiographic changes; group 3, 30 with neither pain nor electrocardiographic changes. Troponin T, CRP, electrocardiogram on admission, and Holter monitoring were analyzed blindly in the core laboratory. Fifteen patients developed AMI: 22% in group 1, 13% in group 2, and 10% in group 3. Twenty-eight patients underwent revascularization: 37% in group 1, 35% in group 2, and 7% in group 3. AMI was more frequent in patients with elevated troponin T (50% vs. 9%) and elevated CRP (24% vs. 4%). Positive troponin T or CRP identified all AMIs in group 3. Only 1 of 46 patients with negative troponin T and CRP developed AMIs. Among the indicators available on admission, multivariate analysis showed that troponin T and CRP were independently associated with AMI. Troponin T had the highest specificity (92%), and CRP the highest sensitivity (87%). Positive results on Holter monitoring were also associated with AMI, but when added to troponin T and CRP, increased specificity and positive predictive value by only 3%. Thus, in patients with class IIIB unstable angina, among data potentially available on admission, serum levels of troponin T and CRP have a significantly greater prognostic accuracy than symptoms and electrocardiograms. Holter monitoring, available 24 hours later, adds no significant information (Table 2-5).

Clinical Trial of Chest-Pain Observation Unit

Farkouh and colleagues[99] evaluated the safety, efficacy, and cost of admission to a chest-pain observation unit located in the emergency department for patients with unstable angina. They performed a community-based, prospective, randomized trial of the safety, efficacy, and cost of admission to a chest-pain unit compared with those of regular hospital admission for patients with

unstable angina who were considered to be at intermediate risk for cardiovascular events in the short term. A total of 424 eligible patients were randomly
assigned to routine hospital admission in a monitored bed under the care of
the cardiology service or admission to the chest-pain unit where patients were
cared for according to a strict protocol, including aspirin, heparin, continuous
ST-segment monitoring, determination of creatine kinase isoenzyme levels, 6
hours of observation, and a study of cardiac function. The chest-pain unit was
managed by the emergency department staff. Patients whose test results were
negative were discharged and the others were hospitalized. Patient outcomes
and the use of resources were compared between the 2 groups. The 212 patients
in the hospital-admission group had 15 primary events (13 AMIs and 2 cases
of CHF) and the 212 patients in the chest-pain unit group had 7 events (5
AMIs, 1 death from cardiovascular causes, and 1 case of CHF). There was no
significant difference in the rate of cardiac events between the 2 groups. No
primary events occurred among the 97 patients who were assigned to the chest-
pain unit and discharged. Resource use during the first 6 months was greater
among patients assigned to hospital admission than among those assigned to
the chest-pain unit (p = 0.003). Thus, these data suggest that a chest-pain unit
located in the emergency department can be a safe, effective, and cost-saving
means of ensuring that patients with unstable angina who are considered at
some risk of cardiovascular events receive appropriate care.

Acute Myocardial Infarction

Evaluation of Seasonal Distribution of Acute Myocardial Infarction

A circadian variation, with a morning predominance of AMI, is well established. Spencer and colleagues[100] from Worcester, Massachusetts, analyzed the
cases of AMI reported to the National Registry of Myocardial Infarction-2 to
evaluate the seasonal distribution of AMI. A total of 259,891 cases of AMI were
analyzed during the study. Approximately 53% more cases were reported in
winter than during the summer. These authors conclude that there is a seasonal
pattern in the occurrence of AMIs that is characterized by a marked peak of
cases in the winter months and a nadir in the summer months. This pattern
was seen in all subgroups analyzed, as well as in different geographic areas,
and indicates that there is a chronobiology of seasonal variation in AMI that
is of importance (Figure 2-36).

Prehospital Delay in Patients with Coronary Artery Disease

Patient-associated delay in seeking medical care in the setting of acute
coronary disease is assuming increasing importance as the benefits of reperfusion therapies become more time dependent. Given the importance of accurate
information concerning prehospital delay, Goldberg and associates[101] from

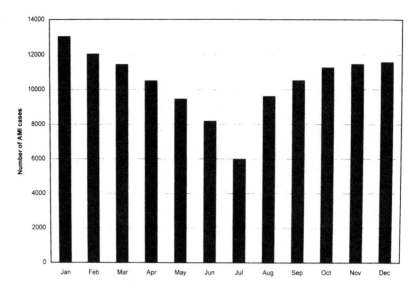

FIGURE 2-36. Seasonal distribution of AMI. Reproduced with permission from Spencer et al.[100]

Worcester, Massachusetts; Minneapolis, Minnesota; and Chapel Hill, North Carolina, examined the extent of concordance between information reported by patients in structured interviews by hospital staff nurses compared with information about time of acute symptom onset as recorded in the medical record. Data were obtained from 1,137 patients with a discharge diagnosis of coronary heart disease who were admitted to 6 coronary care units in the Minneapolis–St. Paul metropolitan area. The average and median durations of prehospital delay were similar as reported in the structured personal interviews and through the the review of medical records for the respective disease groups. The extent of individual level of agreement of delay time was considerably poorer, however. The Pearson correlation coefficients on the logarithmically transformed data were 0.48, 0.50, and 0.59 for persons with AMI, unstable angina, and chronic coronary disease, respectively, in comparing data noted in the medical record with that obtained in the personal interviews concerning prehospital delay time. These results suggest good agreement between personal interviews and medical record accounts in characterizing the average length of prehospital delay at the aggregate level but considerably less agreement at the individual patient level.

Sphygmomanometrically Measured Pressure Pulse as Predictor

Mitchell and colleagues[102] in Boston, Massachusetts, evaluated the relationship between baseline pulse pressure measured by sphygmomanometry 3 to 16 days after AMI and subsequent adverse clinical events in 2,231 patients enrolled in the Survival and Ventricular Enlargement (SAVE) Trial. Increased pulse pressure was associated with increased age, LVEF, female gender, history of prior AMI, diabetes, hypertension, and the use of digoxin and calcium chan-

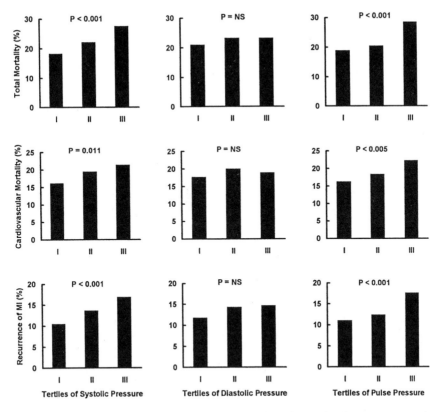

FIGURE 2-37. Relationship between baseline systolic, diastolic, and pulse pressure tertile and subsequent mortality, cardiovascular mortality, and recurrence of myocardial infarction (MI). P values represent a test for linear association. Reproduced with permission from Mitchell et al.[102]

nel blockers. During a 42-month period, there were 503 deaths, 422 cardiovascular deaths, and 303 AMIs. Pulse pressure was significantly related to each of these endpoints as a univariate predictor. In a multivariate analysis, pulse pressure remained a significant predictor of total mortality and recurrent AMI after controlling for age, LVEF, mean arterial pressure, gender, treatment arm, smoking history, history of prior AMI, diabetes, or hypertension, and treatment with β-blockers, calcium channel blockers, digoxin, aspirin, or thrombolytic therapy (Figure 2-37). These data provide evidence for a link between pulse pressure, which is related to conduit vessel stiffness, and subsequent cardiovascular events after AMI in patients with LV dysfunction.

Influence of Personality on Clinical Outcome of Patients with Decreased Left Ventricular Ejection Fraction

Denollet and Brutsaert[103] in Antwerp, Belgium, hypothesized that emotional stress in patients with MI with a decreased LVEF (1) is unrelated to the

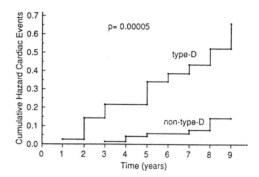

FIGURE 2-38. Cumulative hazard functions for adverse cardiac events (cardiac death or nonfatal myocardial infarction) according to personality type. Type D indicates "distressed" personality type. These curves depict how likely a patient is to experience a cardiac event given he or she has survived without recurrent MI to that time. Number of patients exposed to risk of cardiac events were 27 and 60 at baseline and 20 and 57 at the 5-year interval for type D and non-type D subgroups, respectively. Reproduced with permission from Denollet and Brutsaert.[103]

severity of the cardiac disorder, (2) predicts future cardiac events, and (3) is a function of basic personality traits. Eighty-seven patients with MI ages 41 to 69 years with an LVEF of 50% or less underwent psychological assessment at baseline. Patients and their families were contacted after 6 to 10 years, mean 7.9 years. Cardiac events were defined as cardiac death or nonfatal MI. Emotional distress was unrelated to the severity of cardiac disorder. At follow-up, 21 patients had experienced a cardiac event with 13 fatal events. These events were related to an LVEF of 30% or less, poor exercise tolerance, previous MI, anxiety, anger, and depression (Figure 2-38). Patients with a distressed personality, especially the tendency to suppress negative emotions, were more likely to experience an event over time compared with other individuals. Cox proportional hazards analysis identified LVEF of 30% or less and the distressed personality identified above as independent predictors. Anxiety, anger, and depression did not add to the predictive power. Thus, these data suggest that personality influences the clinical course of patients with a decreased LVEF.

Iron Stores and the Risk of Acute Myocardial Infarction

Tuomainen and colleagues[104] in Kuopio, Finland, investigated the association between the concentration ratio of serum transferrin receptor to serum ferritin, a state-of-the-art measurement of body iron stores, and the risk of AMI in a prospective nested case-control study in 1,931 men from eastern Finland. Transferrin receptor assays were carried out for 99 men who had an AMI during an average of 6.4 years of follow-up and 98 control men. Both the cases and the controls were nested from the Kuopio Ischemic Heart Disease Risk Factor Study cohort of 1,931 men who had no clinical CAD at the baseline evaluation. The controls were matched for age, examination year, and residence. AMIs were registered prospectively. Soluble transferrin receptors were measured by

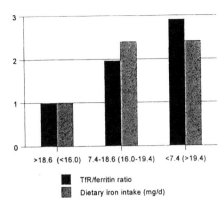

FIGURE 2-39. Risk-factor-adjusted risk of AMI in thirds of serum TfR/ferritin ratio and dietary iron intake. Reproduced with permission from Tuomainen et al.[104]

immunoenzymometric assay and ferritin concentration by radioimmunoassay from frozen baseline serum samples. The mean transferrin receptor assay/ferritin ratio was 15.1 among cases and 21.3 among controls. In logistic regression models adjusting for other strong risk factors for AMI and indicators of inflammation and alcohol intake, men in the lowest and second lowest thirds of the transferrin receptor assay to serum ferritin ratio had a 2.9-fold and 2.0-fold risk of AMI compared with men in the highest third. These data suggest an association between increased body iron stores and risk of AMI, confirming previous epidemiological data (Figure 2-39).

Evaluation of Left Ventricular Thrombosis

No widespread multicenter trials on AMI have provided information about LV thrombus. The protocol of the Gruppo Italiano per lo Studio della Sopravvivenza nell'Infarcto Miocardico (GISSI 3) Study included the search for the presence of LV thrombi in patients from 200 coronary care units that did not specifically focus on LV thrombus. Chiarella and associates on behalf of the GISSI 3 Investigators[105] examined the GISSI 3 database results related to 8,326 patients at low to medium risk for LV thrombi in which a predischarge echocardiogram (9 ± 5 days) was available. LV thrombosis was found in 427 patients (5.1%): 292 of 2,544 patients (11.5%) with anterior AMI and in 135 of 5,782 patients (2.3%) with AMI in other sites. The incidence of LV thrombosis was higher in patients with EF 40% or lower (151 of 1,432 [10.5%] vs. 276 of 6,894 [4%]) both in the total population and in the subgroup with anterior AMI (106 of 597 [17.8%] vs. 186 of 1,947 [9.6%]). Multivariate analysis showed that only the Killip class greater than 1 and early intravenous β-blocker administration were independently associated with higher LV thrombosis risk in the subgroup of patients with anterior AMI. In patients with anterior AMI, oral β-blocker therapy given or not given after early intravenous β-blocker administration does not influence the occurrence of LV thrombosis. The rate of LV thrombosis was similar in patients treated or not treated with nitrates and lisinopril both in the total population and in patients with anterior and nonanterior AMI. In conclusion, in the GISSI-3 population at low to medium risk for LV thrombosis,

TABLE 2-6
LV Thrombi in All Patients Studied and in Patients with Anterior AMI

	Total AMI	LV Thrombus (%)	Anterior AMI	LV Thrombus (%)
Patients				
Total patients	8,326	427 (5.1)	2,544	292 (11.5)
Women	1,614	66 (4.1)	490	42 (8.6)
Men	6,712	361 (5.4)	2,054	250 (12.2)
Age ≤70	6,508	336 (5.2)	2,016	235 (11.7)
Age >70	1,818	91 (5.0)	528	57 (10.8)
Clinical Features				
Killip I	7,305	343 (4.7)	2,160	228 (10.6)
Killip II	946	76 (8.0)	353	57 (16.1)
Killip III	44	6 (13.6)	21	5 (23.8)
Previous AMI	1,018	69 (6.8)	267	35 (13.1)
No previous AMI	7,217	354 (4.9)	2,247	255 (11.3)
Diabetes mellitus	1,181	75 (6.4)	380	50 (13.2)
No diabetes mellitus	6,903	346 (5.0)	2,085	237 (11.4)
Hypertension	3,025	154 (5.1)	894	97 (10.9)
No hypertension	4,949	265 (5.4)	1,539	190 (12.3)
Treatment				
Thrombolysis	6,159	331 (5.4)	1,998	233 (11.7)
No thrombolysis	2,132	96 (4.5)	535	59 (11.0)
Intravenous β blocker	2,683	186 (6.9)	1,048	134 (12.8)
No intravenous β blocker	5,554	238 (4.3)	1,467	155 (10.6)
Intravenous heparin	2,071	101 (4.9)	615	64 (10.4)
No intravenous heparin	6,255	326 (5.2)	1,929	228 (11.8)
Subcutaneous heparin	4,457	246 (5.5)	1,391	164 (11.8)
No subcutaneous heparin	3,869	181 (4.7)	1,153	128 (11.1)
Lisinopril	4,148	213 (5.1)	1,223	142 (11.6)
No lisinopril	4,178	214 (5.1)	1,321	150 (11.4)
Nitrates	4,139	203 (4.9)	1,275	142 (11.1)
No nitrates	4,187	224 (5.3)	1,269	150 (11.8)
Aspirin	7,142	356 (5.0)	2,157	249 (11.5)
No aspirin	1,131	68 (6.0)	370	40 (10.8)

Reproduced with permission from Chiarella et al.[105]

the highest rate of occurrence of LV thrombosis was found among patients with anterior wall AMI and an EF less than 40%. Killip class greater than 1 and the early intravenous β-blocker administration were the only variables independently associated with a higher predischarge incidence of LV thrombi after anterior wall AMI (Table 2-6).

Primary Ventricular Fibrillation in Acute Myocardial Infarction

Primary VF complicating AMI predicts short-term mortality. The broad category of patients with primary VF might include subgroups with different

TABLE 2-7
Characteristics of Patients with Early Primary Ventricular Fibrillation (VF) and of the Reference Group

	Early Primary VF n = 302 (%)	Reference Group n = 7320 (%)	p Value
Mean age (yrs)	58 ± 10	60 ± 11	<0.001
Men	267 (88)	5,874 (80)	<0.001
Current smoking	203 (67)	3,998 (55)	<0.001
Previous angina	40 (13)	1,302 (18)	<0.05
Hypertension treatment	83 (27)	2,023 (28)	NS
Insulin-dependent diabetes	4 (1)	134 (2)	NS
Anterior infarction	88 (29)	2,636 (36)	NS
Inferoposterior infarction	167 (55)	3,428 (47)	<0.01
Non-Q-wave infarction	39 (13)	1,116 (15)	NS
≥6 leads with ST elevation	120 (40)	2,482 (34)	<0.05
Mean admission heart rate (beats/min)	71 ± 18	75 ± 27	<0.05
Mean admission systolic BP (mm Hg)	129 ± 25	137 ± 23	<0.001
Mean serum potassium (mEq/L)	3.8 ± 0.6	4.0 ± 0.6	<0.001

Continuous variables are expressed as mean values ± SD.
BP = blood pressure.
Reproduced with permission from Volpi et al.[106]

outcomes. It is still not certain whether early onset (≤4 hours) primary VF is a risk predictor, and information on correlates of these early VFs is scarce. Volpi and associates[106] on behalf of the Gruppo Italiano per lo Studio della Sopravvivenza nell'Infarcto Miocardico (GISSI 2) investigators sought to prospectively analyze the incidence and prognosis of early as opposed to late (time window >4–48 hours) primary VF and restrospectively identified predisposing factors for early onset primary VF. The authors analyzed the incidence and recurrence rates of early and late primary VF in 9,720 patients with a first AMI, treated with thrombolytics, enrolled in the GISSI 2 trial. The independent prognostic significance of early and late primary VF was assessed by logistic regression analysis. The incidence rates of early and late primary VF were 3.1% and 0.6%, respectively; recurrence rates were 11% and 15%, respectively. The 2 variables most closely related to early primary VF were hypokalemia and systemic BP higher than 120 mm Hg on admission. Patients with early primary VF had a more complicated in-hospital course than matched controls. Both early (odds ratio [OR] 2.47) and late primary VF (OR 3.97) were independent predictors of in-hospital mortality. Postdischarge to 6-month death rates were similar for both primary VF subgroups and controls. Primary VF, irrespective of its timing, was an independent predictor of in-hospital mortality. Postdischarge to 6-month prognosis was unaffected by the occurrence of either early or late primary VF (Tables 2-7, 2-8).

Early Versus Late Recurrent Nonfatal Myocardial Infarction

Recurrent nonfatal myocardial infarction (RNMI) is the most significant risk factor for later outcome after an index infarction. However, little is known

TABLE 2-8
Hospital Course

	Early Primary VF n = 302 (%)	Reference Group n = 7,320 (%)	p Value
Reinfarction	12 (4)	136 (2)	<0.01
Cardiogenic shock	10 (3)	112 (2)	<0.05
Pericarditis	23 (8)	417 (6)	NS
Early postinfarction angina	29 (10)	689 (9)	NS
Left ventricular failure	38 (13)	906 (12)	NS
Stroke	1 (0.3)	60 (0.8)	NS
Sustained ventricular tachycardia*	5 (2)	171 (2)	NS
Atrial fibrillation or flutter	42 (14)	473 (6)	<0.001
Asystole	15 (5)	128 (2)	<0.001
Heart block: 2nd degree	44 (15)	360 (5)	<0.001
Heart block: 3rd degree	54 (18)	333 (5)	<0.001
Pulmonary embolism	1 (0.3)	9 (0.1)	NS
Systemic embolism	3 (1)	20 (0.3)	NS
CK level (> ×6, normal)	250 (83)	4928 (67)	<0.001

* Events occurring from day 3 onward.
Reproduced with permission from Volpi et al.[106]

about the prognosis after RNMIs that occur beyond the first year after the index infarction. In 3,867 nonselected patients younger than 76 years of age with AMI, Sajadieh and associates[107] from Copenhagen, Denmark, studied the rate of and prognosis after a first RNMI, depending on the year of its occurrence after the index infarction. Mortality rate was estimated by the Kaplan-Meier method, and the differences were evaluated by means of the Tarone-Ware test. Four hundred ninety-three (14%) patients had a first RNMI in the first year, 151 (5.4%) in the second, 105 (4.2%) in the third, and 71 (3.8%) in the fourth year after the index infarction (groups 1–4). The 1-year mortality rate after RNMI was 24% in the first group, 24% in the second group, 18% in the third group, and 23% in the fourth group. When all the groups were compared with each other, no significant difference was found between the mortality rates or standardized mortality rates. Late RNMIs have almost the same grave prognosis as do early RNMIs.

Treatment of Acute Myocardial Infarction

Long-Term Intervention with Pravastatin in Ischemic Disease (LIPID) Study Group

The Long-Term Intervention with Pravastatin in Ischemic Heart Disease (LIPID) Study Group[108] compared the effects of pravastatin (40 mg/day) with those of placebo over a mean follow-up period of 6 years in 9,014 patients who were 31 to 75 years of age. The patients had a history of AMI or hospitalization for unstable angina and initial plasma total cholesterol levels of 155 to 271

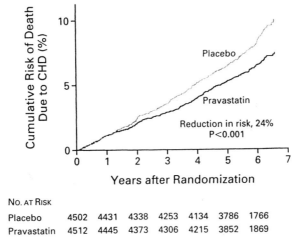

FIGURE 2-40. Kaplan-Meier estimates of mortality due to coronary heart disease (CHD), the primary outcome, in the pravastatin and placebo groups. The relative reduction in risk with pravastatin therapy was derived from the Cox proportional-hazards model. The p value was based on the log-rank test with stratification according to the qualifying event. On the basis of the differences in the proportions of patients who died of CHD during the entire study period, for every 1,000 patients assigned to pravastatin, death from CHD was avoided in 19 patients. Reproduced with permission from the LIPID Study Group.[108]

mg/dL. Both groups received advice on following a cholesterol-lowering diet. The primary study outcome was mortality from CAD. Death from CAD occurred in 8% of the patients in the placebo group and 6% of those in the pravastatin group, a relative reduction in risk of 24%, p<0.001 (Figure 2-40). Overall mortality was 14% in the placebo group and 11% in the pravastatin group for a 22% reduction, p<0.001. The incidence of all cardiovascular outcomes was consistently lower among patients assigned to receive pravastatin, including the risk of AMI, death, or nonfatal AMI, and coronary revascularization (Figure 2-41). The effects of treatment were similar for all predefined subgroups. There were no clinically significant adverse effects of treatment with pravastatin. Thus, pravastatin therapy reduces mortality from CAD and overall mortality, as well as the incidence of cardiovascular events in patients with a history of AMI or unstable angina who have a broad range of initial serum cholesterol values.

Veterans Affairs Non-Q-Wave Infarction Strategies in Hospital (VANQWISH) Trial

Boden and colleagues[109] randomly assigned 920 patients to either invasive management (462 patients) or conservative management, defined as medical therapy and noninvasive testing, with subsequent invasive management if indicated by the development of spontaneous or inducible ischemia (458 patients), within 72 hours of the onset of a non-Q-wave AMI. Death or nonfatal AMI made up the combined primary endpoint. During an average follow-up of 23

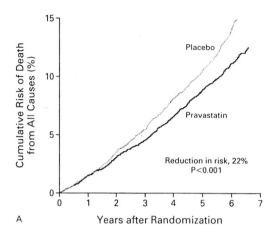

A

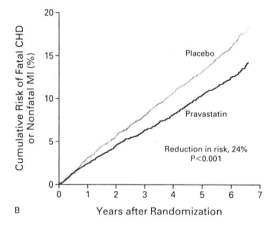

B

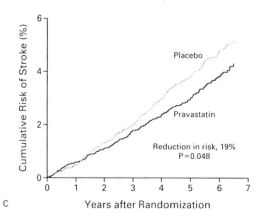

C

FIGURE 2-41. Kaplan-Meier estimates of the incidence of major secondary outcomes in the pravastatin and placebo groups. **A** shows mortality from all causes, **B** shows death due to coronary heart disease (CHD) or nonfatal myocardial infarction (MI), and **C** shows stroke of any type. The relative reductions in risk with pravastatin therapy were derived from the Cox proportional-hazards model. The p values were based on the log-rank test, with stratification according to the qualifying event. On the basis of the differences in the proportions of patients with an event during the entire study period, for every 1,000 patients assigned to pravastatin, death from any cause was avoided in 30 patients, death due to CHD or nonfatal MI was avoided in 35 patients, and stroke was avoided in 8 patients. Reproduced with permission from the LIPID Study Group.[108]

months, 152 events occurred in 138 patients who had been randomly assigned to the invasive strategy and 139 events in patients assigned to the conservative strategy (p=NS). Patients assigned to the invasive strategy had worse clinical outcomes during the first year of follow-up. The number of patients with 1 of the components of the primary endpoint, i.e., death or nonfatal AMI, and the number who died were significantly higher in the invasive strategy group at hospital discharge (36 vs. 15 patients, p=0.004 for the primary endpoint), at 1 month (48 vs. 26, p=0.021), and at 1 year (111 vs. 85, p=0.05). Overall mortality during follow-up did not differ significantly between patients assigned to the conservative strategy group and those assigned to the invasive strategy group. Thus, most patients with non-Q-wave AMI do not benefit from routine, early, invasive management consisting of coronary angiography and revascularization. A conservative, ischemia-guided initial approach is both safe and effective.

Adequate Use of Reperfusion Therapy in the United States

Barron and colleagues[110] determined whether reperfusion therapy is underutilized in patients with AMI in the US. They examined the use of reperfusion therapy in patients with AMI hospitalized at 1,470 hospitals participating in the National Registry of Myocardial Infarction 2. They identified 84,663 patients who were eligible for reperfusion therapy as defined by diagnostic changes on initial 12-lead electrocardiogram, presentation to the hospital within 6 hours from symptom onset, and no contraindications to thrombolytic therapy. Twenty-four percent of these eligible patients did not receive any form of reperfusion therapy (7.5% of all patients). When multivariate analyses were used, LBBB, lack of chest pain at presentation, age 75 years or older, female gender, and various preexisting cardiovascular conditions were independent predictors that the patient would not receive reperfusion therapy. Thus, these data suggest that reperfusion therapy is still underutilized in the US. Increased use of reperfusion therapy could reduce the unnecessarily high mortality rates observed in women, the elderly, and other patient groups with the highest risk of death from an AMI (Figure 2-42).

Effects of Aspirin

There are conflicting reports on the interaction of aspirin with angiotensin-converting enzyme inhibitors in CHF and in systemic hypertension. Oosterga and associates[111] from Nieuwegein, The Netherlands, conducted a post hoc analysis of the Captopril and Thrombolysis Study (CATS) study. At randomization, 94 patients (31.5%) took aspirin. In patients who took aspirin, the cumulative α-hydroxy butyrate dehydrogenase release was $1,151 \pm 132$ IU/L in patients randomized to captopril compared with $1,401 \pm 136$ IU/L in patients randomized to placebo (difference -250 ± 189). This difference was comparable to the difference in patients who did not use aspirin (-199 ± 147). One year after AMI, an increase in LV end-diastolic volume index of 2.2 ± 3.0

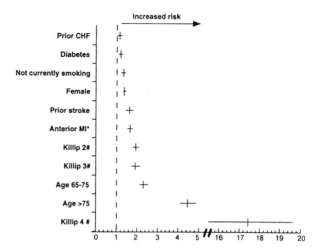

FIGURE 2-42. Multivariate adjusted odds ratio and 95% CI (line) for in-hospital mortality. CHF = congestive heart failure; MI = myocardial infarction. #Reference group is Killip 1; *reference group is inferior wall myocardial infarction. Reproduced with permission from Barron et al.[110]

mL/m^2 in captopril-treated and 1.9 ± 2.9 mL/m^2 in placebo-treated patients was observed in patients who took aspirin (difference 0.4 ± 4.2). This difference was also comparable to the difference in patients who did not take aspirin (2.2 ± 3.8). One year after AMI, patients who did take aspirin had a mean change in LV end-diastolic volume index of 2.1 ± 2.1 mL/m^2 compared with 8.4 ± 1.9 mL/m^2 in patients who did not use aspirin. Thus, aspirin does not attenuate the acute and long-term effects of angiotensin-converting enzyme inhibition after AMI, but independently reduces LV dilation after AMI.

Effect of β-Blockade on Mortality After Acute Myocardial Infarction

The medical records of 201,752 patients with AMI were abstracted by the Cooperative Cardiovascular Project. Using a Cox proportional-hazards model that accounted for multiple factors that might influence survival, Gottlieb and associates[112] compared mortality among patients treated with β-blockers with mortality among untreated patients during the 2 years after AMI. A total of 34% of the patients received β-blockers. The percentage was lower among the elderly, blacks, and patients with the lowest ejection fractions, CHF, chronic obstructive pulmonary disease (COPD), elevated serum creatinine concentrations, or type 1 diabetes mellitus. Mortality was lower in every subgroup of patients treated with β-blockers than in untreated patients. In patients with AMI and no other complications, treatment with β-blockers was associated with a 40% reduction in mortality. Mortality was also reduced by 40% in patients with non-Q-wave AMI and those with COPD. Blacks, patients 80 years old

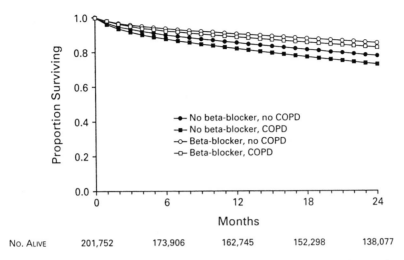

FIGURE 2-43. Adjusted probability of survival among patients with or without a history of chronic obstructive pulmonary disease (COPD) who received or did not receive β-blockers. Patients with COPD had a larger absolute benefit with β-blockade. Reproduced with permission from Gottlieb et al.[112]

or older, and those with an LVEF below 20%, serum creatinine concentrations greater than 1.4 mg/dL, or diabetes mellitus had a lower percentage reduction in mortality. However, given the higher mortality rates in these subgroups, the absolute reduction in mortality was similar to or greater than that among patients with no specific risk factors. Thus, after AMI, patients with conditions that are often considered contraindications to β-blockers, including CHF, COPD, and older age and those with nontransmural AMI benefit from β-blocker therapy (Figure 2-43).

Grampian Region Early Anistreplase Trial

The earlier that thrombolytic therapy is given for AMI, theoretically, there should be greater benefit because of earlier revascularization. Rawles[113] from Aberdeen, Scotland, United Kingdom, presented the 5-year results of the Grampian Region Early Anistreplase Trial (GREAT). In this randomized trial, 30 U anistreplase was given intravenously either before hospital admission or in the hospital at a median time of 105 and 240 minutes. By 5 years, 25% of patients died in the pre-hospital treatment group compared with 36% in the hospital treatment group. Thus, he concluded that the magnitude of the benefit from earlier thrombolysis is such that giving thrombolytic therapy to patients with AMI should be accorded the same degree of urgency as treatment of cardiac arrest. Delaying thrombolytic treatment by 30 minutes reduces the average expectation of life by approximately 1 year. Thus, the early benefits seen in the GREAT trial are sustained at 5 years.

Cholesterol and Recurrent Events Study

Sacks and colleagues[114] for the Cholesterol and Recurrent Events Study (CARE) Investigators compared pravastatin and placebo in patients who had experienced AMI who had average concentrations of total cholesterol less than 240 mg/dL (baseline mean 209 mg/dL) and cholesterols of 115 to 174 mg/dL (mean 139 mg/dL). Pravastatin reduced coronary death or recurrent MI by 24%. In multivariate analysis, the LDL concentration achieved during follow-up was a significant, although nonlinear, predictor of the coronary event rate, whereas the extent of LDL reduction was not significant. The coronary event rate declined as LDL decreased during follow-up from 174 to 125 mg/dL, but no further decline was seen in the LDL range from 125 to 71 mg/dL. In multivariate analysis, serum triglyceride but not HDL concentration during follow-up were weakly but significantly associated with the coronary event rate. Thus, the LDL concentrations achieved during treatment of pravastatin or placebo are associated with reductions in coronary events down to an LDL concentration of approximately 125 mg/dL (Figure 2-44). LDL concentrations less than 125 mg/dL during treatment are not associated with further benefit. Absolute or percentage reduction in LDL has little relationship to future coronary events.

Indications for Angiotensin-Converting Enzyme Inhibitors in the Treatment of Acute Myocardial Infarction

The Angiotensin-Converting Enzyme (ACE) Inhibitor Myocardial Infarction Collaborative Group[115] led by Dr. Franzosi in Milan, Italy, has provided a systematic overview regarding ACE inhibitor therapy started during AMI by obtaining individual patient data from all randomized trials involving more than 1,000 patients in whom ACE-inhibitor therapy was started during the acute phase (0 to 36 hours) of AMI and continued for 4 to 6 weeks. Data were available for 98,496 patients from 4 eligible trials, and the results were consistent among the trials. Thirty-day mortality was 7% among patients treated with ACE inhibitors and 7.6% among control subjects, corresponding to a 7% proportional reduction. This represented avoidance of approximately 5 deaths/1,000 patients with most of the benefit observed during the first week of therapy. The proportional benefit was similar in patients at different underlying risk. The absolute benefit was particularly great in some high-risk groups, including patients with Killip class 2 to 3 CHF, heart rate of 100 or more beats/minute at entry into the study, and in patients with anterior AMI (Figure 2-45). ACE inhibitor therapy reduced the incidence of nonfatal CHF, but it was associated with an excess of persistent hypotension (18% vs. 9%) and renal dysfunction (1% vs. 0.6%). These data support the use of ACE inhibitors early in the treatment of AMI, especially in patients with anterior AMI and in those patients at increased risk of death.

Efficacy and Safety of Subcutaneous Enoxaparin in Non-Q-Wave Coronary Events (ESSENCE) Trial Results

Montalescot and colleagues[116] in Paris, France, and the Efficacy and Safety of Subcutaneous Enoxaparin in Non-Q-Wave Coronary Events (ESSENCE)

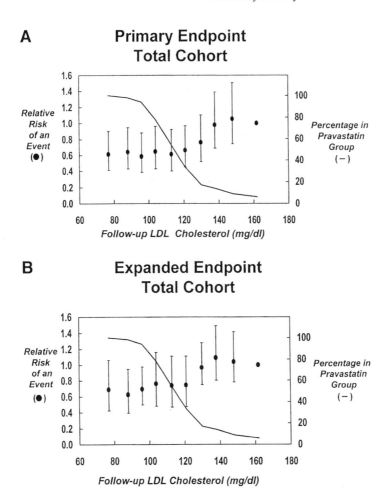

FIGURE 2-44. LDL cholesterol concentration during follow-up and coronary events. Placebo and pravastatin groups combined, n = 4,159 patients. **(A)** Primary endpoint: coronary death or nonfatal MI (n = 486 patients with endpoint, 55 in the 10th decile). **(B)** Expanded endpoint: coronary death, nonfatal MI, CABG, or PTCA (n = 979 patients with endpoint, 111 in 10th decile). Relative risk determined by Cox proportional hazards analysis with time-dependent covariates (see text). Data points show relative risks with 95% confidence intervals for coronary events for deciles of follow-up LDL concentration. Percentages of patients in each decile of LDL concentration who are in the pravastatin group are indicated by the solid line, corresponding to the right vertical axis. Reproduced with permission from Sacks et al.[114]

Investigators studied the predictive value of 5 biological indicators of inflammation, thrombogenesis, vasoconstriction, and myocardial necrosis and examined the effects of enoxaparin and unfractionated heparin on these markers after 48 hours of treatment. Sixty-eight patients with unstable angina or non-Q-wave AMI randomized in the international ESSENCE trial participated in this French substudy. C-reactive protein, fibrinogen, von Willebrand factor antigen, endothelin-1, and troponin I were measured on admission and 48 hours later. The composite endpoint of death, AMI, recurrent angina, or revascularization was significantly lower at 14 and 30 days of follow-up in patients

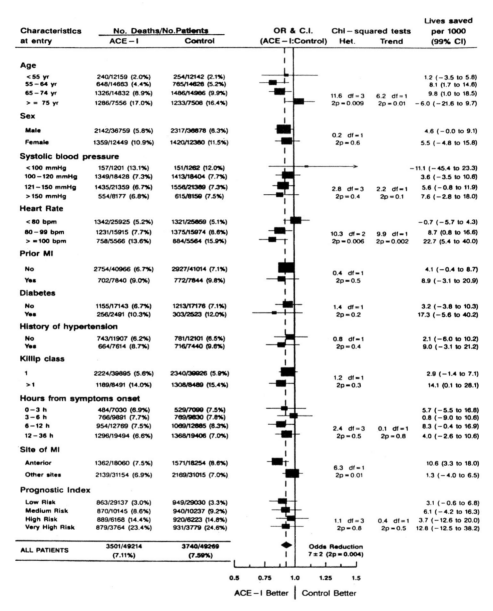

FIGURE 2-45. Effects of ACE-inhibitor therapy on mortality in days 0 to 30 subdivided by presentation features. Odds of death among patients allocated to ACE-inhibitor therapy to that among those allocated to control treatment is derived from "observed minus expected" numbers of death (and variances) calculated within each subdivision of presentation features stratified by trial. Odds ratios within each presentation feature are plotted with their 99% confidence intervals whereas overall result and 95% confidence interval are represented by a diamond. Reproduced with permission from Franzosi et al.[115]

randomized to enoxaparin compared with unfractionated heparin. All acute-phase reactive proteins were elevated on admission and increased further at 48 hours. Multivariate analysis demonstrated that the rise of von Willebrand factor over 48 hours was a significant and independent predictor of the composite endpoint at both 14 days and 30 days. Moreover, the early increase of von Willebrand factor was more frequent and more severe with unfractionated heparin than with enoxaparin. The other clinical and biological variables did not predict outcome. Thus, in patients with unstable angina or non-Q-wave AMI, the acute-phase proteins increase over the first 2 days despite medical therapy. An early rise of von Willebrand factor is an independent predictor of adverse clinical outcome at 14 days and at 30 days. Enoxaparin provides protection as indicated by the reduced release of the von Willebrand factor, which represents a favorable prognostic finding.

Assessment of Enoxaparin Versus Standard Unfractionated Heparin

Mark and colleagues[117] in Durham, North Carolina, have shown in the Efficacy and Safety of Subcutaneous Enoxaparin in Non-Q-Wave Coronary Events (ESSENCE) trial that subcutaneous low-molecular-weight heparin (enoxaparin) reduces the 30-day incidence of death, AMI, and recurrent angina in comparison to intravenous unfractionated heparin in 3,171 patients with acute coronary syndromes of unstable angina or non-Q-wave AMI. There was no increase in major bleeding. Among the 936 ESSENCE patients randomized in the US, 655 had hospital billing data collected. In the remainder, hospital costs were computed with a multivariable linear regression model. Physician fees were estimated from the Medicare Fee Schedule. During the initial hospitalization, major resource use was reduced for enoxaparin patients, with the largest effect seen with PTCA (15% vs. 20% for heparin). At 30 days, these effects persisted, with the largest reductions seen in diagnostic catheterization (57% vs. 63% for heparin) and PTCA (18% vs. 22%) (Figure 2-46). All resource-

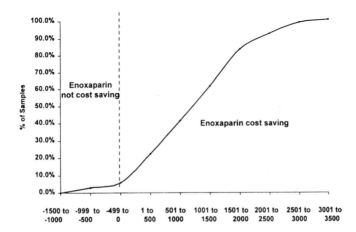

FIGURE 2-46. Cumulative distribution function of mean differences in 30-day medical costs between the enoxaparin arm and the heparin arm in 200 bootstrap samples. In 94% of samples, enoxaparin was cost saving. Reproduced with permission from Mark et al.[117]

use trends seen in the US were also evident in the overall ESSENCE study population. In the US, the mean cost of a course of enoxaparin therapy was $155, whereas that for heparin was $80. The total medical costs for the initial hospitalization were $11,857 for enoxaparin and $12,620 for heparin, a cost advantage for the enoxaparin of $763. At the end of 30 days, the cumulative cost savings associated with enoxaparin was $1,172. Thus, in patients with acute coronary syndromes, low-molecular-weight heparin (enoxaparin) both improves clinical outcomes and saves money relative to therapy with standard unfractionated heparin.

Benefit of Early Postinfarction Reperfusion

Ross and colleagues[118] for the Global Utilization of Streptokinase and Tissue Plasminogen Activator for Occluded Coronary Arteries (GUSTO I) Angiographic Investigators calculated 2-year survival differences among 2,431 AMI patients according to early infarct artery patency and outcome LVEF using Kaplan-Meier curves. Hazard ratios for significant survival determinants were derived from Cox regression models. Two-year vital status was determined in 2,375 patients. A substantial mortality advantage for early complete reperfusion and for preserved LVEF occurred beyond 30 days. The unadjusted hazard ratio for the TIMI 3 flow compared with lesser grades at 30 days was 0.57, and at 30 to 688 or more days it was 0.39. Therefore, early TIMI 3 flow was associated with approximately a 3 patient/100 mortality reduction the first month with an additional 5 lives/100 from 30 days to 2 years. For LVEFs greater than 40% compared with those 40% or less, the unadjusted hazard ratio was 0.25 at 30 days and 0.22 after 30 days through 2 years. Thus, successful reperfusion and myocardial salvage produce significant mortality benefits that are amplified beyond the initial 30 days (Figure 2-47).

Morphology of the Infarct-Related Vessel 1 Month After Acute Myocardial Infarction

Van Belle and colleagues[119] in Lille, France, studied with angioscopy the morphological characteristics of the infarct-related lesion in 56 patients between 24 hours and 4 weeks after AMI. Forty of these patients were initially treated with a thrombolytic agent. Most lesions were complex, including having an ulcerated shape. The predominant color of the plaque was yellow in 79% of cases; only 6% were uniformly white. Angioscopically visible thrombus was found in 77% of cases. Despite angioscopic evidence of instability, only 7% of the patients had post-MI angina. During the 1-month time window since the occurrence of MI, there was no significant difference in the angioscopic appearance of the plaque except for a slight increase in uniformly white plaques. The use of a thrombolytic agent at the onset of MI was associated with a reduction in thrombus size and less protruding thrombus, but not with a decreased frequency of plaque containing thrombi. There was also a trend for more frequently ulcerated plaques with the use of a thrombolytic agent (Figure 2-48).

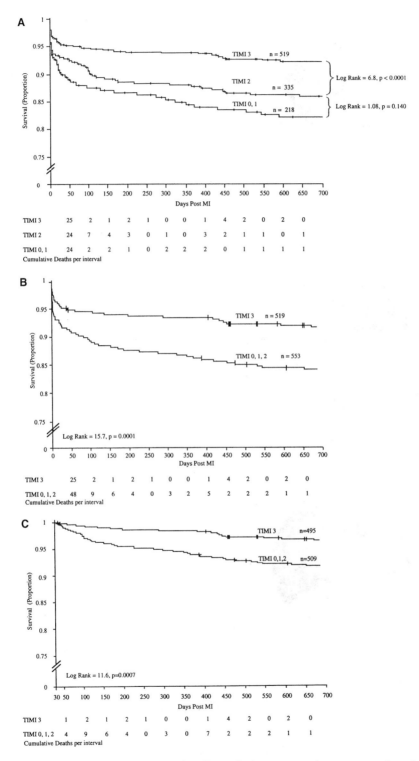

FIGURE 2-47. Two-year survival curves for all enrolled patients with 90-minute Thrombolysis in Myocardial Infarction (TIMI) flow: **(A)** TIMI 3 versus TIMI 2 versus TIMI 0, 1 flow; **(B)** TIMI 3 versus TIMI 0,1,2; **(C)** TIMI 3 versus TIMI 0,1,2 for patients who survived to 30 days. Vertical lines = censored cases; MI = myocardial infarction. Reproduced with permission from Ross et al.[118]

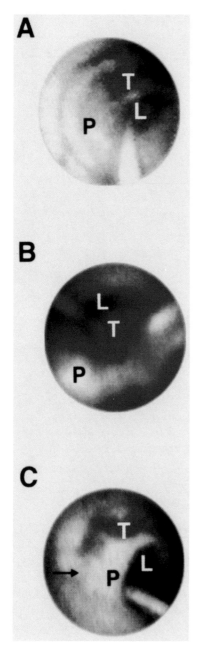

FIGURE 2-48. Coronary angioscopic findings. **(A)** Yellow plaque (P) with a lining thrombus (T). **(B)** Yellow plaque (P) with a large protruding thrombus (T). **(C)** Predominantly white plaque (P) with a localized yellow area (arrow) and an adjacent lining thrombus (T). L = lumen. Reproduced with permission from Van Belle et al.[119]

The authors conclude that these results suggest that healing of the infarct-related lesion requires more than 1 month and that an "unstable" yellow plaque with adherent thrombus is common during that period.

Clinical Outcomes with Atenolol Use

Early intravenous β-blockade is generally recommended after AMI, especially for patients with tachycardia and/or hypertension and for those without heart failure. Pfisterer and colleagues[120] from the multicenter Global Utilization of Streptokinase and Tissue Plasminogen Activator for Occluded Coronary Arteries (GUSTO I) trial evaluated this theory. In addition to 1 of 4 thrombolytic strategies, patients in the GUSTO trial without hypotension, bradycardia, or signs of heart failure were to receive atenolol 5 mg intravenously as soon as possible, another 5 mg intravenously 10 minutes later, and 50–100 mg orally daily during the hospitalization. Patients given any atenolol had a lower baseline risk than those not given atenolol. Adjusted 30-day mortality was significantly lower in atenolol-treated patients, but patients treated with intravenous and oral atenolol treatment versus oral treatment alone were more likely to die. Subgroups had similar rates of stroke, intracranial hemorrhage, and reinfarction but intravenous atenolol use was associated with more heart failure, shock, recurrent ischemia, and pacemaker use than oral atenolol was. These authors conclude that although atenolol appears to improve outcomes after thrombolysis for myocardial infarction, early intravenous atenolol seems of limited value. They recommended that patients begin oral atenolol once stable. This recommendation is different from official recommendations regarding the use of intravenous β-blockers in acute myocardial infarction, but this relatively convincing data in the patient population of the GUSTO trial appear to justify their recommendation.

Spontaneous Reperfusion

This study by Christian and associates[121] from Rochester, Minnesota, sought to determine the prevalence of spontaneous reperfusion of an infarct-related artery (IRA) and associated myocardial salvage in the absence of thrombolysis or angioplasty. Twenty-one patients with AMI received only heparin and aspirin. At a median of 18 hours after presentation, 12 patients (57%) had angiographic patency of the IRA. Technetium-99m sestamibi was injected acutely on presentation and again at hospital discharge. Acute and final perfusion defect sizes were measured. Their difference, myocardial salvage, was calculated along with salvage index (myocardial salvage/acute defect). Comparing patients with a patent versus occluded IRA, myocardium at risk was similar (16% ± 12% vs. 12% ± 9% left ventricle); however, myocardial salvage (9% ± 9% vs. −2% ± 7% left ventricle), and salvage index (0.62 ± 0.37 vs. 0.19 ± 0.33) were greater in patients with spontaneous reperfusion. Resolution of chest pain was greater in patients with a patent IRA (100% vs. 55%). Spontaneous reperfusion of the IRA occurs frequently in patients with AMI and is associated with significant myocardial salvage.

Risk Factors for Acute Myocardial Infarction

Relationship of Acute Myocardial Infarction and the Use of Low-Dose Oral Contraceptives

In this study by Sidney and associates,[122] the estimated risk of AMI in relationship to the use of low-dose oral contraceptive medications was determined in a pooled analysis combining results from 2 sites in women aged 18 to 44 years with incident AMI who had no prior history of CAD or cerebrovascular disease. Women in the case and control groups were interviewed in person regarding oral contraceptive use and cardiovascular risk factors. The analyses included 271 AMI cases and 993 controls. Compared with noncurrent users, the adjusted pooled odds ratio for AMI in current oral contraceptive users was 0.94 after adjustment for major risk factors and sociodemographic factors. Compared with never users, the adjusted pooled odds ratio for AMI was 0.56 in current users and 0.54 in past users. Among past oral contraceptive users, duration and recency of use were unrelated to AMI risk as was current hormone replacement therapy. There was no evidence of an interaction between oral contraceptive use and age, presence of cardiovascular risk factors, including hypercholesterolemia, hypertension, diabetes, obesity, or smoking. Thus, these data suggest that low-dose oral contraceptive use is safe with respect to the risk of AMI in women.

Natural Disasters as Triggers for Cardiac Events

Natural disasters can serve as triggers for AMI. Kloner and associates[123] from Los Angeles, California; Beer-Sheva, Israel; and Research Triangle Park, North Carolina, evaluated the effects of the January 17, 1994, Northridge earthquake on all deaths and causes of death within the entire population of Los Angeles County. There were an average of 73 deaths/day due to ischemic heart disease and atherosclerotic cardiovascular disease in the 16 days preceding the earthquake. This increased to 125 on the day of the earthquake and then decreased to 57 deaths/day for the next 2 weeks. The decrease in deaths during the 14 days after the earthquake overcompensated for the increase on the day of the earthquake. Thus, they conclude that there is an increase due to CAD followed by a decrease that overcompensates for the excessive deaths. This overcompensation may represent a residual population that is more resistant to stress or there may be a possible preconditioning effect of the stress or both. This study supports the concept that cardiovascular events within an entire population can be triggered by a shared stress.

Polymorphisms in a Receptor Mediating Shear Stress-Dependent Platelet Activation

Murata and colleagues[124] in Tokyo, Japan, determined the association between the presence of CAD and polymorphisms in a platelet receptor for von Willebrand factor, the glycoprotein lb/IX complex, which mediates shear stress-dependent platelet activation. Genotypes of the α-chain of the receptor GP lbα [145]Thr/Met were determined in 91 patients with AMI or angina pectoris whose lesions were confirmed by coronary angiography as well as in 105 individuals from the general population with no history of angina or other heart disease and normal resting electrocardiograms. There were no homozygotes for the Met/Met in either the control or the patient groups. The prevalence of the GP Ibα, [145]Thr/Met genotype in all patients was not significantly different from that in the control group. However, the frequency of this genotype was significantly higher in patients aged 60 years or younger (32%) than in control subjects of similar age (16%, p<0.05). An association was also demonstrated between CAD and the other polymorphisms of GP Ibα, a variable number of tandem repeats of the 13-amino acid sequence, which is known to be linked to the [145]Thr/Met polymorphism. There was an association between the frequency of this genotype and the angiographic severity of CAD. There was no difference in the distribution of GP Ibα genotypes between patients with AMI and those with angina. These data suggest that the presence of the Met allele in GP Ibα is a risk factor for the prevalence and severity of CAD in individuals aged 60 years or younger.

Non-Q-Wave Acute Myocardial Infarction in Diabetics Versus Nondiabetics

Risk factors and outcome associated with non-Q-wave AMI in diabetics and nondiabetics were analyzed by Gowda and associates[125] from Kansas City, Missouri, in 376 consecutive patients, 77 with diabetes (20%) and 299 nondiabetics (80%), who had non-Q-wave AMI and PTCA performed before discharge from hospital from January 1992 to February 1996. Diabetics were slightly older (64 ± 10 years vs. 61 ± 12 years), had more prior CABG surgery (27% vs. 12%), and hypertension (77% vs. 49%). There was no significant difference in unstable angina, saphenous vein graft PTCA, single versus multiple vessel disease, or history of AMI. PTCA success rates for diabetics versus nondiabetics were similar (96% vs. 97%). In-hospital complications such as CABG, recurrent AMI, repeat PTCA, stroke, and death were not statistically significant between the 2 groups. At 1-year follow-up, survival in diabetics (92%) was similar to nondiabetics (94%), although event-free survival (PTCA, CABG, AMI, death) was worse in diabetics (55% vs. 67% for nondiabetics). Although diabetic patients with non-Q-wave AMI represent a cohort with more risk factors for poor outcome, aggressive in-hospital revascularization with PTCA results in an excellent short-term outcome as well as 1-year survival similar to the nondiabetic patients. However, total events at 1-year follow-up are more common in the diabetic patients, suggesting that more aggressive screening and therapy in follow-up may be warranted, and that a diabetic with non-Q-wave AMI will require increased utilization of cardiovascular resources in the first year after the event.

Gender Comparison of Early Outcome of Acute Myocardial Infarction

Malacrida and colleagues,[126] as part of the Third International Study of Infarct Survival (ISIS 3), collected information on deaths during days 0 to 35

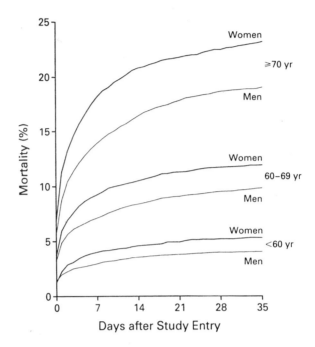

FIGURE 2-49. Cumulative mortality from day 0 to day 35, according to age and sex. Reproduced with permission from Malacrida et al.[126]

and on major clinical events during hospitalization up to day 35 for 9,600 women and 26,480 men with suspected AMI who were considered to have a clear indication for thrombolytic therapy. They compared the outcome among women and men, first without adjustment, then with adjustment for age, and finally with adjustment for other recorded baseline characteristics by means of multiple logistic regression. The unadjusted odds ratio for death among women as compared with men was 1.73. The women were significantly older than the men, and after adjustment for age, the odds ratio was reduced markedly to 1.20. Adjustment for other differences in baseline clinical features reduced further the odds ratio to 1.14. Excesses in other major clinical events among women were generally reduced to a similar extent by adjustment. These data suggest that at most, there is only a small independent association between female gender and early morbidity and mortality after suspected AMI (Figure 2-49).

Utility of C-Reactive Protein in Determining Acute Myocardial Infarction Risk in Women

Ridker and colleagues[127] in Boston, Massachusetts, determined the utility of C-reactive (CRP) protein in predicting risk of AMI and stroke among apparently healthy women. Baseline blood samples were used from 122 participants from the Women's Health Study who subsequently suffered a first cardiovascu-

TABLE 2-9
Relative Risks of Future Cardiovascular Events Among Apparently Healthy Women According to Baseline Concentration of C-Reactive Protein (CRP)

	Quartile of CRP (range, mg/L)				
	1 (<1.5)	**2** (1.5–3.7)	**3** (3.8–7.3)	**4** (>7.3)	**p for Trend**
Any event					
RR (crude)	1.0	2.4	2.5	4.8	0.0001
95% CI	. . .	1.1–5.2	1.1–5.6	2.3–10.1	
p	. . .	0.03	0.02	0.0001	
RR (adjusted)	1.0	2.0	2.3	4.1	0.001
95% CI	. . .	0.8–4.7	1.0–5.6	1.7–9.9	
p	. . .	0.1	0.06	0.002	
MI or stroke					
RR (crude)	1.0	3.5	4.5	7.3	0.0001
95% CI	. . .	1.2–10.0	1.6–12.6	2.7–19.9	
p	. . .	0.02	0.005	0.0001	
RR (adjusted)	1.0	2.7	3.5	5.5	0.002
95% CI	. . .	0.9–8.1	1.1–10.4	1.8–16.6	
p	. . .	0.08	0.03	0.002	

All models age- and smoking-matched. Adjusted models controlled for body mass index, diabetes, hypertension, hypercholesterolemia, exercise, family history, and treatment assignment.
CI = confidence interval.
Reproduced with permission from Ridker et al.[127]

lar event and from 244 age- and smoking-matched control subjects who remained free of cardiovascular disease during a 3-year follow-up period. Women who developed cardiovascular events had higher baseline CRP levels than control subjects, such that those with the highest levels of baseline had a 5-fold increase in risk of any vascular event and a 7-fold increase in risk of MI or stroke (Table 2-9). Risk estimates were independent of other risk factors and prediction models that included CRP provided a better method to predict risk than models that excluded CRP. Thus, CRP was a predictor among subgroups of women with low as well as high risk as defined by other cardiovascular risk factors. In these data, CRP is a strong independent risk factor for cardiovascular disease that adds to the predictive value of risk models based on the usual factors that are analyzed.

Chlamydia Pneumoniae

This study by Mazzoli and associates[128] from Florence, Italy, concerned the possible relation between seroreactivity to *Chlamydia pneumoniae* and MI. A group of 29 patients with AMI, 74 members of a healthy control group, and a subgroup of 24 members of a healthy control group matched for age, gender, and coronary risk factors (HCM) were included in the study. In addition, they evaluated the AMI group in a 1-year patient follow-up study. They used 2 different tests to detect anti-*C. pneumoniae* antibodies: recombinant enzyme immunoassay antilipopolysaccharide antibodies and a reference microimmunofluorescence test. High titers of *C. pneumoniae* microimmunofluorescence antibodies were found in 90% of the AMI group and in 25% of the HCM group. Immunoglobulin A-microimmunofluorescence was 52% in the AMI group and 21% in the HCM group. Immunoglobulin G and immunoglobulin A antilipopolysaccharide titers were 66% and 63% in the AMI group and 21% in the HCM group, respectively. High concentrations of interleukin-6 were found in 86% of the AMI group when compared with the control group. A good correlation between interleukin-6 levels and immunoglobulin A-lipopolysaccharide titers was found. The presence of a high prevalence rate and high titers of immunoglobulin G and immunoglobulin A-specific anti-*C. pneumoniae* antibodies in AMI at admission demonstrates the presence of a specific anti-*C. pneumoniae* immunization in the AMI population.

Inflammation, Pravastatin, and Risk of Coronary Events After Myocardial Infarction

Ridker and colleagues[129] in Boston, Massachusetts, determined whether inflammation after AMI is a risk factor for recurrent coronary events and whether randomized treatment with pravastatin reduces that risk. A nested case-control design was used to compare C-reactive protein (CRP) and serum amyloid A (SAA) levels in prerandomization blood samples from 391 patients in the Cholesterol and Recurrent Events (CARE) Trial who subsequently developed recurrent nonfatal AMI or a fatal coronary event and from an equal number of age- and gender-matched participants who remained free of these events during follow-up. CRP and SAA were higher among cases than control subjects, such that those with levels in the highest quintile had a relative risk of recurrent events of 75% compared with those with levels in the lowest quintile (Figure 2-50). The study group with the highest risk was that with consistent evidence

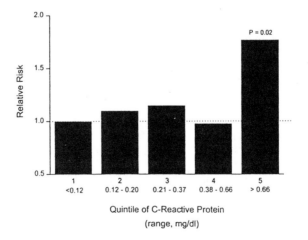

FIGURE 2-50. Relative risks of recurrent coronary events among postmyocardial infarction patients according to baseline plasma concentration of CRP. Reproduced with permission from Ridker et al.[129]

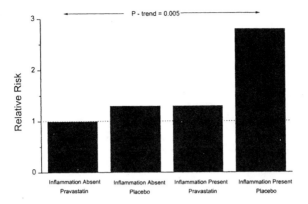

FIGURE 2-51. Relative risks of recurrent coronary events among postmyocardial infarction patients according to presence (both CRP and SAA levels ≥90th percentile or absence (both CRP and SAA levels <90th percentile) of evidence of inflammation and by randomized pravastatin assignment. Reproduced with permission from Ridker et al.[129]

of inflammation; specifically elevation of both CRP and SAA who were randomly assigned placebo. In these individuals, the risk estimate was greater than the product of the individual risks associated with inflammation or placebo assignment alone. In stratified analyses, the association between inflammation and risk was significant among those randomized to placebo, but was attenuated and nonsignificant among those randomized to pravastatin (Figure 2-51). Thus, these data suggest that evidence of inflammation after AMI is associated with increased risk of recurrent coronary events. Therapy with pravastatin may decrease this risk, an observation consistent with an effect beyond the lipid-lowering properties of this agent.

Prognostic Influence of Fibrinogen and C-Reactive Protein Levels

Toss and colleagues[130] in Uppsala, Sweden, evaluated the prognostic influence of fibrinogen and C-reactive protein (CRP) levels in their relation to myocardial damage in unstable coronary syndromes. Fibrinogen and CRP were determined at inclusion and related to outcome after 5 months in 965 patients with unstable angina or non-Q-wave AMI randomized to 5 weeks with low-molecular-weight heparin or placebo. The probabilities of death were 1.6%, 4.6%, and 6.9% (p=0.005) and the probabilities of death and/or AMI were 9.3%, 14.2%, and 19.1% (p=0.002), respectively, in patients stratified by tertiles of fibrinogen. The probabilities of death were 2.2%, 3.6%, and 7.5% (p=0.003) after stratification of patient data by tertiles of CRP level for less than 2, 2-20, and greater than 10 mg/L (Figure 2-52). In logistic multiple regression analysis, increased fibrinogen levels were independently associated with the incidence of death and/or AMI and elevated CRP was associated with the incidence of death. Thus, these data suggest that increased levels of both fibrinogen and CRP are associated with a poorer outcome in patients with unstable CAD.

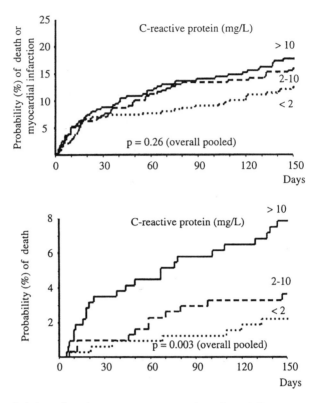

FIGURE 2-52. Probability of cardiac events in groups based on different tertiles of C-reactive protein level. Reproduced with permission from Toss et al.[130]

Diagnosis and Early Testing in Acute Myocardial Infarction

Use of Cardiac Troponins as Predictors of Cardiac Events

Cardiac troponins are being used with increasing frequency to diagnose myocardial necrosis in patients who present with chest pain in the emergency room. Polanczyk and colleagues[131] from Boston, Massachusetts, evaluated the diagnostic and prognostic value of troponin I in 1,047 patients over 30 years old who were admitted for acute chest pain. The sensitivity, specificity, and positive predictive values of troponin I for major cardiac events were 47%, 80%, and 19%, respectively. Elevated troponin I in the presence of ischemia on the electrocardiogram was associated with an adjusted odds ratio of 1.8 for major cardiac events within 72 hours. Among patients without an AMI or unstable angina, troponin I was not an independent correlate of complications. These authors conclude that in patients presenting to the emergency room with acute chest pain, troponin I was an independent predictor of major cardiac events. However, the positive predictive value of an abnormal assay result was not high in this heterogeneous cohort of patients. These data are consistent with other studies that have shown that levels of troponin I can risk stratify patients with acute coronary syndromes.

Early Negative Exercise Tolerance Test

An exercise tolerance test (ETT) is often performed to identify patients for early discharge after observation for acute chest pain, but the safety of this strategy is unproven. Polanczyk and associates[132] from Boston, Massachusetts, prospectively studied 276 low-risk patients who underwent an ETT within 48 hours after presentation to the emergency department with acute chest pain. The ETT was considered negative if subjects achieved at least stage 1 of the Bruce protocol and the electrocardiogram showed no evidence of ischemia. There were no complications associated with ETT performance. The ETT was negative in 195 patients (71%); there were no identifiable subsets of patients at very low probability of an abnormal test. During the 6-month follow-up, patients with a negative ETT had fewer additional visits to the emergency department (17% vs. 21%, respectively), and fewer readmissions to the hospital (12% vs. 17%) than those with positive or inconclusive ETTs. No patient with a negative ETT experienced a major cardiac event (AMI, coronary angioplasty, or bypass) within 6 months. Among these 4 patients, only 1 had an event within 4 months. In conclusion, these results suggest that ETT can be safely used to identify patients at low risk for subsequent events. Patients without a clearly negative test are at increased risk for readmission and cardiac events and should be reevaluated either during the same admission or shortly after discharge.

Dobutamine Echocardiography Versus Single Photon Emission Computed Tomography Thallium-201 Scintigraphy

To directly compare dobutamine echocardiography and resting single photon emission computed tomographic (SPECT) thallium-201 (Tl-201) scintigraphy for the detection of reversible dysfunction, 64 patients underwent dobutamine echocardiography (baseline, low dose 5 and 10 mg/kg/min, and peak dose), rest T1-201 scintigraphy (3mCi-15 minute and 3- to 4-hour SPECT imaging), and coronary angiography during the first week after AMI in this study by Smart and associates[133] from Milwaukee, Wisconsin. Follow-up echocardiography was performed 4 to 8 weeks after discharge. Wall thickening improved at follow-up in 52% (207 of 399) of the dysfunctional segments. By receiver operating characteristic analysis, biphasic responses and sustained improvement during dobutamine echocardiography were more accurate than T1-201 uptake by SPECT scintigraphy for reversible dysfunction. The greater accuracy of dobutamine echocardiography resulted from higher accuracy in akinetic segments, Q-wave infarction, and multivessel CAD. In conclusion, dobutamine echocardiography is more accurate than resting SPECT Tl-201 scintigraphy for reversible dysfunction after AMI.

Sudden Death

Risk Factors for Acute Thrombosis and Sudden Coronary Death in Women

Burke and colleagues[134] at the Armed Forces Institute of Pathology in Washington, DC, examined 51 cases of sudden cardiac death in 15 hearts from women who died of trauma. Coronary deaths were divided into 4 mechanisms of death, including ruptured plaque with acute thrombus (n = 8), eroded plaque with acute thrombus (n = 18), stable plaque with healed infarct (n = 18), and stable plaque without AMI (n = 7). Vulnerable plaques prone to rupture were defined as those with a thin, fibrous cap infiltrated by macrophages and in comparison with control subjects, women with plaque ruptures had elevated total serum cholesterols (270 ± 55 vs. 194 ± 44 mg/dL) and those with erosions were more like to be smokers (78% vs. 33%) (Table 2-10). Women with stable plaque and healed AMI had elevated glycosylated hemoglobin and were more likely to be hypertensive. By multivariate analysis, cigarette smoking was associated with plaque erosion, glycosylated hemoglobin with stable plaque and healed AMI, total cholesterol with plaque rupture, and hypertension with stable

TABLE 2-10
Risk Factors in Women Who Died of Severe Coronary Disease: Multivariate Comparison with Control Subjects by Mechanism of Death

Mechanism of Death	Risk Factor	p vs. Control Subjects	Odds Ratio vs. Control Subjects
Plaque rupture	Total cholesterol	0.02	7†
	Low HDL-C	0.14	
	Age	0.2	
	Others	>0.4	
Plaque erosion	Smoking	0.03	21
	Hypertension	0.2	
	Low HDL-C	0.19	
	Age*	0.17	
	Total cholesterol*	0.2	
	Others	>0.4	
Stable plaque, healed MI	Hypertension	0.02	15
	GlycoHgb	0.03	41‡
	Total cholesterol	0.17	
	Heart weight	0.2	
	Smoking	0.3	
	Others	>0.4	

Multivariate analysis using stepwise logistic regression, p = 0.4 for removing, p = 0.2 for entering. Odds ratios given only if p <0.05.
* Negative association.
† Odds ratio calculated if used as dichotomous variable, cutoff 210 mg/dL for TC, 10%. Odds ratio as continuous variable, 1.04.
‡ Odds ratio calculated if used as dichotomous variable, cutoff 10% glycosylated hemoglobin. Odds ratio as continuous variable, 9.
Reproduced with permission from Burke et al.[134]

plaque with healed AMI. Seven of 8 plaque ruptures occurred in women over 50 years of age versus 3 of 18 erosions. Vulnerable plaques were associated with elevated serum cholesterol and age over 50 years, independent of other risk factors in cases of coronary death in this study. Thus, in women, traditional risk factors have distinct effects on the mechanisms of sudden cardiac death that vary by menopausal status.

Nonuniform Nighttime Distribution of Acute Cardiac Events

Lavery and colleagues[135] examined whether the incidence of AMI, sudden cardiac death, and automatic implantable cardioverter-defibrillator (AICD) discharge was nonuniform to further evaluate the fact that many AMIs and sudden cardiac deaths occur at night. They conducted a review of the circadian pattern of the onset of AMI, sudden cardiac death, and AICD discharge. The nighttime period was chosen *a priori* as midnight to 5:59 AM. They documented 11,633 nocturnal AMIs (20% of the total MIs), 1,981 nocturnal sudden cardiac deaths (14.6% of the total sudden cardiac deaths), and 1,200 nocturnal AICD discharges (15% of the total discharges). The distributions of MI, sudden cardiac death, and AICD discharge were each significantly nonuniform. The peak incidence of AMI and AICD discharge occurred between midnight and 0:59 AM, whereas the peak incidence of sudden cardiac death was between 1:00 and 1:59 AM. The trough in incidence occurred between 4:00 and 4:59 AM for sudden cardiac death and between 3:00 and 3:59 AM for AMI and AICD discharge. These data indicate that nocturnal AMIs, sudden cardiac death, and AICD discharge exhibit nonuniform distributions. The findings are consistent with the hypothesis that sleep-state-dependent fluctuations in autonomic nervous system activity may trigger the onset of major cardiovascular events.

Coronary Stenosis and Sudden Death in Patients with Diabetes

Persons with diabetes are at higher risk for AMI and sudden death than are persons without diabetes. It has been demonstrated that the artery that occludes during AMI generally has less than 75% stenosis on a previous angiogram. The extent of coronary artery stenosis was analyzed for 820 consecutively examined patients who underwent coronary angiography by Henry and associates[136] from Paris and Saint-Denis, France. The patients were categorized according to the presence or absence of diabetes mellitus. The severity of stenosis was taken into consideration. Patients with diabetes had moderate (50% to 75% narrowing) stenosis much more frequently than patients without diabetes (51% vs. 30%). Moreover diabetes mellitus was an independent risk factor for moderate stenosis. The lesions were more frequently located on distal arteries, more frequently had a pattern of 3-vessel disease, and had a trend toward more diffuse disease than described 25 years ago. This greater amount of moderate stenosis may be considered a substrate for future acute plaque rupture. It may explain the high prevalence of AMI and sudden death among patients with diabetes without an increase in the incidence of angina pectoris.

Sudden Coronary Death in Women

The objective of this study by Kannel and associates[137] from Boston and Framingham, Massachusetts, was to examine prospectively the incidence, predisposing cardiovascular conditions, and risk factors for sudden death in women compared with men. The study design was a prospective general population examination of a cohort of 2,873 women for development of sudden coronary death in relation to antecedent overt CAD, cardiac failure, and risk factors for CAD. Participants were women aged 30 to 62 years participating in the Framingham Study, receiving routine biennial examinations for risk factors and cardiovascular conditions. Among women monitored over a period of 38 years, there were 750 initial coronary events, of which 94 (12%) were sudden cardiac deaths. Of the 292 CAD fatalities in women, 32% were sudden cardiac deaths and 37% of the women had a history of CAD. Sudden death incidence in women lagged behind that in men by more than 10 years. However, above age 75, 17% of all CAD events in women were sudden deaths. Sudden death risk in women with CAD was half as high as in men if they had CAD. In both genders, a myocardial infarction conferred twice the risk of angina. Cardiac failure escalated sudden death risk of women 5-fold but was only one fourth that of men with failure or CAD. Ventricular ectopy increased sudden death risk only in women without prior overt CAD. Except for diabetes, CAD risk factors imposed a lower sudden death risk in women than in men. However, even in women, sudden death risk increased over a 17-fold range in relation to their burden of CAD risk factors. Sudden death is a prominent feature of CAD in women as well as men, particularly in advanced age. A higher fraction of sudden deaths in women than men is unexpected occuring in the absence of prior overt CAD. It is subject to the same risk factors and as predictable in women as in men. However, at any level of multivariate risk, women are less vulnerable to sudden death than men.

Prognostic Indicators for Acute Myocardial Infarction

Influence of Polymorphisms of Factor VII Gene on Acute Myocardial Infarction

Iacoviello and colleagues[138] performed a case-control study of 165 patients with MI, mean age 55 ± 9 years, and 225 controls without a personal or family history of cardiovascular disease. The polymorphisms involved R353Q and hypervariable region 4 of the factor VII gene. Factor VII clotting activity and antigen levels were also measured. Patients with the *QQ* or *H7H7* genotype had decreased risk of AMI (odds ratio 0.08). For the R353Q polymorphism, the *RR* genotype was associated with the highest risk followed by the *RQ* genotype and then by the *QQ* genotype. For the polymorphism involving hypervariable region 4, the combined *H7H5* and *H6H5* genotypes were associated with the highest risk followed in descending order by the *H6H6*, *H6H7*, and *H7H7* genotypes. Patients with the *QQ* or *H7H7* genotype had lower levels of both factor VII antigen and factor VII clotting activity than those with the *RR* or *H6H6* genotype. Patients with the lowest level of factor VII clotting activity had a lower risk of AMI than those with the highest level. These data suggest that certain polymorphisms of factor VII gene may influence the risk of AMI. It is possible that this effect may be mediated by alterations in factor VII levels.

Predictive Characteristics at Hospital Admission

Birnbaum and associates[139] from Tel Aviv, Israel, assessed the ability of simple and clinical electrocardiographic variables routinely obtained on admission to identify patients at high risk of developing high-degree AV block during hospitalization in 1,336 patients with inferior wall AMI. Patients were classified into 2 initial electrocardiographic patterns based on the J-point to R-wave amplitude ratio: pattern 1—those with J point/R wave less than 0.5, and pattern 2—patients with J point/R wave 0.5 or more in 2 or more leads of the inferior leads II, III, and aVF. High-degree AV block was found in 6.7% of patients (41 of 615) with pattern 1 versus 11.8% of the patients (85 of 721) with pattern 2 on admission electrocardiogram. Multivariate logistic regression analysis revealed that the only variables found to be independently associated with high-degree AV block were female gender (odds ratio [OR] 1.48; Killip class on admission 2 or more (OR 2.24); initial electrocardiographic pattern 2 versus pattern 1 (OR 1.82); and absence of abnormal Q waves on admission (OR yes vs. no 0.68). A simple electrocardiographic sign (J point/R wave $\geq$0.5 in $\geq$2 leads) is a reliable predictor of the development of advanced AV block among patients receiving thrombolytic therapy for inferior wall AMI (Figure 2-53).

Albumin Excretion Rate Increase as a Predictor of Mortality

Berton and colleagues[140] in Padova, Italy, determined whether albumin excretion rate increases during AMI and whether it predicts in-hospital mortality. The study was performed in 496 patients admitted to the hospital with suspected AMI. Among these, 360 had evidence of AMI and the remaining 136 served as controls for the study. Albumin excretion rate was assessed by radioimmunoassay in 3 24-hour urine collections performed on the first, third, and seventh days after admission. LVEF was measured by 2-dimensional echocardiography in 254 patients. Albumin excretion rate adjusted for several confounders was higher in the patients with AMI than in the non-AMI group on the first and third days, but no difference was present on the seventh day. When subjects with CHF were excluded, the difference between the 2 groups remained significant. In the 26 AMI patients who died in hospital, the mortality rate progressively increased with increasing levels of albumin excretion rate. In a Cox proportional hazards model, albumin excretion rate was a better predictor of in-hospital mortality than Killip class or LVEF determined by echocardiogram. A cutoff value of 50 mg/24 hours for first-day albumin excretion rate and 30 mg/24 hours for the third day yielded a sensitivity of 92% and of 89% and

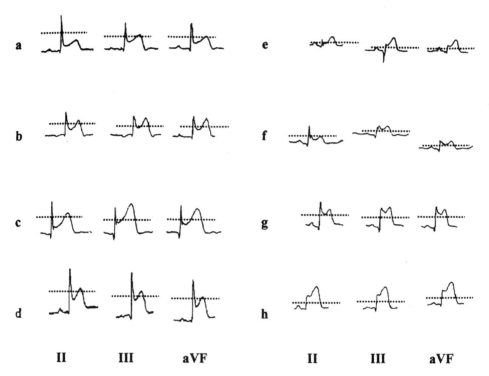

FIGURE 2-53. Leads II, III, and aVF on admission electrocardiograms of 8 patients with inferior wall AMI (recorded at a paper speed of 25 mm/s; sensitivity 1 mV = 10 mm). **(a)** to **(d)** Electrocardiographic pattern 1; despite a different magnitude of total ST-segment elevation, in all 3 leads the J point emerges below 50% of the R-wave height (dashed line). **(e)** to **(h)** Electrocardiographic pattern 2; in ≥2 of the inferior leads, the J point emerges above 50% of the R-wave height (dashed line). Reproduced with permission from Birnbaum et al.[139]

a specificity of 72% and 79%, respectively, for mortality (Table 2-11). Adjusted relative risks for the 2 cutoff values were 17.3 and 8.4. Thus, these data demonstrate that albumin excretion rate increases in patients with AMI and that it yields prognostic information additional to that provided by clinical or echocardiographic evaluation of LV performance.

C-Reactive Protein as a Predictor of Mortality

Several acute phase proteins such as C-reactive protein, which serve as non-specific markers of human inflammation, have been found to be elevated in patients with atherosclerotic CAD. Morrow and colleagues[141] from Boston, Massachusetts, evaluated C-reactive protein together with troponin T for predicting 14-day mortality in patients with unstable angina or non-Q-wave MI. In the TIMI II A trial, a dose-ranging trial of enoxaparin for unstable angina and non-Q-wave MI, serum was obtained for C-reactive protein and troponin T measurements. C-reactive protein was higher among patients who died than those who survived (7.2 vs. 1.3 mg/dL). Among patients with a negative tropo-

TABLE 2-11

In-Hospital Mortality Rate in Patients with AMI Divided According to Whether They Had Normal AER, Microalbuminuria, or Overt Albuminuria on the First and Third Days after Admission to the Hospital

First Day	AER <30 (n = 204)	AER 30–299 (n = 135)	AER ≥300 (n = 21)
Alive, n (%)	202 (99.0)	118 (87.4)	14 (66.7)
In-hospital mortality rate, n (%)	2 (1.0)	17 (12.6)	7 (33.3)

Third Day	AER <30 (n = 268)	AER 30–299 (n = 90)	AER ≥300 (n = 2)
Alive, n (%)	265 (98.9)	68 (75.6)	1 (50)
In-hospital mortality rate, n (%)	3 (1.1)	22 (24.4)	1 (50)

$\chi^2 = 39.0$, p <. 0001 and $\chi^2 = 60.2$, p < .0001 for first and third day, respectively.
Reproduced with permission from Berton et al.[140]
AER = albumin excretion rate.

nin T assay, the mortality was higher among patients with C-reactive protein greater than 1.55 mg/dL (5.8% vs. 0.36%). Patients with both an early positive troponin T and C-reactive protein greater than 1.55 mg/dL had the highest mortality. These authors conclude that elevated C-reactive protein at presentation in patients with unstable angina or non-Q-wave MI is correlated with increased 14-day mortality even in patients with a negative rapid troponin T assay. C-reactive protein and troponin T provide complementary information for stratifying patients with regard to mortality risk.

Single Photon Emission Computed Tomography Myocardial Perfusion Imaging

Patients frequently are seen in the emergency room with chest pain and a nondiagnostic electrocardiogram. Heller and colleagues[142] from multiple US centers and Tel-Aviv, Israel, evaluated the clinical use of acute rest technetium-99m SPECT myocardial perfusion imaging in such patients. Three hundred fifty seven patients presenting to 6 centers with symptoms suggestive of myocardial ischemia and a nondiagnostic electrocardiogram underwent radionuclide testing, during or within 6 hours of symptoms. Fifty seven percent of images were normal and 43% were abnormal. Of 20 patients with an AMI during the hospital period, 18 had abnormal images (sensitivity 90%), whereas only 2 had normal images. Multiple logistic regression analysis demonstrated abnormal single photon emission computed tomography (SPECT) imaging to be the best predictor of AMI and significantly better than clinical data. Using the normal SPECT image as a criterion not to admit patients might also reduce hospital admission rate. These authors conclude that abnormal rest technetium-99m tetrofosmin SPECT imaging accurately predicts AMI in patients with symptoms and a nondiagnostic electrocardiogram whereas a normal study is associated with a very low cardiac event rate. They consider that this technique may be very helpful in the emergency room in deciding who should be admitted to the hospital.

Determinants of Regional Myocardial Infarction

The aim of this study by Mutlak and associates[143] from Haifa, Israel, was to evaluate the effect of collateral flow, stenosis severity, antegrade flow, and location of the lesion on regional myocardial function in patients with chronic LAD. Seventy-four patients who underwent coronary angiography and ventriculography were divided into 3 groups: group A (n=9), patients with normal coronary angiogram and ventriculogram; group B (n=32) patients with LAD stenosis greater than 75%; and group C, 33 patients with LAD occlusion. The effect of collateral flow, stenosis severity, location, and antegrade flow on regional myocardial function in the LAD territory was studied. Regional function was impaired in both groups B and C. In group B, univariate analysis confirmed that antegrade flow had a significant effect on regional function. With the use of multiple regression, none of the other variables had an additional independent effect. In group C, no significant correlation was found between regional function and the study variables by univariate analysis; however, multiple regression analysis revealed a significant correlation among anterobasal function, the lesion site, and collateral flow. In patients with LAD stenosis, antegrade flow has the strongest effect on regional myocardial function, with no additional effect of visible collaterals. In patients with LAD occlusion, both angiographic collateral flow and the site of the lesion have a significant effect on the function of the anterobasal area.

Gender Differences in Symptom Presentation for Myocardial Infarction

This study by Goldberg and associates[144] from Worcester and Amherst, Massachusetts, describes gender differences in symptom presentation after AMI while controlling for differences in age and other potentially confounding factors. Although several studies have examined gender differences in diagnosis, management, and survival after AMI, limited data exist about possible gender differences in symptom presentation in the setting of AMI. Utilized was a community-based study of patients hospitalized with confirmed AMI in all 16 metropolitan Worcester, Massachusetts, hospitals (1990 census population = 437,000). Men (n=810) and women (n=550) hospitalized and validated AMI in 1986 and 1988 comprised the study sample. After simultaneously controlling for age, medical history, and AMI characteristics through regression modeling, men were significantly less likely to complain of neck pain than women. Conversely, men were significantly more likely to report diaphoresis than women. There were no statistically significant gender differences in complaints of chest pain although men were more likely to complain of this symptom. The results of this population-based observational study suggest differences in symptom presentation in men and women hospitalized with AMI. These findings have implications for public and health care provider education concerning recognition of gender differences in AMI-related symptoms and health care seeking behaviors.

Angiographic Characteristics of Stenoses

In patients with CAD, angiographic and postmortem studies have shown that coronary stenoses in infarct-related arteries often have complex morphology. It is not known whether in patients with multivessel disease stenosis morphology in noninfarct-related arteries is different from those of the infarct-related arteries. In 24 consecutive patients, Tousoulis and associates[145] from London, United Kingdom, and Rome, Italy, examined the angiographic characteristics of both the infarct-related stenoses and noninfarct-related stenoses before and after spontaneous AMI, by visual inspection and computerized edge detection of coronary angiograms. Before MI, the severity of the infarct-related stenoses was less than 50% in 14 patients and 50% or more in 10 patients and of noninfarct-related stenoses was less than 50% in 16 and 50% or more in 13. A significantly greater proportion of infarct-related stenoses with severity of 50% or more progressed to non-Q-wave MI (71% vs. 50%). Before MI, the percentage of concentric, eccentric, and irregular infarct-related stenoses was 8%, 13%, and 50%, respectively, whereas in the noninfarct-related stenoses it was 62%, 17%, and 21%, respectively. A similar proportion of irregular morphology progressed to Q-wave or non-Q-wave MI. In patients with stable angina who had AMI develop, the infarct-related and noninfarct-related stenoses on average are similar in severity but different in morphology. Nonsevere stenoses more frequently progress to Q-wave than to non-Q-wave MI.

New Therapeutic Modalities Improve Prognosis of Patients

The reported incidence of non-Q-wave AMI has increased in the thrombolytic era. Data comparing prognosis among these patients before and after the advent of the thrombolytic era are scarce. Haim and associates[146] from Tel Hashomer, Israel, compared the early and late prognosis among 2 cohorts of consecutive patients with a first non-Q-wave AMI hospitalized in the coronary care units operating in Israel: 610 patients from 1981 to 1983 and 225 patients in 1994. The proportion of patients with non-Q-wave AMI increased from 14% in 1981 to 1983 to 32% in 1994. Baseline characteristics in both periods were comparable. In-hospital management of patients differed during the last decade. Patients in 1994 received aspirin, angiotensin-converting enzyme inhibitors, β-blockers, and nitrates more frequently than from 1981 to 1983. Thrombolytic therapy, coronary angiography, and PTCA, or CABG were not used during the index hospitalization in the early 1980s, whereas in 1994 these procedures were used in 28%, 38%, 19%, and 6% of patients, respectively. In-hospital complications, including arrhythmias, conduction disturbances, and heart failure, were less frequent in 1994 compared with the period 1981 to 1983. The 7- and 30-day crude mortality rates were significantly lower in 1994 compared with the early 1980s (5% vs. 9% and 5% vs. 13%, respectively), whereas the 1-year crude mortality rate decreased slightly (15% vs. 19%). Multivariate analyses adjusting for pertinent variables revealed a decreased risk for death in 1994 versus 1981 to 1983; for 7-day (odds ratio = 0.49), 30-day (odds ratio = 0.36) and for 1-year (odds ratio = 0.65). The prognosis of patients with a first non-Q-wave AMI has improved considerably during the last decade. The introduction of new therapeutic modalities, including invasive cardiac procedures and new medications, probably played a major role in the favorable outcome of these patients.

Complications of Acute Myocardial Infarction

Out-of-Hospital Cardiac Arrest Survivors

The incidence, characteristics, and survival of out-of-hospital sudden cardiac arrest remain a challenging problem in the population at large. de Vreede-Swagemakers and associates[147] from Maastricht, The Netherlands, determined the incidence, patient characteristics, and survival rates by prospectively collecting information on all cases of sudden cardiac arrest occurring in the age group 20 to 75 years between January 1, 1991, and December 31, 1994. Five hundred fifteen patients were included (72% men, 28% women). In 44% of men and 53% of women, sudden cardiac arrest was most likely the first manifestation of heart disease. In patients known to have had a previous myocardial infarction, the mean interval between the AMI and arrest was 6.5 years with more than 50% having an LVEF greater than 30%. Nearly 80% of arrests occurred at home. In 60% of all cases, a witness was present. Cardiac resuscitation was attempted in 51% of all subjects resulting in 6% of the 515 patients being discharged alive from the hospital. Survival rates for witnessed arrests were 8% at home and 18% outside the home. These authors conclude that the majority of victims of sudden cardiac arrest cannot be identified before the event. It usually occurs at home when the survival of those with witnessed arrest is low, compared to those outside the home, indicating the necessity of optimizing out-of-hospital resuscitation, especially in the at-home situation.

Mortality Rate After Acute Myocardial Infarction for Patients on Dialysis

Herzog and colleagues[148] undertook a study to assess long-term survival after AMI among patients in the US who were receiving long-term dialysis. Patients on dialysis hospitalized during the period from 1977 to 1995 for a first AMI after the initiation of renal-replacement therapy were retrospectively identified from the US Renal Data System database. Overall mortality and mortality from cardiac causes were estimated by the life-table method. Overall mortality after AMI among 34,189 patients on long-term dialysis was 59% at 1 year, 73% at 2 years, and 90% at 5 years. The mortality from cardiac causes was 41% at 1 year, 52% at 2 years, and 70% at 5 years. Patients who were older or who had diabetes had a higher mortality rate than patients without these characteristics. Adverse outcomes occurred even in patients who had no AMI in 1990 through 1995. Mortality rate after AMI was considerably higher for patients on long-term dialysis than for renal transplant recipients. Thus, patients on dialysis who have AMI have high mortality from cardiac causes and poor long-term survival.

Risk Factors for Left Ventricular Free Wall Rupture

Risk factors for LV free wall rupture during AMI are still not clearly defined. Melchior and associates[149] from Frederiksburg and Hellerup, Denmark, studied 1,408 consecutive patients with AMI to determine a possible relation between diabetes mellitus, systemic hypertension, and LV free wall rupture. The authors analyzed all cases with AMI from 1980 to 1983. AMI was assumed to take place on onset of severe chest discomfort in patients with typical changes in the electrocardiogram. In all patients who survived a few hours after admission to the coronary care unit, diagnosis was confirmed by transient serum elevations of creatine kinase MB. Autopsy was performed routinely in all patients who died from known or suspected AMI during the study. Data were available in 94% (n = 29) of fatal cases. Systemic hypertension was considered to be present if antihypertensive therapy had previously been prescribed. As shown in Tables 2-12 and 2-13, only age and no previous indications of symptomatic myocardial ischemia had independent influence on the occurrence of LV free wall rupture. The presence of diabetes and systemic hypertension were not risk factors for LV free wall rupture. Female gender specifically had no influence on the frequency of LV free wall rupture.

TABLE 2-12
Clinical Data of All Patients with Acute Myocardial Infarction and in the Group of Patients with Left Ventricular (LV) Free Wall Rupture

	LV Free Wall Rupture	
	Negative n = 1,379 (98%)	Positive n = 29 (2.1%)
Men	1,005 (72.9%)	21 (72.4%)
<65 years	828 (60.0%)	10 (34.4%)*
>65 years	551 (40.0%)	19 (65.5%)*
Diabetes mellitus	117 (8.5%)	2 (6.9%)
Systemic hypertension	161 (11.7%)	2 (6.9%)
Previous AMI	412 (29.9%)	5 (17.2%)
Congestive heart failure	576 (41.8%)	9 (31.0%)
In-hospital complications		
Cardiogenic shock	225 (16.3%)	5 (17.2%)
Pulmonary edema	101 (7.3%)	0
Ventricular fibrillation	154 (11.2%)	5 (17.2%)
Asystole	45 (3.3%)	2 (6.9%)

*p = 0.006.
Reproduced with permission from Melchior et al.[149]

TABLE 2-13
Cox Proportional Hazard Model for the Effect of Several Potential Risk Factors on Left
Ventricular Free Wall Rupture in Patients with Acute Myocardial Infarction

Factor	p Value	RR	95% Confidence Limits of RR
Diabetes mellitus	0.76	1.255	0.29–5.52
Systemic hypertension	0.44	1.777	0.41–7.64
Age (per decreasing year)	0.001	0.939	0.90–0.98
No history of coronary artery disease	0.049	4.340	1.01–18.70
Congestive heart failure	0.07	2.207	0.95–5.14
Previous AMI	0.57	0.619	0.31–3.24
Male gender	0.52	0.753	0.32–1.78

RR = risk ratio.
Reproduced with permission from Melchior et al.[149]

Influence of Previous Angina on In-Hospital Deaths Secondary to Acute Myocardial Infarction

There is little information on how previous angina influences in-hospital deaths secondary to AMI. Kobayashi and associates[150] from Osaka, Japan, evaluated the causes of in-hospital deaths in AMI patients with and without previous angina. A total of 2,264 consecutive patients were admitted to their hospital due to AMI. These patients were divided into 2 groups according to the presence or absence of prior AMI. Both groups were further divided according to the presence or absence of previous angina. The causes of in-hospital deaths were classified into 4 categories: (1) cardiogenic shock or CHF, (2) cardiac rupture, (3) arrhythmia, and (4) other causes. In patients with a first AMI, the in-hospital mortality rate was lower in patients with previous angina than those without (6.9% vs. 11.4%). There was no significant difference between these patients with and without previous angina in in-hospital deaths due to cardiogenic shock or CHF, arrhythmia, or other causes. Death due to cardiac rupture was less frequent in patients with previous angina (1.4% vs. 5.0%). In patients with prior AMI, the in-hospital mortality rate was lower in patients with than without previous angina (17.7% vs. 25.3%). In contrast to patients with their first AMI, there was a trend toward a lower incidence of in-hospital death due to cardiogenic shock or CHF in patients with previous angina (12.8% vs. 19.0%). There were no significant differences in in-hospital deaths due to cardiac rupture, arrhythmia, and other causes between the 2 subgroups. In multivariate analysis, previous angina was an independent predictor of in-hospital death. Thus, in-hospital mortality rate after AMI in patients with previous angina is lower because of less cardiac rupture in patients with a first AMI and less cardiogenic shock or CHF in patients with prior AMI (Figures 2-54, 2-55).

Sudden Cardiac Death After Myocardial Infarction

To evaluate the potential prognostic value of the circadian variation of QT intervals in predicting sudden cardiac death (SCD) in patients after AMI, 15

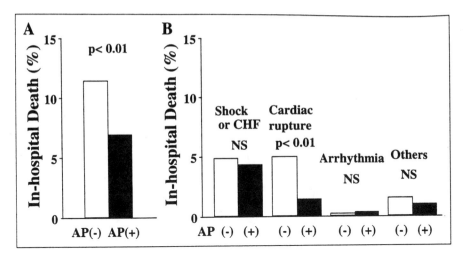

FIGURE 2-54. The in-hospital mortality in patients with a first MI. **(A)** In-hospital mortality rate was lower in patients with previous angina than those without. **(B)** There was no significant difference between patients with and without previous angina in the incidence of in-hospital death due to cardiogenic shock or congestive heart failure, arrhythmia, and other causes except cardiac rupture. AP = previous angina; CHF = congestive heart failure. Reproduced with permission from Kobayashi et al.[150]

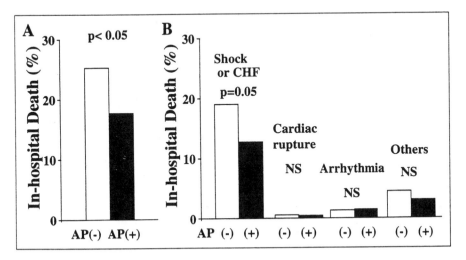

FIGURE 2-55. The in-hospital mortality in patients with prior MI. **(A)** In-hospital mortality rate was lower in patients with previous angina than those without. **(B)** There was a trend toward a lower in-hospital death due to cardiogenic shock or congestive heart failure in patients with previous angina than those without. There were no significant differences in the incidences of in-hospital deaths due to cardiac rupture, arrhythmia, and other causes between the 2 groups. Abbreviations as in Figure 2-54. Reproduced with permission from Kobayashi et al.[150]

pairs of post-AMI patients (15 died suddenly within 1 year after AMI [SCD victims] and 15 remained event free [AMI survivors]) were studied (mean age 60 ± 8 years; 24 men and 6 women) by Yi and associates.[151] The pairs were matched for age, gender, infarct site, presence of Q wave, LVEF, thrombolytic and β-blocker therapy. Fourteen normal subjects served as controls (mean age 55 ± 9 years; 12 men). A 24-hour Holter electrocardiographic recording was obtained from each subject. All recordings were analyzed using a Holter electrocardiogram analyzer. QT, RR, and heart rate-corrected QT intervals (QT_c) were automatically calculated by the analyzer, and hourly and 24-hour mean values of each measurement were derived from each recording. There was a pronounced circadian variation in the QT interval in parallel with the trend in the RR interval in normal subjects and in AMI survivors. Circadian variation in both indexes was blunted in SCD victims. The QT interval was significantly longer at night than during the day in normal subjects (388 ± 28 vs. 355 ± 21 ms) and in AMI survivors (358 ± 25 vs. 346 ± 15 ms), but not in SCD victims (357 ± 32 vs. 350 ± 31 ms). The 24-hour mean value of the QT interval in SCD victims did not differ significantly from that in normal subjects or AMI survivors. The QT interval at night was significantly shorter in SCD victims than in normal subjects (357 ± 32 vs. 388 ± 28 ms), but daytime values were similar. The QT interval in SCD victims did not differ significantly from that of AMI survivors at any time. The QT_c interval exhibited a small circadian variation in normal subjects. This variation was abolished in SCD victims and in AMI survivors. The 24-hour mean value of QT_c was significantly longer in SCD victims than in normal subjects (424 ± 25 vs. 402 ± 21 ms), and in AMI survivors (424 ± 25 vs. 404 ± 32 ms). The QT_c interval of SCD victims differed from that of normal subjects during both the day (421 ± 25 vs. 400 ± 17 ms) and the night (424 ± 26 vs. 403 ± 23 ms). Thus, blunted circadian variation in QT intervals, abolished circadian variation in QT_c intervals, and prolonged QT_c intervals may suggest an increased risk of SCD in patients after AMI.

Cardiac Findings at Necropsy in Different Age Groups

Roberts and Shirani[152] from Dallas, Texas, and New York, New York, described and compared certain clinical and necropsy cardiac findings in 391 octogenarians (80%), in 93 nonagenarians (19%), and in 6 centenarians (1%). The number of men and women was similar (248 [51%] and 242 [49%]). The cause of death was cardiac in 228 patients (47%), vascular but noncardiac in 71 (14%), and noncardiac and nonvascular in 191 (39%). The frequency of a cardiac condition causing death decreased with increasing age groups (51% vs. 32% vs. 0), and the frequency of a noncardiac, nonvascular condition causing death increased with increasing age groups (36% vs. 47% vs. 100%). Among the cardiac conditions causing death, CAD was found in 62% of cases (141 of 228), aortic valve stenosis in 16% (36 of 228), and cardiac amyloidosis in 10% of cases (22 of 228). Calcific deposits were found in necropsy in the coronary arteries in 81% of the patients (398 of 490), in the aortic valve in 47% (228 of 490), in the mitral annular area in 39% of the patients (190 of 490), and in 1 or both LV papillary muscles in 25% of the patients (122 of 490). The calcific deposits tended to be less frequent in the octogenarians. Three hundred (61%) of the 490 patients had 1 or more major coronary artery narrowed 75% or more in cross-sectional area by plaque, and the percent of patients in each of the 3 age groups and the percent of coronary arteries significantly narrowed in each of the 3 age groups were similar (Table 2-14).

Ventricular Late Potentials After First Myocardial Infarction

Ventricular late potentials have been shown to be independent predictors of arrhythmic events after MI. However, many studies have had 1 or more limitations: limited follow-up period, small study group, possible selection bias, inadequate statistical analysis, or inclusion of patients with previous infarction. The purpose of this study by Zimmermann and associates[153] from Geneva, Switzerland, was to assess the long-term prognostic value of ventricular late potentials in a large group of unselected patients after a first AMI. Time-domain signal averaging was performed in 458 patients (380 male, 78 female, mean age 59 ± 11 years) a mean of 10 days (range 7 to 13 days) after a first AMI. The overall prevalence of ventricular late potentials was 20% (90 of 458 patients). By univariate analysis, an LVEF less than 40% and the presence of an occluded infarct-related artery were the only statistically significant predictors for the development of ventricular late potentials. During a median follow-up of 70 months, 21 (5%) patients died suddenly, and 11 (2%) patients had documented sustained VT. The presence of ventricular late potentials, older age, and an occluded infarct-related artery were the only variables significantly associated with the occurrence of serious arrhythmic events during follow-up. The probability of having no arrhythmic events was 99% at 1 year and 96% at 5 years in the absence of ventricular late potentials and 87% at 1 year and 80% at 5 years in the presence of ventricular late potentials (4.6-fold increase in arrhythmic risk). Ventricular late potentials are powerful predictors of serious arrhythmic events in patients after a first AMI, and their prognostic value, although waning with time, persists for at least 7 years. This study also provides further evidence that an open infarct-related artery may reduce the arrhythmic risk after MI.

Remodeling After Acute Myocardial Infarction

Prognostic Implications of Restrictive Left Ventricular Filling

Although diastolic dysfunction is common, its contribution to the prognosis after AMI is not well understood. Nijland and colleagues[154] from Amsterdam, The Netherlands, evaluated 95 patients on days 1, 3, and 7, and 3 months after AMI to determine the potential additional value of measurements of diastolic function over the assessment of systolic dysfunction. Patients were classified into 2 groups: a restrictive group (n = 12) with a peak velocity of early diastolic filling wave (E:A ratio >2 or between 1 and 2, and a deceleration time <140 ms); and a nonrestrictive group (n = 83) with an E:A ratio less than

TABLE 2-14
Certain Clinical and Necropsy Findings in 490 Patients Aged 80 to 103 Years

Variable	Age Group (yrs)		
	80–89 (n = 391)	90–99 (n = 93)	≥100 (n = 6)
1. Mean age (yrs)	84 ± 4	93 ± 4	102
2. Men:women	194 (50%):197 (50%)	52 (56%):41 (44%)	2/4
3. Angina pectoris	137 (35%)	5 (5%)	0
4. Acute myocardial infarction	78 (20%)	18 (18%)	0
5. Chronic congestive heart failure	140 (36%)	23 (25%)	0
6. Systemic hypertension (history)	174 (44%)	50 (54%)	0
7. Diabetes mellitus	56 (14%)	8 (9%)	0
8. Atrial fibrillation	57 (15%)	35 (38%)	0
9. Heart weight (g):range (mean)	185–900 (449)	220–660 (420)	240–410 (328)
Men	230–830 (493)	285–660 (436)	335–410 (372)
Women	185–900 (409)	220–630 (406)	240–385 (306)
10. Cardiomegaly			
Men >400 g	103/154 (67%)	27/49 (55%)	1/2
Women >350 g	133/165 (81%)	23/42 (55%)	1/4
11. Cardiac calcific deposits			
None	43 (11%)	3 (3%)	0
Present	348 (89%)	90 (97%)	6 (100%)
Coronary arteries	304 (78%)	89 (96%)	5
Aortic valve cusps	164 (42%)	59 (63%)	5
Heavy (stenosis)	43 (11%)	8 (9%)	0
Mitral annulus	146 (37%)	42 (45%)	2
Heavy	52 (13%)	11 (12%)	0
Papillary muscle	37 (9%)	42 (45%)	6
12. No. of patients with 0, 1, 2, or 3 major (right, left anterior descending, left circumflex) coronary arteries ↓ >75% in cross-sectional area			
0	159 (41%)	33 (35%)	2
1	67 ⎫	20 ⎫	2 ⎫
2	71 ⎬ 232 (59%)	32 ⎬ 60 (65%)	2 ⎬ 4
3	94 ⎭	8 ⎭	0 ⎭
Mean	1.7	1.5	1.5
13. Number of major coronary arteries (3/patient) ↓ >75% in cross-sectional area by plaque			
0	0/477	0/99	0/6
1	67/201	20/60	2/6
2	142/213	64/96	4/6
3	282/282	24/24	0
Totals	491/1,173 (42%)	108/279 (39%)	6/18 (33%)
14. Left ventricular necrosis/fibrosis			
Necrosis only	54 (14%)	10 (11%)	0
Fibrosis only	101 (26%)	20 (21%)	2
Both	37 (9%)	5 (5%)	0
15. Ventricular cavity dilation			
Neither	222 (57%)	58 (62%)	4
One	84 (21%)	4 (4%)	2
Right ventricle	42	2	2
Left ventricle	42	2	2
Both	85 (22%)	31 (34%)	0
16. Cardiac amyloidosis (massive)	14 (4%)	8 (9%)	0

Reproduced with permission from Roberts and Shirani.[152]

1 or between 1 and 2, and a deceleration time longer than 140 ms. Cardiac death occurred in 10 patients during a mean follow-up interval of 32 months. The survival rate at 1 year was 100% in the nonrestrictive group and only 50% in the restricted group. After 1 year there was a continuing divergence of mortality resulting in a 3-year survival rate of 100% and 22%, respectively. Multivariate analysis showed that restrictive filling added prognostic information to clinical and echo variables of systolic dysfunction. These authors conclude that restrictive left ventricular filling after AMI is the single best predictor of cardiac death and adds significantly to clinical and echocardiographic markers of systolic dysfunction.

Modification of Serum Concentration of Aminoterminal Propeptide of Type III Procollagen

The aim of a study by Modena and associates[155] from Modena and Pavia, Italy, was to evaluate the modification of serum concentration of aminoterminal propeptide of type III procollagen (PIIINP) in 70 patients with previous transmural myocardial infarction. In 38 patients (group 1) PIIINP levels increased at 6 and 12 months after infarction; in 32 patients (group 2) PIIINP increased at 6 months, returning to baseline at 12 months. At the same time, they observed a significant LV enlargement and worsening of the performance in group 1, whereas in group 2, an improvement was seen in LV volumes and performance. In conclusion, rearrangement of collagen myocardial matrix plays an important role in LV postinfarction modification. This process can be easily followed over time in a noninvasive manner by dosing serum PIIINP concentrations.

Cardiovascular Death and Left Ventricular Remodeling 2 Years After Myocardial Infarction

St. John Sutton and colleagues[156] in Philadelphia, Pennsylvania, quantified cardiovascular death and/or LV dilatation in patients from the Survival and Ventricular Enlargement (SAVE) trial to determine whether dilatation continued beyond 1 year, whether angiotensin-converting enzyme inhibitor therapy attenuated late LV dilatation, and whether any baseline descriptors predicted late dilatation. They used 2-dimensional echocardiograms in 512 patients at 11 ± 3 days and 1 and 2 years postinfarction to assess LV size, percentage of the LV that was akinetic/dyskinetic, and LV shape index. LV function was assessed by radionuclide ejection fraction. Two hundred sixty-three patients sustained cardiovascular death and/or LV diastolic dilatation; 279 had cardiovascular death and/or systolic dilatation. In 373 patients with serial echocardiograms, LV end-diastolic and end-systolic sizes increased progressively from baseline to 2 years. In most patients with LV dilatation, there was a decrease in LVEF. Captopril attenuated diastolic LV dilatation at 2 years, but this effect was carried over from the first year of therapy. Changes in LV

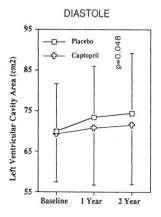
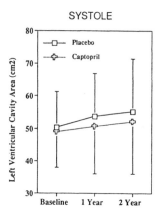

FIGURE 2-56. LV cavity areas at end diastole and end systole in the captopril and placebo treatment groups at 1 and 2 years after MI. p<0.001, for the effect of time (within-subject variable). p = 0.107, for the effect of treatment. p = 0.048, for the time X treatment interaction, reflecting an attenuation in the change in LV size in the captopril-treated group in diastole but not in systole. Reproduced with permission from St. John Sutton et al.[156]

size in patients receiving captopril after 1 year were similar to those receiving placebo. Predictors of cardiovascular death and/or dilatation were age, prior AMI, lower LVEF, angina, CHF, LV size, and infarct size. Thus, cardiovascular disease and/or LV dilatation occurred in >50% of patients by 2 years. This process is progressive, associated with deteriorating LV function, but it is unaffected by captopril after 1 year of therapy (Figure 2-56).

Ventricular Remodeling

To investigate the relation between plasma brain natriuretic peptide (BNP) and progressive ventricular remodeling, Nagaya and associates[157] from Osaka, Japan, measured plasma BNP and atrial natriuretic peptide (ANP) in 30 patients with AMI on days 2, 7, 14, and 30 after the onset. LV end-diastolic volume index (EDVI), end-systolic volume index (ESVI), and EF on admission and 1 month after the onset were assessed by left ventriculography. Changes in EDVI (ΔEDVI), ESVI (ΔESVI), and EF (ΔEF) were obtained by subtracting respective acute-phase values from corresponding chronic-phase values. Plasma ANP on days 2 and 7 showed only weak correlations with ΔEDVI, whereas plasma BNP on day 7 more closely correlated with ΔEDVI. When study patients were divided into 2 groups according to plasma BNP on day 7, the group with BNP higher than 100 pg/mL showed greater increases in LV volume and less improvement in EF compared with the other group with BNP lower than 100 pg/mL. Multiple regression analysis revealed that only plasma BNP on day 7, but not ANP, peak creatine phosphokinase level, LV end-diastolic pressure, or acute-phase EF, correlated independently with ΔEDVI. These results suggest that plasma BNP may be a simple and useful biochemical marker for the prediction of progressive ventricular remodeling within the first 30 days of AMI.

New Neurohormonal Predictors of Left Ventricular Function After Myocardial Infarction

Richards and colleagues[158] in New Zealand measured the N-terminal pro-brain natriuretic peptide (N-BNP) and adrenomedullin and determined their utility in predicting cardiac function and prognosis when compared with previously reported markers in 121 patients with AMI. The association between radionuclide-determined LVEF and N-BNP at 2 and 4 days ($r = -.63$, P<.0001) and 3 to 5 months ($r = -.58$, P<.0001) after AMI was comparable to that for C-terminal BNP and far stronger than for adrenomedullin ($r = -.26$, P<.01), N-terminal atrial natriuretic peptide, C-terminal atrial natriuretic peptide or plasma catecholamine concentrations. In the prediction of death over 24 months of follow-up, an early postinfarction N-BNP serum value of 160 pmol/L or more had sensitivity, specificity, positive predictive value, and negative predictive values of 91%, 72%, 39%, and 97%, respectively, and was superior to any other neurohormone measured and to the LVEF value itself. Only 1 of 21 deaths occurred in a patient with an N-BNP level below the group median (Figure 2-57). For prediction of CHF, plasma N-BNP of 145 pmol/L or higher had sensitivity (85%) and negative predictive value (91%) comparable to the other cardiac peptides and was superior to adrenomedullin, plasma catecholamines, and LVEF. By multivariate analysis, N-BNP, but not adrenomedullin, provided predictive information for death and LV failure independent of pa-

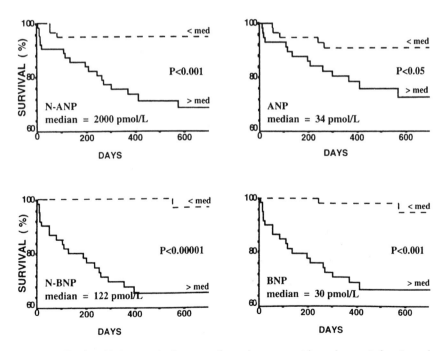

FIGURE 2-57. Kaplan-Meier survival curves for subgroups with early postinfarction plasma peptide (N-ANP, AN, N-BNP, and BNP) concentrations above (solid line) and below (dashed line) the group median in 121 patients with myocardial infarction. Reproduced with permission from Richards et al.[158]

tient age, gender, LVEF, other hormone levels, and previous history of CHF, AMI, hypertension, or diabetes. Thus, the plasma N-BNP value measured 2 to 4 days after AMI independently predicts LV function and 2-year survival.

General Treatment for Acute Myocardial Infarction

Use of Transdermal Nitroglycerin Patch Therapy After Acute Myocardial Infarction

Mahmarian and colleagues[159] in Houston, Texas, performed a randomized, double-blind, placebo-controlled trial investigating the long-term (6 months) efficacy of intermittent transdermal nitroglycerin patches on LV remodeling in 291 survivors of AMI. Patients meeting entry criteria had baseline gated radionuclide ventriculograms followed by randomization to placebo or active nitroglycerin patches delivering 0.4, 0.8, or 1.6 mg/h. The radionuclide evaluation of LV function was repeated at 6 months and 6.5 days after withdrawal of double-blind medication. The primary study endpoint was a change in end-systolic volume index. Both LV end-systolic index and end-diastolic volume index were reduced with 0.4 mg/h nitroglycerin patches (Figure 2-58). This beneficial effect was found primarily in patients with a baseline LVEF 40% or less and only at the 0.4 mg/h dose. After nitroglycerin patch withdrawal, end-systolic volume index increased significantly but did not reach pretreatment values. Thus, these data suggest that transdermal nitroglycerin patches prevent LV dilation in patients surviving AMI. The beneficial effects are limited to patients with depressed LV function and found at the lowest nitroglycerin patch dose.

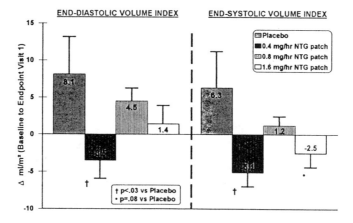

FIGURE 2-58. Changes in LV EDVI and ESVI (mL/m^2) from baseline to end-point visit 1 in the 4 randomized treatment groups. Only the 0.4-mg/h nitroglycerin (NTG) patch dose significantly reduced cardiac volumes. Data are presented at mean ± SEM. Reproduced with permission from Mahmarian et al.[159]

Effect of Lisinopril on Mortality in Diabetic Patients

Zuanetti and colleagues[160] in Milano, Italy, evaluated whether treatment with an angiotensin-converting enzyme (ACE) inhibitor begun within 24 hours from the onset of symptoms is able to decrease mortality and morbidity of diabetic patients with AMI. They performed a retrospective analysis of the data of the Gruppo Italiano per lo Studio della Sopravvivenza nell'Infarcto Miocardico (GISSI-3) study in patients with and without a history of diabetes. Patients with suspected AMI were randomized to treatment with lisinopril (2.5 to 5 up to 10 mg/day) with or without nitroglycerin (5 to 20 μg IV then 10 mg/day) begun within 24 hours and continued for 6 weeks. The main endpoint was mortality at 6 weeks, and the secondary endpoint was a combined evaluation of mortality and severe LV dysfunction. Information on diabetic status was available for 18,131 patients of whom 2,790 had a history of diabetes. Treatment with lisinopril was associated with a decreased 6-week mortality in diabetic patients (Figure 2-59). The survival benefit in the diabetics was mostly maintained at 6 months despite withdrawal from treatment at 6 weeks. Thus, these data suggest that early treatment with an ACE inhibitor, lisinopril, in diabetic patients with AMI is associated with a decreased 6-week mortality.

Effect of Pravastatin on Cardiovascular Events

In the Cholesterol and Recurrent Events (CARE) trial, Lewis and associates[161] found pravastatin was effective overall in reducing morbidity and mortality. Little information, however, is available on the effectiveness of lipid

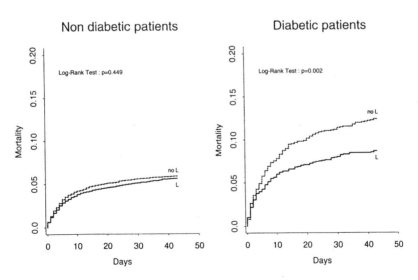

FIGURE 2-59. Mortality curves up to 6 weeks in diabetic and nondiabetic patients treated (solid line; L) and not treated (dotted line; No L) with lisinopril. Reproduced with permission from Zuanetti et al.[160]

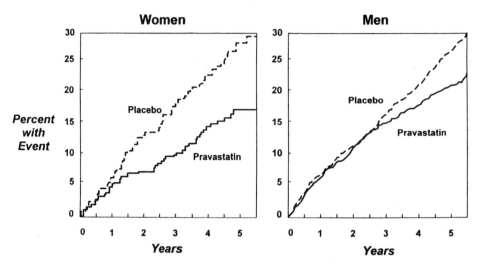

FIGURE 2-60. Effect of pravastatin on cardiovascular events in women after AMI. Reproduced with permission from Lewis et al.[161]

lowering in the secondary prevention of CAD in women who have average cholesterol levels. Therefore, in the CARE trial, 576 postmenopausal women between 3 and 20 months after MI with a total cholesterol less than 240 and an LDL cholesterol level 114 to 174 were randomized to receive either pravastatin 40 mg/day or matching placebo for a median follow-up period of 5 years. The main outcome measures were combined coronary events (coronary death, nonfatal MI, PTCA, or CABG), the primary trial endpoint (coronary death and nonfatal MI), and stroke. Women treated with pravastatin had a risk reduction of 43% for the primary endpoint, 46% for combined coronary events, 48% for PTCA, 40% for CABG, and 56% for stroke. Men in the CARE trial also showed a reduction in risk but the magnitude tended to be less. Pravastatin improved plasma lipids similarly in men and women. There were no differences in risk of coronary events in the placebo group men and women. These authors conclude that pravastatin led to significant early reduction of a wide range of cardiovascular events in post-MI women with average cholesterol levels (Figure 2-60).

Analysis of Clinical Use of Calcium Channel Blockers

As a result of randomized controlled trials with calcium channel blockers after myocardial infarction, concern has developed that these agents are associated with an increased risk of cardiovascular events, particularly in the presence of LV dysfunction. To test the hypothesis that calcium channel blockers increase cardiovascular events in such patients, the incidence of all-cause mortality, cardiovascular death, severe heart failure, and recurrent infarction was examined in 940 patients taking calcium channel blockers and in 1,180 not taking them 24 hours before randomization to placebo or captopril in the Survival and Ventricular Enlargement (SAVE) trial carried out by Hager and associates[162] from Farmington, Connecticut; Houston, Texas; Dearborn, Michigan; Montreal, Quebec, Canada; Miami Beach, Florida; and Boston, Massachusetts. All patients had an EF of 40% or less. Relative risks for calcium channel blocker users versus nonusers and the 95% confidence intervals were computed with univariate and multivariate Cox regressions. Adjustments were made for differences in baseline covariates. For all causes of mortality, the relative risk for calcium channel blocker users versus nonusers was 0.96. In the SAVE placebo and captopril groups, the relative risks for the development of severe heart failure among the calcium channel block users versus nonusers were 0.95 and 1.23. A similar neutral result held for patients with and without a history of hypertension. Furthermore, calcium channel blockers did not alter the benefit of the angiotensin-coverting enzyme inhibitor, captopril. This analysis of the nonrandomized clinical use of calcium channel blockers in the postmyocardial infarction population with LV dysfunction did not identify either a clinical deterioration or improvement with respect to subsequent cardiovascular events.

Diltiazem Therapy

Experimental studies have shown that calcium antagonists protect myocardial cells against the damage caused by coronary artery occlusion and reperfusion. Theroux and colleagues[163] from Montreal, Quebec, Canada, evaluated this concept in patients. Fifty nine patients with an AMI treated with t-PA were randomized, double-blinded to intravenous diltiazem or placebo for 48 hours followed by oral therapy for 4 weeks. Creatinine kinase elevation, Q-wave score, global and regional left ventricular function, and coronary artery patency at 48 hours were not significantly different between the diltiazem and placebo groups. The greater improvement observed in regional perfusion and function of diltiazem was likely explained by initial larger defects. Diltiazem reduced the rate of death, reinfarction, or recurrent ischemia at 35 days from 41% to 13%. The rate of death from myocardial infarction was reduced by 65%. Bradycardia and/or hypotension required transient or permanent discontinuation of the study drug in 27% of patients versus 17% of placebo patients. These authors conclude that a protective effect for clinical events related to early postinfarction ischemia and reperfusion were suggested in this study with the intravenous use of diltiazem followed by 1 month of oral therapy.

Early Assessment and In-Hospital Management of Patients with Acute Myocardial Infarction at Increased Risk for Adverse Outcomes: A Nationwide Perspective of Current Clinical Practice

Therapeutic decision making in critically ill patients requires both prompt and comprehensive analysis of available information. Data derived from randomized clinical trials provide a powerful tool for risk assessment in the setting of AMI; however, timely and appropriate use of existing therapies and resources are the key determinants of outcome among high-risk patients. Demographic, procedural, and outcome data from patients with AMI were collected at 1,073 US hospitals collaborating in the National Registry of MI (NRMI 2) by Becker and associates[164] from Worcester, Massachusetts; Torrance and South San Francisco, California; Portland, Maine; Tempe, Arizona; and Birmingham, Alabama. Patients were classified on hospital arrival as either low risk or high risk according to a modified Thrombolysis in Myocardial Infarction (TIMI) II Risk Scale based on predetermined demographic, electrocardiographic, and clinical features. Among the 170,143 patients enrolled, 115,222 (68%) were classified as low risk and 55,521 (33%) as high risk for in-hospital death, recurrent ischemia, recurrent AMI, CHF, and stroke. Using a composite unsatisfactory outcome measure, in-hospital adverse events were experienced by a greater proportion of patients initially classified as high risk compared with those classified as low risk. By multivariate analysis, age over 70 years, prior AMI, Killip class greater than 1, anterior site of infarction, and the combination of hypotension and tachycardia were independent predictions of poor outcome in patients with or without ST-segment elevation on the presenting electrocardiogram. High-risk patients with ST-segment elevation were treated with thrombolytics (48%), or alternative forms of reperfusion therapy (9.3%) within 62 minutes and 226 minutes of hospital arrival, respectively. High-risk patients offered reperfusion therapy were also more likely to receive aspirin, β-blockers (intravenous or oral), and angiotensin-converting enzyme inhibitors within 24 hours of infarction, and they survived their event (8.4 vs. 21%) and left the hospital sooner than those not reperfused. This large registry experience included more than 150,000 nonselected patients with AMI and suggests that high-risk patients can be identified on initial hospital presentation. The current use of reperfusion and adjunctive therapies among high-risk patients is suboptimal and may directly influence outcome. Randomized trials designed to test the impact of specific management strategies on outcome according to initial risk classification are warranted.

Benefit of Angiotensin-Converting Enzyme Inhibitors After Acute Myocardial Infarction

Clinical trials have demonstrated a significant mortality benefit in patients treated with angiotensin-converting enzyme (ACE) inhibitors after AMI. Numerous studies have also suggested that there is an underuse of ACE inhibitors and other beneficial therapies postmyocardial infarction. Barron and colleagues[165] from San Francisco, California, and Seattle, Washington, evaluated data from 190,000 patients with AMI at 1,470 US hospitals participating in the National Registry of Myocardial Infarction 2. Prescriptions for ACE inhibitor therapy at hospital discharge increased from 25% in 1994 to 31% in 1996. Patients with a reduced EF or evidence of CHF were discharged with ACE inhibitor treatment 43% of the time. Patients experiencing an anterior wall AMI without evidence of CHF were discharged 26% of the time on an ACE inhibitor. Of the remaining patients, 16% received ACE inhibitors at discharge. These authors concluded that physicians are prescribing ACE inhibitors in patients with AMI with increasing frequency. However, there is still considerable benefit to be gained by increasing the percentage of patients who are so treated. These data are very similar to the postmyocardial infarction underuse of aspirin and β-blockers.

Use of Intravenous Adenosine and Lidocaine in Acute Myocardial Infarction

A pilot study was designed by Garratt and associates[166] from Rochester, Minnesota, and Research Triangle Park, North Carolina, to assess the safety of combined intravenous adenosine and lidocaine in patients with AMI and to estimate the likelihood of a beneficial effect on final infarct size. Adenosine plus lidocaine reduces infarct size in animals, but the safety and efficacy in human beings is unknown. Adenosine (70 μg/kg per minute intravenous infusion) plus lidocaine (1 mg/kg intravenous bolus injection and 2 mg/kg/minute infusion) was given to 45 patients with AMI. Patients underwent immediate balloon angioplasty without preceding thrombolytic therapy. Myocardial perfusion defects were measured with serial technetium 99m sestamibi studies. One patient developed persisting hypotension in conjunction with a large inferolateral myocardial infarction. Transient hypotension in 3 other patients resolved with a reduction in adenosine. Advanced AV block was never observed. Other adverse events (including AF, ventricular tachyarrhythmia, bradycardia, and respiratory distress) occurred at low frequencies, as expected for patients with AMI. An initial median perfusion defect of 45% of the left ventricle (60% for anterior infarction, 17% for nonanterior infarction) was observed. At hospital discharge (4.3 ± 2.1 days) the median value was 12% and at 8 ± 4 weeks it was 3% (7% for anterior infarction, 0% for nonanterior infarction); 14 patients had no measurable follow-up. Compared with historical control patients, prehospital discharge measurements were not different but late perfusion defects were improved. Treatment with intravenous adenosine and lidocaine during AMI has sufficient safety and potential for improved myocardial salvage. Randomized studies are justified.

Thrombolysis

Fragmin in Acute Myocardial Infarction Trial

Low-molecular-weight heparin may have a role in certain syndromes similar to heparin or coumadin. Kontny and colleagues[167] from Oslo, Norway, investigated the efficacy and safety of 1 of these agents (dalteparin) in the prevention of arterial thromboembolism after an acute AMI. A total of 776 patients were enrolled in a multicenter, randomized, double-blind, placebo-controlled trial of subcutaneous dalteparin (150 IU/kg body weight every 12 hours in the hospital). Thrombolytic therapy and aspirin were administered in 91.5% and 97.6% of patients, respectively. The primary study endpoint was the composite thrombus formation diagnosed by echocardiography and arterial embolism . on day 9. In patients undergoing echocardiography, thrombus formation or embolism or both were found in 22% of patients in the placebo group and in 14% of patients in the dalteparin group. Dalteparin was associated with increased risk of hemorrhage, (2.9%) versus placebo (0.3%). These authors conclude that dalteparin treatment significantly reduces LV thrombus formation in acute anterior MI but is associated with increased hemorrhagic risk.

Platelet IIb/IIIa in Unstable Angina Receptor Suppression Using Integrilin Therapy (PURSUIT) Trial

The Platelet IIb/IIIa in Unstable Angina Receptor Suppression Using Integrilin Therapy (PURSUIT) Trial Investigators[168] tested the hypothesis that inhibition of platelet aggregation with eptifibatide (Integrilin), a synthetic cyclic heptapeptide selective high-affinity inhibitor of the platelet glycoprotein IIb/IIIa receptors, may have incremental benefit beyond that of heparin and aspirin in reducing the frequency of adverse outcomes in patients with acute coronary syndromes who did not have persistent ST-segment elevation. Patients who had presented with ischemic chest pain within the previous 24 hours and who had either electrocardiographic changes indicative of ischemia, but not persistent ST-segment elevation or high serum concentrations of creatine kinase MB isoenzymes were enrolled in the study. They were randomly assigned in a double-blind manner to receive a bolus infusion of either eptifibatide or placebo for up to 72 hours. The primary endpoint was a composite of death and nonfatal AMI occurring up to 30 days after the index event. A total of 10,948 patients were enrolled between November 1995 and January 1997. The eptifibatide group had a 1.5% absolute reduction in the incidence of the primary endpoint (14% vs. 16%, p = 0.04). The benefit was apparent by 96 hours and persisted through 30 days. The effect was consistent in most major subgroups, except for women. Bleeding was more common in the eptifibatide group, although there was no increase in the incidence of hemorrhagic stroke. Thus, inhibition of platelet aggregation with eptifibatide reduces the incidence of the composite endpoint of death or nonfatal AMI in patients with acute coronary syndromes who do not have persistent ST-segment elevation (Figure 2-61).

Survival After Thrombolysis for Acute Myocardial Infarction

Early patency of an infarct-related artery is a major determinant of survival after thrombolysis for AMI. Some data have suggested that the time to treatment may influence the efficacy of certain thrombolytic agents in restoring early patency. Steg and colleagues[169] from Paris and Clichy, France, performed a retrospective analysis of the cohort of 481 patients receiving thrombolytic

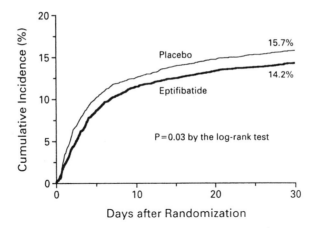

FIGURE 2-61. Kaplan-Meier curves showing the incidence of death or nonfatal myocardial infarction at 30 days. This analysis is based on endpoints as assessed by the central clinical events committee. The percentages shown are for the incidence at 30 days. Reproduced with permission from the PURSUIT Trial Investigators.[168]

therapy for AMI less than 6 hours after pain onset, all of whom underwent 90-minute coronary angiography. Thrombolysis in Myocardial Infarction (TIMI) flow grade 2 or 3 patency rate after streptokinase correlated negatively with time between onset of pain and thrombolysis, whereas the 90-minute patency rate after t-PA was stable as a function of time to treatment. When patients were categorized as having received treatment under 3 or over 3 hours after pain onset, the patency rate was similar with t-PA but significantly higher when streptokinase was administered early rather than late regardless of the TIMI flow grade (87% vs. 59%). These authors conclude that the efficacy of streptokinase but not t-PA in restoring early coronary patency after intravenous thrombolysis is markedly lower when patients are treated later after the onset of pain.

Clinical Markers of Reperfusion

Patients who cannot be reperfused after thrombolytic therapy have a high mortality rate. Noninvasive clinical markers of reperfusion have been widely studied, yet their prognostic significance remains unclear. To assess the prognostic value of commonly used noninvasive clinical markers of early reperfusion, Iparraguirre and associates[170] from Buenos Aires, Argentina, and Durham, North Carolina, studied 327 patients who received intravenous thrombolytic treatment (1.5 MU streptokinase in 1 hour of 100 mg alteplase in 3 hours) within 6 hours of acute infarction. Successful clinical reperfusion was defined as the presence of at least 2 of the following criteria at 2 hours after thrombolytic treatment: (1) significant relief of pain (a 5-point reduction on a 1 to 10 subjective scale), (2) 50% reduction of sum of ST-segment elevation, and (3) abrupt initial increase of creatine kinase levels (more than 2-fold over the upper-normal or baseline elevated values). Clinical variables that were significantly associated by univariate analysis were tested by multivariate analysis to obtain independent predictors of 30-day mortality rate. Successful clinical reperfusion was present in 210 (64%) patients (group 1), and absent in 117 (36%) patients (group 2). The groups were similar for most baseline characteristics, although group 2 patients were slightly older (mean 60 vs. 57 years). Thirty-day outcomes for group 2 patients compared with group 1 patients were heart failure in 23% and 11%, progression to cardiogenic shock in 13% and 0.5%, and death in 16% and 4%, respectively. By multivariate analysis, the Killip class at admission, the absence of successful clinic reperfusion, anterior infarct location, and age were independent predictors of mortality rate, and gender had borderline significance. The absence of successful clinical reperfusion defined a group of patients with a significantly higher mortality rate (odds ratio 4.89). These simple noninvasive clinical criteria of successful reperfusion may be used to identify a group of patients with poor prognosis after thrombolytic therapy in whom alternative strategies could be applied.

Markers of Reperfusion: Results from the Thrombolysis in Myocardial Infarction (TIMI 10A) Trial

The availability of a reliable, noninvasive serum marker of reperfusion may permit early identification of patients with occlusion after thrombolysis who might benefit from further interventions. Tanasijevic and associates[171] from Boston and West Roxbury, Massachusetts, measured myoglobin, creatine kinase MB, and cardiac troponin I concentrations in sera obtained just before thrombolysis (TO) and 60 minutes later (T60) in 30 patients given TNK-t-PA for AMI as part of the Thrombolysis in Myocardial Infarction (TIMI) 10A trial. Angiography at T60 showed reperfusion (TIMI flow grade 2 to 3; n = 19) or occlusion (TIMI flow grade 0 to 1; n = 8). The median serum T60 concentration, the ratio of the T60 and T0 serum concentration, and the slope of increase over a 60-minute period for each serum marker were significantly higher in patients with patent arteries compared with patients with occluded arteries. The areas under the receiver operator characteristics curve for diagnosis of occlusion were 0.96, 0.91, and 0.87 for the T60 concentration of myoglobin, creatine kinase MB and cardiac troponin, respectively. Although the T60 levels of less than 469 ng/mL for myoglobin, less than 11.5 ng/mL for creatine kinase MB, and less than 1.1 ng/mL for cardiac troponin I identified all patients with occlusion, the specificity of myoglobin (94%) was higher than that of creatine kinase (61%) and cardiac troponin I (67%). Similar results were obtained for the 60-minute ratios and 60-minute slopes for each marker, with indexes for myoglobin having the highest specificity. In this study, noninvasive diagnosis of occlusion 60 minutes after thrombolysis was achieved with a high degree of sensitivity and specificity with the myoglobin, creatine kinase MB, and cardiac troponin I concentrations measured at that time point. These findings may permit a new strategy for assessment of the success of reperfusion, with triage to rescue angioplasty for patients in whom the 60-minute cardiac marker values or indexes are consistent with occlusion of the infarct-related artery.

Early Sustained Reperfusion

Brieger and associates[172] for the Global Utilization of Streptokinase and Tissue Plasminogen Activator for Occluded Coronary Arteries (GUSTO-1) Investigators performed a study to characterize a large cohort of patients receiving thrombolytic therapy for AMI with respect to the group with a prior event. Patients were randomly assigned to 1 of 4 thrombolytic strategies. Baseline characteristics, 30-day outcomes, and 1-year mortality were compared in patients with (n = 6,704) and without (n = 34,143) prior AMI. Patients with prior AMI presented to the hospital earlier than those having their first event, but institution of thrombolytic therapy was delayed. Mortality at 30 days (11.7% vs. 5.9%) and 1 year (17.3% vs. 8.2%) was greater among patients with prior infarction, and independent of other demographic variables. Accelerated alteplase was more effective than streptokinase or combination therapy (30-day mortality 10.4% vs. 12.2%; 1-year mortality 15.9% vs. 17.8%). Infarct vessel patency did not differ between those with and without prior AMI (67.3% vs. 67% at 90 minutes); however, recurrent ischemia was more common in patients with prior AMI. Patients with healed myocardial infarction should be educated to ensure early hospital admission if they develop symptoms suggestive of AMI, and upon hospital arrival, should be promptly triaged to receive reperfusion therapy with accelerated alteplase (Table 2-15).

Global Utilization of Streptokinase and Tissue Plasminogen Activator for Occluded Coronary Arteries (GUSTO I) Trial Results

Goodman and colleagues[173] in Toronto, Ontario, Canada, examined 12-lead electrocardiograms, coronary anatomy, LV function, and mortality among 2,046 patients with ST-segment elevation infarction from the Global Utilization of Streptokinase and Tissue Plasminogen Activator for Occluded Coronary Arteries (GUSTO I) trial angiographic subset attempting to gain further insight into pathophysiology and prognosis of Q- versus non-Q-wave infarctions in the thrombolytic era. Non-Q-wave infarction developed in 409 patients (20%) after thrombolytic therapy. Compared with Q-wave patients, non-Q-wave patients were more likely to present with lesser ST-segment elevation in a nonanterior location. The infarct-related artery in non-Q-wave patients was more likely to be nonanterior (67% vs. 58%) and distally located (33% vs. 39%). Early (90 minute, 77% vs. 65%) and complete (54% vs. 44%) infarct-related artery patency was greater among the non-Q-wave group. Non-Q-wave patients had better LVEFs and regional LV function. In-hospital 30-day, 1-year, and 2-year mortality rates were lower among non-Q-wave patients (Figure 2-62). Thus, the excellent prognosis among the subgroup of patients who developed non-Q-wave infarction after thrombolysis is related to early, complete, and sustained infarct-related artery patency.

TABLE 2-15
Angiographic Characteristics

	Overall (n = 1,148)	Prior Myocardial Infarction (n = 151) (%)	No Prior Myocardial Infarction (n = 994) (%)
Multivessel disease	39.9	71.5	35*
Left ventricular ejection fraction (%)	59.5 (48.6, 68.6)	51.9 (37.9, 63.8)	60.3 (49.5, 69.0)*
Infarct artery stenosis (%)	80	80	80
TIMI flow in infarct vessel 90 min after thrombolysis			
0	285 (24.8)	39 (26.0)	246 (24.6)
1	96 (8.3)	10 (6.7)	85 (8.5)
2	336 (29.2)	44 (29.3)	292 (29.3)
3	434 (37.7)	57 (38)	376 (37.7)†
Reocclusion (%)			
From TIMI grade 2 at 90 min to grade 0 or 1 at follow-up‡	13/260 (5.0)	2/31 (6.4)	11/229 (4.8)
From TIMI grade 3 at 90 min to grade 0 or 1 at follow-up‡	15/329 (4.6)	3/38 (7.9)	12/291 (4.1)
Overall reocclusion	28/589 (4.8)	5/69 (7.2)	23/520 (4.4)§

* p <0.001 for comparison of patients with and without a history of prior myocardial infarction.
† p = 0.944 for comparison of this group with the group with prior myocardial infarction.
‡ Five- to 7-day follow-up.
§ p = 0.359 for comparison of this group with the group with prior myocardial infarction.
Values followed by parentheses are medians, with the 25th and 75th percentiles shown inside the parentheses.
Reproduced with permission from Brieger et al.[172]

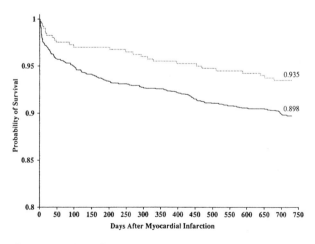

FIGURE 2-62. Kaplan-Meier plot of 2-year survival among patients who developed non-Q-wave (dashed line, n = 409) or Q-wave (solid line, n = 1637) MI after thrombolysis. Reproduced with permission from Goodman et al.[173]

Time to Treatment with Thrombolytic Therapy

Goldberg and associates[174] from several US medical centers examined the association between time to treatment with thrombolytic therapy and hospital outcomes in patients with AMI enrolled in a national registry. A total of 71,253 patients hospitalized with AMI from June 1994 to July 1996 who received tissue plasminogen activator (t-PA) therapy in 1,474 US hospitals were studied. In this study sample, approximately 39% of patients presented to participating hospitals within 2 hours of acute symptom onset and received t-PA; 36% were treated within 2.1 to 4 hours, 12% between 4.1 to 6 hours, and the remaining 13% thereafter. After controlling for potentially confounding factors, in-hospital death rates increased progressively with increasing delays in time of administration of t-PA. The lowest risk for dying during acute hospitalization was seen for those treated with t-PA within 2 hours of acute symptoms. No significant association was seen between time of administration of t-PA and in-hospital risk of recurrent AMI, myocardial ischemia, cardiogenic shock, major bleeding episodes, or stroke and/or intracranial bleeding. The incidence of sustained ventricular arrhythmias declined with progressively longer time to administration of t-PA. The results of this multihospital observational study suggest that patients with AMI treated earlier with t-PA are significantly more likely to survive the acute hospitalization than patients treated later. These data reinforce the benefits to be gained by treatment with t-PA as soon as possible following the onset of acute ischemic symptoms and for community-wide efforts to reduce the duration of prehospital delay in patients with acute CAD.

Thrombolytic Therapy and Risk of Early Reinfarction

The study by Birnbaum and associates[175] from Petah-Teqva, Tel-Hashomer, and Tel Aviv, Israel, assessed the ability of clinical and electrocardiographic variables routinely obtained on admission to identify patients with AMI treated with thrombolytic therapy at risk of early reinfarction. The study included 2,602 patients who received thrombolytic therapy for AMI. Baseline demographic variables and admission clinical electrocardiographic variables were compared between patients with and without reinfarction. Multivariable logistic regression technique was used and included recurrent infarction as the dependent variable, and baseline demographic, clinical, and electrocardiographic variables as independent variables. History of hypertension and diabetes mellitus were associated with a higher risk, and current smoking was associated with a lower risk of early hospital reinfarction. Distortion of the terminal portion of the QRS complex and absence of abnormal Q waves on admission were associated with increased risk of early reinfarction. A simple electrocardiographic sign is a reliable predictor of early reinfarction among patients who receive thrombolytic therapy for AMI.

Clinical Outcomes with Atenolol Use

Early intravenous β-blockade is generally recommended after AMI, especially for patients with tachycardia and/or hypertension, and those without

heart failure. Pfisterer and colleagues[176] from the multicenter Global Utilization of Streptokinase and Tissue Plasminogen Activator for Occluded Coronary
Arteries (GUSTO I) experience evaluated this recommendation. In addition to
1 of 4 thrombolytic strategies, patients in the GUSTO trial without hypotension,
bradycardia, or signs of heart failure were to receive atenolol 5 mg intravenously as soon as possible, another 5 mg intravenously 10 minutes later, and
50–100 mg orally daily during the hospitalization. Patients given any atenolol
had a lower baseline risk than those not given atenolol. Adjusted 30-day mortality was significantly lower in atenolol-treated patients, but patients treated with
intravenous and oral atenolol treatment versus oral treatment alone were more
likely to die. Subgroups had similar rates of stroke, intracranial hemorrhage,
and reinfarction but intravenous atenolol use was associated with more heart
failure, shock, recurrent ischemia, and pacemaker use than oral atenolol was.
These authors conclude that although atenolol appears to improve outcomes
after thrombolysis for myocardial infarction, early intravenous atenolol seems
of limited value. They recommend that patients begin oral atenolol once stable.
This recommendation is different from official recommendations regarding
the use of intravenous β-blockers in acute myocardial infarction, but these
relatively convincing data in the patient population of GUSTO appear to justify
their recommendation.

Early Identification of Failed Reperfusion

In patients undergoing thrombolysis for myocardial infarction, it is difficult noninvasively to know if reperfusion has occurred. Stewart and colleagues[177] from Auckland, New Zealand, and Montreal, Quebec, Canada, evaluated serial blood samples for creatine kinase MB, cardiac troponin T, and
myoglobin to assess this issue. They studied 105 patients with AMI who underwent angiography after intravenous streptokinase. The ratios of the 60- and
90-minute concentrations to prethrombolytic values were used to determine
an index that could identify failure to achieve TIMI grade 3 flow in the infarct-
related artery at 90 minutes. Significant increases in serum concentrations of
markers at 60 minutes were more likely with TIMI grade 3 flow (59 patients)
than with TIMI grade 0–2 flow (467 patients). Ratios less than 5 at 60 minutes
after thrombolysis detected failure to achieve 90-minute TIMI grade 3 flow
(92% to 97% sensitivity and 43% to 60% specificity). Ratios less than 10 at 90
minutes showed 88% to 95% sensitivity and 49% to 65% specificity. The overall
predictive values were similar for all 3 markers. These authors conclude that
in AMI treated with intravenous streptokinase, a simple measurement of increased serum concentrations of creatine kinase MB, troponin T, or myoglobin
at 60 and 90 minutes can accurately predict failure to achieve TIMI grade 3
flow in the infarct-related artery at 90 minutes.

Thrombolytic Therapy in Patients with ST-Segment Elevation

Because the posterior wall is faced by none of the 12 standard electrocardiographic leads, the electrocardiographic diagnosis of posterior infarction is

problematic and has often remained undiagnosed, especially in the acute phase. Matetzky and colleagues[178] from Tel-Hashomer and Tel-Aviv, Israel, examined whether ST-segment elevation in posterior chest leads (V_7–V_9) during acute inferior infarction identifies patients with a concomitant posterior infarction and whether these patients might benefit more from thrombolysis. Eighty seven patients with a first inferior infarct who were treated with t-PA were stratified according to the presence (46 patients) or absence (41 patients) of concomitant ST-segment elevation in posterior chest leads V_7 to V_9. Patients with ST-segment elevation had a higher incidence of posterior lateral wall motion abnormalities on radionuclide ventriculography, a larger infarct was evidenced by higher peak creatinine kinase levels, and a lower LVEF at hospital discharge. Patency of the infarct-related artery in patients with ST-segment elevation resulted in improved LVEF. LVEF was unchanged in patients without ST-segment elevation in the posterior leads. These investigators conclude that ST-segment elevation in leads V_7 to V_9 identifies patients with a larger inferior infarction because of concomitant posterior lateral involvement. Such patients might benefit more from thrombolytic therapy.

Results of the ReoPro and Primary PTCA Organization and Randomized Trial (RAPPORT)

Brener and colleagues[179] in Cleveland, Ohio, and the ReoPro and Primary PTCA Organization and Randomized Trial (RAPPORT) Investigators evaluated the potential benefits of inhibiting platelet aggregation with ReoPro in patients with AMI of less than 12 hours' duration who were randomized on a double-blind basis to placebo or ReoPro if they were deemed candidates for primary PTCA. The primary efficacy endpoint was death, reinfarction, or any target vessel revascularization within 6 months. Other key prespecified endpoints were early death (7 and 30 days after the event), reinfarction, or urgent target vessel revascularization. Baseline clinical and angiographic variables of 483 patients were balanced. There was no difference in the incidence of the primary 6 month endpoint in the 2 groups. However, ReoPro significantly reduced the incidence of death, reinfarction, or urgent target vessel revascularization at all time points assessed, including at 7 days, 30 days, and 6 months (Figure 2-63). Analysis by actual treatment with PTCA and study drug demonstrated a considerable effect of ReoPro with respect to death or reinfarction. The need for unplanned bailout stenting was reduced by 42% in the ReoPro-treated group. Major bleeding occurred significantly more frequently in the ReoPro group, mostly at the arterial access site. There were no intracranial hemorrhages in either group. Thus, aggressive platelet inhibition with ReoPro during primary PTCA for AMI yields a substantial reduction in the acute incidence of death, reinfarction, and urgent target vessel revascularization and the bleeding is not excessive.

Heparin Use as Therapy Before Angioplasty

Thrombolysis, together with heparin, is an effective strategy for producing reperfusion in patients with an AMI. Verheugt and associates[180] in the Heparin

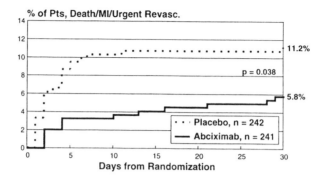

FIGURE 2-63. Probability of death, repeat MI, or urgent TVR (Revasc.) within 30 days in abciximab (solid line) and placebo (dashed line) groups by ITT analysis. Kaplan-Meier plot. Pts = patients. Reproduced with permission from Brener et al.[179]

and Early Patency (HEAP) pilot study evaluated whether heparin alone could induce reperfusion. One hundred eight patients with signs and symptoms of AMI in under 6 hours who were eligible for primary PTCA received a single intravenous bolus of 300 U/kg of heparin together with 160 mg of chewed aspirin in the emergency room. The median dose of bolus heparin was 27,000 U. Patency was assessed by coronary angiography at a mean of 85 minutes after the heparin bolus. In 55 patients, TIMI flow grade 3 was observed in 33 patients, and TIMI flow grade 2 in 22 patients. Thus, 64% of patients with symptoms treated less than 2 hours had TIMI flow grade 2 or 3 versus 48% of patients with symptoms longer than 2 hours. No significant bleeding was seen. One hundred eight patients from a large primary PTCA database who were treated with standard therapy but no intravenous heparin were matched for clinical and angiographic characteristics with the HEAP pilot study patients. The control patients showed an 18% patency rate before primary PTCA. These authors conclude that early therapy with high-dose heparin is associated with full coronary reperfusion in a considerable number of patients with AMI, especially in those treated early (<2 hours). They recommend that this simple, inexpensive first-line treatment of AMI could be used in conjunction with primary PTCA.

Saruplase as a Thrombolytic Agent

The use of thrombolytic agents is well-established treatment for AMI. Saruplase is a recombinant, unglycosolated, human, single chain u-PA of a protein of a known amino acid sequence that is produced through the use of genetically transformed *Eschericia coli* bacteria. There is no risk of allergic reaction or antigenicity as occurs with streptokinase. Tebbe and colleagues[181] in a large, multicenter trial evaluated the equivalence of saruplase and streptokinase in terms of 30-day mortality. Three thousand eighty-nine patients with symptoms compatible with AMI of less than 6 hours entered the study at 104 centers and were randomized to receive streptokinase (1.5 MU infusion over 60 minutes) or saruplase (20 mg bolus and 60 mg infusion over 60 minutes). In the saruplase group, a bolus of heparin (5,000 IU) was administered before saruplase. All patients received intravenous heparin infusions for at least 24 hours starting 30 minutes after the end of the thrombolytic infusions. Death at 30 days occurred in 5.7% of the patients receiving saruplase and in 6.7% of the patients receiving streptokinase (odds ratio 0.84). Hemorrhagic strokes occurred more often in patients receiving saruplase (0.9% vs. 0.3%), whereas thromboembolic strokes were more prevalent in the streptokinase-treated patients (0.5% vs. 1%). The rate of bleeding was similar in the 2 treatment groups (10.4% vs. 10.9%). Hypotension and cardiogenic shock occurred less frequently in the saruplase group. Reinfarction rates were similar. These authors conclude that saruplase is a clinically safe and effective thrombolytic medication. This profile ranks saruplase favorably among the currently available thrombolytic agents.

Abnormal Coronary Flow in Infarct Arteries

Because 25% to 30% of patent infarct-related arteries occlude in the year following thrombolytic therapy for AMI, angiographic factors including corrected Thrombolysis in Myocardial Infarction (TIMI) frame count which may predict abnormal infarct artery flow, require definition. French and associates[182] from Auckland, New Zealand, examined changes in coronary flow and infarct-artery lesion severity by computerized quantitative angiography over 1 year in 154 patients with a patent infarct-related artery 4 weeks after AMI. These patients were randomized to receive either ongoing daily therapy of 50 mg aspirin and 400 mg dipyridamole, or placebo. All angiograms were interpreted blind in our core angiographic laboratory. Infarct-artery flow, assessed by corrected TIMI frame counts, was normal ($\leq$27) in 46% and 45% of patients at 4 weeks and 1 year, respectively. At 4 weeks, patients with corrected TIMI frame counts ($\leq$27) had higher EF (60 $\pm$ 11% vs. 56 $\pm$ 12%) than those with corrected TIMI frame counts (>27). On multivariate analysis, corrected TIMI frame count and stenosis severity were predictive of late abnormal infarct-artery flow (TIMI 0 to 2 flow). Only stenosis severity at 4 weeks predicted reocclusion at 1 year. Aspirin and dipyridamole had no effect on flow or reocclusion. Thus, corrected TIMI frame count and stenosis severity at 4 weeks was highly correlated with infarct-artery flow at 1 year.

Increased T-Wave Amplitude

Increased T-wave amplitude is one of the earliest electrocardiographic changes following coronary occlusion. Therefore, higher T-waves in the presenting electrocardiogram should represent earlier time to treatment and thus be associated with lower mortality following thrombolytic therapy. T-wave amplitude, however, has never been evaluated as a prognostic marker in this setting. Hochrein and colleagues,[183] from multiple international medical centers, evaluated clinical outcomes in 3,317 patients with AMI who underwent thrombolysis and the Global Utilization of Streptokinase and t-PA for Occluded Coro-

TABLE 2-16
Outcomes in Patients with and without High T Waves

	No High T Waves (n = 701)	High T Waves (n = 2,616)	p Value
All patients			
30-d mortality	60 (8.6%)	136 (5.2%)	0.001
Congestive heart failure	170 (24%)	386 (15%)	<0.001
Shock	60 (8.6%)	159 (6.1%)	0.023
Reinfarction	33 (4.7%)	98 (3.8%)	0.259
Recurrent ischemia	157 (22%)	557 (21%)	0.527
Stroke	8 (1.1%)	35 (1.3%)	0.675
Anterior infarction			
30-d mortality	47 (11%)	63 (7.8%)	0.037
Congestive heart failure	129 (32%)	167 (21%)	<0.001
Shock	49 (12%)	65 (8.1%)	0.028
Reinfarction	17 (4.2%)	30 (3.7%)	0.703
Recurrent ischemia	103 (25%)	188 (23%)	0.454
Stroke	4 (1.0%)	11 (1.4%)	0.558
Inferior infarction			
30-d mortality	12 (4.6%)	70 (4.0%)	0.662
Congestive heart failure	37 (14%)	216 (12%)	0.437
Shock	10 (3.8%)	94 (5.4%)	0.266
Reinfarction	15 (5.7%)	68 (3.9%)	0.186
Recurrent Ischemia	50 (19%)	361 (21%)	0.567
Stroke	4 (1.5%)	23 (1.3%)	0.785

Reproduced with permission from Hochrein et al.[183]

nary Arteries (GUSTO I) Study. Patients were classified as either those with high T-waves or those with low T-waves. Higher T-waves were defined as those higher than the 98th percentile of the upper limit of normal. T-wave amplitude was also evaluated as a continuous variable according to infarct location (maximum T-wave amplitude) and as the amount of excess T-wave amplitude above normal (excess T-wave amplitude). Patients with higher T-waves had lower 30-day mortality than those without (5.2% vs. 8.6%) and were less likely to develop CHF (15% vs. 24%) or cardiogenic shock (6.1% vs. 8.6%). Higher maximum T-wave amplitude and excess T-wave amplitude were predictive of lower 30-day mortality (chi-square = 67, and chi-square = 33, respectively). These differences remain significant after controlling for other prognostic baseline electrocardiographic variables. In addition, T-wave amplitude added prognostic significance after controlling for time to treatment. T-wave amplitude, an often overlooked component of the electrocardiogram, can add significant prognostic information in initial evaluation of patients with AMI (Table 2-16).

Thirty-Day Mortality Prediction in Thrombolysis-Related Intracranial Hemorrhage

Sloan and colleagues[184] performed an observational analysis within a randomized trial of 4 thrombolytic therapies, conducted in 1,081 hospitals in 15 countries. Patients presented with ST-segment elevation within 6 hours of symptom onset. The population was composed of 268 patients who had pri-

1. Find Points For Each Risk Factor							
Age, y		Glasgow Coma Scale (GCS) Score		Time from Thrombolysis to Stroke Onset, *h*		Total Hemorrhagic Volume, mm^3	
Age	Points	Score	Points	Time	Points	Volume	Points
≤40	0	3	20	0	100	≤50	0
45	2	4	18	20	93	60	2
50	4	5	16	40	87	80	5
55	5	6	15	60	80	100	9
60	7	7	13	80	73	120	13
65	9	8	12	100	67	140	16
70	11	9	10	120	60	160	20
75	13	10	8	140	53	180	24
80	14	11	7	160	47	200	27
85	16	12	5	180	40	220	31
90	18	13	3	200	33	240	35
		14	2	220	27	260	38
		15	0	240	20	280	42
				260	13	300	46
				280	7		
				≥300	0		

2. Sum Points For All Risk Factors				
___ +	___ +	___ +	___ =	___
Age	GCS score	Time to stroke	Volume	Point Total

3. Look Up Risk Corresponding to Point Total

Points	Risk	Points	Risk	Points	Risk
87	1%	109	30%	128	90%
97	5%	115	50%	132	95%
101	10%	120	70%	142	99%

FIGURE 2-64. Nomogram to predict individual risk of mortality at 30 days in patients with intracranial hemorrhage after thrombolysis. The C-index for the model is 0.923. Reproduced with permission from Sloan et al.[184]

mary intracranial hemorrhage after thrombolysis. With univariate and multivariate analyses, the authors identified clinical and brain imaging characteristics that would predict 30-day mortality among the patients. Computed tomography or magnetic resonance imaging were available for 240 patients. The 30-day mortality rate was 59.7%. Glasgow Coma Scale score, age, time from thrombolysis to symptoms of intracranial hemorrhage, hydrocephalus, herniation, mass effect, intraventricular extension, and volume and location of intracranial hemorrhage were significant univariable predictors. Multivariate analysis of 170 patients with complete data, 98 of whom died, identified the following independent predictors: Glasgow Coma Scale score; time from thrombolysis to intracranial hemorrhage; volume of intracranial hemorrhage; and baseline clinical predictors of mortality in the overall GUSTO I trial (Figure 2-64). These data suggest that a model can be developed that provides excellent discrimination between patients who are likely to live and those who are likely to die after thrombolysis-related intracranial hemorrhage, and this may aid in making decisions about the appropriate level of care in such patients.

Percutaneous Transluminal Coronary Angioplasty and Stents

Early Discharge of Low-Risk Patients

In low-risk patients with AMI treated with primary PTCA, there is a potential for early discharge to reduce hospital costs and length of stay. Grines and colleagues[185] for the Primary Angioplasty in Myocardial Infarction (PAMI II) Investigators evaluated patients with AMI undergoing PTCA who were under 70 years of age, LVEF greater than 45%, 1- or 2-vessel disease, successful PTCA, and no persistent arrhythmias; to receive accelerated care (admission to a non-intensive care unit and day 3 hospital discharge) without noninvasive testing (n = 237) or with traditional care (n = 234). Patients who received accelerated care had similar in-hospital outcomes but were discharged 3 days earlier (4.2 vs. 7.1 days), and had lower hospital costs than the patients who received traditional care. At 6 months, accelerated and traditional care groups had a similar rate of mortality (0.8% vs. 0.4%) and similar rates of unstable ischemia, reinfarction, stroke, CHF, or their combined recurrence. These authors conclude that early identification of low-risk patients with AMI allows safe omission of the intensive care phase and noninvasive testing, and a day 3 hospital discharge strategy, resulting in substantial cost savings.

Assessment of Acute Myocardial Infarction with Myocardial Blush Grade

van 't Hof and colleagues[186] studied 777 patients who underwent primary PTCA during a 6-year period and investigated the value of angiographic evidence of myocardial reperfusion in the form of myocardial blush grade in relation to the extent of ST-segment elevation resolution, enzymatic infarct size, LV function, and long-term mortality. The myocardial blush immediately after the PTCA procedure was graded by 2 experienced investigators who were otherwise blinded to all clinical data: 0, no myocardial blush; 1, minimal myocardial blush; 2, moderate myocardial blush; and 3, normal myocardial blush. The myocardial blush was related to the extent of the early ST-segment elevation resolution on the 12-lead electrocardiogram. Patients with blush grades of 3, 2, and 0/1 had enzymatic infarct sizes of 757, 1143, and 1623, respectively, and LVEFs of 50%, 46%, and 39%, respectively (Figure 2-65). After mean follow-up of 1.9 ± 1.7 years, mortality rates for patients with myocardial blush grades 3, 2, and 0/1 were 3%, 6%, and 23% (p<0.0001), respectively. Multivariate analysis showed that the myocardial blush grade was predictor of long-term mortality, independent of Killip class, TIMI grade flow, LVEF, and other clinical variables. Thus, in patients with reperfusion therapy, the myocardial blush grade as seen on coronary angiogram may be used to describe the effectiveness of myocardial reperfusion and is an independent predictor of long-term mortality.

A Marker of Vascular Inflammation and Restenosis

Plasma levels of soluable intercellular adhesion molecule-1 (s1CAM-1) have been shown to predict activities of inflammatory disorders and malignancies. However, it is unknown whether the plasma level of s1CAM-1 is increased in patients with AMI with coronary intervention and whether the levels have

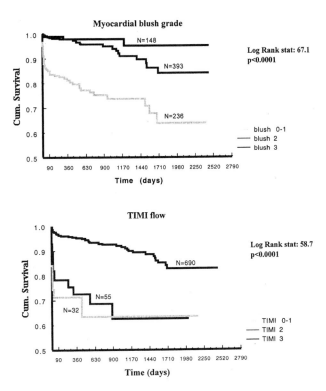

FIGURE 2-65. Kaplan-Meier survival curves for 777 patients with known TIMI flow and myocardial blush grades. Myocardial blush grade 0 or 1 indicates no or minimal blush or contrast density of myocardium supplied by infarct-related vessel on postangioplasty angiogram. Blush grade 2 indicates moderate blush contrast density, and blush grade 3 indicates normal blush or contrast density, comparable with blush obtained during angiography of contralateral or ipsilateral non-infarct-related coronary artery. TIMI flow is defined as previously described. Cum. Survival = comulative survival. Reproduced with permission from van't Hof et al.[186]

any diagnostic or predictive values for vascular disease activity in patients with AMI. Kamijikkoku and associates[187] from Kumamoto, Japan, prospectively observed the time course of the plasma s1CAM-1 levels in 20 patients with AMI whose infarct-related coronary artery was successfully recanalized by emergency balloon angioplasty. s1CAM-1 was measured by enzyme-linked immunoassay. At admission, 48 hours, 1 week, and 2 weeks after angioplasty, s1CAM-1 levels were significantly elevated in patients who had early (3 weeks) restenosis develop compared with those who did not. At the other time points examined, there was a tendency of higher s1CAM-1 levels in patients with than without restenosis. The relation of s1CAM-1 levels and total white blood cell counts, neutrophil counts, or numbers of diseased major coronary artery branches was not statistically significant. A persistent increase in plasma s1CAM-1 levels may indirectly implicate vascular inflammation, which could predict the risk of early coronary restenosis after emergency angioplasty in patients with AMI. Hence, measurements of s1CAM-1 in patients with AMI would serve as a potentially useful predictor of the risk of early postangioplasty restenosis.

The Florence Randomized Elective Stenting in Acute Coronary Occlusions (FRESCO) Trial

Primary PTCA is emerging as an important therapeutic modality for patients with AMI. Antoniucci and colleagues[188] from Florence, Italy, evaluated the potential for acute stenting to provide additional benefit. After successful primary PTCA, 150 patients were randomly assigned to elective stenting or no further interventions. Stenting of the infarct-related artery was successful in all patients randomized to stent treatment. At 6 months, the incidence of the primary endpoint of a combination of death, reinfarction, or repeat target vessel revascularization was 9% in the stent group and 28% in the PTCA group. The incidence of restenosis or reocclusion was 17% in the stent group and 43% in the PTCA group. These authors conclude that primary stenting of the infarct-related artery compared to optimal primary angioplasty results in a lower rate of major adverse events secondary to recurrent ischemia and to a lower rate of angiographically detected restenosis or reocclusion of the infarct-related artery.

Mechanical Recanalization of Total Coronary Occlusions

The mechanical approach in the recanalization of total coronary occlusions by Reimers and associates[189] from Milan, Italy, consisted of the use of a new 0.014-inch standard coronary guidewire with jointless spring coil design that improves steering characteristics and tip stiffness. In addition, a 0.014-inch soft tip wire with hydrophilic coating and low-profile 1.5 mm over-the-wire balloons were used. The first wire was used selectively in 86 patients to treat 95 total occlusions, of which 51 (54%) were older than 3 months. Unfavorable angiographic characteristics were present in 79 (83%) of 95 lesions. Overall crossing success was 71% (67 of 95 lesions). There was 1 coronary perforation with cardiac tamponade necessitating emergency bypass surgery. In conclusion, the mechanical approach with the use of the standard coronary guidewire with jointless spring coil design provides a high success rate in the recanalization of unfavorable total occlusions.

Complications of Cardiogenic Shock

Previous studies have reported encouraging results with PTCA in patients with AMI complicated by cardiogenic shock. Antoniucci and colleagues[190] from Florence, Italy, evaluated 364 consecutive patients undergoing direct PTCA; and in 66 patients, AMI was complicated by cardiogenic shock. In patients with shock, direct PTCA had a success rate of 94%, an optimal angiographic result in 85%; primary stenting of the infarct-related artery was accomplished in 47% and the in-hospital mortality rate was 26%. Survival rate at 6 months was 71%. Comparison of event-free survival in patients with a stented or non-stented infarct-related artery suggested an initial and long-term benefit of pri-

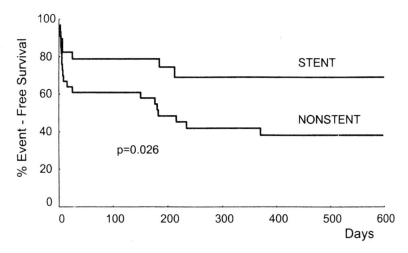

Figure 2-66. Comparison of direct angioplasty and stent-supported direct angioplasty for cardiogenic shock. Reproduced with permission from Antoniucci et al.[190]

mary stenting. These authors conclude that systematic direct PTCA including stent-supported PTCA can establish TIMI grade 3 flow in the great majority of patients presenting with AMI and early cardiogenic shock (Figure 2-66).

Complications of Angioplasty

Acute complications of percutaneous PTCA are more common in patients with unstable coronary syndromes. The objective of this study by Malekianpour and associates[191] from Montreal, Canada, was to prospectively determine the differences between ionic and nonionic low osmolar contrast media (LOCM) on potential risk of acute complications, particularly abrupt vessel closure, in patients with unstable angina undergoing PTCA. A total of 210 patients with 278 lesions were randomized to receive either ionic or nonionic LOCM during PTCA. Quantitative coronary angiographic measurements and assessment of filling defects were made by experienced observers who were blinded to the type of contrast media used. The baseline clinical and angiographic characteristics, the immediate postangioplasty results, and clinical outcome were similar in both groups. Subacute recoil, defined as the difference between minimal luminal diameter (in millimeters) at 0 and 15 minutes after angioplasty, was significantly greater in patients receiving nonionic LOCM (0.17 ± 0.36 mm vs. 0.07 ± 0.18 mm). A filling defect abnormality attributable to dissection, thrombus, or a combination of the 2 was noted in similar proportions of the 2 groups. Although nonsignificant, more thrombus was noted in the nonionic group. The abrupt vessel closure rate was similar in the 2 groups and was only 1.9% in the first 24 hours. However, 17 (8.3%) patients had a repeat PTCA at 15 minutes (9 ionic vs. 8 nonionic). In patients with unstable angina, the choice of ionic or nonionic LOCM does not appear to significantly affect the clinical outcome of PTCA.

Measurement of Cardiac Troponin T

Cardiac troponin T is a sensitive and specific marker for the detection of minor myocardial injury. However, it has been rarely used to monitor myocardial injury after coronary stenting. The purpose of the study by Shyu and associates[192] from Taiwan, Republic of China, was to measure troponin T after apparently successful PTCA with or without coronary stenting and to compare its results with serum creatine kinase and its isoform, CK-MB. The incidence of cardiac troponin T elevation was compared with that of creatine kinase or CK-MB in 120 consecutive patients with symptomatic ischemia undergoing visually successful PTCA with (n = 59) or without stenting (n = 61). Troponin T, creatine kinase, and CK-MB were measured before, immediately after, and 18–24 hours after the procedures were performed. No patient had abnormal troponin T, creatine kinase, or CK-MB levels before and immediately after the procedures, Moreover, no patient showed electrocardiographic evidence of myocardial infarction. Troponin T was elevated in 17 patients at 18 to 24 hours after coronary stenting and in 8 patients after PTCA. Both creatine kinase and CK-MB were elevated in 5 patients after coronary stenting and in 3 patients after PTCA. The frequency of abnormal troponin T levels was significantly higher than that of creatine kinase or CK-MB after coronary interventions (21% vs. 6.7%) and it was significantly higher after stenting when compared with angioplasty alone (29% vs. 13%). Patients with abnormal troponin T levels were more likely to undergo repeat revascularization than those without (24% vs. 6%). Cardiac troponin T is more sensitive than creatine kinase and CK-MB in detecting minor myocardial injury after coronary interventions. The incidence of troponin T release is higher in the patients undergoing stent implantation than in patients treated with angioplasty alone.

Use of Repeat Coronary Angiography After Angioplasty

There is an ongoing controversy as to whether repeat coronary angiography should be routinely performed after successful PTCA. Rupprecht and associates[193] from Mainz and Essen, Germany, examined the 10-year outcome in 400 patients who had or had not undergone an angiographic control 6 months after successful PTCA and a subsequent event-free 6-month period. This comparison was based on data gathered by questionnaire and telephone interview in 315 patients with (group 1) and 85 patients without (group 2) routine 6-month angiographic control. Mutivariate analysis (Cox model) was performed to identify predictors of adverse events. During the 10-year follow-up period, 22 (7%) of the 315 patients in group 1 died, compared with 16 (19%) patients in group 2. In groups 1 and 2, respectively, AMI occurred in 28 (9%) and 10 (12%) patients; CABG was performed in 42 (13%) and 14 (16%) patients; repeat PTCA was performed in 89 (28%) and 11 (13%) patients; and serious adverse events (death, AMI, CABG) occurred in 76 (24%) and 32 (38%) patients. Absence of a 6-month angiographic follow-up was identified as an independent predictor of death associated with a 2.7 times higher mortality rate during the

10-year follow-up period. Previous myocardial infarction increased the risk of death 2.5 times. Any increase of residual diameter stenosis by 10% was combined with a 1.4 times higher mortality rate. The chance of bypass surgery was higher in patients with multivessel disease (2.9 times), in patients with unstable angina (2.1 times), and in case of an increase of residual diameter stenosis by 10% (1.3 times). No predictor for the risk of myocardial infarction was found. Angiographic follow-up increased the likelihood of PTCA 2.5 times. A routinely performed angiographic control 6 months after successful PTCA is associated with a significantly higher rate of repeat PTCA but, most importantly, is correlated with a significantly lower mortality rate during the 10-year follow-up period.

Location of Anginal Pain After Angioplasty

Pasceri and colleagues[194] in Rome, Italy, determined whether a different location of anginal pain after PTCA may help identify patients with a new stenosis on an artery perfusing another myocardial region as opposed to those with restenosis after PTCA. They studied 38 patients with a mean age of 59 years who underwent PTCA for single-vessel disease with recurrence of symptoms requiring repeat coronary angiography during a 3-year follow-up. Angiography showed either a significant restenosis of the dilated lesion with no evidence of lesions in other vessels (n = 26) or a new stenosis in either of the other coronary arteries with no restenosis in the dilated vessel (n = 12). Before each procedure, patients reported the location and radiation of anginal pain. There was no relation between location of pain and site of the coronary stenosis. However, none of the patients with restenosis reported a different location of pain after PTCA, but 6 patients with new stenoses described a radiation of pain into different areas of the body. Location or radiation of pain in a different body area had a specificity of 96% and a sensitivity of 58% in detecting a stenosis in a new artery. Thus, a different location of anginal pain may distinguish patients with a new coronary stenosis from those with restenosis after PTCA for single-vessel disease.

Post-Coronary Artery Bypass Grafting Mortality in Diabetics and Nondiabetics

Cohen and associates[195] for the Israeli Coronary Artery Bypass (ISCAB) Study Consortium from Tel-Aviv and Jerusalem, Israel, identified factors associated with 30-day mortality after CABG among diabetic and nondiabetic patients. A subanalysis of a prospective national cohort study was performed that included patients who underwent CABG in 14 medical centers in Israel during 1994. Data including patient demographic and historical information, co-morbidity, and cardiac catheterization results were collected by trained nurses. Data were derived from direct patient interviews, charts, catheterization reports, surgical reports, and national vital records. Multivariate logistic regression analysis was used to identify factors associated with a 30-day mortality in diabetic and nondiabetic patient populations. The results showed that crude mortality was 5.0% among diabetic patients (n = 1,034) and 2.5% among nondiabetics (n = 3,350). The risk profile in diabetics was found to be worse. Multivariate logistic regression analysis identified female gender, 3-vessel disease, and left main disease as independent risk factors for 30-day, post-CABG mortality *unique to diabetic patients*. LV dysfunction was found to effect a greater risk among diabetic patients, whereas chronic renal failure was associated with greater risk among nondiabetics. In conclusion, the authors found differences in patterns of risk factors for post-CABG mortality between diabetics and nondiabetics. These findings may help physicians to identify patients at high risk for CABG mortality.

Vascular Access Site Complications After Percutaneous Coronary Intervention

Thrombolytic therapy or intense anticoagulation during percutaneous transluminal coronary revascularization (PTCR) increases the risk of vascular access site complications. Blankenship and associates[196] for the Evaluation of c7E3 for the Prevention of Ischemic Complications (EPIC) Investigators evaluated the association of abciximab, a glycoprotein IIb/IIIa receptor blocker, with vascular access site complications after PTCR. Of 2,058 patients who underwent PTCR in the EPIC trial, major vascular access site bleeding (a drop in hematocrit >15%), minor vascular access site bleeding (>10% drop), or surgical repair of the access site occurred in 5%, 12%, and 1.4% of all patients, respectively. Minor and/or major bleeding or surgery occurred in 21.8% of abciximab patients, compared with 9.1% of placebo patients. Logistic regression analysis identified these predictors of minor and/or major bleeding and/or surgical repair, in descending order of importance: abciximab therapy, acute myocardial infarction at enrollment, high baseline hematocrit, time in catheterization laboratory, heavier weight, female gender, maximum in catheterization laboratory activated clotting time, sheath size, and age. Vascular access site complications increased median post-PTCR length of stay from 2 days (no bleeding) to 3 days (minor bleeding) and 6 days (major bleeding). Site-to-site variation in vascular access site complications varied 6-fold. Analyses of subsequent studies of PTCR with abciximab will determine whether discontinuing heparin and removing sheaths early after PTCR reduces the risk of vascular access site complications.

Decline in Morbidity in Women Undergoing Coronary Angioplasty

To determine whether there has been an improvement in the relatively unfavorable outcome of PTCA in women, the 1993 to 1994 National Heart, Lung, and Blood Institute Percutaneous Transluminal Coronary Angioplasty

Registry collected data from 12 clinical centers that participated in the earlier registries. The report, written by Jacobs and colleagues,[197] compared 274 consecutive women in 1993 to 1994 with 545 consecutive women in 1985 to 1986 undergoing PTCA. Women in the 1993 to 1994 registry were older (64.3 vs. 61.0 years) with more diabetes mellitus (34.3% vs. 19.9%), CHF (13.7% vs. 8.6%), and co-morbid disease (19.5% vs. 9.3%). LVF and multivessel CAD were similar between groups. Angiographic success (90.9% vs. 85.1%) and clinical success (89.4% vs. 79.4%) were higher in women undergoing PTCA in 1993 to 1994 than in 1985 to 1986. Whereas there was no difference in in-hospital mortality (1.5% vs. 2.6%), the incidence of nonfatal AMI (1.8% vs. 4.6%), emergency CABG surgery (1.8% vs. 4.6%), and the combined endpoints of death, AMI, and emergency CABG (4.4% vs. 9.7%) were lower in women in 1993 to 1994 than in women in 1985 to 1986, respectively. Multivariate analysis revealed an odds ratio of 0.36 (95% confidence interval 0.18 to 0.72) for major complications and of 2.34 (95% confidence interval, 1.49 to 3.69) for clinical success in the 1993 to 1994 versus 1985 to 1986 registry. Therefore, despite a higher risk profile, women undergoing PTCA in 1993 to 1994 had a higher clinical success and lower major complication rate than women treated with PTCA in 1985 to 1986.

Possibility for Reuse of Balloon Catheters in the United States

Most countries outside the US routinely reuse disposable medical equipment resulting in significant cost savings. Because of quality and legal concerns, reuse in the US has been limited. Browne and colleagues[198] from Lakeland, Florida, investigated the reuse of PTCA balloon catheters restored by a process strictly controlled for bioburden and sterility, in patients undergoing PTCA. Used PTCA balloon catheters were shipped to a central facility and were decontaminated, cleaned, and tested for endotoxin using the LAL gel clot method. Physical testing and quality assurance were performed. The products were packaged and sterilized with ethylene oxide. One hundred seven patients were studied. The indication for PTCA was stable angina pectoris in 69 patients, unstable angina in 22, and AMI in 16. Of the 107 patients enrolled, 106 had a successful laboratory outcome and 1 required CABG after failed rescue stenting. The angiographic failure rate was 7% compared to the 10% rate seen with new balloon and other studies. These authors conclude that restoration of disposable coronary angioplasty catheters using a highly controlled process appears to be safe and effective with success rates similar to those of new products with no detectable sacrifice in performance. Cost analysis suggests that implementation of reused technology for expensive disposable equipment may offer cost savings for US hospitals without sacrifice of quality.

Diabetes Mellitus, Glycoprotein IIb/IIIa Blockade, and Heparin

Kleiman and colleagues[199] determined whether treatment with the monoclonal antibody directed against the platelet glycoprotein IIb/IIIa receptors, abciximab, is effective in reducing major complications and ischemic events after PTCA in diabetics. They used the Evaluation of PTCA to Improve Long-Term Outcome by c7E3 GP IIb/IIIa Receptor Blockade (EPILOG) trial to analyze outcomes in diabetic patients. Of the 2,792 patients enrolled, 638 (23%) were diabetic. The diabetics were older, heavier, more likely to be female and to have 3-vessel CAD, prior CABG, a history of hypertension, or recent AMI, and less likely to be current smokers than their nondiabetic counterparts. During hospitalization, death, AMI, or urgent CABG occurred in 7% of diabetics and 7.5% of nondiabetics. By 6 months, the composite of death and AMI had occurred in 8.8% of diabetics and 7.4% of nondiabetics, whereas death, AMI, or revascularization had occurred in 27% and 22.6%, respectively. Abciximab treatment reduced death or AMI among diabetic and nondiabetic patients at 30 days (Figure 2-67). Abciximab reduced target vessel revascularization among nondiabetics, but not among the diabetic patients. When standard and low-dose heparin adjuncts were compared, diabetics who were receiving abciximab with standard-dose heparin had marginally greater reductions in the composite of death and AMI and in target vessel revascularization than diabetics assigned to abciximab with low-dose heparin. Thus, these data indicate that abciximab treatment in diabetics leads to a reduction in the composite of death and AMI which is at least as great as that seen in nondiabetic patients. However, target vessel revascularization was reduced in nondiabetics but not diabetic patients. Whether this difference is related to the use of a lower dose of heparin is not clear from this study.

The Oral Glycoprotein IIb/IIIa Receptor Blockade to Inhibit Thrombosis (ORBIT) Trial

Kereiakes and colleagues[200] for the Oral Glycoprotein IIb/IIIa Receptor Blockade to Inhibit Thrombosis (ORBIT) trial investigators, conducted a multi-center, placebo-controlled randomized trial of xemilofiban, an oral platelet glycoprotein IIb/IIIa blocking agent, administered to patients after percutaneous coronary intervention. After successful elective percutaneous coronary intervention, 549 patients were randomized to receive either placebo or xemilofiban in a dose of 15 or 20 mg. Stented patients randomized to placebo also received ticlopidine 250 mg orally twice a day for 4 weeks. Patients who received abciximab during the coronary intervention and who were randomized to receive xemilofiban were administered reduced dosage (10 mg 3 times a day for 2 weeks) followed by the randomized maintenance dose of 15 or 20 mg twice a day for 2 more weeks. All patients received 325 mg aspirin. *Ex vivo* platelet aggregation in response to ADP and collagen was measured over time after the initial dose of study drug and at days 14 and 28 of long-term therapy in 230 patients. All patients were followed clinically for 90 days. Xemilofiban inhibited platelet aggregation to both ADP and collagen with peak levels of inhibition that were similar at 14 and 28 days of long-term oral therapy. Plasma levels of xemilofiban correlated with the degree of platelet inhibition. Peak platelet inhibition on day 1 correlated with the subsequent occurrence of insignificant or mild bleeding events. A trend was observed for reduction of cardiovascular events at 3 months in patients not treated with abciximab who re-

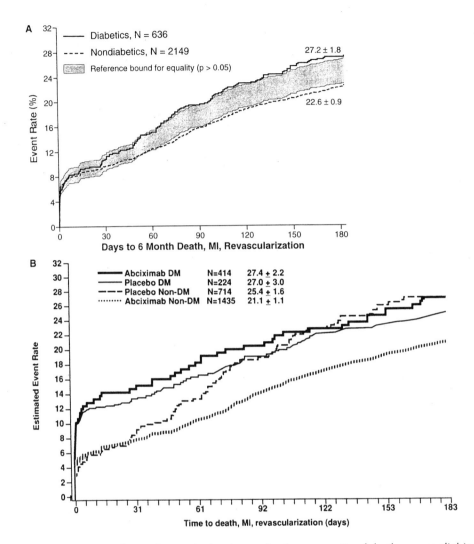

FIGURE 2-67. (A) Kaplan-Meier survival estimates for the composite of death, myocardial infarction (MI), or revascularization according to diabetic status. The shaded area represents the reference bounds for equivalence (p > 0.05) between the 2 groups. (B) Kaplan-Meier survival estimates for the composite endpoint according to diabetic status and treatment assignment among nondiabetics. The curves diverge sharply after 1 month, whereas among diabetics, the curves do not change. DM = diabetes mellitus. Reproduced with permission from Kleiman et al.[199]

ceived the highest dose of xemilofiban studied. Thus, these data suggest that xemilofiban inhibits platelet aggregation and was well tolerated during 28 days of long-term oral therapy.

Effect of Antioxidants on Restenosis After Percutaneous Transluminal Coronary Angioplasty

Antioxidants have an inhibitory effect on smooth muscle cell growth. Yokoi and colleagues[201] from a multicenter trial in Japan evaluated the effects of probucol on the rate of restenosis after PTCA. One hundred one patients were randomly assigned to receive 1,000 mg/day of probucol or control therapy 4 weeks before PTCA. After 4 weeks of pre-medication, both groups underwent PTCA. Probucol was continued until follow-up angiography 24 weeks after PTCA. Dilation was successful in 46 of 50 patients in the probucol group and in 45 of 51 patients in the control group. At follow-up angiography 24 weeks later, angiographic restenosis occurred in 23% of patients in the probucol group and 58% in the control group. Minimum lumen diameter was 1.49 mm in the probucol group and 1.13 mm in the control group. These authors conclude that probucol administered beginning 4 weeks before PTCA appears to reduce the restenosis rate.

Effect of Pravastatin on Restenosis After Percutaneous Transluminal Coronary Angioplasty

There is experimental and preliminary clinical data to suggest that lipid-lowering drugs might have a beneficial effect on restenosis after PTCA. Bertrand and colleagues,[202] for a randomized trial at multiple sites in France, randomized 695 patients to receive pravastatin 40 mg/day or placebo for 6 months after successful PTCA. All patients received aspirin 100 mg/day. At baseline, the patient groups were the same. In patients treated with pravastatin, there was a significant reduction in total and LDL cholesterol and triglyceride levels, and a significant increase in HDL cholesterol. However, there was no significant difference in the mean luminal diameter or restenosis rate (44% in the placebo group and 39% in the pravastatin group). Thus, although pravastatin has documented efficacy in reducing clinical events and angiographic disease progression in patients with CAD, these authors conclude that there is no beneficial effect on angiographic outcome at the target site 6 months after PTCA.

Effect of Verapamil on Patients Undergoing Percutaneous Transluminal Coronary Angioplasty

There are data that calcium entry blockers may have benefit in patients undergoing ischemia and reperfusion. Taniyama and associates[203] from Osaka, Japan, evaluated the effects of verapamil in patients undergoing primary PTCA for AMI. Forty patients with a first AMI were randomly assigned to verapamil or the control group. In the verapamil group, verapamil 0.5 mg was injected into the infarct-related artery shortly after PTCA, followed by oral administration. The low reflow zone was observed shortly after PTCA in 14 verapamil-treated patients and the low reflow ratio decreased after verapamil. The reduction in wall motion score from the acute to the late stage was significantly greater in the verapamil group than in the control group (0.7 vs. 0.2). These authors conclude that intracoronary administration of verapamil after primary PTCA can attenuate microvascular dysfunction and thereby augment myocardial blood flow in patients with AMI, leading to better functional outcome than with PTCA alone.

Abciximab Inhibits $\alpha_V\beta_3$ and Glycoprotein IIb/IIIa-Mediated Cell Adhesion

Tam and colleagues[204] in Malvern, Pennsylvania, evaluated the ability of abciximab (ReoPro, chimeric 7E3 Fab) to block $\alpha_V\beta_3$ receptors and compared this capability to its blocking of glycoprotein (GP) IIb/IIIa receptors on platelets. The data obtained demonstrate that abciximab binds with comparable affinity to $\alpha_V\beta_3$ and GP IIb/IIIa platelet receptors and that it inhibits $\alpha_V\beta_3$ and GP IIb/IIIa-mediated cell adhesion *in vitro* with IC_{50} values approximating K_D values. The experiments also showed a redistribution between GP IIb/IIIa and $\alpha_V\beta_3$ integrins *in vitro*. Thus, these data suggest that ReoPro is an antagonist of not only GP IIb/IIIa but also of $\alpha_V\beta_3$ receptors on platelets and that its additional clinical benefit in preventing thrombin generation, clot retraction, and smooth muscle cell migration and proliferation may, at least in part, relate to its ability to block $\alpha_V\beta_3$ receptors.

Treatment of Saphenous Vein Grafts

Percutaneous treatment of narrowed aortocoronary saphenous vein graft disease represents a viable option for patients with recurrent angina following CABG. Present strategies are limited by high rates of distal embolization, non-Q-wave AMI, and restenosis. Because these complications may be mediated by platelets, inhibition of platelet glycoprotein IIb/IIIa receptor, the final common pathway for aggregation, may improve clinical outcomes. In the evaluation of IIb/IIIa platelet receptor antagonist 7E3 in Preventing Ischemic Complications (EPIC) trial, by Mak and associates,[205] 2,099 patients undergoing high-risk percutaneous coronary revascularization were randomized to receive abciximab bolus and infusion, abciximab bolus followed by placebo infusion, or placebo. A total of 101 patients were treated for narrowing of saphenous vein grafts, 38 in the bolus and infusion group, 34 in the bolus group, and 29 in the placebo group. Clinical endpoints included all-cause mortality, nonfatal AMI, and the need for repeat revascularization at 30 days. Compared with placebo, bolus and infusion therapy resulted in a significant reduction in distal embolization (2% vs. 18%) and a trend toward reduction in early large non-Q-wave AMI (2% vs. 12%). The occurrence of a 30-day composite endpoint was similar among the 3 treatment groups. At 6 months, there was also no difference in the composite endpoint. These results suggest that adjunctive therapy with abciximab during percutaneous treatment of narrowed saphenous vein grafts reduces the occurrence of distal embolization and possibly non-Q-wave AMI.

Balloon Inflation Strategies After Coronary Angioplasty

Balloon inflation during coronary angioplasty results in shear stress-induced vessel wall injury with development of restenosis. This randomized trial by Miketic and associates[206] from Detmold, Germany, compared the impact of 2 different balloon inflation strategies (slow vs. fast) on restenosis after coronary angioplasty. Two hundred seven patients were randomized to undergo either fast or gradually increased slow inflation after successful placement of the balloon catheter inside the target lesion. One hundred six underwent fast, and 101 underwent gradually increased slow balloon inflation. Coronary angiograms were quantitatively analyzed before angioplasty, after angioplasty, and at follow-up 5.9 ± 1.6 months after the initial procedure. Both groups had an identical primary success rate (98% vs. 98%) and a similar minimal luminal diameter before (0.49 ± 0.26 mm vs. 0.48 ± 0.22 mm) and after (2.22 ± 0.97 mm vs. 2.26 ± 0.66 mm) angioplasty. Slow balloon inflation did not significantly reduce late luminal loss (0.58 ± 0.77 mm vs. 0.74 ± 0.87 mm), net gain (1.33 ± 0.84 mm vs. 1.19 ± 0.81 mm), or minimal luminal diameter at follow-up (1.80 ± 0.97 mm vs. 1.72 ± 1.0 mm). Restenosis, defined as more than 50% diameter stenosis at follow-up, occurred in 24% in the slow inflation group versus 36% in the fast inflation group. Clinical events during 6-month follow-up were similar in both groups (repeat angioplasty, fast 5.6% vs. slow 4.8%; nonfatal myocardial infarction, fast 2.2% vs. slow 1.2%; or death, fast 1.1% vs. slow 0%). The present randomized trial of 2 different balloon inflation strategies shows no statistically significant difference in net gain, minimal luminal diameter, or restenosis after coronary angioplasty. The difference in net gain, minimal luminal diameter, and restenosis rate were not statistically significant, but may represent a trend toward a reduction of smooth muscle cell proliferation and intimal hyperplasia induced by careful dilation of the stenotic lesion with gradually increased slow balloon inflation and reduction of shear stress-related vessel wall injury.

Influence of Coronary Remodeling on the Mechanism of Balloon Angioplasty

Intracoronary ultrasonography was used to assess coronary arteries before and after balloon PTCA to determine whether the mode of coronary atherosclerotic remodeling affects the mechanism of balloon dilation in this study by Timmis and associates[207] from Chicago, Illinois, and Indianapolis, Indiana. Coronary arteries may enlarge or shrink in response to atherosclerotic plaque development. The effect of coronary remodeling on the mechanism of balloon PTCA has not yet been studied. Forty-one patients with 47 native *de novo* coronary artery lesions were studied with a 30-MHz intracoronary ultrasound catheter before and after balloon PTCA. Images were analyzed at the lesion site and the adjacent reference segments. At each site the lumen, vessel, and plaque area and the percent area stenosis were measured. Lesions were separated into 2 groups based on relative vessel area (lesions vessel area/reference vessel area). A relative vessel area larger than 1.0 defines adaptive enlargement (group 1, n = 25), whereas a relative vessel area ≤1.0 reflects coronary shrinkage (group 2, n = 22). Regression analysis examined whether elastic recoil and the PTCA balloon/vessel area ratio correlated. After balloon PTCA was performed, both the enlargement and shrinkage groups had similar gains in luminal area (2.3

± 1.8 mm² vs. 2.8 ± 1.7 mm²), reduction in percent stenosis (− 19% ± 12% vs. − 14 ± 13), and final lumen area (4.9 ± 1.7 mm² vs. 4.7 ± 1.9 mm²). However, the mechanism of luminal enlargement was different in each group. Reduction in plaque area was significantly greater in the enlargement group (group 1, − 2.0 ± 1.7 mm² vs. group 2, 0.04 ± 2.2 mm²), whereas increased vessel area was more important in the shrinkage group (group 1, 0.8 ± 1.5 mm² vs. group 2, 2.4 ± 2.3 mm²). Positive correlation was seen between elastic recoil and the balloon/vessel area ratio in lesions with vessel enlargement. No such correlation was observed in shrinkage vessels. In conclusion, the acute luminal gain after balloon PTCA is similar regardless of the type of coronary remodeling. However, the mode of remodeling affects the mechanism of balloon dilation such that enlargement vessels exhibit plaque compression, whereas shrinkage arteries demonstrate vessel stretch. The post-PTCA elastic recoil correlates linearly to the balloon/vessel area ratio in arteries that have undergone adaptive enlargement.

Angioplasty in Patients Younger Than 40 Years

Ellis and associates[208] from Auckland, New Zealand, examined factors influencing the outcome of PTCA in patients under 40 years of age. The authors followed 86 patients (mean age 37) treated from 1982 to 1994. The primary procedural success was 90%. At follow-up of 83 patients (97%) at a mean of 48 ± 33 months (range 5–147), there had been 3 late deaths. Actuarial survival at 5 and 10 years was 95% and 91%, respectively. At review only 5% of patients had class III angina and no patient had class IV angina. Repeat revascularization (PTCA alone in 21 [25%], surgery in 8 [10%], or both in 10 [12%] patients) was performed for restenosis in 29 patients (35%) and for disease progression at other sites in 10 patients (12%). On multivariate analysis, a history of diabetes mellitus was the only factor associated with death or a subsequent cardiovascular event (AMI, stroke, or hospital admission with unstable angina). At follow-up, 20 patients (24%) still smoked, 64 (77%) had a total cholesterol level of 200 mg/dL or higher, 20 (24%) had a body mass index of 30 or greater, and 15 (18%) were not taking aspirin. In conclusion, PTCA in adults under 40 years of age has excellent early results with a low morbidity and mortality. The medium-term prognosis and control of symptoms was good, although by 5 years, further revascularization was required in almost half of the patients (Figure 2-68).

Impact of Stents on Clinical Outcome

Despite effective treatment of LMCA disease by CABG, there is still need for treatment of LMCA disease due to progression of atherosclerosis or bypass graft failure. Kornowski and associates[209] from Washington, DC, compared the in-hospital and 1-year follow-up outcomes of patients with LMCA disease treated with stents (n=88), with a matched group of patients undergoing LMCA nonstent procedures (n=36). Ninety-seven percent of patients in each

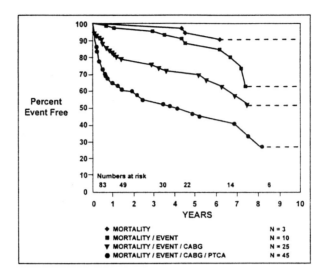

FIGURE 2-68. Actuarial outcomes after PTCA. Cumulative percent free from death, cardiovascular (CVS) events (stroke, myocardial infarction, unstable angina requiring hospitalization), subsequent bypass surgery, and further PTCA. CABG = coronary artery bypass graft surgery. Reproduced with permission from Ellis et al.[208]

group underwent previous coronary bypass. Procedural success (angiographic success without major in-hospital complications) tended to be higher in stent patients than in their nonstent counterparts (98% vs. 92%), and overall procedural complications were higher for the nonstent group (5.4% vs. 0%). The incidence of non-Q-wave AMI was higher in patients with the LMCA disease treated with stents than in nonstent patients (13% vs. 2.7%). There was no difference in death rate or Q-wave AMI between the 2 groups during follow-up. Overall target lesion revascularization at 1 year was 15% after LMCA stenting, and 18% in nonstent patients. Also, any cardiac event-free survival (including death, Q-wave AMI, coronary bypass, or angioplasty) was similar for both groups (78% for stents vs. 76% for nonstents). The authors conclude that in patients undergoing LMCA interventions, stents reduce major hospital complications, but may not significantly reduce repeat revascularization or major cardiac events at 1 year compared with nonstent LMCA procedures (Table 2-17).

Use of Coronary Blood Flow Reserve to Predict Recovery

The aim of the study by Mazur and associates[210] from Houston, Texas, was to determine whether the recovery of global and regional LV function after successful PTCA could be predicted by measuring coronary flow reserve before performing the intervention. Thirty-two patients underwent PTCA 6.9 ± 3.4 days after a recent myocardial infarction. Coronary flow reserve was determined in the infarct-related artery before PTCA by using an intracoronary Doppler tipped wire. Global and regional wall motion were determined by 2-

TABLE 2-17
In-Hospital Events and 1-Year Follow-up Outcome

	Stent (n = 88)	Non-Stent (n = 36)	p Value
In-hospital results			
Angiographic success	87 (99%)	35 (97%)	0.52
Procedural success	86 (98%)	33 (92%)	0.12
Major complications	0 (0%)	2 (5.4%)	0.03
Death	0 (0%)	1 (2.7%)	0.12
Q-wave myocardial infarction	0 (0%)	1 (2.7%)	0.12
Emergency coronary bypass	0 (0%)	1 (2.7%)	0.12
Use of intraaortic balloon pump			
Emergency	0 (0%)	1 (2.7%)	0.12
Prophylactic	10 (12%)	4 (11%)	0.35
Non-Q myocardial infarction	11 (13%)	1 (2.7%)	0.09
Stent thrombosis	1 (1.1%)	—	—
One-year follow-up events			
Death	0 (0%)	0 (0%)	—
Q-wave myocardial infarction	2 (2.3%)	1 (2.7%)	0.84
Target lesion revascularization			
Coronary bypass surgery	4 (4.6%)	0 (0%)	0.20
Coronary angioplasty	11 (13%)	8 (18%)	0.48
Overall	13 (15%)	8 (18%)	0.71
Cardiac event-free survival	69 (78%)	27 (76%)	0.85

Reproduced with permission from Kornowski et al.[209]

dimensional echocardiography before the Flowire study and again 7 weeks after the angioplasty. Whereas the global and regional wall motion score indices improved in 20 patients (recovery group), they deteriorated or did not change in 9 patients (nonrecovery group). Coronary flow reserve distal to the lesion in the infarct-related artery was significantly higher in the recovery group (1.43 ± 0.57 vs. 0.98 ± 0.70). Coronary flow reserve distal to the lesion in the infarct-related artery was less than 1.1 in patients whose global or regional LV function did not improve at follow-up, whereas flow reserve ranged between 1.1 and 1.8 in patients in whom LV function improved. These results suggest that the absence of inducible coronary flow reserve may predict failure of LV systolic function to improve between the first and sixth week after infarction. Measurement of flow reserve with a Flowire at the time of diagnostic angiography after recent myocardial infarction may ultimately prove helpful in deciding whether to proceed with revascularization.

Evaluation of Prolonged Heparin Use After Coronary Interventions

Continuous heparin infusion after PTCA procedures prolongs the hospital stay and could increase the occurrence of bleeding complications. The aim of this randomized trial by Garachemani and associates[211] from Bern, Switzerland, was to evaluate whether omission of heparin infusion after uncomplicated coronary interventions in patients with stable and unstable angina with or without stent implantation increased the incidence of acute cardiac complications. A total of 191 consecutive patients who underwent successful PTCA were randomly assigned to receive either prolonged heparin (heparin group) or no postprocedure heparin (control group). The 2 treatment groups were comparable with respect to clinical and angiographic characteristics. Stents were used in 36% of the control group and in 33% of the heparin group. Cardiac complications occurred in 8 (4%) patients. Four (4%) patients in the control group and 3 (3%) patients in the heparin group had a myocardial infarction. One patient in the control group died 3 days after the intervention. No patient in either group needed a repeat revascularization during the target hospitalization. Peripheral vascular complications in the control and heparin groups occurred in 1% and 3% of the patients, respectively. Omission of heparin after successful PTCA with or without stent implantation in patients with stable and unstable angina did not significantly increase the incidence of acute cardiac complications. It allows for early sheath removal and patient discharge and saves costs. This study, combined with other small studies in the field, provides strong evidence that heparin should not be used routinely.

Preventing Early Reocclusion After Angioplasty

PTCA for AMI achieves high patency rates. Conversely, it has been shown that after thrombolysis, early reocclusion of the infarct-related coronary artery is associated with substantial morbidity and mortality. Garot and associates[212] from Paris, France, retrospectively studied the incidences, prognostic implications, and clinical risk factors for in-hospital reocclusion of the infarct-related artery after successful PTCA for AMI. The authors studied 399 consecutive patients (aged 59 ± 14 years, 52% with anterior wall infarction) admitted less than 6 hours after AMI onset, of whom 374 (94%) were successfully treated with primary (n = 297) or rescue (n = 77) PTCA with a stenting rate of 8%. Predischarge angiography was performed in 306 (82%). Early reocclusion of the infarct-related artery occurred in 28 patients (9%) and was silent in 6 (2%). The reocclusion rate was 10% for primary PTCA and 8% for rescue PTCA. Twenty-two of 28 patients (6%) underwent repeat emergency coronary angiography because of early recurrent ischemia and most (n = 18) were treated with emergency PTCA. Early recurrent ischemia occurred mostly (86%) within 5 days of AMI onset. There was a higher prevalence of on-site hemorrhage (18% vs. 5%), blood transfusion (11% vs. 2%), pulmonary edema (21% vs. 4%), and in-hospital death (21% vs. 1%) in patients with predischarge reocclusion. On multivariate analysis, cardiogenic shock on admission and absence of dyslipidemia were strong and independent predictors of infarct-related artery reocclusion. In conclusion, early reocclusion after emergency PTCA occurred in 9% of the patients and was associated with substantial morbidity and mortality. This warrants attempts to decrease its incidence, e.g., with more frequent use of stents.

Angioplasty Versus New Device Intervention

Because of the shortcomings of PTCA, a number of new devices have been developed for performing coronary interventions in an attempt to improve clinical outcomes. King and associates[213] in a multicenter study evaluated the NHBLI registry for PTCA and a second NHBLI-funded registry, the NACI, which collected data on newer interventions. Patients enrolled in the NACI registry were older, had undergone more previous CABG, and had more stenoses located in bypass grafts than patients in the PTCA registry. Procedural success was achieved in 72% and 83% of patients in the PTCA and NACI registries. However, the in-hospital and 1-year mortality rates were 1% versus 1.8% and 3.1% versus 5.9%, respectively. After risk adjustment, there was no difference in 1-year mortality. These authors conclude that this comparative study found no overall superiority of these new devices in terms of patient survival or freedom from additional target lesion revascularization. Since these registries predated the use of stents, it is unclear whether these large databases will be similar for the use of stent placement which has appeared to be helpful in reducing morbidity.

Healthcare Cost and Utilization Project

It is estimated that more than 400,000 PTCA procedures are performed in the US annually. Maynard and colleagues[214] from Seattle, Washington, reported patient characteristics and outcomes for 163,527 PTCAs performed in 214 hospitals in 17 states from 1993 to 1994. These hospitals were a 20% random sample of hospitals in the Healthcare Cost and Utilization Project, which was designed to reflect hospitalization in the US, generally. Cases with International Classification Modification procedure codes 36.01, 36.02, and 36.05 were defined as PTCA and were categorized as to whether AMI was the principal discharge diagnosis. The average age of 44,270 AMI discharges (27%) was 62 ± 12 years and that of 119,257 no-AMI cases (73%) was 64 ± 11 years; 1/3 of both groups were women, 88% were white, and almost 90% had Medicare or private insurance as the primary payer. The states contributing the most cases were Florida (26%), California (12%), and Wisconsin (10%). Hospital mortality was 1.7% overall and was 3.8% for AMI and 0.8% for no-AMI cases. Bypass surgery performed during the same admission was 3.4% overall and was 4.5% and 3.0% for AMI and no-AMI cases, respectively. Multivariate analysis showed that advanced age, diabetes, female gender, and Medicaid payer status were associated with increased risk of mortality. National estimates from this 20% sample indicate that more than 850,000 PTCAs were performed in the 2 years, with 452,319 cases estimated for 1994. In 1994 there were an estimated 2,789 deaths and 9,903 bypass surgeries in the no-AMI subset of 327,856 procedures. For the AMI group of 124,463 procedures, there were 4,486 deaths and 5,799 bypass surgeries in 1994. This study of PTCA outcomes contains the largest

TABLE 2-18
Demographic Characteristics in the Healthcare Cost and Utilization Project, 1993–1994

Characteristics	AMI (n = 44,270)	No AMI (n = 119,257)	All (n = 163,527)
Age	62 ± 12	64 ± 11	63 ± 12
Women	32%	33%	33%
Race			
White	87%	88%	88%
Black	5%	4%	5%
Hispanic	5%	6%	6%
Asian	1%	1%	1%
Native American	<1%	<1%	<1%
Other	2%	2%	2%
Primary payer			
Medicare	43%	51%	49%
Medicaid	4%	3%	3%
Private	44%	40%	41%
Self-pay	5%	3%	3%
Other	4%	3%	3%
Admission source			
Emergency department	42%	17%	24%
Other hospital	33%	19%	22%
Long term care/other	3%	2%	2%
Routine	22%	62%	52%
Admission type			
Emergency	56%	26%	34%
Urgent	35%	36%	35%
Elective	9%	38%	30%
Median income			
<15K	2%	1%	1%
15–20	6%	5%	5%
20–25	19%	17%	18%
25–30	22%	22%	22%
30–35	18%	18%	18%
35–40	12%	13%	13%
40–45	8%	9%	9%
>45	13%	15%	14%
Region			
West	18%	18%	18%
East	28%	24%	27%
Midwest	24%	28%	25%
South	29%	30%	30%

Reproduced with permission from Maynard et al.[214]

number of cases as well as the most representative sample reported to date (Tables 2-18–2-22).

Long-Term Outcome of Coronary Angioplasty

To examine the long-term outcome of coronary angioplasty, lesions that remained patent after 3 to 12 months were monitored angiographically at 3-

TABLE 2-19
**Medical History Characteristics in the Healthcare Cost and Utilization Project,
1993–1994**

Characteristics	AMI (n = 44,270)	No AMI (n = 119,257)	All (n = 163,527)
Diabetes with chronic complications	1%	2%	2%
Diabetes	15%	18%	17%
Chronic pulmonary disease	10%	8%	8%
Cerebrovascular disease	1%	1%	1%
Peripheral vascular disease	2%	3%	3%
Renal disease	1%	1%	1%
Rheumatic disease	1%	1%	1%
Hypertension	36%	42%	40%
Unstable angina	4%	55%	41%
Multivessel angioplasty	9%	13%	12%

Reproduced with permission from Maynard et al.[214]

year intervals by Kitazume and associates[215] from Tokyo, Japan. There were 252 lesions successfully dilated (from 83% + 13% preprocedural stenosis to 19% + 14% residual stenosis) between 1983 and 1986 that remained patent on follow-up angiography (23% + 15% stenosis) and were monitored further at the outpatient department. Repeat angiography was done for 186 lesions at 2 to 4 years and showed that 179 were patent (0% to 50% stenosis), 1 had mild stenosis (55% to 70% stenosis), and 6 had severe stenosis (75% to 100% stenosis). Angiography was repeated for 138 lesions at 5 to 7 years, showing that 127 were patent, 4 had mild stenosis, and 7 had severe stenosis. Finally, angiography was performed for 78 lesions at 8 to 10 years, showing that 63 were patent, 4 had mild stenosis, and 11 had severe stenosis. Although numerous lesions were lost to follow-up, most appeared to remain patent for 4 years, after which a significant number developed restenosis.

Determinants of Long-Term Outcome After Angioplasty

Halon and associates[216] from Haifa, Israel, examined the 10-year outcome in a cohort of 227 unselected, consecutive patients (age 58 ± 10 years) undergo-

TABLE 2-20
Outcomes of the Healthcare Cost and Utilization Project, 1993–1994

Outcome	AMI (n = 44,270)	No AMI (n = 119,257)	All (n = 163,527)
Hospital death	3.8%	0.8%	1.7%
Same admission CABG	4.5%	3.0%	3.4%
Hospital death and/or same admission CABG	8.0%	3.7%	4.9%
Length of stay (d)	7.0 ± 5.6	4.3 ± 4.9	5.0 ± 5.2
Total charges (thousands)	$27.1 ± 23.3	$19.3 ± 18.2	$21.4 ± 20.0

Reproduced with permission from Maynard et al.[214]

TABLE 2-21
Predictors of Outcomes of Coronary Angioplasty Odds Ratios
and 95% Confidence Intervals

	AMI		No AMI	
Variable	Death (n = 44,105)*	Same Admission Surgery (n = 44,270)†	Death (n = 118,807)‡	Same Admission Surgery (n = 118,852)§
Age (per 10-year increase)	1.91 (1.82–2.01)	NS	1.98 (1.84–2.12)	0.89 (0.87–0.92)
Systemic hypertension	0.51 (0.45–0.57)	0.88 (0.80–0.96)	0.56 (0.49–0.64)	0.92 (0.86–0.99)
Renal disease	3.94 (2.97–5.22)	NS	3.40 (2.47–4.68)	NS
Women	1.42 (1.28–1.57)	NS	1.38 (1.21–1.57)	1.22 (1.13–1.31)
Unstable angina	0.49 (0.35–0.70)	1.53 (1.24–1.88)	0.52 (0.46–0.59)	1.12 (1.05–1.20)
Diabetes mellitus	1.25 (1.10–1.41)	NS	1.17 (1.00–1.37)	0.78 (0.71–0.85)
Cerebrovascular disease	1.74 (1.15–2.63)	NS	NS	NS
Chronic pulmonary disease	NS	1.22 (1.06–1.41)	NS	1.47 (1.32–1.64)
Multivessel procedure	NS	0.84 (0.71–0.99)	NS	0.63 (0.56–0.70)
Medicaid	1.61 (1.22–2.13)	NS	1.84 (1.26–2.68)	NS
Geographic region (South is reference category)				
West	0.82 (0.70–0.95)	0.98 (0.86–1.12)	0.91 (0.76–1.09)	1.00 (0.91–1.09)
East	0.79 (0.69–0.92)	0.71 (0.62–0.81)	0.75 (0.63–0.89)	0.73 (0.67–0.80)
Midwest	1.05 (0.93–1.19)	1.09 (0.97–1.22)	0.96 (0.82–1.14)	0.88 (0.81–0.97)

* Model 1 variables included in order of entry: age, hypertension, renal disease, gender, unstable angina, region, diabetes, Medicaid, and cerebrovascular disease.
† Model 2 variables included in order of entry: region, unstable angina, hypertension, chronic pulmonary disease, and multivessel angioplasty.
‡ Model 3 variables included in order of entry: age, unstable angina, renal disease, hypertension, gender, Medicaid, region, and diabetes.
§ Model 4 variables included in order of entry: multivessel angioplasty, chronic pulmonary disease, region, age, diabetes, gender, unstable angina, and hypertension.
Reproduced with permission from Maynard et al.[214]

ing PTCA between 1984 and 1986 and followed in a single cardiac center. In particular, the authors sought to identify the relative importance of the systemic risk factors diabetes mellitus and systemic hypertension and the extent of CAD in contrast to procedure-related technical variables, the immediate success of the procedure, or completeness of revascularization. By life-table analysis (99% follow-up), 94% of the patients were alive at 5 years, and 77%

TABLE 2-22
National Estimates of Coronary Angioplasty Outcomes, 1993–1994

	1993 (n = 420,472)	1994 (n = 452,319)
Deaths	6,963 (1.7%)	7,275 (1.6%)
Same admission bypass surgery	14,414 (3.4%)	15,702 (3.5%)
Acute myocardial infarction	113,226	124,463
Deaths	4,439 (3.9%)	4,486 (3.6%)
Same admission bypass surgery	5,043 (4.5%)	5,799 (4.7%)
No acute myocardial infarction	307,246	327,856
Deaths	2,524 (0.8%)	2,789 (0.9%)
Same admission bypass surgery	9,371 (3.0%)	9,903 (3.0%)

Reproduced with permission from Maynard et al.[214]

at 10 years after angioplasty. Ten-year survival was reduced in patients with diabetes mellitus (59% vs. 83%), in patients with previous AMI (68% vs. 85%), in patients with EF less than 50% (55% vs. 82%), and in patients with 3-vessel disease (58% vs. 84% and 86% for 1- and 2-vessel disease, respectively). Diabetes mellitus was the major independent predictor of poor survival (adjusted odds ratio 3.1). Survival at 10 years was identical in 199 patients in whom angioplasty was complete and in 25 in whom the balloon catheter did not cross the lesion, although bypass surgery was more frequent in the latter group (45% vs. 21%). Incomplete revascularization did not predict poor survival (72% vs. 79%) with complete angioplasty. Event-free survival at 10 years for the whole group was 29% and 49% of patients survived with no event other than a single repeat angioplasty procedure. Multivessel disease, hypertension, and diabetes mellitus were independent predictors of decreased event-free survival, but incomplete revascularization was not. Thus, long-term outcome after coronary balloon angioplasty was related to diabetes mellitus, systemic hypertension, and extent of CAD, but not to the immediate success of the procedure or completeness of revascularization (Figures 2-69, 2-70).

Stenting Versus Percutaneous Transluminal Coronary Angioplasty to Reduce Restenosis

Erbel and colleagues[217] conducted a prospective, randomized, multicenter study to determine whether intracoronary stenting as compared with standard PTCA reduces the recurrence of luminal narrowing in restenotic lesions. A total of 383 patients who had undergone at least 1 PTCA and had clinical and angiographic evidence of restenosis after the procedure were randomly assigned to undergo standard PTCA or repeat PTCA (192 patients) or intracoronary stenting with a Palmaz-Schatz stent (191 patients). The primary endpoint was angiographic evidence of restenosis, defined as stenosis of more than 50% of the luminal diameter at 6 months. The secondary endpoints were death, Q-wave AMI, CABG, and revascularization of the target vessel. The rate of restenosis was significantly higher in the angioplasty group than in the stent group

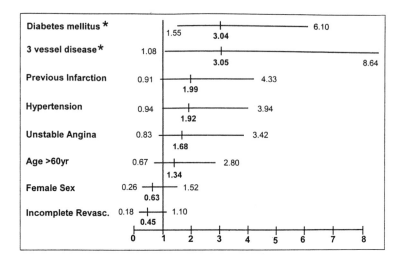

FIGURE 2-69. Adjusted odds ratios and 95% confidence intervals for predictors of 10-year survival after PTCA. The numbers are those at entry into the Cox multivariate model before exclusion of nonsignificant variables by backward elimination. Asterisks denote variables that remained significant predictors after nonsignificant variables were eliminated. Revasc. = revascularization. Reproduced with permission from Halon et al.[216]

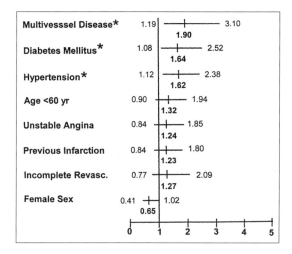

FIGURE 2-70. Adjusted odds ratios and 95% confidence intervals for 10-year survival free from myocardial infarction, CABG, or repeat PTCA. The numbers are those at entry into the Cox multivariate model before exclusion of nonsignificant variables by backward elimination. Asterisks denote variables that remained significant predictors of outcome after nonsignificant variables were eliminated. Revasc. = revascularization. Reproduced with permission from Halon et al.[216]

(32% as compared with 18%, p=0.03). Revascularization of the target vessel at 6 months was required in 27% of the PTCA group, but in only 10% of the stent group (p=0.001). This difference resulted from a smaller mean minimal luminal diameter in the PTCA group (1.85 ± 0.56 mm) than in the stent group (2.04 ± 0.66 mm) (p=0.01). Subacute thrombosis occurred in 0.6% of the PTCA group and in 3.9% of the stent group. The rate of event-free survival at 250 days was 72% in the PTCA group and 84% in the stent group (p=0.04). Thus, elective coronary stenting is effective in the treatment of restenosis after PTCA. Stenting results in a lower rate of recurrent stenosis despite a higher incidence of subacute thrombosis.

Restenosis Rate After Repeat Intervention

Bauters and colleagues[218] from Lille, France, studied 103 consecutive patients and 107 vessels in patients undergoing repeat PTCA for the treatment of in-stent restenosis in a prospective angiographic follow-up program. Repeat PTCA was performed in 93 lesions and additional stenting in 14 lesions (13%). The primary success rate was 98%. Six-month angiographic follow-up was obtained in 85% of eligible patients. Restenosis was determined by quantitative arteriography. Restenosis defined as a less than 50% diameter stenosis at follow-up occurred in 22% of lesions. The rate of target-lesion revascularization at 6 months was 17%. Diffuse in-stent restenosis and severe stenosis before repeat intervention were both associated with significantly higher rates of recurrent restenosis (Table 2-23). Thus, the overall restenosis rate after repeat intervention for in-stent restenosis is low and the subgroup of patients with diffuse or severe in-stent restenosis appear to be at the highest risk.

Use of Probucol to Prevent Restenosis

Rodés and colleagues[219] in Montreal, Quebec, Canada, had demonstrated previously that multivitamins and probucol, a potent antioxidant, reduces restenosis after balloon angioplasty. In the present study, they wished to determine whether the benefit of probucol is maintained in the subgroup of patients with smaller coronary vessels, i.e., those smaller than 3.0 mm in diameter. They studied a subgroup of 189 patients included in the MultiVitamins and Probucol (MVP) trial who underwent successful balloon angioplasty of at least 1 coronary segment with a reference diameter smaller than 3.0 mm. One month before PTCA, patients were randomly assigned to 1 of 4 treatments: placebo, probucol (500 mg), multivitamins, including β-carotene, vitamin C, and vitamin E, or probucol plus multivitamins twice daily. Treatment was maintained until follow-up angiography at 6 months. The mean reference diameter of this study population was 2.49 ± 0.34 mm. Late lumen loss was 0.12 ± 0.34 mm for probucol, 0.25 ± 0.43 mm for the combined treatment, 0.35 ± 0.56 mm for vitamins, and 0.39 ± 0.51 mm for placebo (p=0.005 for probucol) (Figure 2-71). Restenosis rates per segment were 20% for probucol, 28.6% for the combined treatment, 41% for vitamins, and 37% for placebo (p=0.006 for probu-

TABLE 2-23
Predictors of Recurrent In-Stent Restenosis

	Restenosis (n = 19)	No Restenosis (n = 68)	p
Age, yr	59 ± 9	59 ± 11	NS
Men, n (%)	16 (84)	61 (90)	NS
Diabetes mellitus, n (%)	5 (26)	16 (24)	NS
Hypercholesterolemia, n (%)	6 (32)	37 (54)	NS
Interval from stent implantation to repeat intervention, mo	5.1 ± 1.3	5.8 ± 2.4	NS
Unstable angina, n (%)	8 (42)	15 (22)	NS
Vessel treated, n (%)			
Left anterior descending artery	6 (32)	37 (54)	
Left circumflex	4 (21)	10 (15)	NS
Right coronary artery	7 (37)	19 (28)	
Saphenous vein graft	2 (10)	2 (3)	
Ostial location	3 (16)	3 (4)	NS
Type of stent, n (%)			
Palmaz-Schatz	15 (79)	37 (55)	
Wiktor	4 (21)	24 (35)	NS
Others	0	7 (10)	
Number of stents	1.5 ± 0.8	1.4 ± 0.6	NS
Inflation pressure at stent implantation, atm	14.7 ± 3.3	14.5 ± 3.9	NS
Type of stent restenosis, n (%)			
Focal	9 (47)	54 (79)	.006
Diffuse	10 (53)	14 (21)	
Location of stent restenosis, n (%)			
Body	17 (89)	54 (79)	NS
Edge	2 (11)	14 (21)	
Repeat treatment, n (%)			
Balloon only	17 (89)	57 (84)	NS
Stent	2 (11)	11 (16)	
Inflation pressure at repeat intervention, atm	12.8 ± 3.3	12.6 ± 3.7	NS
Reference diameter, mm	2.69 ± 0.64	2.93 ± 0.57	NS
Percent stenosis before repeat intervention	77 ± 14	68 ± 11	.004
Percent stenosis after repeat intervention	25 ± 17	21 ± 12	NS

Reproduced with permission from Bauters et al.[218].

col). Probucol appears to reduce lumen loss and restenosis rate after balloon angioplasty in small coronary arteries.

Plasma Activity and Insertion/Deletion Polymorphism of Angiotensin-Converting Enzyme Gene

Plasma angiotensin-converting enzyme (ACE) levels are largely controlled by the insertion/deletion (I/D) polymorphism of the enzyme gene. The association among restenosis within coronary stents, plasma ACE level, and the I/D polymorphism was analyzed by Ribichini and colleagues[220] in Torino, Italy. One hundred seventy-six consecutive patients with successful, high-pressure,

A

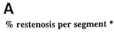

% restenosis per segment *

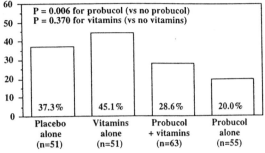

P = 0.006 for probucol (vs no probucol)
P = 0.370 for vitamins (vs no vitamins)

Placebo alone (n=51)	Vitamins alone (n=51)	Probucol + vitamins (n=63)	Probucol alone (n=55)
37.3%	45.1%	28.6%	20.0%

* P Values are based on multiple logistic regression adjusted for target vessels and for 15 min post-angioplasty luminal diameter using the Generalized Estimating Equations (GEE) technique.

B

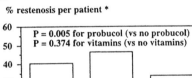

% restenosis per patient *

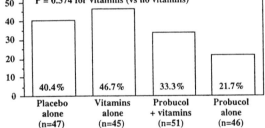

P = 0.005 for probucol (vs no probucol)
P = 0.374 for vitamins (vs no vitamins)

Placebo alone (n=47)	Vitamins alone (n=45)	Probucol + vitamins (n=51)	Probucol alone (n=46)
40.4%	46.7%	33.3%	21.7%

FIGURE 2-71. Restenosis rates for the 4 study groups of the intent-to-treat population. **(A)** Restenosis rates per segment. **(B)** Restenosis rates per patient. Reproduced with permission from Rodés et al.[219]

elective stenting of *de novo* lesions in the native coronary arteries were considered. Recurrence was observed in 35 patients (19.9%). Baseline clinical and demographic variables, plasma glucose and serum fibrinogen levels, lipid profile, descriptive and quantitative angiographic data, and procedural variables were not different in patients with and without restenosis. Mean plasma ACE levels were 40.8 ± 3.5 and 20.7 ± 1.0 U/L, respectively. Diameter stenosis percentage and minimal lumen diameter at 6 months showed statistically significant correlations with plasma ACE level. Twenty-one of 62 patients with D/D genotype, 13 of 80 (16%) with I/D genotype, and 1 of 34 (2.9%) with I/I genotype showed recurrence of restenosis. The restenosis rate for each genotype was consistent with a co-dominant expression of the D allele. Thus, in a selected cohort of patients, both the D/D genotype of the ACE gene and high plasma activity of the enzyme were significantly associated with in-stent restenosis (Figure 2-72).

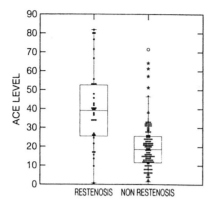

FIGURE 2-72. ACE plasma levels (U/L) observed in patients with or without restenosis represented by a box plot. The box bounds the first and the third quartiles (interquartile range); encompasses 50% of the data, and includes the median (line within the box). Dispersion of the data above and below this range is marked by "whiskers" that extend to the most extreme values within a "fence" at 1.5 times the interquartile range. Mild outliers (*) are found within 3 times the interquartile range, and extreme outliers (open circles) are found outside of this boundary. Reproduced with permission from Ribichini et al.[220]

Impact of Diabetes Mellitus on In-Stent Restenosis

Diabetic patients have increased restenosis and late morbidity following PTCA. The impact of diabetes mellitus on in-stent restenosis was evaluated by Abizaid and colleagues[221] from Washington, DC. They studied 954 consecutive patients with native coronary artery lesions treated with elective Palmaz-Schatz stent implantation. In-hospital mortality was 2% in insulin-dependent diabetes which was significantly higher compared with those without diabetes (.3%). Stent thrombosis did not differ among groups with insulin-dependent diabetes and those with non-insulin-dependent diabetes. Target lesion revascularization was 20% in insulin-dependent diabetics compared with 18% in non-insulin-dependent diabetics and 16% in nondiabetics. Late cardiac event-free survival was significantly lower in insulin-dependent diabetes (60%) compared with non-insulin-dependent diabetes (70%) and nondiabetic patients (76%). By multivariate analysis, insulin-dependent diabetes mellitus was an independent predictor for any late cardiac event (odds ratio = 2). These authors conclude that insulin-dependent diabetics are at higher risk for in-hospital mortality and subsequent target lesion revascularization. On the other hand, acute and long-term procedural outcome was found to be similar for non-insulin-dependent diabetics compared with nondiabetic patients.

Mechanisms of Restenosis After Coronary Angioplasty

Mechanisms of restenosis after PTCA have not been yet defined. Experimental studies by Salvioni and associates[222] show that thrombin, by stimulating platelet growth factor secretion and smooth muscle cell proliferation, can play a major role. In 34 patients with single-vessel CAD undergoing PTCA, thrombin activity was evaluated through serial fibrinopeptide A (FPA) plasma determinations. Samples were performed before PTCA, immediately after and 24 hours, 72 hours, and 6 months later. Patients were grouped according to the development (group 1, n = 13) or nondevelopment (group 2, n = 21) of restenosis at a 6-month angiographic control. No difference in the 2 groups was found concerning baseline FPA values. Soon after PCTA, patients in group 1 had higher FPA levels (27 ± 14 ng/mL) than those in group 2 (9.2 ± 5.6 ng/mL). No differences in FPA levels were detected at the other steps between the 2 groups. These data suggest that thrombin plays a role in the process of restenosis after PTCA; acute FPA response to the procedure seems to have a predictive value.

Prediction of Restenosis

Serum lipoprotein(a) level is a known risk factor for atherosclerotic CAD. However, its association with restenosis after PTCA is controversial. Alaigh and colleagues[223] in Stony Brook, New York, hypothesized that the lipoprotein(a) level is a significant risk factor for restenosis after angioplasty through a pathophysiological mechanism leading to excess thrombin generation or inhibition of fibrinolysis. The investigators designed a prospective study of the relation of lipoprotein(a) to outcome after angioplasty, in which they measured selected laboratory variables at entry and collected clinical, procedural, lesion-related, and outcome data pertaining to restenosis. Restenosis was defined as greater than 50% stenosis of the target lesion by angiography or as ischemia in the target vessel distribution by radionuclide perfusion scan. Before the patients underwent angioplasty, blood was obtained by venipuncture for measurement of lipoprotein(a), total cholesterol, thrombin-antithrombin complex, α_2-antiplasmin-plasmin complex, and plasminogen activator inhibitor-1. Evaluable outcome data were obtained on 162 patients who formed a basis of the report. Restenosis occurred in 61 patients (38%). The lipoprotein(a) level was not correlated significantly with thrombin-antithrombin complex, α_2-antiplasmin/plasmin, plasminogen activator inhibitor-1 or the thrombin-antithrombin-α_2-antiplasmin/plasmin ratio. Levels of these blood measurements were not statistically different in patients with versus those without restenosis. The median ratio of thrombin-antithrombin to α_2-antiplasmin/plasmin was 2-fold higher in the restenosis group, and this difference approached statistical significance (p = 0.07). Univariate analysis was performed for the association of clinical, lesion-related, and procedural risk factors with restenosis. Lipoprotein(a) levels did not differ significantly in the restenosis versus no restenosis group, whether assessed categorically or as a continuous variable by the Mann-Whitney U test. The number of lesions dilated and the lack of family history of premature heart disease were significantly associated with restenosis. A history of diabetes mellitus was of borderline significance. By multiple logistic regression analysis, the number of lesions dilated was the only variable significantly associated with restenosis. The investigators conclude that the number of lesions dilated during PTCA is a significant risk factor for restenosis, whereas the serum lipoprotein(a) level was not a significant risk factor for restenosis in the patient population. The thrombin-antithrombin to α_2-antiplasmin/plasmin ratio appears to merit further study as a possible risk factor for restenosis.

Restenosis After Coronary Angioplasty

Randomized trials have demonstrated that planned coronary stenting may lower restenosis rate in patients with *de novo* short lesions. In a prospective study, Antoniucci and associates[224] from Florence, Italy, sought to determine the frequency of restenosis, reocclusion, and adverse cardiovascular events after coronary stenting in a series of 258 consecutive nonselected patients, including those with complex lesions not fulfilling past and ongoing randomized trial criteria for stent implantation. Criteria for stenting were as follows: (1) dissection associated with occlusion or threatened closure, (2) a residual percentage stenosis less than 30% or nonocclusive dissection, and (3) restenotic lesion or chronic total occlusion. In most cases (89%) the target lesion had 2 or more unfavorable morphologic characteristics, whereas only 11% of target lesions could be classified as type A or B 1 lesions. Overall, the 6-month restenosis rate was 23%. By use of subgroup analysis, restenosis rate was found to range widely, from 11% to 46%. With multivariate analysis, only 4 variables were found to be independently related to restenosis: age older than 63 years, female gender, lesion length longer than 12 mm, and type C lesion. Results from randomized trials on coronary stenting cannot be extrapolated to current clinical practice because most of the treated lesions do not fulfill the criteria adopted in these studies for stent implantation. The restenosis rate is nearly 4 times greater for long and complex lesions treated by multiple stent implantation as compared with simple lesions, and additional studies need to be performed to evaluate the efficacy of stenting on these lesions.

Predictors of Restenosis After Angioplasty

Previous studies have suggested that restenosis and reocclusion occur frequently in patients with acute coronary syndromes. The study by van 't Hof and associates[225] from Zqolle, The Netherlands, was undertaken to assess the incidence and predictors of restenosis in a cohort of patients who underwent successful primary coronary angioplasty for AMI. Three hundred twelve patients who underwent successful primary angioplasty of a native coronary vessel were candidates for follow-up coronary angiography. This was performed in 284 patients (92%) at the 3- or 6-month follow-up. Quantitative coronary angiography was performed and multivariate analysis was performed to determine dependent predictors of restenosis. Restenosis, defined as a diameter stenosis of greater than 50% occurred in 27% of patients at 3 months and in 37% of patients at 6-month follow-up. Reocclusion occurred in 4% and 6%, respectively. Reference diameter (vessel size) was related to restenosis. Age and lumen diameter immediately after angioplasty were independent predictors of restenosis. Young patients (<50 years) and patients with a minimal luminal diameter of more than 2.5 mm had restenosis rates of less than 25%. The radionuclide EF was 46% in patients with restenosis compared with 47% in patients without restenosis. The incidence of restenosis after successful primary coronary angioplasty for AMI is comparable to the reported incidence after elective coronary angioplasty for stable angina. Restenosis is related to age and the lumen diameter after angioplasty and does not affect LV function in this population.

Evaluation the Success of Coronary Angioplasty

Historically, restenosis after coronary angioplasty has been assessed angiographically at about 6 months. The desirability of avoiding routine follow-up angiography, as well as the recognition that angiographic and clinical assessments are not necessarily the same, has prompted greater interest in following patients clinically after angioplasty. Clinical restenosis has been defined as the composite of death, AMI, CABG, or additional angioplasty within 6 months of the index procedure. Weintraub and colleagues[226] in Atlanta, Georgia, observed clinical restenosis in 2,340 of 11,473 patients (20.4%). The mortality at 6 months was 1%. Although there was somewhat more AMI and CABG, the most frequent event was additional angioplasty. Angiographic restenosis was noted in 30% of patients without clinical restenosis and in 87% of patients with clinical restenosis. Patients with clinical restenosis were less likely to be women, had more systemic hypertension, diabetes mellitus, more severe angina originally, fewer prior myocardial infarctions, more multivessel and LAD CAD, more multisite procedures, more branch site procedures, and longer and tighter stenoses both before and after the procedure. The year of the procedure did not correlate with restenosis. Clinical restenosis is less common than angiographic restenosis and the most common event is additional angioplasty. Although clinical restenosis is rarely fatal, it does result in inconvenience and additional resource consumption (Figures 2-73, 2-74; Table 2-24).

Use of Endovascular β-Radiation to Reduce Restenosis

King and colleagues[227] in Atlanta, Georgia, evaluated the feasibility of the delivery of 12, 14, or 16 Gy at 2 mm after PTCA of stenoses of native coronary

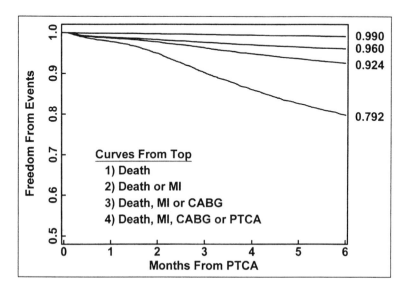

FIGURE 2-73. Kaplan-Meier curves showing the incidence of events after coronary angioplasty. The bottom composite curve represents clinical restenosis. Reproduced with permission from Weintraub et al.[226]

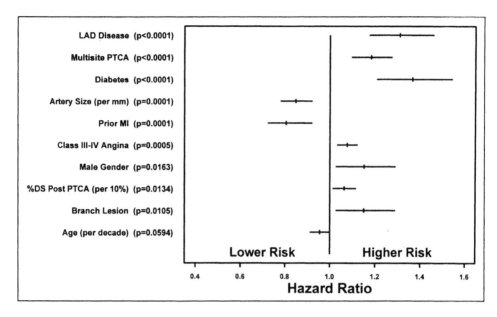

FIGURE 2-74. Multivariate correlates of clinical restenosis, with p values and hazard ratios with 95% confidence intervals. LAD = left anterior descending; MI = myocardial infarction; PTCA = percutaneous transluminal coronary angioplasty. Reproduced with permission from Weintraub et al.[226]

TABLE 2-24
Clinical and Angiographic Characteristics

	Clinical Restenosis Absent (n = 9,113)	Clinical Restenosis Present (n = 2,340)	p Value
Age (yr)	59 ± 11	59 ± 11	0.99
Women	2,548 (28%)	603 (26%)	0.04
Systemic arterial hypertension	4,035 (44%)	1,128 (48%)	0.0006
Diabetes mellitus	1,230 (14%)	434 (19%)	<0.0001
Class III to IV angina	5,579 (65%)	1,577 (71%)	<0.0001
	(n = 8,571)	(n = 2,231)	
Congestive failure	256 (3%)	72 (3%)	0.6
Prior myocardial infarction	3,252 (36%)	744 (32%)	0.0004
Multivessel coronary disease	2,704 (30%)	870 (37%)	<0.0001
Left anterior descending narrowing	5,273 (58%)	1,545 (66%)	<0.0001
Ejection fraction (%)	57 ± 11	58 ± 11	0.19
	(n = 6,537)	(n = 1,854)	

Reproduced with permission from Weintraub et al.[226]

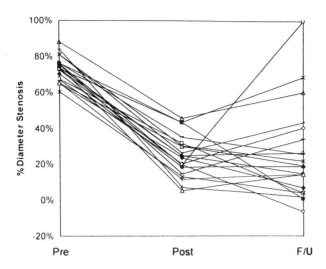

Figure 2-75. Percent diameter stenosis preangioplasty, postangioplasty, and at 6 months in patients in BERT. F/U = follow-up. Reproduced with permission from King et al.[227]

vessels. The delivery of β-radiation was attempted in 23 patients after successful PTCA. Source delivery was successful in 21 of the 23 patients (91%). There was no in-hospital or 30-day morbidity or mortality. Follow-up quantitative coronary angiography in 20 patients demonstrated a late loss of 0.05 mm, a late loss index of 4%, and a restenosis rate of 15%. The use of a β-emitter ^{90}Sr/Y significantly reduced treatment time and operator exposure compared with previous trials with the γ-emitter ^{192}Ir. Thus, in this study, the administration of endovascular β-radiation after PTCA was safe and feasible and substantially altered the postangioplasty late lumen loss, resulting in a lower than expected rate of restenosis (Figure 2-75).

Prediction of Restenosis

To determine predictive factors of the development of restenosis after PTCA, Osanai and associates[228] from Nagoya and Toyota, Japan, subjected 25 nondiabetic nonobese patients under 80 years old and 57 consecutive patients with successful direct PTCA with AMI to a 75-gm oral glucose tolerance test (OGTT) and underwent follow-up coronary angiography 4 months later. The relation between the development of restenosis (late loss index: the decrease in the absolute minimal lumen diameter at follow-up coronary angiography divided by minimal lumen diameter measured 1 day after PTCA) and the results of OGTT together with basic patient characteristics including age, body mass index, plasma levels of cholesterol, triglycerides, and HDL cholesterol were analyzed. Spearman's rank correlation analysis revealed that age, body mass index, and plasma lipids did not correlate with late loss index, but only insulin area and insulin area/glucose area significantly correlated with the development of restenosis; a stepwise multiple regression analysis revealed that the insulin area was the only independent predictor of restenosis. These results suggest that enhanced insulin secretion in response to glucose plays an important role in the development of restenosis after direct PTCA in nondiabetic patients, which may be through the direct action of insulin on smooth muscle cells of the coronary artery. This study also suggests the importance of performing OGTT for patients undergoing PTCA for the prediction of the development of restenosis.

Intravascular Ultrasound Study

Before balloon dilation, failure of compensatory enlargement and even arterial shrinkage are frequently observed at the lesion site in response to plaque accumulation. Balloon angioplasty may be regarded as artificial remodeling to enlarge the artery. The prevalence of the different types of arterial wall remodeling after applied stretch by balloon angioplasty is unknown. An intravascular ultrasound study was performed in 181 patients after coronary balloon angioplasty (n = 200 lesions) in this investigation by Pasterkamp and associates[229] from Utrecht and Amsterdam, The Netherlands. The vessel area was measured at a proximal and distal reference site and at the lesion site. Subsequently, the relative vessel area [(vessel area lesion site)/vessel area reference site) × 100] was calculated. Lesions were classified in 3 groups on the basis of their relative vessel areas: greater than or equal to 105%, less than 105% but greater than 95%, and less than or equal to 95%. A relative vessel area greater than or equal to 105%, indicating enlargement compared with the reference site, was observed in 84 (44%) lesions. A relative vessel area less than 105% but greater than 95% was observed in 43 (22%) lesions. A relative vessel area less than or equal to 95%, indicating shrinkage compared with the reference site, was observed in 66 (34%) lesions. In conclusion, after balloon angioplasty, the vessel area was found to be smaller compared with the reference site in 34% of the lesions. This small vessel area at the lesion site compared with a reference site may be a reflection of insufficient stretch by balloon angioplasty.

Accurate Measurement of Lumen Dimension

The accurate measurement of lumen dimensions is essential for guidance of interventional procedures and the assessment of acute and late results. Hoffmann and associates[230] from Washington, DC, and Dusseldorf, Germany, compared intravascular ultrasound (IVUS) with quantitative coronary angiography (QCA) in the assessment of lumen dimensions before and after intervention and follow-up. Two hundred thirty-one consecutive patients treated with Palmaz-Schatz stents and evaluated using serial (before and after intervention, and follow-up) IVUS and QCA were screened. Because IVUS cannot measure dimensions smaller than the imaging catheter, patients having an angiographic minimal lumen diameter less than the IVUS catheter (1.0 mm) during any study were excluded, leaving 71 patients in the final study group. IVUS and

QCA measurements (reference dimensions and minimal lumen diameter) and calculations (percent diameter restenosis rates) were compared. Correlation coefficients ranged from 0.641 to 0.816 for measured variables and from 0.280 to 0.680 for calculated variables. Reference lumen dimensions were consistently larger by IVUS than by QCA: 0.50 ± 0.52 mm before intervention, 0.46 ± 0.45 mm after intervention, and 0.38 ± 0.53 mm at follow-up. Minimal lumen diameters measured by IVUS were larger before intervention (0.17 ± 0.28 mm), smaller after intervention (0.17 ± 0.34), and larger at follow-up (0.14 ± 0.41). This resulted in a smaller acute gain and late loss measured by IVUS (0.33 ± 0.39 and 0.30 ± 0.47 mm, respectively, both). Although measures of restenosis (i.e., loss index and restenosis rates) were similar, the classification of lesions in individual patients (as restenotic vs. nonrestenotic) was significantly different (concordance rate = 73%). There are systematic differences between IVUS and QCA in the measurement of reference and lesion lumen dimensions. Although indexes of restenosis were similar, classification of lesions in individual patients was different.

Competence of Interventional Cardiologists

The American College of Cardiology/American Heart Association recommendations state that 75 interventions per year are required to assure competency for interventional cardiologists. Klein and colleagues[231] from Chicago, Illinois, assessed the relation between individual operator coronary interventional volume and incidence of complications at a single urban academic center over a 3-year period. Average yearly operator volume ranged from 26 to 83 cases. Each operator had performed a total of 590 coronary interventions with 10 years of coronary interventional experience. The in-hospital major complication rate overall was 1.4% for all coronary interventions including death in 3 patients, bypass surgery in 13, arrhythmia in 3, and Q-wave MI in 2. These results were comparable or better than those of 4 large standard registries. These authors note that despite individual operator volumes falling below those currently being considered for credentialing, the overall institution outcome is excellent in a diverse and complex patient population.

Relationship of Operator Outcome to Volume of Procedures

In 1993, the American College of Cardiology/American Heart Association (ACC/AHA) guidelines stated that cardiologists should perform at least 75 procedures/year to maintain competency in percutaneous coronary interventions. McGrath and associates in New England[232] collected data from 12,988 interventions performed by 31 cardiologists in 5 hospitals in New England. After adjustment for case mix, higher angiographic and clinical success rates and fewer referrals to CABG were seen as operator volume increase. There was a trend toward higher AMI rates for high-volume operators, and all groups had similar in-hospital mortality rates. These authors conclude that there is a significant relation between operator volume and outcomes in interventional cardiology. This study supports the concept that higher volume operators have a better performance record and that the previous ACC/AHA guidelines were reasonable.

Pathogenesis of Restenosis

Decreases in programmed cell death (apoptosis) may contribute to restenotic hyperplasia by prolonging the life span of intimal cells. Apoptotic events were compared by Bauriedel and coinvestigators[233] in Bonn, Germany, in restenotic versus primary lesions by using atherectomy samples from 16 restenotic and 30 primary human peripheral and coronary lesions from patients presenting with stable angina. The investigators used transmission electron microscopy to identify apoptosis, quantify its frequency, distinguish apoptosis from necrosis, and relate these events to cellular composition. Smooth muscle cell density was higher in restenotic versus primary lesions, whereas the number of macrophages was significantly reduced and the number of lymphocytes was lower, but not significantly. As the main finding, restenotic lesions contained fewer apoptotic cells compared with primary lesions, whereas no differences were found for cellular necrosis (Figure 2-76). With regard to cell type, the lower frequency of apoptotic cells observed in restenotic tissue was attributed to both smooth muscle cells and macrophages. The key finding of less apoptosis

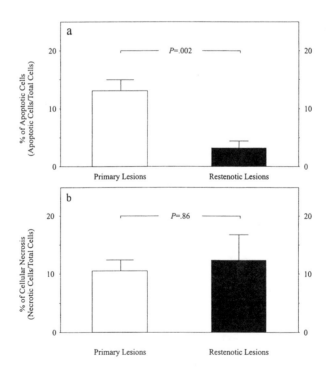

FIGURE 2-76. Frequency of smooth muscle cell/macrophage apoptosis (a) and necrosis (b) in 30 primary versus 16 restenotic lesions. All values are given as mean ± SEM. Reproduced with permission from Bauriedel et al.[233]

in restenotic versus primary lesions was in agreement with terminal deoxy-nucleotidyl transferase-mediated dUTP nick-end labeling analysis. For all lesions analyzed, significant inverse correlations were observed between the density of smooth muscle cells and the frequency of apoptotic cell death, as well as the density of smooth muscle cells and that of macrophages. No relationship was seen between the frequency of apoptosis and the density of macrophages. In conclusion, the data of the study indicate that a low level of apoptosis may be an important mechanism leading to restenotic intimal lesion development after interventional procedures.

The Evaluation of Platelet IIb/IIIa Inhibitor for Stenting (EPISTENT) Investigation

The Evaluation of Platelet IIb/IIIa Inhibitor for Stenting (EPISTENT) Investigators[234] performed a randomized, controlled trial to assess the role of platelet glycoprotein IIb/IIIa blockade for use in elective stenting at 63 hospitals in the US and Canada and in 2,399 patients with CAD and suitable coronary artery lesions. The patients were randomized to stenting plus placebo (n = 809), stenting plus abciximab, a IIb/IIIa inhibitor (n = 794), or PTCA plus abciximab (n = 796). The primary endpoint was a combination of death, AMI, or need for urgent revascularization in the first 30 days. All patients received heparin, aspirin, and standard pharmacological therapy. The primary endpoint occurred in 87 (10.8%) of 809 patients in the stent plus placebo group, 42 (5.3%) of 794 in the stent plus abciximab group (hazard ratio 0.48, p<0.001), and 55 (6.9%) of 796 in the balloon plus abciximab group (0.63, p = 0.007). The main outcomes that occurred less with abciximab were death and large AMI, 7.8% in the placebo group, 3.0% for stent plus abciximab, and 4.7% for PTCA plus abciximab. Major bleeding complications occurred in 2% of patients assigned stent plus placebo, in 1.5% assigned stent plus abciximab, and in 1.4% assigned PTCA plus abciximab. Thus, platelet glycoprotein IIb/IIIa blockade with abciximab substantially improves the safety of coronary stenting procedures. PTCA with abciximab is safer than stenting without abciximab (Figure 2-77).

The Belgium Netherlands Stent Trial (BENESTENT II)

The multicenter, randomized Belgium Netherlands Stent Trial (BENESTENT II) by Serruys and associates[235] investigated a strategy of implantation of a heparin-coated Palmaz-Schatz stent plus antiplatelet drugs compared with the use of PTCA in selected patients with stable or stabilized unstable angina, with 1 or more *de novo* lesions less than 18 mm long, in vessels of diameter 3 mm or more. There were 827 patients randomly assigned to stent implantation (414 patients) or PTCA (413 patients). The primary clinical endpoint was event-free survival at 6 months, including death, AMI, and the need for revascularization. The secondary endpoints were the restenosis rate at 6 months and the cost-effectiveness at 12 months. There was also 1-to-1 subrandomization to either clinical and angiographic follow-up or clinical follow-up alone. Analyses

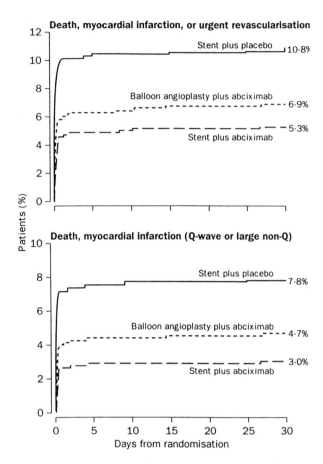

FIGURE 2-77. Cumulative event rate for endpoints for stent plus placebo versus balloon angio-plasty plus abciximab. Reproduced with permission from the EPISTENT Investigators.[234]

were by intention to treat. Four patients were excluded from analysis since no lesion was found. At 6 months, a primary clinical endpoint had occurred in 53 (12.8%) of 413 patients in the stent group and in 79 (19.3%) of 410 in the PTCA group (p = 0.013). This significant difference in clinical outcome was maintained at 12 months (Figure 2-78). In the subgroup assigned angiographic follow-up, the mean minimum lumen diameter was greater in the stent group than in the balloon angioplasty group (1.89 vs. 1.66 mm, p = 0.0002), which corresponds to restenosis rates of 16% and 13%, respectively (p = 0.0008). Thus, in the group assigned clinical follow-up alone, event-free survival at 12 months was higher in the stent group than in the PTCA group at a cost of an additional 2,085 Dutch guilders (US $1,020) per patient.

Clinical Trial of 3 Antithrombotic Drug Regimens After Stenting

Leon and associates[236] compared the efficacy and safety of 3 antithrombotic drug regimens: aspirin alone, aspirin and warfarin, and aspirin and ticlopi-

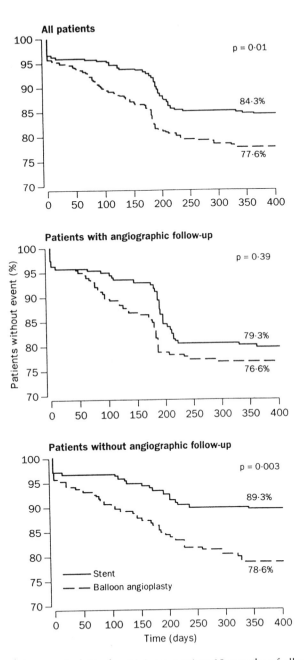

FIGURE 2-78. Event-free survival (Kaplan-Meier curves) at 12 months of all patients (n = 823) included in intention-to-treat analysis and of patients assigned clinical and angiographic follow-up or clinical follow-up alone. Reproduced with permission from Serruys et al.[235]

dine after coronary stenting. Among 1,965 patients who underwent coronary stenting at 50 centers, 1,653 (84%) met angiographic criteria for successful placement of the stent and were randomly assigned to 1 of 3 regimens: aspirin alone (557 patients), aspirin and warfarin (550 patients), or aspirin and ticlopidine (546 patients). All clinical events reflecting stent thrombosis were included in the prespecified primary endpoint: death, revascularization of the target lesion, angiographically evident thrombosis, or AMI within 30 days. The primary endpoint was observed in 38 patients: 20 (3.6%) assigned to receive aspirin alone, 15 (2.7%) assigned to receive aspirin and warfarin, and 3 (0.5%) assigned to receive aspirin and ticlopidine (p=0.001 for the comparison of all 3 groups). Hemorrhagic complications occurred in 10 patients who received aspirin alone, in 34 who received aspirin and warfarin, and in 30 who received aspirin and ticlopidine (p<0.001). The incidence of vascular surgical complications was slightly greater in the aspirin and ticlopidine group as well (p=0.02). There were no significant differences in the incidence of neutropenia or thrombocytopenia among the 3 groups. Thus, compared with aspirin alone and a combination of aspirin and warfarin, treatment with aspirin and ticlopidine results in a lower rate of stent thrombosis, although there are more hemorrhagic complications than with aspirin alone.

Clinical Outcome After Placement of 3 or More Stents in Single Lesion

Kornowski and colleagues[237] from Washington, DC, evaluated procedural success, major complications, and clinical outcomes for more than 1 year in a consecutive series of patients treated with multiple (≥3) contiguous stents in single lesions. They evaluated in-hospital and long-term clinical outcomes in 117 consecutive patients treated with more than 3 coronary stents compared with a concurrent series of patients treated with 1 or more stents (n=1,673) between January 1, 1994, and December 31, 1995. Multiple stents were implanted more often in larger vessels, in the right coronary artery or saphenous vein grafts, and for unfavorable lesion characteristics, including those larger than 20 mm, calcified, ulcerated, thrombotic, and/or flow-obstructing lesions. Overall procedural success was obtained in 97% of patients and was similar whether 1 or 2 versus 3 or more stents were used. Non-Q-wave MI was more frequent after 3 or more stents. Target lesion revascularization was 14.6% for 1 or 2 stents and 13.3% for 3 or more stents. There were no differences in death between the 2 groups, and overall cardiac event-free survival was similar during follow-up. Thus, patients treated with multiple (≥3) contiguous stents compared with 1 or 2 stents have (1) similar in-hospital procedural success and major complications, (2) a higher rate of procedural non-Q-wave MI, and (3) similar target lesion revascularization and overall major cardiac event rates during 1-year follow-up (Figure 2-79).

Multivessel Stenting

Moussa and colleagues[238] in Milan, Italy, tested the hypothesis that multivessel stenting is safe and effective in reducing the need for repeat interven-

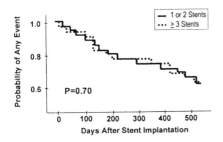

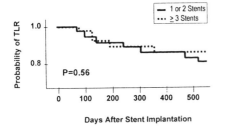

FIGURE 2-79. Actuarial event-free survival curves for any adverse event (death, Q-wave MI, PTCA, and CABG, top) or TLR (bottom) for 550 days after ≥3 vs. 1 or 2 stents. Reproduced with permission from Kornowski et al.[237]

tions, especially the need for CABG. One hundred consecutive patients with 243 lesions had multivessel coronary stenting between March 1993 and June 1995. High-pressure stent optimization was used in all patients. Procedural success was achieved in 97% of lesions. Two patients required emergent CABG. Angiographic follow-up was obtained in 89% of patients at 5 ± 2.5 months after the procedure. Angiographic restenosis occurred in 22% of the lesions, but 37% of patients had 1 or more lesions with restenosis. Clinical follow-up was obtained in all patients at 21 ± 10 months and target lesion revascularization was needed in 30 patients (30%). Repeat PTCA was required in 28 patients (28%) and CABG in 2 patients (2%). The overall survival rate was 96% with 2% noncardiac deaths. Thus, multivessel coronary artery stenting may be performed with a high success rate and a low need for emergent CABG; however, there is a correlation between the number of stented lesions per patient and the number of restenotic lesions per patient in subsequent follow-up (Figure 2-80).

Primary Angioplasty in Myocardial Infarction (PAMI) Stent Pilot Trial

Primary PTCA has been an effective technique for managing patients with AMI. There appear to be superior reperfusion rates and improved clinical outcomes with the invasive approach. In the elective setting, stents on top of PTCA have appeared to be more valuable than PTCA alone. Accordingly, Stone and colleagues[239] in a multicenter trial evaluated the safety and feasibility of primary stenting in acute myocardial infarction. Three hundred twelve consecutive patients treated with primary PTCA at 9 centers were prospectively enrolled. After PTCA, stenting was attempted in all eligible lesions. Patients with stents were treated with aspirin, ticlopidine, and a 60-hour tapering heparin

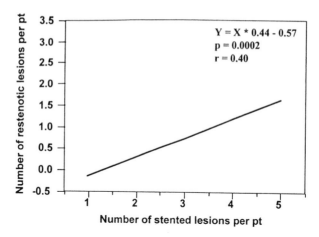

FIGURE 2-80. Simple linear regression analysis showing the correlation between the number of stented lesions (per patient) and the number of restenotic lesions (per patient). Reproduced with permission from Moussa et al.[238]

regimen. Stenting was attempted in 77% of patients and accomplished success-fully in 98%, with TIMI grade 3 flow restored in 96%. Patients with stents had low rates of in-hospital death (0.8%), reinfarction (1.7%), recurrent ischemia (3.8%), and pre-discharge target vessel revascularization for ischemia (1.3%). At 30 days' follow-up, no additional deaths or reinfarction occurred among patients with stents, and target vessel revascularization was required in only 1 additional patient (0.4%). These authors conclude in the Primary Angioplasty in Myocardial Infarction (PAMI) stent pilot trial that primary stenting is safe and feasible in the majority of patients with AMI and results in excellent short-term outcome.

Comparison of Radial Versus Femoral Access Sites

In patients undergoing catheterization with acute coronary syndromes, aggressive anticoagulation increases the risk of femoral vascular complica-tions. Mann and colleagues[240] from Raleigh, North Carolina, compared the radial approach with the femoral approach for coronary stenting in patients with acute coronary syndromes. One hundred forty two patients undergoing coronary stenting with acute coronary syndromes were prospectively random-ized to have their procedure performed from either the radial or the femoral access site. Nine of 74 patients randomized to the radial group crossed over to the femoral group. The primary success rate was the same in both groups (96%). There were no procedural myocardial infarctions or deaths and no pa-tient was referred for emergency bypass surgery. There were no access site bleeding complications in the radial group compared with 4% in the femoral group. Postprocedure length of stay was 1.4 days in the radial group versus 2.3 in the femoral group. Similarly, total hospital days were 3.0 in the radial group versus 4.5 in the femoral group. This reduced hospital stay led to a

15% reduction in total hospital charges. These authors conclude that coronary stenting from the radial approach is efficacious in patients with acute coronary syndromes. Access site bleeding complications are fewer and early ambulation results in a shorter hospital length of stay.

Impact of Intravascular Ultrasound Guided Stent Implantation

There remains uncertainty about the impact of intravascular ultrasound guided stent implantation on the subsequent course of patients who have CAD and undergo the procedure. Schiele and colleagues[241] from Besancon, Nancy, and Grenoble, France, evaluated 155 patients who were randomized into 2 groups. Group A had no further dilation and group B had additional balloon dilation until achievement of intravascular ultrasound criteria for stent expansion was reached. Overdilation was carried out in 39% of the group B patients with the intravascular ultrasound (IVUS) criteria being achieved in 80%. No significant difference was noted in the minimal lumenal diameter, but the stent lumenal cross-sectional area was significantly larger in group B (7.95 vs. 7.16). At 6 months, there was no significant difference in the restenosis rate. Thus, there was a 6.3% absolute reduction and a nonsignificant difference in minimal lumenal diameter observed in this study. Since the power of this study was only 40%, it is possible that IVUS guidance will provide improved results over standard stent placement. Since there was a significant increase in immediate and 6-month lumen size as detected by IVUS, there is the potential for benefit with this procedure. Nevertheless, the data do not yet support the routine use of IVUS post-stent placement.

Stent Implantation After Angioplasty

PTCA in chronic total occlusions is associated with a higher rate of angiographic restenosis and reocclusion than PTCA in subtotal stenoses. Preliminary reports have suggested a decreased restenosis rate after stent implantation in coronary total occlusions. Rubartelli and colleagues[242] from several centers in Italy randomly assigned 110 patients with recanalized total occlusion to Palmaz-Schatz stent implantation, followed by 1 month of anticoagulant therapy versus no other treatment. The primary endpoint was the minimal lumen diameter of the treated segment at follow-up as determined by quantitative angiography at a core laboratory. At 9 months, the minimal lumen diameter at follow-up was 1.74 mm in patients assigned to stent implantation and 0.85 mm in patients assigned to PTCA. Stent implantation was associated with a lower incidence of restenosis and reocclusion than balloon PTCA. Likewise, stent-treated patients had less recurrent ischemia and target lesion revascularization, but experienced a longer hospital stay. These authors conclude in this multicenter study that stent implantation after successful PTCA of chronic total occlusions improves the mid-term angiographic and clinical outcome and could be the preferred treatment option in selected patients with occluded vessels.

Benefit of Stenting After Angioplasty

Chronic coronary artery occlusions remain a challenge for the interventional cardiologist. In the Stenting In Chronic Coronary Occlusion (SICCO) study, Sirnes and colleagues[243] from Feiring and Oslo, Norway; and Goteborg, Sweden, randomized patients to additional stent implantation or not after successful recanalization and dilation of the chronic coronary occlusion. Six-month angiographic follow-up results showed reduction of the restenosis rate from 74% to 32%. Late clinical follow-up was obtained in all patients at an average of 33 months. Major adverse cardiac events occurred in 24% of the stent group compared with 59% in PTCA group. Target vessel revascularization was performed in 24% of the stent group and in 53% of the PTCA group. There were no events in the stent group after 8 months, whereas events continued to occur in the PTCA group. These authors conclude that stenting after opening up a chronic coronary occlusion provides considerable clinical benefit. These data add to the body of literature suggesting that stenting provides an incremental benefit over PTCA alone.

Stent Implantation in the Most Proximal Left Anterior Descending Coronary Artery

Balloon angioplasty of the proximal LAD artery is associated with a high rate of restenosis. Phillips and associates[244] from Madrid, Spain, hypothesized that the significant reduction in restenosis rates demonstrated by stent implantation in the coronary arteries in general would be especially prominent in the most proximal LAD coronary artery. They reviewed 65 consecutive patients in whom stents were placed in the most proximal LAD artery between March 1990 and July 1995 and compared them with 56 consecutive patients with angioplasty. Minimum luminal diameter was measured angiographically before, after, and 6 months after the intervention. They compared the change in minimum luminal diameter and restenosis rate between the patients with stents and the patients with angioplasty to clarify the response of this important artery to these different procedures. There was 6-month angiographic follow-up of the treated lesion in 99% of the patients. The post-procedure minimum luminal diameter, acute gain, and minimum luminal diameter at follow-up were greater in arteries treated with stents than in those treated with balloons. Of importance, late loss was not significantly different between the 2 groups after treatment at this site. Thus, the restenosis rate after angioplasty was 52% compared with 20% after stent implantation. Stent implantation in the most proximal LAD artery is associated with an even greater reduction in restenosis rate than implantations elsewhere in the coronary arteries. This enhanced reduction in restenosis appears to be due to an unusually large amount of late loss after angioplasty at this site.

Evaluation of Therapy After Coronary Stent Implantation

Antiplatelet therapy has been shown to be superior to oral anticoagulation after coronary stent implantation. Different regimens for post-interventional antiplatelet therapy have been proposed. A combination of ticlopidine and aspirin has gained the most widespread use. The relative merit of the different compounds in this combination remains unclear. There are several, partly conflicting, reports on coronary stent implantation followed by aspirin alone, but data on ticlopidine monotherapy are scarce. Elsner and associates[245] from Frankfurt, Germany, conducted a prospective trial of elective coronary stenting followed by ticlopidine monotherapy in 263 consecutive, unselected patients. One-, 2-, and 3-vessel CAD was present in 43%, 43%, and 14% of patients, respectively. The authors deployed a total of 322 stents. All patients received 250 mg of ticlopidine twice daily for up to 6 months. The clinical endpoints encountered during the hospital stay and at 5.9 ± 2.9 months, respectively, were: death (2 [0.8%] and 2 [0.8%]); AMI (5 [1.9%] and 4 [1.5%]); target vessel occlusion (2 [0.8%]); and repeat angioplasty (2 [0.8%] and 52 [19.8%]). There was 1 vascular surgery (0.4%) and 4 (1.5%) nonprocedure-related ischemic cerebrovascular events at follow-up. The authors conclude that coronary stent deployment followed by ticlopidine monotherapy is safe and effective in an unselected population. The overall clinical outcome at 6 months is good and comparable to that of patients treated with combined antiplatelet therapy. Ticlopidine monotherapy may be a safe alternative for patients with contraindications to aspirin.

Kissing Stents

Mendelsohn and associates[246] from Durham, North Carolina, and Washington DC, report the first series of simultaneously delivered stents used to treat stenosis of the aortic bifurcation. Surgical treatment of aortoiliac occlusive disease carries up to a 3% mortality rate. Percutaneous balloon techniques to treat aortic bifurcation stenosis, although safer, are still associated with up to a 9% incidence of dissection, thrombosis, or significant residual stenosis. Kissing stent insertion should decrease the incidence of these complications. Twenty patients underwent kissing stent insertion. Suitable candidates included patients with symptoms of lower limb ischemia and significant atherosclerotic lesions in both ostial common iliac arteries (n = 15) or with extremely complex single ostial iliac stenoses (n = 5). Palmaz stents were delivered simultaneously to both limbs of aortic bifurcation. Kissing stent insertion was successfully performed in all 20 patients without acute complications. Mean percent stenosis decreased from 46% ± 25% to −6.8% ± 13% in the right iliac artery, 42% ± 23% to −1.6% ± 18% in the left iliac artery, and 19% ± 17% to 2.3% ± 16% in the distal aorta. Intermittent claudication symptoms were improved in 18 (95%) of 19 patients with 12 (63%) of 19 patients becoming totally asymptomatic. The strongest predictor of clinical outcome after kissing stent insertion was the pre-procedural extent of femoropopliteal disease: 8 (89%) of 9 patients with femoropopliteal narrowing less than 75% bilaterally became completely asymptomatic at follow-up compared with only 3 (30%) of 10 patients with more severe stenoses. This study demonstrates in 20 patients that stenoses of the aortic bifurcation can be treated effectively with kissing stents with few serious adverse events.

Evaluation of Changes in Neointimal Thickness After Stenting

Asakura and colleagues[247] evaluated the changes in neointimal thickness and appearance of neointima by a series of angiographic and angioscopic observations for 3 years after stent implantation in 12 patients who received a Wiktor coronary stent. They underwent serial angiographic and angioscopic examinations beginning immediately, at 2 to 4 weeks, 3 months, 6 months, and after 3 years following stenting without repetition of PTCA. Neointimal thickness was determined by angiography as the difference between stent and luminal diameters. The angioscopic appearance of neointima over the stent was classified as transparent or nontransparent according to the visibility of the majority of the stent. Neointimal thickness increased significantly at 3 months (0.75 ± 0.32 mm) without further changes at 6 months. Thereafter, it decreased significantly over 3 years (0.51 ± 0.26 mm). The angioscopic appearance was classified as transparent in 8 patients immediately after stenting, in 6 patients at 2 to 4 weeks, in 2 patients at 3 months, in 2 patients at 6 months, and in 7 patients at 3 years. The neointima became thick and nontransparent until 6 months and then thin and transparent by 3 years. These data suggest that neointimal remodeling exists after stenting and plays an important role in the alteration of the coronary lumen after stenting.

Late Coronary Artery Stenting After Acute Myocardial Infarction

The safety and efficacy of late coronary artery stenting of the infarct-related artery after AMI have not been evaluated previously. In this report by Hsieh and associates[248] from Taiwan, Republic of China, coronary artery stenting was performed in 117 consecutive patients with AMI who were receiving a ticlopidine/aspirin regimen without coumarin. There were 97 men and 18 women, aged 58 ± 11 years. A total of 136 Palmaz-Schatz stents were successfully implanted in 130 lesions 15 ± 8 days after AMI (median 9 days) in 115 of 117 (98%) patients. The minimal luminal diameter increased from 0.66 ± 0.46 to 3.14 ± 0.53 mm, with an acute gain of 2.49 ± 0.61 mm. One patient had acute thrombosis requiring further stenting and another patient received emergency CABG. There were no subacute thromboses or other complications. During a follow-up duration of 14 ± 3 months, 2 patients developed angina pectoris and 1 died suddenly. Sixty-two patients underwent follow-up coronary angiography 195 ± 36 days after stenting. Restenosis was noted in 8 patients (13%); the minimal luminal diameter was 2.19 ± 0.73 mm, the late loss was 0.96 ± 0.65 mm, the loss index was 0.39 ± 0.28, and the net gain was 1.56 ± 0.79 mm. The angiographic LVEF increased from 47% ± 12% to 55% ± 12%. Late coronary stenting of the infarct-related artery in patients with AMI is safe and effective late reperfusion therapy, and may be beneficial to these patients.

Stent Placement in Diabetic Versus Nondiabetic Patients

It remains controversial whether diabetes is associated with an increased risk of restenosis after intracoronary stenting. Lau and associates[249] from Singapore selected 42 diabetic patients and an equal number of nondiabetic patients with follow-up angiographic restudy after single-vessel stenting, matched for 4 important stent-related and angiographic variables (stent design, reference vessel size and expanded stent diameter, coronary vessel treated, and poststent residual diameter stenosis). The 2 patient groups did not differ in their baseline lesion severity and acute luminal gain. At 5-month angiographic assessment, the observed in-stent restenosis rate was significantly higher in diabetic than in nondiabetic patients (41% vs. 17%). It was highest in diabetic patients who received stents smaller than 3.0 mm in diameter and intermediate in diabetic patients who received larger stent sizes (55% vs. 27%). The frequency of restenosis in nondiabetic patients, however, was low; it was 18% and 15% in those who received small stents and larger stents, respectively. These data suggest that diabetes predisposes to an increased risk of in-stent restenosis, particularly in small vessels.

Late Clinical Angiographic Follow-Up After Stenting

A study by Le May and associates[250] from Ottawa, Canada, sought to assess the late clinical angiographic outcomes of patients who received stents within the first week of AMI. Recent studies have demonstrated that stenting of the infarct-related artery is a useful adjunct to balloon angioplasty in patients with AMI. However, there are limited data on the late clinical and angiographic outcomes of these patients. Between January 1994 and September 1995, 32 patients underwent stenting of the infarct-related artery within 1 week of AMI: 13 within 14 hours (evolving group) and 19 between days 2 and 7 (recent AMI group). Late clinical follow-up was obtained on all survivors. Quantitative angiographic measurements were recorded on the stented segments before stenting, immediately after stenting, and on the follow-up angiograms. At 13 ± 6.4 months from the time of stenting, 3 patients died and 3 required repeat angioplasty, but no patient had reinfarction or required bypass surgery. At follow-up, 26 (81%) of 32 patients remained free of major cardiac events; of these, 24 (92%) were free of angina. Repeat angiography performed at 11 ± 7.5 months in 26 (87%) of 30 discharged patients showed that all infarct-related arteries were patent and the restenosis rate was low: 22% in the 13 patients with evolving AMI (<14 hours) and 12% in the 19 patients with recent AMI (days 2 through 7). In this study, stenting of the infarct-related artery in patients with evolving and recent AMI was associated with a favorable late clinical outcome. Patency of the infarct-related artery was well maintained, and the restenosis rate was low.

Direct Brachial Approach for Stent Implantation

Implantation of stents in selected patients improves outcome after coronary angioplasty. Newer antiplatelet regimes limit access site complications associated with stenting by the percutaneous femoral approach, but a substantial proportion of patients will require anticoagulant therapy for concomitant disease or will have peripheral vascular disease that prevents access from the leg. Nolan and associates[251] from Leeds, United Kingdom, investigated procedural success rates and outcome in consecutive patients undergoing elective stent implantation. In 73 patients who were receiving anticoagulation therapy and were stented by a direct approach to the left brachial artery, 99% of stents were successfully deployed, with a major vascular access site complication rate of 1.4%. Equipment consumption, procedural success rate, and fluoroscopy time were similar in patients stented by the direct brachial or percutaneous femoral approach. In cases where the percutaneous femoral approach is precluded or patients are anticoagulated, stent procedures can be successfully performed by the direct brachial approach with a low rate of access site complications, even when large-caliber guiding catheters are required.

Total Occlusions Versus Subtotal Occlusions

Moussa and associates[252] from New York, New York, assessed the short- and long-term outcome of patients undergoing coronary stenting for chronic total occlusions compared with a control patient population with nonocclusive stenoses. A total of 789 consecutive patients (1,043 lesions) underwent coronary stenting using a high-pressure stent optimization technique. The study population was divided into total occlusion group (94 consecutive patients [95 lesions] with chronic total occlusions) and subtotal occlusion group (695 consecutive patients [948 lesions] with nonocclusive stenoses). There was no difference in post-procedure angiographic minimum lumen diameter (3.13 ± 0.48 vs. 3.15 ± 0.57 mm) and minimum intrastent cross-sectional area by intravascular ultrasound (7.31 ± 2.06 vs. 7.64 ± 2.53 mm^2) between the total and subtotal groups, respectively. Subacute thrombosis occurred in 2 patients (2.1%) in the total group compared with 9 patients (1.3%) in the subtotal group. Angiographic restenosis occurred in 27% versus 22% and repeat angioplasty in 15% versus 13% in the total and subtotal groups, respectively. Thus, coronary stenting of chronic total occlusions after successful recanalization could be performed with a high success rate. In addition, the incidence of stent thrombosis, angiographic restenosis, and the need for target lesion revascularization is comparable to that of an unselected cohort of patients with nonocclusive stenoses.

Use of Single Long or Multiple Short Stents

Recently, long (≥20 mm) coronary stents were introduced for clinical use. They are intended as an alternative to multiple conventional stents to treat extensive dissections or suboptimal results of long lesions after balloon angioplasty. In a total of 113 such consecutive vessels in 107 patients, the flexible Freedom stent was implanted in this study by DeScheerder and associates[253] from Leuven, Belgium. In 60 of these vessels, because of anatomic constraints, multiple overlapping short (16 mm) stents were implanted. The other 53 vessels were treated with a single long (≥20 mm) stent. In the single stent group there were 4 implantation failures (8%) successfully managed by crossover to multiple overlapping short stents. During early follow-up, in-stent thrombosis was not observed, but 3 patients with a single long stent and 2 patients with multiple overlapping stents suffered myocardial infarction as a result of long-lasting myocardial ischemia during a difficult angioplasty procedure. At 6-month follow-up, 50% or more restenosis was measured in 29% and 35% of the patients with a single long stent and in those with multiple overlapping stents, respectively. Compared with the alternative treatment modality (implantation of multiple short stents), no difference between in-hospital and 6-month outcome was observed. However, implantation of a single long stent, when technically feasible, reduces catheterization time, dye volume for the patient, and radiation exposure for both patient and operator during these embarrassing angioplasty procedures.

Intracoronary Stenting and the Risk of Adverse Cardiac Events

Schühlen and colleagues[254] in Munich, Germany, analyzed the risk for procedure failure of attempted stenting and the risk for major cardiac events after success and to develop a risk stratification protocol for successful coronary artery stenting. Stenting was attempted in 2,894 procedures during a 5-year study period with a success rate of 98% among 3,815 lesions. After failure, the major adverse cardiac event rate was 42.6%. The risk for failure was higher for lesions in the left circumflex coronary artery and in venous bypass grafts and after an acute occlusion before stenting. It increased with stenosis length or grade and decreased with vessel size and growing institutional experience in stenting. After successful procedures, death occurred in 0.8%, death or AMI in 2%, and a major adverse cardiac event in 3.6%. Independent risk factors for major adverse cardiac events were older age, diabetes, AMI, unstable angina, impaired LV function, residual dissection, stent overlap, longer stented segments, and a post-procedural regimen without ticlopidine. Procedural factors were substantially stronger predictors than operator-independent variables available before procedures. The risk declined after the first 3 days following stenting. Two major factors exhibited time-dependent variations of their influence: residual dissections were the dominant risk factor within the first 3 days with a reduction after that, and no protective effect of ticlopidine could be identified after day 3 (Figure 2-81). The results of this study emphasize the importance of optimal angiographic results and the need for antiplatelet regimens with immediate onset in patients who are to undergo coronary artery stenting.

Costs of Intracoronary Stents

As stenting practice has evolved to include greater numbers of stents and adjunctive balloon catheters per case, concern has focused on the increasing costs of equipment for the delivery of stents. To evaluate temporal changes in costs of intracoronary stenting, Vaitkus and associates[255] from Burlington,

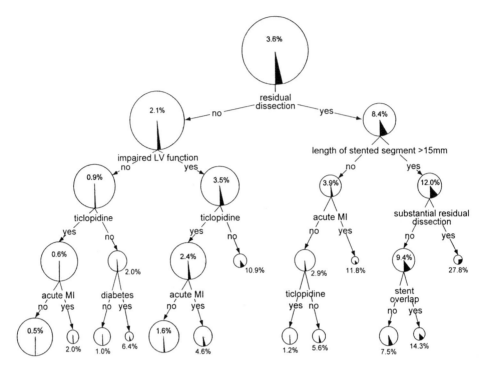

FIGURE 2-81. CART model constructed with independent risk factors for major adverse cardiac events. Knots identify subgroups of procedures with different major adverse cardiac event rates. Area of a circle indicates size of a subgroup relative to whole group (n = 2,833). Discriminating factors of knots are indicated; the group with a higher event rate is always positioned on right branch. Reproduced with permission from Schühlen et al.[254]

Virginia, examined total costs, catheterization laboratory equipment costs, equipment utilization, and nonlaboratory hospital costs for stent cases for 2 time periods: period 1 (n=46; 3 months in 1995 involving routine warfarin anticoagulation) and period 2 (n=129; 4 months during which warfarin was being abandoned). Overall costs declined from period 1 ($11,293 ± $7,672) to period 2 ($9,819 ± $3,636) (p=0.074). Catheterization laboratory equipment expenditures rose (period 1, $3,823 ± $1,394 vs. period 2, $4,278 ± $1,533), whereas noncatheterization laboratory hospital costs declined significantly (period 1, $7,281 ± $7,179 vs. period 2, $5,560 ± $3,420). The difference in costs was most notable when taking into account the deletion of warfarin anticoagulation. Costs declined by $2,428 for patients in period 2 in whom warfarin was not prescribed. It is concluded that despite the increasing costs for equipment of stent cases, overall costs of providing stents decline as warfarin anticoagulation is abandoned.

Stenting After Chronic Total Occlusions

Coronary angioplasty of chronic total occlusions has been limited by a relatively low success rate and a high average restenosis rate of 53%. Suttorp and associates[256] from Nieuwegein, The Netherlands, prospectively assessed the immediate and long-term outcome of primary stenting after performing successful recanalization of chronic total occlusions in 38 consecutive patients. Thirty-three men and 5 women (mean age 56 ± 11 years) in whom 39 total occlusions were stented with a successful stent delivery of 97% were evaluated. After stent deployment, quantitative angiography demonstrated the mean reference diameter to be 3.42 ± 0.44 mm with a mean residual stenosis of 6% ± 9%. Immediately after the stent was implanted, no major complications occurred. Patients underwent clinical and angiographic follow-up at a mean of 6 ± 1 months after stent implantation. At 6 months after stent implantation, 74% of the patients had no symptoms and remained free of death, myocardial infarction, or target lesion revascularization. Quantitative follow-up angiography was performed in 90% of the patients. The angiographic restenosis rate (>50% diameter stenosis) was 40% (14 of 35 lesions). In 8 (23%) of these lesions a reocclusion was noted. Repeat uneventful angioplasty was performed in 5 (14%) patients with symptomatic restenosis at the stent site, and 2 (5%) patients had elective CABG surgery. In conclusion, intracoronary stent implantation is a safe and effective technique in patients with chronic total coronary occlusions. The angiographic restenosis rate of 40% after stenting compares favorably with that in historical balloon angioplasty control series. However, further improvement of this technique is required to reduce the relatively high restenosis rate in patients with chronic total occlusions.

Abciximab Therapy and Unplanned Coronary Stent Deployment

In this study, Kereiakes and his colleagues[257] evaluated the effect of abciximab in patients with unplanned coronary stent deployment during an interventional procedure to determine whether this platelet glycoprotein IIb/IIIa receptor altered clinical outcomes during 6 months of follow-up. After randomization in the Evaluation of PTCA to Improve Long-Term Outcome by c7E3 GP IIb/IIIa Receptor Blockade (EPILOG) double-blind, placebo-controlled trial of abciximab therapy during percutaneous coronary interventions, 326 (12%) of 2,792 patients required unplanned coronary stent deployment. Although stented patients were not distinguished by clinical variables, they had greater coronary lesion complexity by ACC/AHA criteria and greater lesion length (>10 mm), lesion eccentricity, irregular lesion contour, and bifurcation involvement than nonstented patients. Unplanned stents were required less often in patients treated with abciximab and low-dose, weight-adjusted heparin than in patients receiving placebo and standard-dose heparin (Figure 2-82). Although adverse clinical outcomes, including target-vessel revascularization and bleeding events, were more frequent in patients requiring unplanned stent deployment, abciximab therapy reduced adverse outcomes in these patients at 30 days and 6 months to a greater extent than was observed in patients not requiring stent placement. Among the stented patients, abciximab therapy did not increase bleeding events. Thus, in patients requiring unplanned coronary stent deployment with more complex coronary lesion morphology, abciximab

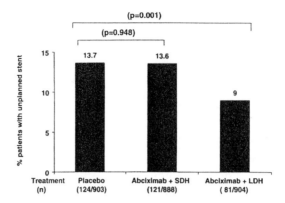

FIGURE 2-82. Incidence of unplanned stent deployment by pharmacological treatment regimen. Patients treated with abciximab and low-dose, weight-adjusted heparin were less likely to require an unplanned coronary stent. SDH = standard-dose heparin; LDH = low-dose heparin. Reproduced with permission from Kereiakes et al.[257]

therapy reduces the need for unplanned stent deployment and provides clinical benefits requiring a previously unplanned stent.

Early Lumen Loss After Treatment of In-Stent Restenosis

Shiran and colleagues[258] in Washington, DC, performed quantitative coronary angiographic and intravascular ultrasound studies in 37 patients with lesions with Palmaz-Schatz stents enrolled in a study of intracoronary radiation for in-stent restenosis. Primary treatment was at the discretion of the operator: PTCA was used in 8 patients and ablation plus adjunctive PTCA in 29 patients. Lesions were studied before intervention, immediately after primary intervention, and 42 minutes later. Quantitative coronary arteriographic measurements included minimal lumen diameter and diameter stenosis. Planar intravascular ultrasound measurements included arterial, stent, lumen and in-stent tissue areas. Stent, lumen, and in-stent tissue volumes were calculated by Simpson's rule. Compared with immediately after intervention, the delayed minimal lumen area decreased by 20% and the late lumen volume by 12%. Ten lesions had a 2.0 mm^2 or more decrease in minimum lumen area. Lumen loss resulted from increased tissue within the stent, and it correlated with lesion length and pre-intervention in-stent tissue. It was not seen angiographically. Thus, there is significant tissue reintrusion soon after catheter-based treatment of in-stent restenosis. This is greater in longer lesions and in those with larger in-stent tissue burden, and it was not reflected in the quantitative coronary arteriographic measurements.

Full Anticoagulation Versus Aspirin and Ticlopidine (FANTASTIC) Study

Bertrand and colleagues[259] in Lille, France, randomized patients to conventional anticoagulation or to treatment with antiplatelet therapy alone to determine the safety and efficacy of these forms of therapy. In 13 centers, 237 patients were randomized to anticoagulation and 249 to antiplatelet therapy. Patients randomized to anticoagulation were started on oral anticoagulant immediately after stent implantation. They received a bolus of heparin followed by continuous infusion of heparin adjusted to achieve a partial thromboplastin time 2.0 to 2.5 times control immediately after removal of sheaths and obtaining of hemostasis. The daily dose of oral anticoagulant was adjusted to achieve stable oral anticoagulation at an international normalized ratio (INR) between 2.5 and 3.0. When the target INR had been documented on 2 consecutive days, heparin was discontinued. Patients receiving antiplatelet therapy received ticlopidine 500 mg in the catheterization laboratory and they were discharged on ticlopidine 250 mg twice a day for 6 weeks and aspirin 100 to 325 mg daily for life. Stenting was elective in 58% of patients and unplanned in 42%. Stent implantation was successfully achieved in 99% of patients. A primary endpoint occurred in 33 patients (13.5%) in the antiplatelet group and in 48 patients (21%) in the anticoagulation group (p = 0.03). Major cardiac events in electively stented patients were less common in the antiplatelet-treated group than in the anticoagulation group. Hospital stay was significantly shorter in the antiplatelet group (Table 2-25). Thus, after coronary stenting, antiplatelet therapy significantly reduces the rate of bleeding and subacute stent occlusion compared with conventional anticoagulation.

Use of Abciximab After Stent Placement

Although adjunctive abciximab therapy improves outcome after coronary angioplasty or atherectomy, there are few data demonstrating its benefit for intracoronary stent implantation. Hasdai and associates[260] from Rochester, Minnesota, characterized patients receiving abciximab for stent placement and determined the impact of abciximab on outcome. Abciximab was introduced to our practice in April 1995 for percutaneous revascularization. Demographic, clinical, and angiographic variables that were independently associated with the use of abciximab for stent placement through 1996 (abciximab era) were examined. We then examined among all patients receiving stents from 1992 through 1996 (pre-abciximab and abciximab eras) whether the use of abciximab was independently associated with improved outcome (death, nonfatal Q-wave AMI, CABG, or target vessel percutaneous revascularization) in the hospital and at 30 days. The 30-day event rate was 7% for those who did or did not receive abciximab. The following characteristics were independently associated with the use of abciximab for stent placement: more than 2 stents implanted, stent in venous graft, calcific lesion, and hypertension. Among all patients receiving stents in the pre-abciximab and abciximab eras (n = 1,859), the presence of these characteristics were independently associated with worse outcome. Abciximab, however, did not improve outcome in the hospital (odds ratio = 0.96) or at 30 days (odds ratio = 0.87), even after adjusting for these characteristics. Abciximab for stent placement was used in high-risk patients but was not associated with improved outcome.

TABLE 2-25
**Major Cardiac Clinical Events: Effects of Indication for Stenting and Immediate
Angiographic Results**

	Antiplatelet Therapy, n (%)	Conventional Anticoagulation, n (%)	p
Elective stenting	(n = 123)	(n = 110)	
Death	1 (0.8)	1 (0.9)	
Acute myocardial infarction	2 (1.6)	10 (9)	
Q wave	0 (0)	4 (3.6)	
Non-Q wave	2 (1.6)	6 (5.4)	
Total cardiac-related events	3 (2.4)	11 (9.9)	0.01
Unplanned stenting	(n = 120)	(n = 120)	
Death	1 (0.8)	4 (3.3)	
Acute myocardial infarction	10 (6.9)	5 (4.1)	
Q wave	3 (2.5)	2 (1.7)	
Non-Q wave	7 (5.8)	3 (2.7)	
Total cardiac-related events	11 (8.9)	9 (8.1)	0.6
Optimal result after stenting	(n = 225)	(n = 209)	
Death	2 (0.9)	4 (1.9)	
Acute myocardial infarction	10 (4.5)	13 (6.2)	
Q wave	3 (1.3)	6 (2.9)	
Non-Q wave	7 (3.1)	7 (3.3)	
Total cardiac-related events	12 (5.3)	17 (8.1)	0.24
Suboptimal result after stenting	(n = 18)	(n = 21)	
Death	0 (0)	0 (0)	
Acute myocardial infarction	2 (11.1)	2 (9.5)	
Q wave	0 (0)	0 (0)	
Non-Q wave	2 (11.1)	2 (9.5)	
Total cardiac-related events	2 (11.1)	2 (9.5)	0.87

Optimal result after stenting: residual stenosis <30%, no residual dissection, and no evidence of thrombus. Suboptimal result after stenting (any of the following): residual stenosis >30%, presence of residual dissection, or presence of thrombus.
Reproduced with permission from Bertrand.[259]

Dependence of Restenosis Between Lesions in Multilesional Intervention

Kastrati and colleagues[261] in Munich, Germany, tested the hypothesis that there is an intrapatient dependence of restenosis between lesions in patients who undergo coronary artery stenting. Quantitative analysis was carried out on angiograms obtained before, immediately after, and at 6 months after coronary stent placement in 1,734 lesions in 1,244 patients. They used a specialized logistic regression that not only accounted for intraclass correlation, but also in the form of odds ratio as the change in risk of lesion to develop restenosis if another companion lesion had restenosis. The model was based on 23 patient- and lesion-related variables with binary restenosis with a diameter stenosis of 50% or greater as the endpoint. The overall restenosis rate was 27.5%: 24.4% for single lesions, 28.6% for double lesions, and 33.8% for 3 or more lesion interventions (Figure 2-83). After adjustment for the influence of significant clinical factors, including lipids, blood pressure, diabetes mellitus, previ-

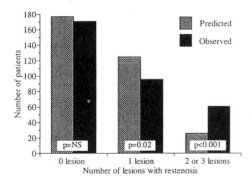

FIGURE 2-83. Assuming independence of lesions to develop restenosis, this graph compares predicted with observed incidence of restenosis for patients with intervention in 2 or 3 lesions. Prediction is based on analysis of restenosis in single-lesion interventions. This graph signifies that assumption of independence overestimates number of patients who develop restenosis at only 1 lesion but underestimates number of patients developing multiple-lesion restenosis. Reproduced with permission from Kastrati et al.[261]

ous PTCA, ostial lesions and lesions in the LAD, number of stents placed, vessel size, stenosis severity, etc., the analysis demonstrated a significant intrapatient correlation indicating that in patients with multilesion interventions, the risk of a lesion to develop restenosis is 2.5 times higher if a companion lesion has restenosis, independent of the presence or absence of analyzed patient risk factors. Thus, this study demonstrates that there is a dependence of restenosis between coronary lesions in patients who undergo a multilesional intervention.

Frequency of Adverse Clinical Events

Little is known about the frequency of adverse events in the year following stent placement in patients treated with aspirin and ticlopidine without warfarin. Berger and colleagues[262] analyzed the first study of 234 consecutive patients treated at their hospital between October 1994 and December 1995. Their mean age was 62 ± 12 years; 40% had had a prior AMI, 22% had undergone CABG, and 65% had multivessel disease. The indication for stent placement was dissection or abrupt closure in 24% of patients and suboptimal balloon angioplasty results in 14%; placement was elective in 62% of patients. Three hundred forty-five coronary segments were treated in the 234 patients; 305 stents (1.3 stents/patient) were placed. Palmaz-Schatz coronary stents (75%), Gianturco-Roubin stents (21%), and Johnson & Johnson biliary stents (4%) were used. Mean nominal stent size was 3.4 ± 0.4 mm. High-pressure inflations (≥14 atm, mean 17 ± 2) were performed in all patients. The mean residual stenosis was 3% ± 5% by visual estimate. Intravascular ultrasound was utilized to facilitate stent placement in 53% of patients. Mean follow-up was 1.6 ± 0.5 years. There were no deaths, Q-wave myocardial infarctions, coronary artery bypass operations, or repeat angioplasty procedures required during the remainder of the hospitalization or in 30 days after stent placement; stent thrombosis did not occur. Kaplan-Meier analysis of adverse events in the 6 months following the procedure revealed a mortality rate of 0.9%; the rate of AMI (Q-wave or non-Q-wave) was 1.3%. Bypass surgery was performed in 0.9% and angioplasty for in-stent restenosis was performed in 9.5% of patients. Any 1 of these events occurred in 11.7% of patients in the 6 months after the procedure. The corresponding event rates at 1 year were 1.3%, 2.2%, 3.5%, and

12.2%, respectively; any 1 of these events occurred in 16.5% of patients. In patients receiving intracoronary stents of varying designs followed by high-pressure post-deployment inflations in whom an excellent visual angiographic result is achieved, antithrombotic therapy with aspirin and ticlopidine is associated with a very low frequency of adverse cardiovascular events in the 12 months following the procedure regardless of the indication for stent placement.

Detection of Restenosis After Coronary Angioplasty

Exercise-induced ST-segment changes 3 months after angioplasty may sometimes show a false positive result. Michaelides and associates[263] from Athens, Greece, therefore analyzed the ST-segment changes observed during the exercise tests performed before and 3 months after angioplasty in 118 patients with single-vessel CAD. Ninety-two (78%) of the 118 patients had ST-segment changes in the same lead before and after angioplasty, whereas the remaining 26 (22%) patients had ST-segment changes in other leads in the post-angioplasty test when compared with the pre-angioplasty exercise test. Restenosis was found in 44 (48%) of the 92 patients with ST-segment changes in the same lead but in only 4 (15%) of the 26 patients with ST-segment changes in other leads. In conclusion, exercise-induced ST-segment changes are not reliable markers of restenosis 3 months after angioplasty. ST-segment changes observed in other leads after angioplasty compared with the pre-angioplasty exercise test may show a false positive result.

Directional Coronary Atherectomy

Tranilast

Tranilast is an antiallergic drug used widely in Japan that also inhibits the migration and proliferation of vascular smooth muscle cells. The study by Kosuga and associates[264] from Shiga, Japan, was undertaken to determine the effectiveness of tranilast on restenosis after successful directional coronary atherectomy. After the procedure, 40 patients (56 lesions, tranilast group) were treated with oral tranilast for 3 months, and 152 patients (188 lesions, control group) did not receive tranilast. Angiographic and clinical variables were compared between the 2 groups. The minimal lumen diameter was significantly larger in the tranilast group than in the control group at both 3- (2.08 vs. 1.75 mm) and 6-month follow-ups (2.04 vs. 1.70 mm). The diameter stenosis in the tranilast group was smaller than that in the control group both 3 months (28% vs. 40%) and 6 months (30% vs. 43%) after the procedure, with a lower restenosis rate (percent diameter stenosis ≥ 50) in the tranilast group at 3 months (11% vs. 26%). The number of clinical events over the 12-month period after the procedure was significantly reduced by tranilast administration. These findings suggest that the oral administration of tranilast strongly prevents re-stenosis after directional coronary atherectomy.

Balloon Versus Optimal Atherectomy Trial (BOAT) Results

Baim and colleagues[265] in Boston, Massachusetts, led the Balloon versus Optimal Atherectomy Trial to evaluate whether optimal directional coronary atherectomy provides short- and long-term benefits compared with balloon angioplasty. One thousand patients with single *de novo* native lesions were randomized to either directional coronary atherectomy or PTCA at 37 partici-pating centers. Lesion success was obtained in 99% versus 97% of patients to a final residual diameter stenosis of 15% versus 28% for the directional coronary atherectomy and PTCA, respectively. Stents were placed in 9% of the patients with PTCA. There was no increase in major complications, death, Q-wave MI, or emergent CABG, although creatine kinase MB more than 3 times normal was more common with directional coronary atherectomy (16% vs. 6%). Angio-graphic restudy in 80% of eligible patients at a median of 7 months showed a significant reduction in the prespecified primary endpoint of angiographic restenosis by directional coronary atherectomy (31% vs. 39.8%, p = 0.016) (Fig-ure 2-84). Clinical follow-up to 1 year showed nonsignificant reductions for mortality, target vessel revascularization, target site revascularization, and tar-get vessel failure. Thus, optimal directional coronary atherectomy provides significantly greater short-term success, lower residual stenosis, and lower an-giographic restenosis than conventional PTCA.

Stenting After Directional Atherectomy

Moussa and colleagues[266] in Milan, Italy, tested the hypothesis that plaque removal with directional atherectomy before stent implantation may lower the intensity of late neointimal hyperplasia, reducing the incidence of in-stent restenosis. Seventy-one patients with 90 lesions underwent directional atherec-tomy before coronary stenting. Intravascular ultrasound-guided stenting was performed in 73 lesions (81%). Clinical success was achieved in 96% of patients. Procedural complications included emergency CABG in 1 patient who died 2 weeks later, Q-wave AMI in 2 patients, and non-Q-wave AMI in 8 patients. None of the patients had stent thrombosis at follow-up. Angiographic follow-up was performed in 89% of eligible patients at 5.7 months. Loss index was 0.33, and angiographic restenosis was 11%. Clinical follow-up was performed in all patients at 18 ± 3 months. Target lesion revascularization was 7%. Thus, directional atherectomy followed by coronary stenting can be performed with good clinical success. The data obtained in this study suggest a possible reduc-tion in angiographic restenosis and a significant reduction in the need for repeated coronary interventions. The authors recommend a randomized clini-cal trial to evaluate the validity of this approach.

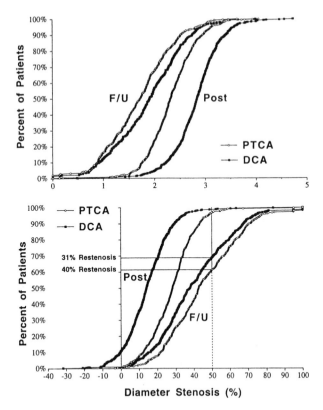

FIGURE 2-84. Acute and follow-up angiographic results. **Top:** Cumulative distribution of minimal lumen diameter (MLD) immediately after the procedure (Post) and at angiographic follow-up (F/U). Despite greater absolute late loss, the F/U MLD for DCA patients remained larger as a result of the significantly greater acute post-procedural lumen diameter. **Bottom:** Cumulative distribution of percent diameter stenosis immediately after the procedure and at angiographic F/U. F/U diameter stenosis remains lower for direct coronary atherectomy patients, with significantly lower (31.4% vs. 39.8%; p = 0.016) binary angiographic restenosis (defined as F/U diameter stenosis >50%). Reproduced with permission from Baim et al.[265]

Percutaneous Transluminal Coronary Angioplasty/Atherectomy Stenting/Thrombolysis/Coronary Artery Bypass Grafting

The Randomised Interventional Trial of Angina (RITA 1) Results

PTCA and CABG are both effective strategies for patients with CAD. Henderson and colleagues[267] from Nottingham, United Kingdom, report comparative long-term clinical and health service cost findings for these interventions in the first Randomised Interventional Trial of Angina (RITA 1) trial. One thousand eleven patients with CAD (45% single vessel, 55% multivessel) were randomly assigned into initial treatment strategies of PTCA or CABG. Information on clinical events, subsequent intervention, symptomatic status, exercise testing, and use of health care resources was available for a median of 6.5 years of follow-up. The predefined primary endpoint of death or nonfatal AMI occurred in 87 (17%) PTCA-treated patients and in 80 (16%) CABG-treated patients (p=NS). There was no significant treatment difference in deaths alone. In both groups, the risk of cardiac death or AMI was more than 5 times higher in the first year than in subsequent years of follow-up. Twenty-six of the patients assigned to PTCA subsequently had CABG and a further 19% required nonrandomized PTCA. Most of these reinterventions occurred within 1 year of randomization and from 3 years onward, the reintervention rate averaged 4%/year. In the CABG group, the reintervention rate averaged 2%/year. The prevalence of angina was consistently higher in the PTCA group with an absolute average 10% excess compared with the CABG group (p<0.001). Total health service costs over 5 years showed no significant difference between initial strategies of PTCA and CABG. Thus, initial strategies of PTCA and CABG led to similar long-term results in terms of survival and avoidance of AMI and to similar long-term health care costs.

Results from a Multicenter Registry Analysis

Ellis and colleagues[268] in Cleveland, Ohio, assessed the results of PTCA and unprotected left main coronary artery stenoses from a wide variety of experienced interventional centers. They requested data on consecutive patients treated after January 1, 1994, from 25 centers. One hundred seven patients were identified who were treated either electively (n=91) or for AMI (n=16). Among patients treated electively, 25% were considered inoperable and 27% were considered at high risk for CABG. Primary treatment included stents in 50% of the patients, directional atherectomy in 24%, and PTCA alone in 20%. Follow-up was 98.8% complete at 15 ± 8 months. The results varied considerably, depending on presentation and treatment. For patients with AMI, technical success was achieved in 75% and survival to hospital discharge was 31%. For elective patients, technical success was achieved in 98.9% and in-hospital survival was strongly correlated with LVEF. Longer-term events, including death, AMI, or CABG-free survival was correlated with LVEF and was inversely related to presentation with progressive or rest angina (Figure 2-85). Surgical candidates with LVEFs of 40% or higher had an in-hospital survival of 98% and a 9-month event-free interval of 86% ± 5%, whereas patients with LVEFs of less than 40% had 67% and 22% ± 12% in-hospital and 9-month event-free survivals, respectively. Nine hospital survivors (10.6%) experienced death within 6 months of hospital discharge. Thus, while the results for selected patients appear promising, until early post-hospital discharge cardiac death can be better understood and minimized, percutaneous revascularization of unprotected left main stenosis should not be considered an alternative to CABG for most patients. When percutaneous revascularization of unprotected left main coronary artery stenoses are required, directional atherectomy and stenting appear to be preferred techniques, and follow-up angioplasty 6 to 8 weeks after treatment is probably advisable.

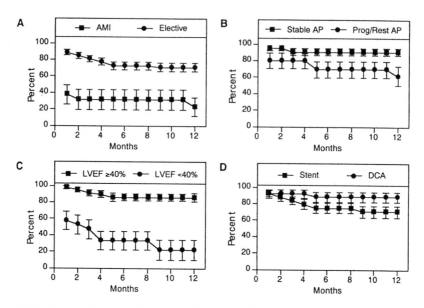

FIGURE 2-85. Kaplan-Meier survival curves for selected patient subsets. **(A)** Patients presenting with acute myocardial infarction (AMI) or noninfarct (elective) patients. **(B)** Patients with stable angina pectoris (AP) and rest or progressive angina pectoris. **(C)** Patients with left ventricular ejection fraction (LVEF) ≥40% or <40%. **(D)** Patients treated with stent or directional coronary atherectomy (DCA). Reproduced with permission from Ellis et al.[268]

Randomized Efficacy Study of Tirofiban for Outcomes and Restenosis (RESTORE)

Tirofiban is a highly selective, short-acting inhibitor of fibrinogen binding to platelet glycoprotein IIb/IIIa. The Randomized Efficacy Study of Tirofiban for Outcomes and Restenosis (RESTORE), by Gibson and associates[269] from Roxbury, Massachusetts, was a randomized, double-blind, placebo-controlled trial of tirofiban in patients undergoing PTCA or directional atherectomy within 72 hours of presentation with either unstable angina pectoris or AMI. All patients received an initial bolus followed by a 36-hour infusion of either tirofiban or placebo. At 6 months, the composite endpoint (either death from any cause, new myocardial infarction, bypass surgery for angioplasty failure, recurrent ischemia, repeat target vessel angioplasty, or stent insertion for actual or threatened abrupt closure) occurred in 27.1% of the placebo patients and in 24.1% of the tirofiban patients. This 3% absolute reduction in the incidence of the composite endpoint at 6 months was similar to that at 2 days (8.7% vs. 5.4%) and there does not appear to be any late effect of tirofiban on clinical endpoints between day 2 and 6 months. Tirofiban did not reduce the incidence of restenosis at 6 months.

The Coronary Angioplasty Versus Excisional Atherectomy Trial (CAVEAT)

The Coronary Angioplasty Versus Excisional Atherectomy (CAVEAT I) Trial tested the hypothesis that directional coronary atherectomy (DCA) was superior to PTCA for treating native primary coronary lesions amenable to either intervention. The study showed that DCA resulted in higher rates of early complications at a higher cost and with no clinical benefit. Omoigui and associates[270] from Columbia, South Carolina; Cleveland, Ohio; and Durham, North Carolina, examined the subsequent practice patterns among the investigators participating in the CAVEAT I trial. At these sites, balloon angioplasty decreased from 84% to 69%, and DCA increased from 10.8% to 14.1%. Similarly, the use of other devices increased from 5.4% to 17.5%. Stand-alone balloon use was more prevalent at nonparticipating control sites than at sites that took part in CAVEAT I. Thus, paradoxically, despite the negative findings of CAVEAT I, there was a trend toward an increase in the use of DCA and other devices at CAVEAT I sites. These investigators conclude that there was a lack of influence of trial data on clinical practice patterns 1 year after publication of the results.

Comparison of Percutaneous Transluminal Coronary Angioplasty and Coronary Artery Bypass Grafts in Diabetic Patients with Multivessel Disease

Data from the Bypass Angioplasty Revascularization Investigation (BARI) and CABRI trials have suggested that diabetic patients treated with oral hypoglycemic agents or insulin have a higher mortality with PTCA than with CABG. In a single-center study, Weintraub and associates[271] from Atlanta, Georgia, compared the outcome of PTCA and CABG in diabetic patients with multivessel CAD from an observational database. After CABG there were more in-hospital deaths (0.36% vs. 4.99%) and a trend toward more Q-wave myocardial infarctions than after PTCA. Five- and 10-year survival rates were 78% and 45% after PTCA and 76% and 48% after CABG, respectively. At 5 and 10 years, insulin-requiring patients had lower survival rates of 72% and 31% after PTCA versus 70% and 48% after CABG, respectively. Multivariate correlates of long-term mortality were older age, low LVEF, CHF, and hypertension. In the insulin-requiring subgroup of patients, the hazard ratio was 1.35 for PTCA versus CABG. These authors conclude that there is a high incidence of events in diabetic patients and raise further questions about the use of PTCA in insulin-requiring diabetic patients with multivessel disease.

Left Main Coronary Artery Disease

Left main CAD carries a high morbidity and mortality. Initial therapy with PTCA was mixed in terms of the risk/benefit ratio. Park and colleagues[272] from Seoul, Korea, and Washington, DC, examined the immediate and long-term outcomes after stenting of unprotected left main coronary artery (LMCA) stenoses in patients with normal LV function. Forty two consecutive patients with unprotected LMCA stenosis and normal LV function were treated with stents. The post-stent antithrombotic regimens were aspirin and ticlopidine; 14 patients also received warfarin. The procedural success rate was 100% with no episodes of subacute thrombosis regardless of anticoagulation regimen. At 6 months' follow-up, angiographic restenosis occurred in 22% of patients. Five patients subsequently underwent elective CABG and 2 patients were treated with rotational atherectomy plus adjunct PTCA. The only death occurred 2 days after elective CABG for treatment of in-stent restenosis. These authors conclude that stenting of unprotected LMCA stenoses may be a safe and effective alternative to CABG in carefully selected patients with normal LV function. Further studies in larger patient populations are needed to assess the late outcome.

Trial Comparing Stenting with Balloon Angioplasty in Patients with Acute Myocardial Infarction

Suryapranata and colleagues[273] from Zwolle, The Netherlands, conducted a prospective randomized trial comparing primary stenting with PTCA in patients with AMI. Patients with AMI were randomly assigned to receive either primary stenting (n=112) or PTCA (n=115). The clinical endpoints were death, recurrent AMI, subsequent CABG, or repeat PTCA of the infarct-related vessel. The overall mortality rate at 6 months was 2%. Recurrent AMI occurred in 8 patients after PTCA and in 1 after stenting. Subsequent target vessel revascularization was necessary in 19 and 4, respectively (Figure 2-86). The cardiac event-free survival rate in the stent group was higher than the PTCA group (95% vs. 80%). Thus, in selected patients with AMI, primary stenting can be applied safely and effectively, resulting in a lower incidence of recurrent AMI and a significant reduction in the need for target revascularization subsequently.

Comparison of Thrombolysis and Angioplasty

Several comparisons have been made between thrombolysis and PTCA as therapies for AMI. Tiefenbrunn and colleagues[274] from multiple centers evalu-

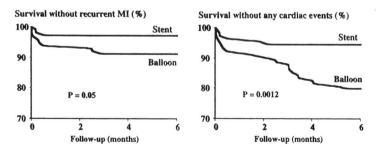

FIGURE 2-86. Kaplan-Meier cardiac event-free survival curves in both study groups during the 6-month follow-up period. The left panel represents patients without death or recurrent myocardial infarction (MI) and the right panel represents those without any cardiac events (death, recurrent MI, or subsequent target-vessel revascularization). Reproduced with permission from Suryapranata et al.[273]

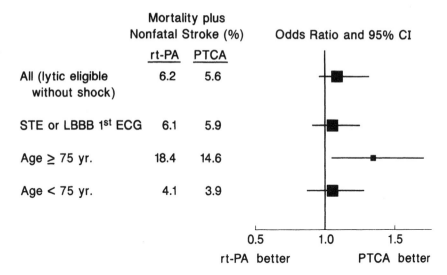

	Mortality plus Nonfatal Stroke (%)		Odds Ratio and 95% CI
	rt-PA	PTCA	
All (lytic eligible without shock)	6.2	5.6	
STE or LBBB 1st ECG	6.1	5.9	
Age ≥ 75 yr.	18.4	14.6	
Age < 75 yr.	4.1	3.9	

FIGURE 2-87. Clinical experience with PTCA and rt-PA. Reproduced with permission from Tiefenbrunn et al.[274]

ated the second National Registry of Myocardial Infarction to compare the results of these two modalities of treatment. Over a 16-month period, 4,939 nontransfer patients underwent primary PTCA within 12 hours of symptom onset and 24,705 patients received rt-PA. The median time from presentation to rt-PA in the thrombolytic group was 42 minutes; the median time to first balloon inflation in the primary PTCA group was 111 minutes. In-hospital mortality was higher in patients in shock after rt-PA than after PTCA (52% vs. 32%). In-hospital mortality was the same in lytic-eligible patients not in shock: 5.4% versus 5.2%. The stroke rate was higher after lytic therapy (1.6% vs. 0.7%) but the combined endpoint of death and nonfatal stroke was not significantly different between the 2 groups. There was no difference in the rate of reinfarction between the 2 groups (2.9% vs. 2.5%). These authors conclude that in lytic-eligible patients not in shock, PTCA and rt-PA were comparable alternative methods of reperfusion when analyzed in terms of in-hospital mortality, mortality plus nonfatal stroke, and reinfarction. These results, of course, are limited somewhat by the lack of a prospective, randomized, comparative trial (Figure 2-87).

The Bypass Angioplasty Revascularization Investigation (BARI)

Jacobs and colleagues[275] from Boston, Massachusetts, evaluated 1,829 patients with symptomatic multivessel CAD randomized to CABG or PTCA in the Bypass Angioplasty Revascularization Investigation (BARI), of whom 27% were women. Women were older, they had more CHF, hypertension, treated diabetes mellitus, and unstable angina than men, but had similar preservation of LV function and extent of multivessel CAD. Women assigned to surgery received the same number of total grafts but fewer internal mammary artery grafts and those assigned to PTCA had more intended lesions successfully dilated than men. At an average of 5.4 years' follow-up, crude mortality rates were similar in women (12.8%) and men (12%). The Cox regression model adjusting for baseline differences revealed that women had a significantly lower risk of death, but not a significantly lower risk of death plus AMI than men. Although unadjusted mortality rate suggests that women and men undergoing CABG and PTCA have a similar 5-year mortality rate, women have higher risk profiles in this study. Therefore, and contrary to previous reports, female gender is an independent predictor of improved 5-year survival after controlling for multiple risk factors.

Evaluation of Integrated Coronary Revascularization

Cohen and colleagues[276] in Pittsburgh, Pennsylvania, retrospectively reviewed the first 31 consecutive patients treated at their institution with integrated coronary revascularization, including a minimally invasive direct coronary artery bypass to the LAD through a small left anterior thoracotomy using the left internal mammary artery combined with PTCA of the other diseased vessels in patients with multivessel CAD. Postoperative angiography in 84% of patients revealed a patent anastomosis and normal flow in the graft and bypassed vessel. Thirty-eight (97%) of 39 vessels were successfully treated by PTCA. At a mean follow-up of 7 months, all patients were asymptomatic. There were 2 adverse clinical events, both related to PTCA; in 1 patient, subacute stent thrombosis due to failure of the patient to take ticlid was successfully treated with repeat PTCA and ultimately with CABG because of recurrent symptoms. In the second patient, an AMI occurred 3 months after integrated coronary revascularization with an acute occlusion of the proximal right coronary artery remote from the stent placed in the mid-right coronary artery during the initial procedure. The average length of stay in the hospital for all of the patients was 2.79 ± 1.05 days. These preliminary results with integrated coronary revascularization are encouraging and suggest further evaluation of this approach in patients with multivessel CAD.

The Stent Restenosis Study (STRESS 1)

George and colleagues[277] from Pittsburgh, Pennsylvania, presented the completed 1-year follow-up results of the original Stent Restenosis Study (STRESS 1), in which 407 patients with symptomatic CAD and new narrowings of the native coronary arteries were randomly assigned to treatment with either the Palmaz-Schatz coronary stent or conventional PTCA. They compared the safety of elective stenting to PTCA in terms of freedom from clinical events up to 1 year after treatment. Patients were enrolled and treated from January 1991 through February 1993, and follow-up data were collected and verified until July 1995. Ninety-seven percent of all patients had complete follow-up (decreased or alive with known clinical status) beyond 8 months, and 94% beyond 11 months. Anginal status between 9 to 15 months post-procedure was available for 78% of patients. At 1 year, 154 patients (75%) assigned to stent implantation and 141 (70%) to PTCA were free of all clinical events (death, AMI, or any revascularization procedure), and 162 stent patients (79%) and 149 PTCA patients (74%) were free from death, AMI, or target lesion revascularization. Symptom-driven target lesion revascularization occurred in 12% of the stent group versus 17% of the PTCA group. None of these differences in clinical events were statistically significant. Only 2 patients in the stent group and 7 in the PTCA group had a first event after 239 days, and freedom from angina at 1 year was reported in equal frequency in both groups (84%). There appear to be no late adverse effects of stent implantation. However, these results are limited by low statistical power, narrow patient selection, and the anticoagulation regimen used in the early experience with this device.

Stenting in Patients 75 Years of Age or Older

CABG is associated with increased morbidity and mortality in elderly patients. Similarly, it has been shown that PTCA is associated with a higher risk of complications in the elderly than in younger patients. Lefèvre and associates[278] from Massy, France, evaluated the 1-month outcome of patients 75 years of age or older who were included in the Stenting without Coumadin French Registry. From December 1992 to March 1995, 2,900 patients (mean age 61 ± 11 years) were included in this registry. All patients were treated with ticlopidine (250 to 500 mg/day) for 1 month from the day of PTCA, aspirin (100 to 250 mg/day) for over 6 months, and low-molecular-weight heparin (antiXa 0.5 to 1 IU/mL) for 1 month in phase III, 15 days in phase II, and 7 days in phase IV. No heparin was given in phase V. The study group included 233 patients (8.0%) 75 years of age or older (mean age 79 ± 4), 44 (18%) of whom were women. All patients underwent dilatation of a native coronary vessel. One hundred seventeen had unstable angina (50.2%), 20 had post-AMI ischemia (8.6%), and 6 had AMI (2.6%). Indications for stenting were *de novo* lesion in 63 patients (27.0%), restenosis in 38 (16.3%), suboptimal result in 48 (20.6%), nonocclusive dissection in 56 (24.0%), and occlusive dissection in 28 (12.0%), respectively. Stented coronary arteries were the LAD in 109 (46.8%), the right in 80 (34.3%), the LC in 40 (17.2%), and the LM in 4 (1.7%). Palmaz-Schatz stents were used in 228 patients (82.0%), AVE microstents in 38 (13.7%), and other stents in 12 (4.3%). More than 1 stent was used in 48 patients (17.3%). The mean diameter of the balloon used for stenting was 3.31 ± 0.38 mm and maximal inflation pressure was 12.2 ± 2.9 atm. At 1-month follow-up, vascular complications occurred in 5 patients, requiring surgery in 2 (1.3%), acute closure occurred in 1 (0.4%), subacute closure in 3 (1.3%), emergency or planned CABG in none, AMI in 4 (1.7%), stroke in 1 (0.4%), and death in 8 (3.4%). The composite endpoint of a major cardiac event was observed in 13 cases (5.6%). Coronary stenting using ticlopidine and aspirin appears to be a particularly safe approach in this high-risk subset.

Stenting Compared with Angioplasty and Stent Bailout

Mahdi and associates[279] from Boston, Massachusetts, compared the immediate and long-term outcomes of a primary coronary stenting strategy with primary balloon angioplasty with stent bailout in the treatment of patients with AMI: 147 consecutive patients underwent primary balloon angioplasty with stent bailout (n=94) or primary stenting (n=53) for AMI and were followed for 8 ± 6 and 8 ± 4 months, respectively. Immediate results, as well as in-hospital and long-term ischemic events (death, reinfarction, and repeat revascularization), were compared between both groups. Angiographic success was 91.5% in the balloon angioplasty group and 94% in the stent group. In-hospital and late follow-up combined ischemic events were 22 of 94 (23%) versus 0 of 53 (0%); less than 0.001 and 33 of 78 (42%) versus 13 of 53 (25%) for the balloon angioplasty and stent groups, respectively. At 6 months, the cumulative probability of repeat target lesion revascularization was higher in the balloon angioplasty group (47% vs. 18%) as was the probability of late target revascularization (36% vs. 18%); the cumulative event-free survival after 6 months was significantly lower in the balloon angioplasty group (44% vs. 80%). This study demonstrates that a primary stent placement strategy in patients with AMI is safe, feasible, and superior to primary balloon angioplasty with stent bailout. Primary stenting results in a larger post-procedural minimal luminal diameter, a lower early and late recurrent ischemic event rate, and a lower incidence of target lesion revascularization.

The Gianturco-Roubin in Acute Myocardial Infarction (GRAMI) Trial

Rodriguez and colleagues[280] from Spain on behalf of The Gianturco-Roubin in Acute Myocardial Infarction (GRAMI) Trial investigators randomized 104 patients presenting with AMI less than 24 hours after onset into 2 groups: group 1 (n=52) were treated with balloon angioplasty followed electively with Gianturco-Roubin II stents, and group 2 were treated with conventional balloon angioplasty alone (n=52). All lesions were suitable for stenting. Baseline clinical, demographic, and angiographic characteristics were similar in the 2 groups. Procedural success was defined as no laboratory death or emergent coronary bypass, Thrombolysis In Myocardial Infarction (TIMI) trial 2 or 3 flow after the procedure in a culprit vessel, and a residual stenosis less than 30% for coronary angioplasty and less than 20% for stent. Procedural success was 98% in group 1 versus 94.2% in group II. Thirteen patients in group II (25%) had bailout stenting during the initial procedure. Adverse in-hospital events including either death, nonelective coronary bypass, recurrent ischemia, and reinfarction occurred in 3.8% in group I versus 19.2% in group II. Repeat angiography performed routinely before hospital discharge revealed TIMI 3 flow in the infarct-related artery in 98% in group I versus 8.3% in group II. At late follow-up, event-free survival was significantly better in the stent (83%) than in the coronary angioplasty (65%) group. The procedural in-hospital and

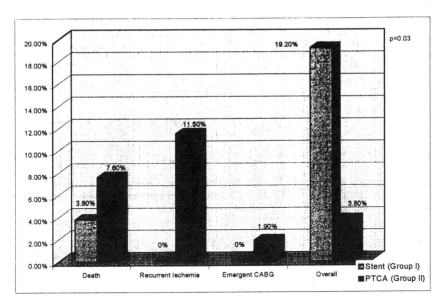

FIGURE 2-88. Hospital major complications in patients assigned to stent (group I) or percutaneous transluminal coronary angioplasty (PTCA) (group II). There were significantly fewer overall complications in group I. CABG = coronary artery bypass graft. Reproduced with permission from Rodriguez et al.[280]

late outcomes of this randomized study demonstrate that balloon angioplasty followed electively by coronary stents can be used as the primary modality for patients undergoing coronary interventions for AMI, increasing TIMI 3 flow, reducing in-hospital adverse events, and improving late outcome compared with balloon angioplasty alone (Figure 2-88, Table 2-26).

Preferred Treatment for Favorable Late Clinical Responses

Hoffmann and colleagues[281] from Washington, DC, determined the preferred treatment modality for calcified narrowings in large (>3mm) coronary arteries, resulting in the largest luminal dimensions and the most favorable late clinical responses. Three hundred six narrowings in 306 patients (223 men, mean age 66 ± 11 years) were treated with either rotational atherectomy plus adjunct balloon angioplasty (n = 147), Palmaz-Schatz stents (n = 103), or a combination of rotational atherectomy plus adjunct Palmaz-Schatz stents (n = 56). The procedural success rate was 98.0% to 98.6% for each treatment modality. Minimal lumen diameter (MLD) before therapy was similar for all therapies. Final MLD after combination of rotational atherectomy plus Palmaz-Schatz stents was larger than after stent therapy or rotational atherectomy plus balloon angioplasty (3.21 ± 0.49 mm, 2.88 ± 0.51 mm, and 2.29 ± 0.55 mm, respectively). Correspondingly, final percent diameter stenosis was lowest after the combination of rotational atherectomy plus stent therapy, and significantly higher for stents or rotational atherectomy plus balloon angioplasty (4.2 ±

TABLE 2-26
In-Hospital Outcome of Patients in the Stent and Angioplasty-Only Groups

	Stent (n = 52)	Angioplasty Only (n = 52)	p Value
Death*	2 (3.8)	4 (7.6)	NS
Recurrent ischemia	0	6 (11.5)	0.049
Reinfarction	0	4 (7.6)	NS
Any clinical event	2 (3.8)	10 (19.2)	0.03
Repeat PTCA	0	3 (5.7)	NS
Emergent CABG*	0	1 (1.9)	NS
Elective CABG	1 (1.9)	1 (1.9)	NS
Major bleeding			
Intracranial hemorrhage	0	0	
Vascular repair	1 (1.9)	1 (1.9)	NS
Renal failure	2 (3.8)	3 (5.7)	NS
TIMI 3 at discharge	51 (98)	40/48 (83)	<0.03
Length of hospitalization (d)	6.2 ± 2	5.6 ± 6	NS

* Including procedural complications.
All results are expressed as number (%).
CABG = coronary artery bypass graft; PTCA = percutaneous transluminal coronary angioplasty.
Reproduced with permission from Rodriguez et al.[280]

15.3%, 14.1 ± 13.3%, and 26.7% ± 16.9%, respectively). Event-free survival at 9 months was higher for patients treated with the combination of rotational atherectomy plus stents than either stent therapy or rotational atherectomy alone (85%, 77%, and 67%, respectively). The only significant independent predictor of an event during the 9-month follow-up period was the MLD after intervention. The authors conclude that pre-atheroablation using rotational atherectomy, followed by adjunct stent placement for calcified lesions in large arteries, is associated with infrequent complications, the largest acute angiographic results, and the most favorable late clinical event rates.

Inhibition of Platelet Glycoprotein IIb/IIIa Receptor in Patients with Coronary Heart Disease and Acute Coronary Syndrome

Pharmacodynamic Profile of Short-Term Abciximab Treatment

Mascelli and colleagues[282] in Malvern, Pennsylvania, determined the pharmacodynamic profile and platelet-bound life span of the monoclonal antibody directed against the platelet glycoprotein IIb/IIIa receptor, abciximab, in 41 individuals who were randomized to receive a 0.25-mg/kg bolus and a 12-hour infusion of either 10 μg/min or 0.125 μg/kg/min of the antiplatelet agent. The amount and distribution of platelet-bound abciximab were monitored by flow cytometry. The Evaluation of 7E3 in Preventing Ischemic Complications and

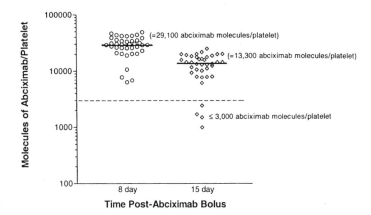

FIGURE 2-89. Abciximab molecules per platelet for individual subjects at 8 and 15 days after treatment. Values were extrapolated from fluorescence calibration curve. Line and value to right of data points represent corresponding median values for test population. Reproduced with permission from Mascelli et al.[282]

Evaluation of PTCA to Improve Long-Term Outcome by c7E3 GP IIb/IIIa Receptor Blockade (EPILOG) (EPIC) infusion regimens as described above, respectively, exhibited equivalent blockade of both GP IIb/IIIa receptors and platelet aggregation throughout the duration of treatment. Flow cytometry revealed a single, highly fluorescent platelet population during treatment, consistent with complete saturation and homogeneous distribution of abciximab on circulating platelets. For 15 days after treatment, the fluorescence histograms remained unimodal with gradually diminishing fluorescence intensity, indicating decreasing levels of platelet-bound abciximab. At 8 and 15 days, which exceeds the normal circulating life span of platelets, median relative fluorescence intensity corresponded to a level of GP IIb/IIIa receptor blockade of 29%. These data are consistent with a continuous re-equilibration of abciximab among circulating platelets and may explain the gradual recovery of platelet function and longer-term prevention of ischemic complications by abciximab after coronary intervention (Figure 2-89).

Thrombolysis in Myocardial Infarction (TIMI 12) Trial Results

Cannon and colleagues[283] in Boston, Massachusetts, used an oral, peptidomimetic, selective antagonist of the glycoprotein IIb/IIIa receptor, sibrafiban, to determine whether effective, long-term platelet inhibition may be provided by this oral inhibitor of platelet glycoprotein IIb/IIIa receptors. The Thrombolysis in Myocardial Infarction (TIMI) 12 trial was a phase II, double-blind, dose-ranging trial designed to evaluate the pharmacokinetics, pharmacodynamics, and tolerability of sibrafiban in 329 patients after acute coronary syndromes. One hundred six patients were randomized to receive 1 of 7 dosing regimens of sibrafiban, ranging from 5 mg daily to 10 mg twice daily for 28 days. In the safety cohort, 223 patients were randomized to 1 of 4 dosing regi-

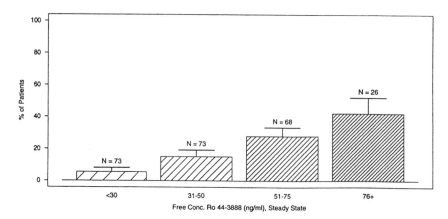

Figure 2-90. Rate of major and minor hemorrhage versus peak blood concentration of the active drug at steady state (day 28). Reproduced with permission from Cannon et al.[283]

mens of sibrafiban, ranging from 5 mg twice daily to 15 mg once daily or aspirin for 28 days. High levels of platelet inhibition were achieved with mean peak values ranging from 47% to 97% inhibition of 20 μmol/L ADP-induced platelet aggregation on day 28 with all 7 doses. Twice-daily dosing provided more sustained platelet inhibition (mean inhibition 36% to 86% on day 28), but platelet inhibition returned to baseline values by 24 hours with once-daily dosing. Major hemorrhage occurred in 1.5% of patients treated with sibrafiban and in 1.9% of patients treated with aspirin. Minor bleeding, including mucocutaneous bleeding, occurred in various sibrafiban groups, but in none of the patients treated with aspirin. Minor bleeding was related to total daily dose, once versus twice daily dosing, renal function, and presentation with unstable angina (Figure 2-90). These data suggest that the oral glycoprotein IIb/IIIa antagonist, sibrafiban, achieves effective and long-term platelet inhibition with a clear dose-response but at the expense of a relatively high incidence of minor bleeding.

Platelet Receptor Blockade Reduces Ischemic Complications

Ghaffari and associates[284] for the EPILOG Investigators determined the efficacy of abciximab, a platelet glycoprotein IIb/IIIa receptor antagonist, combined with low-dose weight-adjusted heparin, in reducing myocardial ischemic complications in patients undergoing directional atherectomy (DCA). The Evaluation of IIb/IIIa platelet receptor antagonist 7E3 in Preventing Ischemic Complications (EPIC) trial demonstrated a reduction in the incidence of non-Q-wave AMI in DCA patients who were treated with abciximab bolus and infusion plus heparin. This benefit, however, was associated with increased bleeding complications. Of the 2,792 patients who had coronary intervention in the Evaluation of PTCA to Improve Long-term Outcome by c7E3 GP IIb/IIIa receptor blockade (EPILOG) trial, 144 (5%) underwent DCA. Patients were randomly assigned to 3 treatment groups: placebo with standard-dose, weight-adjusted heparin; abciximab with low-dose weight-adjusted heparin; or abciximab with standard-dose weight-adjusted heparin. Study endpoints included 30-day and 6-month composite incidence of death, AMI, or revascularization. Compared with those undergoing PTCA, DCA patients had a higher rate of AMI (11.1% vs. 4.9%) and predominantly non-Q-wave AMI (9.7% vs. 4.4%). Abciximab was associated with a 57% lower combined rate of death, AMI, or urgent revascularization within 30 days following DCA (20% placebo vs. 8.7% abciximab with low-dose heparin) without excess risk of bleeding complications. A combined analysis of data from the EPIC and EPILOG trials demonstrates a reduction in the rate of death or AMI (19.9% vs. 8.4%) at 30 days that was sustained for up to 6 months in the abciximab-treated patients. These findings support the premise that non-Q-wave AMI in DCA patients are platelet mediated (Table 2-27; Figure 2-91).

TABLE 2-27
Procedural Features of Patients Undergoing Directional Coronary Atherectomy (DCA) or Percutaneous Transluminal Coronary Angioplasty (PTCA) in the EPILOG Trial

	DCA (n = 144)	PTCA (n = 2,483)
Treated vessel		
Vein graft	3 (2%)	99 (4%)
Left anterior descending only	81 (56%)	770 (31%)
Left circumflex only	17 (12%)	621 (25%)
Right only	30 (21%)	795 (32%)
>1 artery	13 (9%)	224 (9%)
Preprocedural diameter stenosis (mean)	90%	90%
Preprocedural TIMI grade flow		
0	2 (1%)	180 (7%)
1	2 (1%)	113 (5%)
2	11 (8%)	232 (10%)
3	128 (90%)	1,903 (78%)
ACC/AHA lesion morphology		
A–B1	29 (20%)	722 (29%)
B2	105 (73%)	1,333 (54%)
C	10 (7%)	428 (17%)
Ostial lesion	31 (22%)	219 (9%)
Eccentric lesion	123 (85%)	1,613 (65%)
Median duration of procedure (min)	44	27
Postprocedural diameter stenosis (mean)	10%	20%
Dissection		
None	114 (79%)	1,690 (68%)
Minor	22 (15%)	599 (24%)
Major	8 (6%)	193 (8%)
Bailout stent	9 (6%)	323 (13%)
Thrombus	8 (6%)	164 (7%)
Distal embolization	5 (4%)	34 (1%)

Data presented are number (%) of patients.
ACC/AHA = American College of Cardiology/American Heart Association.
Reproduced with permission from Ghaffari et al.[284]

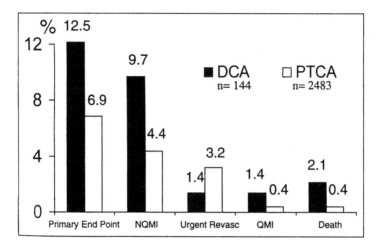

FIGURE 2-91. Thirty-day outcomes in the DCA and PTCA groups in the EPILOG trial. NQMI = non-Q-wave myocardial infarction; QMI = Q-wave myocardial infarction; Revasc = revascularization. Reproduced with permission from Ghaffari et al.[284]

Coronary Artery Bypass Grafting

Mortality in Elderly Patients Undergoing Coronary Artery Bypass Grafting

Ivanov and colleagues[285] examined trends in risk severity and operative mortality in 3,330 consecutive patients aged 70 years and older who underwent isolated CABG between 1982 and 1996. The proportion of elderly patients increased significantly over time. Operative mortality rates among the elderly was 7.2% in 1982 to 1986, fell to 4.4% in 1987 to 1991, but did not improve from 1986 to 1996. Logistic regression analysis of operative mortality was used to construct relative risk group, the prevalence of high-risk elderly patients rose over time from 16% in 1982 to 1986 to 19.5% in 1987 to 1991 and 26.9% in 1992 to 1996. Operative mortality in high-risk patients fell significantly from 17% in 1982 to 1986 to 9% in 1987 to 1991 and 8.9% in 1992 to 1996. Independent predictors of operative mortality among elderly patients were poor LV function, previous CABG, female gender, peripheral vascular disease, and diabetes. Prior angioplasty was protective. These data suggest that operative mortality in the elderly patients has declined significantly in recent years despite an increase in the prevalence and severity of the risk factors. The authors suggest that advanced age alone should not determine who is offered CABG. However, poor ventricular function and prior CABG have the greatest impact on operative mortality in elderly patients.

Evaluation of Early Discharge after Coronary Artery Bypass Grafting

Medical plans are encouraging earlier discharge of patients who have had CABG. Cowper and colleagues[286] from Durham, North Carolina, examined the prevalence of early discharge among 83,347 non-HMO Medicare patients who underwent CABG in the US in 1992. Six percent of Medicare patients undergoing CABG were discharged within 5 days of the operation. The prevalence of early discharge varied considerably among states, ranging from 1% to 21%. Patients discharged early tended to be younger and male, and have fewer co-morbid illnesses. Risk-adjusted rates of death and cardiovascular readmission was lowest among patients discharged early. These authors conclude that as of 1992, early discharge of elderly patients treated with CABG in non-HMO settings was not associated with higher 60-day rates of death or readmission. This suggests that physicians are able to identify low-risk candidates for early discharge. Variation across the nation in early discharge rates along with the percentage of patients without major risk factors or adverse outcomes, suggests that higher rates of early discharge might be safely achieved.

Veterans Affairs Cooperative Study of Coronary Artery Bypass Surgery

Peduzzi and associates[287] for The Veterans Affairs Coronary Artery Bypass Study Cooperative Study Group evaluated the 22-year results of initial CABG with saphenous vein grafts compared with initial medical therapy on survival, incidence of AMI, reoperation, and symptomatic status in 686 patients (average 51 years) with stable angina in the VA Cooperative Study of Coronary Artery Bypass Surgery. Between 1972 and 1974, 354 patients were assigned to medical treatment and 332 to surgical revascularization. In the surgical cohort, 312 patients underwent operation (operative mortality 5.8%) and 25% subsequently underwent repeat operation (operative mortality 10.3%). In the medical cohort, 160 patients crossed over to surgery (operative mortality 4.4%) and 21% of these patients had reoperation (operative mortality 9.1%). Neither crossover nor reoperation was predictable by angiographic or clinical risk factors measured at baseline. The overall 22-year cumulative survival rates were 25% and 20% in the medical and surgical cohorts. Corresponding rates in low-risk patients who had 1 or 2 diseased vessels, or 3 diseased vessels with normal LVF were 31% and 24%. Although significant at 10 years, there was also no long-term survival benefit for high-risk patients assigned to bypass surgery. The probabilities of remaining free of AMI and of being alive without infarction were significantly higher with initial medical therapy: 57% versus 41% and 18% versus 11%, respectively. This trial provides strong evidence that initial bypass surgery did not improve survival for low-risk patients and that it did not reduce the overall risk of AMI. Although there was an early survival benefit with surgery in high-risk patients (up to a decade), long-term survival rates became comparable in both treatment groups. In total, there were twice as many bypass procedures performed in the group assigned to surgery without any long-term survival or symptomatic benefit (Figures 2-92, 2-93, 2-94).

Prediction of Outcome After Coronary Artery Bypass Grafting

Past studies have examined the predictors of outcome in medically treated patients with CAD. There is limited information on predictors of outcome after

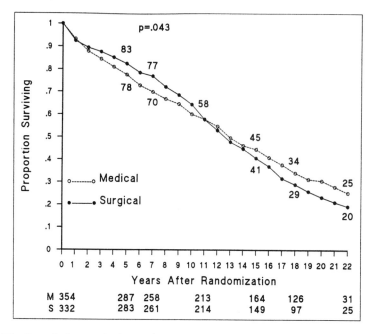

FIGURE 2-92. Cumulative survival rates by treatment assigned. Numbers of patients at risk are indicated at bottom of figure. M = medical; S = surgical. Reproduced with permission from Peduzzi et al.[287]

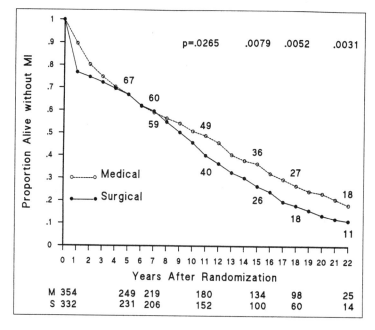

FIGURE 2-93. Cumulative probability of being alive without myocardial infarction (MI) by treatment assigned. Numbers of patients at risk are indicated at bottom of figure. Abbreviations as in Figure 92. Reproduced with permission from Peduzzi et al.[287]

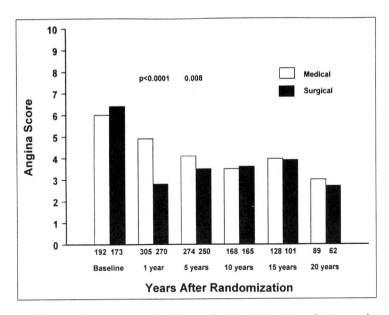

Figure 2-94. Mean angina scores at baseline and at 1, 5, 10, 15, and 20 years by treatment assigned. Numbers of patients evaluated are given at bottom of figure. Reproduced with permission from Peduzzi et al.[287]

CABG. Nallamothu and associates[288] from Philadelphia, Pennsylvania, examined the predictors of outcome of 255 patients with CAD at a mean time of 5 years after CABG for angina pectoris. The 255 patients underwent coronary angiography and stress single-photon emission computed tomography (SPECT) myocardial perfusion imaging after CABG. During a mean follow-up of 41 ± 28 months after stress testing, there were 34 hard events (24 cardiac deaths and 10 nonfatal AMIs). The hemodynamics during stress testing, and age and gender were not predictors of events. The SPECT variables of multivessel perfusion abnormality, perfusion deficit size, and increased lung thallium uptake were predictors of death and total events by uni- and multivariate survival analysis. There were 14 events in 45 patients (31%) with multivessel abnormality and increased lung thallium uptake, 14 events in 101 patients (14%) with either multivessel abnormality or increased lung uptake, and 6 events in 109 patients (6%) with neither of these 2 variables. The annual mortality and total event rates were 7.5% and 9.5% with both variables, 3.4% and 4.3% with either variable, and 0.6% and 1.7% with neither of the variables. Thus, stress SPECT perfusion imaging is useful to stratify patients after CABG into low, intermediate, and high-risk groups for future cardiac events.

Obesity and Risk of Adverse Outcomes After Bypass Surgery

Birkmeyer and colleagues[289] in Burlington, Vermont, and Portland, Maine, evaluated the impact of obesity on risk of adverse outcomes after CABG among 11,101 consecutive patients. Body mass index was used as the measure of obe-

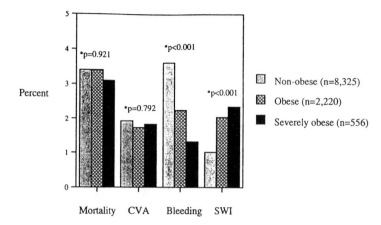

FIGURE 2-95. Incidence of in-hospital adverse outcomes (mortality, CVA), bleeding, and sternal wound infection (SWI) of CABG. $*\chi^2$ test for association. Reproduced with permission from Birkmeyer et al.[289]

sity and was categorized as nonobese in the 1st to 74th percentile, obese in the 75th to 94th percentile, or severely obese in the 95th to 100th percentile. Adverse outcomes occurring in-hospital, including mortality, intraoperative/postoperative cerebrovascular accident, postoperative bleeding, and sternal wound infection were defined prospectively. The associations between obesity and postoperative outcomes were assessed by use of logistic regression to adjust for confounding variables. In this assessment, obesity was not associated with increased mortality or postoperative cerebrovascular accident, but risks of sternal wound infection were substantially increased in the obese and severely obese patients (Figure 2-95). Rates of postoperative bleeding were lower in the obese and severely obese patients. Thus, with the exception of sternal wound infection, the perception among clinicians that obesity predisposes to various postoperative complications after CABG is not supported by these data.

Risk Assessment with Positron Emission Tomography Before Surgery

Patients with CAD and severe LV dysfunction are at higher risk for periop-erative complications associated with CABG. Therefore, the selection of pa-tients who will benefit from CABG becomes critical. Haas and colleagues[290] from Munich, Germany, sought to investigate whether determination of tissue viability by means of positron emission tomography before CABG affects clini-cal outcome with respect to both in-hospital mortality and 1-year survival rate. Seventy six patients were evaluated retrospectively who had advanced CAD and LV dysfunction (ejection fraction <.35) who were considered candidates for CABG. Thirty five patients were selected for CABG on the basis of clinical presentation and angiographic data (group A) and 34 of 41 patients were selected according to extent of viable tissue determined by PET (group B) in addition to the clinical presentation and angiographic data. There were 4 in-hospital deaths (11.4%) in group A and none in group B. After 12 months the survival rate was 79% in group A and 97% in group B. Postoperatively, group B patients had a less complicated recovery, required lower doses of catecholamines, and demonstrated a significantly decreased incidence of low output syndrome. These authors conclude that the selection of patients with impaired LV function on the basis of extent of viability is supplementary to clinical and angiographic data and may lead to postoperative recovery with a low early mortality and promising short-term survival.

Improvement of Left Ventricular Global Function

A number of different techniques have been used to predict improvement of LV global function after surgical revascularization in patients with stable CAD. Cornel and colleagues[291] from Alkmaar, Leiden, and Rotterdam, The Netherlands, and Udine, Italy, evaluated the accuracy of dobutamine echocardiography for predicting improvement after CABG. Sixty one patients with chronic ischemic LV dysfunction were prospectively selected. They underwent dobutamine echocardiography and radionuclide ventriculography, both preoperatively and at 3 months' follow-up. At 14 months, another evaluation of LV function was obtained. Of the 61 patients, LVEF improved in 12 in 3 months and in 19 at late follow-up (32 to 42). The frequency and time course of improvement of ejection fraction were similar in patients with mild and severe LV dysfunction. A biphasic response to dobutamine was predictive of recovery in 63% at 3 months and in 75% at late follow-up. The sensitivity and specificity for improvement of global function on a patient basis were 89% and 81%, respectively, at late follow-up. These authors conclude that dobutamine echocardiography may have a role in predicting improvement of global LV function after CABG.

Electrical Stimulation Versus Coronary Artery Bypass Surgery

Mannheimer and colleagues[292] determined whether spinal cord stimulation may be used as an alternative to CABG in selected patient groups, especially in patients with no proven prognostic benefit from CABG and an increased surgical risk. One hundred four patients were randomized, including 53 to spinal cord stimulation and 51 to CABG. The patients were assessed with respect to symptoms, exercise capacity, ischemic electrocardiogram changes during exercise, rate-pressure product, mortality, and cardiovascular morbidity before and 6 months after the operation. Both groups had adequate symptom relief, and there was no difference between those receiving spinal cord stimulation and CABG. The CABG group, however, had an increase in exercise capacity, less ST-segment on maximum and comparable workloads, and an increase in the rate-pressure product both at maximum and at comparable workloads compared with the spinal cord stimulation group. Eight deaths occurred during the follow-up period: 7 in the CABG group, and 1 in the spinal cord stimulation group. On an intention-to-treat basis, the mortality rate was lower in the spinal cord stimulation group. Cerebrovascular morbidity was also lower in the spinal cord stimulation group. Thus, CABG and spinal cord stimulation appear to be equivalent methods in terms of symptom relief in the patients that were studied. However, CABG has a more beneficial effect on exercise capacity and in the prevention of myocardial ischemia during exercise.

Measurement of Psychological Status Before Bypass Surgery

The inclusion of large, heterogeneous groups of patients for CABG surgery has resulted in a more mixed treatment outcome. Thus, it becomes important to identify patients who are less likely to benefit from surgery or who may require additional support to improve treatment outcome. The aim of the present study by Perski and associates[293] from Stockholm, Sweden, was to examine whether psychological status measured before CABG can contribute to prediction of short- and long-term outcomes of this surgery. One hundred seventy-one consecutive patients from 2 large university hospitals in Stockholm completed a psychosocial questionnaire before being scheduled for surgery. One year after CABG, patients again completed the questionnaire. Follow-up of medical charts was conducted during the first 3 years after surgery. All major cardiac events (cardiac death, definite myocardial infarction, revascularization, and unstable angina verified by angiography or myocardial scintigraphy) were recorded. Although the overall effect of surgery was excellent in the majority of cases, the patients exhibiting a high degree of distress (anxiety, depression, and tiredness) before surgery assessed their status as being much worse both before the operation and at the 1-year follow-up. Equally important was the fact that patients considered distressed before surgery had significantly higher rates of cardiac events (16%) in the 3-year follow-up period compared with nondistressed patients (5%). Systematic evaluation and treatment of emotional distress in the candidates for coronary revascularization may be expected to result in more optimal subjective results and a reduction in the number of serious cardiac events after surgery.

Comparison of Atherosclerosis in Native Coronary Arteries and Saphenous Vein Grafts

Coronary vein grafts develop accelerated atherosclerosis after aortocoronary bypass surgery. Previous pathologic studies have suggested that the morphologic appearance of atherosclerotic lesions in saphenous vein grafts may have subtle differences compared with those of native coronary arteries and may be more prone to disruption and thrombus formation. However, a comparative *in vivo* assessment of the angioscopic morphology differences between these 2 types of vessels has not been reported previously. Silva and associates[294] from New Orleans, Louisiana, compared the angioscopic lesion morphology of native coronary arteries and saphenous vein grafts in patients with unstable angina. Percutaneous coronary angioscopy was performed in 60 consecutive patients with unstable angina. Plaque color, texture, friability, and the presence of atherosclerotic plaque ulceration or intracoronary thrombus were noted in the culprit lesion. The culprit lesion was located in native coronary arteries in 42 (70%) patients and in a saphenous vein graft in 18 (30%) patients. There were no significant differences in age, gender, and coronary risk factors including tobacco use, hypertension, hypercholesterolemia, or diabetes mellitus between the 2 populations. There were also no significant differences between the 2 groups in terms of plaque color, surface texture, or the incidence of complex plaque morphology (plaque ulceration and intracoronary thrombosis). Loosely adherent, friable plaque, detected by angioscopy, was absent in native coronary arteries and was present in 44% of the saphenous vein grafts. The results of this angioscopic study indicate that other than a high incidence of plaque friability in vein grafts, the surface morphology of culprit lesions in unstable angina patients is similar for saphenous vein grafts and native coronary arteries.

Conduction Defects

The incidence of permanent AV conduction defects (CDs) caused by CABG varies from 5% to 43% if cold crystalloid or blood cardioplegia is used for myocardial preservation. The long-term effects of CDs on clinical outcomes are not well known. Mustonen and colleagues[295] from Kuopio, Finland, compared the outcome of 52 patients with permanent CAD-associated CDs to 47 patients without CDs after a 3-year follow-up. Recovery of CDs was found in 2 patients during the follow-up. There were no significant differences between groups in late mortality, cardiac or neurological events, or capability to work. Although exercise capacity was similar, the exercise-limiting symptom more often was chest pain or dyspnea in the CD+ group than in the CD− group. LVEFs at rest and at 50-W workload level were lower in the CD+ group. In addition, CD+ patients with left bundle branch block or cardiac pacemaker had significantly lower EFs at maximal workload level than patients without CDs. No significant differences were observed between the groups in the potential risk for ventricular arrhythmias according to signal-averaged electrocardiograms. In conclusion, the clinical outcome of patients with CDs after CABG operations is almost comparable to those without CDs during a 3-year follow-up. However, patients with CDs have lower LV systolic function and more often have chest pain or dyspnea as the exercise-limiting symptom than patients without CDs (Table 2-28).

Miscellaneous

Pain Sensitivity in Patients with Syndrome X

In patients with syndrome X, previous studies have reported an increased sensitivity to potentially painful cardiac stimuli. It is unclear, however, whether

TABLE 2-28
General Outcome Measures and Electrocardiographic Findings in Patients with (CD+ group, n=52) and without (CD− group, n=47) CABG-Associated Conduction Defects After 3-Year Follow-Up

	CD+	CD−	p Value
General Outcome Measures			
NYHA class (mean)	1.9 ± 0.8	1.6 ± 0.6	0.22
Subjective outcome of CABG	27/22/3	31/16/0	0.27
Good/satisfactory/poor	(52/42/6)	(66/34/0)	
Working status	9/1/42	11/0/36	0.49
Employed/sick leave/retired	(17/2/81)	(23/0/77)	
Medication			
β-blocker	30 (58)	37 (79)	0.03
Calcium antagonist	16 (31)	9 (19)	0.18
Digoxin	8 (15)	6 (13)	0.71
Diuretic	7 (13)	4 (9)	0.43
Electrocardiographic Findings			
Rhythm			
Sinus rhythm/atrial fibrillation	46/4/2	45/2/0	0.27
or flutter/pacemaker	(88/8/4)	(96/4/0)	
PQ interval (ms)	185 ± 29	174 ± 22	0.07
QT_c interval (ms)	435 ± 34	399 ± 23	0.01
QRS duration (ms)	150 ± 20	107 ± 13	0.001
RMS_{40} (μV)	24 ± 17	39 ± 22	0.001
LAS (ms)	42 ± 22	26 ± 11	0.001

Values are expressed as mean ±SD or number (%).
LAS = terminal vector magnitude complex <40 μV; RMS_{40} = root-mean-square voltage of the terminal 40 ms of the filtered QRS; CD = conduction defect.
Reproduced with permission from Mustonen et al.[295]

this is an increased perception of pain or a psychological response. Accordingly, Pasceri and colleagues[296] from Rome, Italy, assessed cardiac sensitivity to pain in 16 patients with syndrome X and in 15 control subjects by performing right atrial and ventricular pacing with increased stimulus intensity (1–10 mA) at a rate 5 to 10 beats higher than the patient's heart rate. False and true pacing were performed in random sequence with both patients and investigators having no knowledge of the type of stimulation being administered. No control subject had pacing-induced pain while 8 patients with syndrome X reported angina during atrial pacing and 15 during ventricular pacing. During atrial stimulation, both true and false pacing caused chest pain in a similar proportion of patients (50% vs. 63%), whereas during ventricular stimulation, true pacing caused chest pain in a higher proportion of patients (94% vs. 50%). Pain threshold and severity of pain were similar during true and false atrial pacing whereas true ventricular pacing resulted in a lower pain threshold and a higher level of pain severity than did false pacing. These authors conclude that patients with syndrome X frequently report chest pain even in the absence of cardiac stimulation. In addition to this increased tendency to complain, however, they also exhibit a selective enhancement of ventricular painful sensitivity to electrical stimulation.

Multivariate Associates of QT Dispersion

QT dispersion (QTd; Qt interval maximum minus minimum) has been shown to reflect regional variations in ventricular repolarization and is increased in patients with life-threatening ventricular arrhythmias. To determine correlates of QTd in patients who had had myocardial infarction, 207 patients (158 men, age 57 ± 11 years) with AMI who were treated with alteplase or anistreplase within 2.7 ± 0.9 hours of symptom onset were studied by Karagounis and associates[297] from Salt Lake City, Utah. Angiograms at a median of 27 hours after thrombolysis showed reperfusion (Thrombolysis in Myocardial Infarction [TIMI] flow grade ±2) in 184 (88%) patients. QT was measured in 10 ± 2 leads on discharge electrocardiograms with a computerized analysis program interfaced with a digitizer. Associations of QTd with 24 variables related to patient characteristics, AMI angiography, interventions, and radionuclide ventriculography were evaluated by univariate and multivariate regression. Univariate associations with QTd were TIMI flow grade 0/1 versus 2/3, minimal luminal diameter, LVEF at discharge, reinfarction, number of leads with ST elevation, end-systolic volume at discharge, and time to peak creatine kinase. Independent associates of QTd were TIMI flow grade 0/1 versus 2/3, reinfarction, and EF. Successful thrombolysis is associated with less QTd in patients after AMI. These results support the hypothesis that QTd after AMI depends on reperfusion status, reinfarction, and LV function. Reduction in QTd may be an additional mechanism by which the benefit of thrombolytic therapy is realized.

Heart Rate Variability During Smoking Cessation

Heart rate variability (HRV) is known to increase after smoking cessation. However, no work has been performed concerning HRV immediately after smoking cessation. Yotsukura and associates[298] from Tokyo, Japan, studied HRV before and from 1 day to 1 month after smoking cessation and also determined whether there is a relation between HRV and the withdrawal syndrome immediately after smoking cessation. They determined HRV by using a 2-channel 24-hour ambulatory electrocardiogram system before and 1, 2, 3, 7, 14, 21, and 28 days after smoking cessation in 20 healthy male volunteers who had smoked 1 or more packs/day for 2 or more years. One day after smoking cessation, heart rate decreased significantly, and all 24-hour time and frequency domain indices of HRV increased except the standard deviations of the normal R-R intervals and the 5-minute mean R-R. The magnitude of increase in these indices peaked 2 to 7 days after smoking cessation and gradually decreased thereafter. The increase in HRV persisted 1 month after smoking cessation. In the 16 subjects with signs of withdrawal syndrome and in the 4 subjects without evidence of withdrawal before and immediately and 1 month after smoking cessation, HRV increased immediately after smoking cessation and remained elevated after 1 month. HRV increases immediately after smoking cessation and gradually declines thereafter, which suggests that the effect of smoking on autonomic activity rapidly disappears immediately after smoking cessation. HRV remains unaffected by the presence or absence of the withdrawal syndrome.

Appropriateness of Blood Transfusions

Increased awareness of the risk of blood-borne infections has recently led to profound changes in the practice of transfusion medicine. These changes include among others the development of guidelines by the American College of Physicians (ACP) for transfusion. Although the incidence and predictors of vascular complications of percutaneous interventions have been well defined, there currently are no data on frequency, risk factors, and appropriateness of blood transfusions. Moscucci and associates[299] from Darlinghurst, Australia, performed a retrospective of analyses of 628 consecutive percutaneous coronary revascularization procedures. Predictors of blood transfusion were identified using multivariate logistic regression analyses. Appropriateness of transfusions was determined using modified ACP guidelines. Transfusions were administered after 8.9% of interventions (56 of 628). Multivariate analysis identified age 70 years or older, female gender, procedure duration, coronary stenting, AMI, post-procedural use of heparin and intra-aortic balloon, post-procedural use of heparin, and intra-aortic balloon pump placement as independent predictors of blood transfusions. According to the ACP guidelines, 36 of 56 patients (64%) received transfusions inappropriately. Transfusion reactions (fever) occurred in 10% of patients who received transfusions appropriately and in 5% of patients who received transfusions inappropriately.

Early Behavior of Biochemical Markers

Biochemical markers have been suggested for the noninvasive diagnosis of reperfusion early after thrombolysis. Their ability to discriminate between Thrombolysis in Myocardial Infarction (TIMI) 2 and 3 flow grades remains unknown. In 97 patients with myocardial infarction 6 hours or less, myoglobin, troponin T, creatine kinase MB and MM isoforms were measured before thrombolysis and after 90 minutes in a study by Laperche and associates[300] from Clichy and Paris, France. A 90-minute coronary angiography ascertained the patency status of the infarct-related artery in all patients according to the TIMI grade flow (group A: TIMI 0–1 (n = 35), group B: TIMI 2 (n = 17), and group C: TIMI 3 (n = 45). For each marker the absolute rate of increase and the relative increase 90 minutes after thrombolysis were studied. Both absolute values and absolute rate of increase at 90 minutes of myoglobin were higher in group B than in groups A and C. Relative increases were consistently higher in group C than in other groups with statistical significance for myoglobin in the subset of patients treated after 3 hours of symptom onset. Diagnostic indexes based on relative increases tend to discriminate between patients with TIMI 2 and 3 flow, and the best performance is obtained when the relative increase of myoglobin at 90 minutes is used in patients treated later than 3 hours after onset of symptoms.

Estimation of Infarct Size

Estimation of infarct size with serum-time activity curves of creatine kinase (or CK-MB) or α-hydroxybutyrate dehydrogenase (HBDH) is widely used in clinical trials. However, an independent variable, such as LV function has not been directly compared with creatine kinase and HBDH infarct size measurements in the same group of patients. In this study by Dissmann and associates[301] from Berlin, Germany, infarct size was calculated by the creatine kinase area under the curve (AUC) and by the cumulative release of HBDH in 90 patients with AMI undergoing early thrombolysis. Infarct size estimates by creatine kinase AUC and HBDH release were closely correlated. HBDH release was significantly better correlated to angiographically assessed EF 8 days after infarction than to creatine kinase AUC, as was maximum HBDH compared with creatine kinase maximum. In contrast to creatine kinase, maximum levels of HBDH only slightly overestimated myocardial damage in patients with early reperfusion. Data reanalyzed from the former placebo-controlled Intravenous Streptokinase in Acute Myocardial Infarction (ISAM) study revealed significant differences in favor of streptokinase for creatine kinase and CK-MB AUC and for HBDH maximum, but no difference for creatine kinase and CK-MB maximums. For comparative clinical trials, HBDH appears to be the preferable marker enzyme for estimates of infarct size and measure of reperfusion effectiveness. In clinical practice, 1 routine measure of HBDH serum activity on the second day after infarction may be a useful approximate value of infarct size.

Activated Coagulation Time

The activated coagulation time (ACT) is a rapid measurement of a patient's level of heparin anticoagulation during cardiac catheterization. Patients receiving warfarin therapy occasionally are seen at the catheterization laboratory for emergency procedures. The effects of warfarin on ACT activity have not been previously described. Chang and associates[302] from Torrance, California, compared ACT and the international normalization ratios (INR) in 77 patients receiving warfarin and in 57 patients who were not receiving an anticoagulant (controls). Both the mean ACT (131 ± 17 seconds) and the INR (2.5 ± 0.90 seconds) of the anticoagulation patients differed from the controls (ACT = 115 ± 15 seconds, INR = 1.0 ± 0.10 seconds). ACT increased linearly with INR in the warfarin group. There was no relation between ACT and INR in the control group. Patients receiving warfarin therapy will have a linear increase in ACT develop similar to patients receiving heparin therapy.

Influence of Exercise Training on Blood Viscosity

Exercise training has recently become an accepted therapeutic modality in chronic heart failure after myocardial infarction. Because the therapeutic mechanism behind it is controversial and not well understood, Reinhart and associates[303] from Chur, Switzerland, and Palo Alto, California, analyzed the influence of exercise training on blood viscosity. Twenty-five patients with chronic heart failure (EF<40%) after myocardial infarction were randomly assigned to either an 8-week intensive exercise program at a residential rehabilitation center or 8 weeks of sedentary life at home. Exercise consisted of 2 1-hour walking sessions/day and 4 intensive bicycle ergometer training sessions of 40 minutes at 70% to 80% peak exercise capacity/week. Whole blood viscosity, viscosity at standardized hematocrit at 45% (P_{45}) at high and low shear rates, and plasma viscosity were measured in a Couette-type viscometer before, during, and at the end of the study period. Exercise training, which significantly increased maximal cardiac output and oxygen uptake, did not change plasma viscosity, whole blood viscosity, and P_{45} significantly. Sedentary controls, however, had a higher whole blood viscosity and P_{45} after 8 weeks. No statistical difference was found, however, between the 2 groups. It was concluded that blood rheology remains unaffected by exercise training in patients with chronic heart failure. The improvement of blood viscosity remains an interesting therapeutic option for the symptoms of these patients, which must be achieved by methods other than exercise training.

Effect of Cocaine Use Specificity of Cardiac Markers

Hollander and associates[304] from Philadelphia, Pennsylvania; Oakland, California; Hauppauge, New York; and Toronto, Canada, evaluated whether recent cocaine use alters the specificity of creatine kinase (CK) MB CK-MB, myoglobin, and cardiac troponin I for AMI in patients who are seen in the emergency department for chest pain. Patients less than 60 years old with potential myocardial ischemia underwent a standardized history and physical examination and routine CK-MB assays every 8 to 12 hours and had study serum obtained at presentation for CK-MB, myoglobin, and cardiac troponin I immunoassays, as well as benzoylecgonine, cocaine's main metabolite. They enrolled 97 patients, 19 (20%) of whom had recently used cocaine. Patients with and without cocaine use were similar with regard to gender, race, renal and muscular disease, diabetes, family history, and hypertension and rate of AMI (12% vs. 11%). In patients without AMI, the mean myoglobin level was higher in cocaine users than in noncocaine users (179 vs. 74 ng/mL), but the mean values were similar for CK-MB (2.2 vs. 2.1 ng/mL) and for cardiac troponin I (0.02 vs. 0.02 ng/mL). The specificities of the markers in patients with and without cocaine use were as follows: cardiac troponin I, 94% versus 94%; CK-MB, 75% versus 88%; and myoglobin, 50% versus 82%, respectively. These data demonstrate that the specificity of myoglobin is altered by recent cocaine use. The specificity of CK-MB is affected less and the specificity of cardiac troponin I is not affected by recent cocaine use.

Effects of Spontaneous Respiration on Doppler Flow Patterns

The potential effects of spontaneous respiration on Doppler mitral inflow patterns in patients with abnormal LV diastolic function are poorly understood. The respiratory changes of Doppler transmitral flow velocity indexes were investigated in 20 healthy subjects and 20 patients with CAD in this study by Tsai and associates[305] from Taiwan, Republic of China. All patients had a mitral inflow pattern of abnormal LV relaxation (reversal of early/late diastolic peak flow velocity ratio). The Doppler mitral inflow signals were measured at end-expiration and end-inspiration. In both groups, the early diastolic peak flow velocity and flow velocity integral, the ratio of early/late diastolic peak flow velocity, and the ratio of early/late diastolic flow velocity integral at end-inspiration were significantly lower than those at end-expiration. However, the late diastolic peak flow velocity and flow velocity integral were not significantly different between end-inspiration and end-expiration. During inspiration, the early diastolic peak flow velocity and the ratio of early/late diastolic peak flow velocity were reduced by an average of 23% and 22%, respectively, in normal subjects and were reduced by an average of 19% and 17%, respectively, in the patient group. LV early diastolic filling can be substantially reduced by inspiration in normal subjects and in patients with abnormal LV diastolic function. The potential effects of respiratory cycle should be taken into account when assessing LV diastolic function by using Doppler echocardiography.

1. Schumacher B, Pecher P, von Specht BU, Stegmann Th: Induction of neoangiogenesis in ischemic myocardium by human growth factors: First clinical results of a new treatment of coronary heart disease. Circulation 1998 (February 24);97: 645–650.
2. Hakim AA, Petrovitch H, Burchfiel CM, Ross GW, Rodriguez BL, White LR, Yano K, Curb JD, Abbott RD: Effects of walking on mortality among nonsmoking retired men. N Engl J Med 1998 (January 8);338:94–99.
3. Caulin-Glaser T, Farrell WJ, Pfau SE, Zaret B, Bunger K, Setaro JF, Brennan JJ, Bender JR, Cleman MW, Cabin HS, Remetz MS: Modulation of circulating cellular adhesion molecules in postmenopausal women with coronary artery disease. JACC 1998 (June);31:1555–1560.
4. Klein RM, Schwartzkopff B, Strauer BE: Endothelial dysfunction of epicardial coronary arteries in immunohistochemically proven myocarditis. Am Heart J 1998 (September);136:389–397.
5. Smith FB, Lee AJ, Fowkes FGR, Price JF, Rumley A, Lowe GDO: Hemostatic factors as predictors of ischemic heart disease and stroke in the Edinburgh Artery Study. Arterioscler Thromb Vasc Biol 1997 (November);17:3321–3325.
6. Cannon RO III, Curiel RV, Prascad A, Quyyumi AA, Panza JA: Comparison of coronary endothelial dynamics with electrocardiographic and left ventricular contractile responses to stress in the absence of coronary artery disease. Am J Cardiol 1998 (September 15);82:710–714.
7. Stone PH, Chaitman BR, Forman S, Andrews TC, Bittner V, Bourassa MG, Davies RF, Deanfield JE, Frishman W, Goldberg AD, MacCallum G, Ouyang P, Pepine CJ, Pratt CM, Sharaf B, Steingart R, Knatterud GL, Sopko G, Conti CR, for the ACIP Investigators: Prognostic significance of myocardial ischemia detected by ambulatory electrocardiography, exercise treadmill testing, and electrocardiogram at rest to predict cardiac events by one year (The Asymptomatic Cardiac Ischemia Pilot [ACIP] study). Am J Cardiol 1997 (December 1);80:1395–1401.
8. Katzel LI, Fleg JL, Busby-Whitehead MJ, Sorkin JD, Becker LC, Lakatta EG, Gold-

berg AP: Exercise-induced silent myocardial ischemia in master athletes. Am J Cardiol 1998 (February 1);81:261–265.

9. Hikita H, Etsuda H, Takase B, Satomura K, Kurita A, Nakamura H: Extent of ischemic stimulus and plasma β-endorphin levels in silent myocardial ischemia. Am Heart J 1998 (May);135:813–818.

10. van Boven Ad J, Jukema JW, Haaksma J, Zwinderman AH, Crijns HJGM, Lie KI, on behalf of the REGRESS Study Group: Depressed heart rate variability is associated with events in patients with stable CAD and preserved LV function. Am Heart J 1998 (April);135:571–576.

11. Chuah S-C, Pellikka PA, Roger VL, McCully RB, Seward JB: Role of dobutamine stress echocardiography in predicting outcome in 860 patients with known or suspected coronary artery disease. Circulation 1998 (April 21);97:1474–1480.

12. Kuivenhoven JA, Jukema JW, Zwinderman AH, de Knijff P, McPherson R, Bruschke AVG, Lie KI, Kastelein JJP, for the Regression Growth Evaluation Statin Study Group: The role of a common variant of the cholesteryl ester transfer protein gene in the progression of coronary atherosclerosis. N Engl J Med 1998 (January 8);338:86–93.

13. Achenbach S, Moshage W, Ropers D, Nossen J, Daniel WG: Value of electron-beam computed tomography for the noninvasive detection of high-grade coronary-artery stenoses and occlusions. N Engl J Med 1998 (December 31);339:1964–1971.

14. Guerci AD, Spadaro LA, Goodman KJ, Lledo-Perez A, Newstein D, Lerner G, Arad Y: Comparison of electron beam computed tomography scanning and conventional risk factor assessment for the prediction of angiographic coronary artery disease. JACC 1998 (September);32:673–679.

15. Kontos MC, Jesse RL, Schmidt KL, Ornato JP, Tatum JL: Value of acute rest sestamibi perfusion imaging for evaluation of patients admitted to the emergency department with chest pain. JACC 1997 (October);30:976–982.

16. Colon PJ III, Mobarek SK, Milani RV, Lavie CJ, Cassidy MM, Murgo JP, Cheirif J: Prognostic value of stress echocardiography in the evaluation of atypical chest pain patients without known coronary artery disease. Am J Cardiol 1998 (March 1);81:545–551.

17. Lloyd-Jones DM, Camargo CA, Jr., Lapuerta P, Giugliano RP, O'Donnell CJ: Electrocardiographic and clinical predictors of acute myocardial infarction in patients with unstable angina pectoris. Am J Cardiol 1998 (May 15);81:1182–1186.

18. Hachamovitch R, Berman DS, Shaw LJ, Kiat H, Cohen I, Cabico JA, Friedman J, Diamond GA: Incremental prognostic value of myocardial perfusion single photon emission computed tomography for the prediction of cardiac death: Differential stratification for risk of cardiac death and myocardial infarction. Circulation 1998 (February 17);97:535–543.

19. Wagdy HM, Hodge D, Christian TF, Miller TD, Gibbons RJ: Prognostic value of vasodilator myocardial perfusion imaging in patients with left bundle-branch block. Circulation 1998 (April 28);97:1563–1570.

20. Schmermund A, Baumgart D, Adamzik M, Ge J, Grönemeyer D, Seibel R, Sehnert C, Görge G, Haude M, Erbel R: Comparison of electron-beam computed tomography and intracoronary ultrasound in detecting calcified and noncalcified plaques in patients with acute coronary syndromes and no or minimal to moderate angiographic coronary artery disease. Am J Cardiol 1998 (January 15);81:141–146.

21. Senior R, Khattar R, Lahiri A: Value of dobutamine stress echocardiography for the detection of multivessel coronary artery disease. Am J Cardiol 1998 (February 1);81:298–301.

22. Alfonso F, Fernandez-Ortiz A, Goicolea J, Hernandez R, Segovi Phillips P, Banuelos C, Macaya C: Angioscopic evaluation of angiographically complex coronary lesions. Am Heart J 1997 (October);134:703–711.

23. Afridi I, Main ML, Parrish DL, Kizilbash A, Levine BD, Grayburn PA: Usefulness of isometric hand grip exercise in detecting coronary artery disease during dobutamine atropine stress echocardiography in patients with either stable angina pectoris or another type of positive stress test. Am J Cardiol 1998 (September 1);82:564–568.

24. Pitts WR, Lange RA, Cigarroa JE, Hillis LD: Repeat coronary angiography in patients with chest pain and previously normal coronary angiogram. Am J Cardiol 1997 (October 15);80:1086–1087.

25. Laurienzo JM, Cannon RO III, Quyyumi AA, Dilsizian V, Panza JA: Improved specificity of transesophageal dobutamine stress echocardiography compared to standard tests for evaluation of coronary artery disease in women presenting with chest pain. Am J Cardiol 1997 (December 1);80:1402–1407.

26. Gadallah S, Thaker KB, Kawanishi D, Mehra A, Lau S, Rashtia Chandraratna ANT: Comparison of intracoronary Doppler guide wire and transesophageal echocardiography in measurement of flow velocity and coronary flow reserve in the LAD coronary artery Am Heart J 1998 (January);135:38–42.

27. Guerci AD, Spadaro LA, Goodman KJ, Lledo-Perez A, Newstein D, Lerner G, Arad Y: Comparison of electron-beam computed tomography scanning and conventional risk factor assessment for the prediction of angiographic coronary artery disease. JACC 1998 (September);32:673–679.

28. Sobel BE, Woodcock-Mitchell J, Schneider DJ, Holt RE, Marutsuka K, Gold H: Increased plasminogen activator inhibitor type 1 in coronary artery atherectomy specimens from type 2 diabetic compared with nondiabetic patients: A potential factor predisposing to thrombosis and its persistence. Circulation 1998 (June 9); 97:2213–2221.

29. Friedlander Y, Siscovick DS, Weinmann S, Austin MA, Psaty BM, Lemaitre RN, Arbogast P, Raghunathan TE, Cobb LA: Family history as a risk factor for primary cardiac arrest. Circulation 1998 (January 20);97:155–160.

30. Narkiewicz K, van de Borne PJH, Hausberg M, Cooley RL, Winniford MD, Davison DE, Somers VK: Cigarette smoking increases sympathetic outflow in humans. Circulation 1998 (August 11);98:528–534.

31. Stevens MJ, Raffel DM, Allman KC, Dayanikli F, Ficaro E, Sandford T, Wieland DM, Pfeifer MA, Schwaiger M: Cardiac sympathetic dysinnervation in diabetes. Implications for enhanced cardiovascular risk. Circulation 1998 (September 8); 98:961–968.

32. Cantin B, Gagnon F, Moorjani S, Despres J-P, Lamarche B, Lupien P-J, Dagenais GR: Is lipoprotein(a) an independent risk factor for ischemic heart disease in men? The Quebec Cardiovascular Study. JACC 1998 (March 1);31:519–525.

33. Gaudet D, Vohl M-C, Perron P, Tremblay G, Gagné C, Lesiège D, Bergeron J, Moorjani S, Després J-P: Relationships of abdominal obesity and hyperinsulinemia to angiographically assessed coronary artery disease in men with known mutations in the LDL receptor gene. Circulation 1998 (March 10);97:871–877.

34. Holvoet P, Vanhaecke J, Janssens S, Van de Werf F, Collen D: Oxidized LDL and malondialdehyde-modified LDL in patients with acute coronary syndromes and stable coronary artery disease. Circulation 1998 (October 13);98:1487–1494.

35. Hopkins PN, Wu LL, Hunt SC, James BC, Vincent GM, Williams RR: Lipoprotein (a) interactions with lipid and nonlipid risk factors in early familial coronary artery disease. Arterioscler Thromb Vasc Biol 1997 (November);17:2783–2792.

36. Evans RW, Shaten BJ, Hempel JD, Cutler JA, Kuller LH, for the MRFIT Research Group: Homocyst(e)ine and risks of cardiovascular disease in the Multiple Risk Factor Intervention Trial. Arterioscler Thromb Vasc Biol 1997 (October);17: 1947–1953.

37. Kuller L, Fisher L, McClelland R, Fried L, Cushman M, Jackson S, Manolio T: Differences in prevalence of and risk factors for subclinical vascular disese among black and white participants in the Cardiovascular Health Study. Arterioscler Thromb Vasc Biol 1998 (February);18:283–293.

38. Strachan DP, Mendall MA, Carrington D, Butland BK, Yarnell JWG, Sweetnam PM, Elwood PC: Relation of *Helicobacter pylori* infection to 13-year mortality and incident ischemic heart disease in the Caerphilly prospective heart disease study. Circulation 1998 (September 29);98:1286–1290.

39. Pasceri V, Cammarota G, Patti G, Cuoco L, Gasbarrini A, Grillo RL, Fedeli G, Gasbarrini G, Maseri A: Association of virulent *Helicobacter pylori* strains with ischemic heart disease. Circulation 1998 (May 5);97:1675–1679.

40. Folsom AR, Nieto FJ, Sorlie P, Chambless LE, Graham DY, for the Atherosclerosis Risk in Communities (ARIC) Study Investigators: *Helicobacter pylori* seropositivity and coronary heart disease incidence. Circulation 1998 (September 1);98:845–850.

41. Davidson M, Kuo C-C, Middaugh JP, Campbell LA, Wang S-P, Newman WP III, Finley JC, Grayston JT: Confirmed previous infection with *Chlamydia pneumoniae* (TWAR) and its presence in early coronary atherosclerosis. Circulation 1998 (August 18);98:628–633.

42. Zama T, Murata M, Matsubara Y, Kawano K, Aoki N, Yoshino H, Watanabe T, Ishikawa K, Ikeda Y: A^{192} Arg variant of the human paraoxonase (HUMPONA) gene polymorphism is associated with an increased risk for coronary disease in the Japanese. Arterioscler Thromb Vasc Biol 1997 (December);17:3565–3569.

43. Penninx BWJH, Guralnik JM, de Leon CFM, Pahor M, Visser M, Corti M-C, Wallace RB: Cardiovascular events and mortality in newly and chronically depressed persons >70 years of age. Am J Cardiol 1998 (April 15);81:988–994.

44. Junker R, Heinrich J, Ulbrich H, Schulte H, Schoenfeld R, Kohler E, Assmann G: Relationship between plasma viscosity and the severity of coronary artery disease. Arterioscler Thromb Vasc Biol 1998 (June);18:870–875.

45. Allen JK, Blumental RS: Risk factors in the offspring of women with premature CAD. Am Heart J 1998 (March);135:428–434.

46. Tracy RP, Psaty BM, Macy E, Bovill EG, Cushman M, Cornell ES, Kuller LH: Lifetime smoking exposure affects the association of C-reactive protein with cardiovascular disease risk factors and subclinical disease in healthy elderly subjects. Arterioscler Thromb Vasc Biol 1997 (October);17:2167–2176.

47. Anderson JL, Carlquist JF, Muhlestein JB, Horne BD, Elmer SP: Evaluation of C-reactive protein, an inflammatory marker, and infectious serology as risk factors for coronary artery disease and myocardial infarction. JACC 1998 (July);32:35–41.

48. Hayano J, Kimura K, Hosaka T, Shibata N, Fukinishi I, Yamas Mono H, Maeda S: Members of the type A behavior pattern coronary disease-prone behavior among Japanese men: Job, lifestyle and social dominance. Am Heart J 1997 (December); 134:1029–1036.

49. Sheu WHH, Lee WJ, Jeng CY, Young MS, Ding YA, Chen YT: Angiotensinogen gene polymorphism is associated with insulin resistance in nondiabetic men with or without coronary heart disease. Am Heart J 1998 (July);136:125–131.

50. Merz CNB, Kop W, Krantz DS, Helmers KF, Berman DS, Rozanski A: Cardiovascular stress response and CAD: Evidence of an adverse postmenopausal effect in women. Am Heart J 1998 (May);135:881–887.

51. VanDenBrink AM, Reekers M, Bax WA, Ferrari MD, Saxena PR: Coronary side-effect potential of current and prospective antimigraine drugs. Circulation 1998 (July 7);98:25–30.

52. Rywik TM, Zink RC, Gittings NS, Khan AA, Wright JG, O'Connor FC, Fleg JL: Independent prognostic significance of ischemic ST-segment response limited to recovery from treadmill exercise in asymptomatic subjects. Circulation 1998 (June 2);97:2117–2122.

53. Belardinelli R, Georgiou D, Ginzton L, Cianci G, Purcato A: Effects of moderate exercise training on thallium uptake and contractile response to low-dose dobutamine of dysfunctional myocardium in patients with ischemic cardiomyopathy. Circulation 1998 (February 17);97:553–561.

54. Pilote L, Pashkow F, Thomas JD, Snader CE, Harvey SA, Marwick TH, Lauer MS: Clinical yield and cost of exercise treadmill testing to screen for coronary artery disease in asymptomatic adults. Am J Cardiol 1998 (January 15);81:219–224.

55. Sheps DS, McMahon RP, Pepine CJ, Stone PH, Goldberg AD, Taylor H, Cohen JD, Becker LC, Chaitman B, Knatterud GL, Kaufmann PG: Heterogeneity among cardiac ischemic and anginal responses to exercise, mental stress, and daily life. Am J Cardiol 1998 (July 1);82:1–6.

56. Parisi AF, Hartigan PM, Folland ED: Evaluation of exercise thallium scintigraphy versus exercise electrocardiography in predicting survival outcomes and morbid cardiac events in patients with single- and double-vessel disease: Findings from the angioplasty compared to medicine (ACME) study. JACC 1997 (November 1); 30:1256–1263.

57. Lauer MS, Pashkow FJ, Snader CE, Harvey SA, Thomas JD: Gender and diagnostic evaluation of possible CAD after exercise treadmill testing. Am Heart J 1997 (November);134:807–813.
58. Kaprielian RR, Gunning M, Dupont E, Sheppard MN, Rothery SM, Underwood R, Pennell DJ, Fox K, Pepper J, Poole-Wilson PA, Severs NJ: Downregulation of immunodetectable connexin43 and decreased gap junction size in the pathogenesis of chronic hibernation in the human left ventricle. Circulation 1998 (February 24);97:651–660.
59. Kitsiou AN, Srinivasan G, Quyyumi AA, Summers RM, Bacharach SL, Dilsizian V: Stress-induced reversible and mild-to-moderate irreversible thallium defects: Are they equally accurate for predicting recovery of regional left ventricular function after revascularization? Circulation 1998 (August 11);98:501–508.
60. Takiuchi S, Ito H, Iwakura K, Taniyama Y, Nishikawa N, Masuyama T, Hori M, Higashino Y, Fujii K, Minamino T: Ultrasonic tissue characterization predicts myocardial viability in early stage of reperfused acute myocardial infarction. Circulation 1998 (February 3);97:356–362.
61. Geskin G, Kramer CM, Rogers WJ, Theobald TM, Pakstis D, Hu Y-L, Reichek N: Quantitative assessment of myocardial viability after infarction by dobutamine magnetic resonance tagging. Circulation 1998 (July 21);98:217–223.
62. Srinivasan G, Kitsiou AN, Bacharach SL, Bartlett ML, Miller-Davis C, Dilsizian V: [^{18}F]Fluorodeoxyglucose single photon emission computed tomography: Can it replace PET and thallium SPECT for the assessment of myocardial viability? Circulation 1998 (March 10);97:843–850.
63. Picano E, Sicari R, Landi P, Cortigiani L, Bigi R, Coletta C, Galati A, Heyman J, Mattioli R, Previtali M, Mathias W Jr., Dodi C, Minardi G, Lowenstein J, Seveso G, Pingitore A, Salustri A, Raciti M, for the EDIC Study Group: Prognostic value of myocardial viability in medically treated patients with global left ventricular dysfunction early after an acute uncomplicated myocardial infarction: A dobutamine stress echocardiographic study. Circulation 1998 (September 15);98: 1078–1084.
64. Dendale P, Franken PR, Block P, Pratikakis Y, DeRoos A: Contrast enhanced and functional magnetic resonance imaging for the detection of viable myocardium after AMI. Am Heart J 1998 (May);135:875–880.
65. Hennessey T, Diamond P, Holligan B, O'Keane C, Hurley J, Codd M, McCarthy C, McCann H, Sugre D: Correlation of myocardial histologic changes in hibernating myocardium with dobutamine stress echocardiographic findings. Am Heart J 1998 (June);135:952–959.
66. Vernon S, Kaul S, Powers ER, Camarano G, Gimple LW: Ragos Myocardial viability in patients with chronic CAD and previous comparison of myocardial contrast echocardiography and myocardial perfusion scintigraphy. Am Heart J 1997 (November);134:835–840.
67. Knudsen AS, Darwish AZ, Norgaard A, Gotzsche O: Time course of myocardial viability after AMI: An echocardiographic study. Am Heart J 1998 (January);135: 51–57.
68. Baliga RR, Rosen SD, Camici PG, Kooner JS: Regional myocardial blood flow redistribution as a cause of postprandial angina pectoris. Circulation 1998 (March 31);97:1144–1149.
69. Chareonthaitawee P, Christian TF, O'Connor MK, Berger PB, ST, O'Keefe JH, Spain MG, Grines CL, Gibbons RJ: Noninvasive prediction of residual blood flow within the risk area during AMI: Multicenter validation study of patients undergoing direct coronary angioplasty. Am Heart J 1997 (October);134:639–646.
70. Lerman A, Burnett JC Jr., Higano ST, McKinley LJ, Holmes DR Jr: Long-term L-arginine supplementation improves small-vessel coronary endothelial function in humans. Circulation 1998 (June 2);97:2123–2128.
71. Kaski JC, Cox ID, Crooke JR, Salomone OA, Frederics S, Hann C, Holt D: Differential plasma endothelin levels in subgroups of angina and angiographically normal coronary arteries. Am Heart J 1998 (September);136:412–417.
72. Shemesh J, Stroh CI, Tenenbaum A, Hod H, Boyko V, Fisman EZ, Motro M:

Comparison of coronary calcium in stable angina pectoris and in first acute myocardial infarction utilizing double helical computerized tomography. Am J Cardiol 1998 (February 1);81:271–275.

73. Lupi A, Lanza GA, Lucente M, Crea F, Proietti I, Maseri A: The "warm-up" phenomenon occurs in patients with chronic stable angina but not in patients with syndrome X. Am J Cardiol 1998 (January 15);81:123–127.

74. Braun S, Boyko V, Behar S, Reicher-Reiss H, Laniado S, Kaplinsky E, Goldbourt U: Calcium channel blocking agents and risk of cancer in patients with coronary heart disease. JACC 1998 (March 15);31:804–808.

75. Russell MW, Huse DM, Drowns S, Hamel EC, Hartz SC: Direct medical costs of coronary artery disease in the United States. Am J Cardiol 1998 (May 1);81:1110–1115.

76. Davey PJ, Schulz M, Gliksman M, Dobson M, Aristides M, Stephens NG: Cost-effectiveness of vitamin E therapy in the treatment of patients with angiographically proven coronary narrowing (CHAOS trial). Am J Cardiol 1998 (August 15);82:414–417.

77. McGrath BP, Liang Y-L, Teede H, Shiel LM, Cameron JD, Dart A: Age-related deterioration in arterial structure and function in post menopausal women: Impact of hormone replacement therapy. Arterioscler Thromb Vasc Biol 1998 (July);18:1149–1156.

78. Abu-Halawa SA, Thompson K, Kirkeeide RL, Vaughn WK, Rosales O, Fujisi K, Schroth G, Smalling R, Anderson HV: Estrogen replacement therapy and outcome of balloon angioplasty in postmenopausal women. Am J Cardiol 1998 (August 15);82:409–413.

79. McLaughlin VV, Hoff JA, Rich S: Relation between hormone replacement therapy in women and CAD estimated by electron beam tomography. Am Heart J 1997 (December);134:1115–1119.

80. Richards MJ, Edwards JR, Culver DH, Gaynes RP, and the National Nosocomial Infections Surveillance System: Nosocomial infections in coronary care units in the United States. Am J Cardiol 1998 (September 15);82:789–793.

81. Valles J, Santos T, Aznar J, Osa A, Lago A, Cosin J, Sanchez E, Broekman J, Marcus AJ: Erythrocyte promotion of platelet reactivity decreases the effectiveness of aspirin as an antithrombotic therapeutic modality: The effect of low-dose aspirin is less than optimal in patients with vascular disease due to prothrombotic effects of erythrocytes on platelet reactivity. Circulation 1998 (February 3);97:350–355.

82. Haim M, Shotan A, Boyko V, Reicher-Reiss H, Benderly M, Goldbourt U, Behar S, for The Bezafibrate Infarction Prevention (BIP) Study Group: Effect of beta-blocker therapy in patients with coronary artery disease in New York Heart Association classes II and III. Am J Cardiol 1998 (June 15);81:1455–1460.

83. Pepine CJ, Lopez LM, Bell DM, Handberg-Thurmond EM, Marks RG, McGorray S: Effects of intermittent transdermal nitroglycerin on occurrence of ischemia after patch removal: Results of the second Transdermal Intermittent Dosing Evaluation Study (TIDES-II). JACC 1997 (October);30:955–961.

84. Dunselman PHJM, van Kempen LHJ, Bouwens LHM, Holwerda KJ, Herweijer AH, Bernink PJLM: Value of the addition of amlodipine to atenolol in patients with angina pectoris despite adequate beta blockade. Am J Cardiol 1998 (January 15);81:128–132.

85. Heitzer T, Just H, Brockhoff C, Meinertz T, Olschewski M, Munzel T: Long-term nitroglycerin treatment is associated with supersensitivity to vasoconstrictors in men with stable coronary artery disease: Prevention by concomitant treatment with captopril. JACC 1998 (January);31:83–88.

86. Knight CJ, Fox KM, on behalf of the Centralized European Studies in Angina Research (CESAR) Investigators: Amlodipine versus diltiazem as additional antianginal treatment to atenolol. Am J Cardiol 1998 (January 15);81:133–136.

87. Yazdani S, Simon AD, Vidhun R, Gulotta C, Schwartz A, Rabbani LE: Inflammatory profile in unstable angina versus stable angina in patients undergoing percutaneous interventions. Am Heart J 1998 (August);136:357–361.

88. Lin SS, Lauer MS, Marwick TH: Risk stratification of patients with medically

treated unstable angina using exercise echocardiography. Am J Cardiol 1998 (September 15);82:720–724.

89. Olatidoye AG, Wu AHB, Feng Y-J, Waters D: Prognostic role of troponin T versus troponin I in unstable angina pectoris for cardiac events with meta-analysis comparing published studies. Am J Cardiol 1998 (June 15);81:1405–1410.

90. Ritchie ME: Nuclear factor-κB is selectively and markedly activated in humans with unstable angina pectoris. Circulation 1998 (October 27);98:1707–1713.

91. Terres W, Kummel P, Sudrow A, Reuter H, Meinertz T: Enhanced coagulation activation in troponin T-positive unstable angina pectoris. Am Heart J 1998 (February);135:281–286.

92. Al-Kadra AS, Salem R, Rand WM, Udelson JE, Smith JJ, Konstam MA: Antiplatelet agents and survival: A cohort analysis from the Studies of Left Ventricular Dysfunction (SOLVD) Trial. JACC 1998 (February);31:419–425.

93. Borzak S, Cannon CP, Kraft PL, Douthat L, Becker RC, Palmeri ST, Henry T, Hochman JS, Fuchs J, Antman EM, McCabe C, Braunwald E, for the TIMI 7 Investigators: Effects of prior aspirin and anti-ischemic therapy on outcome of patients with unstable angina. Am J Cardiol 1998 (March 15);81:678–681.

94. Andersen K, Dellborg M, on behalf of the Thrombin Inhibition in Myocardial Ischemia (TIMI) Study Group: Heparin is more effective than inogatran, a low-molecular weight thrombin inhibitor in suppressing ischemia and recurrent angina in unstable coronary disease. Am J Cardiol 1998 (April 15);81:939–944.

95. The PARAGON Investigators: International, randomized, controlled trial of lamifiban (a platelet glycoprotein IIb/IIIa inhibitor), heparin, or both in unstable angina. Circulation 1998 (June 23);97:2386–2395.

96. Anand SS, Yusuf S, Pogue J, Weitz JI, Flather M, for the OASIS Pilot Study Investigators: Long-term oral anticoagulant therapy in patients with unstable angina or suspected non-Q-wave myocardial infarction: Organization to Assess Strategies for Ischemic Syndromes (OASIS) pilot study results. Circulation 1998 (September 15);98:1064–1070.

97. Klootwijk P, Meij S, Melkert R, Lenderink T, Simoons ML: Reduction of recurrent ischemia with abciximab during continuous ECG-ischemia monitoring in patients with unstable angina refractory to standard treatment (CAPTURE). Circulation 1998 (October 6);98:1358–1364.

98. Rebuzzi AG, Quaranta G, Liuzzo G, Caligiuri G, Lanza GA, Gallimore JR, Grillo RL, Cianflone D, Biasucci LM, Maseri A: Incremental prognostic value of serum levels of troponin T and C-reactive protein on admission in patients with unstable angina pectoris. Am J Cardiol 1998 (September 15);82:715–719.

99. Farkouh ME, Smars PA, Reeder GS, Zinsmeister AR, Evans RW, Meloy TD, Kopecky SL, Allen M, Allison TG, Gibbons RJ, Gabriel SE, for the Chest Pain Evaluation in the Emergency Room (CHEER) Investigators: A clinical trial of a chest-pain observation unit for patients with unstable angina. N Engl J Med 1998 (December 24);339:1882–1888.

100. Spencer FA, Goldberg RJ, Becker RC, Gore JM: Seasonal distribution of acute myocardial infarction in the second National Registry of Myocardial Infarction. JACC 1998. (May);31:1226–1233.

101. Goldberg RJ, McGovern PG, Guggina T, Savageau J, Rosamon Luepker RV: Prehospital delay in patients with acute coronary heart disease: Concordance between patient interviews and medical records. Am Heart J 1998 (February);135:293–299.

102. Mitchell GF, Moyé LA, Braunwald E, Rouleau J-L, Bernstein V, Geltman EM, Flaker GC, Pfeffer MA, for the SAVE Investigators: Sphygmomanometrically determined pulse pressure is a powerful independent predictor of recurrent events after myocardial infarction in patients with impaired left ventricular function. Circulation 1997 (December 16);96:4254–4260.

103. Denollet J, Brutsaert DL: Personality, disease severity, and the risk of long-term cardiac events in patients with a decreased ejection fraction after myocardial infarction. Circulation 1998 (January 20);97:167–173.

104. Tuomainen T-P, Punnonen K, Nyyssönen K, Salonen JT: Association between body iron stores and the risk of acute myocardial infarction in men. Circulation 1998 (April 21);97:1461–1466.

105. Chiarella F, Santoro E, Domenicucci S, Maggioni A, Vecchio C, on behalf of the GISSI-3 Investigators: Predischarge two-dimensional echocardiographic evaluation of left ventricular thrombosis after acute myocardial infarction in the GISSI-3 study. Am J Cardiol 1998 (April 1);81:822–827.

106. Volpi A, Cavalli A, Santoro L, Negri E, on behalf of the GISSI-2 investigators: Incidence and prognosis of early primary ventricular fibrillation in acute myocardial infarction: Results of the Gruppo Italiano per lo Studio della Sopravvivenza nell'Infarto Miocardico (GISSI-2)* database. Am J Cardiol 1998 (August 1);82:265–271.

107. Sajadieh A, Hansen JF, Mortensen LS, and the DAVIT Study Group: Comparison of the prognosis after early versus late recurrent nonfatal myocardial infarction. Am Heart J 1998 (July);136:164–168.

108. The Long-Term Intervention with Pravastatin in Ischaemic Disease (LIPID) Study Group: Prevention of cardiovascular events and death with pravastatin in patients with coronary heart disease and a broad range of initial cholesterol levels. N Engl J Med 1998 (November 5);339:1349–1357.

109. Boden WE, O'Rourke RA, Crawford MH, Blaustein AS, Deedwania PC, Zoble RG, Wexler LF, Kleiger RE, Pepine CJ, Ferry DR, Chow BK, Lavori PW, for the Veterans Affairs Non-Q-Wave Infarction Strategies in Hospital (VANQWISH) Trial Investigators: Outcomes in patients with acute non-Q-wave myocardial infarction randomly assigned to an invasive as compared with a conservative management strategy. N Engl J Med 1998 (June 18);338:1785–1792.

110. Barron HV, Bowlby LJ, Breen T, Rogers WJ, Canto JG, Zhang Y, Tiefenbrunn AJ, Weaver WD, for the National Registry of Myocardial Infarction 2 Investigators: Use of reperfusion therapy for acute myocardial infarction in the United States: Data from the National Registry of Myocardial Infarction 2. Circulation 1998 (March 31);97:1150–1156.

111. Oosterga M, Anthonio RL, de Kam P-J, Kingma JH, Crijns HJGM, van Gilst WH: Effects of aspirin on angiotensin-converting enzyme inhibition and left ventricular dilation one year after acute myocardial infarction. Am J Cardiol 1998 (May 15);81:1178–1181.

112. Gottlieb SS, McCarter RJ, Vogel RA: Effect of beta-blockade on mortality among high-risk and low-risk patients after myocardial infarction. N Engl J Med 1998 (August 20);339:489–497.

113. Rawles JM: Quantification of the benefit of earlier thrombolytic therapy: Five-year results of the Grampian Region Early Anistreplase Trial (GREAT). JACC 1997 (November 1);30:1181–1186.

114. Sacks FM, Moyé LA, Davis BR, Cole TG, Rouleau JL, Nash DT, Pfeffer MA, Braunwald E: Relationship between plasma LDL concentrations during treatment with pravastatin and recurrent coronary events in the cholesterol and recurrent events trial. Circulation 1998 (April 21);97:1446–1452.

115. ACE Inhibitor Myocardial Infarction Collaborative Group: Indications for ACE inhibitors in the early treatment of acute myocardial infarction: Systematic overview of individual data from 100,000 patients in randomized trials. Circulation 1998 (June 9);97:2202–2212.

116. Montalescot G, Philippe F, Ankri A, Vicaut E, Bearez E, Poulard JE, Carrie D, Flammang D, Dutoit A, Carayon A, Jardel C, Chevrot M, Bastard JP, Bigonzi F, Thomas D, for the French Investigators of the ESSENCE Trial: Early increase of von Willebrand factor predicts adverse outcome in unstable coronary artery disease: Beneficial effects of enoxaparin. Circulation 1998 (July 28);98:294–299.

117. Mark DB, Cowper PA, Berkowitz SD, Davidson-Ray L, DeLong ER, Turpie AGG, Califf RM, Weatherly B, Cohen M: Economic assessment of low-molecular-weight heparin (enoxaparin) versus unfractionated heparin in acute coronary syndrome patients: Results from the ESSENCE randomized trial. Circulation 1998 (May 5);97:1702–1707.

118. Ross AM, Coyne KS, Moreyra E, Reiner JS, Greenhouse SW, Walker PL, Simoons ML, Draoui YC, Califf RM, Topol EJ, Van de Werf F, Lundergan CF, for the GUSTO-I Angiographic Investigators: Extended mortality benefit of early postinfarction reperfusion. Circulation 1998 (April 28);97:1549–1546.

119. Van Belle E, Lablanche J-M, Bauters C, Renaud N, McFadden EP, Bertrand ME: Coronary angioscopic findings in the infarct-related vessel within 1 month of acute myocardial infarction: Natural history and the effect of thrombolysis. Circulation 1998 (January 6/13);97:26–33.

120. Pfisterer M, Cox JL, Granger CB, Brener SJ, Naylor CD, Califf RM, van de Werf F, Stebbins AL, Lee KL, Topol EJ, Armstrong PW: Atenolol use and clinical outcomes after thrombolysis for acute myocardial infarction: The GUSTO-I experience. JACC 1998 (September);32:634–640.

121. Christian TF, Milavetz JJ, Miller TD, Clements IP, Holmes DR, Gibbons RJ: Prevalence of spontaneous reperfusion and associated myocardial salvage in patients with AMI. Am Heart J 1998 (March);135:421–427.

122. Sidney S, Siscovick DS, Petitti DB, Schwartz SM, Quesenberry CP, Psaty BM, Raghunathan TE, Kelaghan J, Koepsell TD: Myocardial infarction and use of low-dose oral contraceptives: A pooled analysis of 2 US studies. Circulation 1998 (September 15);98:1058–1063.

123. Kloner RA, Leor J, Poole WK, Perritt R: Population-based analysis of the effect of the Northridge earthquake on cardiac death in Los Angeles county. JACC 1997 (November 1);30:1174–1180.

124. Murata M, Matsubara Y, Kawano K, Zama T, Aoki N, Yoshino H, Watanabe G, Ishikawa K, Ikeda Y: Coronary artery disease and polymorphisms in a receptor mediating shear stress-dependent platelet activation. Circulation 1997 (November 18);96:3281–3286.

125. Gowda MS, Vacek JL, Hallas D: One-year outcomes of diabetic versus nondiabetic patients with non-Q-wave acute myocardial infarction treated with percutaneous transluminal coronary angioplasty. Am J Cardiol 1998 (May 1);81:1067–1071.

126. Malacrida R, Genoni M, Maggioni AP, Spataro V, Parish S, Palmer A, Collins R, Moccetti T, for the Third International Study of Infarct Survival Collaborative Group: A comparison of the early outcome of acute myocardial infarction in women and men. N Engl J Med 1998 (January 1);338:8–14.

127. Ridker PM, Buring JE, Shih J, Matias M, Hennekens CH: Prospective study of C-reactive protein and the risk of future cardiovascular events among apparently healthy women. Circulation 1998 (August 25);98:731–733.

128. Mazzoli S, Tofani N, Fantini A, Semplici F, Bandini F, Salvi A, Vergassola R: *Chlamydia pneumoniae* antibody response in patients with AMI and their follow-up Am Heart J 1998 (January);135:15–20.

129. Ridker PM, Rifai N, Pfeffer MA, Sacks FM, Moye LA, Goldman S, Flaker GC, Braunwald E, for the Cholesterol and Recurrent Events (CARE) Investigators: Inflammation, pravastatin, and the risk of coronary events after myocardial infarction in patients with average cholesterol levels. Circulation 1998 (September 1); 98:839–844.

130. Toss H, Lindahl B, Siegbahn A, Wallentin L, for the FRISC Study Group: Prognostic influence of increased fibrinogen and C-reactive protein levels in unstable coronary artery disease. Circulation 1997 (December 16);96:4204–4210.

131. Polanczyk CA, Lee TH, Cook EF, Walls R, Wybenga D, Printy-Klein G, Ludwig L, Guldbrandsen G, Johnson PA: Cardiac troponin I as a predictor of major cardiac events in emergency department patients with acute chest pain. JACC 1998 (July); 32:8–14.

132. Polanczyk CA, Johnson PA, Hartley LH, Walls RM, Shaykevich S, Lee TH: Clinical correlates and prognostic significance of early negative exercise tolerance test in patients with acute chest pain seen in the hospital emergency department. Am J Cardiol 1998 (February 1);81:288–292.

133. Smart S, Stoiber T, Hellman R, Duchak J, Wynsen J, Kitapci M, Isitman A, Krasnow A, Collier D, Sagar K: Low-dose dobutamine echocardiography is more predictive of reversible dysfunction after AMI than resting single photon emission computed tomographic thallium-201 scintigraphy Am Heart J 1997 (November); 134:822–824.

134. Burke AP, Farb A, Malcom GT, Liang Y, Smialek J, Virmani R: Effects of risk factors on the mechanism of acute thrombosis and sudden coronary death in women. Circulation 1998 (June 2);97:2110–2116.

135. Lavery CE, Mittleman MA, Cohen MC, Muller JE, Verrier RL: Nonuniform night-time distribution of acute cardiac events: A possible effect of sleep states. Circulation 1997 (November 18);96:3321–3327.

136. Henry P, Makowski S, Richard P, Beverelli F, Casanova S, Loua Boughalem K, Battaglia S, Guize L, Guermonprez JL: Increased incidence of moderate coronary stenosis among patients with diabetes: Possible substrate for AMI. Am Heart J 1997 (December);134:1037–1043.

137. Kannel WB, Wilson PWF, D'Agostino RB, Cobb J: Sudden coronary death in women. Am Heart J 1998 (August);136:205–212.

138. Iacoviello L, Di Castelnuovo A, de Knijff P, D'Orazio A, Amore C, Arboretti R, Kluft C, Donati MB: Polymorphisms in the coagulation factor VII gene and the risk of myocardial infarction. N Engl J Med 1998 (January 8);338:79–85.

139. Birnbaum Y, Sclarovsky S, Herz I, Zlotikamien B, Chetrit A, Olmer L, Barbash GI: Admission clinical and electrocardiographic characteristics predicting in-hospital development of high-degree atrioventricular block in inferior wall acute myocardial infarction. Am J Cardiol 1997 (November 1);80:1134–1138.

140. Berton G, Citro T, Palmieri R, Petucco S, De Toni R, Palatini P: Albumin excretion rate increases during acute myocardial infarction and strongly predicts early mortality. Circulation 1997 (November 18);96:3338–3345.

141. Morrow DA, Rifai N, Antman EM, Weiner DL, McCabe CH, Cannon CP, Braunwald E: C-reactive protein is a potent predictor of mortality independently of and in combination with troponin T in acute coronary syndromes: A TIMI 11A substudy. JACC 1998 (June);31:1460–1465.

142. Heller GV, Stowers SA, Hendel RC, Herman SD, Daher E, Ahlbert AW, Baron JM, Wachers FJT: Clinical value of acute rest technetium-99m tetrofosmin tomographic myocardial perfusion imaging in patients with acute chest pain and nondiagnostic electrocardiograms. JACC 1998 (April);31:1011–1017.

143. Mutlak DM, Habib S, Markiewicz W, Beyar R: Determinants of regional myocardial function in patients with chronic significant coronary stenosis or occlusion. Am Heart J 1998 (July);136:169–175.

144. Goldberg RJ, O'Donnell C, Yarzebski J, Bigelow C, Savageau J, Gore JM: Sex difference symptom presentation associated with AMI: A population-based perspective. Am Heart J 1998 (August);136:189–195.

145. Tousoulis D, Davies G, Crake T, Lefroy DC, Rosen S, Maser A: Angiographic characteristics of infarct-related and non-infarct-related stenoses in stable angina progressing to AMI. Am Heart J 1998 (September);136:382–388.

146. Haim M, Gottlieb S, Boyko V, Reicher-Reiss H, Hod H, Kaplinsky E, Mandelzweig L, Goldbourt U, Behar S, for the SPRINT and the Israeli Thrombolytic Survey Groups: Prognosis of patients with a first non-Q-wave myocardial infarction before and in the reperfusion era. Am Heart J 1998 (August);136:245–251.

147. de Vreede-Swagemakers JJM, Gorgels APM, Dubois-Arbouw WI, van Ree JW, Daemen MJAP, Houben LGE, Wellens HJJ: Out-of-hospital cardiac arrest in the 1990s: A population-based study in the Maastricht area on incidence, characteristics and survival. JACC 1997 (November 15);30:1500–1505.

148. Herzog CA, Ma JZ, Collins AJ: Poor long-term survival after acute myocardial infarction among patients on long-term dialysis. N Engl J Med 1998 (September 17);339:799–805.

149. Melchior T, Hildebrant P, Køber L, Jensen G, Torp-Pederson C: Do diabetes mellitus and systemic hypertension predispose to left ventricular free wall rupture in acute myocardial infarction? Am J Cardiol 1997 (November 1);80:1224–1225.

150. Kobayashi Y, Miyazaki S, Itoh A, Daikoku S, Morii I, Matsumoto T, Goto Y, Nonogi H: Previous angina reduces in-hospital death in patients with acute myocardial infarction. Am J Cardiol 1998 (January 15);81:117–122.

151. Yi G, Guo X-H, Reardon M, Gallagher MM, Hnatkova K, Camm AJ, Malik M: Circadian variations of the QT interval in patients with sudden cardiac death after myocardial infarction. Am J Cardiol 1998 (April 15);81:950–956.

152. Roberts WC, Shirani J: Comparison of cardiac findings at necropsy in octogenarians, nonagenarians, and centenarians. Am J Cardiol 1998 (September 1);82:627–631.

153. Zimmermann M, Sentici A, Adamec R, Metzger J, Mermillod B, Rutishauser W: Long-term prognostic significance of ventricular late potentials after a first AMI. Am Heart J 1997 (December);134:1019–1028.

154. Nijland F, Kamp O, Karreman AJP, van Eenige MJ, Visser CA: Prognostic implications of restrictive left ventricular filling in acute myocardial infarction: A serial Doppler echocardiographic study. JACC 1997 (December);30:1618–1624.

155. Modena MG, Molinari R, Rossi R, Muia Jr N, Castelli A, Matti Bacchella L, Gobba F: Modification in serum concentrations of aminoterminal propeptide type III procollagen in patients with previous transmural AMI Am Heart J 1998 (February); 135:287–292.

156. St. John Sutton M, Pfeffer MA, Moye L, Plappert T, Rouleau JL, Lamas G, Rouleau J, Parker JO, Arnold MO, Sussex B, Braunwald E, for the SAVE Investigators: Cardiovascular death and left ventricular remodeling two years after myocardial infarction. Baseline predictors and impact of long-term use of captopril: information from the Survival and Ventricular Enlargement (SAVE) trial. Circulation 1997 (November 18);96:3294–3299.

157. Nagaya N, Nishikimi T, Goto Y, Miyao Y, Kobayashi Y, Morri Daikoku S, Matsumoto T, Miyazaki S, Matsuoka H, Takishita S, Kangawa K, Matsuo H, Nonogi H: Plasma brain natriuretic peptide is a biochemical marker for the prediction of progressive ventricular remodeling after AMI. Am Heart J 1998 (January);135: 21–28.

158. Richards AM, Nicholls MG, Yandle TG, Frampton C, Espiner EA, Turner JG, Buttimore RC, Lainchbury JG, Elliott JM, Ikram H, Crozier IG, Smyth DW: Plasma N-terminal pro-brain natriuretic peptide and adrenomedullin: New neurohormonal predictors of left ventricular function and prognosis after myocardial infarction. Circulation 1998 (May 19);97:1921–1929.

159. Mahmarian JJ, Moyé LA, Chinoy DA, Sequeira RF, Habib GB, Henry WJ, Jain A, Chaitman BR, Weng CSW, Morales-Ballejo H, Pratt CM: Transdermal nitroglycerin patch therapy improves left ventricular function and prevents remodeling after acute myocardial infarction: Results of a multicenter prospective randomized, double-blind, placebo-controlled trial. Circulation 1998 (May 26);97: 2017–2024.

160. Zuanetti G, Latini R, Maggioni AP, Franzosi MG, Santoro L, Tognoni G, for the GISSI-3 Investigators: Effect of the ACE inhibitor lisinopril on mortality in diabetic patients with acute myocardial infarction: Data from the GISSI-3 study. Circulation 1997 (December 16);96:4239–4245.

161. Lewis SJ, Sacks FM, Mitchell JS, East C, Glasser S, Kell S, Letterer R, Limacher M, Moye LA, Rouleau JL, Pfeffer MA, Braunwald E: Effect of pravastatin on cardiovascular events in women after myocardial infarction: The cholesterol and recurrent events (CARE) trial. JACC 1998 (July);32:140–146.

162. Hager WD, Davis BR, Riba A, Moyé LA, Wun CC, Rouleau JL, Lamas GA, Pfeffer MA, for the SAVE Investigators: Absence of a deleterious effect of calcium channel blockers in patients with LV dysfunction after myocardial infarction: The SAVE study experience. Am Heart J 1998 (March);135:406–413.

163. Theroux P, Gregoire J, Chin C, Pelletier G, de Guise P, Juneau M: Intravenous diltiazem in acute myocardial infarction: Diltiazem as adjunctive therapy to activase (DATA) trial. JACC 1998 (September);32:620–628.

164. Becker RC, Burns M, Gore JM, Spencer FA, Ball SP, French W, Lambrew C, Bowlby L, Hilbe J, Rogers WJ for the National Registry of Myocardial Infarction (NRMI-2): Am Heart J 1998 (May);135:786–796.

165. Barron HV, Michaels AD, Maynard C, Every NR: Use of angiotensin-converting enzyme inhibitors at discharge in patients with acute myocardial infarction in the United States: Data from the national register of myocardial infarction 2. JACC 1998 (August);32:360–367.

166. Garrett KN, Holmes DR, Molina-Viamonte V, Reeder GS, Hodge DO, Bailey KR, Libl JK, Laudon DA, Gibbons RJ: Intravenous adenosine and lidocaine in AMI patients. Am Heart J 1998 (August);136:196–204.

167. Kontny F, Dale J, Abildgaard U, Pedersen TR: Randomized trial of low-molecular-

weight heparin (dalteparin) in prevention of left ventricular thrombus formation and arterial embolism after acute anterior myocardial infarction: The Fragmin in Acute Myocardial Infarction (FRAMI) study. JACC 1997 (October);30:962–969.

168. The PURSUIT Trial Investigators: Inhibition of platelet glycoprotein IIb/IIIa with eptifibatide in patients with acute coronary syndromes. N Engl J Med 1998 (August 13);339:436–443.

169. Steg PG, Laperche T, Golmard J-L, Juliard J-M, Benamer H, Himbert D, Aubry P: Efficacy of streptokinase, but not tissue-type plasminogen activator, in achieving 90-minute patency after thrombolysis for acute myocardial infarction decreases with time to treatment. JACC 1998 (March 15);31:776–779.

170. Iparraguirre HP, Conti C, Grancelli H, Ohman EM, Calandrelli Volman S, Garber V: Prognostic value of clinical markers of reperfusion in patients with AMI treated by thrombolytic therapy. Am Heart J 1997 (October);134:631–638.

171. Tanasijevic ML, Cannon CP, Wybenga DR, Fischer GA, Grudzi Gibson CM, Winkelman JW, Antman EM, Braunwald E. Myoglobin, creatine kinase MG, and cardiac troponin-I to assess reperfusion after thrombolysis for AMI: Results from TIMI 10A. Am Heart J 1997 (October);134:622–630.

172. Brieger DB, Mak K-H, White HD, Kleiman NS, Miller DP, Vahanian A, Ross AM, Califf RM, Topol EJ, for the GUSTO-I Investigators: Benefit of early sustained reperfusion in patients with prior myocardial infarction (The GUSTO-I Trial). Am J Cardiol 1998 (February 1);81:282–287.

173. Goodman SG, Langer A, Ross AM, Wildermann NM, Barbagelata A, Sgarbossa EB, Wagner GS, Granger CB, Califf RM, Topol EJ, Simoons ML, Armstrong PW, for the GUSTO-I Angiographic Investigators: Non-Q-wave versus Q-wave myocardial infarction after thrombolytic therapy: Angiographic and prognostic insights from the Global Utilization of Streptokinase and Tissue Plasminogen Activator for Occluded Coronary Arteries-I Angiographic Substudy. Circulation 1998 (February 10);97:444–450.

174. Goldberg RJ, Mooradd M, Gurwitz JH, Rogers WJ, French WJ, Barron HV, Gore JM: Impact of time to treatment with tissue plasminogen activator on morbidity and mortality following acute myocardial infarction (the second national registry of myocardial infarction) Am J Cardiol 1998 (August 1);82:259–264.

175. Birnbaum Y, Herz I, Sclarovsky S, Zlotikamien B, Chetrit A, Olmer L, Barbash GI: Admission clinical and electrocardiographic characteristics predicting an increased risk for early reinfarction after thrombolytic therapy in AMI. Am Heart J 1998 (May);135:805–812.

176. Pfisterer M, Cox JL, Granger CB, Brener SJ, Naylor CD, Califf RM, van de Werf F, Stebbins AL, Lee KL, Topol EJ, Armstrong PW: Atenolol use and clinical outcomes after thrombolysis for acute myocardial infarction: The GUSTO-I experience. JACC 1998 (September);32:634–640.

177. Stewart JT, French JK, Theroux P, Ramanathan K, Solymoss BC, Johnson R, White HD: Early noninvasive identification of failed reperfusion after intravenous thrombolytic therapy in acute myocardial infarction. JACC 1998 (June);31:1499–1505.

178. Matetzky S, Freimark D, Chouraqui P, Rabinowitz B, Rath S, Kaplinsky E, Hod H: Significance of ST segment elevations in posterior chest leads (V_7 to V_9) in patients with acute inferior myocardial infarction: Application for thrombolytic therapy. JACC 1998 (March 1);31:506–511.

179. Brener SJ, Barr LA, Burchenal JEB, Katz S, George BS, Jones AA, Cohen ED, Gainey PC, White HJ, Cheek HB, Moses JW, Moliterno DJ, Effron MB, Topol EJ, on behalf of the ReoPro and Primary PTCA Organization and Randomized Trial (RAPPORT) Investigators: Randomized, placebo-controlled trial of platelet glycoprotein IIb/IIIa blockade with primary angioplasty for acute myocardial infarction. Circulation 1998 (August 25);98:734–741.

180. Verheugt FWA, Liem A, Zijlstra F, Marsh RC, Veen G, Bronzwaer JGF: High-dose bolus heparin as initial therapy before primary angioplasty for acute myocardial infarction: Results of the heparin in early patency (HEAP) pilot study. JACC 1998 (February);31:289–293.

181. Tebbe U, Michels R, Adgey J, Boland J, Caspi A, Charbonnier B, Windeler J, Barth H, Groves R, Hopkins GR, Fennell W, Betriu A, Ruda M: Randomized, double-blind study comparing saruplase with streptokinase therapy in acute myocardial infarction: The COMPASS equivalence trial. JACC 1998 (March 1);31:487–493.

182. French JK, Ellis CJ, Webber BJ, Williams BF, Amos DJ, Ramanathan K, Whitlock RML, White HD: Abnormal coronary flow in infarct arteries 1 year after myocardial infarction is predicted at 4 weeks by corrected thrombolysis in myocardial infarction (TIMI) frame count and stenosis severity. Am J Cardiol 1998 (March 15);81:665–671.

183. Hochrein J, Sun F, Pieper KS, Lee KL, Gates KB, Armstrong PW, Weaver WD, Goodman SG, Topol EJ, Califf RM, Granger CB, Wagner GS: Higher T-wave amplitude associated with better prognosis in patients receiving thrombolytic therapy for acute myocardial infarction (a GUSTO-I Substudy). Am J Cardiol 1998 (May 1);81:1078–1084.

184. Sloan MA, Sila CA, Mahaffey KW, Granger CB, Longstreth WT Jr., Koudstaal P, White HD, Gore JM, Simoons ML, Weaver WD, Green CL, Topol EJ, Califf RM, for the GUSTO-I Investigators: Prediction of 30-day mortality among patients with thrombolysis-related intracranial hemorrhage. Circulation 1998 (October 6);98:1376–1382.

185. Grines CL, Marsalese DL, Brodie B, Griffin J, Donohue B, Costantini CR, Balestrini C, Stone G, Wharton T, Esente P, Spain M, Moses J, Nobuyoshi M, Ayres M, Jones D, Mason D, Grines LL, O'Neill W: Safety and cost-effectiveness of early discharge after primary angioplasty in low-risk patients with acute myocardial infarction. JACC 1998 (April);31:967–972.

186. van 't Hof AWJ, Liem A, Suryapranata H, Hoorntje JCA, de Boer M-J, Zijlstra F, on behalf of the Zwolle Myocardial Infarction Study Group: Angiographic assessment of myocardial reperfusion in patients treated with primary angioplasty for acute myocardial infarction: Myocardial blush grade. Circulation 1998 (June 16);97:2302–2306.

187. Kamijikkoku S, Murohara T, Tayama S, Matsuyama K, Honda T, Ando M, Hayasaki K: AMI and increased soluable intercellular adhesion molecule-1: A marker of vascular inflammation and a risk of early restenosis after PTCA. Am Heart J 1998 (August);136:231–236.

188. Antoniucci D, Santoro GM, Bolognese L, Valenti R, Trapani M, Fazzini PF: A clinical trial comparing primary stenting of the infarct-related artery with optimal primary angioplasty for acute myocardial infarction: Results from the Florence Randomized Elective Stenting in Acute Coronary Occlusions (FRESCO) trial. JACC 1998 (May);31:1234–1239.

189. Reimers B, Camassa N, DiMario C, Akiyama T, DiFrancesco L, Finci L, Colombo: Mechanical recanalization of total coronary occlusions with the use of a new guide wire. Am Heart J 1998 (April);135:726–731.

190. Antoniucci D, Valenti R, Santoro GM, Bolognese L, Trapani M, Moschi G, Fazzini PF: Systematic direct angioplasty and stent-supported direct angioplasty therapy for cardiogenic shock complicating acute myocardial infarction: In-hospital and long-term survival. JACC 1998 (February);31:294–300.

191. Malekianpour M, Bonan R, Lesperance J, Gosselin G, Hudon G, Doucet S, Laurier J, Duval D: Comparison of ionic and nonionic low osmolar contrast media in relation to thrombotic complications of angioplasty in patients with unstable angina. Am Heart J 1998 (June);135:1067–1075.

192. Shyu KG, Kuan PL, Cheng JJ, Hung CR: Cardiac troponin T, creatine kinase, and its isoform release after successful PTCA with or without stenting. Am Heart J 1998 (May);135:862–867.

193. Rupprecht HJ, Espinola-Klein C, Erbel R, Nafe B, Brennecke R, Dietz U, Meyer J: Impact of routine angiographic follow-up after PTCA. Am Heart J 1998 (October);136:613–619.

194. Pasceri V, Patti G, Maseri A: Changing features of anginal pain after PTCA suggest a stenosis on a different artery rather than restenosis. Circulation 1997 (November 18);96:3278–3280.

195. Cohen Y, Raz I, Merin G, Mozes B, for the Israeli Coronary Artery Bypass (ISCAB) Study Consortium: Comparison of factors associated with 30-day mortality after coronary artery bypass grafting in patients with versus without diabetes mellitus. Am J Cardiol 1998 (January 1);81:7–11.

196. Blankenship JC, Hellkamp AS, Aguirre FV, Demko SL, Topol EJ, Califf RM, for the EPIC Investigators: Vascular access site complications after percutaneous coronary intervention with abciximab in the Evaluation of c7E3 for the Prevention of Ischemic Complications (EPIC) trial. Am J Cardiol 1998 (January 1);81:36–40.

197. Jacobs AK, Kelsey SF, Yeh W, Holmes DR, Jr., Block PC, Cowley MJ, Bourassa MG, Williams DO, King SB, III, Faxon DP, Myler R, Detre KM: Documentation of decline in morbidity in women undergoing coronary angioplasty (a report from the 1993–94 NHLBI Percutaneous Transluminal Coronary Angioplasty Registry). Am J Cardiol 1997 (October 15);80:979–984.

198. Browne KF, Maldonado R, Telatnik M, Vlietstra RE, Brenner AS: Initial experience with reuse of coronary angioplasty catheters in the United States. JACC 1997 (December);30:1735–1740.

199. Kleiman NS, Lincoff AM, Kereiakes DJ, Miller DP, Aguirre FV, Anderson KM, Weisman HF, Califf RM, Topol EJ, for the EPILOG Investigators: Diabetes mellitus, glycoprotein IIb/IIIa blockade, and heparin: Evidence for a complex interaction in a multicenter trial. Circulation 1998 (May 19);97:1912–1920.

200. Kereiakes DJ, Kleiman NS, Ferguson JJ, Masud ARZ, Broderick TM, Abbottsmith CW, Runyon JP, Anderson LC, Anders RJ, Dreiling RJ, Hantsbarger GL, Bryzinski B, Topol EJ, for the Oral Glycoprotein IIb/IIIa Receptor Blockade to Inhibit Thrombosis (ORBIT) Trial Investigators: Circulation 1998 (September 29);98:1268–1278.

201. Yokoi H, Daida H, Kuwabara Y, Nishikawa H, Takatsu F, Tomihara H, Nakata Y, Kutsumi Y, Ohshima S, Nishiyama S, Seki A, Kato K, Nishimura S, Kanoh T, Yamaguchi H: Effectiveness of an antioxidant in preventing restenosis after percutaneous transluminal coronary angioplasty: The Probucol Angioplasty Restenosis trial. JACC 1997 (October);30:855–862.

202. Bertrand ME, McFadden EP, Fruchart J-C, van Belle E, Commeau P, Grollier G, Bassand J-P, Machecourt J, Cassagnes J, Mossard J-M, Vacheron A, Castaigne A, Danchin N, Lablanche J-M: Effect of pravastatin on angiographic restenosis after coronary balloon angioplasty. JACC 1997 (October);30:863–869.

203. Taniyama Y, Ito H, Iwakura K, Masuyama T, Hori M, Takiuchi S, Nishikawa N, Higashino Y, Fujii K, Minamino T: Beneficial effect of intracoronary verapamil on microvascular and myocardial salvage in patients with acute myocardial infarction. JACC 1997 (November 1);30:1193–1199.

204. Tam SH, Sassoli PM, Jordan RE, Nakada MT: Abciximab (ReoPro, chimeric 7E3 Fab) demonstrates equivalent affinity and functional blockade of glycoprotein IIb/IIIa and $\alpha_v\beta_3$ integrins. Circulation 1998 (September 15);98:1085–1091.

205. Mak K-H, Challapalli R, Eisenberg MJ, Anderson KM, Califf RM, Topol EJ, for the EPIC Investigators: Effect of platelet glycoprotein IIb/IIIa receptor inhibition on distal embolization during percutaneous revascularization of aortocoronary saphenous vein grafts. Am J Cardiol 1997 (October 15);80:985–988.

206. Miketic S, Carlsson J, Tebbe U: Influence of gradually increased slow balloon inflation on restenosis after coronary angioplasty. Am Heart J 1998 (April);135:709–713.

207. Timmis SB, Burns WJ, Hermiller JB, Parker MA, Meyers SN: Influence of coronary atherosclerotic remodeling on the mechanics of balloon angioplasty. Am Heart J 1997 (December);134:1099–1106.

208. Ellis CJ, French JK, White HD, Ormiston JA, Whitlock RML, Webster MWI: Results of percutaneous coronary angioplasty in patients under 40 years of age. Am J Cardiol 1998 (July 15);82:135–139.

209. Kornowski R, Klutstein M, Satler LF, Pichard AD, Kent KM, Abizaid A, Mintz GS, Hong MK, Popma JJ, Mehran R, Leon MB: Impact of stents on clinical outcomes in percutaneous left main coronary-artery revascularization. Am J Cardiol 1998 (July 1);82:32–37.

210. Mazur W, Bitar JN, Lecin M, Grinstead C, Khalil A, Khan MM, Sekili S, Zoghbi WA, Raizner AE, Kleiman NS: Coronary flow reserve may predict myocardial recovery after myocardial infarction in patients with TIMI grade 3 flow. Am Heart J 1998 (August);136:335–344.
211. Garachemani AR, Kaufmann U, Fleisch M, Meier B: Prolonged heparin after uncomplicated coronary interventions: A prospective, randomized trial. Am Heart J 1998 (August);136:352–356.
212. Garot P, Himbert D, Juliard J-M, Golmard J-L, Steg PG: Incidence, consequences, and risk factors of early reocclusion after primary and/or rescue percutaneous transluminal coronary angioplasty for acute myocardial infarction. Am J Cardiol 1998 (September 1);82:554–558.
213. King SB III, Yeh W, Holubkov R, Baim DS, Sopko G, Desvigne-Nickens P, Holmes DR, Cowley MJ, Bourassa MG, Margolis J, Detre KM: Balloon angioplasty versus new device intervention: Clinical outcomes. JACC 1998 (March 1);31:558–566.
214. Maynard C, Chapko MK, Every NR, Martin DC, Ritchie JL: Coronary angioplasty outcomes in the healthcare cost and utilization project, 1993–1994. Am J Cardiol 1998 (April 1);81:848–852.
215. Kitazume H, Kubo I, Iwama T: Long-term angiographic prognosis of lesions dilated by coronary angioplasty. Am Heart J 1998 (June);135:1076–1080.
216. Halon DA, Merdler A, Flugelman MY, Shifroni G, Khader N, Shiran A, Shala J, Lewis BS: Importance of diabetes mellitus and systemic hypertension rather than completeness of revascularization in determining long-term outcome after coronary balloon angioplasty (the LDCMC registry). Am J Cardiol 1998 (September 1);82:547–553.
217. Erbel R, Haude M, Höpp HW, Franzen D, Rupprecht HJ, Heublein B, Fischer K, de Jaegere P, Serruys P, Rutsch W, Probst P, for the Restenosis Stent Study Group: Coronary artery stenting compared with balloon angioplasty for restenosis after initial balloon angioplasty. N Engl J Med 1998 (December 3);339:1672–1678.
218. Bauters C, Banos J-L, Van Belle E, McFadden EP, Lablanche J-M, Bertrand ME: Six-month angiographic outcome after successful repeat percutaneous intervention for in-stent restenosis. Circulation 1998 (February 3);97:318–321.
219. Rodés J, Côté G, Lespérance J, Bourassa MG, Doucet S, Bilodeau L, Bertrand OF, Harel F, Gallo R, Tardif J-C: Prevention of restenosis after angioplasty in small coronary arteries with probucol. Circulation 1998 (February 10);97:429–436.
220. Ribichini F, Steffenino G, Dellavalle A, Matullo G, Colajanni E, Camilla T, Vado A, Benetton G, Uslenghi E, Piazza A: Plasma activity and insertion/deletion polymorphism of angiotensin I-converting enzyme: A major risk factor and a marker of risk for coronary stent restenosis. Circulation 1998 (January 20);97:147–154.
221. Abizaid A, Kornowski R, Mintz GS, Hong MK, Abizaid AS, Mehran R, Pichard AD, Kent KM, Satler LF, Wu H, Popma JJ, Leon MB: The influence of diabetes mellitus on acute and late clinical outcomes following coronary stent implantation. JACC 1998 (September);32:584–589.
222. Salvioni A, Galli S, Marenzi G, Lauri G, Perego GB, Assanelli E, Guazzi MD: Thrombin activation and late restenosis after PTCA. Am Heart J 1998 (March);135:503–509.
223. Alaigh P, Hoffman CJ, Korlipara G, Neuroth A, Dervan JP, Lawson WE, Hultin MB: Lipoprotein(a) level does not predict restenosis after percutaneous transluminal coronary angioplasty. Arterioscler Thromb Vascular Biol 1998 (August);18:1281–1286.
224. Antoniucci D, Valenti R, Santoro GM, Bolognese L, Trapani M, Cerisano G, Boddi V, Fazzini PF: Restenosis after coronary stenting in current clinical practice. Am Heart J 1998 (March);135:510–518.
225. van't Hof AWJ, de Boer MJ, Suryapranata H, Hoorntje JCA, Zijlstra F: Incidence and predictors of restenosis after successful primary coronary angioplasty for AMI: The importance of age and procedural result. Am Heart J 1998 (September);136:518–527.
226. Weintraub WS, Ghazzal ZMB, Douglas JS, Jr., Morris DC, King SB III: Usefulness of the substitution of nonangiographic end points (death, acute myocardial infarc-

tion, coronary bypass and/or repeat angioplasty) for follow-up coronary angiography in evaluating the success of coronary angioplasty in patients with angina pectoris. Am J Cardiol 1998 (February 15);81:382–386.

227. King SB, Williams DO, Chougule P, Klein JL, Waksman R, Hilstead R, MacDonald J, Anderberg K, Crocker IR: Endovascular β-radiation to reduce restenosis after coronary balloon angioplasty: Results of the Beta Energy Restenosis Trial (BERT). Circulation 1998 (May 26);97:2025–2030.

228. Osanai H, Kanayama H, Miyazaki Y, Fukushima A, Shinoda M, Ito T: Usefulness of enhanced insulin secretion during an oral glucose tolerance test as a predictor of restenosis after direct percutaneous transluminal coronary angioplasty during acute myocardial infarction in patients without diabetes mellitus. Am J Cardiol 1998 (March 15);81:698–701.

229. Pasterkamp G, Peters RJG, Kok WEM, Van Leeuwen TG, for the PICTURE Investigators: Arterial remodeling after balloon angioplasty of the coronary artery intravascular ultrasound study. Am Heart J 1997 (October);134:680–684.

230. Hoffmann R, Mintz GS, Popma JJ, Satler LF, Kent KM, Pichard AD, Leon MB: Overestimation of acute lumen gain and late lumen loss by quantitative coronary angiography (compared with intravascular ultrasound) in stented lesions. Am J Cardiol 1997 (November 15);80:1277–1281.

231. Klein LW, Schaer GL, Calvin JE, Palvas B, Allen J, Loew J, Uretz E, Parrillo JE: Does low individual operator coronary interventional procedural volume correlate with worse institutional procedural outcome? JACC 1997 (October);30:870–877.

232. McGrath PD, Wennberg DE, Malenka DJ, Kellett MA, Ryan TJ, Jr, O'Meara JR, Bradley WA, Hearne MJ, Hettleman B, Robb JF, Shubrooks S, VerLee P, Watkins MW, Lucas FL, O'Connor GT: Operator volume and outcomes in 12,988 percutaneous coronary interventions. JACC 1998 (March 1);31:570–576.

233. Bauriedel G, Schluckebier S, Hutter R, Welsch U, Kandolf R, Luderitz B, Prescott MF: Apoptosis and restenosis versus stable angina atherosclerosis: Indications for the pathogenesis of restenosis. Arterioscler Thromb Vasc Biol 1998 (July);18:1132–1139.

234. The EPISTENT Investigators: Randomised placebo-controlled and balloon-angioplasty-controlled trial to assess safety of coronary stenting with use of platelet glycoprotein-IIb/IIIa blockade. The Lancet 1998 (July 11);352:87–92.

235. Serruys PW, van Hout B, Bonnier H, Legrand V, Garcia E, Macaya C, Sousa E, van der Giessen W, Colombo A, Seabra-Gomes R, Kiemeneij F, Ruygrok P, Ormiston J, Emanuelsson H, Fajadet J, Haude M, Klugmann S, Morel M-A, for the BENESTENT Study Group: Randomised comparison of implantation of heparin-coated stents with balloon angioplasty in selected patients with coronary artery disease (BENESTENT II). The Lancet 1998 (August);352:673–681.

236. Leon MB, Baim DS, Popma JJ, Gordon PC, Cutlip DE, Ho KKL, Giambartolomei A, Diver DJ, Lasorda DM, Williams DO, Pocock SJ, Kuntz RE, for the Stent Anticoagulation Restenosis Study Investigators: A clinical trial comparing three antithrombotic-drug regimens after coronary artery stenting. N Engl J Med 1998 (December 3);339:1665–1671.

237. Kornowski R, Mehran R, Hong MK, Satler LF, Pichard AD, Kent KM, Mintz GS, Waksman R, Laird JR, Lansky AJ, Bucher TA, Popma JJ, Leon MB: Procedural results and late clinical outcomes after placement of three or more stents in single coronary lesions. Circulation 1998 (April 14);97:1355–1361.

238. Moussa I, Reimers B, Moses J, Di Mario C, Di Francesco L, Ferraro M, Colombo A: Long-term angiographic and clinical outcome of patients undergoing multivessel coronary stenting. Circulation 1997 (December 2);96:3873–3879.

239. Stone GW, Brodie BR, Griffin JJ, Morice MC, Costantini C, St. Goar FG, Overlie PA, Popma JJ, McDonnell J, Jones D, O'Neill WW, Grines CL: Prospective, multicenter study of the safety and feasibility of primary stenting in acute myocardial infarction: In-hospital and 30-day results of the PAMI stent pilot trial. JACC 1998 (January);31:23–30.

240. Mann T, Cubeddu G, Bowen J, Schneider JE, Arrowood M, Newman WN, Zellinger

MJ, Rose GC: Stenting in acute coronary syndromes: A comparison of radial versus femoral access sites. JACC 1998 (September);32:572–376.

241. Schiele F, Meneveau N, Vuillemenot A, Zhang DD, Gupta S, Mercier M, Danchin N, Bertrand B, Bassand J-P: Impact of intravascular ultrasound guidance in stent deployment on 6-month restenosis rate: A multicenter, randomized study comparing two strategies—with and without intravascular ultrasound guidance. JACC 1998 (August);32:320–328.

242. Rubartelli P, Niccoli L, Verna E, Giachero C, Zimarino M, Fontanelli A, Vassanelli C, Campolo L, Martuscelli E, Tommasini G: Stent implantation versus balloon angioplasty in chronic coronary occlusions: Results from the GISSOC trial. JACC 1998 (July);32:90–96.

243. Sirnes PA, Golf S, Myreng Y, Molstad P, Albertsson P, Mangschau A, Endresen K, Kjekshus J: Sustained benefit of stenting chronic coronary occlusion: Long-term clinical follow-up of the stenting in chronic coronary occlusion (SICCO) study. JACC 1998 (August);32:305–310.

244. Phillips PS, Segovia J, Alfonso F, Goicolea J, Hernandez R, Banuelos C, Fernandez-Ortiz A, Perez-Vizcayno MJ, Kimura BJ, Macaya C: Advantage of stents in the most proximal LAD coronary artery. Am Heart J 1998 (April);135:719–725.

245. Elsner M, Peifer A, Drexler M, Wenzel C, Hebbeker C, Kasper W: Clinical outcome at six months of coronary stenting followed by ticlopidine monotherapy. Am J Cardiol 1998 (January 15);81:147–151.

246. Mendelsohn FO, Santos RM, Crowley JJ, Lederman RJ, Cobb FR, Phillips HR, Weissman NJ, Stack RS: Kissing stents in the aortic bifurcation. Am Heart J 1998 (October);136:600–605.

247. Asakura M, Ueda Y, Nanto S, Hirayama A, Adachi T, Kitakaze M, Hori M, Kodama K: Remodeling of in-stent neointima, which became thinner and transparent over 3 years: Serial angiographic and angioscopic follow-up. Circulation 1998 (May 26);97:2003–2006.

248. Hsieh IC, Chang HJ, Chern MS, Hung KCC, Lin FC, Wu D: Late coronary artery stenting in patients with AMI. Am Heart J 1998 (October);136:606–612.

249. Lau KW, Ding ZP, Johan A, Lim YL: Midterm angiographic outcome of single-vessel intracoronary stent placement in diabetic versus nondiabetic patients. Am Heart J 1998 (July);136:150–155.

250. Le May MR, Libinaz M, Marquis JF, O'Brien ER, Beanlands RS, Laramee LA, Williams WL, Davies RF, Kearns SA, Higginson LA: Late clinical and angiographic follow-up after stenting in evolving and recent myocardial infarction. Am Heart J 1998 (April);135:714–718.

251. Nolan J, Batin P, Welsh C, Lindsay S, McLenachan J, Cowan C, Perrins J: Feasibility and applicability of coronary stent implantation with the direct brachial approach. Am Heart J 1997 (November);134:939–944.

252. Moussa I, Di Mario C, Moses J, Reimers B, Di Francesco L, Blengino S, Colombo A: Comparison of angiographic and clinical outcomes of coronary stenting of chronic total occlusions versus subtotal occlusions. Am J Cardiol 1998 (January 1);81:1–6.

253. De Scheerder IK, Wang K, Kostopoulos K, Dens J, Desmet W, Piessens JH: Treatment of long dissections by use of a single long or multiple short stents: Clinical and angiographic follow-up. Am Heart J 1998 (August);136:345–351.

254. Schühlen H, Kastrati A, Dirschinger J, Hausleiter J, Elezi S, Wehinger A, Pache J, Hadamitzky M, Schömig A: Intracoronary stenting and risk for major adverse cardiac events during the first month. Circulation 1998 (July 14);98:104–111.

255. Vaitkus PT, Adele C, Wells SK, Zehnacker JP: The evolving costs of intracoronary stents. Am Heart J 1998 (July);136:132–135.

256. Suttorp M, Mast EG, Plokker HWT, Kelder JC, Ernest SMPG: Primary coronary stenting after successful balloon angioplasty of chronic total occlusions. Am Heart J 1998 (February);135:318–322.

257. Kereiakes DJ, Lincoff AM, Miller DP, Tcheng JE, Cabot CF, Anderson KM, Weisman HF, Califf RM, Topol EJ, for the EPILOG Trial Investigators: Abciximab therapy and unplanned coronary stent deployment: Favorable effects on stent use,

clinical outcomes, and bleeding complications. Circulation 1998 (March 10);97: 857–864.

258. Shiran A, Mintz GS, Waksman R, Mehran R, Abizaid A, Kent KM, Pichard AD, Satler LF, Popma JJ, Leon MB: Early lumen loss after treatment of in-stent restenosis: An intravascular ultrasound study. Circulation 1998 (July 21);98:200–203.

259. Bertrand ME, Legrand V, Boland J, Fleck E, Bonnier J, Emmanuelson H, Vrolix M, Missault L, Chierchia S, Casaccia M, Niccoli L, Oto A, White C, Webb-Peploe M, Van Belle E, McFadden EP: Randomized multicenter comparison of conventional anticoagulation versus antiplatelet therapy in unplanned and elective coronary stenting: The full anticoagulation versus aspirin and ticlopidine (FANTASTIC) study. Circulation 1998 (October 20);98:1597–1603.

260. Hasdai D, Rihal CS, Bell MR, Berger PB, Grill DE, Garratt KN, Holmes DR, Jr: Abciximab administration and outcome after intracoronary stent implantation. Am J Cardiol 1998 (September 15);82:705–709.

261. Kastrati A, Schömig A, Elezi S, Schühlen H, Wilhelm M, Dirschinger J: Interlesion dependence of the risk for restenosis in patients with coronary stent placement in multiple lesions. Circulation 1998 (June 23);97:2396–2401.

262. Berger PB, Bell MR, Grill DE, Melby S, Holmes DR, Jr: Frequency of adverse clinical events in the 12 months following successful intracoronary stent placement in patients treated with aspirin and ticlopidine (without warfarin). Am J Cardiol 1998 (March 15);81:713–718.

263. Michaelides AP, Dilaveris PE, Psomadaki ZD, Aggelakas S, Stefanadis C, Cokkinos D, Gialafos J, Toutouzas: Reliability of exercise-induced ST-segment changes to detect restenosis 3 months after coronary angioplasty. Am Heart J 1998 (March); 135:449–456.

264. Kosuga K, Tamai H, Ueda K, Hsu YS, Ono S, Tanaka S, Doi T, W, Motohara S, Uehata H: Effectiveness of tranilast on restenosis after directional coronary atherectomy. Am Heart J 1997 (October);134:712–718.

265. Baim DS, Cutlip DE, Sharma SK, Ho KKL, Fortuna R, Schreiber TL, Feldman RL, Shani J, Senerchia C, Zhang Y, Lansky AJ, Popma JJ, Kuntz RE, for the BOAT Investigators: Final results of the balloon vs optimal atherectomy trial (BOAT). Circulation 1998 (February 3);97:322–331.

266. Moussa I, Moses J, Di Mario C, Busi G, Reimers B, Kobayashi Y, Albiero R, Ferraro M, Colombo A: Stenting after Optimal Lesion Debulking (SOLD) Registry: Angiographic and clinical outcome. Circulation 1998 (October 20);98:1604–1609.

267. Henderson RA, Pocock SJ, Sharp SJ, Nanchahal K, Sculpher MJ, Buxton MJ, Hampton JR, for the Randomised Intervention Treatment of Angina (RITA-1) trial participants: Long-term results of RITA-1 trial: Clinical and cost comparisons of coronary angioplasty and coronary artery bypass grafting. The Lancet 1998 (October 31);352:1419–1425.

268. Ellis SG, Tamai H, Nobuyoshi M, Kosuga K, Colombo A, Holmes DR, Macaya C, Grines CL, Whitlow PL, White HJ, Moses J, Teirstein PS, Serruys PW, Bittl JA, Mooney MR, Shimshak TM, Block PC, Erbel R: Contemporary percutaneous treatment of unprotected left main coronary stenoses. Initial results from a multicenter registry analysis 1994–1996. Circulation 1997 (December 2);96:3867–3872.

269. Gibson CM, Goel M, Cohen DJ, Piana RN, Deckelbaum LI, Harris KE, King SB: Six-month angiographic and clinical follow-up of patients prospectively randomized to receive either tirofiban or placebo during angioplasty in the RESTORE trial. JACC 1998 (July);32:28–34.

270. Omoigui NA, Silver MJ, Rybicki LA, Rosenthal M, Berdan LG, Pieper K, King SV, Califf RM, Topol EJ: Influence of a randomized clinical trial on practice by participating investigators: Lessons from the coronary angioplasty versus excisional atherectomy trial (CAVEAT) JACC 1998 (February);31:265–272.

271. Weintraub WS, Stein B, Kosinski A, Douglas JS Jr, Ghazzal ZMB, Jones EL, Morris DC, Guyton RA, Craver JM, King SP III: Outcome of coronary bypass surgery versus coronary angioplasty in diabetic patients with multivessel coronary artery disease. JACC 1998 (January);31:10–19.

272. Park S-J, Park S-W, Hong M-K, Cheong S-S, Lee CW, Kim J-J, Hong MK, Mintz

GS, Leon MB: Stenting of unprotected left main coronary artery stenosis: Immediate and late outcomes. JACC 1998 (January);31:37–42.

273. Suryapranata H, van't Hof AWJ, Hoorntje JCA, de Boer M-J, Zijlstra F: Randomized comparison of coronary stenting with balloon angioplasty in selected patients with acute myocardial infarction. Circulation 1998 (June 23);97:2502–2505.

274. Tiefenbrunn AJ, Chandra NC, French WJ, Gore JM, Rogers WJ: Clinical experience with primary percutaneous transluminal coronary angioplasty compared with alteplase (recombinant tissue-type plasminogen activator) in patients with acute myocardial infarction: A report from the second National Registry of Myocardial Infarction (NRMI-2). JACC 1998 (May);31:1240–1245.

275. Jacobs AK, Kelsey SF, Brooks MM, Faxon DP, Chaitman BR, Bittner V, Mock MB, Weiner BH, Dean L, Winston C, Drew L, Sopko G: Better outcome for women compared with men undergoing coronary revascularization: A report from the Bypass Angioplasty Revascularization Investigation (BARI). Circulation 1998 (September 29);98:1279–1285.

276. Cohen HA, Zenati M, Smith AJC, Lee JS, Chough S, Jafar Z, Counihan P, Izzo M, Burchenal JE, Feldman AM, Griffith B: Feasibility of combined percutaneous transluminal angioplasty and minimally invasive direct coronary artery bypass in patients with multivessel coronary artery disease. Circulation 1998 (September 15);98:1048–1050.

277. George CJ, Baim DS, Brinker JA, Fischman DL, Goldberg S, Holubkov R, Kennard ED, Veltri L, Detre KM: One-year follow-up of the stent restenosis (STRESS 1) study. Am J Cardiol 1998 (April 1);81:860–865.

278. Lefèvre T, Morice M-C, Eltchaninoff H, Chabrillat Y, Amor M, Juliard JM, Gommeaux A, Cattan S, Dumas P, Benveniste E: One-month results of coronary stenting in patients ≥75 years of age. Am J Cardiol 1998 (July 1);82:17–21.

279. Mahdi NA, Lopez J, Leon M, Pathan A, Harrell L, Jang I-K, Palacios IF: Comparison of primary coronary stenting to primary balloon angioplasty with stent bailout for the treatment of patients with acute myocardial infarction. Am J Cardiol 1998 (April 15);81:957–963.

280. Rodríquez A, Bernardi V, Fernández M, Mauvecín C, Ayala F, Santaera O, Martínez J, Mele E, Roubin GS, Palacios I, Ambrose JA, on behalf of the GRAMI Investigators: In-hospital and late results of coronary stents versus conventional balloon angioplasty in acute myocardial infarction (GRAMI trial). Am J Cardiol 1998 (June 1);81:1286–1291.

281. Hoffmann R, Mintz GS, Kent KM, Pichard AD, Satler LF, Popma JJ, Hong MK, Laird JR, Leon MB: Comparative early and nine-month results of rotational atherectomy, stents, and the combination of both for calcified lesions in large coronary arteries. Am J Cardiol 1998 (March 1);81:552–557.

282. Mascelli MA, Lance ET, Damaraju L, Wagner CL, Weisman HF, Jordan RE: Pharmacodynamic profile of short-term abciximab treatment demonstrates prolonged platelet inhibition with gradual recovery from GP IIb/IIIa receptor blockade. Circulation 1998 (May 5);97:1680–1688.

283. Cannon CP, McCabe CH, Borzak S, Henry TD, Tischler MD, Mueller HS, Feldman R, Palmeri ST, Ault K, Hamilton SA, Rothman JM, Novotny WF, Braunwald E, for the TIMI 12 Investigators: Randomized trial of an oral platelet glycoprotein IIb/IIIa antagonist, sibrafiban, in patients after an acute coronary syndrome: Results of the TIMI 12 trial. Circulation 1998 (February 3);97:340–349.

284. Ghaffari S, Kereiakes DJ, Lincoff AM, Kelly TA, Timmis GC, Kleiman NS, Ferguson JJ, Miller DP, Califf RA, Topol EJ, for the EPILOG Investigators: Platelet glycoprotein IIb/IIIa receptor blockade with abciximab reduces ischemic complications in patients undergoing directional coronary atherectomy. Am J Cardiol 1998 (July 1);82:7–12.

285. Ivanov J, Weisel RD, David TE, Naylor CD: Fifteen-year trends in risk severity and operative mortality in elderly patients undergoing coronary artery bypass graft surgery. Circulation 1998 (February 24);97:673–680.

286. Cowper PA, Peterson ED, DeLong ER, Jollis JG, Muhlbaier LH, Mark DB: Impact of early discharge after coronary artery bypass graft surgery on rates of hospital readmission and death. JACC 1997 (October);30:908–913.

287. Peduzzi P, Kamina A, Detre K, for The VA Coronary Artery Bypass Surgery Cooperative Study Group: Twenty-two-year follow-up in the VA Cooperative Artery Bypass Surgery for Stable Angina. Am J Cardiol 1998 (June 15);81:1393–1399.

288. Nallamothu N, Johnson JH, Bagheri B, Heo J, Iskandrian AE: Utility of stress single-photon emission computed tomography (SPECT) perfusion imaging in predicting outcome after coronary artery disease grafting. Am J Cardiol 1997 (December 15);80:1517–1521.

289. Birkmeyer NJO, Charlesworth DC, Hernandez F, Leavitt BJ, Marrin CAS, Morton JR, Olmstead EM, O'Connor GT, for the Northern New England Cardiovascular Disease Study Group: Obesity and risk of adverse outcomes associated with coronary artery bypass surgery. Circulation 1998 (May 5);97:1689–1694.

290. Haas F, Haehnel CJ, Pick W, Nekolla S, Martinoff S, Meisner H, Schwaiger M: Preoperative positron emission tomographic viability assessment and perioperative and postoperative risk in patients with advanced ischemic heart disease. JACC 1997 (December);30:1693–1700.

291. Cornel JH, Bax JJ, Elhendy A, Maat APWM, Kimman G-JP, Geleijnse ML, Rambaldi R, Boersma E, Fioretti PM: Biphasic response to dobutamine predicts improvement of global left ventricular function after surgical revascularization in patients with stable coronary artery disease. JACC 1998 (April);31:1002–1010.

292. Mannheimer C, Eliasson T, Augustinsson L-E, Blomstrand C, Emanuelsson H, Larsson S, Norrsell H, Hjalmarsson Å: Electrical stimulation versus coronary artery bypass surgery in severe angina pectoris: The ESBY Study. Circulation 1998 (March 31);97:1157–1163.

293. Perski A, Feleke E, Anderson G, Samad BA, Westerlund H, Ericsson CG, Rehnquist N: Emotional distress before CABG limits the benefits of surgery. Am Heart J 1998 (September);136:510–517.

294. Silva JA, White CJ, Collins TJ, Ramee SR: Morphologic comparison of atherosclerotic lesions in native coronary arteries and saphenous vein grafts with intracoronary angioscopy in unstable angina. Am Heart J 1998 (July);136:156–163.

295. Mustonen P, Hippeläinen M, Vanninen E, Rehnberg S, Tenhunen-Eskelinen M, Hartikainen J: Significance of coronary artery bypass grafting-associated conduction defects. Am J Cardiol 1998 (March 1);81:558–563.

296. Pasceri V, Lanza GA, Buffon A, Montenero AS, Crea F, Maseri A: Role of abnormal pain sensitivity and behavioral factors in determining chest pain in syndrome X. JACC 1998 (January);31:62–66.

297. Karagounis LA, Anderson JL, Moreno FL, Sorensen SG, TEAM-3 Investigators: Multivariate associates of QT dispersion in patients with AMI: Primacy of patency status of the infarct-related artery. Am Heart J 1998 (June);135:1027–1035.

298. Yotsukura, M, Koide Y, Fujii K, Tomono Y, Katayama A, Ando H, Suzuki J, Ishikawa K: Heart rate variability during the first month of smoking cessation. Am Heart J 1998 (June);135:1004–1009.

299. Moscucci M, Ricciardi M, Eagle KA, Kline E, Bates ER, Werns SW, Karavite D, Muller DWM: Frequency, predictors, and appropriateness of blood transfusion after percutaneous coronary interventions. Am J Cardiol 1998 (March 15);81:702–707.

300. Laperche T, Golmard JL, Steg PG, for the PERM Study Group: Early behavior of biochemical markers in patients with Thrombolysis in Myocardial Infarction grade 2 flow in the infarct artery as opposed to other flow grades after intravenous thrombolysis for Am Heart J 1997 (December);134:1044–1051.

301. Dissmann R, Linderer T, Schroder R: Estimation of enzymatic infarct size: Direct comparison of the marker enzymes creatine kinase and alpha-hydroxybutyrate dehydrogenase. Am Heart J 1998 (January);135:1–9.

302. Chang RJ, Doherty TM, Goldberg SL: Mechanism of warfarin effect on the activated coagulation time. Am Heart J (September) 1998;136:477–479.

303. Reinhart WH, Dziekan G, Goebbels U, Myers J, Dubach P: Influence of exercise training on blood viscosity in patients with CAD and impaired LV function. Am Heart J 1998 (March);135:379–382.

304. Hollander JE, Levitt MA, Young GP, Briglia E, Wetli CV: Effect of recent cocaine use on the specificity of cardiac markers for diagnosis of AMI. Am Heart J 1998 (February);135:245–252.
305. Tsai LM, Kuo KJ, Chen JH: Effects of spontaneous respiration on transmitral Doppler flow patterns in normal subjects and CAD patients. Am Heart J 1998 (July);136:99–102.

3

Congestive Heart Failure

Congestive Heart Failure (General Topics)

Assessment of Hospital Admission for Heart Failure

Heart failure is one of the most common reasons for admission to acute care hospitals. A proportion of these admissions are probably low risk and could be managed in subacute facilities, resulting in substantial costs savings. To investigate the proportion of low-risk hospital admissions for heart failure, Butler and associates[1] from Nashville, Tennessee, identified all admissions for heart failure to Vanderbilt University Medical Center between July 1993 and June 1995 (n = 743); 120 of these admissions were randomly selected, reviewed, and classified into high-risk or low-risk groups on admission based on the severity of heart failure and the presence of life-threatening complications. Of the 120 admissions, 57 (48%) were classified as high risk based on the presence of moderate to severe heart failure for the first time or recurrent heart failure with a major complicating factor. Sixteen admissions (28%) were associated with adverse outcomes, including AMI in 5 (9%), intubation in 6 (11%), and death in 4 (7%). Sixty-three admissions (52%) were classified as low risk based on the presence of new-onset mild heart failure with no complicating factors. Most of these admissions were for dyspnea without any life-threatening complication; 57 (91%) had no evidence of interstitial or alveolar pulmonary edema, and arterial oxygen saturation averaged 95 ± 3%. Only 3 of these low-risk admissions (5%) were associated with adverse cardiovascular events. None of the patients died. These data suggest that over half of the patients admitted to an acute care facility for heart failure are at low risk and probably could be managed in a subacute care setting, resulting in large cost savings.

Resuscitation Preferences Among Patients with Congestive Heart Failure

Krumholz and colleagues[2] sought to identify the resuscitation preferences of patients hospitalized with an exacerbation of severe CHF, perceptions of those preferences by their physicians, and the stability of the preferences. Among 936 patients in this study, 215 (23%) explicitly stated that they did not want to be resuscitated. Significant correlates of not wanting to be resuscitated included older age, perception of a worse prognosis, poorer functional status,

363

and a higher income. The physician's perception of the patient's preference disagreed with the patient's actual preference in 24% of the cases overall. Only 25% of the patients reported discussing resuscitation preferences with their physicians, but discussion of preferences was not significantly associated with higher agreement between the patient and physician. Among 600 patients who responded to the resuscitation question again 2 months later, 19% had changed their preferences, including 14% of those who initially wanted resuscitation and 40% of those who initially did not. The physician's perception of the patient's hospital resuscitation preference was correct for 84% of patients who had a stable preference and for 68% of those who did not. Thus, almost 25% of patients hospitalized with severe CHF expressed a preference not to be resuscitated. The physician's perception of the patient's preference was not accurate in almost 25% of the cases.

Cardiac Arrest Survivors

Thompson and associates[3] from Royal Oak and Detroit, Michigan, reviewed the hospital records of 127 consecutive patients who were resuscitated from cardiac arrest in a retrospective cohort analysis. A cardiac arrest score was calculated utilizing time to return of spontaneous circulation, systolic blood pressure at the time of presentation, and initial neurological exam. This score was analyzed with 39 other clinical variables for significance with regard to mortality or neurological survival using multivariate analysis. Combining these variables into a cardiac arrest score (levels 0, 1, 2, 3, from least to most favorable) allowed prediction of neurological outcomes and mortality from a single variable in an independent fashion. Logistic regression models found scores of 0, 1, 2, and 3 predicted in-hospital mortality rates of 90%, 71%, 42%, 18%, and neurological recovery in 3%, 17%, 57%, and 89%, respectively. The cardiac arrest score was able to predict in-hospital mortality and neurological outcomes in those who survived to emergency department arrival. This scoring scheme may aid in selection of patients for early aggressive measures, including triage coronary angiography and angioplasty.

Endothelin Receptors in the Failing and Nonfailing Human Heart

Pönicke and colleagues[4] in Halle/Saale, Germany, determined whether cardiac endothelin receptors were altered in patients with CHF; they obtained slices from the right atria and left ventricles in 6 potential heart transplant donors and in 15 patients with end-stage CHF. They studied endothelin-induced inhibition of isoprenaline- and forskolin-stimulated adenylyl cyclase and endothelin-receptor density. Endothelin increased inositol phosphate formation in the right atria and left ventricles through ET_A-receptor stimulation in a concentration-dependent manner with no difference in potency or efficacy between the potential heart transplant donors and patients with heart failure.

Endothelin-1 binding revealed the coexistence of ET_A and ET_B receptors in both tissues, but the density of ET_A receptors was not significantly different between the transplant donors and CHF hearts. Thus, in the human heart, ET_A and ET_B receptors coexist, but only ET_A receptors appear to be of functional importance. In the right atria, ET_A receptors couple to inositol phosphate formation and inhibition of adenylyl cyclase; in the left ventricles, they couple only to an inositol phosphate formation. In end-stage CHF, the functional responsiveness of the cardiac ET_A receptor system is not altered.

Basal Nitric Oxide Activity on Pulmonary Vascular Resistance

Increased pulmonary resistance may reduce survival and treatment options in patients with CHF. NO is a determinant of normal pulmonary resistance vessel tone. Cooper and associates[5] from Boston, Massachusetts, tested the hypothesis that loss of NO function contributes to increased pulmonary vascular resistance index (PVRI) in CHF. Pulmonary arterial resistance vessel function was studied in 25 conscious adults. Three groups were studied: 8 controls, 9 patients with CHF and normal PVRI, and 8 patients with CHF and raised PVRI. Segmental arterial flow was determined with a Doppler wire and quantitative angiography. N^G-monomethyl-L-arginine (L-NMMA) was used to inhibit NO, whereas phenylephrine was used as an endothelium-independent control. The response to inhibition of NO with L-NMMA was less in patients with CHF and elevated PVRI than in patients with CHF and normal PVRI. The difference in response between the CHF groups was specific to NO-dependent regulation because the response to the endothelium-independent constrictor phenylephrine was not different. There was no difference in response to L-NMMA between controls and patients with CHF and normal PVRI. In adults with CHF, NO appears to play an important role in maintaining normal pulmonary resistance.

Evaluation of Oxidant Stress on Ventricular Remodeling

Mallat and colleagues[6] have evaluated oxidant stress in the heart by measuring pericardial fluid levels of 8 iso-prostaglandin $F_{2\alpha}$, a specific and quantitative marker of oxidant stress *in vivo* in a series of 51 consecutive patients with ischemic and/or valvular heart disease referred for cardiac surgery. Pericardial levels of 8-iso-$PGF_{2\alpha}$ were correlated with the functional severity of CHF and with echocardiographic indices of ventricular dilatation measured by independent physicians. Pericardial levels of 8-iso-$PGF_{2\alpha}$ were increased in patients with symptomatic CHF compared with asymptomatic patients. They gradually increased with increasing functional severity of heart failure (Figure 3-1). Pericardial levels of 8-iso-$PGF_{2\alpha}$ were significantly correlated with LV end-diastolic and end-systolic diameters. Thus, pericardial levels of 8-iso-$PGF_{2\alpha}$ increased with the functional severity of CHF and are associated with ventricular dilatation. These data suggest a potentially important role for *in vivo* oxidant stress on ventricular remodeling and the progression to CHF.

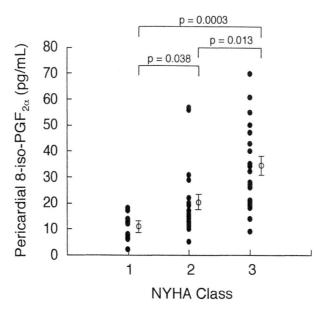

FIGURE 3-1. Pericardial levels of 8-iso-PFG$_{2\alpha}$ in patients with ischemic and/or valvular heart disease referred for cardiac surgery. Pericardial levels of 8-iso-PGF$_{2\alpha}$ significantly increased with the functional severity of heart failure assessed using the NYHA classification. Reproduced with permission from Mallat et al.[6]

Tachycardia-Induced Cardiomyopathy

Left ventricular function was assessed in a series of 59 consecutive patients with successful radiofrequency ablation of atrial flutter before and after the procedure. Luchsinger and Steinberg[7] from New York, New York, attempted to evaluate the potential of tachycardia-induced cardiomyopathy in this group of patients and its response to direct catheter ablation. All patients were male and 59 years old. The preablation LVEF was 31% and improved to 41% when measured 7 months after successful ablation. New York Heart Association class improved from 2.6 to 1.6. Six of 11 patients had normalization of their EF with complete resolution of CHF symptoms. A lower initial EF and functional class predicted nonresolution of dilated cardiomyopathy. These authors conclude that restoration of normal sinus rhythm in patients with chronic atrial flutter and cardiomyopathy substantially improved LV function. This suggests that tachycardia-induced cardiomyopathy may be a more common mechanism of LV dysfunction in patients with atrial flutter than expected and that aggressive treatment of this arrhythmia should be considered.

Vasodilatory Effects of Peptides

B-type natriuretic peptide (BNP) and atrial natriuretic peptide (ANP) are secreted from the heart and are thought to be equally important factors in the regulation of vascular tone in health and in CHF. However, no studies directly compare vasodilatory effects of these peptides in healthy subjects and in patients with CHF. Makamura and associates[8] used plethysmography to determine the vasodilatory effects of BNP and to compare these to the effects of ANP in patients with CHF (n = 15) and in age-matched healthy subjects (n = 16). Graded doses of ANP and BNP (8, 16, 32, and 48 pmol/min/100 mL of tissue volume for both) were administered randomly into the brachial arterial. Forearm blood flow (FBF) was measured, and cyclic GMP (cGMP) spillover was calculated. Responses in FBF to both peptides in CHF were significantly lower than those of healthy subjects. Similarly, forearm spillover of cGMP was significantly lower in CHF than in healthy subjects. When vascular responses in healthy subjects were compared between BNP and ANP, BNP-induced changes in FBF and forearm cGMP spillover were significantly less than changes induced by ANP. In CHF, FBF change and cGMP spillover induced by the 2 peptides were not significantly different. These results suggest that the metabolism and action of these natriuretic peptides in CHF may differ from the healthy state.

Plasma Brain Natriuretic Peptide

Plasma atrial natriuretic peptide (ANP), mainly from the atrium, brain natriuretic peptide (BNP), mainly from the ventricle, norepinpehrine (NE), and endothelin-1 (ET-1) levels are increased with the severity of CHF. Although a close correlation between the LV end-diastolic pressure (LVEDP) and plasma ANP in patients with LV dysfunction has been reported, it is not yet known which cardiac natriuretic peptide is a better predictor of high LVEDP in patients with CHF. To investigate the biochemical predictors of the high LVEDP in patients with LV dysfunction, Maeda and associates[9] from Otsu, Japan, measured plasma ANP, BNP, NE, and ET-1 levels and the hemodynamic parameters in 72 patients with symptomatic LV dysfunction. Stepwise multivariate regression analyses were also used to determine whether the plasma levels of ANP, BNP, NE, and ET-1 could predict high LVEDP. Although significant positive correlations were found among the plasma levels of ANP, BNP, ET-1, and NE and the LVEDP, only BNP was an independent and significant predictor of high LVEDP in patients with CHF. In all 8 patients with severe CHF measured for hemodynamics before and after the treatments, the plasma BNP levels decreased in association with the decrease of LVEDP, whereas other factors increased in some patients despite the decrease of LVEDP. These findings suggest that plasma BNP is superior to ANP as a predictor of high LVEDP in patients with symptomatic LV dysfunction.

Cellular Expression and Activity of eNOS and iNOS in Congestive Heart Failure

Fukuchi and colleagues[10] in Montreal, Quebec, Canada, investigated the cellular expression and activity of endothelial NO synthase and inducible NO synthase in human hearts with CHF. Myocardial tissues were obtained from 28 hearts with CHF with various etiologies and 4 nonfailing hearts as controls. Only weak or focal expression of both eNOS and INOS were seen in ventricles of nonfailing hearts. However, in failing hearts, immunoreactivity and hybridization signals for eNOS were increased only in cardiac myocytes of subendocardial areas. Signals for iNOS in cardiac myocytes were consistently seen in CHF of various etiologies and were apparent in both infarcted and noninfarcted regions of ischemic cardiomyopathy. Apparent signals for iNOS were also seen in infiltrating macrophages in infarcted regions of ischemic cardiomyopathy, myocarditis, and septic hearts. The expression of eNOS, but not iNOS, in the myocytes was intimately associated with β-adrenergic therapy before the operation, being more abundant in patients on β-blockers compared with diminished presence in patients on β-agonists. The iNOS activity was more variable than constitutive NOS activity and correlated significantly with the density of infiltrating macrophages. Thus, these data suggest that whereas increased eNOS and/or iNOS expression in failing cardiac myocytes may contribute to myocardial dysfunction, myocardial injury, or death associated with inflammatory lesions may be caused in part by abundant iNOS expression within infiltrating macrophages rather than the cardiac myocytes (Figure 3-2).

Elevated Circulating Levels of C-C Chemokines

Aukrust and colleagues[11] in Oslo, Norway, measured circulating levels of 3 C-C chemokines in 44 patients with CHF and in 21 healthy control subjects. Immunologic and inflammatory responses appear to play a pathogenic role in the development of CHF and activation and migration of leukocytes to areas of inflammation are important factors in these responses. C-C chemokines are potent chemoattractants of monocytes and lymphocytes, and they modulate functions of these cells. Levels of macrophage chemoattractant protein-1 (MCP-1), macrophage inflammatory protein-1α and RANTES (regulated on activation normally T cell expressed and secreted) were measured by enzyme immunoassays. CHF patients had significantly elevated levels of all chemokines with the highest levels in New York Heart Association class IV and MCP-1 and MIP-1α levels were significantly inversely correlated with LVEF. Elevated C-C chemokine levels were found independent of the cause of heart failure, but MCP-1 levels were particularly raised in patients with CAD (Figure 3-3). Studies on cells isolated from peripheral blood suggested that platelets, CD3 + lymphocytes, and monocytes might contribute to the elevated C-C chemokine levels in CHF. The increased MCP-1 levels in CHF were correlated with increased monocyte activity, reflecting an enhancing effect of serum from CHF patients. This is a first demonstration of increased circulating levels of C-C chemokines in patients with CHF.

Effect of Tumor Necrosis Factor in Congestive Heart Failure Patients

Kubota and colleagues[12] studied the prevalence of tumor necrosis factor-α gene polymorphisms in CHF patients and their correlation of genotypes to

Infarcted myocardial wall

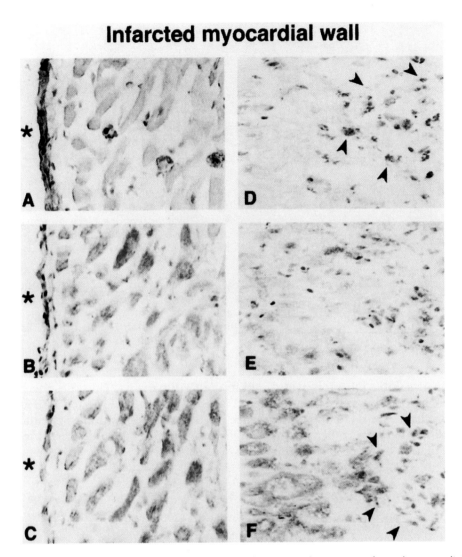

FIGURE 3-2. Immunohistochemical localization of eNOS and iNOS in infarcted myocardial wall of ischemic cardiomyopathy. **(A–F)** Different areas of the same infarcted myocardial wall: subendothelial area **(A–C)** and scarred area of deep myocardial layer **(D–F)** immunostained for von Willebrand factor **(A)**, macrophage-specific marker CD68 **(D)**, eNOS **(B and E)**, and iNOS **(C and F)** in serial sections. Note that increased immunoreactivity for eNOS was localized only in subendocardial myocytes, whereas apparent iNOS immunoreactivity was found in most surviving myocytes and infiltrating macrophages (arrowheads) of infarcted myocardial wall. Asterisk indicates intracardiac cavity. Magnification × 400. Reproduced with permission from Fukuchi et al.[10]

in vivo TNF-α levels. TNFA and TNFB genotypes were determined by the polymerase chain reaction, restriction fragment length polymorphism technique. There were no differences in the TNF allele frequencies between CHF (n = 229) patients and control subjects (n = 139). In 211 with CHF, circulating levels of TNF-α and the soluble receptors type I and type II were measured and no correlations between TNFA or TNFB genotypes and circulating levels of TNF-

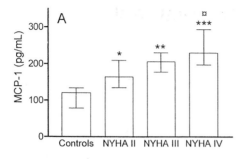
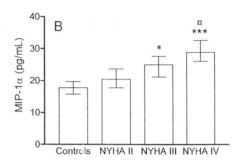
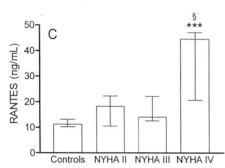

FIGURE 3-3. Circulating levels of MCP-1 **(A)**, MIP-1α **(B)**, and RANTES **(C)** in 44 CHF patients and 21 healthy control subjects as a function of severity of symptoms according to NYHA functional class (NYHA class II, n = 11; NYHA class III, n = 18; NYHA class IV, n = 15). ***p < 0.001 vs. control subjects, **p < 0.01 vs. control subjects, *p < 0.05 vs. control subjects, □ p < 0.05 vs. NYHA class II, §p < 0.05 vs. both NYHA class II and III. Data are given as medians and 25th to 75th percentiles. Reproduced with permission from Aukrust et al.[11]

α or its soluble receptors was found in the CHF patients. Thus, despite their association with other inflammatory diseases, neither TNFA nor TNFB polymorphisms are related to the presence of CHF or the elevation of circulating TNF-α. Therefore, other factors may be more important in determining the circulating levels of TNF-α in patients with CHF.

Evaluation of Anergy

Skin tests to recall antigens are performed as indicators of clinical outcomes in CHF. A diminution in the response to recall antigens, termed "anergy," is regarded as an indication of poor clinical prognosis, although little analysis has been done to support that conclusion. Vredevoe and associates[13] from Los Angeles, California, studied 222 patients with advanced CHF in New York Heart Association classes III and IV with complete data sets for all the variables. The sample was 77% men, mean age 52 ± 12 years, and LVEF, 21 ± 7. Patients with ischemic (n = 113) and idiopathic (n = 109) disease were analyzed separately. The relation of energy to 1-year mortality and selected hemodynamic factors, blood chemistries, medications, and nutritional status markers was analyzed. Anergy was present in 45% (47% idiopathic and 42% ischemic) of patients. Anergy was related to 1-year mortality (univariate) and patients with ischemic CHF had shorter survival times. Lower cholesterol, HDL, LDL, and triglycerides were predictors of mortality in idiopathic CHF. In ischemic CHF, LDL and triglycerides were univariate predictors of skin test anergy, but not mortality. Thus, there were distinct differences in clinical correlates of skin test anergy in patients with idiopathic and ischemic CHF.

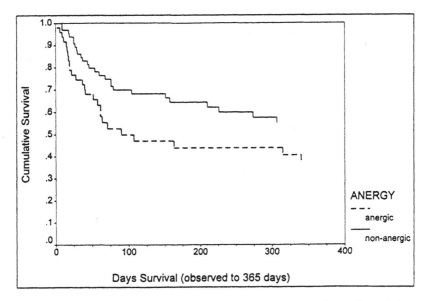

FIGURE 3-4. Survival curves for anergic noncoronary patients with ischemic heart failure. Mantel Cox test showed a significantly shorter (p = 0.035) survival for anergic patients. Reproduced with permission from Vredevoe et al.[13]

This study supports evaluation of anergy to skin tests as one of the markers of mortality in patients with ischemic CHF (Figure 3-4; Table 3-1).

Study of Heart Rate Variability and Mortality in Congestive Heart Failure

Nolan and colleagues[14] in a prospective study powered for mortality, recruited 433 patients with a mean age of 62 years with CHF (NYHA functional class I to III and with a mean LVEF of 41%). Time-domain heart rate variability indices and conventional prognostic indicators were related to death by multivariate analysis. During 482 ± 161 days of follow-up, cardiothoracic ratio, LV end-systolic diameter, and serum sodium were significant predictors of all-cause mortality. The risk ratio for a reduction in SDNN was 1.62. SDNN was defined as the standard deviation of all normal-to-normal RR intervals in the entire 24-hour recording period and represented an index of the total amount of heart rate variability present in the 24-hour recording period. The annual mortality rate for the study population in SDNN subgroups was 5.5% for greater than 100 ms, 12.7% for 50 to 100 ms, and 51.4% for less than 50 ms. SDNN, creatinine, and serum sodium were related to progressive CHF death. Cardiothoracic ratio, LV end-diastolic diameter, the presence of nonsustained VT, and serum potassium were related to sudden cardiac death. A reduction in SDNN was the most powerful predictor of the risk of death due to progressive CHF. Thus, CHF is associated with autonomic dysfunction, which can be quantified by measuring heart rate variability. A reduction in SDNN identifies pa-

Table 3-1
Comparison of Anergic and Nonanergic Groups

	Nonanergic (n = 123)	Anergic (n = 99)	p Value
Gender			
Male	93 (76)	77 (78)	0.705
Female	30 (24)	22 (22)	
New York Heart Association functional class			
III	61 (50)	29 (29)	0.002*
IV	62 (50)	70 (71)	
Etiology			
Idiopathic	58 (47)	51 (52)	0.518
Ischemic	65 (53)	48 (48)	
Angiotensin-converting enzyme inhibitors			
No	19 (15)	17 (17)	0.729
Yes	104 (85)	82 (83)	
Age	50.2 ± 11.6	53.4 ± 11.4	0.038*
Ejection fraction	21.1 ± 6.7	20.4 ± 7.3	0.550
Right atrial pressure (mm Hg)	11.3 ± 6.1	12.5 ± 6.6	0.158
Cardiac output (L/min)	3.9 ± 1.1	3.6 ± 1.3	0.112
Pulmonary capillary wedge pressure	24.4 ± 9.5	25.9 ± 9.3	0.234
Serum sodium	135.1 ± 4.6	133.4 ± 4.6	0.006*
Cholesterol	182.0 ± 58.4	156.7 ± 48.3	<0.001*
HDL	33.1 ± 13.1	30.4 ± 12.1	0.121
LDL	124.4 ± 47.5	106.0 ± 39.1	0.002*
Triglycerides	125.3 ± 74.1	104.7 ± 68.4	0.034*
Body mass index	26.1 ± 7.0	25.0 ± 8.0	0.252

* Anergy groups significantly different at $\alpha < 0.05$ using chi-square test for percentage and t test for means.
Values are expressed as number (%) or mean ± SD.
Reproduced with permission from Vredevoe et al.[13]

tients at high risk of death and is a better predictor of death due to progressive CHF than other conventional measurements (Figure 3-5).

Sleep Apnea in Patients with Stable Heart Failure

Javaheri and colleagues[15] in Cincinnati, Ohio, determined the prevalence, consequences, and differences in various sleep-related breathing disorders in ambulatory patients with stable CHF in the prospective study of 81 of 92 eligible patients with CHF and an LVEF less than 45%. There were 40 patients without and 41 patients with sleep apnea. Sleep disruption and arterial oxyhemoglobin desaturation were significantly more severe in the prevalence of atrial fibrillation, and ventricular arrhythmias were greater in the patients with sleep apnea than in those without. Forty percent of all patients had central sleep apnea and 11% had obstructive sleep apnea. The latter patients had significantly greater mean body weight and prevalence of habitual snoring (112 ± 30 vs. 75 ± 16 kg and 78% vs. 28%, respectively). However, the hourly rates of episodes of apnea and hypopnea, episodes of arousal, and desaturation were similar in patients with the different types of apnea. Thus, 51% of male patients

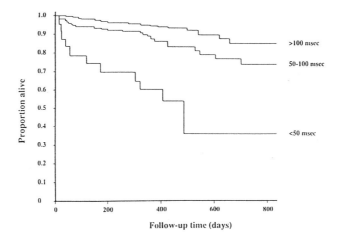

FIGURE 3-5. Kaplan-Meier survival curves in patients categorized into SDNN subgroups. P < 0.0001 for difference in survival. Reproduced with permission from Nolan et al.[14]

with stable CHF had sleep-related breathing disorders in this study: 40% from central and 11% from obstructive sleep apnea. Both types of sleep apnea resulted in sleep disruption and arterial oxyhemoglobin desaturation. Patients with sleep apnea had a higher prevalence of atrial fibrillation and ventricular arrhythmias in this study.

Amyloidosis and Congestive Heart Failure

Primary Amyloidosis

In this investigation by Dubrey and associates[16] from Boston, Massachusetts, 133 patients with biopsy-proven AL (immunocyte-derived) amyloidosis were studied with echocardiography, Holter recording, 12-lead electrocardiography, and signal-averaged electrocardiograms. Features from these tests were analyzed in relation to their effect on mortality. Late potentials were more frequent in patients with echocardiographic evidence of cardiac amyloidosis (31%) compared with patients with normal echocardiograms (9%). One hundred six of the 133 patients died during follow-up, of which 34 were nonsudden cardiac deaths and 33 were sudden deaths. Abnormal echocardiograms and signal-averaged electrocardiograms were each predictive of all-cause cardiac death and sudden cardiac death. Abnormal signal-averaged electrocardiograms were also independently predictive of sudden death in the subgroup of patients with an abnormal echocardiogram. Thus, late potentials are predictive of sudden death in patients with AL amyloidosis and provide independent prognostic information in patients with echocardiographic evidence of amyloid involvement.

Treatment

Evaluation of the Use of Vesnarinone in Congestive Heart Failure

Cohn and colleagues[17] in Minneapolis, Minnesota, enrolled 3,833 patients who had New York Heart Association class III or IV CHF and a LVEF of 30% or less despite optimal treatment to evaluate the longer-term effects of daily doses of 60 mg or 30 mg of vesnarinone as compared with placebo on mortality and morbidity. There were significantly fewer deaths in the placebo group (18.9%) than in the 60-mg vesnarinone (22.9%) and longer survival (Figure 3-6). The increase in mortality with vesnarinone was attributed to an increase in sudden death, presumed to be due to an arrhythmia. The quality of life had improved significantly more in the 60-mg vesnarinone group than in the placebo group at 8 weeks and 16 weeks after randomization. Trends in mortality and in measures of the quality of life in the 30-mg vesnarinone group were similar to those in the 60-mg group but not significantly different from those in the placebo group. Agranulocytosis occurred in 1.2% of the patients given 60 mg of vesnarinone/day and 0.2% of those given 30 mg of vesnarinone. Thus, vesnarinone is associated with a dose-dependent increase in mortality among patients with severe CHF, an increase that is probably related to an increase in arrhythmic deaths. This occurs in a situation in which there is short-term benefit in terms of the quality of life from vesnarinone.

Combined Therapy for Treatment of Severe Heart Failure

Patients with severe class IV heart failure who receive standard medical therapy exhibit a 1-year mortality rate greater than 50%. Positive inotropic agents including phosphodiesterase inhibitors are frequently given to these patients short-term although an increased mortality has been noted over the

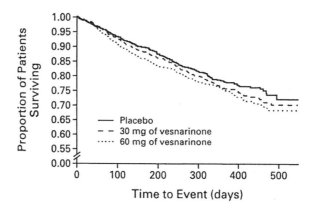

FIGURE 3-6. Survival in the 3 groups. Reproduced with permission from Cohn et al.[17]

long term. The addition of a β-blocker to positive inotropic therapy might attenuate the adverse effects. Shakar and colleagues[18] from Denver, Colorado, and Salt Lake City, Utah, evaluated 30 patients with severe CHF who were treated with a combination of oral enoximone and oral metoprolol. Enoximone was given in a dose of 1 mg/kg body weight 3 times/day. After stabilization, metoprolol was initiated at 6.25 mg twice a day and slowly titrated up to a target dose of 100–200 mg/day. Ninety six percent of the patients tolerated enoximone and 80% tolerated the addition of metoprolol. Of the 23 patients receiving the combination therapy, 48% were weaned off enoximone over the long term. LVEF increased significantly from 17.7% to 27.6% and the New York Heart Association functional class improved from 4 to 2.8. The estimated probability of survival at 1 year was 81% and heart transplantation was performed successfully in 30% of patients. These authors conclude that combination therapy with a positive inotrope and a β-blocker appear to be useful in the treatment of severe class IV heart failure. It may be used as a palliative measure when transplantation is not an option or as a bridge to heart transplantation.

Differential Effects of Fosinopril and Enalapril

To investigate the efficacy and safety of fosinopril in the treatment of chronic heart failure, Zannad and associates[19] from Nancy, France, randomly assigned patients with mild to moderate CHF and an LVEF less than 40% in a double-blind manner to receive fosinopril 5 to 20 mg every day (n = 122) or enalapril 5 to 20 mg every day (n = 132) for 1 year. The event-free survival time was longer (1.6 vs. 1.0 months) and the total rate of hospitalizations plus deaths was lower with fosinopril than with enalapril (20% vs. 25%). There was consistently better symptom improvement with fosinopril. The incidence of orthostatic hypotension was lower in the fosinopril group. Fosinopril 5 to 20 mg every day is more effective in improving symptoms and delaying events related to worsening of CHF and produces less orthostatic hypotension than enalapril 5 to 20 mg every day.

Clinical Effect of β-Blockers in Congestive Heart Failure

Lechat and colleagues[20] combined the results of all 18 published double-blind, placebo-controlled, parallel-group trials of β-blockers in patients with CHF. From this combined database of 3,023, they evaluated the strength of evidence supporting an effect of treatment on LVEF, NYHA functional class, hospitalizations for CHF and death. β-blockers exerted their most persuasive effects on LVEF and on the combined risk of death and hospitalization for CHF. β-blockade increased the LVEF by 29% and reduced the combined risk of death or hospitalization for CHF by 37%. Both effects remained significant even if more than 90% of the trials were eliminated from analysis or if a larger number of trials with a neutral result were added. In contrast, the effect of β-blockade on NYHA functional class was of borderline significance and disap-

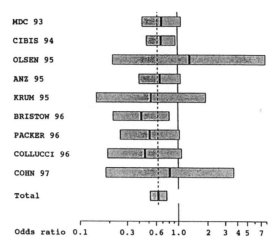

Figure 3-7. Effect of β-blockade on combined risk of all-cause mortality and hospitalizations for heart failure. Overall, β-blockers reduced risk of death or hospitalization for heart failure by 37% (p < 0.001). Reproduced with permission from Lechat et al.[20]

peared with the addition or removal of only 1 moderate-sized study. Although β-blockade reduced all-cause mortality by 32%, this effect is only modestly robust and varied according to the type of β-blocker tested, i.e., the reduction of mortality risk was greater for nonselected β-blockers than for β_1-selective agents (49% vs. 18%). However, selective and nonselective β-blockers did not differ in their effects on other measures of clinical efficacy. Thus, pooled analyses indicate that there is persuasive evidence supporting a favorable effect of β-blockade on LVEF and the combined risk of death and hospitalization for CHF (Figure 3-7).

Prospective Randomized Study of Ventricular Function and Efficacy of Digoxin (PROVED) and Randomized Assessment of Digoxin and Inhibitors of Angiotensin-Converting Enzyme (RADIANCE) Trials

Although digoxin, diuretics, and ACE-inhibitors are considered by some as standard triple therapy for heart failure, others are uncertain about the value of digoxin in this combination. Young and colleagues[21] evaluated the multicenter PROVED and RADIANCE trials to look at the potential benefit of single, double, and triple therapy in patients with CHF. A total of 266 patients comprising the 4 treatment groups of the combined PROVED and RADIANCE trials were analyzed. Worsening heart failure occurred in only 4 of the 85 patients on triple therapy (4.7%) compared to 19% on digoxin and diuretic therapy, 25% on ACE-inhibitor and diuretic therapy, and 39% on diuretics alone. Life-table and multivariate analysis also demonstrated that worsening heart failure was least likely in patients with triple therapy. These combined data provide important evidence arguing that triple therapy is the appropriate initial

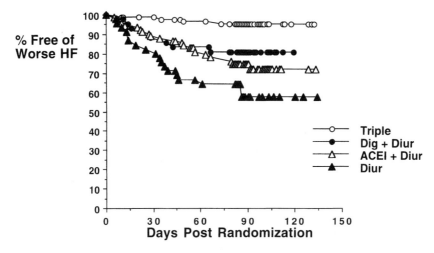

FIGURE 3-8. Superiority of triple drug therapy in heart failure. Reproduced with permission from Young et al.[21]

management of patients with symptomatic heart failure due to systolic dysfunction (Figure 3-8).

Improved Exercise Tolerance After Losartan and Enalapril in Congestive Heart Failure

Vescovo and colleagues[22] in Brescia, Italy, evaluated the impact on exercise capacity in patients with CHF treated with an angiotensin receptor antagonist (losartan) and an ACE inhibitor (enalapril). Eight patients with CHF, New York Heart Association functional classes I through IV were treated for 6 months with enalapril 20 mg/day and another 8 with losartan 50 mg/day. Exercise capacity was assessed with maximal cardiopulmonary exercise testing at baseline and after treatment. Myosin heavy chain composition of the gastrocnemius muscle was studied after electrophoretic separation of slow MHC1, fast oxidative MHC2a, and fast glycolytic MHC2b isoforms from needle biopsies obtained at baseline and after 6 months. Exercise capacity improved in both groups. Peak oxygen consumption increased from 21.0 to 27.6 mL $\cdot$ kg^{-1} $\cdot$ min^{-1} in the losartan group and from 17.5 to 25.0 mL $\cdot$ kg^{-1} $\cdot$ min^{-1} in the enalapril treated group. Ventilatory threshold changed from 15 to 20 mL with losartan and from 12 to 15 mL with enalapril. MCH1 increased from 61 to 75 with losartan and from 61 to 80 with enalapril. Similarly, MHC2a decreased with losartan and enalapril therapy. MHC2b also decreased with losartan and enalapril therapy. There was a significant correlation between net changes in MHC1 and absolute changes in peak oxygen consumption. These data suggest that 6 months after treatment with losartan and enalapril, there is an improvement in exercise capacity of similar magnitude in patients with CHF. These changes are accompanied by a reshift of myosin heavy chain of leg skeletal muscle toward the slow, more fatigue-resistant isoforms.

Losartan Versus Enalapril

In CHF, some of the effects of ACE inhibitors, such as an increase in oxygen uptake (VO_2), are mediated through prostaglandins. Angiotensin (AT_1) receptor blockers apparently do not share potentiation of this biosystem. Guazzi and associates[23] from Milano, Italy, tested whether losartin improves exercise VO_2 in CHF and if the effect is the same as for enalapril. Sixteen men with CHF and 8 volunteers, all nonsmokers and not taking ACE, AT_1 receptor, or cyclooxygenase inhibitors, were randomized to receive placebo, enalapril (10 mg 2 times daily), losartan (50 mg/day), each of these 2 drugs plus aspirin (325 mg/day), aspirin, or the same preparations in a reverse order, each for 3 weeks, with a 3-week washout period between treatments. Pulmonary function and VO_2 were assessed at the end of each treatment. In CHF, losartan and enalapril caused a similar improvement of VO_2 and exercise tolerance, which was absent in controls and was counteracted by aspirin (prostaglandin inhibitions) when obtained with enalapril and not with losartan. While on enalapril, we also detected an increase in the diffusing lung capacity for carbon monoxide, which correlated with changes in VO_2 and was antagonized by aspirin, suggesting the possibility that a prostaglandin-mediated functional improvement of the alveolar capillary membrane contributes to the rise in VO_2. Thus, losartan is as effective as enalapril for exercise VO_2 and exercise tolerance, but the mechanism seems to be dissociated from a prostaglandin biosystem activation. Losartan may represent an advancement in CHF because its efficacy on VO_2 is similar to that of enalapril, but is not antagonized by aspirin (Figure 3-9).

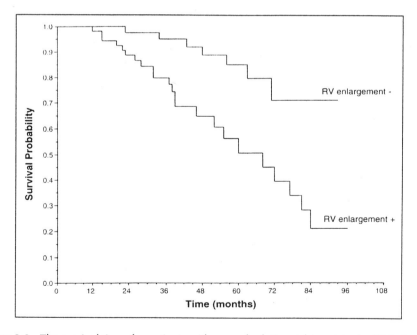

FIGURE 3-9. The survival times for patients with normal relative right ventricular (RV) chamber size (RV enlargement− group) were significantly better ($p = 0.001$) than those for patients with RV enlargement RV enlargement+ group by Kaplan-Meier survival analysis. Reproduced with permission from Guazzi et al.[23]

Comparative Effects of Losartan and Enalapril in Congestive Heart Failure

Losartan is an angiotensin receptor blocker agent that may have benefit in patients with heart failure. Lang and colleagues[24] in a multicenter trial evaluated the effects of losartan and enalapril on treadmill exercise time and the 6-minute walk test. One hundred sixteen patients with CHF classes II–IV and LVEF less than 45% were studied. After replacement of an open-label ACE inhibitor with losartan or enalapril, there was no difference in the treadmill exercise time or 6-minute walk test. These authors conclude that losartan was well tolerated and comparable to enalapril in terms of exercise tolerance in this short-term (12-week) study of patients with heart failure.

Interaction of Aspirin and Ticlopidine with Enalapril

Spaulding and colleagues[25] evaluated potential interactions between aspirin and ACE inhibitors compared to interactions between ticlopidine and ACE inhibitors. The objective of this study was to compare the influence of co-administration of ticlopidine or aspirin on the hemodynamic effects of an ACE inhibitor (enalapril) in patients with CHF. Twenty patients with severe CHF were enrolled in a double-blind comparative trial and randomized to ticlopidine (500 mg daily) or aspirin (325 mg daily). Hemodynamic evaluation was performed after 7 days of treatment, every hour for 4 hours after an oral administration of 10 mg of enalapril. Significant reductions in systemic vascular resistance were observed in the ticlopidine group in contrast to no significant decrease in the aspirin group. A significant time-by-treatment interaction indicated significant aspirin–enalapril drug interaction. Total pulmonary resistance decreased significantly in both groups with no differences between patients assigned to aspirin or ticlopidine. Thus, enalapril reduces systemic vascular resistance more effectively when given in combination with ticlopidine than with aspirin (Figure 3-10). Negative aspirin-enalapril prostaglandin synthesis presumably alters vasodilatation in systemic vessels, whereas prostaglandin-independent actions of ACE inhibition, such as pulmonary arterial vasodilatation, may be maintained.

Digitalization for Systolic Heart Failure

The efficacy of short-term digitalization on exercise tolerance may, in part, reflect enhanced diastolic performance. However, cardiac glycosides can impair ventricular relaxation from cytosolic Ca^{++} overload. To detect any time-dependent adverse effect, Hassopoyannes and associates[26] from Columbia, South Carolina, assessed the diastolic function after long-term use of digitalis in patients with mild to moderate systolic LV failure. From a cohort of 80 patients who received long-term, randomized, double-blind treatment with digitalis versus placebo, 38 survivors were evaluated at the end of follow-up (mean

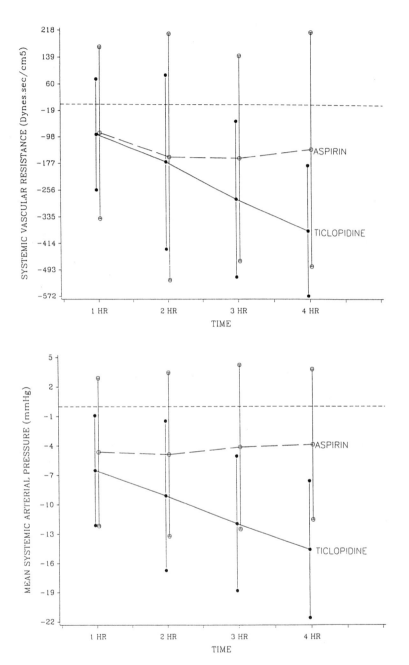

FIGURE 3-10. Summary plots of mean changes in systemic vascular resistance and MPA. Values plotted are mean change from baseline with 95% nonadjusted confidence intervals. Resistance is expressed in dyne · s · cm⁻⁵, pressure in mm Hg, and time in hours after administration of enalapril. Consistent decrease in systemic vascular resistance was noted in patients receiving ticlopidine, with significant reductions 3 and 4 hours after enalapril intake. In contrast, nonsignificant decreases in systemic vascular resistance were noted in the aspirin group, with a significant time-by-treatment interaction (p = 0.03), indicating significant aspirin-enalapril drug interaction. Consistent significant decrease in mean systemic arterial pressure was noted in the ticlopidine group, with no significant reductions in the aspirin group, resulting in a significant difference between the 2 groups (p = 0.02). Reproduced with permission from Spaulding et al.[25]

48 months) with evaluators blinded to treatment used. Each survivor underwent equilibrium scintigraphic and echocardiographic assessment of diastolic function. Peak and mean filling rates normalized with filling volume, diastolic phase durations normalized with duration of diastole, and filling fractions were measured from the time–activity curve. The isovolumic relaxation period and ventricular dimensions were computed echocardiographically. By actual-treatment-received analysis, treated versus untreated patients manifested a trend toward longer isovolumic relaxation but a markedly lower peak rapid filling rate despite comparable loading conditions. In addition, treated patients exhibited a lower mean rate of rapid filling in the absence of a longer rapid filling duration. However, the end-diastolic ventricular dimension did not differ between the 2 groups. Similar results were obtained by intention-to-treat analysis. Importantly, the mortality rate from worsening heart failure in the inception cohort was lower in the digitalis group versus the placebo group with no difference in total cardiac or all-cause mortality. After long-term digitalization for systolic LV failure, cross-sectional comparison with a control group from the same inception cohort shows a decrease in the rate and degree of ventricular relaxation. This effect did not interfere with the overall ventricular filling or with a favorable impact on outcome from worsening heart failure.

Effect of Digitalis on Brain Natriuretic Peptide

Ouabain can cause increased secretion of atrial natriuretic peptide (ANP) from atrial cardiocyte culture, but the effects of digitalis in a therapeutic range on the secretion of cardiac natriuretic peptide, including ANP and brain natriuretic peptide (BNP), mainly from the ventricle, in patients with CHF remain to be investigated. Therefore, Tsutamoto and associates[27] from Otsu, Japan, studied the acute effects of intravenous infusion of a relatively low dose of digitalis or placebo on hemodynamics and neurohumoral factors including the plasma levels of ANP and BNP and cyclic guanosine monophosphate, a second messenger of cardiac natriuretic peptide, in 13 patients with severe CHF. No significant change in the hemodynamic parameters or neurohumoral factors was observed with placebo. After 1 hour of intravenous administration of deslanoside (0.01 mg/kg), there was a significant decrease of plasma renin activity and angiotensin II, aldosterone, and norepinephrine levels, but no significant change of plasma levels of vasopressin. There was a significant decrease of the PA wedge pressure but no significant change in cardiac index. In addition, plasma levels of ANP (217 ± 47 vs. 281 ± 70 pg/mL), BNP (628 ± 116 vs. 689 ± 132 pg/mL), and cyclic guanosine monophosphate (9.7 ± 1.1 vs. 11 ± 1.5 pmol/mL) increased despite the decrease of PA wedge pressure (20 ± 2.3 vs. 17 ± 2.3 mm Hg). These results indicate that the acute intravenous low dose of digitalis resulted in a significant increase in plasma levels of ANP, BNP, and cyclic guanosine monophosphate concomitant with the significant decrease of PA wedge pressure, suggesting the acute direct action of digitalis on the cardiac natriuretic peptides released from the heart in patients with severe CHF.

Digoxin Withdrawal

Previous work provides limited information concerning predictors of clinical deterioration after digoxin withdrawal. Adams and associates[28] from Chapel Hill, North Carolina; Chicago, Illinois; Galveston, Texas; Cleveland, Ohio; and New York, New York, investigated the association between selected baseline clinical characteristics and symptomatic deterioration in 2 similarly designed trials: Prospective Randomized Study of Ventricular Function and Efficacy of Digoxin (PROVED) and Randomized Assessment of Digoxin and Inhibitors of Angiotensin-Converting Enzyme (RADIANCE). Cox proportional hazards analysis found the following independent predictors of worsening heart failure during follow-up in the combined PROVED and RADIANCE patients: heart failure score, LVEF, cardiothoracic ratio, use of an angiotensin-converting enzyme inhibitor, use of digoxin, and age. When these factors, except for digoxin use, were tested in the subgroup of patients withdrawn from digoxin, they all were significant independent predictors of worsening heart failure. In contrast, only use of angiotensin-converting enzyme inhibitor predicted deterioration in patients who continued digoxin. Patients with more congestive symptoms, worse ventricular function, greater cardiac enlargement, or who were not taking an angiotensin-converting enzyme inhibitor were significantly more likely to worsen early after digoxin discontinuation than patients without these characteristics.

Warfarin Anticoagulation and Survival

In patients who have AF or who have had a large AMI, anticoagulation with warfarin appears to play an important clinical role. Al-Khadra and associates[29] from Boston, Massachusetts, evaluated the potential of warfarin anticoagulation in patients with LV dysfunction. They reviewed data on warfarin use in 6,797 patients enrolled in the studies of LV dysfunction (SOLVD) and analyzed the relation between warfarin use and all-cause mortality. On multivariate analysis, use of warfarin was associated with a significant reduction in all-cause mortality and in the risk of death or hospital readmission for CHF. Risk reduction was observed when each trial or randomization arm was analyzed separately, as well as in both genders. It was not significantly influenced by the presence of AF, age, EF, New York Heart Association functional class, or etiology. These authors conclude that in patients with LV systolic dysfunction, warfarin use is associated with improved survival and reduced morbidity. This association is due primarily to a reduction in cardiac events and does not appear to be limited to any particular subgroup (Figure 3-11).

Emotional Support for Elderly Heart Failure Patients

Krumholz and colleagues[30] in New Haven, Connecticut, attempted to determine whether emotional support is associated with fatal and nonfatal

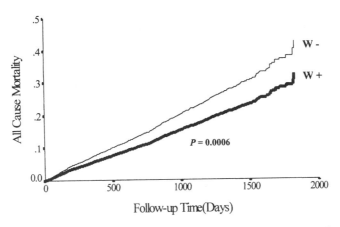

FIGURE 3-11. Use of warfarin anticoagulant in LV dysfunction. Reproduced with permission from Al-Khadra et al.[29]

cardiovascular events in elderly patients hospitalized with CHF. They reviewed the medical records of 292 subjects aged 65 years or older, hospitalized with clinical CHF and who were part of the New Haven, Connecticut, cohort of the Established Population for the Epidemiologic Study of the Elderly, a longitudinal, community-based study of aging that included a comprehensive assessment of psychosocial support. Lack of emotional support was significantly associated with the 1-year risk of fatal and nonfatal cardiovascular outcome. After adjustment for demographic factors, clinical severity, co-morbidity, and functional status, social ties, and instrumental support, the absence of emotional support remained associated with a significantly higher risk (Figure 3-12). The test for interaction between emotional support and gender was significant. In the fully adjusted model, the odds ratio for women was 8.2 compared with 1.0 for men. Among elderly patients hospitalized with clinical CHF, the absence of emotional support measured before admission is a strong indepen-

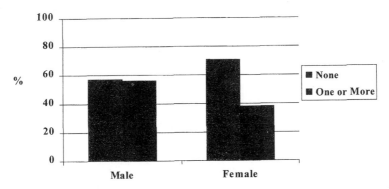

FIGURE 3-12. The association between emotional support (none vs. 1 or more) and the incidence of 1-year cardiovascular events, by gender. Reproduced with permission from Krumholz et al.[30]

dent predictor of the occurrence of fatal and nonfatal cardiovascular events in the year after admission. In this study, the associated was restricted to women.

Evaluation of Pacing Sites in Heart Failure Patients

Blanc and colleagues[31] compared the acute hemodynamic changes associated with pacing the RV apex or outflow tract alone, LV pacing alone, or biventricular pacing of the RV apex and the left ventricle together in 27 patients with severe CHF despite optimal therapy in either first degree AV block and/or an intraventricular conduction defect. In the 23 patients with a high pulmonary capillary wedge pressure greater than 15 mm Hg, data were collected after transvenous pacing at different ventricular sites in either the AV sequential or the ventricular pacing mode. The latter was used in patients with atrial fibrillation and included 6 patients. The mean baseline cardiac index was 1.82 L/min, pulmonary capillary wedge pressure 26 ± 6.6 mm Hg, and V-wave amplitude 39 ± 14.6 mm Hg, and they were similar before and after either pacing from the RV apex or from the RV outflow tract. In contrast, LV-based pacing, either LV pacing alone or both RV and LV pacing, resulted in higher systolic blood pressure and lower pulmonary capillary wedge pressure and V-wave amplitude than either baseline or RV pacing measurements (Figure 3-13). With LV pacing alone, systolic blood pressure, pulmonary capillary wedge pressure, and V waves were 126.5 ± 15.1, 20.7 ± 5.9, and 25.5 ± 8.1 mm Hg, respectively. The results with LV pacing alone were similar to those obtained with biventricular

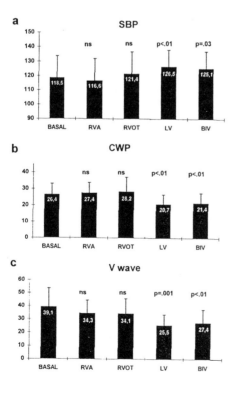

FIGURE 3-13. Changes in hemodynamic parameters induced by pacing at each ventricular site (RVA = right ventricular apex; RVOT = right ventricular outflow tract; LV = left ventricular free wall; BIV = biventricular) compared with baseline. Values are mean ± SD: systolic blood pressure (SBP) (a), capillary wedge pressure (CWP) (b), and V-wave amplitude (c). Reproduced with permission from Blanc et al.[31]

pacing. Thus, in patients with severe CHF, both LV pacing alone and biventricular pacing result in a similar and significant improvement in cardiac hemodynamics. These results provide a basis for initiating longer-term studies examining the chronic effects of these pacing modalities in patients with severe CHF.

Effect of Amlodipine in Chronic Heart Failure

The role of calcium antagonists in patients with ischemic heart failure is currently unclear. Walsh and associates[32] from Nottingham, United Kingdom, examined the effects of amlodipine on exercise capacity and central and regional hemodynamics in 32 patients with mild to moderate chronic heart failure in a single-center, double-blind, randomized placebo-controlled trial. All were taking at least 40 mg of furosemide daily with an angiotensin-converting enzyme inhibitor. Ischemic heart disease was the most common cause of heart failure, but no patient had symptom-limiting angina. Mean treadmill exercise capacity in patients taking amlodipine increased by 96 seconds and 50 seconds in the placebo group; mean difference in change between treatments was 70 seconds. Active treatment with amlodipine did not affect self-paced corridor walking times. Similarly, there were no significant effects on cardiac output, oxygen uptake, heart rate, and mean arterial pressure at rest or during exercise. Calf and renal blood flow were also unchanged by treatment. The lack of significant effect demonstrated by these data suggests a limited role for amlodipine in patients with ischemic cardiomyopathy, although it may prove beneficial in those with nonischemic disease. More data are required before amlodipine can be recommended for all patients with chronic heart failure.

Trends in Treatment of Heart Failure

Since 1987, publications in widely circulated medical journals have reported improved survival and lower hospital readmission rates when patients with heart failure and systolic dysfunction are treated with ACE inhibitors. McDermott and associates[33] from Chicago, Illinois, describe changes in ACE inhibitor use among patients hospitalized with heart failure between 1986 and 1993. Simultaneous trends in readmissions and survival rates are reported. Subjects were 612 consecutive patients hospitalized with a principal diagnosis of heart failure at an academic medical center during the period of September 1, 1986, to December 31, 1987 (interval I), or during the period August 1, 1992, to November 30, 1993 (interval II). Medical records were reviewed for 434 patients, consisting of all patients hospitalized with heart failure during interval II and a randomly selected 50% subset of patients hospitalized during interval I. Among 145 patients with systolic dysfunction whose medical records were reviewed, ACE inhibitor prescriptions significantly increased between interval I and interval II (43% vs. 71%). Prescriptions of ACE inhibitors combined with digoxin and a diuretic also increased (37% vs. 56%). Among all 612 patients, 6-month heart failure readmission rates increased from 13% to 21%.

There was no significant change in survival rate between interval I and interval II; however, survival rate was marginally significantly improved among patients with systolic dysfunction. These results suggest that drug-prescribing practices have significantly changed between 1986 and 1993. The absence of observed improvement in outcomes may result from changes in hospital admission criteria for heart failure.

Effects of Dopamine Usage in Congestive Heart Failure

van de Borne and colleagues[34] in Iowa City, Iowa, determined the effects of dopamine given as 5 μg/kg/min and placebo infusion on oxygen saturation, minute ventilation, and sympathetic nerve activity during normoxia and 5 minutes of hypoxia in 10 normal young subjects. They further investigated the effects of dopamine and placebo on minute ventilation during normoxic breathing in 8 patients with severe CHF and in 8 age-matched controls. Dopamine did not decrease minute ventilation during normoxia in normal subjects. During hypoxia, minute ventilation was 12.9 $\pm$ 1.3 L/min on dopamine and 15.8 $\pm$ 1.5 L/min on placebo. Oxygen saturation during hypoxia was lower with dopamine than with placebo. Sympathetic nerve activity during hypoxia was not enhanced with dopamine despite the lower oxygen saturation. Subjects were able to maintain a voluntary apnea to a lower oxygen saturation on dopamine than on placebo. In patients with CHF breathing room air, but not in age-matched control subjects, dopamine decreased minute ventilation despite decreased oxygen saturation and increased PETCO$_2$ during dopamine. Thus, dopamine inhibits chemoreflex responses during hypoxic breathing in normal humans, preferentially affecting the ventilatory response more than the sympathetic response. Dopamine also depresses ventilation in normoxic patients with CHF breathing room air (Figure 3-14). Ventilatory inhibition by low-dose dopamine may adversely influence outcome in hypoxic patients, especially in those with CHF.

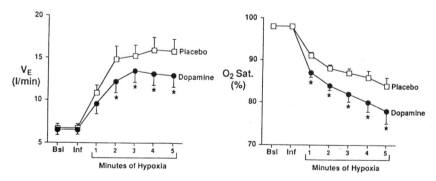

FIGURE 3-14. Effects of dopamine on responses to hypoxia. Values are mean $\pm$ SEM for placebo □ and dopamine ●. Measurements are shown for baseline values before start of infusion (Bsl), during infusion (Inf), and during all 5 minutes of hypoxia. Measurements are shown for minute ventilation (V$_E$, **left**) and oxygen saturation (O$_2$ sat, **right**). Dopamine depressed ventilatory response to hypoxia and was associated with lower levels of oxygen saturation during hypoxia versus placebo (*p < 0.008). Reproduced with permission from van de Borne et al.[34]

Effects of Intracoronary Infusion of Cocaine

Pitts and colleagues[35] in Dallas, Texas, assessed the influence of a high intracoronary cocaine concentration on LV systolic and diastolic function in 20 patients, 14 men and 6 women ranging in ages from 39 to 72 years, referred for cardiac catheterization for the evaluation of chest pain. They measured heart rate, systemic arterial pressure, LV pressure and its first derivative (dP/dt), and LV volumes and ejection fraction before and during the final 2 to 3 minutes of a 15-minute intracoronary infusion of saline (n = 10 control subjects) or cocaine hydrochloride 1 mg/min (n = 10). No variable changed with saline. With cocaine, the drug concentration in blood obtained from the coronary sinus was 3.0 ± 0.4 (mean ± SD) mg/L, and similar in magnitude to the blood cocaine concentration reported in abusers dying of cocaine intoxication. Cocaine induced no significant change in heart rate, LV dP/dt, or LV end-diastolic volume, but it caused an increase in LV systolic and mean arterial pressures, LV end-diastolic pressure, and LV end-systolic volume, as well as a decrease in ejection fraction. Thus, in humans, the intracoronary infusion of cocaine in amounts similar to those obtained in humans using cocaine, cause a deterioration of LV systolic and diastolic performance (Figure 3-15).

Heart Rate Variability in Congestive Heart Failure Patients

Some antiarrhythmic agents that may increase mortality rates have been shown to reduce heart rate variability in patients with heart failure. Amiodarone is a potent antiarrhythmic agent that may reduce mortality rates in heart failure, but little is known about its effects on heart rate variability. The purpose of this study by Rohde and associates[36] from Porto Alegre, Brazil, was to evalu-

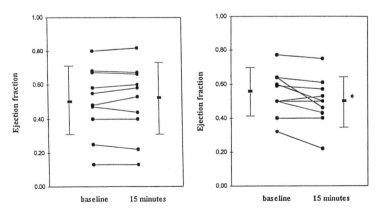

FIGURE 3-15. Left ventricular ejection fraction before and after an intracoronary saline **(left)** or cocaine **(right)** infusion. Each line represents the data from 1 patient, and mean ± 1 SD values are shown on either side of each set of lines. Left ventricular ejection fraction decreased with intracoronary cocaine (*p = 0.03 compared with baseline). Reproduced with permission from Pitts et al.[35]

ate the effect of partial arrhythmia suppression by amiodarone on indexes of heart rate variability in patients with heart failure. Ten clinically stable patients in New York Heart Association class II–III received amiodarone during a 4-week period (600 mg/day for 14 days and 300 mg/day for 16 days), and 24-hour Holter recordings were performed before and after treatment. Heart rate variability indexes were calculated by a semiautomatic method that applies a 20% filter to the temporal series, excluding ectopy and compensatory pauses. After amiodarone administration, there was a significant reduction in pNN50 from 8% ± 7% to 3% ± 2% and there was a trend toward reduction in rMSSD. Other time domain indexes did not change significantly. Special analysis demonstrated a significant reduction of low-frequency components and total power. Multivariate analysis showed that the observed reduction in pNN50 was strongly associated with the number and the reduction of ventricular premature contractions before and after amiodarone administration. These findings indicate that despite the use of software corrections for arrhythmia, short-term domain indexes of heart rate variability may be affected by partial suppression of ectopy.

Elevation of Neurohormones in Patients with Congestive Heart Failure

Many neurohormones have been reported to be elevated in patients with CHF and to have prognostic significance. Tsutamoto and colleagues[37] from Otsu, Japan, evaluated the levels of interleukin-6 in the peripheral circulation in patients with CHF. Plasma IL-6 levels increased significantly from the femoral artery to the femoral vein in normal subjects and in patients with CHF. IL-6 spillover in the leg increased with the severity of the heart failure. Among the hemodynamic variables and various neurohumoral factors, the plasma norepinephrine level showed an independent and significant positive relation with plasma IL-6 level in patients with CHF. Moreover, treatment with β-adrenergic blocking agents showed an independent and significant negative relation with plasma IL-6 levels. In 100 patients, plasma IL-6, norepinephrine, and LVEF were significant independent prognostic predictors. These authors conclude that IL-6 spillover in the peripheral circulation increases with the severity of CHF and the increase in plasma IL-6 is mainly associated with activation of the sympathetic nervous system. High plasma levels of IL-6 can provide prognostic information in patients with CHF (Figure 3-16).

Exercise and Congestive Heart Failure

Improvement of Exercise Capacity

In patients with LV dysfunction, one of the aims of therapy may be to improve functional capacity. This study by Williams and associates[38] from Cleveland, Ohio, compared the improvement of functional capacity in response

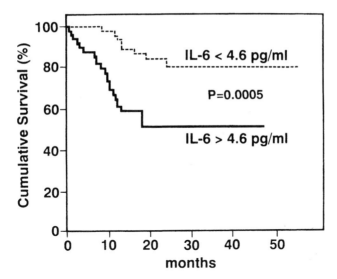

FIGURE 3-16. Interleukin-6 spillover in the peripheral circulation of patients with CHF. Reproduced with permission from Tsutamoto et al.[37]

to medical therapy with that caused by revascularization. Fifty-two patients with severe LV dysfunction were divided into groups with ischemic cardiomyopathy undergoing revascularization (group A, n = 20) or incremental medical treatment (group B, n = 16) and a control group receiving maximal medical therapy at the start of the study (group C, n = 16). All patients underwent a baseline metabolic exercise test with evaluation of peak oxygen consumption and derived exercise capacity in metabolic equivalents (METS) with standard electrocardiographic and hemodynamic monitoring. Therapy was then optimized in the medical treatment group, whereas the revascularization group underwent coronary bypass grafting. All patient subsequently underwent follow-up metabolic exercise testing. In groups A, B, and C, resting LVEFs were comparable, as were results of initial metabolic exercise tests. At follow-up, group A improved exercise capacity from 4.7 to 5.6 METS. Groups B (4.7 to 5.0 METS) and C (5.2 to 5.6 METS) had no significant improvement. The mean respiratory exchange ratio improved significantly in group A, as did LVEF (26% to 31%). However, neither parameter changed significantly in groups B or C. In patients with severe LV dysfunction, improvements of exercise capacity are more marked after coronary revascularization than may be obtained after maximization of medical therapy.

Exercise Training to Improve Left Ventricular Function

Exercise training can improve LV function as well as functional capacity in patients with a previous AMI and LV dysfunction. If the magnitude of this improvement is related to the extent of hibernating myocardium, it is possible that tests demonstrating hibernating myocardium might be helpful in predicting which patients will improve after exercise training. Belardinelli and colleagues[39] from Ancona, Italy, studied 71 consecutive patients with CHF secondary to ischemic cardiomyopathy. Thirty six patients underwent exercise training 3 times/week for 10 weeks whereas 35 patients did not exercise. Low-dose dobutamine stress echocardiography was positive in 317 of 576 patients who underwent exercise training and 291 of 560 patients who did not. The presence of a positive test at baseline was associated with a sensitivity of 70% and a specificity of 77% for predicting an increase in functional capacity after exercise training. Positive and negative predictive values of dobutamine stress echocardiography were 84% and 59%, respectively. These authors conclude that the presence of hibernating myocardium as demonstrated by low-dose dobutamine stress echocardiography can predict the magnitude of improvement in functional capacity after moderate exercise training in the patients with CHF. Similarly, a significant increase in functional capacity after exercise training is associated with a lower incidence of cardiac events during follow-up.

Hypertrophic Cardiomyopathy

Hypertrophy in Athletes

Douglas and associates[40] from 3 US medical centers examined 235 athletes participating in the Hawaii Ironman Triathlon between 1985 and 1995. Each was studied within 1 week of competition at the peak of their training. All athletes were white and were selected on the basis of their willingness to volunteer for the study. The study evaluated 168 men, mean age 40 ± 1, and 67 women, mean age 39 ± 1. The athletes trained an average of 21 hours per week, including approximately 8 km swimming, 330 km cycling, and 75 km running. Fifty-eight percent of the athletes supplemented swim-bike-run training with weight lifting, usually 2 or 3 sessions/week. All subjects underwent M-mode, 2-dimensional, and Doppler echocardiography. Comparison of men and women revealed similar heart rates and higher systolic but not diastolic blood pressures in men. Average values for all cardiac dimensions were within normal limits for all groups. Most values were greater in men than in women. Older athletes had slightly but significantly lower early-late diastolic flow velocities and slower deceleration of rapid filling than did younger athletes. Although mild elevations in cardiac dimensions were common, marked increases were rare except for LV mass. Left ventricular cavity size was increased more often than wall thickness. About one-fourth of the athletes met gender-specific cutoffs for LV hypertrophy. The prevalence of LV hypertrophy was greater among women compared to men. Thus, LV wall thickness more than 1.3 cm, septal-2-posterior wall thickness ratios more than 1.5, diastolic LV size more than 6.0 cm, and eccentric or concentric remodeling were rare in the athletes. Values outside of these cutoffs in an athlete of any age probably represent a pathologic state (Tables 3-2, 3-3).

TABLE 3-2
Demographics, Left Ventricular Dimensions, and Mass

	All Subjects (n = 235)	Men (n = 168)	Women (n = 67)	Age <40 (n = 140 [102 m, 38 w])	Age ≥40 (n = 95 [66 m, 29 w])
Age (yr)	39 ± 1 (18–74)	40 ± 1 (18–74)	39 ± 1 (20–62)	30 ± 1 (18–39)	53 ± 1 (40–74)
Heart rate (beat/min)	57 ± 1 (36–92)	57 ± 1 (36–92)	56 ± 2 (36–76)	57 ± 1 (38–92)	56 ± 2 (36–76)
SBP (mm Hg)	122 ± 1 (85–156)	124 ± 1 (85–156)	116 ± 2* (90–156)	122 ± 1 (85–156)	122 ± 2 (85–155)
DBP (mm Hg)	74 ± 1 (40–100)	75 ± 1 (40–100)	73 ± 2 (40–100)	74 ± 1 (40–100)	74 ± 1 (40–100)
BSA (m²)	1.81 ± 0.01 (1.38–2.24)	1.91 ± 0.01 (1.59–2.24)	1.62 ± 0.01* (1.38–1.94)	1.85 ± 0.02 (1.45–2.24)	1.80 ± 0.02 (1.38–2.16)
Height (m)	1.76 ± 0.01 (1.39–2.11)	1.79 ± 0.01 (1.47–2.11)	1.67 ± 0.01* (1.40–1.83)	1.77 ± 0.01 (1.54–2.11)	1.73 ± 0.01† (1.39–1.93)
Left atrium (cm)	3.5 ± 0.3 (2.3–5.2)	3.7 ± 0.3 (2.3–4.6)	3.2 ± 0.05* (2.4–5.2)	3.5 ± 0.04 (2.4–5.2)	3.58 ± 0.05 (2.3–4.6)
Septum (cm)	1.0 ± 0.01 (0.6–1.4)	1.0 ± 0.01 (0.6–1.4)	0.9 ± 0.02* (0.6–1.2)	1.0 ± 0.01 (0.6–1.2)	1.0 ± 0.02 (0.6–1.4)
PW (cm)	0.9 ± 0.01 (0.7–1.4)	0.9 ± 0.01 (0.7–1.4)	0.8 ± 0.01* (0.7–1.1)	0.6 ± 0.1 (0.7–1.4)	0.9 ± 0.01 (0.7–1.1)
Septum/PW ratio	1.07 ± 0.01 (0.8–1.5)	1.07 ± 0.01 (0.8–1.5)	1.07 ± 0.01 (0.9–1.3)	1.08 ± 0.01 (0.8–1.4)	1.06 ± 0.01 (0.8–1.5)
LVID diastole (cm)	5.2 ± 0.4 (4.0–6.5)	5.4 ± 0.3 (4.2–6.5)	4.8 ± 0.05* (4.0–5.5)	5.2 ± 0.04 (4.0–6.4)	5.1 ± 0.05 (4.0–6.5)
RWT	0.35 ± 0.003 (0.24–0.54)	0.35 ± 0.003 (0.24–0.54)	0.36 ± 0.01 (0.27–0.54)	0.35 ± 0.004 (0.27–0.47)	0.35 ± 0.005 (0.24–0.54)
LV mass (g)	232 ± 4 (105–480)	249 ± 5 (105–480)	189 ± 5* (111–291)	237 ± 5 (110–480)	225 ± 6 (105–384)
LV mass/BSA	127 ± 2 (64–219)	131 ± 2 (64–219)	115 ± 3* (68–170)	127 ± 2 (68–219)	126 ± 3 (64–203)
LV mass/height	132 ± 2 (64–249)	140 ± 2 (64–249)	113 ± 3* (68–168)	134 ± 3 (68–249)	130 ± 3 (64–216)

* p <0.05 versus men; †p <0.05 versus age <40.
Values are expressed as mean ± SEM (range).
BSA = body surface area; DBP = diastolic blood pressure; LV = left ventricular; LVID = left ventricular internal dimension; PW = posterior wall; RWT = relative wall thickness; SBP = systolic blood pressure.
Reproduced with permission from Douglas et al.[40]

Use of Handgrip Apexcardiographic Test

Manolas and associates[41] from Athens, Greece, have previously shown that the handgrip apexcardiographic test (HAT) is a useful method for detecting LV diastolic abnormalities in patients with CAD and in those with systemic hypertension. In the present study, they evaluated the use of HAT for assessing the prevalence and types of exercise-induced LV diastolic abnormalities in patients with obstructive (n = 31) and nonobstructive (n = 35) hypertrophic cardiomyopathy (HC), as well as its potential value for separating healthy subjects and athletes from patients with HC. The authors obtained an HAT in 66 consecutive patients with HC and in 72 controls (52 healthy volunteers and 20 athletes). A positive HAT was defined by the presence of 1 of the following: (1) relative A wave to total height (A/H) during or after handgrip greater than 21% (compliance type), (2) total apexcardiographic relaxation time (TART) greater

TABLE 3-3
Prevalence of Abnormal Left Ventricular Dimension and Mass

	All Subjects	Men	Women	Age <40 (all)	Age ≥40 (all)	Age <40 (men)	Age ≥40 (men)	Age ≤40 (women)	Age ≥40 (women)
LA >4.0 cm	34 (17%)	33 (22%)	1 (2%)§	16 (11%)	18 (19%)	15 (16%)	18 (32%)	1 (3%)	0
Septum >1.1 cm	32 (16%)	29 (20%)	3 (5%)§	20 (14%)	12 (13%)	19 (20%)	10 (17%)	1 (3%)	2 (8%)
Septum ≥1.3 cm	2 (1%)	2 (1%)	0	0	2 (1%)	0	2 (3%)	0	0
PW >1.1 cm	7 (3%)	5 (3%)	2 (4%)	6 (4%)	1 (1%)	5 (5%)	0	1 (3%)	1 (4%)
PW ≥1.3 cm	1 (0.5%)	1 (0.5%)	0	1 (0.5%)	0	1 (1%)	0	0	0
Septum/PW >1.3	4 (2%)	3 (2%)	1 (2%)	3 (2%)	1 (1%)	2 (2%)	1 (2%)	1 (3%)	0
LVID >5.5 cm	61 (30%)	60 (41%)	1 (2%)§	43 (30%)	18 (19%)	42 (46%)	18 (32%)	1 (3%)	0
LVID >6.0 cm	14 (7%)	14 (10%)	0§	10 (7%)	4 (4%)	10 (11%)	4 (7%)	0	0
RWT <0.30	15 (7%)	13 (9%)	2 (4%)	11 (9%)	4 (5%)	9 (10%)	4 (7%)	1 (3%)	1 (4%)
RWT ≥0.45	4 (2%)	3 (2%)	1 (1%)	3 (2%)	1 (1%)	3 (3%)	0	0	1 (4%)
LV mass*	49 (24%)	25 (17%)	24 (43%)§	29 (24%)	20 (24%)	19 (20%)	6 (11%)	10 (33%)	14 (54%)
LV mass/BSA†	55 (27%)	33 (22%)	22 (39%)§	30 (25%)	25 (30%)	22 (24%)	11 (20%)	8 (27%)	14 (54%)
LV mass/height‡	45 (22%)	25 (17%)	20 (36%)§	26 (21%)	19 (23%)	18 (20%)	7 (12%)	8 (27%)	12 (46%)

* Left ventricular mass >294 g in men or >198 g in women.
† Left ventricular mass body surface area >150 g in men or >120 g in women.
‡ Left ventricular mass/hour >163 g/m in men or >121 g/m in women.
§ p ≤0.05 women versus men.
Reproduced with permission from Douglas et al.[40]

than 143 ms or the heart rate corrected TART (TART1) during handgrip greater than 0.14, (relaxation type), (3) both types present (mixed type), and (4) diastolic amplitude time index (DATI = TART1/[A/D]) during handgrip greater than 0.27. Of the controls, only 1 of 52 healthy subjects and 1 of 20 athletes showed a positive HAT, whereas of the total HC cohort, 63 of 66 patients (95%) had a positive result. There was no significant difference in the distribution of these types between obstructive and nonobstructive HC. Further, no LV diastolic abnormalities were present in 10 of 35 patients (29%) with nonobstructive HC at rest and 3 of 35 patients (9%) during handgrip, whereas of the patients with obstructive HC, only 1 of 31 (3%) had no LV diastolic abnormalities at rest and none during handgrip. Based on HAT data, our study demonstrates that in HC (1) LV diastolic abnormalities are very frequent during handgrip; (2) patients with nonobstructive HC show significantly fewer LV diastolic abnormalities at rest than those with obstructive HC; and (3) no significant difference exists between obstructive and nonobstructive HC in the prevalence of types of handgrip-induced LV diastolic abnormalities. Consequently, HAT appears to be of clinical value as an additional tool for separating normal patients and athletes from patients with HC.

Prognostic Value of Dipyridamole-Induced Ischemia

Lazzeroni and colleagues[42] in Pisa, Italy, assessed the relative prevalence and the prognostic value of dipyridamole-induced ischemia in 79 patients with

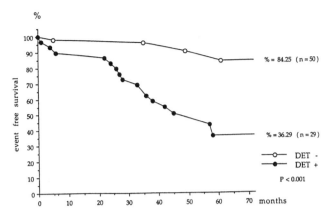

%

FIGURE 3-17. Kaplan-Meier curve indicating the cumulative event-free survival rates in patients with a positive dipyridamole echocardiographic–ECG test (DET +) and in patients with a negative test (DET –). Reproduced with permission from Lazzeroni et al.[42]

HC and without concomitant CAD, including 53 men with a mean age of 46 ± 15 years. They underwent a high-dose dipyridamole test with 12-lead electrocardiography and 2-dimensional echo monitoring and were followed for a mean of 6 years. Twenty-nine patients (37%) showed electrocardiographic signs of myocardial ischemia, including ST segment depression ≥2 mV. Fifty patients had a negative test. No patient had transient wall motion abnormalities during the dipyridamole test. During the follow-up, 16 events occurred in 29 patients among those with electrocardiographic evidence of ischemia during dipyridamole testing and in 5 of 50 patients who had no evidence of ischemia during dipyridamole testing. Patients with a positive dipyridamole test showed a poorer 72-month event-free survival rate compared with patients with a negative test (Figure 3-17). A forward stepwise event-free survival analysis identified dipyridamole test positivity by electrocardiographic criteria, rest gradient, and age as independent and additive predictors of subsequent events. Thus, these data indicate that electrocardiographic signs of myocardial ischemia elicited by dipyridamole are frequent in patient with HC and identify patients at higher risk for future cardiac events.

Prognosis of Patients with Phe110lle Mutation in the cTnT Gene

Anan and colleagues[43] in Kagoshima, Japan, examined patients with mutations in the cardiac troponin gene to determine whether the characteristics and prognosis of patients with the Phe110lle mutation in the cTnT gene occur. Forty-six probands with familial HC were screened for mutations in cTnT gene. The Phe110lle missense mutation was found in 6 probands. Individuals in the 6 families were analyzed genetically and clinically. Haplotype analysis was performed with markers encompassing the cTnT gene. LV hypertrophy was classified. The Phe110lle mutation in the cTnT gene was found in 16 individu-

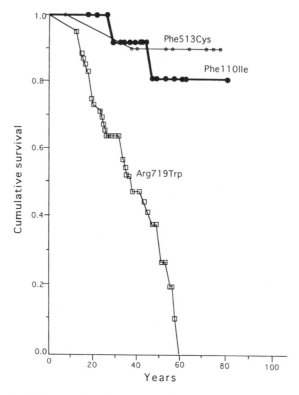

FIGURE 3-18. Kaplan-Meier product-limit curves for survival of individuals with Phe110Ile mutation and 2 other mutations in β-cardiac myosin heavy chain gene. Survival was good in patients with Phe110Ile mutation in cTnT gene and similar to that for benign Phe513Cys β-cardiac myosin heavy chain gene mutation. A significant difference (p = 0.002) in life expectancy was observed in individuals with Phe110Ile versus malignant Arg719Trp mutation of β-cardiac myosin heavy chain gene. Reproduced with permission from Anan et al.[43]

als. Two of the 6 families shared the same flanking haplotype and 4 were different from each other. Affected individuals exhibited different cardiac morphologies: 4 had type II, 6 had type III, and 3 had type IV hypertrophy with apical involvement. Three individuals with disease-causing mutations did not fulfill clinical criteria for the disease. The survival curve analysis demonstrated a favorable prognosis (Figure 3-18). Thus, multiple independent mutations of residue 340 in the cTnT gene have been described, suggesting that this may be an important location for such events. The Phe110Ile substitution causes HC with variable cardiac morphologies and a more favorable prognosis.

Benefit From VDD Pacing in the Hypertrophied Heart

Pak and colleagues[44] in Baltimore, Maryland, hypothesized that pacing generates discoordinate contraction and a rightward shift of the end-systolic pressure–volume relation and that benefits from this mechanism do not depend on the presence of resting outflow pressure gradients or obstruction. They studied 11 patients with New York Heart Association class III symptoms, 5 with HC, and 6 with hypertensive hypertrophy and cavity obliteration. Invasive conductive catheter methods were used. No patient had CAD or primary valvular disease. Pressure–volume relations were recorded before and during VDD pacing. LV cavity pressure was recorded simultaneously at basal and apical sites with pressure at the basal site used to generate the end-systolic pressure–volume relations. VDD pacing shifted the end-systolic pressure–volume relation rightward, increasing end-systolic volume by 45%. Resting and provokable gradients declined by 20% and 30%, respectively (Figure 3-19). Preload declined by 3% to 10% because of the short RT interval. Preload-corrected contractility indexes and myocardial workload declined by about 10%. Diastolic compliance and relaxation times were unchanged. Pacing made apical pressure–volume loops discoordinate, limiting cavity obliteration and reducing distal systolic pressures. Thus, VDD pacing shifts the end-systolic pressure–volume relationship rightward in HC patients with cavity obliteration with or without obstruction, increasing end-systolic volumes and reducing apical cavity compression and cardiac work. These effects are likely to contribute to reduced metabolic demand and improved symptoms.

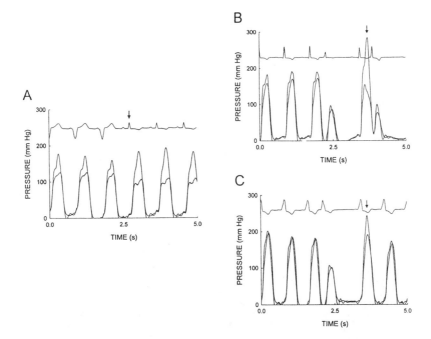

FIGURE 3-19. Effect of VDD pacing on rest and provokable pressure gradients. Pressure tracings from the LV base and apex are plotted along with the ECG. (A) Hypertrophic cardiomyopathy patient with rest gradient. Note the sharp increase in the pressure gradients on cessation of pacing (arrow). (B) HH-CO patient with a small rest gradient but a provokable gradient > 100 mm Hg at baseline. The gradient was provoked by pulmonary end-systolic pressure (arrow). (C) Same patient as in B. With VDD pacing, the provokable gradient (arrow) is much reduced. Note the similar coupling intervals before and after the extrasystole. Reproduced with permission from Pak et al.[44]

Echocardiography-Guided Ethanol Septal Reduction for Hypertrophic Obstructive Cardiomyopathy

Lakkis and colleagues[45] enrolled 33 symptomatic patients with hypertrophic obstructive cardiomyopathy with LV outflow gradients 40 mm Hg or greater at rest or 60 mm Hg or greater when provoked by dobutamine. By contrast echocardiography, the bulging septum was localized and infarcted by injection of 2 to 5 mL of absolute ethanol into the septal arteries supplying the hypertrophied area. Baseline echocardiograms with Doppler, myocardial perfusion tomograms, and treadmill exercise or pharmacological testing were compared with those at 6 weeks and 6 months. The mean rise in serum CK was 1,964 ± 796 units. All patients experienced symptomatic relief. New York Heart Association functional class decreased from 3.0 to 0.9. Exercise time increased from 286 to 421 seconds. The resting and dobutamine-provoked gradients decreased from 49 ± 33 and 96 ± 34 mm Hg to 9 ± 19 and 24 ± 31 mm Hg, respectively. Echocardiograms repeated at 6 weeks after the procedure showed a 28% reduction in septal thickness and 17% reduction in LV mass. Myocardial perfusion showed a "septal amputation pattern" with scarring in the upper and middle septal areas. Complete heart block developed in 11 patients who then required a permanent pacemaker. Thus, echocardiography-guided ethanol septal reduction in patients with hypertrophic obstructive cardiomyopathy is a safe, minimally invasive procedure that provides symptomatic relief with improved hemodynamic and LV parameters (Figure 3-20).

Percutaneous Transluminal Septal Myocardial Ablation

In the treatment of hypertrophic cardiomyopathy, DDD pacemaker therapy and surgical myectomy are standard extensions to drug therapy with negatively inotropic agents. An alternative to surgery for reducing the LV outflow tract gradient is septal myocardial ablation. Seggewiss and colleagues[46] from

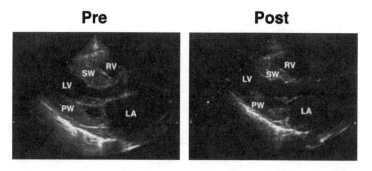

FIGURE 3-20. Parasternal long-axis view showing reduction of septal thickness after ethanol septal infarction. Septal basal thickness decreased from 2.1 cm (left) to 1.2 cm at 6 weeks (right). PW = posterior wall; SW = septal wall; RV = right ventricle; LV = left ventricle; LA = left atrium. Reproduced with permission from Lakkis et al.[45]

Bad Oeynhausen, Germany, performed percutaneous transluminal septal myocardial ablation in 25 symptomatic patients with hypertrophic obstructive cardiomyopathy. Septal branches were occluded and then an injection of 4.1 mL of alcohol was used to create a controlled infarct and ablate the hypertrophied intraventricular septum. The invasively determined LV outflow tract gradients were reduced in 88% of patients, with a mean reduction from 62 to 30 mm Hg. All patients had angina pectoris for 24 hours with an increase in creatinine kinase to a maximum of 780 U/liter. Fifty two percent of patients developed a trifascicular block for 5 minutes to 8 days (32%) or permanent DDD pacemaker implantation (20%). An 86-year-old woman died 8 days after successful intervention with uncontrolled ventricular fibrillation in conjunction with β agonists used for chronic obstructive pulmonary disease. The remaining patients were discharged after 11.3 days after an uncomplicated hospital course. Eighty-eight percent of patients showed clinical improvement with a further reduction in LV outflow tract gradient in 58%. These authors conclude that percutaneous transluminal septal myocardial ablation in patients with hypertrophic cardiomyopathy is a promising nonsurgical technique for septal myocardial reduction and reduction in the LV outflow tract gradient. Possible complications are trifascicular block requiring permanent pacemaker implantation and rhythm disturbances. It is obvious that larger numbers of patients need to be followed for a longer period of time to fully assess the relative role of this new procedure compared to more standard procedures.

Predictors of Sudden Cardiac Death

Patients with HC die suddenly. Proposed risk factors for sudden cardiac death (SCD) in patients with HC are youth, a family history of SCD, syncope, and ventricular tachycardia. Hemodynamic variables have not convincingly proved to be risk factors for CAD. Makl and associates[47] from Kurume, Japan, designed a study to examine predictors of SCD in a large number of patients with HC during long-term follow-up periods. The relation of studied variables (clinical, electrocardiographic, echocardiographic, hemodynamic, and exercise test findings) to SCD in 309 patients with HC who were initially diagnosed during 1971 through 1994 (mean follow-up 9.4 years) was examined by multivariate analysis, SCD occurred in 28 patients. Independent predictors of SCD were a smaller difference between peak and rest systolic BP during exercise testing and higher LV outflow tract pressure gradient at rest. Exercise-related SCD occurred in 8 patients and exercise-unrelated SCD in 20 patients (mean age 28 vs. 47 years). Thus, patients of exercise-related SCD were younger and had smaller increases in systolic BP during exercise testing, whereas patients with exercise-unrelated SCD were older and had higher LV outflow tract pressure gradients.

Mechanism of Mitral Regurgitation in Hypertrophic Cardiomyopathy

Schwammenthal and colleagues[48] in Boston, Massachusetts, evaluated mechanisms responsible for mitral regurgitation in patients with HC. They have noted that in the individual patient, mitral systemic anterior motion and regurgitation vary in parallel, but that clinically greater interindividual differences in mitral regurgitation (MR) can occur for comparable degrees of systolic anterior motion. They hypothesized that these differences relate to variations in posterior leaflet length and mobility, restricting its ability to following the anterior leaflet and coapt effectively. Different mitral geometries produced surgically in porcine valves were studied *in vitro*. Comparable degrees of systolic anterior motion resulted in more severe MR for geometries characterized by limited posterior leaflet excursion. Mitral geometry was also analyzed in 23 patients with HC, by intraoperative transesophageal echocardiography. All had typical systolic anterior motion with significant outflow tract gradients but considerably more variable MR. Thus, MR did not correlate with obstruction. In contrast, MR correlated inversely with the length over which the leaflets coapted, the most severe regurgitation occurring with a visible gap. MR increased with increasing mismatch of anterior to posterior leaflet length and decreasing posterior leaflet mobility. Thus, systolic anterior motion produces greater MR if the posterior leaflet is limited in its ability to move anteriorly, participate in systolic anterior motion, and coapt effectively. The spectrum of leaflet length and mobility that affects subaortic obstruction also influences MR in patients with systolic anterior motion.

Benefit of Negative Inotropes in Hypertrophic Cardiomyopathy

In this report, Sherrid and colleagues[49] in New York, New York, used M-mode, 2-dimensional, and pulsed Doppler echocardiography to study 11 patients with obstructive HC before and after medical elimination of LV outflow obstruction. They measured 148 digitized pulsed Doppler tracings recorded in the LV cavity 2.5 cm apical of the mitral valve. Successful treatment slowed average acceleration of LVEF by 34%. Mean time to peak velocity in the LV was prolonged 31%. Mean time to an ejection velocity of 60 cm/s was prolonged 91%. Before treatment, LV ejection velocity peaked in the first half of systole, but after successful treatment, it peaked in the second half. In contrast, after treatment, they found no change in peak LV ejection velocity. They also found no change in the distance between mitral coaptation point and the septum, indicating no treatment-induced alteration of this anatomic relationship. Medical treatment in this study included intravenous metoprolol at a dose of 15 mg unless contraindicated. If the Doppler gradient was reduced within 30 minutes to less than 30 mm Hg, oral β-blockers were continued as sole therapy. If a greater than 30 mm Hg gradient persisted, oral disopyramide was administered. In patients with a contraindication to disopyramide, oral verapamil was begun at 240 to 360 mg/day in divided doses. Treatment failures defined as persistent gradient greater than 30 mm Hg were identified by Doppler within 48 hours, and combination regimens were begun. From the data obtained above, the authors conclude that medical treatment eliminates mitral-septal contact and obstruction by decreasing LV ejection acceleration. By slowing acceleration, the treatment reduces the hydrodynamic forces on the protruding mitral leaflet and delays mitral-septal contact, resulting in a lower final pressure gradient.

Cardiac Angiotensin-Converting Enzyme Inhibition Versus Circulatory Angiotensin-Converting Enzyme Inhibition in Hypertrophic Cardiomyopathy

Kyriakidis and colleagues[50] in Athens, Greece, evaluated the influence of ACE inhibition on LV diastolic function and coronary blood flow in 20 patients with hypertrophic obstructive cardiomyopathy. Intracoronary enalaprilat (0.05 mg/min infused into the LAD for 15 minutes) followed by circulatory ACE inhibition with 25 mg sublingual captopril was studied in these patients. Contrast ventriculography, pressure, and coronary flow measurements were performed at baseline, after enalaprilat infusion, and 45 minutes after sublingual captopril. Heart rate was not affected by these interventions, but mean arterial pressure dropped slightly after the intracoronary enalaprilat and significantly after sublingual captopril. Compared with baseline, intracoronary enalaprilat resulted in a decrease in the LV end-diastolic pressure, time constant of isovolumic LV pressure relaxation, and outflow obstruction and in an increase in coronary blood flow and coronary flow reserve (Figures 3-21, 3-22). After sublingual captopril, the isovolumic LV pressure relaxation was prolonged and LV outflow gradient, coronary blood flow, and coronary flow reserve values returned to baseline. These data suggest that activation of the cardiac renin–angiotensin system contributes to LV diastolic dysfunction and to decreased coronary blood flow and coronary flow reserve in patients with hypertrophic ob-

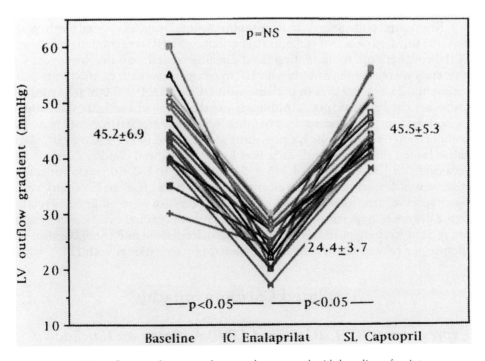

FIGURE 3-21. LV outflow gradient was decreased compared with baseline after intracoronary (IC) enalaprilat and returned to baseline after sublingual (SL) captopril. Reproduced with permission from Kyriakidis et al.[50]

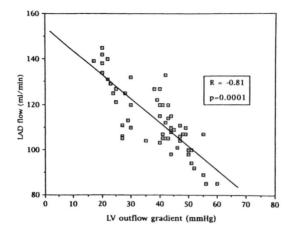

FIGURE 3-22. Inverse relationship between LV outflow gradient and coronary blood flow. Reproduced with permission from Kyriakidis et al.[50]

structive cardiomyopathy. Cardiac ACE inhibition restores and circulatory ACE inhibition aggravates the above abnormalities.

Decreased Coronary Flow Reserve in Hypertrophic Cardiomyopathy

Krams and colleagues[51] in Rotterdam, Netherlands, evaluated the hypothesis that the occurrence of ischemia in patients with HC is related to remodeling of the coronary microcirculation. End-diastolic septal wall thickness was significantly increased in patients with HC in comparison with cardiac transplant recipients, 25.8 ± 2.9 mm in patients with HC and 11.4 ± 3.0 mm in controls following cardiac transplant. Although the diameter of the LAD was similar in both groups, the coronary resistance reserve corrected for extravascular compression (end-diastolic LV pressure) was reduced to 1.5 ± 0.6 in HC. Arteriolar lumen divided by wall area was lower in HC and capillary density decreased from 1,824 ± 424 to 1,445 ± 513 per mm² in HC. Coronary resistance reserve was linearly related to normalized arteriolar lumen. Coronary resistance reserve, arteriolar lumen, and capillary density were all linearly related to the degree of hypertrophy. Thus, decrements in coronary resistance reserve are related to changes in the coronary microcirculation and these changes are themselves related to the degree of hypertrophy in patients with HC.

Dilated Cardiomyopathy

Expression of B7-1, B7-2, and CD40 Antigens on Cardiac Myocytes

Seko and colleagues[52] in Tokyo, Japan, investigated the role of the costimulatory molecules B7-1, B7-2, and CD40 in the development of acute myo-

carditis and dilated cardiomyopathy by analyzing the expression of these antigens in myocardial tissues of patients with acute myocarditis and dilated cardiomyopathy. These authors had previously reported that antigen-specific T cells
infiltrate the heart and play an important role in the myocardial damage. In
order for antigen-specific T-cell activation to occur, it is necessary for T cells
to receive a co-stimulatory signal provided by co-stimulatory molecules expressed on antigen-presenting cells as well as a main signal provided by binding
of T-cell receptors to the antigen. In this study, they also examined the expression of cytolytic factor, perforin, in the infiltrating cytotoxic T lymphocytes and
natural killer cells. Killer lymphocytes are thought to damage B7-1 expressing
antigen-presenting cells. They found that B7-1, B7-2, and CD40 were moderately to strongly expressed in the cardiac myocytes of patients with acute myocarditis. Weak to moderate expression of these antigens was found in the cardiac myocytes of patients with dilated cardiomyopathy. There was infiltration
of perforin-expressing cytotoxic T lymphocytes and natural killer cells in the
myocardial tissues of patients with acute myocarditis and dilated cardiomyopathy. These results suggest that expression of B7-1, B7-2, and CD40 antigens
on cardiac myocytes may make them antigen-presenting cells for infiltrating
cytotoxic T lymphocytes and natural killer cells and they may play an important
role in the direct myocardial damage by these killer cells in acute myocarditis
and dilated cardiomyopathy (Figures 3-23, 3-24).

Increased Sensitivity to Nitric Oxide Synthase Inhibition in Congestive Heart Failure

Hare and colleagues[53] in Boston, Massachusetts, tested the hypothesis that
inhibition of cardiac NO potentiates the positive inotropic response to β-adren-

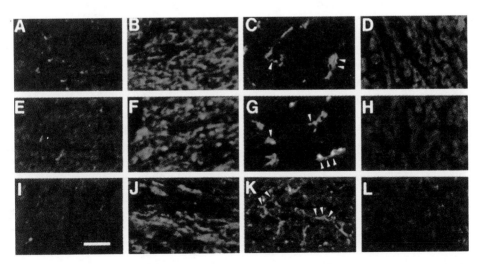

FIGURE 3-23. Immunohistochemical study for B7-1, B7-2, and CD40 antigens in ventricular
tissues of patients with acute myocarditis and dilated cardiomyopathy. Ventricular tissues
of a normal subject (A, E, and I) and patients with acute myocarditis (B, F, and J), dilated
cardiomyopathy (C, G, and K), and congestive heart failure due to doxorubicin cardiotoxicity
(D, H, and L) were stained with anti-B7-1 mAb (A, B, C, and D), anti-B7-2 mAb (E, F, G, and
H), or anti-CD40 mAb (I, J, K, and L) by immunofluorescence by use of tyramide signal
amplification technology. Bar = 20 μm. Reproduced with permission from Seko et al.[52]

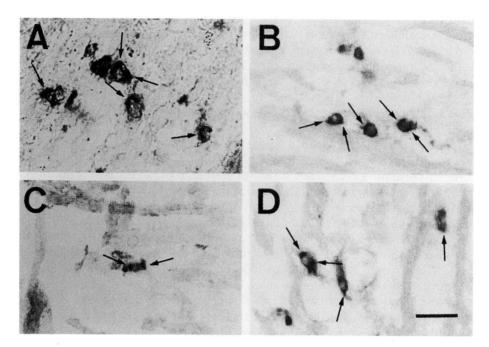

FIGURE 3-24. Expression of perforin in infiltrating CTLs and NK cells in the hearts of patients with acute myocarditis and dilated cardiomyopathy. Myocardial tissues of patients with acute myocarditis **(A and C)** and dilated cardiomyopathy **(B and D)** were double stained by enzyme antibody method for perforin (blue, arrows) and surface markers (brown) CD8 **(A and B)** and CD16 **(C and D),** respectively. Bar = 10 μm. Reproduced with permission from Seko et al.[52]

ergic stimulation in patients with symptomatic LV CHF, but not in subjects with normal LV function. They studied 11 patients with LV CHF due to idiopathic dilated cardiomyopathy and 7 control subjects with normal LV function. The β-adrenergic agonist dobutamine was infused intravenously before and during concomitant intracoronary infusion of acetylcholine, which activates the agonist-coupled isoforms of NO synthase, and N^G-monomethyl-L-arginine, which inhibits all isoforms of NO synthase. Changes in LV contractility were assessed by measuring the peak rate of rise of LV pressure (+ dP/dt). Dobutamine increased + dP/dt by 40% ± 6% and 73% ± 14% in patients with CHF and control subjects, respectively. Acetylcholine inhibited the + dP/dt response to dobutamine to a similar degree in patients with CHF and control subjects. Infusion of N^G-monomethyl-L-arginine potentiated the + dP/dt response to dobutamine by 51% ± 15% in patients with CHF, but had no effect on control subjects. Thus, inhibition of cardiac NO augments a positive inotropic response to β-adrenergic receptor stimulation in patients with CHF due to idiopathic dilated cardiomyopathy (Figure 3-25).

Relationship of Human Immunodeficiency Virus and Dilated Cardiomyopathy

Barbaro and colleagues[54] performed a prospective, long-term clinical and echocardiographic follow-up study of 952 asymptomatic HIV-positive patients

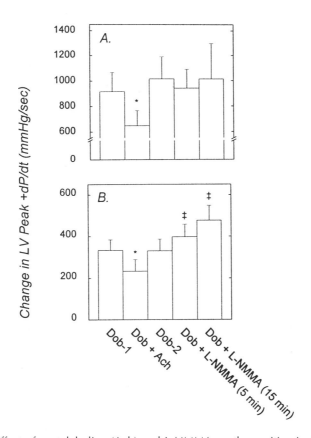

FIGURE 3-25. Effect of acetylcholine (Ach) and L-NMMA on the positive inotropic response to dobutamine (Dob) in subjects with normal LV function **(A)** and patients with LV failure due to idiopathic dilated cardiomyopathy **(B)**. Dob was infused via a systemic vein. Ach was infused into the left main coronary artery for 5 minutes and L-NMMA was infused for 5 or 15 minutes. Depicted is the absolute change in LV peak $+dP/dt$ from baseline. Baseline $+dP/dt$ was 838 ± 58 and $1,366 \pm 152$ mm Hg/s in the patients with heart failure and control subjects, respectively. *$p < 0.01$ versus Dob-1; ‡$p < 0.05$ versus Dob-2. Reproduced with permission from Hare et al.[53]

to assess the incidence of dilated cardiomyopathy and to analyze clinical variables associated with the development of cardiomyopathy. All patients with an echocardiographic diagnosis of dilated cardiomyopathy underwent endomyocardial biopsy for histologic, immunohistologic, and virologic evaluations. During a mean follow-up period of 60 ± 5 months, an echocardiographic diagnosis of dilated cardiomyopathy was made in 76 patients (8%), with a mean annual incidence rate of 15.9 cases per 1,000 patients. The incidence of dilated cardiomyopathy was higher in patients with a CD4 count of less than 400 cells/cumm as compared with a CD4 count of 400 or more cells/cumm and in those who received therapy with zidovudine. A histologic diagnosis of myocarditis was made in 63 of the patients with dilated cardiomyopathy (83%). Inflammatory infiltrates were predominantly composed of CD3 and CD8 lymphocytes with staining for major histocompatibility complex class I antigens in 71% of the patients. In the myocytes of 58 patients, HIV nucleic acid sequences were detected by *in situ* hybridization, and active myocarditis was documented in 36 of the 58 patients. Among these 36 patients, 6 were also infected with coxsackievirus group B (17%), 2 with cytomegalovirus (6%), and 1 with Epstein-Barr virus (3%). Thus, dilated cardiomyopathy may be related either to a direct action of HIV on the myocardial tissue or to an autoimmune process induced by HIV, possibly in association with other cardiotropic viruses.

Home Ambulatory Inotropic Therapy

Some patients with dilated cardiomyopathy who are inotrope-dependent but remain well by undergoing infusions can be managed by ambulatory infusions at home. Sindone and associates[55] from Sydney, Australia, report their results in 20 patients awaiting heart transplantation, unable to be weaned from intravenous inotropic therapy on 2 or more occasions, but who were well while receiving inotropes and received home ambulatory infusions. The patients were treated with ACE inhibitors, digoxin, diuretics, vasodilators, close electrolyte management, and low-dose amiodarone for those with more than 4-beat VT. Infusions were delivered by a tunneled subclavian catheter and syringe driver. Thirteen patients received dopamine, 4 received dobutamine, and 3 received both. Mean duration of inotropic therapy was 5 months, with 70% of the time spent as an outpatient. Eleven patients received transplants, 2 remain on the waiting list, and 7 died after being removed from the list because of general deterioration or renal dysfunction. There were no sudden deaths. Actuarial survival was 71% at 3 months, which is not less than that expected for an inotrope-dependent population. All patients with idiopathic dilated cardiomyopathy survived to transplantation. In contrast, all 3 with right heart failure caused by pulmonary vascular disease and 4 of 7 with ischemic cardiomyopathy died. Inpatient days were reduced by 70%, leading to considerable cost savings. Home ambulatory inotropic therapy is safe, cost-effective, best suited to those with idiopathic dilated cardiomyopathy, and dramatically reduces inpatient hospital duration.

Increased Mast Cell Density in Cardiomyopathies

Patella and colleagues[56] in Naples, Italy, compared cardiac mast cell density and the immunological and nonimmunological release of mediators from mast cells isolated from heart tissue of patients with idiopathic dilated (n = 24) and ischemic cardiomyopathy (n = 10) undergoing heart transplantation and from control subjects (n = 10) without cardiovascular disease. Cardiac mast cell density in patients with dilated cardiomyopathies and ischemic cardiomyopathies was higher than in control hearts (Figure 3-26). The histamine and tryptase contents of the hearts of patients with dilated and ischemic cardiomyopathies were also higher than control hearts. The histamine content of the hearts correlated with mast cell density (r = .91). Protein A/gold staining of heart tissue revealed stem cell factor, the principal growth, differentiating, and activating factor of human mast cells, in the cardiac mast cell secretory gran-

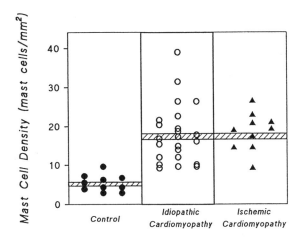

FIGURE 3-26. Mast cell density of human heart from control subjects (●) and patients with DCM (○) and ICM (▲). Each point represents the value from a single donor. The hatched area represents the mean ±SEM. Reproduced with permission from Patella et al.[56]

ules. Histamine release from cardiac mast cells caused by immunological and nonimmunological stimuli was higher in patients with dilated and ischemic cardiomyopathies compared with controls. Thus, these data indicate that histamine and tryptase content and mast cell density are higher in patients with dilated and ischemic cardiomyopathies and CHF than in control patients.

Familial Dilated Cardiomyopathy

Familial disease is present in 9% to 20% of patients with dilated cardiomyopathy. The ability to identify early disease in such people may improve patient management and aid in the understanding of pathogenesis. Baig and colleagues[57] from London, England, and Padua, Italy, prospectively assessed 408 asymptomatic relatives of 110 consecutive patients with dilated cardiomyopathy by means of history, physical examination, 2-dimensional echocardiography, 12-lead and signal-averaged electrocardiography, and metabolic exercise testing. Twenty nine percent of relatives had abnormal results on the electrocardiogram, 20% had LV enlargement, 6% had depressed fractional shortening, and 3% had frank dilated cardiomyopathy. The greater number of relatives with LV enlargement had an abnormal metabolic exercise test as compared to normal relatives. The QRS duration on the signal-averaged electrocardiogram was prolonged in relatives with LV enlargement compared with that of normal relatives. Over a mean 39-month follow-up period, 12 relatives with LV enlargement (27%) developed symptomatic dilated cardiomyopathy. One patient with LV enlargement died suddenly and another underwent heart transplantation. These authors conclude that nearly ⅓ of asymptomatic relatives (29%) have echocardiographic abnormalities, and 27% of such relatives progressed to development of overt dilated cardiomyopathy. Early identification of such people would permit appropriate intervention that might influence the serious complications and mortality of this disease.

Differential Expression of Tissue Inhibitors of Metalloproteinases in Congestive Heart Failure

Li and colleagues[58] in Pittsburgh, Pennsylvania, hypothesized that expression of matrix metalloproteinases (MMPs) and the family of tissue inhibitors of metalloproteinases (TIMPs) might be differentially regulated in the failing human heart. They obtained ventricular tissue from patients with ischemic cardiomyopathy (n = 16) or idiopathic dilated cardiomyopathy (n = 15) and nonfailing control hearts (n = 15) to study their hypothesis. TIMP-1 to 4 and MMP-9 proteins were quantified by ELISA and/or Western blot, and the total gelatinolytic activity was studied by gelatin zymography. The results demonstrate that cardiac expression of TIMP-1 and -3 transcripts and proteins was significantly reduced in the hearts of patients with ischemic cardiomyopathy and dilated cardiomyopathy. No significant difference was observed in TIMP-2 and -4 transcripts. However, TIMP-4 protein was significantly reduced in ischemic cardiomyopathy. MMP-9 protein content and total gelatinolytic activity were upregulated in the same samples. These studies demonstrate a selective downregulation of TIMPs along with upregulation of MMP-9 and gelatinolytic activity in the failing hearts, suggesting that matrix degradation and turnover may be related to the expression of selected metalloproteinases and decreases in their intrinsic tissue inhibitors (Figure 3-27).

Angiotensin-Converting Enzyme Binding Sites and AT_1 Receptor Density

Zisman and colleagues[59] in Chicago, Illinois, evaluated the regulation and interaction of ACE and the angiotensin II receptors in the failing human heart in 36 patients with dilated cardiomyopathy, 8 with primary pulmonary hypertension, and 32 organ donors with normal cardiac function. Angiotensin II formation was measured in a subset of hearts. AT_1 and AT_2 receptor binding was determined with the AT_1 receptor antagonist losartan. Maximal ACE binding was 578 ± 47 fmol/mg in patients with idiopathic dilated cardiomyopathy, 713 ± 97 fmol/mg in patients with primary pulmonary hypertension, and 325 ± 27 fmol/mg in nonfailing human myocardium. There was selective downregulation of the AT_1 receptor subtype in failing primary pulmonary hypertension ventricles (Figure 3-28). Thus, ACE binding sites are increased in the hearts of patients with CHF, and idiopathic dilated cardiomyopathy and nonfailing primary pulmonary hypertension ventricles. In primary pulmonary hypertension hearts, the AT_1 receptor is also downregulated in the failing RV.

Right Ventricular Dilation

Sun and colleagues[60] from Cleveland, Ohio, assessed the influence of RV dilation on the progression of LV dysfunction and survival in patients with

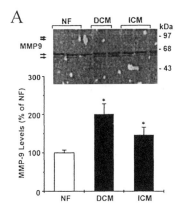

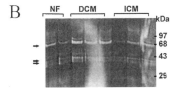

A

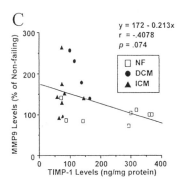

B

C

$$y = 172 - 0.213x$$
$$r = -.4078$$
$$p = .074$$

□ NF
● DCM
▲ ICM

FIGURE 3-27. MMP-9 protein content and total gelatino-lytic activity in nonfailing (NF) and failing human hearts. **(A)** Western blot analysis of MMP-9 in human hearts. Bar graph shows summary of quantitative results of 8 NF control hearts and 6 DCM and 8 ICM patients. *P < 0.01. **(B)** Gelatin zymography of 30 μg of myocardial extracts demonstrating increased total gelatinolytic activities in failing human hearts versus NF control hearts. **(C)** Correlation of reduced TIMP-1 levels with increased MMP-9 levels. Reproduced with permission from Li et al.[58]

idiopathic dilated cardiomyopathy (IDC). Using transthoracic echocardiography, the authors studied 100 patients with IDC aged 20 to 80 years (mean 55 ± 14); 67% were men. In the apical 4-chamber view, diastolic LV and RV chamber area measurements classified patients into 2 groups: group RV enlargement + (RV area/LV area >0.5) included 54 patients; group RV enlargement − (no RV enlargement) had RV area/LV area of 0.5 or more. Echocardiographic studies were repeated in all patients after a mean of 33 ± 16 months. At the time of the initial study, the 2 groups did not differ in age, gender, incidence of AF and diabetes, LV mass, and LVEF, but the RV enlargement + group had more severe tricuspid regurgitation and less LV enlargement. After 47 ± 22 months (range 12 to 96), patients in group RV enlargement + had lower LVEF (29% vs. 34%) than patients with initial RV enlargement −. At clinical follow-up, mortality was higher (43%) in patients with initial RV enlargement than in those without initial RV enlargement (15%). For survivors,

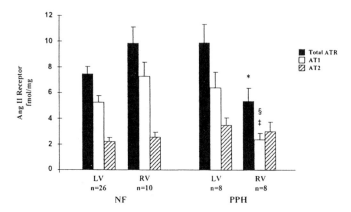

FIGURE 3-28. Total Ang II receptor (ATR) B_{max} was lower in PPH RVs than in PPH LVs or NF RVs. Decrease in total Ang II receptor density was explained by selective downregulation of AT_1 receptor subtype (*$p < 0.05$ vs. PPH LV or NF RV; ‡$p < 0.05$ vs. PPH LV; §$p < 0.001$ vs. NF RV). Reproduced with permission from Zisman et al.[59]

the mitral deceleration time averaged 157 ± 36 ms; for nonsurvivors or patients who required transplant, the mitral deceleration time averaged 97 ± 12 ms. With use of a multivariate Cox model adjusting for LVEF, LV size, and age, the relative risk ratio of mortality from initial RV enlargement + was 4.4 (95% confidence limits 1.7 to 11.1). Thus, patients with significant RV dilation had nearly triple the mortality over 4 years and more rapidly deteriorating LV function than patients with less initial RV dilation. In IDC, RV enlargement is a strong marker for adverse prognosis that may represent a different morphologic subset.

Induction of COX-2 and Activation of NF-κB in the Myocardium

Wong and colleagues[61] in Montreal, Quebec, Canada, determined the expression of COX-2 and activation of NF-κB in patients with CHF by obtaining myocardial tissue from 27 patients with end-stage CHF of varying etiologies, including CAD, idiopathic dilated cardiomyopathy, and valvular heart disease and from normal control subjects. The tissue was immunostained with antisera to COX-2 and NF-κB. Western blotting was performed and showed high anti-COX-2 antibody specificity and the presence of COX-2 protein in the sample tissues. *In situ* hybridization and immunohistochemistry showed little or no expression of COX-2 and NF-κB in the control hearts. However, there was abundant expression of COX-2 mRNA and protein in myocytes and inflammatory cells in areas of fibrotic scar compared with regions of normal morphology in all cases of CHF. Sites of NF-κB activation were associated with those of COX-2 expression. Thus, these data demonstrate induction of COX-2 and activation of NF-κB in the myocardium of failing human hearts.

Idiopathic Myocarditis

Evidence of Myocyte Injury

It is frequently difficult to demonstrate myocyte injury in patients with clinically suspected myocarditis. Lauer and colleagues[62] from Leipzig, Dusseldorf, and Berlin, Germany, investigated whether the use of cardiac troponin T could predict the results of histologic and immunohistologic analysis of endomyocardial biopsy specimens of patients suspected of acute myocarditis. Eighty patients with clinically suspected myocarditis were screened for CK-MB activity, and troponin T. In the myocardial biopsy, specimens were examined histologically and immunohistologically. Troponin T was elevated in 28 of 80 patients with clinically suspected myocarditis, CK in 4, and CK-MB in 1. Histologic analysis of the endomyocardial biopsy specimen revealed evidence of myocarditis in only 5 patients, all with elevated troponin T levels. Twenty three of 28 patients with elevated troponin T levels had histologic negative findings for myocarditis. Additional immunohistologic analysis revealed evidence of myocarditis in 26 of 28 patients with elevated troponin T levels, and in 23 of 52 patients with normal troponin T levels. Mean troponin T levels were higher with myocarditis proved histologically or immunohistologically or both than in patients without myocarditis (0.59 vs. 0.04). These authors conclude that measurement of serum levels of troponin T provides evidence of myocyte injury in patients with clinically suspected myocarditis more sensitively than does conventional determination of cardiac enzyme levels. Myocardial cell damage may be present even in the absence of histologic signs of myocarditis.

Assessment of Left Ventricular Systolic Function

Changes in the importance of LV systolic dysfunction and CHF with time after AMI after the introduction of thrombolytic therapy have not been studied. Køber and associates[63] on behalf of the TRACE Study Group assessed LV systolic function, measured as wall motion index (WMI) by echocardiography in 6,676 consecutive patients with an enzyme-confirmed AMI. So that changes in the prognostic value of WMI or CHF could be studied, separate analyses were performed at selected time periods. Average monthly mortality (deaths/100 patients/month) was determined from life-table analyses, with groups divided by WMI above and below 1.2 (a WMI > 1.2 corresponds to an EF > .035) or by presence and/or absence of CHF. Relative risk was determined by proportional hazard models, including baseline characteristics. In patients with LV dysfunction or CHF, monthly mortality was high during the first month (18.3% ± 1.6% and 20.2% ± 1.6%, respectively), decreased during the first year, and was stable thereafter (0.8% ± 0.1% and 1.0% ± 0.1%, respectively, average monthly mortality after year 3). The relative risk of LV dysfunction decreased from 2.4 to 1.3 in the same period. The relative risk of CHF decreased from 2.9 to 1.6. In patients without LV dysfunction or CHF, monthly mortality was relatively high during the first month (5.2% ± 0.7% and 3.4% ± 0.6%, respectively) but decreased within the first year to low, stable values (0.6% ± 0.1%

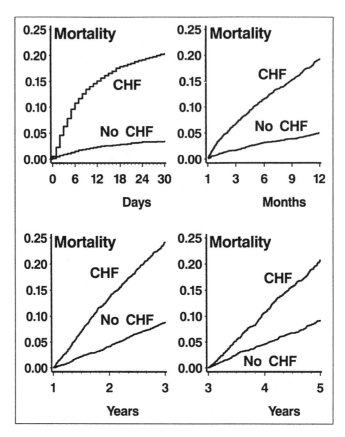

Figure 3-29. Mortality curves in 4 different time periods for 6,676 patients with a myocardial infarction in relation to the presence of CHF. Reproduced with permission from Køber et al.[63]

and 0.4% ± 0.1%, respectively, average monthly mortality after year 3). In patients who received thrombolytic therapy, the relative risk associated with a WMI of 1.2 or more decreased from 3.0 to 1.3 and from 3.2 to 1.7 in patients with CHF. The risk of dying decreases steeply with time after an AMI with or without LV dysfunction or CHF and stabilizes at low values after 1 year. This is in contrast to the relative importance of these risk factors, which is maintained for 5 or more years but decreases with time (Figures 3-29, 3-30).

Left Ventricular Assist Device

Myocyte Recovery After Left Ventricular Assist Device in End-Stage Congestive Heart Failure

Dipla and colleagues[64] in Philadelphia, Pennsylvania, determined whether circulatory support with a left ventricular assist device (LVAD) influenced the functional properties of myocytes in the failing heart. Myocytes were isolated from human explanted failing hearts and failing hearts with antecedent LVAD

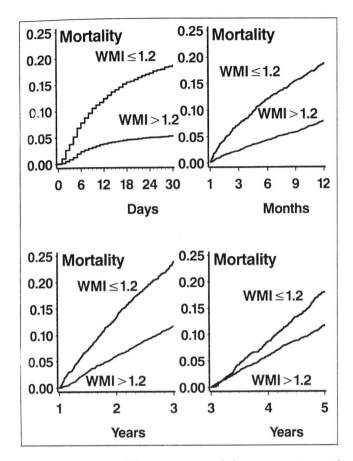

FIGURE 3-30. Mortality curves in 4 different time periods for 6,232 patients with a myocardial infarction in relation to LV systolic dysfunction (WMI ≤ 1.2). Reproduced with permission from Kⓞber et al.[63]

support. Studies of myocyte function indicated that the magnitude of contraction was greater, the time to peak contraction was significantly shorter, and the time to 50% relaxation was reduced in the heart failure–LVAD myocytes compared with the heart failure–myocytes (Figure 3-31). The heart failure–LVAD myocytes had larger contractions than the heart failure–myocytes at all frequencies of stimulation tested. The negative force–frequency relationship of the heart failure–myocytes was improved in heart failure–LVAD myocytes, but it was not reversed. Responses to β-adrenergic stimulation by isoproterenol were greater in the heart failure–LVAD myocytes versus the heart failure–myocytes. Thus, the results of this study support the hypothesis that circulatory support with an LVAD improves myocyte contractile properties and increases β-adrenergic responsiveness.

Exercise Performance in Patients with Congestive Heart Failure and Left Ventricular Assist Device

Mancini and colleagues[65] in New York, New York, compared the exercise performance of patients on left ventricular assist devices (LVADs) with that

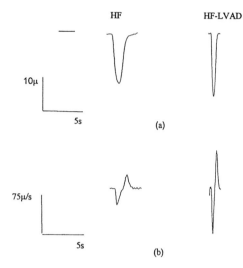

HF   HF-LVAD

10μ

5s

(a)

75μ/s

5s

(b)

FIGURE 3-31. (a) Steady-state contractions (at 0.2 Hz) from an HF and an HF LVAD myocyte; (b) corresponding derivatives. Solid line represents zero shortening; contractions from myocytes with similar RCLs are shown (HF myocyte length = 162 μm; HF LVAD-myocyte length = 160 μm). Reproduced with permission from Dipla et al.[64]

of ambulatory patients with CHF. Exercise testing with hemodynamic and respiratory gas measurements was performed on 65 patients with CHF with a mean age of 53 years and 20 LVAD patients with a mean age of 49 years. Peak Vo₂ was significantly higher in the LVAD than the CHF patients as was the Vo₂ at the anaerobic threshold. At rest, mean arterial blood pressure and cardiac output were increased, but mean pulmonary artery pressure and pulmonary artery wedge pressure were reduced. At peak exercise, HR, BP, and CO were higher, whereas mean pulmonary artery pressure and mean pulmonary capillary wedge pressure were lower in the LVAD group. Fick determined cardiac output was higher than LVAD flow sensor measurements. Thus, in this study, hemodynamic measurements at rest and during exercise are significantly improved in patients with LVAD, compared with results obtained in ambulatory CHF patients awaiting cardiac transplantation (Figure 3-32).

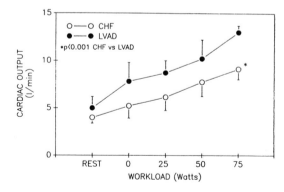

FIGURE 3-32. Cardiac output response at rest and throughout exercise in CHF and LVAD patients. Reproduced with permission from Mancini et al.[65]

Regression of Cellular Hypertrophy After Left Ventricular Assist Device Support

Zafeiridis and colleagues[66] wished to determine the effects of left ventricular assist device (LVAD) support on cardiac myocyte size and shape. Thus, isolated myocytes were obtained at cardiac transplantation from 30 failing hearts (12 ischemic, 18 nonischemic) without LVAD support, from 10 failing hearts that received LVAD support for 75 ± 15 days, and from 6 nonfailing hearts. Cardiac myocyte volume, length, width, and thickness were determined by use of previously validated techniques. Isolated myocytes from myopathic hearts exhibited increased volume, length, width, and length-to-thickness ratio compared with normal myocytes. There were no differences in any variable between myocytes from ischemic and nonischemic cardiomyopathic hearts. Long-term LVAD support resulted in a 28% reduction in myocyte volume, 20% reduction in cell length, 20% reduction in cell width, and 32% reduction in cell length-to-thickness ratio (Figure 3-33). LVAD support was associated with no change in cell thickness. These cellular changes were associated with reductions in LV dilation and LV mass measured echocardiographically in 6 of 10 LVAD-supported patients. Thus, these data suggest that regression of cellular hypertrophy is a major contributor to the "reverse remodeling" of the heart after LVAD implantation.

Left Ventricular Assist Devices as Permanent Treatment

The experience with inpatient left ventricular assist device (LVAD) support as a bridge to transplantation has proven the efficacy of such therapy. With miniaturization of the power supplies and controllers, such mechanical circulatory support can now be accomplished in an outpatient setting. DeRose and colleagues[67] from New York, New York, reported on 32 patients who under-

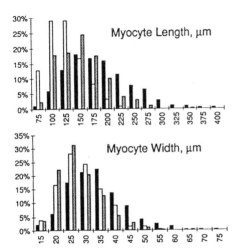

FIGURE 3-33. Frequency distributions of individual cardiac myocyte dimensions for length and average width, from HF (solid bars, 1050 cells), HF/LVAD (shaded bars, 350 cells), and nonfailing (open bars, 210 cells) groups. In each plot, abscissa indicates percent of cells in each size range. Reproduced with permission from Zafeiridis et al.[66]

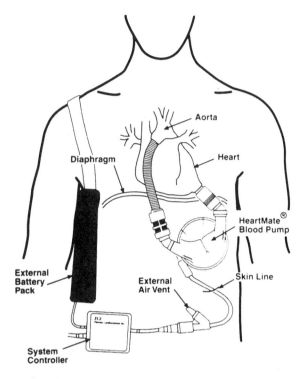

Aorta

Diaphragm

Heart

HeartMate®
Blood Pump

External
Battery
Pack

External
Air Vent

Skin Line

System
Controller

FIGURE 3-34. The implantable LVAD. Reproduced with permission from DeRose et al.[67]

went implantation of the Heartmate vented electric LVAD. This LVAD is powered by batteries worn on shoulder holsters and is operated by a belt-mounted system controller, allowing unrestricted patient ambulation and hospital discharge. The mean duration of support was 122 days with a survival rate to transplantation or explantation of 78%. Nineteen patients were discharged from the hospital on mean postoperative day 41 for an outpatient support time of 108 days. Four patients underwent early transplantation and could not participate in the discharge program. The complication rate was not statistically different from that encountered in 52 previous patients with a pneumatic LVAD. These authors conclude that outpatient LVAD support is safe and provides improved quality of life for patients awaiting transplantation. Wearable and totally implantable LVADs should be studied as permanent treatment options for patients who are not candidates for heart transplantation (Figure 3-34).

1. Butler J, Hanumanthu S, Chomsky D, Wilson JR: Frequency of low-risk hospital admissions for heart failure. Am J Cardiol 1998 (January 1);81:41–44.
2. Krumholz HM, Phillips RS, Hamel MB, Teno JM, Bellamy P, Broste SK, Califf RM, Vidaillet H, Davis RB, Muhlbaier LH, Connors AF Jr., Lynn J, Goldman L, for the SUPPORT Investigators: Resuscitation preferences among patients with severe congestive heart failure: Results from the SUPPORT project. Circulation 1998 (August 18);98:648–655.

3. Thompson RJ, McCullough PA, Kahn JK, O'Neill WW: Prediction of death and neurologic outcome in the emergency department of out-of-hospital cardiac arrest survivors. Am J Cardiol 1998 (January 1);81:17–21.

4. Pönicke K, Vogelsang M, Heinroth M, Becker K, Zolk O, Böhm M, Zerkowski H-R, Brodde O-E: Endothelin receptors in the failing and nonfailing human heart. Circulation 1998 (March 3);97:744–751.

5. Cooper CJ, Jevnikar FW, Walsh T, Dickinson J, Mouhaffel A, Selwyn AP: The influence of basal nitric oxide activity on pulmonary vascular resistance in patients with congestive heart failure. Am J Cardiol 1998 (September 1);82:609–614.

6. Mallat Z, Philip I, Lebret M, Chatel D, Maclouf J, Tedgui A: Elevated levels of 8-iso-prostaglandin $F_{2\alpha}$ in pericardial fluid of patients with heart failure: A potential role for *in vivo* oxidant stress in ventricular dilatation and progression to heart failure. Circulation 1998 (April 28);97:1536–1539.

7. Luchsinger JA, Steinberg JS: Resolution of cardiomyopathy after ablation of atrial flutter. JACC 1998 (July);33:205–210.

8. Nakamura M, Arakawa N, Yoshida H, Makita S, Niinuma H, Hiramori K: Vasodilatory effects of B-type natriuretic peptide are impaired in patients with chronic heart failure. Am Heart J 1998 (March);135:414–420.

9. Maeda K, Tsutamoto T, Wada A, Hisanaga T, Kinoshita M: Plasma brain natriuretic peptide as a biochemical marker of high LV end-diastolic pressure in symptomatic LV dysfunction. 1998 (May);135:825–832.

10. Fukuchi M, Hussain SNA, Giaid A: Heterogeneous expression and activity of endothelial and inducible nitric oxide synthases in end-stage human heart failure: Their relation to lesion site and β-adrenergic receptor therapy. Circulation 1998 (July 14);98:132–139.

11. Aukrust P, Ueland T, Müller F, Andreassen AK, Nordøy I, Aas H, Kjekshus J, Simonsen S, Frøland SS, Gullestad L: Elevated circulating levels of C-C chemokines in patients with congestive heart failure. Circulation 1998 (March 31);97:1136–1143.

12. Kubota T, McNamara DM, Wang JJ, Trost M, McTiernan CF, Mann DL, Feldman AM, for the VEST Investigators for TNF Genotype Analysis: Effects of tumor necrosis factor gene polymorphisms in patients with congestive heart failure. Circulation 1998 (June 30);97:2499–2501.

13. Vredevoe DL, Woo MA, Doering LV, Brecht ML, Hamilton MA, Fonarow GC: Skin test anergy in advanced heart failure secondary to either ischemic or idiopathic dilated cardiomyopathy. Am J Cardiol 1998 (August 1);82:323–328.

14. Nolan J, Batin PD, Andrews R, Lindsay SJ, Brooksby P, Mullen M, Baig W, Flapan AD, Cowley A, Prescott RJ, Neilson JMM, Fox KAA: Prospective study of heart rate variability and mortality in chronic heart failure: Results of the United Kingdom heart failure evaluation and assessment of risk trial (UK-Heart). Circulation 1998 (October 13);98:1510–1516.

15. Javaheri S, Parker TJ, Liming JD, Corbett WS, Nishiyama H, Wexler L, Roselle GA: Sleep apnea in 81 ambulatory male patients with stable heart failure: Types and their prevalences, consequences, and presentations. Circulation 1998 (June 2);97:2154–2159.

16. Dubrey SW, Bilazarian S, La Valley M, Reisinger J, Skinner M: Signal-averaged electrocardiography in patients with AL primary amyloidosis. Am Heart J 1997 (December);134:994–1001.

17. Cohn JN, Goldstein SO, Greenberg BH, Lorell BH, Bourge RC, Jaski BE, Gottlieb SO, McGrew F III, DeMets DL, White BG, for the Vesnarinone Trial Investigators: A dose-dependent increase in mortality with vesnarinone among patients with severe heart failure. N Engl J Med 1998 (December 17);339:1810–1816.

18. Shakar SF, Abraham WT, Gilbert EM, Robertson AD, Lowes BD, Zisman LS, Ferguson DA, Bristow MR: Combined oral positive inotropic and beta-blocker therapy for treatment of refractory class IV heart failure. JACC 1998 (May);31:1336–1340.

19. Zannad F, Chati Z, Guest M, Plat F, and the Fosinopril in Heart Failure Study Investigators: Differential effects of fosinopril and enalapril in mild to moderate chronic heart failure. Am Heart J 1998 (October);136:672–680.

20. Lechat P, Packer M, Chalon S, Cucherat M, Arab T, Boissel J-P: Clinical effect of β-adrenergic blockade in chronic heart failure: A meta-analysis of double-blind, placebo-controlled, randomized trials. Circulation 1998 (September 22);98: 1184–1191.

21. Young JB, Gheorghiade M, Uretsky BJ, Patterson JH, Adams KF, Jr: Superiority of "triple" drug therapy in heart failure: Insights from the PROVED and RADIANCE trials. JACC 1998 (September);33:686–692.

22. Vescovo G, Dalla Libera L, Serafini F, Leprotti C, Facchin L, Volterrani M, Ceconi C, Ambrosio GB: Improved exercise tolerance after losartan and enalapril in heart failure: Correlation with changes in skeletal muscle myosin heavy chain composition. Circulation 1998 (October 27);98:1742–1749.

23. Guazzi M, Melzi G, Agostoni P: Comparison of changes in respiratory function and exercise oxygen uptake with losartan versus enalapril in congestive heart failure secondary to ischemic or idiopathic dilated cardiomyopathy. Am J Cardiol 1997 (December 15);80:1572–1576.

24. Lang RM, Elkayam U, Yellen LG, Krauss D, McKelvie RS, Vaughan DE, Ney DE, Makris L, Chang PI: Comparative effects of losartan and enalapril on exercise capacity and clinical status in patients with heart failure. JACC 1997 (October);30: 983–991.

25. Spaulding C, Charbonnier B, Cohen-Solal A, Juillière Y, Kromer EP, Benhamda K, Cador R, Weber S: Acute hemodynamic interaction of aspirin and ticlopidine with enalapril: Results of a double-blind, randomized, comparative trial. Circulation 1998 (August 25);98:757–765.

26. Hassapoyannes CA, Bergh ME, Movahed MR, Easterling BM, Omoigui NA: Diastolic effects of chronic digitalization in systolic heart failure. Am Heart J 1998 (October);136:688–695.

27. Tsutamoto T, Wada A, Maeda K, Hisanaga T, Fukai D, Maeda M, Mabuchi N, Kinoshita M: Digitalis increases brain natriuretic peptide in patients with severe CHF. Am Heart J 1997 (November);134:910–916.

28. Adams KF, Gheorghiade M, Uretsky BF, Young JB, Patterson JH, Tomasko L, Packer M: Clinical predictors of worsening heart failure during withdrawal from digoxin therapy. Am Heart J 1998 (March);135:389–397.

29. Al-Khadra AS, Salem DN, Rand WM, Udelson JE, Smith JJ, Konstam MA: Warfarin anticoagulation and survival: A cohort analysis from the studies of left ventricular dysfunction. JACC 1998 (March 15);31:749–753.

30. Krumholz HM, Butler J, Miller J, Vaccarino V, Williams CS, Mendes de Leon CF, Seeman TE, Kasi SV, Berkman LF: Prognostic importance of emotional support for elderly patients hospitalized with heart failure. Circulation 1998 (March 17); 97:958–964.

31. Blanc J-J, Etienne Y, Gilard M, Mansourati J, Munier S, Boschat J, Benditt DG, Lurie KG: Evaluation of different ventricular pacing sites in patients with severe heart failure: Result of an acute hemodynamic study. Circulation 1997 (November 18);96:3273–3277.

32. Walsh JT, Andrews R, Curtis S, Evans A: Effects of amlodipine in patients with chronic CHF Am Heart J 1997 (November);134:872–878.

33. McDermott MM, Feinglass J, Lee P, Mehta S, Schmitt B, Lefevr Puppala J, Gheorghiade M: Heart failure between 1986 and 1994: Temporal trends in drug-p academic medical center. Am Heart J 1997 (November);134:901–909.

34. van de Borne P, Oren R, Somers VK: Dopamine depresses minute ventilation in patients with heart failure. Circulation 1998 (July 14);98:126–131.

35. Pitts WR, Vongpatanasin W, Cigarroa JE, Hillis LD, Lange RA: Effects of the intracoronary infusion of cocaine on left ventricular systolic and diastolic function in humans. Circulation 1998 (April 7);97:1270–1273.

36. Rohde LEP, Polanczykj CA, Moraes RS, Ferlin E, Ribeiro JP: Effect of partial arrhythmia suppression with amiodarone on heart rate variability of CHF patients. Am Heart J 1998 (July);136:31–36.

37. Tsutamoto T, Hisanaga T, Wada A, Maeda K, Ohnishi M, Fukai D, Mabuchi N, Sawaki M, Kinoshita M: Interleukin-6 spillover in the peripheral circulation in-

creases with the severity of heart failure, and the high plasma level of interleukin-6 is an important prognostic predictor in patients with congestive heart failure. JACC 1998 (February);31:391–398.

38. Williams MJ, Luthern L, Blackburn G, Lytle BW, Marwick TH: Relative efficacy of medical therapy and revascularization for improving exercise capacity in patients with chronic LV dysfunction. Am Heart J 1998 (July);136:57–62.

39. Belardinelli R, Georgiou D, Purcaro A: Low dose dobutamine echocardiography predicts improvement in functional capacity after exercise training in patients with ischemic cardiomyopathy: Prognostic implication. JACC 1998 (April);31:1027–1034.

40. Douglas PS, O'Toole ML, Katz SE, Ginsburg GS, Hiller WDB, Laird RH: Left ventricular hypertrophy in athletes. Am J Cardiol 1997 (November 15);80:1384–1388.

41. Manolas J, Kyriakidis M, Anastasakis A, Pegas P, Rigopoulos A, Theopistou A, Toutouzas P: Usefulness of noninvasive detection of left ventricular diastolic abnormalities during isometric stress in hypertrophic cardiomyopathy and in athletes. Am J Cardiol 1998 (February 1);81:306–313.

42. Lazzeroni E, Picano E, Morozzi L, Maurizio AR, Palma G, Ceriati R, Iori E, Barilli A, for the Echo Persantine Italian Cooperative (EPIC) study group, subproject hypertrophic cardiomyopathy: Dipyridamole-induced ischemia as a prognostic marker of future adverse cardiac events in adult patients with hypertrophic cardiomyopathy. Circulation 1997 (December 16);96:4268–4272.

43. Anan R, Shono H, Kisanuki A, Arima S, Nakao S, Tanaka H: Patients with familial hypertrophic cardiomyopathy caused by a Phe110Ile missense mutation in the cardiac troponin T gene have variable cardiac morphologies and a favorable prognosis. Circulation 1998 (August 4);98:391–397.

44. Pak PH, Maughan L, Baughman KL, Kieval RS, Kass DA: Mechanism of acute myocardial benefit from VDD pacing in hypertrophied heart: Similarity of responses in hypertrophic cardiomyopathy and hypertensive heart disease. Circulation 1998 (July 21);98:242–248.

45. Lakkis NM, Nagueh SF, Kleiman NS, Killip D, He Z-X, Verani MS, Roberts R, Spencer WH III: Echocardiography-guided ethanol septal reduction for hypertrophic obstructive cardiomyopathy. Circulation 1998 (October 27);98:1750–1755.

46. Seggewiss H, Gleichmann U, Faber L, Fassbender D, Schmidt HK, Strick S: Percutaneous transluminal septal myocardial ablation in hypertrophic obstructive cardiomyopathy: Acute results and 3-month follow-up in 25 patients. JACC 1998 (February);31:252–258.

47. Maki S, Ikeda H, Muro A, Yoshida N, Shibata A, Koga Y, Imaizumi T: Predictors of sudden cardiac death in hypertrophic cardiomyopathy. Am J Cardiol 1998 (September 15);82:774–778.

48. Schwammenthal E, Nakatani S, He S, Hopmeyer J, Sagie A, Weyman AE, Lever HM, Yoganathan AP, Thomas JD, Levine RA: Mechanism of mitral regurgitation in hypertrophic cardiomyopathy: Mismatch of posterior to anterior leaflet length and mobility. Circulation 1998 (September 1);98:856–865.

49. Sherrid MV, Pearle G, Gunsburg DZ: Mechanism of benefit of negative inotropes in obstructive hypertrophic cardiomyopathy. Circulation 1998 (January 6/13);97:41–47.

50. Kyriakidis M, Triposkiadis F, Dernellis J, Androulakis AE, Mellas P, Kelepeshis GA, Gialafos JE: Effects of cardiac versus circulatory angiotensin-converting enzyme inhibition on left ventricular diastolic function and coronary blood flow in hypertrophic obstructive cardiomyopathy. Circulation 1998 (April 14);97:1342–1347.

51. Krams R, Kofflard MJM, Duncker DJ, Von Birgelen C, Carlier S, Kliffen M, ten Cate FJ, Serruys PW: Decreased coronary flow reserve in hypertrophic cardiomyopathy is related to remodeling of the coronary microcirculation. Circulation 1998 (January 27);97:230–233.

52. Seko Y, Takahashi N, Ishiyama S, Nishikawa T, Kasajima T, Hiroe M, Suzuki S, Ishiwata S, Kawai S, Azuma M, Yagita H, Okumura K, Yazaki Y: Expression of costimulatory molecules B7-1, B7-2, and CD40 in the heart of patients with acute myocarditis and dilated cardiomyopathy. Circulation 1998 (February 24);97:637–639.

53. Hare JM, Givertz MM, Creager MA, Colucci WS: Increased sensitivity to nitric oxide synthase inhibition in patients with heart failure: Potentiation of β-adrenergic inotropic responsiveness. Circulation 1998 (January 20);97:161–166.
54. Barbaro G, Di Lorenzo G, Grisorio B, Barbarini G, for the Gruppo Italiano per lo Studio Cardiologico dei Pazienti Affetti da AIDS: Incidence of dilated cardiomyopathy and detection of HIV in myocardial cells of HIV-positive patients. N Engl J Med 1998 (October 15);339:1093–1099.
55. Sindone AP, Keogh AM, Macdonald PS, McCosker CJ, Kann A: Continuous home ambulatory intravenous inotropic drug therapy for severe CHF: Safety and cost efficacy. Am Heart J 1997 (November);134:889–900.
56. Patella V, Marino I, Arbustini E, Lamparter-Schummert R, Verga L, Adt M, Marone G: Stem cell factor in mast cells and increased mast cell density in idiopathic and ischemic cardiomyopathy. Circulation 1998 (March 17);97:971–978.
57. Baig KM, Goldman JH, Caforio ALP, Coonar AS, Keeling PJ, McKenna WJ: Familial dilated cardiomyopathy: Cardiac abnormalities are common in asymptomatic relative and may represent early disease. JACC 1998 (January);31:195–201.
58. Li YY, Feldman AM, Sun Y, McTiernan CF: Differential expression of tissue inhibitors of metalloproteinases in the failing human heart. Circulation 1998 (October 27);98:1728–1734.
59. Zisman LS, Asano K, Dutcher DL, Ferdensi A, Robertson AD, Jenkin M, Bush EW, Bohlmeyer T, Perryman MB, Bristow MR: Differential regulation of cardiac angiotensin converting enzyme binding sites and AT_1 receptor density in the failing human heart. Circulation 1998 (October 27);98:1735–1741.
60. Sun JP, James KB, Yang XS, Solankhi N, Shah MS, Arheart KL, Thomas JD, Stewart WJ: Comparison of mortality rates and progression of left ventricular dysfunction in patients with idiopathic dilated cardiomyopathy and dilated versus nondilated right ventricular cavities. Am J Cardiol 1997 (December 15);80:1583–1587.
61. Wong SCY, Fukuchi M, Melnyk P, Rodger I, Giaid A: Induction of cyclooxygenase-2 and activation of nuclear factor-κB in myocardium of patients with congestive heart failure. Circulation 1998 (July 14);98:100–103.
62. Lauer B, Niederau C, Kuhl U, Schannwell M, Pauschinger M, Strauer B-E, Schultheiss H-P: Cardiac troponin T in patients with clinically suspected myocarditis. JACC 1997 (November 1);30:1354–1359.
63. Køber L, Torp-Pederson C, Jørgensen S, Eliasen P, Camm AJ, on behalf of the TRACE Study Group: Changes in absolute and relative importance in the prognostic value of left ventricular systolic function and congestive heart failure after acute myocardial infarction. Am J Cardiol 1998 (June 1);81:1292–1297.
64. Dipla K, Mattiello JA, Jeevanandam V, Houser SR, Margulies KB: Myocyte recovery after mechanical circulatory support in humans with end-stage heart failure. Circulation 1998 (June 16);97:2316–2322.
65. Mancini D, Goldsmith R, Levin H, Beniaminovitz A, Rose E, Catanese K, Flannery M, Oz M: Comparison of exercise performance in patients with chronic severe heart failure versus left ventricular assist devices. Circulation 1998 (September 22);98:1178–1183.
66. Zafeiridis A, Jeevanandam V, Houser SR, Margulies KB: Regression of cellular hypertrophy after left ventricular assist device support. Circulation 1998 (August 18);98:656–662.
67. DeRose JJ, Umana JP, Argenziano M, Catanese KA, Gardocki MT, Flanner M, Levin HR, Sun BC, Rose EA: Implantable left ventricular assist devices provide an excellent outpatient bridge to transplantation and recovery. JACC 1997 (December);30:1773–1777.

Hypertension

Hypertension (General Topics)

Left Ventricular Performance

To investigate whether and how frequently LV systolic performance assessed with endocardial and midwall measurement is depressed in young subjects with mild systemic hypertension, Palatini and colleagues[1] on behalf of the Hypertension and Ambulatory Recording Venetia Study (HARVEST) Group studied 722 borderline to mild hypertensive patients mean age 33 ± 0.3 years, mean office BP 146/94 mm Hg) enrolled in the HARVEST trial and 50 normotensive controls with similar age and gender distribution. BP was measured with 24-hour ambulatory monitoring. LV dimensional and functional indexes were assessed by M-mode echocardiography and sympathetic activity from 24-hour urinary catecholamines. In 64 hypertensive subjects (8.9%) the LV midwall shortening-stress relation was less than 95% of the confidence interval in 50 normotensive controls. Subjects with depressed LV myocardial function had age, duration of hypertension, and LV mass similar to those of hypertensives with normal performance, and greater relative wall thickness (0.42 vs. 0.37). Stroke volume and cardiac output were lower in the former group. Among these 64 subjects, endocardial performance was depressed in 35 (group 1) and normal in 29 (group 2). Group 2 subjects had greater posterior wall (10.0 vs. 9.5 mm), ventricular septum (10.6 vs. 10.1 mm), and relative wall (0.44 vs. 0.40) thicknesses than group 1 subjects. Urinary norepinephrine was 50% higher in group 2 subjects (106 vs. 70 g/24 hours). Stroke volume and cardiac output were similar in both groups. In conclusion, these results show that LV contractility may be depressed in young subjects with borderline to mild hypertension.

Endothelial Dysfunction Due to Abnormal Synthesis of Nitric Oxide

Cardillo and colleagues[2] in Bethesda, Maryland, investigated whether the endothelial dysfunction of hypertensive patients is related to a selective defect in NO synthesis by studying forearm blood flow responses to intra-arterial infusion of acetylcholine, an endothelial agonist linked to NO synthase through the calcium signaling pathway, and isoproterenol, a β-adrenergic agonist that stimulates NO production by increasing intracellular cyclic AMP in 12 normotensive subjects and 12 hypertensive patients. The infusion of isoproterenol was repeated during the concurrent blockade of NO synthesis by N^G-mono-

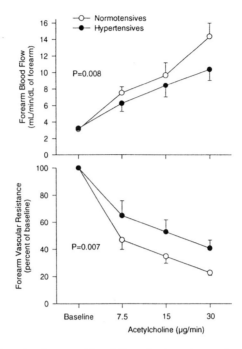

FIGURE 4-1. Graphs showing forearm blood flow **(top)** and vascular resistance **(bottom)** responses to acetylcholine in normotensive subjects and hypertensive patients. Values represent mean ±SEM. The probability values refer to the comparison of blood flow and vascular resistance at the 3 doses of acetylcholine between the 2 curves. Reproduced with permission from Cardillo et al.[2]

methyl-L-arginine. The vasodilator response to acetylcholine was significantly reduced in hypertensive individuals compared with normotensive ones. However, the vasodilator effect of isoproterenol was similar in normotensives and hypertensives and was significantly and equally blunted by L-NMMA in both groups. The vasodilator response to sodium nitroprusside, an exogenous NO donor, was similar in both groups and not modified by L-NMMA. Thus, hypertensive patients have an impaired endothelium-dependent vasodilatation in response to acetylcholine, but have preserved NO activity in response to β-adrenergic stimulation. These data suggest that endothelial dysfunction in essential hypertension is due to a selective abnormality of NO synthesis (Figure 4-1).

Prognostic Significance of Reduction in Left Ventricular Mass in Essential Hypertension

Verdecchia and colleagues[3] in Perugia, Italy, determined the relationship between changes in LV mass and antihypertensive treatment and the influence of increased LV mass in predicting an adverse outcome in patients with essential hypertension. They used echocardiography and 24-hour ambulatory BP monitoring in 430 patients with essential hypertension before therapy and after

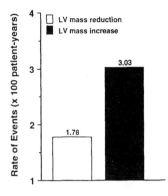

FIGURE 4-2. Event rate in the 2 groups with LV mass reduction (open column) or increase (solid column) from baseline to follow-up visit. Reproduced with permission from Verdecchia et al.[3]

1,217 patient-years. Months or years after the follow-up visit, 31 patients suffered a first cardiovascular morbid event. The patients with a decrease in LV mass from baseline to follow-up visit were compared with those with an increase in LV mass. There were 15 events in the group with a decrease in LV mass and 16 events in the group with an increase in LV mass (p=0.029). In a Cox model, the lesser cardiovascular risk in the group with a decrease in LV mass remained significant after adjustment for age, and baseline LVH on the ECG. In the subset with LV mass greater than 125 g/m² at the baseline visit, the event rate was lower among the subjects who had regression of LVH than in those who did not (p=0.002) (Figure 4-2). The authors conclude that in essential hypertension, a reduction in LV mass during treatment is a favorable prognostic marker that predicts a lesser risk for subsequent cardiovascular morbid events.

Vitamin C Improves Endothelium-Dependent Vasodilation

Taddei and colleagues[4] in Rome, Italy, tested the hypothesis that antioxidant vitamin C would restore relatively normal NO responsiveness in vascular endothelium vasodilator responses in patients with essential hypertension. It has been known that essential hypertension is associated with impaired endothelium-dependent vasodilation and that inactivation of endothelium-derived NO by oxygen free radicals is a contributing factor to endothelial dysfunction in experimental hypertension. The authors studied 14 healthy subjects with a mean age of 47 years and 14 patients with essential hypertension with a mean age of 47 years. They evaluated forearm blood flow using intrabrachial acetylcholine infusion or sodium nitroprusside. In hypertensive patients, but not in control subjects, vitamin C increased the impaired vasodilation to acetylcholine, but the response to sodium nitroprusside was unaffected (Figure 4-3). In another 14 hypertensive patients of similar age, the facilitating effect of vitamin C on vasodilation to acetylcholine was reversed by N^G-monomethyl-L-arginine, an NO synthase inhibitor, suggesting that in essential hypertension, superoxide anions impair endothelium-dependent vasodilation by NO breakdown. However, a cyclooxygenase inhibitor was also studied in an additional 7 hypertensive patients, and it prevented the potentiating effect of vitamin C on vasodila-

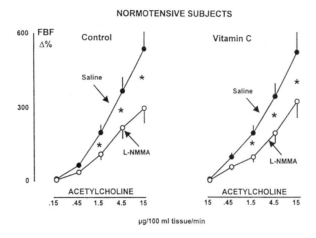

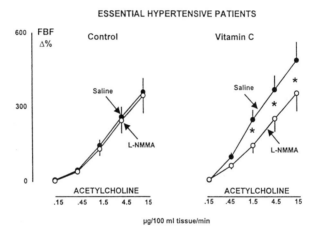

FIGURE 4-3. Acetylcholine-induced increase in forearm blood flow (FBF) in the absence (left) and presence (right) of vitamin C (2.4 mg/100 mL forearm tissue/min) under control conditions (saline at 0.2 mL/min) and in the presence of L-NMMA (100 µg/100 mL forearm tissue/min) in normotensive subjects (n = 14; top) and essential hypertension patients (n = 14; bottom). Data are shown as mean ± SD and, because L-NMMA modifies basal FBF, are expressed as percent increase above basal. *Significant difference between infusion with and without L-NMMA (p < 0.05). Reproduced with permission from Taddei et al.[4]

tion to acetylcholine, suggesting that in patients with essential hypertension, a main source of superoxide anions could be the cyclooxygenase pathway. Thus, impaired endothelium vasodilation can be improved by the antioxidant vitamin C, an effect that can be reversed by the NO synthase in N^G-mono-methyl-L-arginine. These data support the hypothesis that NO inactivation by oxygen free radicals contributes to endothelial dysfunction in patients with essential hypertension.

Effects of Exercise on Hypertension

The prevalence of systemic hypertension and its cardiovascular consequences is higher in African-Americans than in whites. Low to moderate intensity aerobic exercise lowers blood pressure in African-American patients with severe hypertension. It is not known whether such exercise can improve lipid metabolism in these patients. Kokkinos and colleagues[5] from Washington, DC, randomly assigned to exercise (n=17) or no exercise (n=19) a group of 36 African-American men with established systemic hypertension. They were aged 35 to 76 years. The exercise group exercised for 16 weeks, 3 times/week at 60% to 80% of maximum heart rate. After 16 weeks, peak oxygen uptake in the exercise group improved (21 ± 4 vs. 23 ± 3 mL/kg/min). Body weight did not change. Exercise intensity correlated with HDL cholesterol changes from baseline to 16 weeks (r=0.65) and was the strongest predictor of these changes (R^2=0.4). Lipoprotein-lipid changes in the 2 randomized groups did not differ significantly. A 10% increase in HDL cholesterol (42 ± 19 vs. 46 ± 19 mg/dL) noted in 10 patients who exercised at 75% or more of maximal heart rate suggested the existence of an exercise intensity threshold. Thus low to moderate intensity aerobic exercise may not be adequate to modify lipid profiles favorably in patients with severe hypertension. However, substantial changes in HDL cholesterol were noted in patients who exercised at 75% or more intensity of age-predicted maximum heart rate, suggesting an exercise-intensity threshold.

Treatment

Comparative Effects of Medication Administration

White and colleagues[6] from multiple US medical centers assessed the differential affects of a chronotherapeutic agent (controlled-onset extended release [COER] verapamil) administered at bedtime versus a conventional, homeostatic, (nifedipine gastrointestinal therapeutic system [GITS]) taken in the morning on early morning and 24-hour BP, heart rate (HR) and the heart rate x systolic BP product. The study was a multicenter (n=51), randomized, double-blind prospective clinical trial with a 10-week treatment period. Dose titration was performed by study investigators based on systolic and diastolic BP values at the doctor's office. Ambulatory BP monitoring was performed at placebo baseline, after 4 weeks of stable double-blind therapy, and at the end of the study. Twenty-four hour BP profiles were studied in 557 hypertensive patients. Changes in BP, HR, slope of the rate of rise of BP and HR, and the HR-systolic BP product during the 4 hours from 1 hour before to 3 hours after awakening were evaluated. The study was powered to show equivalence between the 2 regimens, predefined as a difference between treatment groups in mean change from baseline in early morning BP of ±5 mm Hg systolic and ±3 mm Hg diastolic. Changes in the early morning BP fell within the definition of equivalence for the 2 treatment strategies (−12.0/−8.2 mm Hg for COER-verapamil and −13.9/−7.3 mm Hg for nifedipine GITS). Changes in both the early morning HR and rate-pressure product were significantly greater following COER-verapamil therapy versus nifedipine GITS (HR, −3.8 beats/min versus +2.6 beats/min, and HR-systolic BP product, −1,437 beats/min · mm Hg versus −703 beats/min · mm Hg, respectively.) Changes in ambulatory BP demonstrated clinically similar reductions for the awake period, but nifedipine

GITS lowered systolic BP to a greater extent than the COER-verapamil during sleep (-11.0 vs. -5.8 mm Hg). COER-verapamil and nifedipine GITS had equivalent effects ($\pm 5/3$ mm Hg) on early morning BP. In addition, both extended-release calcium antagonists effectively lowered 24-hour BP. However, COER-verapamil had greater effects than nifedipine GITS on early morning hemodynamics (HR, HR-systolic BP products, rate of rise of BP and HR) and lesser effects during sleep due to its intrinsic pharmacological properties and chronotherapeutic delivery system.

Calcium Antagonists and Hypertension

To evaluate the effects of calcium antagonists on sympathetic activity in patients with systemic hypertension, Grossman and Messerli[7] conducted a MEDLINE search for English language articles published between 1975 and May 1996 using the terms calcium antagonists, sympathetic nervous system, and catecholamines. Clinical studies reporting only the effects of calcium antagonists on BP, heart rate, and plasma norepinephrine (NE) levels in patients with hypertension were included. Data were combined and analyzed according to class of calcium antagonist (dihydropyridine vs. nondihydropyridine), their duration of action (short-acting vs. long-acting) and treatment duration. They identified 63 studies involving 1,252 patients. Acutely after single dosing, short-acting calcium antagonists decreased mean arterial pressure by 13.7% ± 1.1% and increased heart rate by 13.7% ± 1.4% and NE levels by 28.6% ± 2.5%. Change in NE levels correlated with change in heart rate ($r = 0.59$), and inversely with change in arterial pressure ($r = 0.46$) in patients taking dihydropyridine calcium antagonists acutely. With sustained therapy, both classes of short-acting calcium antagonists increased NE levels. Whereas NE levels remained slightly elevated and heart rate unchanged with long-acting dihydropyridine calcium antagonists, both heart rate and NE levels decreased with long-acting nondihydropyridine calcium antagonists. Short-acting calcium antagonists stimulate sympathetic activity when given acutely and over the long term, irrespective of their molecular structure. Sympathetic activation is less pronounced with long-acting dihydropyridine calcium antagonists and decreases with long-acting nondihydropyridine calcium antagonists. These data offer a possible pathophysiological explanation for the increase in morbidity and mortality observed in some studies using short-acting calcium antagonists.

Safety of Calcium Channel Blockers

Issues raised recently concerning the safety of calcium channel blockers prompted an analysis of the occurrence of cardiovascular events and death in the Pfizer Inc. hypertension clinical trial databases for amlodipine (Norvasc) and nifedipine in the gastrointestinal therapeutic system (GITS) formulation (Procardia XL). Prospectively defined analyses of data from comparative and noncomparative trials of amlodipine and nifedipine GITS were conducted by Kloner and associates.[8] Outcome measures included cardiovascular and noncardiovascular deaths, and adverse cardiovascular events including new/worsened angina, AMI, serious arrhythmia, stroke, CHF, and bleeding. Among all amlodipine-treated patients (n = 32,920), the incidence rates for all-cause death, AMI, and new/worsened angina were 3.0, 3.3., and 1.6/1,000 patient-years of exposure, respectively. Among those in comparative trials alone (n = 4,126), the all-cause death rate was 4.1/1,000 patient-years, which was comparable to that of other non-calcium channel blocker agents and significantly less than that of other calcium channel blockers (23.8/1,000) patient-years, although the difference in rates represents only 2 deaths. Among all nifedipine-GITS-treated patients (n = 2,645), the rate of all-cause death was 4.1/1,000 patient-years, of AMI 6.5/1,000 patient-years, and of new/worsened angina 5.7/1,000 patient-years. The incidence rates for AMI and other cardiac events were low in these hypertension trials, and did not differ among treatment groups in either the amlodipine or nifedipine GITS comparative analyses. In the clinical trial databases analyzed, there is no signal suggesting excessive risk of death or cardiovascular events for hypertensive patients treated with amlodipine or nifedipine GITS.

Relationship Between Use of Calcium Channel Blockers and Mortality in Women

Michels and associates[9] explored the relationships between prescribed calcium channel blocker use and mortality in the Nurses' Health Study, which included 14,617 women who reported hypertension and the regular use of diuretics, β-blockers, calcium channel blockers, ACE inhibitors, or a combination in 1988. Cardiovascular events and deaths were determined through May 1, 1994. The authors documented 234 cases of AMI. Calcium channel blocker monodrug users had an age-adjusted relative risk of AMI of 2.36 compared with those receiving thiazide diuretics. Women prescribed calcium channel blockers had a higher prevalence of CAD. After adjustment for other coronary risk factors, the relative risk was 1.64. Comparing the use of any calcium channel blocker with that of any other antihypertensive agent, the adjusted relative risk was 1.42. An association between calcium channel blocker use and AMI was apparent among women who had ever smoked cigarettes, but not among never smokers. These data suggest a significant increase in relative risk of AMI among women who used calcium channel blockers compared with those who did not. However, after adjustment for co-morbidity and other covariates, the relative risk was reduced. Whether the remaining observed elevated risk is real or a result of residual confounding by indication or chance was not established by these data.

Treatment for Severe Pulmonary Hypertension

Severe pulmonary hypertension is associated with high morbidity and mortality rates despite the use of new vasodilator drugs such as prostacyclin. Sandoval and colleagues[10] from Mexico City, Mexico, investigated whether graded balloon dilation atrial septostomy would be helpful in such patients by inducing a controlled right-to-left shunt. They studied 15 patients with severe primary pulmonary hypertension wherein atrial septostomy dilatation was performed by crossing the interatrial septum with a Brockenbrough needle, followed by progressive dilation of the orifice with a Mansfield balloon in a hemodynamically controlled, step-by-step manner. There was a significant fall in right ventricular end-diastolic pressure and in systemic arterial oxygen saturation, together with an increase in cardiac index. One patient died and 14 survived. There was a modest reduction in pulmonary artery pressure. In the 14 patients who survived the procedure, there was an improvement in mean functional class from 3.57 to 2.07. Exercise endurance (6-minute walk) also improved from 107 to 217 meters. The survival rate among patients who survived the procedure was 92% at 1, 2 and 3 years which is slightly better than historical controls. These authors conclude that graded balloon dilation atrial septostomy is a potentially useful palliative treatment for selected patients with severe primary pulmonary hypertension.

1. Palatini P, Visentin P, Mormino P, Pietra M, Piccolo D, Cozzutti E, Mione V, Bocca P, Perissinotto F, Pessina AC, on behalf of the HARVEST Study Group: Left ventricular performance in the early stages of systemic hypertension. Am J Cardiol 1998 (February 15);81:418–423.
2. Cardillo C, Kilcoyne CM, Quyyumi AA, Cannon RO III, Panza JA: Selective defect in nitric oxide synthesis may explain the impaired endothelium-dependent vasodilation in patients with essential hypertension. Circulation 1998 (March 10);97: 851–856.
3. Verdecchia P, Schillaci G, Borgioni C, Ciucci A, Gattobigio R, Zampi I, Reboldi G, Porcellati C: Prognostic significance of serial changes in left ventricular mass in essential hypertension. Circulation 1998 (January 6/13);97:48–54.
4. Taddei S, Virdis A, Ghiadoni L, Magagna A, Salvetti A: Vitamin C improves endothelium-dependent vasodilation by restoring nitric oxide activity in essential hypertension. Circulation 1998 (June 9);97:2222–2229.
5. Kokkinos PF, Narayan P, Colleran J, Fletcher RD, Lakshman R, Papademetriou V: Effects of moderate intensity exercise on serum lipids in African-American men and with severe systemic hypertension. Am J Cardiol 1998 (March 15);81:732–735.
6. White WB, Black HR, Waber MA, Elliott WJ, Bryzinski B, Fakouhi TD: Comparison of effects of controlled onset extended release verapamil at bedtime and nifedipine gastrointestinal therapeutic system on arising on early morning blood pressure, heart rate, and the heart rate-blood pressure product. Am J Cardiol 1998 (February 15);81:424–431.
7. Grossman E, Messerli FH: Effect of calcium antagonists on plasma norepinephrine levels, heart rate and blood pressure. Am J Cardiol 1998 (December 1);80: 1453–1458.
8. Kloner RA, Vetrovec GW, Materson BJ, Levenstein M: Safety of long-acting dihydropyridine calcium channel blockers in hypertensive patients. Am J Cardiol 1998 (January 15);81:163–169.
9. Michels KB, Rosner BA, Manson JE, Stampfer MJ, Walker AM, Willett WC, Hennekens CH: Prospective study of calcium channel blocker use, cardiovascular disease, and total mortality among hypertensive women: The Nurses' Health Study. Circulation 1998 (April 28);97:1540–1548.
10. Sandoval J, Gaspar J, Pulido T, Bautista E, Martinez-Guerra ML, Zeballos M, Palomar A, Gomez A: Graded balloon dilation atrial septostomy in severe primary pulmonary hypertension: A therapeutic alternative for patients nonresponsive to vasodilator treatment. JACC 1998 (August);32:297–304.

5
Valvular Heart Disease

Valvular Heart Disease (General Topics)

Cardiac Valvular Insufficiency in Patients Taking Appetite-Suppressant Drugs

Khan and colleagues[1] examined patients who had taken dexfenfluramine alone, dexfenfluramine and phentermine, or fenfluramine and phentermine for various periods. They enrolled obese subjects who had taken or were taking these drugs during open-label trial from January 1994 through August 1997. They recruited subjects who had not taken appetite suppressants and who were matched to the patients for gender, height, and pretreatment age and body mass index. The presence of cardiac valve abnormalities, defined by the Food and Drug Administration and Centers for Disease Control and Prevention as at least mild aortic valve or moderate mitral valve insufficiency was determined independently by at least 2 cardiologists. Multivariate logistic regression analysis was used to identify factors associated with cardiac valve abnormalities. Echocardiograms were available for 257 patients and 239 control individuals. The association between the use of any appetite suppressant and cardiac valve abnormalities was analyzed in a final matched group of 233 pairs of patients and controls. A total of 1.3% of the controls and 22.7% of the patients met the case definition for cardiac valve abnormalities. The odds ratio for such cardiac valve abnormalities was 12.7 with the use of dexfenfluramine alone, 24.5 with the use of dexfenfluramine and phentermine, and 26.3 with the use of fenfluramine and phentermine. Thus, obese patients who took fenfluramine and phentermine, dexfenfluramine alone, or dexfenfluramine and phentermine had a significantly higher prevalence of cardiac valvular insufficiency than a matched group of control subjects.

Study of Dexfenfluramine

Weissman and colleagues[2] modified a randomized, double-blind, placebo-controlled study of dexfenfluramine to include echocardiographic examinations of 1,072 overweight patients within a median of 1 month after discontinuation of treatment. The patients, most of whom were women, had been randomly assigned to receive dexfenfluramine (366 patients), investigational sustained release dexfenfluramine (352 patients), or placebo (352 patients). The average duration of treatment was 71 to 72 days in each of the 3 groups. Echocardiograms were evaluated in a blinded fashion. When all degrees of valvular regurgitation were considered and when the 2 dexfenfluramine groups were combined, there was a higher prevalence of any degree of aortic regurgitation (17 vs. 12%, p=0.03) and any degree of mitral regurgitation (61% vs. 54%, p=0.01) in the active treatment group than in the placebo group. These differences were due primarily to a higher prevalence of physiological, trace, or mild regurgitation. Further analyses showed that aortic regurgitation of mild or greater severity occurred in 5% of the patients in the dexfenfluramine group, in 5.8% of those in the sustained release dexfenfluramine group, in 5.4% of those in the 2 active treatment groups combined, and in 3.6% of those in the placebo group. Mitral regurgitation of moderate or greater severity occurred in 1.7, 1.8, 1.8, and 1.2%, respectively. Thus, the authors found a small increase in the prevalence of aortic and mitral regurgitation in patients treated with dexfenfluramine, and the degree of regurgitation was in most cases classified as physiological, trace, or mild. However, in this study, the duration of therapy was short, and whether therapy of longer duration would yield the same or different results is not known.

Study of Appetite-Suppressant Drugs

Jick and colleagues[3] conducted a population-based follow-up study and a nested case-control analysis of 6,532 subjects who received dexfenfluramine, 2,371 who received fenfluramine, and 862 who received phentermine to assess the risk of a subsequent clinical diagnosis of a valvular disorder of uncertain origin. They identified a group of 9,281 obese subjects who had not taken appetite suppressants who were matched to the treated subjects for age, gender, and weight. All subjects were free of diagnosed cardiovascular disease at the start of follow-up. The average duration of follow-up for all subjects was approximately 4 years. There were 11 cases of newly diagnosed idiopathic valvular disorders, 5 after the use of dexfenfluramine, and 6 after the use of fenfluramine. There were 6 cases of aortic regurgitation, 2 cases of mitral regurgitation, and 3 cases of combined aortic and mitral regurgitation. There were no cases of idiopathic cardiac valve abnormalities among the subjects who had not taken appetite suppressants or among those who took only phentermine. Five-year cumulative incidence of idiopathic cardiac valve disorders was 0 per 10,000 subjects among those who had not taken appetite suppressants and among those who had taken phentermine alone, 7.1/10,000 subjects among those who had taken fenfluramine or dexfenfluramine for less than 4 months, 3.6 to 17.8 for the comparison with subjects who had not taken appetite suppressants, and 35/10,000 subjects among those who received either of these medications for more than 4 months. The use of fenfluramine or dexfenfluramine, especially for 4 months or longer, is associated with an increased risk of newly diagnosed cardiac valve disorders.

Mitral Valvular Disease

Percutaneous Balloon Versus Surgical Closed and Open Mitral Commissurotomy

Farhat and colleagues[4] in Monastir, Tunisia, conducted a prospective, randomized trial comparing the results of percutaneous balloon mitral commis-

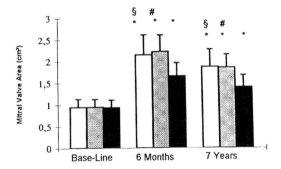

FIGURE 5-1. Mitral valve area determined by 2-dimensional echocardiography at baseline and at follow-up in the 3 groups. BMC (□), OMC (▨), CMC (■). *p < 0.001 for comparison of the baseline value with its change at 6 months within each group. §P < 0.001 for comparison of BMC versus CMC. #P < 0.001 for comparison of OMC versus CMC. Reproduced with permission from Farhat et al.[4]

surotomy (BMC), to surgical closed mitral commissurotomy (CMC) and open mitral commissurotomy (OMC) for the management of rheumatic mitral valve stenosis (MS) comparing the results of the 3 procedures in 90 patients with 30 patients in each group with severe pliable MS. Cardiac catheterization was performed in all patients before and at 6 months after the procedure. All patients had clinical and echocardiographic evaluation initially and throughout the 7-year follow-up period. Gorlin mitral valve area increased much more after BMC (from 0.9 to 2.2 cm^2) and OMC (0.9 to 2.2 cm^2) and after CMC (0.9 to 1.6 cm^2) (Figure 5-1). Residual MS, i.e., mitral valve area smaller than 1.5 cm^2, was 0% after BMC or OMC and 27% after CMC. There was no early or late mortality and there were no thromboembolic events among the 3 groups. At 7 years' follow-up, echocardiographic mitral valve area was similar and greater after BMC and OMC (1.8 ± 0.4 cm^2) than after CMC (1.3 ± 0.3 cm^2). Restenosis rates were 6.6% after BMC or OMC versus 37% after CMC. Residual atrial septal defect was present in 2 patients and severe grade 3 mitral regurgitation was present in 1 patient in the BMC group. Eighty-seven percent of patients after BMC and 90% of patients after OMC were in New York Heart Association functional class I versus 33% after CMC. Freedom from reintervention was 90% after BMC, 93% after OMC, and 50% after CMC. Thus, BMC and OMC produce excellent and comparable early hemodynamic improvement and are associated with a lower rate of residual stenosis and restenosis and need for reintervention than CMC. The comparable results between BMC and OMC and the elimination of thoracotomy and cardiopulmonary bypass suggest that BMC should be the treatment of choice for patients with tight pliable rheumatic MS.

Tricuspid Annuloplasty

Between September 1989 and December 1991, modified De Vega tricuspid annuloplasty was performed in 43 patients who survived surgery for mitral or mitral plus aortic valve replacement at Baragwanath Hospital in Johannesburg,

TABLE 5-1
Pre- and Postoperative Left Ventricular Dimensions and Function, Tricuspid Annulus Diameter,
Pulmonary Artery Systolic Pressure, and Significant TR

| | Tricuspid Annuloplasty | | | | | |
| | No (n=77) | | | Yes (n=43) | | |
Parameter	Before	After	p Value	Before	After	p Value
Tricuspid annulus diameter (mm)	30 ± 6	28 ± 5	<0.05	37 ± 5	24 ± 6	<0.05
Pulmonary artery pressure (mm Hg)	61 ± 18 (n=13)	32 ± 8	<0.05	53 ± 21 (n=16)	39 ± 16	<0.05
Tricuspid regurgitation ≥2+	3	8	NS	33	5	<0.05
Left ventricular end-diastolic dimension (mm)	57 ± 12	48 ± 8	<0.05	55 ± 11	54 ± 9*	NS
Left ventricular end-systolic dimension (mm)	38 ± 8	33 ± 8	<0.05	39 ± 10	39 ± 10*	NS
Left ventricular ejection fraction (%)	61 ± 12	58 ± 13	NS	57 ± 14	51 ± 15*	<0.05

* p <0.05 comparing patients with and without tricuspid annuloplasty after operation.
Reproduced with permission from Tager et al.[5]

South Africa. The results of these procedures were reported by Tager and colleagues.[5] The preoperative indications for tricuspid annuloplasty were moderate to severe TR in 33 patients and mild or no TR but with a dilated tricuspid
annulus (≥30mm) as measured by 2-dimensional echocardiography at end-
diastole in 10 patients. The mean age was 31 ± 13 years. The mean duration
of follow-up was 57 ± 18 months. Overall long-term mortality was 12%. On
Doppler color flow mapping, postoperative severe TR was present in 1 patient
and moderate TR in 4 patients at latest follow-up. The tricuspid annulus diameter decreased from 37 ± 5 mm preoperatively to 24 ± 6 mm at latest follow-
up. During the study period, an additional 77 patients underwent mitral valve
replacement or double valve replacement, but without tricuspid annuloplasty.
Within this group, 38 patients had a preoperative tricuspid annulus diameter
of 30 mm or greater and 5 of these patients (13%) developed moderate or severe
TR in the postoperative period, which may have been prevented had clinicians
adhered to the preoperative indications for tricuspid annuloplasty. Thus, preoperative echocardiography documented moderate or severe TR or a tricuspid
annulus diameter of 30 mm or greater are valid indications for performing
tricuspid annuloplasty; modified De Vega tricuspid annuloplasty is a durable
procedure in rheumatic patients. It appears that reducing the diastolic tricuspid annulus diameter to 24 mm is adequate to prevent residual TR in the long
term (Table 5-1).

Aortic Valvular Disease

Noncardiac Surgery in Patients with Aortic Stenosis

Aortic stenosis (AS) is a major risk factor, of course, for perioperative
cardiac events in patients undergoing noncardiac surgery. It has been shown

previously that some patients with AS who are not candidates for, or refused, aortic valve replacement could undergo noncardiac surgery with acceptable risks. Torsher and associates[6] from Rochester, Minnesota, extended these previous experiences over a subsequent 5-year period by retrospectively analyzing the perioperative course of all patients with severe AS (aortic valve area index less than 0.5 cm^2/m^2 or mean pressure gradient greater than 50 mm Hg), determined by Doppler echocardiography or cardiac catheterization, who underwent noncardiac surgery. Nineteen patients underwent 28 surgical procedures: 22 elective and 6 emergency. The types of these procedures were 12 orthopedic, 6 intra-abdominal, 4 vascular, 4 urologic, 1 otolaryngologic, and 1 thoracic. Mean age was 75 $\pm$ 8 years. Of the 19 patients, 16 (84%) had more than 1 symptom: dyspnea, angina, syncope, or presyncope. Mean LVEF was 61% $\pm$ 11%. The type of anesthesia was general in 26 procedures and continuous spinal in 2. Intra-arterial monitoring of blood pressure was used in 20 of the 28 surgical procedures. Intraoperative hypotensive events were treated promptly, primarily with phenylephrine. In all cases the anesthesia team was aware of the severity of the AS and integrated this into the anesthetic plan. Two patients (elective operation in 1 and emergency in 1) had complicated postoperative courses and died. There were no other intraoperative or postoperative events in any of the other patients. Although aortic valve replacement remains the primary treatment for patients with severe AS, selected patients with severe AS who are otherwise not candidates for aortic valve replacement can undergo noncardiac surgery with acceptable risk when appropriate intraoperative and postoperative management is used. Only 5 of these 19 patients had pressure gradients determined at cardiac catheterization. The rest was by echocardiography.

Heart Failure After Aortic Valve Replacement

The objective of this study by Tornos and associates[7] from Barcelona and Tarragona, Spain, was to assess the probability of development of heart failure during a long-term follow-up in patients submitted for aortic valve replacement for aortic regurgitation on the basis of preoperative findings. Eighty-seven consecutive patients with pure aortic regurgitation and normal coronary arteries were submitted for aortic valve replacement and prospectively followed up. Clinical examination, echocardiography, and radionuclide EF were performed before surgery and at 1, 2, 5, and 10 years after surgery. Operative mortality rate was 2.2% (2 patients). The follow-up period was 1 to 12 years (mean 6 years). Overall survival rate was 87% at 5 years and 81% at 10 years. During follow-up, 19 patients had heart failure develop, and there were 14 deaths (6 caused by heart failure). Probability of heart failure was 16% at 5 years and 24% at 10 years. Age was the single independent preoperative predictor of both death and heart failure. Age 50 or older, preoperative EF less than 40%, and end-systolic diameter less than 50 mm were independently related to the postoperative development of heart failure. Aortic valve replacement can be performed safely in patients with severe aortic regurgitation by following current recommendations. Age older than 50, end-systolic diameter greater than 50 mm, and radionuclide ejection fraction less than 40% were independent preoperative predictors of postoperative heart failure. The only independent predictor of both postoperative death and heart failure was age older than 50 years.

Aortic Valve Replacement in Older Patients

Asimakopoulos and colleagues[8] in London, England, evaluated the results of aortic valve replacement in patients 80 years of age and older by extracting data from the UK Heart Valve Registry between January 1986 to December 1995. One thousand one hundred patients 80 years of age or older had aortic valve replacement and were reported to the registry. Six hundred eleven patients (56%) were women. The mean follow-up time was 38.9 months. The 30-day mortality was 6.6%. Among 73 early deaths, 42 were due to cardiac reasons. The actuarial survival was 89%, 79%, 69%, and 46% at 1, 3, 5, and 8 years, respectively. In the first 30 postoperative days, 144 of the 205 deaths were due to noncardiac reasons. Malignancy, stroke, and pneumonia were the most common causes of late death. Bioprosthetic valves were implanted in 969 patients (88%) and mechanical valves in 131 (12%) patients. There were no differences in early mortality and actuarial survival between the 2 groups. These data suggest that under the selection criteria currently applied in the UK for aortic valve replacement in patients 80 years of age or older, there is a satisfactory early postoperative outcome and moderate medium-term survival benefit (Figure 5-2).

Predictions of Indications for Valve Replacement

Borer and colleagues[9] in New York City, New York, tested prospectively the hypothesis that objective noninvasive measures of LV size and performance

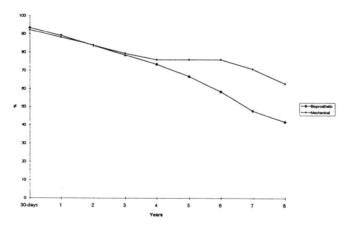

FIGURE 5-2. Actuarial survival in patients 80 years of age or older undergoing AVR: bioprosthetic versus mechanical implant. Reproduced with permission from Asimakopoulos et al.[8]

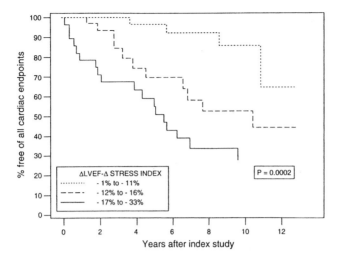

FIGURE 5-3. Relation of △LVEF-△ESS index at study entry to occurrence of any cardiac endpoint (cardiac death, operable symptoms, and/or subnormal LV performance at rest) during follow-up. Population of 88 patients with evaluable data for this analysis has been divided statistically into terciles. △LVEF-△ESS index boundaries for each tercile are boxed. Reproduced with permission from Borer et al.[9]

and of load-adjusted variables, assessed at rest and during exercise, predict the development of currently accepted indications for operation for patients with aortic insufficiency in an 18 year study. Clinical variables and measures of LV size, performance, and end-systolic wall stress were assessed annually in 104 patients by radionuclide cineangiography at rest and maximal exercise and by echocardiography at rest. End-systolic wall stress was derived during exercise. During an average 7.3-year follow-up among patients who had not been operated on, 39 of 104 patients either died suddenly (n=4), developed operable symptoms only (n=22), or subnormal LV performance with or without symptoms (n=13) (progression rate=6.2%/year). By multivariate Cox model analysis, changes in LVEF from rest to exercise, normalized for changes in end-systolic wall stress from rest to exercise, was the strongest predictor of progression to any endpoint or to sudden cardiac death alone (Figure 5-3). The unadjusted change in LVEF was almost as efficient. The population tercile at highest risk by change in LVEF minus change in end-systolic wall stress progressed to endpoints at a rate of 13.3%/year, and the lowest-risk tercile progressed at 1.8%/year. Thus, currently accepted symptom and LV performance indications for valve replacement as well as sudden cardiac death can be predicted in asymptomatic/minimally symptomatic patients with aortic insufficiency by load-adjusted change in LVEF minus change in end-systolic wall index, including data obtained during exercise (Figure 5-4).

Paget's Disease

Hultgren[10] investigated the prevalence of calcific aortic valve stenosis in Paget's disease (osteitis deformans) by reviewing autopsy data of severe cases

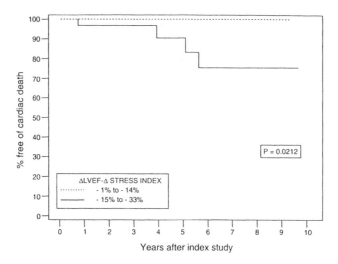

FIGURE 5-4. Relation of $\triangle$LVEF-$\triangle$ESS index at study entry to cardiac death during follow-up. Because of small number of end points, group is divided on basis of a binary split for this figure. Reproduced with permission from Borer et al.[9]

($\geq$75% involvement of 3 or more major bones, the femur, tibia, skull, and pelvis) and moderate cases ($\geq$75% involvement of only 1 or 2 major bones) of Paget's disease. Comparisons were made with normal age-matched controls. As was present in 24% of 27 autopsies of severe Paget's disease compared with 3.5% in 201 controls. Clinical signs of AS were present in 39% of 102 patients with severe Paget's disease compared with 4% in 417 controls. The prevalence of AS in 18 cases of moderate Paget's disease was similar to that of controls. Electrocardiograms were received in 45 cases of Paget's disease and compared with 80 controls of similar age. Complete AV block, incomplete AV block, BBB, and LV hypertrophy were present in 11%, 11%, 20%, and 13% of the Paget's cases and in only 2.5%, 1.3%, 2.5%, and 3.8% in the control cases. The author concludes that in severe Paget's disease there is a high prevalence of AS, heart block, and BBB, but these are not present in moderate degrees of bone involvement.

1. Khan MA, Herzog CA, St. Peter JV, Hartley GG, Madlon-Kay R, Dick CD, Asinger RW, Vessey JT: The prevalence of cardiac valvular insufficiency assessed by trans-thoracic echocardiography in obese patients treated with appetite-suppressant drugs. N Engl J Med 1998 (September 10);339:713–718.
2. Weissman NJ, Tighe JF Jr., Gottdiener JS, Gwynne JT, for the Sustained-Release Dexfenfluramine Study Group: An assessment of heart-valve abnormalities in obese patients taking dexfenfluramine, sustained-release dexfenfluramine, or placebo. N Engl J Med 1998 (September 10);339:725–732.
3. Jick H, Vasilakis C, Weinrauch LA, Meier CR, Jick SS, Derby LE: A population-based study of appetite-suppressant drugs and the risk of cardiac-valve regurgitation. N Engl J Med 1998 (September 10);339:719–724.
4. Farhat MB, Ayari M, Maatouk F, Betbout F, Gamra H, Jarrar M, Tiss M, Hammami S, Thaalbi R, Addad F: Percutaneous balloon versus surgical closed and open mitral commissurotomy: Seven-year follow-up results of a randomized trial. Circulation 1998 (January 27);97:245–250.

5. Tager R, Skudicky D, Mueller U, Essop R, Hammond G, Sareli P: Long-term follow-up of rheumatic patients undergoing left-sided valve replacement with tricuspid annuloplasty—validity of preoperative echocardiographic criteria in the decision to perform tricuspid annuloplasty. Am J Cardiol 1998 (April 15);81:1013–1016.

6. Torsher LC, Shub C, Rettke SR, Brown DL: Risk of patients with severe aortic stenosis undergoing noncardiac surgery. Am J Cardiol 1998 (February 15);81: 448–452.

7. Tornos MP, Olona M, Permanyer-Miralda G, Evangelista A, Candell J, Padilla F, Soler JS: Heart failure after aortic valve replacement for AR: Prospective 20-year study. Am Heart J 1998 (October);36:681–687.

8. Asimakopoulos G, Edwards M-B, Taylor KM: Aortic valve replacement in patients 80 years of age and older. Survival and cause of death based on 1100 cases: Collective results from the UK Heart Valve Registry. Circulation 1997 (November 18);96: 3403–3408.

9. Borer JS, Hochreiter C, Herrold EMcM, Supino P, Aschermann M, Wencker D, Devereux RB, Roman MJ, Szulc M, Kligfield P, Isom OW: Prediction of indications for valve replacement among asymptomatic or minimally symptomatic patients with chronic aortic regurgitation and normal left ventricular performance. Circulation 1998 (February 17);97:525–534.

10. Hultgren HN: Osteitis deformans (Paget's Disease) and calcific disease of the heart valves. Am J Cardiol 1998 (June 15);81:1461–1464.

6

Arrhythmias

Ventricular Arrhythmias

Angiotensin II Type 1a Receptor in Induction of Ventricular Arrhythmias

Harada and colleagues[1] in Tokyo, Japan, determined whether the renin-angiotensin system plays a role in ischemia-reperfusion injury by examining infarct size and arrhythmias after ischemia and reperfusion using angiotensin II type 1a receptor knockout mice. The LAD was occluded for 30 minutes followed by reperfusion for 120 minutes. There were no significant differences in infarct size between the wild type and knockout mice determined by dual staining with triphenyltetrazolium chloride and Evans blue dye. The number of premature ventricular beats after reperfusion in knockout mice, however, was much less than in wild type mice (Figure 6-1). Nonsustained VT occurred in all wild type mice, but there was no VT or VF in the knockout mice or in the mice treated with an AT1 antagonist. There were no significant differences in infarct size expressed as a percentage of the left ventricle or as a percentage of the area at risk. The AT1 antagonist, CV-11974, given before ischemia, blocked reperfusion arrhythmias in wild type mice but had no effect on infarct size. Thus, these data suggest that angiotensin II may be involved in the induction of ventricular arrhythmias, but not in the determination of infarct size after reperfusion.

Occurrence of Ventricular Arrhythmias After Acute Myocardial Infarction

Prognostic studies after AMI have been performed mainly in the prethrombolytic era. Despite the fact that modern management of AMI has reduced mortality rates, the occurrence of malignant ventricular arrhythmias late after AMI continues. De Chillou and associates[2] from Nancy, France, prospectively studied 244 consecutive patients (97 treated with thrombolytics) who survived a first AMI. All patients underwent time domain signal-averaged electrocardiography (vector magnitude: measurements of total QRS duration, terminal low (<40 μV) amplitude signal duration, and root-mean-square voltage of the last 40 ms of the QRS complex), Holter electrocardiographic monitoring, and cardiac catheterization. Late life-threatening ventricular arrhythmias were recorded. Eighteen arrhythmic events occurred during a mean follow-up period of 57 ± 18 months. Three independent factors were associated with a higher risk of arrhythmic events: (1) LVEF (odds ratio 1.9/0.10 decrease), (2)

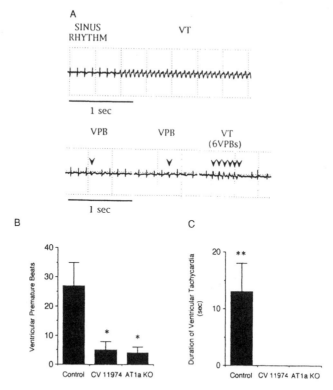

FIGURE 6-1. Examples of ventricular arrhythmias in wild type mice. Paper speed: 25 mm/s during sinus rhythm **(A)** and episodes of VT and VPBs (arrowheads). **(B)** The incidence of VPBs during 10 minutes of reperfusion; p < 0.01 versus controls. **(C)** Duration of VT. *p < 0.01 versus AT1a KO mice and CV-11974. VF = ventricular fibrillation; Control = control wild type mice; and CV-11974 = CV-11974-treated WT mice. Reproduced with permission from Harada et al.[1]

terminal low-amplitude signal duration (odds ratio 1.5/5 ms increase), and (3) absence of thrombolytic therapy (odds ratio 3.9). Low-amplitude signal duration sensitivity for sudden cardiac death was low (30%). LVEF had the highest positive predictive value for sudden cardiac death (10%). Thus, thrombolysis decreases both the incidence of VT and sudden cardiac death with a higher reopening rate of the infarct-related vessel. Signal averaging predicts the occurrence of VT and an impaired LVEF predicts the occurrence of sudden cardiac death.

Electrical Alternans as Predictors

Estes and associates[3] from multiple US medical centers performed a study to evaluate the feasibility of detecting repolarization alternans with the heart rate elevated during a bicycle exercise protocol. Sensitive spectral signal-processing techniques are able to detect beat-to-beat alternations of the amplitude of the T wave, which is not visible on a standard electrocardiogram. Previous animal and human investigations using atrial or ventricular pacing have dem-

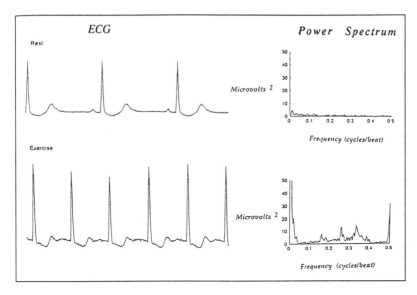

FIGURE 6-2. Representative alternans positive result from a patient with a history of clinical sustained. VT and the absence of visible T-wave alternans at rest or with exercise. Note the development of a discrete spike at 0.5 cycles/beat, indicating alternating amplitude of the T wave on a beat-to-beat basis. Reproduced with permission from Estes et al.[3]

onstrated that T wave alternans is a marker of vulnerability to ventricular arrhythmias. Using a spectral analysis technique incorporating noise reduction signal-processing software, the authors evaluated electrical alternans at rest and with the heart rate elevated during a bicycle exercise protocol. They defined optimal criteria for electrical alternans to separate patients from those without inducible arrhythmias. Alternans and signal-averaged electrocardiographic results were compared with the results of vulnerability to ventricular arrhythmias as defined by induction of sustained VT or fibrillation at electrophysiological evaluation. In 27 patients, alternans recorded at rest and with exercise had a sensitivity of 89%, specificity of 75%, and overall clinical accuracy of 80%. In this patient population, the signal-averaged electrocardiogram was not a significant predictor of arrhythmia vulnerability. This is the first study to report that repolarization alternans can be detected with heart rate elevated during a bicycle exercise protocol. The authors conclude that electrical alternans measured using this technique is an accurate predictor of arrhythmia inducibility (Figure 6-2).

Circadian Variations in the Occurrence of Cardiac Arrests

Peckova and associates[4] explored temporal variations in 6,603 out-of-hospital cardiac arrests attended by the Seattle Fire Department in Seattle, Washington, to determine whether there are diurnal variations in the frequency of cardiac arrest. The data exhibit diurnal variation with a low incidence at night and 2 peaks of approximately the same size at 8 to 11 AM and 4 to 7 PM. The

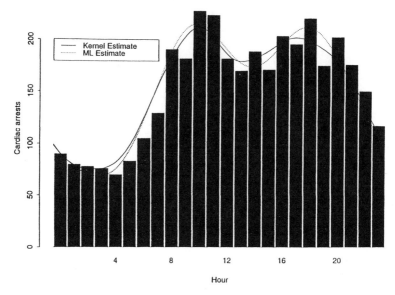

FIGURE 6-3. Distribution of time of 3,690 episodes of out-of-hospital cardiac arrests that were witnessed or ALS-treated. ML = maximum likelihood. Reproduced with permission from Peckova et al.[4]

evening peak is attributed primarily to the patients found in VF, whereas arrests that show other rhythms exhibit mainly a morning peak. Cardiac arrests associated with survival have more pronounced diurnal variation than episodes in which survival did not occur. This difference persisted after adjustment for rhythm. In 597 patients who had at least 2 separate cardiac arrests, the authors found no overall association between the time of day of the recurrent arrests. In women, however, the time of the day of the first and second arrests were closer to each other than one would have expected if the times were unrelated. Cardiac arrests do not occur randomly during the day, but follow certain periodic patterns. These patterns are most likely associated with selected daily activities (Figure 6-3).

Patients with Sick Sinus Syndrome Randomized to Pacing

Nielsen and colleagues[5] in Aarhus, Denmark, evaluated 225 consecutive patients with sick sinus syndrome and intact AV conduction who were randomized to either single-chamber atrial pacing (n = 110) or single-chamber ventricular pacing (n = 115). Clinical assessment included New York Heart Association classification, medication, and M-mode echocardiography before pacemaker implantation, after 3 months, and subsequently once every year. At long-term follow-up, New York Heart Association functional class was higher in the ventricular group than in the atrial group. Increase in New York Heart Association class during follow-up was observed in 35 of 113 patients in the ventricular group versus 10 of 109 in the atrial group (p < 0.0005). Increase in dose of

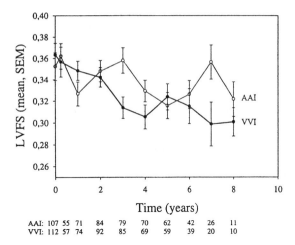

Figure 6-4. Left ventricular fractional shortening (LVFS) during follow-up of patients randomized to atrial (AAI) (n = 110) or ventricular (VVI) (n = 115) pacing. Numbers below abscissa indicate number of patients examined in the 2 treatment groups. Reproduced with permission from Nielsen et al.[5]

diuretics from randomization to last follow-up was significantly higher in the ventricular group than in the atrial group. The LV fractional shortening decreased significantly in the ventricular group, but not in the atrial group (Figure 6-4). The left atrial diameter increased significantly in both treatment groups, but the increase was higher in the ventricular group. Thus, these data suggest that during long-term follow-up, ventricular pacing is associated with a higher incidence of CHF and consumption of diuretics than atrial pacing in association with a decrease in LV fractional shortening and increased dilatation of the left atrium in the ventricular paced patients.

Association of Supraventricular Tachycardias with Ventricular Tachycardias in Arrhythmogenic Right Ventricular Dysplasia

SVT may occur in patients with the arrhythmogenic RV dysplasia (ARVD). The purpose of the study by Brembilla-Perrot and associates[6] from Vandoeuvre les Nancy, France, was to evaluate the incidence of SVT in 47 patients with ARVD proved by RV angiography. Thirty-three men and 14 women, aged 21 to 72 years (mean 44 ± 18) were admitted for nonsustained or sustained VT. Eight patients had a history of spontaneous SVT several years before VT occurrence. Protocol of the study consisted of programmed atrial stimulation with 1 and 2 extrastimuli delivered during sinus rhythm and 2 driven rhythms (600 and 400 ms); programmed ventricular stimulation with up to 3 extrastimuli was performed in the control state and after infusion of isoproterenol. The results of programmed atrial stimulation were compared with those obtained in 36 asymptomatic subjects without heart disease with a mean age of 50 ± 18 years (control group). Sustained SVT (>1 minute) was induced in 7 of 8 patients with spontaneous SVT, in 27 (69%) of those with ARVD who did not have spontaneous SVT, and in 2 control subjects (5.5%). SVT was inducible in the control state, but VT induction required isoproterenol in 11 of 27 patients. Two patients without SVT history but with inducible SVT developed later spontaneous SVT. ARVD was associated with a significantly higher incidence of inducible SVT than in a control population. Supraventricular tachycardias may precede ventricular tachycardias. This association argues for a diffuse myocardial disorder in ARVD.

Survivors of Sudden Cardiac Arrest

Mewis and colleagues[7] from Tübingen, Germany, described clinical, hemodynamic, and electrophysiological characteristics of 18 consecutive survivors of sudden cardiac arrest due to idiopathic VF. Long-term data in relation to the prescribed therapy were presented. The mean age of the 18 patients was 48 ± 14 years (median 49). Electrophysiologic studies showed a low inducibility of sustained VT in 4 patients (22%). Treatment consisted of class III agents, β-blockers, or implantable cardioverter-defibrillators. Two patients were discharged without any therapy. Therapy control was undertaken either by serial drug testing or by the empirical approach. Serious complications of therapy occurred in 2 patients: 1 patient experienced a proarrhythmic effect of antiarrhythmic drug therapy, and the other patient received multiple inadequate defibrillator discharges due to a defect in the transvenous lead. All but 1 patient (94%) remained free of recurrences of sudden cardiac arrest during a follow-up time of 45 ± 29 months (median 41). One patient died 2 weeks after surviving cardiac arrest due to intractable VF while receiving sotalol treatment. Therapy guided by electrophysiological studies did not have any impact on survival. Adverse effects or noncompliance led to discontinuation of drug therapy in 7 patients after a mean period of 31 ± 30 months. Without any treatment 9 patients remained without recurrences over 45 ± 33 months. Because of the absence of risk factors for arrhythmia recurrence and criteria to select therapy, randomized prospective studies are warranted to assess the optimal therapies in these young, ostensibly healthy patients.

Precordial QT Dispersion

Lee and associates[8] from New York, New York, compared the performance of precordial QT dispersion, late potentials on the signal-averaged electrocardiogram, and reduced LVEF for identification of inducible VT in 162 patients undergoing electrophysiologic study. QT_{apex} dispersion in 56 patients with inducible VT (72 ± 55 ms) was greater than that in 106 patients without inducible VT (55 ± 36 ms); dispersion was greater in both groups than in 144 normal subjects (33 ± 19 ms). A QT_{apex} dispersion partition of more than 68 ms, the upper 95th percentile in normal subjects, identified inducible VT with a specificity of 75% and a sensitivity of 45%. Although the performances of late potentials (specificity 82%, sensitivity 59%) and reduced EF (specificity 86%, sensitivity 54%) were each stronger than QT dispersion alone for identification of inducible VT, abnormal QT_{apex} dispersion remained a significant additional predictor of inducible VT in a logistic regression model that included the 3 variables (specificity 78%, sensitivity 75%).

QT Interval Dispersion

An increased spatial dispersion of ventricular repolarization during QT dispersion is associated with an increased vulnerability to arrhythmias. This study by Roukema and associates[9] from Oxford, United Kingdom, was designed to examine the effect of exercise on QT dispersion in ischemic heart disease (IHD). QT dispersion, corrected QT dispersion, and percentage change in uncorrected and corrected QT dispersion between rest and peak exercise were examined in 14 members of a control group, 17 patients with IHD, and 14 patients with IHD who were receiving β-blockers (IHD-B). All subjects had undergone a standard Bruce protocol exercise test, and QT intervals were measured at rest and peak exercise with a digitizing table interfaced to a personal computer. QT dispersion at rest was markedly increased in the IHD group compared with that in the control and IHD-B groups, respectively (corrected QT dispersion in milliseconds 74 ± 7, 40 ± 4, and 49 ± 5). The corrected QT dispersion at peak exercise was greater in the IHD group compared with that in the control group (57 ± 5 vs. 26 ± 3 ms). The percentage change in QT dispersion with exercise was significantly higher in the IHD group ($52\% \pm 5\%$) compared with that in both the control group and the IHD-B group ($30\% \pm 3\%$). A larger mean QT dispersion at peak exercise and an increased percentage change in QT dispersion with exercise may help explain the increased susceptibility of the IHD group for arrhythmias. The cardioprotective action of β-blockers may be explained by their blunting effect on exercise-related changes in QT dispersion.

Torsades de Pointes

Antihistamine Overdose

QT interval prolongation and torsades de pointes VT have been reported after therapeutic doses and overdosage of second generation antihistamines, such as terfenadine and astemizol. Diphenhydramine (DPHM), a first generation H_1 antagonist, is the most common widely used antihistaminic drug. Despite its widespread use, there are no data about cardiac action and electrocardiographic consequences of DPHM overdose. Zareba and associates[10] from Rochester, New York, evaluated by 12-lead electrocardiogram 126 patients (mean age 26 ± 11 years) who had DPHM overdose. The ingestion of large doses of DPHM (in most cases the dose was >500 mg) was primarily suicidal. Repolarization duration, dispersion, and morphology were evaluated in DPHM overdose patients and compared with those of healthy subjects. Mean heart rate of DPHM overdose patients was 103 ± 25 beats/min. The QT duration was significantly longer (453 ± 43 vs. 416 ± 35 ms, respectively, and mean T-wave amplitude significantly lower (0.20 ± 0.10 vs. 0.33 ± 0.15 mV, respectively, in DPHM-overdose patients than in control subjects. Dispersion of repolarization was significantly lower in DPHM-overdose patients than in control subjects (42 ± 25 vs. 52 ± 21 ms, respectively). None of the DPHM-overdose patients experienced torsades de pointes. In conclusion, DPHM overdose is associated with a significant increase in heart rate and a significant but moderate QTc prolongation. None of the studied patients, including those who had apparent QTc prolongation, experienced torsades de pointes VT.

The Survival with Oral D-Sotalol (SWORD) Trial

The Survival With Oral D-Sotalol (SWORD) trial tested the hypothesis that the prophylactic administration of oral d-sotalol would reduce total mortality in patients surviving AMI with an LVEF of 40% or less. The study was reported by Pratt and associates[11] for the SWORD Investigators. Two index AMI groups were included: recent (6–42 days) and remote (>42 days) with clinical CHF (n = 915 and 2,206, respectively). The trial was discontinued when the statistical boundary for harm was crossed (RR = 1.65). All baseline variables known to be associated with mortality risk (e.g., LVEF, CHF class, age) as well as variables related to torsades de pointes (e.g., time from beginning of therapy, QTc, gender, potassium, renal function, dose of d-sotalol) were assessed for interaction of each variable with treatment assignment, computing RR from Cox regression models. The d-sotalol-associated mortality was greatest in the group with remote AMI and LVEFs of 31% to 40% (RR = 7.9). Most variables known to be associated with torsades de pointes were not differentially predictive of d-sotalol-associated risk, except female gender (RR = 4.7). These findings suggest that (1) most of the d-sotalol-associated risk was in patients remote from AMI with an LVEF of 31% to 40%; comparable placebo patients had a very low mortality (0.5%); and (2) very little objective data support torsades de pointes or any specific proarrhythmic mechanism as an explanation for d-sotalol-associated mortality risk.

Syncope

Determination of the Vasovagal Origin of Syncope

Head-up tilt testing is used extensively to determine the vasovagal origin of syncope in patients with otherwise unexplained loss of consciousness, although issues remain regarding the method of the test. The diagnostic value of a shortened head-up tilt test potentiated with sublingual nitroglycerin was assessed in patients with unexplained syncope by Del Rosso and associates[12] from Florence, Italy. Two hundred two patients (mean age 49 ± 19 years) with syncope of unknown origin and 34 subjects in a control group (mean age 45 ± 17 years) were studied. The patients and the subjects in the control group were tilted upright to 60° for 20 minutes. If syncope did not occur, sublingual nitroglycerin (400 μg) was administered and observation was continued for 25 more minutes. During the unmedicated phase, syncope occurred in 22 (11%) patients and in 1 member of the control group. After nitroglycerin was administered, syncope occurred in 119 (59%) patients and in 1 (3%) member of the control group. False-positive response (exaggerated response) was observed in 8 (4%) patients and in 4 (12%) subjects in the control group. The total positivity rate of the test was 70% with a specificity rate of 94%. Short-duration head-up tilt test potentiated with sublingual nitroglycerin provides an adequate specificity and positivity rate in patients with unexplained syncope.

Long QT Syndrome

Gene Mutation in Long QT Syndrome

The long QT syndrome is a disorder of ventricular repolarization characterized by a prolonged QT interval, often associated with seizures, syncope, and sometimes sudden death. Three forms of long QT syndrome have been shown to result from mutations in potassium or sodium ion channels: *KVLQT1* for LQT1, *HERG* for LQT2, and *SCN5A* for LQT3. IsK, an apparent potassium channel subunit encoded by *KCNE1* on chromosome 21, regulates both *KVLQT1* and *HERG*. This relationship makes *KCNE1* a likely candidate gene, because mutations of these genes are known to cause both autosomal dominant Romano-Ward and recessive Jervell and Lange-Nielsen forms of LQTS. Duggal and associates[13] screened 84 unrelated patients with Romano-Ward and 4 with Jervell and Lange-Nielsen syndromes for possible mutations in *KCNE1*. They identified 1 homozygous mutation in a patient with Jervell and Lange-Nielsen syndrome that results in the nonconservative substitution of Asn for Asp at amino acid 76. The patient was congenitally deaf–mute, with recurrent syncopal events and a prolonged QT interval. The proband's mother and half-sister are both heterozygous for this mutation. Both of these family members have prolonged QT intervals and would have been classified as having Romano-Ward syndrome if not for the proband's diagnosis of Jervell and Lange-Nielsen syndrome. This mutation was not identified in more than 100 control individuals. Thus, these data provide strong evidence that *KCNE1* mutations represent a fifth LQTS locus.

Pregnancy and Cardiac Risk in Women with Long QT Syndrome

Rashba and colleagues[14] in Rochester, New York, evaluated the effects of pregnancy on women with hereditary long QT syndrome. A retrospective analysis of 422 women (111 probands affected with the long QT syndrome and 311 first-degree relatives) enrolled in the long QT syndrome registry who had 1 or more pregnancies were included in the study. The first-degree relatives were classified as affected, borderline, and unaffected. Affected patients had QTc greater than 0.47. Cardiac events were defined as the combined incidence of long QT syndrome-related death, aborted cardiac arrest, and syncope. The incidence of cardiac events was compared during equal prepregnancy, pregnancy, and postpartum intervals of 40 weeks each. Multivariate logistic regression analysis was performed by use of a mixed-effects model to identify independent predictors of cardiac events among probands. The pregnancy and postpartum intervals were not associated with cardiac events among first-degree relatives. Postpartum interval was independently associated with cardiac events among probands; the pregnancy interval was not associated with cardiac events. Treatment with β-adrenergic blockers was independently associated with a decrease in the risk for cardiac events among probands. The postpartum interval is associated with a significant increase in risk for cardiac events among probands with a long QT syndrome, but not among first-degree relatives. Prophylactic treatment with β-adrenergic blockers should be continued during pregnancy and the postpartum period.

Findings from the International LQTS Registry

Locati and colleagues[15] Perugia, Italy, evaluated age- and gender-related differences in events among patients with a long QT syndrome. They analyzed data in 479 probands (70% females) and 1,041 affected family members with QTc greater than 440 ms (58% females). Long QTS gene mutations were identified in 162 patients. Male probands were younger than females at first events and had higher event rates than females by age 15 years (74% vs. 51%). Affected family members had similar findings. By Cox analysis adjusting for QTc duration, the hazard ratio for female probands of experiencing events by age 15 years was 0.48 and it was 1.87 by age 15 to 40 years. In female family members, the hazard ratio was 0.58 by age 15 years and it was 3.25 by ages 15 to 40 years. The event rate was higher in males than in female long QTS carriers. No age–gender differences in event rate were detected in long QT2 and long QT3 carriers. Thus, among patients with a long QT syndrome, the risk of cardiac events was higher in males until puberty and higher in females during adulthood (Figure 6-5).

Identification of Gene Mutations in the KVLQT1 Potassium Channel

Li and colleagues[16] from Houston, Texas, used single-strand conformation polymorphism and DNA sequence analysis to identify mutations in the cardiac potassium channel gene, *KVLQT1*. Long QT syndrome is an inherited cardiac arrhythmia that causes sudden death in young, otherwise healthy people. Four genes for LQTS have been mapped to chromosome 11p15.5 (*LQT1*), 7q35–36 (*LQT2*), 3p21-24 (*LQT3*), and 4q25-27 (*LQT4*). Genes responsible for *LQT1*, *LQT2*, *LQT3* have been identified as cardiac potassium channel genes

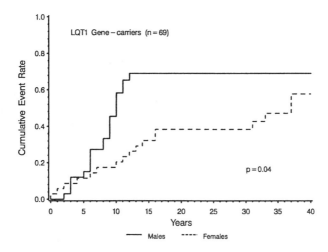

FIGURE 6-5. Cumulative age-related probability of first cardiac event (syncope or death) using birth as time of origin by Kaplan-Meier life-table analysis for LQT1 carriers (40 events among 69 LQT1 carriers). Cumulative probability of having already experienced a first cardiac event by age 15 years was higher in LQT1 males (solid line) than in females (dashed line) (70% vs. 30%, p=0.04). Reproduced with permission from Locati et al.[15]

(*KVLQT1, HERG*) and the cardiac sodium channel gene (*SCN5A*). The authors studied 115 families with LQTS, and affected members of 7 LQTS families were found to have new, previously unidentified mutations, including 2 identical missense mutations, 4 identical splicing mutations, and 1 3-bp deletion. An identical splicing mutation was identified in affected members of 4 unrelated families leading to an alternatively spliced form of *KVLQT1*. The 3-bp deletion arose *de novo* and occurred at an exon-intron boundary. This resulted in a single based deletion in the *KVLQT1* cDNA sequence and altered splicing, leading to the truncation of *KVLQT1* protein. These data suggest that the authors have identified LQTS-causing mutations of *KVLQT1* in 7 families. Five *KVLQT1* mutations cause the truncation of *KVLQT1* protein. These data provide further confirmation that *KVLQT1* mutations cause LQTS. The location and character of these mutations expand the type of mutations, confirm a mutational hot spot, and suggest that they act through a loss-of-function mechanism or a dominant-negative mechanism (Figure 6-6).

Phenotypic Characteristics of the R1623Q Mutation

Kambouris and colleagues[17] in Baltimore, Maryland, characterized the R1623Q mutation in the human cardiac sodium channel using both whole-cell and single-channel recordings. A sporadic SCN5A mutation had been identified in a Japanese girl afflicted with the long QT syndrome earlier. This externally positioned domain, S4 mutation (R1623Q) neutralized a charged residue critically involved in activation-inactivation coupling. In contrast to the autosomal dominant LQT3 mutations of long-QT syndrome, R1623Q increased the probability of long openings and caused early reopenings, producing a 3-fold prolon-

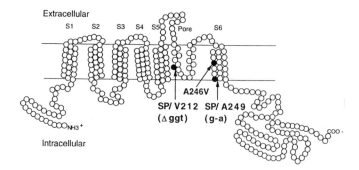

FIGURE 6-6. Model for *KVLQT1* potassium channel and location of LQT mutations. Channel consists of 6 putative membrane-embedded homologous domains (S1 to S6). Reproduced with permission from Li et al.[16]

gation of sodium current decay. Lidocaine restored rapid decay of the R1623Q macroscopic current. The R1623Q mutation produces inactivation gating defects that differ mechanistically from those caused by long QT3 mutations. The authors suggest that these data provide a biophysical explanation for the severe long QT phenotype and extend the understanding of the mechanistic role of the S4 segment in cardiac sodium channel inactivation gating and class I antiarrhythmic drug actions.

Excessive Caffeine Intake in the Genesis of Arrhythmias

Although moderate caffeine ingestion has not been shown to be arrhythmogenic, caffeine toxicity can cause severe cardiac arrhythmias, including AF and VT. AF and VT have been associated with prolongation of P-wave and QRS complex durations on signal-averaged electrocardiograms. This study by Donnerstein and associates[18] from Tucson, Arizona, investigated acute effects of caffeine ingestion on signal-averaged P-wave and QRS complexes. Signal-averaged electrocardiograms were obtained from 12 normal subjects (6 men, 6 women; ages 21 to 26 years) before and after ingestion of caffeine (5 mg/kg body weight) or placebo in a randomized, double-blind, crossover fashion. Electrocardiograms for signal averaging were recorded from electrodes left in a constant location. After bandpass filtering (30 to 300 Hz) and amplification, signals were sampled over 7.2 minutes at 2,000 Hz. Signal-averaged P-wave and QRS complex durations did not significantly change after placebo ingestion. After caffeine ingestion, QRS duration prolonged in 9 of 11 subjects at 90 minutes and in 8 of 9 after 3 hours. No significant change in P-wave duration or heart rate was found after caffeine ingestion at any test interval. Average caffeine level in saliva 90 minutes after ingestion was 6.6 ± 1.6 μg/dL. Although probably not arrhythmogenic in normal subjects, moderate caffeine ingestion does produce a small but statistically significant prolongation of signal-averaged QRS complexes. Further prolongation caused by excessive caffeine intake may be a factor in the genesis of arrhythmias associated with caffeine toxicity.

Antiarrhythmic Medication and Other Interventions

Inpatient Versus Outpatient Therapy

Simons and associates[19] from Durham, North Carolina, assessed the cost effectiveness of inpatient antiarrhythmic therapy initiation for SVT using a meta-analysis of proarrhythmic risk and a decision analysis that compared inpatient to outpatient therapy initiation. A Medline search of trials of antiarrhythmic therapy for SVTs was performed, and episodes of cardiac arrest, sudden or unexplained death, syncope, and sustained or unstable ventricular arrhythmias were recorded. A weighted average event rate, by sample size, was calculated and applied to a clinical decision model of therapy initiation in which patients were either hospitalized for 72 hours or treated as outpatients. Fifty-seven drug trials involving 2,822 patients met study criteria. Based on a 72-hour weighted average event rate of 0.63% (95% confidence interval, 0.2% to 1.2%), inpatient therapy initiation cost $19,231/year of life saved for a 60-year-old patient with a normal life expectancy. Hospitalization remained cost effective when event rates and life expectancies were varied to model hypothetical clinical scenarios. For example, cost-effectiveness ratios for a 40-year-old without structural heart disease and a 6-year-old with structural heart disease were $37,510 and $33,310, respectively, per year of life saved. Thus, a 72-hour hospitalization for antiarrhythmic therapy initiation is cost effective for most patients with SVT.

Comparison of Intravenous Quinidine and Procainamide

Intravenous procainamide hydrochloride is frequently used in the acute care setting and during electrophysiological testing, but intravenous quinidine gluconate is rarely used because of concerns about its safety. This study by Holzberger and associates[20] from Lebanon, New Hampshire, prospectively compared the hemodynamic and electrophysiological effects of these agents in patients undergoing electrophysiological testing. Sixty-five consecutive patients with inducible ventricular tachyarrhythmias were prospectively treated with either intravenous quinidine gluconate or intravenous procainamide hydrochloride in an alternating unblinded fashion. The hemodynamic and electrophysiological effects of these 2 drugs were compared. Seven (22%) patients assigned to intravenous quinidine gluconate and 8 (24%) patients assigned to intravenous procainamide hydrochloride were rendered noninducible for ventricular tachyarrhythmias. Four (13%) patients assigned to intravenous quinidine gluconate were unable to complete the infusion compared with none assigned to intravenous procainamide hydrochloride. Otherwise, the overall hemodynamic and electrophysiological effects of the 2 drugs were similar. Intravenous quinidine gluconate is a reasonable alternative to intravenous procainamide hydrochloride in patients requiring a parenteral type IA antiarrhythmic agent.

Use of Ibutilide in Treatment of Ventricular Tachycardia

Recent studies suggest that class III antiarrhythmic agents may have enhanced efficacy in the treatment of VT. This study by Wood and associates[21] from Richmond, Virginia, and Kalamazoo, Michigan, describes the first clinical assessment of the new class III agent, ibutilide, to suppress inducible monomorphic VT in human beings. Fifty-five patients with CAD and inducible sustained monomorphic VT at baseline received either low-dose (0.005 mg/kg + 0.001 mg/kg, load and maintenance infusion, respectively), middle-dose (0.01 mg/kg + 0.002 mg/kg), or high-dose (0.02 mg/kg + 0.004 mg/kg) infusions of ibutilide followed by repeat programmed ventricular stimulation. The mean age of the study group was 66 ± 9.5 years and mean LVEF was 36% ± 11%. Of 48 evaluable patients, 21 (44%) were rendered noninducible after ibutilide, with no difference in efficacy among the 3 dosing groups (p = 0.83). Ventricular effective refractory periods, QTc interval, and ventricular monophasic action potential duration were prolonged over baseline at all tested cycle lengths. The QTc and action potential prolongation were dose related. Serious drug-related adverse reactions included sustained polymorphic VT in 2 patients (3.6%), spontaneous monomorphic VT in 1 patient (1.8%), heart block in 1 patient (1.8%), and hypotension in 1 patient (1.8%). Ibutilide prolongs ventricular repolarization in humans and demonstrates efficacy in suppressing inducible monomorphic VT. Significant cardiovascular side effects occurred in 13% of patients.

Pacemakers

A Meta-Analysis of Trials to Evaluate Antibiotic Prophylaxis

Da Costa and colleagues[22] performed a meta-analysis of all available randomized trials to evaluate the effectiveness of antibiotic prophylaxis to reduce infection rates after permanent pacemaker implantation. Reports of trials were identified through Medline, Embase, Current Contents, and an extensive bibliography search. Trials that met the following criteria were included: (1) prospective, randomized, controlled, open or blind trials; (2) patients assigned to a systemic antibiotic group or a control group; (3) endpoint events related to any infection after pacemaker implantation: wound infection, septicemia, pocket abscess, purulent secretion, infective endocarditis, inflammatory signs, a positive culture, septic pulmonary embolism, or repeat operation for an infective complication. Seven trials met the inclusion criteria. They included 2,023 patients with established permanent pacemaker implantation, i.e., new implants or replacements. The incidence of endpoint events in control groups ranged from 0% to 12%. The meta-analysis suggested a consistent protective

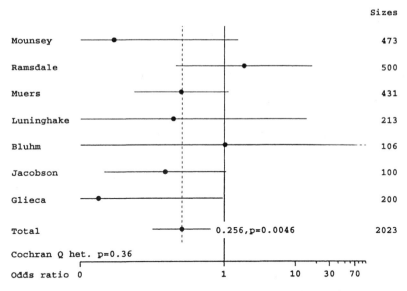

FIGURE 6-7. Antibiotic prophylaxis efficacy for permanent pacemaker implantation. Graphical representation shows odds ratio and 95% confidence interval. Data are based on the longest follow-up. Line graph shows odds ratio and 95% confidence intervals for the reduction of pacemaker infection with antibiotic administration. Reproduced with permission from Da Costa et al.[22]

effect of antibiotic therapy (p=0.0046) (Figure 6-7). Thus, the results of this meta-analysis suggest that systemic antibiotic prophylaxis significantly reduces the incidence of potentially serious infective complications after permanent pacemaker implantation.

Role of Bacteriologic Flora in Pacemaker Infections

Da Costa and colleagues[23] performed a prospective study to evaluate the role of bacteriologic flora and its occurrence. Specimens were collected at the site of implantation for culture from the skin and the pocket before and after insertion in a consecutive series of patients who had elective permanent pacemaker implantation. Microorganisms isolated both at the time of insertion of the pacemaker and of potentially infective complication were compared by using conventional speciation and ribotyping. There were 103 patients with 67 men, with a total group of patients age ranging from 16 to 93 years. At the time of pacemaker implantation, a total of 267 isolates were identified. Most of these (85%) were staphylococci. During a mean follow-up of 16.5 months, infection occurred in 4 patients (3.9%). In 2 of them, an isolate of *Staphylococcus schleiferi* was recognized by molecular method as identical to the one previously found in the pacemaker pocket. In 1 patient, *Staphylococcus aureus,* an organism that was absent at the time of the pacemaker insertion, was isolated. In another patient, *Staphylococcus epidermidis* was identified both at the time of pacemaker insertion and when erosion occurred, but their antibiotic resistance profiles were different. These data support the hypothesis that pacemaker-related infections are due mainly to local contamination during implantation. *S. schleiferi* appears to play an underestimated role in infectious colonization of implanted biomaterials and should be regarded as an important opportunistic pathogen.

Pacemaker Infective Endocarditis

Cacoub and colleagues[24] from Paris, France, identified 33 patients with pacemaker endocarditis. Most patients (75%) were 60 years of age or older (mean 66 ± 3; range 21 to 86). Pouch hematoma or inflammation was common (58%), but other predisposing factors for endocarditis were rare. At the time that pacemaker endocarditis was found, the mean number of leads was 2.4 ± 1.1 (range 1 to 7). The interval from the last procedure to diagnosis of endocarditis was 20 ± 4 months (range 1 to 72). Endocarditis appeared early (<3 months) after pacemaker implantation in 10 patients and late (≥3 months) in 23 patients. Fever was the most common symptom, being isolated in 36%, associated with a poor general condition in 24%, and associated with septic shock in 9%. Transthoracic echocardiography showed vegetations in only 2 of 9 patients. Transesophageal echocardiography demonstrated the presence of lead vegetations (n = 20) or tricuspid vegetations (n = 3) in 23 of 24 patients (96%). Pulmonary scintigraphy showed a typical pulmonary embolus in 7 of 17 patients (41%). Pathogens were isolated mainly from blood (82%) and lead (91%) cultures. The major pathogens causing pacemaker endocarditis were *Staphylococcus epidermidis* (n = 17) and *S. aureus* (n = 7). *S. epidermidis* was found more often in early than in late endocarditis (90% vs. 50%). All patients were treated with prolonged antibiotic regimens before and after electrode removal. Electrode removal was achieved by surgery (n = 29) or traction (n = 4). Associated procedures were performed in 9 patients. After the intensive care period, only 17 patients needed a new permanent pacemaker. Overall mortality was 24% after a mean follow-up period of 22 ± 4 months (range 1 to 88). Eight patients (significantly older [74 ± 3 vs. 63 ± 3 years]) died in 2 months or less after electrode removal, whereas 25 were alive and asymptomatic.

Implantable Cardioverter-Defibrillators

Benefit of Implantable Cardioverter-Defibrillator Therapy

Böcker and colleagues[25] in Münster, Germany, investigated whether New York Heart Association functional class had an impact on the potential benefit from implantable cardioverter-defibrillator therapy (ICD) as assessed from the data stored in the memory of ICDs. Between 1989 and 1996, 603 patients, including 77% men, 59% of whom had CAD and 16% dilated cardiomyopathy with a mean LVEF of 44% ± 18% were treated with an ICD with extended memory function. The stages of heart failure as related to NYHA functional class I through III at implantation were correlated with overall mortality and the recurrence of fast ventricular arrhythmias greater than 240 bpm during follow-up. The potential benefit of the device was estimated as the difference between overall mortality and the hypothetical death rate had the device not been implanted. The latter was based on the recurrence of fast, and without termination by the device, presumably fatal ventricular tachyarrhythmias. In the overall group, a significant difference between hypothetical death rate and overall mortality was observed and was 13.9%, 23.5%, and 26.6% at 1, 3, and 5 years, respectively, suggesting a benefit from ICD implantation. In patients in NYHA class I, the estimated benefit, which increased over time was 15.2%, 29%, and 36% after 1, 3, and 5 years, respectively. In patients in NYHA classes II or III, the estimated benefit increased until the third year (22% and 22%, respectively) and then remained constant until the fifth year (23% and 24%, respectively). Even those patients in NYHA class III with a history of decompensated heart failure benefited from ICD implantation (Figure 6-8). Thus, analysis

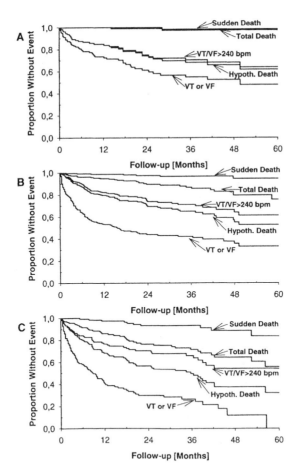

FIGURE 6-8. Actuarial survival rates for freedom from death of any cause, sudden death, fast ventricular tachyarrhythmia (>240 bpm), VTs of any rate, and hypothetical death rate (Hypoth. Death). **(A)** patients in NYHA functional class I; **(B)** patients in NYHA class II; and **(C)** patients in NYHA class III. Reproduced with permission from Böcker et al.[25]

of stored ECG data suggests that in patients with a history of VT or VF, ICD therapy may lead to a prolongation of life in NYHA functional classes I–III.

The Multicenter Automatic Defibrillator Implantation Trial (MADIT) Results

Mushlin and colleagues for the MADIT (Multicenter Automatic Defibrillator Implantation Trial) Investigators[26] determined the economic consequences of defibrillator management in selected asymptomatic patients with CAD and nonsustained VT who had shown improvement as a result of defibrillator implantation. Patients were followed to quantify their use of health care services, including hospitalizations, physician visits, medications, laboratory tests, and procedures during the trial. The costs of these services, including the costs of the defibrillator, were determined in patients randomized to defibrillator and nondefibrillator therapy. Incremental cost-effectiveness ratios were calculated by relating these costs to the increased survival associated with the use of the defibrillator. The average survival for the defibrillator group over a 4-year period was 3.7 years compared with 2.8 years for conventionally treated patients. Accumulated net costs were $97,560 for the defibrillator group compared with $75,980 for individuals treated with medications alone. The resulting incremental cost-effectiveness ratio of $27,000/life-year saved compares favorably with other cardiac interventions. Sensitivity analyses showed that the incremental cost-effectiveness ratio would be reduced to approximately $23,000/life-year saved if transvenous defibrillators were used instead of the older device, which required thoracic surgery for implantation. Thus, an implanted cardiac defibrillator is cost-effective in selected individuals at increased risk for ventricular arrhythmias (Figure 6-9).

The Atrioverter

Wellens and colleagues[27] in Maastricht, The Netherlands, evaluated 51 patients with recurrent AF who had not responded to antiarrhythmic drugs. They were in New York Heart Association functional class I or II and they were at low risk for ventricular arrhythmias. The atrial defibrillation threshold had to be 240 V or less in this study. Wellens et al. tested the safety and efficacy of a system called the Atrioverter in a prospective, multicenter study. The Atrioverter is an implantable defibrillator connected to right atrial and coronary sinus defibrillation leads, allowing prompt restoration of sinus rhythm by low energy shock. AF detection, R-wave shock synchronization, and defibrillation threshold were tested at implantation and during follow-up. Shock termination of spontaneous episodes of AF was performed under physician observation. During a follow-up of 72 to 613 days, mean 259 ± 138 days, 96% of 227 spontaneous episodes of AF in 41 patients were successfully converted to sinus rhythm by the Atrioverter. In 27% of episodes, several shocks were required because of early recurrence of AF. Shocks did not induce ventricular arrhythmias. Most

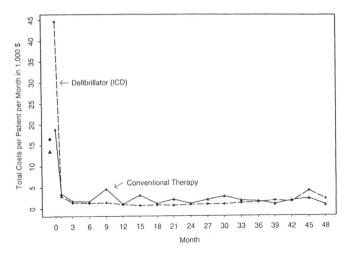

Figure 6-9. Total medical costs per patient per month, according to assigned treatment. For each month indicated (1 through 48), total medical costs during the preceding period were averaged over the available surviving patients in the study, in the indicated treatment group, and converted to a per month basis. Costs at month 0 represent costs for the initial hospitalization, averaged over patients. Before month 0, the diamond represents hospital costs during the prior year averaged over the defibrillator group and the triangle represents hospital costs during the prior year averaged over the conventional therapy group. Total costs include all hospital, emergency room, physician, and specialist visits; prescription medications; outpatient diagnostic tests and procedures; community services; and medical supplies. Reproduced with permission from Mushlin et al.[26]

patients received antiarrhythmic medication during follow-up. In 4 patients, the Atrioverter was removed because of infection in 1, cardiac tamponade in 1, and frequent episodes of AF requiring His bundle ablation in another. Thus, with the Atrioverter, prompt and safe restoration of sinus rhythm is possible in patients with recurrent AF (Figure 6-10).

Antitachycardia Pacing

Schaumann and colleagues[28] in Göttingen, Germany, evaluated whether testing of antitachycardia pacing for induced VT at predischarge examination predicts antitachycardia success from automatic implantable cardioverter-defibrillators (AICDs) during subsequent follow-up. The study involved 200 consecutive patients who received AICD implants from June 1991 through December 1995. All of these patients underwent electrophysiological testing. In 54 patients, antitachycardia pacing terminated induced VT successfully. In 146 patients, only VF could be induced, including 18 with unsuccessful antitachycardia pacing attempts for induced VT. Disregarding the results of antitachycardia pacing testing, the same scheme was programmed in all patients: 3 attempts of autodecremental ramp with 81% of the VT cycle length, with 8 to 10 pulses. During a follow-up of 20 ± 10 months, 95% of 3,819 spontaneous VTs were terminated successfully with antitachycardia pacing in 42 patients

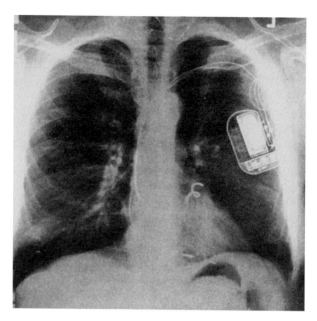

FIGURE 6-10. Chest roentgenogram showing Atrioverter with leads in right atrium, coronary sinus, and apex of right ventricle. Right atrium and coronary sinus leads are used for arrhythmia recognition and defibrillation. Right ventricle lead is used for shock synchronization and, if needed, ventricular pacing. Reproduced with permission from Wellens et al.[27]

of group T. In another group (E), 90% of 1,346 spontaneous VTs in 81 patients were terminated with antitachycardia pacing. Acceleration after antitachycardia pacing occurred in 2% of patients in group T compared to 5% in group E. The success for all episodes in the individual patients was 90% or more in more than 60% of the antitachycardia pacing tested and empirically programmed patients. The results of this 200-patient prospective study comparing tested versus empirical antitachycardia pacing showed high success for VT termination, with low rates of acceleration. Antitachycardia pacing is safe and effective and should be programmed "on" in all patients regardless of the predischarge electrophysiology inducibility.

Risk of Syncope with Implantable Cardioverter-Defibrillators

Implantable cardioverter-defibrillators are effective in terminating VT and VF, although syncope may still occur. This latter problem can be considerable in patients, for example, who drive automobiles. Bansch and colleagues[29] from Munster and Bielefeld, Germany, retrospectively analyzed 421 patients followed for 26 months. Fifty-four percent had recurrent VT/VF and 14.7% had syncope. The actuarial survival rate free of VT/VF was 58%, 45%, and 37% and that for survival from syncope was 90%, 85%, and 81% at 1, 2, and 3 years after implantation. A low baseline LVEF, induction of fast VT during program stimulation, and chronic AF were associated with increased risk of syncope.

If the LVEF was greater than 40%, fast VT had not been induced and patients had no chronic AF, 96%, 92%, and 92% remain free of syncope after 1, 2, and 3 years, respectively. Once patients had a VT recurrence, syncope during the first VT and a high VT rate were the strongest risk predictors of future syncope. These authors conclude that identification of a low and high risk of syncope seems to be feasible in patients with an implantable defibrillator.

Comparison of Metoprolol and Sotalol

Seidl and associates[30] from Lugwigshafen, Germany, evaluated prospectively on an intention-to-treat basis the efficacy of d,l-sotalol and metoprolol with regard to the recurrence of arrhythmic events after implantable cardioverter-defibrillator (ICD) implantation. After ICD implantation, 70 patients were randomly assigned to treatment with either metoprolol (mean dosage 104 ± 37 mg/day in 35 patients) or d,l-sotalol (mean dosage 242 ± 109 mg/day in 35 patients). During follow-up, VT, fast VT, and VF episodes were calculated. Metoprolol treatment led to a marked reduction in the recurrence of arrhythmic events. Actuarial rates for absence of VT recurrence at 1 and 2 years were significantly higher in the metoprolol group compared with the d,l-sotalol group (83% and 80% vs. 57% and 51%, respectively). The actuarial rates for absence of fast VT or VF were 80% in the metoprolol group compared with 46% in the d,l-sotalol group. During a follow-up of 26 ± 16 months, there were 3 deaths in the metoprolol group compared with 6 deaths in the d,l-sotalol group. Actuarial rates of overall survival were not significantly different in the 2 groups (91% vs. 83%). In this prospective, randomized, controlled study, the recurrence rate of VT in patients treated with metoprolol was lower than in patients treated with d,l-sotalol.

Digital Cellular Telephone Interaction with Implantable Cardioverter-Defibrillators

There has been a concern that various environmental energy signals could trigger adverse interactions with implantable cardioverter-defibrillators (ICDs). Fetter and colleagues[31] from Minneapolis, Minnesota, examined the effects of cellular phone interference on the operation of various models of market-released ICDs from a single manufacturer, Medtronic, Inc. None of the ICDs tested in 41 patients were affected by oversensing of the electromagnetic field of cellular telephones during the *in vivo* study. These authors conclude that TDMA-10 cellular telephones did not interfere with these types of implantable defibrillators. As a precautionary measure, however, the authors recommend that the patient not carry or place the digital cellular telephone within 6 inches of the ICD.

Adverse Events with Implantable Cardioverter-Defibrillators

Rosenqvist and colleagues[32] in Stockholm, Sweden, monitored adverse events during prospective clinical evaluation of the Medtronic model 7219

Jewel ICD and classified them according to the definitions of the ISO 14155 standard for device clinical trials into 3 groups: severe and mild device-related and severe non-device-related adverse events. In addition, events were related to the surgical procedure, treatment with the device, or cardiac function. Seven hundred seventy-eight patients were followed for an average of 4.0 months after ICD implantation. Three hundred fifty-six adverse events were observed in 259 patients. At 1, 3, and 12 months after ICD implantation, 99%, 98%, and 97% of the patients, respectively, survived 95%, 93%, and 92%, respectively, free of surgical reintervention, and 79%, 68%, and 51%, respectively, free of any adverse event. Twenty patients died; 6 deaths were related to the surgical procedure. Twelve deaths were considered unrelated to ICD treatment and 2 patients died of unknown causes. Among 111 nonlethal serious adverse device effects, 47 required surgical intervention, 19 times for correction of a dislodged lead. Inappropriate delivery of therapy was observed 128 times in 111 patients; these events were resolved usually by reprogramming the device. Thus, approximately 50% of patients experience an adverse event within the first year after ICD implantation. The incidence of inappropriate therapy emphasizes the need for improved detection algorithms.

Radiofrequency Catheter Ablation

Atrial Mapping and Radiofrequency Catheter Ablation

Gaita and colleagues[33] in Asti, Italy, evaluated the electrophysiological features of idiopathic AF and their relationship to the results of radiofrequency catheter ablation of AF and the safety and effectiveness of this procedure in 16 patients who underwent atrial mapping during AF and then RF ablation in the right atrium. Atrial activation was recorded in 4 regions in the right atrium: high lateral wall, low lateral wall, high septum, and low septum and in the left atrium through the coronary sinus. In these regions, the AF intervals and the morphological features of AF recordings were evaluated by Wells' classification. There were no complications during RF ablation. Among 16 patients, 9 (56%) without AF recurrences during the follow-up of 11 ± 4 months were considered successfully ablated. These patients demonstrated a significantly shorter mean AF interval in the high septum and the low septum than in the high lateral wall and low lateral wall. Moreover, the septum had more irregular electrical activity with greater beat-to-beat changes in AF intervals and a higher prevalence of type III AF in the lateral region. The coronary sinus had similar behavior to the septum. Thus, patients with unsuccessful ablation had an irregular atrial activity in the lateral wall, septum, and coronary sinus with no significant differences between the different sites. Right atrial endocardial catheter ablation of AF is a safe procedure and may be effective in some patients with idiopathic AF. Atrial mapping during AF showed a more disorganized right atrial activation in the septum than in the lateral wall in patients with successful ablation.

Ablation of Type 1 Atrial Flutter

Paydak and colleagues[34] in Chicago, Illinois, examined the time to onset, the determinants, and clinical course of AF after ablation of type I atrial flutter in 110 consecutive patients. AF was documented in 28 (25%) during a mean follow-up of 20 ± 9 months for a cumulative probability of 12% at 1 month, 23% at 1 year, and 30% at 2 years. Among 17 clinical and procedural variables, only a history of spontaneous AF and LVEF of less than 50% were significant and independent predictors of subsequent AF. The presence of both of these characteristics identified a high-risk group with a 74% occurrence of AF (Figure 6-11). Patients with only 1 of these characteristics were at intermediate risk (20%), and those with neither characteristic were at lowest risk (10%). The determinants and clinical course of AF did not differ between an early (≤1 month) compared with a later onset. AF was persistent and recurrent, requiring long-term therapy in 18 patients, including 12 of 19 (63%) with prior AF and LV dysfunction. AF after type I atrial flutter ablation is determined primarily by the presence of a preexisting structural and electrophysiological substrate. These data should be considered in planning postablation management.

Assessment of Treatment in Chronic Atrial Fibrillation

Brignole and colleagues[35] conducted a multicenter, controlled, randomized, 12-month evaluation of the clinical effects of atrioventricular junction ablation and VVIR pacemaker versus pharmacological treatment in 66 patients with chronic AF who had clinically manifest CHF and heart rate faster than 90 bpm on 3 standard electrocardiograms recorded at rest during stable conditions on different days. Before completion of the study, withdrawals occurred in 8 patients in the drug group and in 4 patients with the ablation pacing. At

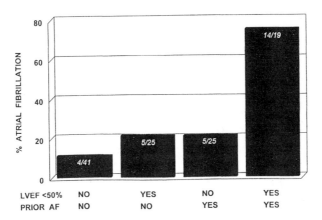

Figure 6-11. Risk of AF during follow-up as a function of a prior history of AF and LV dysfunction. Bars indicate the proportion of each of 4 patient subgroups that developed AF. Numerical proportions are in italics within each bar. AF = atrial fibrillation; LVEF = left ventricular ejection fraction. Reproduced with permission from Paydak et al.[34]

the end of 12 months, the 28 ablation pacing patients who completed the study showed lower scores in palpitations than the patients in the drug-treated group. Lower scores were also observed for exercise intolerance, easy fatigue, and New York Heart Association functional classification, and activity scale. The intrapatient comparison between enrollment and month 12 showed that in the ablation pacing group, all variables except easy fatigue improved significantly from 14% to 82%. However, because an improvement was also observed in the drug-treated group, the difference between the 2 groups was significant only for palpitations, effort dyspnea, exercise intolerance, easy fatigability, and chest discomfort. Cardiac performance, evaluated by a standard echocardiogram and exercise test, did not differ significantly between the 2 groups. Thus, in patients with CHF and chronic AF, ablation pacing treatment is effective and superior to drug therapy in controlling symptoms, although its efficacy appears to be less than observed in uncontrolled studies because some improvement can also be expected in medically treated patients.

Use of Irrigated-Tip Catheter Ablation

Jaïs and colleagues[36] in Bordeaux-Pessac, France, investigated the use of irrigated-tip catheters in a small subset of patients who failed isthmus ablation with conventional radiofrequency ablation attempts of their typical right atrial flutter. Among 170 patients referred for ablation of common atrial flutter, conventional ablation of the cavotricuspid isthmus with more than 21 applications failed to create a bidirectional block in 13 (7.6%). An irrigated-tip catheter ablation was performed on identified gaps in the ablation line according to a protocol found to be safe in animals: a moderate flow rate of 17 mL/min and temperature-controlled radiofrequency delivery with a target temperature of 50°C with a power limit of 50 W. Bidirectional isthmus block was achieved in 12 of these 13 patients by use of a mean delivered power of 40 ± 6 W with a single application in 6 patients and 2 to 6 applications in the remaining 6 individuals. There were no important side effects identified during or after the procedure. Thus, irrigated-tip catheter ablation is safe and effective for achieving cavotricuspid isthmus block when conventional radiofrequency energy has failed.

Radiofrequency Catheter Ablation of Ventricular Tachycardia After Myocardial Infarction

Stevenson and colleagues[37] in Boston, Massachusetts, assessed the feasibility of ablation of VT in patients selected without regard to the presence of multiple VTs by targeting all VTs that allowed EP mapping. Radiofrequency catheter ablation targeting all inducible monomorphic VTs that allowed mapping was performed in 52 patients with prior AMI. Antiarrhythmic drug therapy had failed in 41 (79%) patients, including amiodarone in 36 (69%) patients. An average of 3.6 morphologies of VT were induced per patient. More than 1

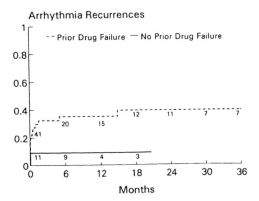

Arrhythmia Recurrences

FIGURE 6-12. Arrhythmia recurrences are shown for the 41 patients who had previously failed antiarrhythmic therapy (dashed line) and 11 patients who had not previously failed antiarrhythmic drug therapy (solid line). Number of patients remaining at each point in time is shown below the curves. Reproduced with permission from Stevenson et al.[37]

ablation session was required in 16 (31%) patients. Complications occurred in 5 (10%) patients, including 1 (2%) death caused by AMI. During a follow-up, 59% of patients continued to receive amiodarone. Twenty-three (45%) had implantable defibrillators. During a mean follow-up of 18 ± 15 months, 1 patient died suddenly, 2 died from uncontrollable VT, and 5 died from heart failure. The three-year survival rate was 70% ± 10%, and rate of risk of VT recurrence was 33% ± 7%. Radiofrequency catheter ablation controls VT that is sufficiently stable to allow mapping in 67% of patients despite failure of antiarrhythmic drug therapy and multiple inducible VTs. However, the ablation was largely adjunctive to amiodarone and defibrillators in this referral population (Figure 6-12).

Radiation Exposure During Catheter Ablation Procedures

Rosenthal and associates[38] from Baltimore, Maryland, identified factors that predict fluoroscopy duration and radiation exposure during catheter ablation procedures. They studied 859 patients who participated in the Atakr Ablation System clinical trial at 1 of 9 centers (398 male and 461 female patients, aged 36 ± 21 years). Each patient underwent catheter ablation of an accessory pathway, the atrioventricular junction, or atrioventricular nodal reentrant tachycardia using standard techniques. The duration of fluoroscopy was 53 ± 50 minutes. Factors identified as independent predictors of fluoroscopy duration included patient age and gender, the success or failure of the ablation procedure, and the institution at which the ablation was performed. Catheter ablation in adults required longer fluoroscopy exposure than it did in children. Men required longer durations of fluoroscopy exposure than did women. The mean estimated "entrance" radiation dose was 1.3 ± 1.3 Sv. The dose needed to cause radiation skin injury was exceeded during 22% of procedures. The overall mean effective absorbed dose from catheter ablation procedures was

0.025 Sv for female patients and 0.017 Sv for male patients. This degree of radiation exposure would result in an estimated 1,400 excess fatal malignancies in female patients and 2,600 excess fatal malignancies in male patients/1 million patients.

Atrioventricular Nodal Reentry Tachycardia

Use of Adenosine-5'-Triphosphate in Diagnosis of Dual Atrioventricular Node Physiology

Belhassen and colleagues[39] in Tel-Aviv, Israel, determined whether administration of adenosine-5'-triphosphate (ATP) during sinus rhythm may be useful in the noninvasive diagnosis of dual AV nodal pathways. During electrophysiological study, they intravenously administered incremental doses of ATP from 10 to 50 mg during sinus rhythm to patients with spontaneous and inducible sustained AV nodal reentrant tachycardia in a study group of 42 patients and to patients with no evidence of dual AV nodal physiology or inducible AV node reentrant tachycardia (21 patients). Signs suggestive of dual AV nodal physiology after ATP administration during sinus rhythm were observed in 32 (76%) of 42 study patients, but in only 1 (5%) of the 21 control patients. Similar results were observed when only surface lead recordings were evaluated. Signs suggestive of dual AV nodal physiology by the ATP test were observed in 29 (80.5%) of 36 patients who had electrophysiological demonstration of dual AV nodal physiology and in 3 (50%) of 6 patients without AV nodal duality. Signs suggestive of dual physiology according to the ATP test disappeared in 11 (92%) of the 12 patients who underwent successful slow AV nodal ablation but persisted in 8 (62%) of 13 patients who underwent AV nodal modification. These data suggest that the administration of ATP during sinus rhythm may be a useful bedside test for identifying patients with dual AV nodal pathways who are prone to AV nodal reentrant tachycardia.

Effects of Adenosine on Antegrade and Retrograde Fast Pathway Conduction

Although adenosine depresses antegrade AV nodal conduction, the effects of adenosine on antegrade and retrograde fast pathway conduction in AV nodal reentry have not been determined. In 17 patients (5 men, 12 women, mean age 49 ± 12 years) with common slow–fast AV nodal reentrant tachycardia, the antegrade slow pathway conduction was selectively and completely ablated by radiofrequency catheter ablation, while the antegrade and retrograde fast pathway conduction remained intact in this study by Lee and associates[40] from Taiwan, Republic of China, and Gainesville, Florida. During high RA pacing at a mean pacing cycle length of 474 ± 36 ms, adenosine was rapidly injected intravenously at an initial dose of 0.5 mg followed by stepwise increases of 0.5 mg or 1.0 mg given at 5-minute intervals until second-degree AV block developed. During RV apical pacing at the same pacing cycle lengths (mean 474 ± 36 m) as those in the study of antegrade conduction, intravenous injection of incremental doses of adenosine was repeated until ventriculoatrial block occurred. The adenosine-induced prolongation of ventriculoatrial conduction was also determined in the presence of verapamil (loading dose 0.15 mg/kg, maintenance dose 0.005 mg/kg/min) in 7 of 17 patients. The dose of adenosine required to produce AV block, the increase in the atrio-His interval by 50% and the maximal response were 3.4 ± 1.4 mg, 1.8 ± 0.6 mg, and 58 ± 5%, respectively. On the other hand, the dose of adenosine required to produce ventriculoatrial block, the increase in the ventriculoatrial interval by 50% and the maximal response were 8.2 ± 2.9 mg, 3.4 ± 0.6 mg, and 20% ± 5%, respectively, in the control and 3.7 ± 0.5 mg, 3.5 ± 0.7 mg, and 23% ± 5%, respectively, in the presence of verapamil. In conclusion, adenosine has a differential potency to depress AV and ventriculoatrial conduction in patients with AV nodal reentry, with greater potency for slowing antegrade fast than retrograde fast pathway conduction. Verapamil had an additive effect to adenosine on slowing retrograde ventriculoatrial conduction, which further supports the evidence that the retrograde fast pathway in part involves an AV nodal-like structure.

Right and Left Bundle Branch Block

Gender Differences in Ventricular Function in Right Bundle Branch Block

LV function in patients with right BBB is variable and depends on the population under study. This study by Allen and associates[41] from Rochester, Minnesota, assessed the implications of right BBB for the estimation of resting LV function in patients with right BBB and suspected CAD. Seventy-four patients with right BBB, symptoms suggestive of CAD, and no electrocardiographic Q waves were compared with 649 patients with entirely normal electrocardiograms to assess the implications of right BBB on resting LV function. Resting EF was determined by radionuclide ventriculography. Patients with right BBB were older (mean 65 ± 10 years vs. 54 ± 11) and had a lower mean EF (60% ± 11% vs. 63% ± 9%) compared with patients with normal electrocardiograms. There was a highly significant interaction between right BBB and gender with respect to resting EF. The mean EF for men with right BBB was 57% ± 10% (17% with abnormal resting EF) compared with 62% ± 8% (7% with abnormal resting EF) for normal men. In contrast, the mean EF for women with right BBB was 68% ± 9% (0% with abnormal resting EF) compared with 65% ± 9% (5% with abnormal resting EF) for normal women. Male patients with right BBB and symptoms suggestive of CAD have a lower resting EF than male patients with normal electrocardiograms. This difference is not seen in female patients.

Right Bundle Branch Block and ST Segment Elevation in Leads V_1–V_3

Brugada and colleagues[42] in Barcelona, Spain, described a specific electrocardiographic pattern of right BBB and ST segment elevation in leads V_1 through V_3 associated with sudden death in patients without demonstrable structural heart disease. Information on long-term outcome had recently become available at 33 centers worldwide, including in 63 patients, 57 men with a mean age of 38 years with the described electrocardiographic pattern. Subsequent arrhythmic events and sudden death were identified and events were analyzed for patients with at least 1 episode of aborted sudden death or syncope of unknown origin before recognition of the syndrome (symptomatic patients, n = 41) and for patients in whom the electrocardiographic pattern was recognized by chance or because of screening related to sudden death or relative asymptomatic patients (n = 22). During a mean follow-up of 34 months, an arrhythmic event occurred in 14 symptomatic patients (34%) and 6 asymptomatic patients (27%). An automatic defibrillator was implanted in 35 patients; 15 received pharmacological therapy with β-blockers and/or amiodarone, and 13 did not receive treatment. The incidence of arrhythmic events was similar in all therapy groups, but total mortality was 0% in the implantable defibrillator group, 26% in the pharmacologically treated groups, and 31% in the no treatment group (Figure 6-13). All mortality was due to sudden death. Patients without demonstrable structural heart disease and an electrocardiographic pattern of right BBB and ST segment elevation in leads V_1 through V_3 are at risk for sudden death. Amiodarone and/or β-blockers do not protect them and an implantable defibrillator appears to be the treatment of choice.

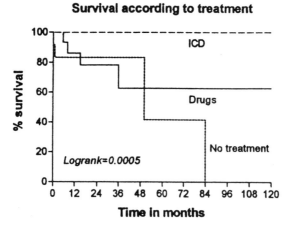

FIGURE 6-13. Kaplan-Meier curves of mortality depending on treatment. Mortality was significantly different during follow-up in patients with an implantable cardioverter defibrillator (ICD) compared with patients with medical therapy or no therapy. Reproduced with permission from Brugada et al.[42]

Atrial Fibrillation/Flutter

Cardiac Performance After Cardioversion

The mechanism for early improvement in cardiac function after cardioversion from AF is unknown. Raymond and associates[43] from Farmington, Connecticut, and Boston, Massachusetts, measured ventricular volumes and load-independent contractility during AF and within 24 hours after cardioversion to sinus rhythm in 15 adult patients (10 men, 5 women; mean age 63 ± 4 years, range 31 to 81 years). Duration of AF ranged from under 1 day to 6 months. After cardioversion, LVEF increased from 51% ± 4% to 61% ± 4%, stroke volume increased from 57 ± 4 mL to 76 ± 6 mL, and mean cycle length increased from 0.77 ± .04 seconds in AF to 1.02 ± 0.04 seconds in sinus rhythm. Cardiac contractility, as expressed by the slope and the intercept of the relation between rate-corrected circumferential velocity of fiber shortening and end-systolic wall stress, remained unaltered in 13 of 15 patients, suggesting that intrinsic inotropic state was unchanged immediately after return of normal sinus rhythm. Finally, a significant correlation was observed between improvement in stroke volume and peak A-wave velocity. Both LV stroke volume and EF increase immediately after cardioversion, whereas intrinsic cardiac contractility is largely unchanged. These data suggest that the mechanism of this increase is enhanced LV diastolic filling due mostly to increased cycle length and return of LA mechanical function.

Reduction in Internal Atrial Defibrillation Thresholds

Cooper and colleagues[44] in Birmingham, Alabama, tested the ability of sequential shocks delivered through dual-current pathways to lower the atrial defibrillation threshold (ADFT) compared with a biphasic shock through a standard single-current pathway. Electrodes were placed in the right atrial appendage, left subclavian vein, proximal coronary sinus, and distal coronary sinus in 14 patients with chronic AF. Using a step-up protocol, the authors compared ADFTs for a single-current pathway that used a single 7.5/2.5 ms biphasic shock from a 150-μF capacitor with those for a dual-current pathway system followed by using sequential biphasic shocks with capacitor discharge waveforms for 150-μF and 600-μF capacitors. Both dual-current pathway configurations had a significantly lower ADFT than the single-current higher pathway. Whereas the dual-current pathway with 150-μF capacitor shocks had a significantly lower energy threshold, there was no statistical difference in terms of leading-edge voltage compared with the dual-current pathway with 600 μF. There were no ventricular arrhythmias induced with appropriately synchronized shocks. Thus, for internal atrial defibrillation in humans, sequential biphasic waveforms delivered over dual-current pathways resulted in a markedly reduced ADFT compared with a single shock over a single-current pathway.

Impact of Atrial Fibrillation on the Risk of Death

In this study, Benjamin and colleagues[45] in the Framingham Heart Study examined the mortality of subjects 55 to 94 years of age who developed AF during 40 years of follow-up of the original Framingham Heart Study cohort. Of the original 5,209 subjects, 296 men and 325 women with mean ages 74 and 76 years, respectively, developed AF. By pooled logistic regression, after adjustment for age, hypertension, smoking, diabetes, LVH, MI, CHF, valvular heart disease, and stroke or transient ischemic attack, AF was associated with an odds ratio for death of 1.5 in men. The risk of mortality conferred by AF did not vary significantly by age. There was a significant AF-gender interaction: AF diminished the female advantage. In secondary multivariate analyses, in subjects free of valvular heart disease and preexisting cardiovascular disease, AF remained significantly associated with excess mortality with an approximate doubling of mortality in both genders. In subjects from the original cohort of the Framingham Heart Study, AF was associated with a 1.5- to 1.9-fold mortality risk after adjustment for the preexisting cardiovascular conditions with which AF was related. Decreased survival seen with AF was present in men and women and across a wide range of ages (Figure 6-14).

Effects of Class I and Class III Drugs on Atrial Flutter

Tai and colleagues[46] in Taipei, Taiwan, evaluated the effects of class I and class III antiarrhythmic agents on the reentrant circuit of typical atrial flutter in 36 patients with a mean age of 53 ± 17 years with clinically documented typical atrial flutter. A 20-pole "halo" catheter was positioned around the tricuspid annulus. Incremental pacing was performed to measure the conduction velocity along the isthmus and lateral wall, and extrastimulation was performed to evaluate atrial refractory period in the baseline state and after intravenous infusion of ibutilide, propafenone, and amiodarone. The efficacy of these drugs in the conversion of typical atrial flutter and patterns of termination were determined. Ibutilide significantly increased the atrial refractory period and decreased conduction velocity in the isthmus at short pacing cycle length. It terminated atrial flutter in 8 (67%) of 12 patients after prolongation of flutter cycle length due to an increase of 86% ± 19% in conduction time in the isthmus. Propafenone predominantly decreased conduction velocity with use dependency and significantly increased atrial refractory period, but it only converted atrial flutter in 4 (33%) of 12 patients. Amiodarone had fewer effects on atrial refractory period and conduction velocity than did ibutilide and propafenone, and it terminated atrial flutter in only 4 (33%) of 12 patients. Termination of typical atrial flutter was due to failure of wavefront propagation through the isthmus, which occurred with cycle length oscillation, abruptly without variability of cycle length, or after premature activation of the reentrant circuit.

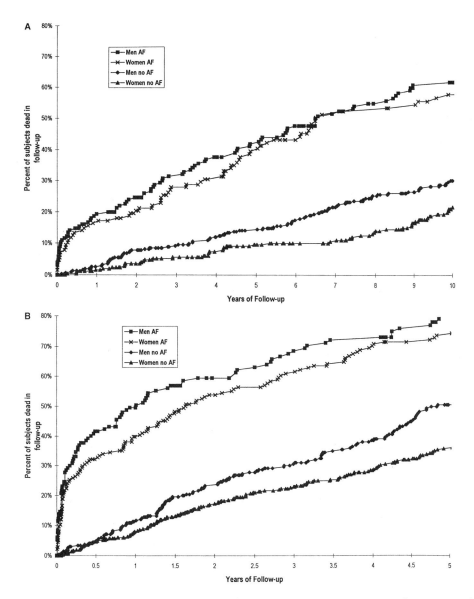

FIGURE 6-14. **(A)** Kaplan-Meier mortality curves for subjects 55 to 74 years of age. Vertical axis shows percent of subjects dead at follow-up (0% to 80%); horizontal axis, up to 10 years of follow-up. Subjects included men with AF (n=159), men without AF (n=318), women with AF (n=133), and women without AF (n=266). Both men and women with AF had significantly higher mortality than age-, gender-, and calendar year-matched non-AF subjects. Log rank test for men gave $\chi^2 = 42.90$ (p < 0.0001); for women, $\chi^2 = 70.93$ (p < 0.0001). **(B)** Kaplan-Meier mortality curves for subjects 75 to 94 years of age. Vertical axis shows percent of subjects dead at follow-up (0% to 80%); horizontal axis, up to 5 years of follow-up. Results are shown for men with AF (n=137), men without AF (n=274), women with AF (n=192), and women without AF (n=384). Both men and women with AF had significantly higher mortality than age-, gender-, and calendar year-matched non-AF subjects. Log rank test for men gave $\chi^2 = 51.44$ (p < 0.0001); for women, $\chi^2 = 101.51$ (p < 0.0001). Reproduced with permission from Benjamin et al.[45]

Mitral Regurgitation and Reduced Stroke Risk in Atrial Flutter

Significant MR is protective against LA spontaneous echo contrast formation that is associated with an increased thromboembolic risk. However, the
effects of MR on the risk of stroke in patients with nonrheumatic AF have been
unknown. Nakagami and associates[47] from Tochigi, Japan, studied whether
or not MR was associated with a decreased risk of stroke in patients with
nonrheumatic AF. The investigators performed an observational analysis of
retrospectively collected data on 290 patients with nonrheumatic AF. Left atrial
diameter (LAD) and the degree of MR were estimated by transthoracic echocardiography. Risk factors for stroke were assessed by univariate and multivariate
analyses. The mean follow-up was 7.4 years. Among these patients, 68 had a
stroke during the follow-up (rate of stroke/year of follow-up 3.2%). In 95 patients with LAD of 48 mm or more, the incidence of stroke (9%) in the severe
MR group (moderate or severe, n = 43) was significantly lower than that (25%)
of the mild MR group (none, trivial, or mild; n = 52). The relative risk of stroke
for increase in MR from mild to severe groups, for every 10 mm increment in
LA size, for gender, and for every increase of 10 years of age was 0.45, 1.06, 0.98,
and 1.33, respectively. In patients with nonrheumatic AF, age is an independent
predictor of an increased risk of stroke, and MR may be protective against
stroke, especially in those patients with LA enlargement.

Prediction of Paroxysmal Idiopathic Atrial Fibrillation

The prolongation of intra-atrial and interatrial conduction time and the
inhomogeneous propagation of sinus impulses are well known electrophysiological characteristics in patients with paroxysmal atrial fibrillation (PAF). To
search for possible electrocardiographic markers that could serve as predictors
of idiopathic PAF, Dilaveris and associates[48] from Athens, Greece, measured
the maximum P-wave duration (P maximum) and the difference between the
maximum and the minimum P-wave duration (P dispersion) from the 12-lead
surface electrocardiogram of 60 patients with a history of idiopathic PAF and
40 age-matched healthy control subjects. P maximum and P dispersion were
found to be significantly higher in patients with idiopathic PAF than in control
subjects. A P maximum value of 110 ms and a P dispersion value of 40 ms
separated patients from control subjects, with a sensitivity of 88% and a specificity of 75% and 85%, respectively. P maximum and P dispersion are simple
electrocardiographic markers that could be used for the prediction of idiopathic PAF.

Left Atrial Appendage Function

Although several flow patterns in the LA appendage have been described,
mechanical determinants of its function have not been elucidated in human
beings. Ito and associates[49] from Osaka, Japan, attempted to investigate

changes in LA appendage function after cardioversion of AF and examine the potential relation between appendage function and LA mechanical function. Twenty patients without mitral valvular disease underwent transesophageal and transthoracic echocardiography at 24 hours and 1 week after cardioversion of AF. LA appendage function was assessed by the pulsed Doppler measurements of LA appendage emptying and filling velocities corresponding to early and late ventricular diastole, respectively. LA mechanical function was evaluated by the transmitral A-wave velocity, percent atrial contribution of the total LV filling (percent atrial filling), and the pulmonary venous A-wave velocity. LV function was also estimated with conventional M-mode echocardiography. The late appendage emptying and filling velocities markedly increased during 1 week after cardioversion. This finding was associated with an increase in LA mechanical function. Changes in the late emptying and filling velocities significantly correlated with changes in the transmitral A-wave velocity, percent atrial filling, and the pulmonary venous A-wave velocity. In contrast, little change was observed in the early emptying and filling velocities. There was no relation between the indexes of LV function and those of appendage function. In conclusion, unless there is an alteration of the loading conditions, LA appendage function improves over several days after cardioversion, and its function is related to LA mechanical function.

Atrial Stunning After Ablation of Atrial Flutter

Atrial stunning and the development of spontaneous echocardiographic contrast is a consequence of electrical cardioversion of atrial flutter to sinus rhythm. This phenomenon may be associated with thrombus formation and embolic stroke. At present, radiofrequency ablation is considered an important definitive treatment for chronic atrial flutter, but evidence regarding the importance of left atrial stunning is inconclusive. Sparks and colleagues[50] from Parkville, Victoria, Australia, examined the effect of radiofrequency ablation on left atrial and left atrial appendage function in patients with chronic atrial flutter. Fifteen patients with chronic atrial flutter underwent transesophageal echocardiography to evaluate left atrial and left atrial appendage function and spontaneous echo contrast before and immediately, 30 minutes, and 3 weeks after radiofrequency ablation. The controls were 7 patients undergoing ablation for paroxysmal atrial flutter. In this group, radiofrequency energy was delivered in sinus rhythm and echocardiographic parameters were assessed before, immediately, and 30 minutes following radiofrequency ablation. The mean arrhythmia duration of the patients with chronic atrial flutter averaged 17 months. Eighty percent of these patients developed spontaneous echo contrast following radiofrequency ablation and conversion to sinus rhythm. Left atrial appendage velocities decreased significantly from 54 in atrial flutter to 18 in sinus rhythm after arrhythmia termination. These changes persisted for 30 minutes. Following 3 weeks of sustained sinus rhythm, significant improvement in left atrial velocities and mitral A-wave velocities were evident and spontaneous echo contrast had resolved in all patients. Radiofrequency energy delivered in sinus rhythm to the control patients with paroxysmal atrial flutter had no significant effect on any of the above indices. These authors conclude that radiofrequency ablation of chronic atrial flutter is associated with significant left atrial stunning and the development of spontaneous echo contrast. Sustained sinus rhythm for 3 weeks leads to resolution of these acute phenomena. This left atrial stunning occurs in the absence of direct current shock or antiarrhythmic drugs. These data are consistent with giving a several-week treatment of coumadin after ablation as has been previously done with patients who are converted from atrial fibrillation to sinus rhythm.

Biochemical Marker of Atrial Pressures

Atrial filling pressures are increased in acute AF, which stimulates the release of atrial natriuretic factor pro-hormone, proANF. In a randomized trial comparing digoxin with placebo in 216 patients, Hornestam and associates[51] from Sweden and Norway investigated whether the baseline plasma level of N-terminal proANF is a predictor for conversion to sinus rhythm and the relation among N-terminal proANF, conversion to sinus rhythm, and changes in heart rate. N-terminal proANF was increased at baseline and decreased significantly in patients converting to sinus rhythm, whereas it was mainly unchanged in nonconverters. N-terminal proANF was not a predictor of conversion to sinus rhythm. A relation was found between relative changes in heart rate and N-terminal proANF in nonconverters. The level of N-terminal proANF does not predict conversion to sinus rhythm, which indicates that hemodynamics *per se* is not important. There is a correlation between relative changes in heart rate and N-terminal proANF in nonconverters.

Analyzing Mechanisms of Atrial Fibrillation Onset

This study by Hnatkova and associates[52] from London, United Kingdom, seeks to elucidate whether there was a common mode of initiation of paroxysmal atrial fibrillation (PAF) episodes that might suggest new therapies. A library of 177 digitized and analyzed 24-hour Holter recordings from PAF pharmacotherapy trials was studied. Noise-free PAF episodes of 0.5 or more minutes were identified. PAF episodes and the preceding 2 minutes of sinus rhythm were printed as tachograms and visually inspected. Heart rate and ectopic beat behavior were used to characterize modes of PAF onset for comparing half-minute segments of the final 2 minutes of sinus rhythm. Thirty-four recordings (from 19 patients, aged 62 ± 12 years) provided 231 PAF episodes suitable for analysis. No patient had a consistent mode of PAF onset. This was confirmed by systematic analysis of the 5 patients with the most episodes. Overall, a highly significant increase in ectopic beats, from 1.34 to 6.52 min^{-1} was found, but heart rate did not significantly change (mean heart rate at onset = 64 beats/min). PAF was initiated by a solitary ectopic beat in more than half of the cases. No consistent evidence for short-long-short sequences, seen in ventricular arrhythmias, was found. The mode of onset of AF is inconsistent, both across a population with PAF and within individuals. This has implications for understanding the mechanisms of AF onset in human beings and for the treatment of the disorder.

Atrial Fibrillation After Cardiovascular Surgery

AF is one of the most frequent complications after cardiovascular surgery. It may result in thromboembolic events, hemodynamic deterioration, and an increased length and cost of hospitalization. Solomon and associates[53] from Washington, DC, retrospectively studied 504 consecutive adult patients undergoing cardiovascular surgery to determine whether patients with new-onset postoperative AF could be safely discharged in AF after ventricular rate had been controlled and anticoagulation initiated. Postoperative AF occurred in 79 (16%) of the 487 survivors. Of these patients, 67 were discharged in sinus rhythm, whereas the remaining 12 were discharged in AF. Patients discharged in AF tended to be older, have higher Parsonnet risk scores, and have an increased incidence of valvular heart surgery. Despite this result, this cohort had a shorter length of hospital stay (7.3 ± 2.0 days vs. 11 ± 9.3 days), decreased hospital costs ($14,188 ± $2,635 vs. $23,016 ± $21,963), and decreased hospital charges ($37,878 ± $7,420 vs. $58,289 ± $50,980) compared with patients with AF discharged in sinus rhythm. In the 12 persons discharged home in AF, no repeat hospitalizations, bleeding complications, or thromboembolic events occurred. A strategy of early discharge of patients with persistent postoperative AF appears promising and deserves prospective testing on a larger scale.

Time of Onset of Atrial Fibrillation

Sakata and associates[54] from Tokyo, Japan, investigated the clinical significance of the time of onset of AF in patients with AMI. Among 1,039 patients with AMI, 100 (9.6%) had AF. These patients were divided into 3 groups: AF group 1 (n = 45), who developed AF within 24 hours of the onset of AMI; AF group 2 (n = 41), who developed AF more than 24 hours after the onset of AMI; and AF group 3 (n = 14), who developed AF before the onset of AMI. The infarct-related lesions were most frequent (67%) in the proximal right coronary artery in AF group 1. RA pressure was most significantly increased in AF group 1. The LA dimension and pulmonary arterial wedge pressure were most significantly increased, and LVEF was most significantly decreased in AF group 2. In the acute phase, the frequencies of heart failure, cardiogenic shock, and in-hospital mortality were higher for all 3 AF groups than for the sinus group. The long-term survival rate was significantly lower in AF group 1 and AF group 2 than in the sinus group. AF was an independent predictor of cardiac death in both AF group 1 (odds ratio 2.5) and AF group 2 (odds ratio 3.7), but not in AF group 3. The onset time of AF appears to be a useful parameter for evaluating the cardiac status and prognosis of patients with AMI.

Recurrent Symptomatic Atrial Fibrillation

To compare the safety and efficacy of amiodarone and sotalol in the treatment of patients with recurrent symptomatic AF, Kochiadakis and colleagues[55] from Crete, Greece, entered 70 patients into a randomized, double-blind study. Of these, 35 received amiodarone and 35 received sotalol. There were no significant differences in baseline clinical characteristics between groups. Patients with EF less than 40% or clinically significant heart disease were excluded. Patients randomized to amiodarone began with 800 to 1,600 mg/day for 7 to 14 days orally. After the initial loading phase, the drug dose was tapered to maintenance levels over 7 to 12 days; thereafter, therapy was generally maintained at a dosage of 200 mg/day. The sotalol dosage was 80 to 360 mg twice daily, as tolerated. Follow-up clinical evaluations were conducted at 1, 2, 4, 6, 9, and 12 months. The proportion of patients remaining in sinus rhythm on each agent was calculated for the 2 groups using the Kaplan-Meier method. Ten of the 35 patients who were taking amiodarone developed AF during the 12-month observation period, compared with 21 of the 35 who were taking sotalol. No significant effect of gender, age, left atrial size, or type of AF could be detected that increased the risk of development of AF. The authors conclude that both amiodarone and sotalol can be used for the maintenance of normal sinus rhythm in patients with recurrent symptomatic AF, but that amiodarone is the more effective of the 2 drugs for this purpose.

Use of Repeated Doses of Ibutilide in Atrial Flutter

This study was conducted by Abi-Mansour and associates[56] from Oaklawn, Illinois; Kalamazoo, Michigan; Charleston, West Virginia; and Cincinnati Ohio, to determine the efficacy and safety of ibutilide fumarate versus placebo in the acute termination of atrial flutter and AF. Two hundred sixty-two patients aged 28 to 88 years with atrial flutter or AF duration of 3 hours to 90 days were randomly assigned in a 5:1 ratio (ibutilide: placebo) to receive 2 10-minute infusions, 10 minutes apart, of ibutilide (1 mg) or placebo. Patients were hospitalized and monitored by telemetry for 24 hours, with follow-up 72 hours later. Seventy-three (35%) of 209 evaluable ibutilide recipients had termination of atrial flutter or AF within 1.5 hours compared with 0 (0%) of 41 placebo recipients. Those with atrial flutter had a higher success rate. At hour 24, 86% remained in normal or alternative sinus rhythm. Of the patients who received ibutilide, 2.3% experienced drug-related sustained polymorphic or monomorphic VT and recovered after intervention. Additionally, 7.3% experienced nonsustained polymorphic or monomorphic VT. Other frequent medical events in ibutilide recipients were generally also noted in the placebo group. Ibutilide is effective and safe for acute termination of AF or atrial flutter.

Evaluation of P Wave Signal-Averaged Electrocardiograms

The purpose of this study by Ehlert and associates[57] from New York, New York, was to evaluate the signal processing and analysis methods currently in use for the P-wave signal-averaged electrocardiogram and to define optimal parameters for its use. P-wave signal-averaged electrocardiograms using the QRS as a trigger for alignment of the analysis window were obtained in 15 subjects with prior AF and 15 controls. Five methods of signal filtering (unidirectional, bidirectional, finite impulse response, least squares fit, and spectral fast-Fourier transform) and 3 filter frequencies (14, 29, and 60 Hz) were compared with logistic regression analysis. Analysis techniques, including P-wave vector duration, individual orthogonal lead duration, and terminal root mean square voltage were also evaluated for the strength of their association with the occurrence of AF. The least-squares fit filter with bandwidth filtering of 29 to 250 Hz produced the strongest association with AF (odds ratio 26). A high correlation was noted among the individual orthogonal leads; however, neither individual leads nor total atrial activation determined from individual leads demonstrated a superior association with AF when compared with total vector P-wave duration. Terminal P-wave RMS voltages were not significantly different between patients with prior AF and controls.

Amiodarone and Acute Heart Rate Control

Control of heart rate in critically ill patients who develop AF or atrial flutter can be difficult. Amiodarone may be an alternative agent for heart rate control if conventional measures are ineffective. Clemo and colleagues[58] from Richmond, Virginia, retrospectively studied intensive care patients (n = 38) who received intravenous amiodarone for heart rate control in the setting of hemodynamically destabilizing atrial tachyarrhythmias resistant to conventional heart rate control measures. AF was present in 33 patients and atrial flutter in 5 patients. Onset of rapid heart rate (mean 149 ± 13 beats/min) was associated with a decrease in systolic BP of 20 ± 5 mm Hg. Intravenous diltiazem (n = 34), esmolol (n = 4), or digoxin (n = 24) had no effect on heart rate, while reducing systolic BP by 6 ± 4 mm Hg. The infusion of amiodarone (242 ± 137 mg over 1 hour) was associated with a decrease in heart rate by 37 ± 8 beats/min and an increase in systolic BP of 24 ± 6 mm Hg. Both of these changes were significantly improved from onset of rapid heart rate or during conventional therapy. Beneficial changes were also noted in pulmonary artery occlusive pressure and cardiac output. There were no adverse effects secondary to amiodarone therapy. Intravenous amiodarone is efficacious and hemodynamically well tolerated in the acute control of heart rate in critically ill patients who develop atrial tachyarrhythmias with rapid ventricular response refractory to conventional treatment. Cardiac electrophysiological consultation should be obtained before using intravenous amiodarone for this purpose.

Thromboembolism in Chronic Atrial Flutter

Some individuals assume that thromboembolic events are rare after cardioversion of atrial flutter. Lanzarotti and Olshansky[59] from Maywood, Illinois, conducted a retrospective analysis of 110 consecutive patients referred to the electrophysiological laboratory for cardioversion of chronic atrial flutter from 1986 to 1996. Flutter was present for at least 6 months. Mean LVEF was 42%. Thirteen patients (13%) had a thromboembolic event. Of these, 7 were attributable to causes other than atrial flutter. In the remaining 6 patients, thromboembolic events occurred during the rhythm of atrial flutter or after cardioversion to sinus rhythm. Other causes of thromboembolism were excluded. Effective anticoagulation was associated with a decreased risk of thromboembolism. These authors conclude that patients with chronic atrial flutter are at an increased risk of thromboembolic events. Effective anticoagulation may decrease this risk.

Spontaneous Conversion of Atrial Fibrillation to Sinus Rhythm

Clinical experience has shown that new-onset AF frequently spontaneously converts back to sinus rhythm. Danias and colleagues[60] from Farmington, Connecticut, and Boston, Massachusetts, prospectively identified 356 patients with AF of less than 72 hours' duration. Spontaneous conversion to sinus rhythm occurred in 68% of the study group. Among patients with spontaneous conversion, the total duration was less than 24 hours in 66%. Logistic regression analysis of the clinical data identified presentation less than 24 hours from onset of symptoms as the only predictor of spontaneous conversion. Normal left ventricular systolic function was more common among the patients with spontaneous conversion but it was not an independent predictor of conversion. Left atrial dimension was similar in the 2 groups. These authors conclude that spontaneous conversion to sinus rhythm occurs in almost 70% of patients presenting with AF less than 72 hours' duration. Presentation with symptoms of less than 24 hours' duration is the best predictor of spontaneous conversion.

Spontaneous Initiation of Atrial Fibrillation by Ectopic Beats

Haïssaguerre and colleagues[61] studied 45 patients with frequent episodes of AF refractory to drug therapy. The spontaneous initiation of AF was mapped with the use of multielectrode catheters designed to record the earliest electrical activity preceding the onset of AF and associated atrial ectopic beats. The accuracy of the mapping was confirmed by the abrupt disappearance of triggered atrial ectopic beats after ablation with local radiofrequency energy. A single point of origin of atrial ectopic beats was identified in 29 patients, 2 points of origin were identified in 9 patients, and 3 or 4 points of origin were identified in 7 patients for a total of 69 ectopic foci. Three foci were in the right atrium, 1 in the posterior left atrium, and 65 in the pulmonary veins. The earliest activation was found to have occurred 2 to 4 cm inside the veins, marked by a local depolarization preceding the atrial ectopic beats on the surface electrocardiogram by 106 ± 24 ms. AF was initiated by a sudden burst of rapid depolarization. A local depolarization could also be recognized during sinus rhythm and abolished by radiofrequency ablation. During a follow-up period of 8 ± 6 months and after ablation, 28 patients had no recurrence of AF.

Thus, the pulmonary veins are an important source of ectopic beats, initiating frequent paroxysms of AF. These foci respond to treatment with radiofrequency ablation.

Three-Dimensional Mapping of Atrial Flutter Circuit

Shah and colleagues[62] in Bordeaux-Pessac, France, performed 3-dimensional right atrial endocardial activation mapping during common counterclockwise atrial flutter in 17 patients, including 16 men with a mean age of 53 ± 11 years, using the Cordis-Biosense EP Navigation System and assessed the distribution of estimated conduction velocities and double and fractionated potentials. Electrocardiographic flutter wave morphologies were compared with activation patterns. Points were sequentially acquired covering 88% ± 11% of the flutter cycle length of 239 ± 22 ms. A wide and variable posterior zone of double and fractionated potentials coincided with blocking and colliding wavefronts and formed the posterior limit of the circuit. A progressively widening septal wavefront ascending from just beyond the coronary sinus ostium passed cranially as a broader front anterior to the superior vena cava in 14 patients, whereas fusion around the SVC formed the superior limb of the circuit in 3 (Figure 6-15). Bounded anteriorly by the tricuspid valve, the wavefront descended down the lateral aspect of the right atrium before completing the circuit in all cases through the inferior vena cava–tricuspid annulus isthmus. The estimated conduction velocity in the medial isthmus was lower than in the other limbs of the circuit. Double and fractionated potentials were constant and more prevalent in the posterior right atrium. Electrocardiographic flutter wave morphology did not correlate with 3-dimensional activation maps. Thus, interindividual variations occur in the right atrial circuit of common atrial flutter with constant activation through the cavotricuspid isthmus. A variable zone of block forms the posterior limit. Fusion around the SVC can occur and ascending medial septal activation does not follow a consistent pattern. These data should be helpful in developing schemes for ablation of this arrhythmia in the future.

Thrombosis in Atrial Fibrillation

Paroxysmal Atrial Fibrillation in the Thrombolytic Era

Eldar and colleagues[63] in Tel Hashomer, Israel, attempted to define the incidence, associated clinical variables, and short- and long-term prognostic significance of paroxysmal atrial fibrillation (PAF) in patients with AMI in the thrombolytic era. A prospective, nationwide study was conducted in 2,866 consecutive patients admitted with AMI in all 25 coronary care units in Israel during January and February of 1992, 1994, and 1996. The data were compared with the previous Israeli study of 5,803 patients with AMI hospitalized in 1981 through 1983, which was considered the prethrombolytic era. Patients in the

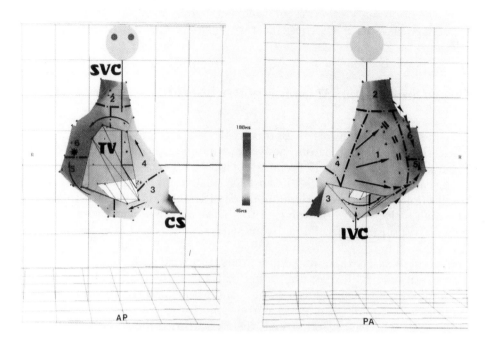

Figure 6-15. Depiction of the 6 segments of the right atrium (RA) (1, posterior RA; 2, superior vena cava [SVC]; 3, pericoronary sinus region; 4, septal region; 5, inferior anterolateral segment; and 6, superior anterolateral segment) superimposed on a reconstructed 3-dimensional electroanatomic RA map obtained during pacing from the coronary sinus (CS) in sinus rhythm at a cycle length of 550 ms: anteroposterior (AP) and posteroanterior (PA) views. Activation in the reconstructed chamber is depicted in the colors of the spectrum, with red representing the earliest (in the coronary sinus region) and violet the latest activation. The color bar in the center indicates the mapped activation times relative to the reference (46 to 188 ms, total activation time of 142 ms) and their corresponding color coding. Note the typical dual front activation pattern with conduction through the cavotricuspid isthmus and collision (*) in the anterior lateral RA in this study group patient before ablation. There is an activation delay of 50 ms longitudinally along the posterior RA (corresponding to the position of the crista terminalis) except at the bottom near the inferior vena cava (IVC), where there appears to be relatively rapid and homogeneous activation with wavefronts from the posterobasal RA and IVC–tricuspid annulus isthmus fusing and ascending upward, as indicated by the arrows. Reproduced with permission from Shah et al.[62]

thrombolytic era with PAF were older and had a worse risk profile than those without PAF. PAF in the thrombolytic era was independently associated with increased 30-day and 1-year mortality rates. The incidence of PAF and the 30-day and 1-year mortality rates of patients with PAF were similar in the thrombolytic era and prethrombolytic era, although PAF in the thrombolytic era occurred in older and sicker patients than in the prethrombolytic era. PAF in the thrombolytic era was associated with significantly lower 30-day and 1-year mortality rates compared with the prethrombolytic era. Patients with AMI who developed PAF in the thrombolytic era have a significantly worse short- and long-term prognosis than patients without PAF, mostly due to their poorer

TABLE 6-1
**Patients With Acute Embolic Events or Any Embolic Event During Follow-Up (n = 12*)
Compared With Those Without Events (n = 169)**

Characteristics	Patients Without Embolism	Patients With Embolism	p Value
Mean age (yrs ± SD)	64 ± 13	66 ± 10	0.61
Men/women	121/48	9/3	1.0
Organic heart disease	111 (72%)	12 (100%)	0.037
History of atrial flutter (mos ± SD)	6 ± 7	5 ± 9	0.27
Additional atrial fibrillation	57 (34%)	4 (33%)	1.0
Diabetes mellitus	31 (18%)	7 (58%)	0.0038
Systemic hypertension	64 (38%)	10 (83%)	0.004
Mean ejection fraction (% ± SD)	53 ± 10	48 ± 9	0.02
Left atrial diameter (mm ± SD)	43 ± 6	46 ± 7	0.13
Recurrence of atrial flutter	56 (33%)	4 (33%)	1.0
Follow-up duration (mos ± SD)	30 ± 20	26 ± 18	0.52

* One patient had an acute and chronic embolic event.
Reproduced with permission from Seidl et al.[64]

risk profile. After adjustment for confounding factors, patients with PAF in the thrombolytic era have a better overall outcome than their counterparts in the prethrombolytic era, probably reflecting the better management of patients with AMI in the more recent time periods.

Based on multiple studies, clear, guided anticoagulation therapy is recommended for patients with AF. The value of anticoagulation therapy in patients with atrial flutter, however, is less well established. Little is known about the incidence of thromboembolism in patients with atrial flutter. Seidl and associates[64] from Ludwigshafen, Germany, evaluated the risk of thromboembolism in 191 consecutive unselected patients referred for treatment of atrial flutter. A history of embolic events was noted in 11 patients. Acute embolism (<48 hours) occurred in 4 patients (3 after direct current cardioversion, 1 after catheter ablation). During follow-up of 26 ± 18 months, 9 patients experienced thromboembolic events. During the follow-up, the average embolic event rate (including acute embolism and thromboembolic events during follow-up) was 7% in this patient population. Risk indicators for an embolic event in a univariate analysis were organic heart disease, depressed LVF, history of systemic hypertension, and diabetes mellitus. Using multivariate analysis, a history of hypertension was the only independent predictor for elevated embolic risk in this patient population. Thus, the thromboembolic risk is higher than previously recognized for patients with atrial flutter. Anticoagulation therapy may decrease this risk (Table 6-1).

1. Harada K, Komuro I, Hayashi D, Sugaya T, Murakami K, Yazaki Y: Angiotensin II type 1a receptor is involved in the occurrence of reperfusion arrhythmias. Circulation 1998 (February 3);97:315–317.
2. De Chillou C, Sadoul N, Bizeau O, Feldmann L, Gazakuré E, Ismaïl M, Magnin-Poull I, Blankoff I, Aliot E: Prognostic value of thrombolysis, coronary artery patency, signal-averaged electrocardiography, left ventricular ejection fraction, and

Holter electrocardiographic monitoring for life-threatening ventricular arrhythmias after a first acute myocardial infarction. Am J Cardiol 1997 (October 1);80: 852–858.

3. Estes NA III, Michaud G, Zipes DP, El-Sherif N, Venditti FJ, Rosenbaum DS, Albrecht P, Wang PJ, Cohen RJ: Electrical alternans during rest and exercise as predictors of vulnerability to ventricular arrhythmias. Am J Cardiol 1997 (November 15); 80:1314–1318.

4. Peckova M, Fahrenbruch CE, Cobb LA, Hallstrom AP: Circadian variations in the occurrence of cardiac arrests. Initial and repeat episodes. Circulation 1998 (July 7);98:31–39.

5. Nielsen JC, Andersen HR, Thomsen PEB, Thuesen L, Mortensen PT, Vesterlund T, Pedersen AK: Heart failure and echocardiographic changes during long-term follow-up of patients with sick sinus syndrome randomized to single-chamber atrial or ventricular pacing. Circulation 1998 (March 17);97:987–995.

6. Brembilla-Perrot B, Jacquemin L, Houplon P, Houriez P, Beurrier D, Berder V, Terrier de la Chaise A, Louis P: Increased atrial vulnerability in arrhythmogenic RV disease. Am Heart J 1998 (May);135:748–754.

7. Mewis C, Kühlkamp V, Spyridopoulos I, Bosch RF, Seipel L: Late outcome of survivors of idiopathic ventricular fibrillation. Am J Cardiol 1998 (April 15);81:999–1003.

8. Lee KW, Okin PM, Kligfield P, Stein KM, Lerman BB: Precordial QT dispersion and inducible VT. Am Heart J 1997 (December);134:1005–1013.

9. Roukema G, Singh JP, Meijs M, Carvalho C, Hart G: Effect of exercise-induced ischemia on QT interval dispersion. Am Heart J 1998 (January);135:88–92.

10. Zareba W, Moss AJ, Rosero SZ, Hajj-Ali R, Konecki J, Andrews M: Electrocardiographic findings in patients with diphenhydramine overdose. Am J Cardiol 1997 (November 1);80:1168–1173.

11. Pratt CM, Camm AJ, Cooper W, Friedman PL, MacNeil DJ, Moulton KM, Pitt B, Schwartz PJ, Veltri EP, Waldo AL, for the SWORD Investigators: Mortality in the Survival with Oral D-Sotalol (SWORD) trial: why did patients die? Am J Cardiol 1998 (April 1);81:869–876.

12. Del Rosso A, Bartoli P, Bartoletti A, Brandinelli-Geri A, Bonechi F, Maioli M, Mazza F, Michelucci A, Russo L, Salvetti E, Sansoni M, Zipoli A, Fierro A, Ieri A: Shortened head-up tilt testing potentiated with sublingual nitroglycerin in patients with unexplained syncope. Am Heart J 1998 (April);135:564–570.

13. Duggal P, Vesely MR, Wattanasirichaigoon D, Villafane J, Kaushik V, Beggs AH: Mutation of the gene for IsK associated with both Jervell and Lange-Nielsen and Romano-Ward forms of long-QT syndrome. Circulation 1998 (January 20);97: 142–146.

14. Rashba EJ, Zareba W, Moss AJ, Hall WJ, Robinson J, Locati EH, Schwartz PJ, Andrews M, for the LQTS Investigators: Influence of pregnancy on the risk for cardiac events in patients with hereditary long QT syndrome. Circulation 1998 (February 10);97:451–456.

15. Locati EH, Zareba W, Moss AJ, Schwartz PJ, Vincent GM, Lehmann MH, Towbin JA, Priori SG, Napolitano C, Robinson JL, Andrews M, Timothy K, Hall WJ: Age- and sex-related differences in clinical manifestations in patients with congenital long-QT syndrome: Findings from the International LQTS Registry. Circulation 1998 (June 9);97:2237–2244.

16. Li H, Chen Q, Moss AJ, Robinson J, Goytia V, Perry JC, Vincent GM, Priori SG, Lehmann MH, Denfield SW, Duff D, Kaine S, Shimizu W, Schwartz PJ, Wang Q, Towbin JA: New mutations in the KVLQT1 potassium channel that cause long-QT syndrome. Circulation 1998 (April 7);97:1264–1269.

17. Kambouris NG, Nuss HB, Johns DC, Tomaselli GF, Marban E, Balser JR: Phenotypic characterization of a novel long-QT syndrome mutation (R1623Q) in the cardiac sodium channel. Circulation 1998 (February 24);97:640–644.

18. Donnerstein RI, Zhu D, Samson R, Bender AM, Goldberg SJ: Acute effects of caffeine ingestion on signal-averaged electrocardiogram. Am Heart J 1998 (October); 136:643–646.

19. Simons GR, Eisenstein EL, Shaw LJ, Mark DB, Pritchett ELC: Cost effectiveness

of inpatient initiation of antiarrhythmic therapy for supraventricular tachycardias. Am J Cardiol 1997 (December 15);80:1551–1557.

20. Holzberger PT, Greenberg ML, Paicopolis MC, Ozahowski TP, Ho PC, O'Connor GT: Prospective comparison of intravenous quinidine and intravenous procainamide in patients undergoing electrophysiologic testing. Am Heart J 1998 (July);36:49–56.

21. Wood MA, Stambler BS, Ellenbogen KA, Gilligan DM, Perry KT, Wakefield LK, VanderLugt JT, and the Ibutilide Investigators: Suppression of inducible ventricular tachycardia by ibutilide in patients with coronary artery disease. Am Heart J 1998 (June);135:1048–1054.

22. Da Costa A, Kirkorian G, Cucherat M, Delahaye F, Chevalier P, Cerisier A, Isaaz K, Touboul P: Antibiotic prophylaxis for permanent pacemaker implantation: A meta-analysis. Circulation 1998 (May 12);97:1796–1801.

23. Da Costa A, Lelièvre H, Kirkorian G, Célard M, Chevalier P, Vandenesch F, Etienne J, Touboul P: Role of the preaxillary flora in pacemaker infections: A prospective study. Circulation 1998 (May 12);97:1791–1795.

24. Cacoub P, Leprince P, Nataf P, Hausfater P, Dorent R, Wechsler B, Bors V, Pavie A, Plette JC, Gandjbakhch I: Pacemaker infective endocarditis. Am J Cardiol 1998 (August 15);82:480–484.

25. Böcker D, Bänsch D, Heinecke A, Weber M, Brunn J, Hammel D, Borggrefe M, Breithardt G, Block M: Potential benefit from implantable cardioverter-defibrillator therapy in patients with and without heart failure. Circulation 1998 (October 20); 98:1636–1643.

26. Mushlin AI, Hall WJ, Zwanziger J, Gajary E, Andrews M, Marron R, Zou KH, Moss AJ, for the MADIT Investigators: The cost-effectiveness of automatic implantable cardiac defibrillators: Results from MADIT. Circulation 1998 (June 2);97: 2129–2135.

27. Wellens HJJ, Lau C-P, Lüderitz B, Akhtar M, Waldo AL, Camm AJ, Timmermans C, Tse H-F, Jung W, Jordaens L, Ayers G, for the METRIX Investigators: Atrioverter: An implantable device for the treatment of atrial fibrillation. Circulation 1998 (October 20);98:1651–1656.

28. Schaumann A, von zur Mühlen F, Herse B, Gonska B-D, Kreuzer H: Empirical versus tested antitachycardia pacing in implantable cardioverter defibrillators: A prospective study including 200 patients. Circulation 1998 (January 6/13);97:66–74.

29. Bansch D, Brunn J, Castrucci M, Weber M, Gietzen F, Borggrefe M, Breithardt G, Block M: Syncope in patients with implantable cardioverter-defibrillator: Incidence, prediction and implications for driving restriction. JACC 1998 (March);31: 608–615.

30. Seidl K, Hauer B, Schwick NG, Zahn R, Senges J: Comparison of metoprolol and sotalol in preventing ventricular tachyarrhythmias after the implantation of a cardioverter/defibrillator. Am J Cardiol 1998 (September 15);82:744–748.

31. Fetter JG, Ivans V, Benditt DG, Collins J: Digital cellular telephone interaction with implantable cardioverter-defibrillators. JACC 1998 (March 1);31:623–628.

32. Rosenqvist M, Beyer T, Block M, den Dulk K, Minten J, Lindemans F, on behalf of the European 7219 Jewel ICD Investigators: Adverse events with transvenous implantable cardioverter-defibrillators: A prospective multicenter study. Circulation 1998 (August 18);98:663–670.

33. Gaita F, Riccardi R, Calò L, Scaglione M, Gargeroglio L, Antolini R, Kirchner M, Lamberti F, Richiardi E: Atrial mapping and radiofrequency catheter ablation in patients with idiopathic atrial fibrillation: Electrophysiological findings and ablation results. Circulation 1998 (June 2);97:2136–2145.

34. Paydak H, Kall JG, Burke MC, Rubenstein D, Kopp DE, Verdino RJ, Wilber DJ: Atrial fibrillation after radiofrequency ablation of type 1 atrial flutter: Time to onset, determinants, and clinical course. Circulation 1998 (July 28);98:315–322.

35. Brignole M, Menozzi C, Gianfranchi L, Musso G, Mureddu R, Bottoni N, Lolli G: Assessment of atrioventricular junction ablation and VVIR pacemaker versus pharmacological treatment in patients with heart failure and chronic atrial fibrillation: A randomized, controlled study. Circulation 1998 (September 8);98:953–960.

36. Jaïs P, Haïssaguerre M, Shah DC, Takahashi A, Hocini M, Lavergne T, Lafitte S,

Le Mouroux A, Fischer B, Clémenty J: Successful irrigated-tip catheter ablation of atrial flutter resistant to conventional radiofrequency ablation. Circulation 1998 (September 1);98:835–838.

37. Stevenson WG, Friedman PL, Kocovic D, Sager PT, Saxon LA, Pavri B: Radiofrequency catheter ablation of ventricular tachycardia after myocardial infarction. Circulation 1998 (July 28);98:308–314.

38. Rosenthal LS, Mahesh M, Beck TJ, Saul JP, Miller JM, Kay N, Klein LS, Huang S, Gillette P, Prystowsky E, Carlson M, Berger RD, Lawrence JH, Yong P, Calkins H: Predictors of fluoroscopy time and estimated radiation exposure during radiofrequency catheter ablation procedures. Am J Cardiol 1998 (August 15);82:451–458.

39. Belhassen B, Fish R, Glikson M, Glick A, Eldar M, Laniado S, Viskin S: Noninvasive diagnosis of dual AV node physiology in patients with AV nodal reentrant tachycardia by administration of adenosine-5′-triphosphate during sinus rhythm. Circulation 1998 (July 7);98:47–53.

40. Lee CS, Lai WT, Wu JC, Sheu SH, Wu SN, Berlardinelli L: Differential effects of adenosine on antegrade and retrograde fast pathway conduction in A-V nodal reentry. Am Heart J 1997 (November);134:799–806.

41. Allen MR, Gibbons RJ, Zinsmeister AR: Sex differences in ventricular function in right BBB. Am Heart J 1998 (September);136:418–424.

42. Brugada J, Brugada R, Brugada P: Right bundle-branch block and ST-segment elevation in leads V_1 through V_3; A marker for sudden death in patients without demonstrable structural heart disease. Circulation 1998 (February 10);97:457–460.

43. Raymond RJ, Lee AJ, Messineo FC, Manning WJ, Silverman DI: Cardiac performance early after cardioversion from AF. Am Heart J 1998 (September);136:435–442.

44. Cooper RAS, Plumb VJ, Epstein AE, Kay GN, Ideker RE: Marked reduction in internal atrial defibrillation thresholds with dual-current pathways and sequential shocks in humans. Circulation 1998 (June 30);97:2527–2535.

45. Benjamin EJ, Wolf PA, D'Agostino RB, Silbershatz H, Kannel WB, Levy D: Impact of atrial fibrillation on the risk of death: The Framingham Heart Study. Circulation 1998 (September 8);98:946–952.

46. Tai C-T, Chen S-A, Feng A-N, Yu W-C, Chen Y-J, Chang M-S: Electropharmacologic effects of class I and class III antiarrhythmic drugs on typical atrial flutter: Insights into the mechanism of termination. Circulation 1998 (May 19);97:1935–1945.

47. Nakagami H, Yamamoto K, Ikeda U, Mitsuhashi T, Goto T, Shimada K: MR reduces the risk of stroke in patients with nonrheumatic AF. Am Heart J 1998 (September);136:528–532.

48. Dilaveris PE, Gialafos EJ, Sideris SK, Theopistou AM, Andrikopoulos GK, Kyriakidis M, Gialafos JE, Toutouzas PK: Simple electrocardiographic markers for the prediction of paroxysmal idiopathic AF. Am Heart J 1998 (May);135:733–738.

49. Ito T, Suwa M, Otake Y, Kobashi A, Hirota Y, Ando H, Kawamura K: Assessment of left atrial appendage function after cardioversion of atrial fibrillation: Relation to left atrial mechanical function. Am Heart J 1998 (June);135:1020–1026.

50. Sparks PB, Jayaprakash S, Vohra JK, Mond HG, Yapanis AG, Grigg LE, Kalman JM: Left atrial "stunning" following radiofrequency catheter ablation of chronic atrial flutter. JACC 1998 (August);33:468–475.

51. Hornestam B, Hall C, Held P, Carlsson T, Falk L, Karlson BW, Lundstrom T, Peterson M for the Digitalis in Acute Atrial Fibrillation (DAAF) Trial Group: N-terminal proANF in acute AF: A biochemical marker of atrial pressures but not a predictor for conversion to sinus rhythm. Am Heart J 1998 (June);135:1040–1047.

52. Hnatkova K, Waktare JEP, Murgatroyd FD, Guo X, Baiyan X, Camm AJ, Malik M: Analysis of the cardiac rhythm preceding episodes of paroxysmal AF. Am Heart J 1998 (June);35:1010–1019.

53. Solomon AJ, Kouretas PC, Hopkins RA, Katz NM, Wallace RB, Hannan RL: Early discharge of patients with new-onset AF after cardiovascular surgery. Am Heart J 1998 (April);135:557–563.

54. Sakata K, Kurihara H, Iwamori K, Maki A, Yoshino H, Yanagisawa A, Ishikawa K: Clinical and prognostic significance of atrial fibrillation in acute myocardial infarction. Am J Cardiol 1997 (December 15);80:1522–1527.

55. Kochiadakis GE, Igoumenidis NE, Marketou ME, Solomou MC, Kanoupakis EM, Vardas PE: Low-dose amiodarone versus sotalol for suppression of recurrent symptomatic atrial fibrillation. Am J Cardiol 1998 (April 15);81:995–998.
56. Abi-Mansour P, Carberry PA, McCowan RJ, Henthorn RW, Dunn GH, Perry KT, and the Study Investigators: Conversion efficacy and safety of repeated doses of ibutilide in atrial flutter and AF. Am Heart J 1998 (October);136:632–642.
57. Ehlert FA, Korenstein D, Steinberg JS: Evaluation of P wave signal-averaged electrocardiographic filtering and analysis methods. Am Heart J 1997 (December);134: 985–993.
58. Clemo HF, Wood MA, Gilligan DM, Ellenbogen KA: Intravenous amiodarone for acute heart rate control in the critically ill patient with atrial tachyarrhythmias. Am J Cardiol 1998 (March 1);81:594–598.
59. Lanzarotti CJ, Olshansky B: Thromboembolism in chronic atrial flutter: Is the risk underestimated? JACC 1997 (November 15);30:1506–1511.
60. Danias PG, Caulfield TA, Weigner MJ, Silverman DI, Manning WJ: Likelihood of spontaneous conversion of atrial fibrillation to sinus rhythm. JACC 1998 (March 1);31:588–592.
61. Haïssaguerre M, Jaïs P, Shah DC, Takahashi A, Hocini M, Quiniou G, Garrigue S, Le Mouroux A, Le Métayer P, Clémenty J: Spontaneous initiation of atrial fibrillation by ectopic beats originating in the pulmonary veins. N Engl J Med 1998 (September 3);339:659–66.
62. Shah DC, Jaïs P, Haïssaguerre M, Chouairi S, Takahashi A, Hocini M, Garrigue S, Clémenty J: Three-dimensional mapping of the common atrial flutter circuit in the right atrium. Circulation 1997 (December 2);96:3904–3912.
63. Eldar M, Canetti M, Rotstein Z, Boyko V, Gottlieb S, Kaplinsky E, Behar S, for the SPRINT and Thrombolytic Survey Groups: Significance of paroxysmal atrial fibrillation complicating acute myocardial infarction in the thrombolytic era. Circulation 1998 (March 17);97:965–970.
64. Seidl K, Hauer B, Schwick NG, Zellner D, Zahn R, Senges J: Risk of thromboembolic events in patients with atrial flutter. Am J Cardiol 1998 (September 1);82:580–583.

7

Peripheral Vascular Disease

Peripheral Atherothrombosclerosis

Aortic Plaque Morphology and Vascular Events

Cohen and colleagues[1] in Paris, France, evaluated the impact of plaque morphology, including ulceration, hypoechoic plaque, or calcification on the risk of subsequent vascular events. They and others have shown that atherosclerotic plaques in the aorta of 4 mm or greater in thickness, especially in the ascending aorta and proximal arch, detected by transesophageal echocardiography are a risk factor for ischemic stroke. They followed a cohort of 334 patients 60 years or older for a period of 2 to 4 years who were consecutively admitted with brain infarction and who had transesophageal echocardiography. The risk of vascular events in patients with plaques in the aortic arch according to the presence of surface ulceration, calcification, and sessile or mobile thrombus was estimated during a total of 788 person-years of follow-up. Hypoechoic plaques, calcifications, and ulcerations were found more frequently in patients with plaques of 4 mm or greater as compared to those with plaques of less than 4 mm. The presence of ulceration did not increase the relative risk of vascular events in patients with plaque of 4 mm or greater. The lack of calcification increased the risk of vascular events in patients with plaque of 4 mm or greater. The highest relative risk of events was found among patients with noncalcified plaques (relative risk 10.3), and the risk of events was systematically higher in patients without calcification (Figure 7-1). Thus, these data suggest that in patients with brain infarction, the relative risk associated with aortic plaque thickness of 4 mm or greater is increased by the absence of plaque calcifications.

Increased Levels of C-Reactive Protein and Risk of Peripheral Vascular Disease

Ridker and colleagues[2] in Boston, Massachusetts, determined whether increased levels of C-reactive protein (CRP) are associated with the development of symptomatic peripheral arterial disease. Using a prospective, nested, case-control design, they measured baseline levels of CRP in 144 apparently healthy men participating in the Physicians' Health Study who developed symptomatic peripheral arterial disease with intermittent claudication or need for revascu-

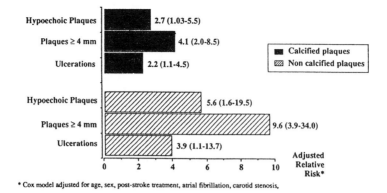

Hypoechoic Plaques — 2.7 (1.03-5.5)
Plaques ≥ 4 mm — 4.1 (2.0-8.5)
Ulcerations — 2.2 (1.1-4.5)

■ Calcified plaques
▨ Non calcified plaques

Hypoechoic Plaques — 5.6 (1.6-19.5)
Plaques ≥ 4 mm — 9.6 (3.9-34.0)
Ulcerations — 3.9 (1.1-13.7)

Adjusted Relative Risk*

* Cox model adjusted for age, sex, post-stroke treatment, atrial fibrillation, carotid stenosis,

FIGURE 7-1. Risk of vascular events during follow-up according to plaque features and the presence of calcification. Reproduced with permission from Cohen et al.[1]

larization and in an equal number of control subjects matched on the basis of age and smoking habit who remained free of vascular disease during a follow-up period of 60 months. Median CRP levels at baseline were higher among those who subsequently developed peripheral arterial disease (Figure 7-2). This risk of developing peripheral arterial disease increased within each increasing quartile of baseline CRP concentrations, such that the relative risks of peripheral arterial disease from lowest to highest quartile of CRP were 1.0, 1.3, 2.0, and 2.1. Compared to patients with no evidence of disease, the subgroup of case patients who required revascularization had the highest CRP levels. Risk estimates were similar after additional control for body mass index, hypercholesterolemia, hypertension, diabetes, and a family history of premature athero-

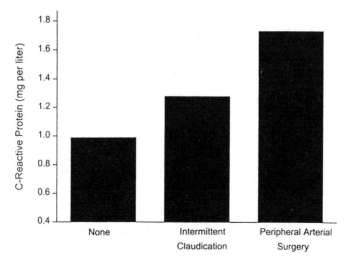

FIGURE 7-2. Median levels of CRP at baseline among study participants who subsequently developed intermittent claudication or who required peripheral arterial revascularization (case subjects) and for those who remained free of vascular disease during follow-up (control subjects). Reproduced with permission from Ridker et al.[2]

sclerosis. These data suggest that among apparently healthy men, baseline levels of CRP predict future risk of developing symptomatic peripheral arterial disease.

Noncoronary Vascular Disease

In the general population, peripheral atherosclerosis is a strong predictor of cardiovascular disease and death. In patients with known CAD, it is unclear whether the presence of additional noncoronary atherosclerosis is of further prognostic value. In the Bypass Angioplasty Revascularization Investigation (BARI), 5-year outcome was compared between patients with and without clinical evidence of noncoronary atherosclerosis, and Sutton-Tyrrell and colleagues[3] for the BARI investigators reported the results. Within the subgroup with noncoronary atherosclerosis, surgery and angioplasty treatment strategies were compared. Noncoronary atherosclerosis was defined as claudication, peripheral vascular surgery, abdominal aortic aneurysm, history of cerebral ischemia, or carotid disease. Among 1,816 patients, 303 (17%) had noncoronary atherosclerosis. These patients were more likely to have a history of CHF, diabetes, and hypertension, and were more likely to smoke. Coronary angiographic variables were similar between the 2 groups. Five-year survival was 75.8% for patients with noncoronary atherosclerosis and 90.2% for those without. The adjusted relative risk of death was 1.7 for any noncoronary atherosclerosis, 1.5 for lower extremity disease alone, 1.7 for cerebral disease alone, and 2.3 for both conditions. Among the 303 patients with noncoronary atherosclerosis, the adjusted relative risk of death for surgery versus angioplasty was 0.87. However, the study has limited power to detect a treatment effect in this small subgroup. Thus, patients with combined coronary and clinically evident noncoronary atherosclerosis are a high-risk group with significantly worse long-term outcome compared to patients with isolated coronary disease (Figures 7-3, 7-4).

Physical Exertion and Increased Risk of Cardiac Events

Sudden extreme physical stress is associated with an increased risk of myocardial infarction mainly in people with preexisting atherosclerosis. Mustonen and colleagues[4] in Helsinki, Finland, compared the effect of submaximal exercise on coagulation and fibrinolysis in patients with peripheral arterial occlusive disease with that in healthy controlled subjects. Fifteen patients with peripheral arterial occlusive disease with intermittent claudication and 15 healthy control subjects, matched for age, gender, medication use, smoking habit, and conditioning, were studied. Thrombin-antithrombin III complex, D-dimer, tissue plasminogen activator, as well as plasma catecholamines were measured before and after a treadmill test. In patients, but not in control subjects, exercise of similar intensity elevated circulating concentrations of thrombin–antithrombin III complex. Exercise caused a parallel increase in the D-dimer, tissue plasminogen activator, plasminogen activator inhibitor antigens,

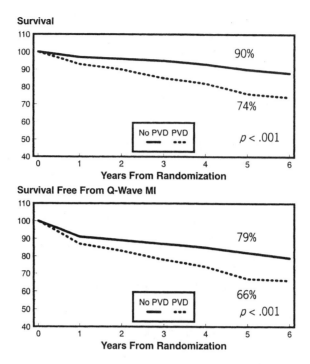

FIGURE 7-3. Long-term survival (top panel) and survival free from Q-wave myocardial infarction (MI) (bottom panel) in BARI patients with (hatched line) and without (solid line) clinically evident noncoronary atherosclerosis (peripheral vascular disease [PVD]). Reproduced with permission from Sutton-Tyrrell et al.[3]

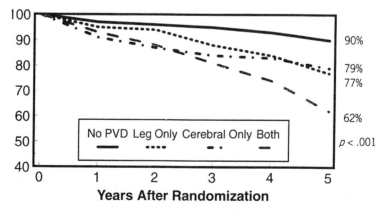

FIGURE 7-4. Long-term survival in BARI patients without noncoronary atherosclerosis (solid line), lower extremity atherosclerosis alone (small hatched line), carotid/cerebral disease alone (dot/hatched line), and those with both conditions (large hatched line). Reproduced with permission from Sutton-Tyrrell et al.[3]

plasmin–α_2–antiplasmin complex, and catecholamines in both groups, whereas plasminogen activator inhibitor antigens remained stable. Plasma lactic acid was significantly higher in patients after exercise and was associated with lower limb ischemia. Compared with healthy control subjects, patients with peripheral arterial occlusive disease showed higher plasminogen activator and inhibitor antigens and D-dimer levels both at rest and after exercise. Notably, submaximal exercise on a treadmill enhanced thrombin formation in patients with peripheral arterial occlusive disease but not in the control subjects. Sudden catecholamine release and local ischemia during exercise may accelerate the preexisting prothrombotic potential of the atherosclerotic vessel wall.

Peripheral Arterial Disease

To assess the age and gender-specific prevalence of peripheral arterial disease and intermittent claudication in an elderly population, Meijer and colleagues[5] in Utrecht, The Netherlands, performed a population-based study in 7,715 subjects (40% men, 60% women) age 55 years and over. The presence of peripheral arterial disease and intermittent claudication was determined by measuring the ankle–arm systolic blood pressure index and by means of the World Health Organization Rose questionnaire, respectively. Peripheral arterial disease was considered present when the ankle–arm index was less than 0.90 in either leg (Figure 7-5). The prevalence of peripheral arterial disease was 19%: 17% in men and 21% in women. Symptoms of intermittent claudication were reported by 2% of the study population. Of those with peripheral arterial disease, 6% reported symptoms of intermittent claudication (9% men,

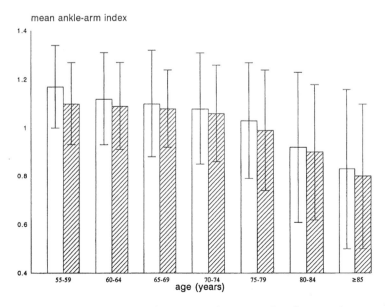

Figure 7-5. AAI (and 95% CI) according to age for men (white bars) and women (shaded bars). Reproduced with permission from Meijer et al.[5]

5% women) whereas in 69% of those with intermittent claudication an ankle–arm index below 0.90 was found. Subjects with an ankle–arm index less
than 0.90 were more likely to be smokers, to have hypertension, and to have
symptomatic or asymptomatic cardiovascular disease compared with subjects
with an ankle–arm index of 0.90 or higher. The authors conclude that the
prevalence of peripheral arterial disease in the elderly was high, whereas the
prevalence of intermittent claudication was rather low, although both prevalences clearly increased with advancing age. The vast majority of peripheral
arterial disease patients reported no symptoms of intermittent claudication.

Carotid Atherosclerosis

Polymorphisms at the β-fibrinogen locus have been shown to be associated
with plasma concentration of fibrinogen and CAD. The effect of genetic heterogeneity of fibrinogen on carotid atherosclerosis has not been reported. Schmidt
and coinvestigators[6] in Graz, Austria, examined the influence of the ($C_{148}{\rightarrow}T$)
polymorphism on carotid disease in a large cohort of middle-aged elderly subjects without evidence of neuropsychiatric disease. This polymorphism is located close to the consensus sequence of the interleukin-6 element and may
represent a functional sequence variant. The genotype of 399 randomly selected
neurologically asymptomatic individuals, aged 45–75 years, was determined
by denaturing gradient gel electrophoresis. Carotid atherosclerosis was assessed by color-coded duplex scanning and was graded on a 5-point scale ranging from 0 (normal) to 5 (complete luminal obstruction). The C/C, C/T, and
T/T genotypes were noted in 226, 148, and 25 individuals, respectively. The
T/T genotype group demonstrated higher grades of carotid atherosclerosis than
did the C/C and the C/T genotypes. Logistic regression analysis created a model
of independent predictors of carotid atherosclerosis that included apolipoprotein B (odds ratio 1.17), age (odds ratio 2.46), lifetime tobacco consumption
(odds ratio 1.03), presence of the β-fibrinogen promoter T-T genotype (odds
ratio 6.17), plasma fibrinogen concentration (odds ratio 1.05), and cardiac
disease (odds ratio 1.80). These data suggest that the β-fibrinogen promoter
T/T 148 genotype represents a genetic risk factor for carotid atherosclerosis in
the middle-aged to elderly population.

Atherosclerosis in the Aorta, Carotid, and Femoral Arteries

Khoury and associates[7] from Jerusalem, Israel, conducted a prospective
study to correlate the presence of angiographically significant CAD and atherosclerotic disease in the aorta, carotid, and femoral arteries as measured by
ultrasound. One hundred two consecutive patients admitted for coronary angiography for suspected CAD participated in the study. All patients underwent
transesophageal echocardiography for the evaluation of thoracic aortic atherosclerosis and B-mode ultrasound for evaluation of carotid and femoral atherosclerosis. Intimal-medial thickness greater than 1 mm in the thoracic aorta or
peripheral vessels was considered as evidence of atherosclerosis. Patients with

CAD (n = 64) had a significantly higher incidence of atherosclerotic plaques in the thoracic aorta, carotid, and femoral arteries than subjects with normal coronary arteries: 91%, 72%, and 77% vs. 31%, 47%, and 42%, respectively. Extracoronary plaque was a stronger predictor of CAD than conventional risk factors. Evidence of plaque in patients younger than median age (64 years) had a higher specificity than in patients above median age (77% vs. 40%, respectively). Plaque score of the extracardiac vessels was significantly higher in patients with multivessel CAD than in patients with 1-vessel CAD disease and in subjects with normal coronary arteries. Thus, atherosclerotic plaques in the aortic and femoral arteries and, to a lesser extent, in the carotid arteries are strong predictors of atherosclerosis.

Lower Extremity Artery Disease

Patients with lower extremity artery disease (LEAD) are at an increased risk of having CAD. Diabetics are at especially high risk for having LEAD with concomitant CAD. This study by Barzilay and associates[8] from Atlanta, Georgia; Seattle, Washington; Birmingham, Alabama; Marshfield, Wisconsin; and Albany, New York, was undertaken (1) to define the clinical and arteriographic features associated with CAD among diabetics and nondiabetics with LEAD and (2) to determine the long-term survival and predictors of mortality of diabetics and nondiabetics with LEAD and CAD. Two hundred sixty-three diabetics and 1,137 nondiabetics from the Coronary Artery Surgery Study who had evidence of LEAD, who were 50 years and older, and who had arteriographically proven CAD were monitored for a mean of 13 years. Among all the subjects with LEAD there was a high prevalence of current and past smoking, history of previous myocardial infarction, systemic hypertension CAF, high degrees of angina pectoris and unstable angina pectoris, and use of β-blockers. On arteriographic evaluation, a high prevalence of 3-vessel epicardial coronary disease and involvement of multiple coronary segments with 50% or more diameter narrowing was found. Multivariate analysis showed the number of coronary segments with 50% or greater occlusion, the presence of cerebrovascular disease, the use of digitalis, and elevated systolic BP were independently associated with diabetes. On follow-up, diabetics had a significantly higher mortality rate (mostly cardiac) than nondiabetics: median survival, 8.1 years and 13 years, respectively. At 15 years, the mortality rates were 77% and 62%, respectively. On multivariate analysis, age, number of coronary occlusions, number of significantly narrowed epicardial arteries, diminished myocardial contractility, hypertension, and smoking were significant predictors of mortality in the total group and in each subgroup. CABG was protective. The presence of diabetes was an independent risk factor for mortality. The presence of LEAD is associated with multivessel epicardial and multiple coronary segment occlusion. On long-term follow-up there is a high mortality rate. In patients with LEAD and diabetes, CAD is especially severe and prognosis is poor.

Risk Stratification of Peripheral Revascularization Patients

Patients with advanced peripheral vascular disease have increased cardiac morbidity and mortality rates. Rossi and colleagues[9] from Rome, Italy, assessed the predictive value of rest and stress echocardiography for perioperative and late cardiac events in 110 patients undergoing limb revascularization. All patients underwent preoperative clinical and echocardiographic evaluation at rest and by dipyridamole stress testing to assess cardiac risk. Patients with 3 or more clinical Eagle markers, low LVEF at rest, or positive dipyridamole stress test results were considered at high cardiac risk. To record adverse cardiac events, all patients were monitored during and after surgery, and followed for at least 1 year after hospital discharge. Cardiac complications occurred in 10 patients (9.7%) perioperatively (2 fatal AMIs), and in 13 (13%) at 1-year follow-up (7 fatal AMIs). Echocardiographic evaluation was the best predictor of early and late cardiac complications. No patients with a negative dipyridamole stress test result and good LVEF had cardiac complications, either postoperatively or during follow-up. Clinical evaluation does not appear sufficiently sensitive for predicting perioperative cardiac events, but was valuable in predicting late cardiac complications. Our data show that echocardiographic evaluation of resting dysfunction and of the ischemic response to dipyridamole is a good predictor of perioperative cardiac risk and is superior to generally available clinical data. Echocardiographic evaluation is useful in defining a low-risk group of patients who can safely undergo limb revascularization, whichever surgical procedure is proposed.

Cerebrovascular Disease

Risk Profile and Prediction of Long-Term Stroke Mortality

Tanne and colleagues[10] assessed the role of ethnicity and estimated the cumulative effect of multiple risk factors on long-term ischemic stroke mortality. Civil servants and municipal employees in Israel (n = 9,734 men with a mean age ≥42 years) chosen by stratified sampling in 6 prespecified areas of birth were included in the Israeli Ischemic Heart Disease project. Over a 21-year follow-up period, age-adjusted mortality rates per 10,000 person-years attributed to ischemic stroke (n = 282) were higher among immigrants to Israel from northern Africa and the Mideast than from 3 parts of Europe. Crude rates per 1,000 subjects observed in those born in Asia or Africa exceeded rates predicted by risk factor profiles. Adjusted hazard ratios were 3.0 for age, 2.15 for LV hypertrophy, 1.69 for systolic BP, 1.86 for diabetes mellitus, 1.83 for peripheral vascular disease, 1.79 for smoking, 1.51 for CAD, 1.16 for percent cholesterol contained in the HDL fraction, and 1.88 for diastolic BP. Accounting for regression dilution bias and assessed from repeated measurements, the authors found that hazard ratio estimates associated with diastolic BP, systolic BP, and percent HDL increased to 3.22, 2.23, and 1.23, respectively. Ischemic stroke mortality rates were 30-fold higher among subjects at the highest versus the lowest quintile of predicted probability according to risk factor profiles (81 vs. 2.6/1,000 subjects). Thus, assessment of multiple risk factors provides useful quantitative prediction of long-term ischemic stroke mortality risk. Regional ethnic variations are consistent with a hypothesis that other, undetermined inherent genetic or sociocultural factors act to increase ischemic stroke mortality rates in immigrants to Israel from the Mideast and northern Africa above that predicted by conventional risk factors.

Association Between Methylenetetrahydrofolate Reductase Gene and Ischemic Stroke

Hyperhomocysteinemia has been identified as an independent risk factor for atherosclerotic and thromboembolic diseases such as CAD, cerebral artery disease, and venous thrombosis. Recently, the alanine/valine (A/V) gene polymorphism of 5,10-methylenetetrahydrofolate reductase (MTHFR), 1 of the key enzymes that catalyzes the re-methylation of homocysteine, was reported. The V/V genotype is correlated with increased plasma homocysteine levels as a result of the reduced ability and increased thermolability of this enzyme. In a recent study, Morita and coworkers[11] in Tokyo, Japan, examined the association between the V allele of the MTHFR gene and ischemic stroke in an elderly Japanese population. The diagnosis of cerebral infarction of all study patients was confirmed by CT scan of the brain. The MTHFR genotype was analyzed by polymerase chain reaction followed by HinfI digestion. In 256 stroke patients and 325 control subjects, the frequencies of the valine allele were 0.45 and 0.32, respectively. The odds ratios of 95% intervals adjusted for the other risk factors were, respectively, 1.51 for the A/V genotype and 3.35 for the V/V genotype compared with the A/A genotype. Both of these effects were statistically significant. In patients with multiple infarctions, in particular, the allele frequency of the V mutation was 0.56, and the association between the V allele and stroke was highly significant. Plasma homocysteine levels were significantly higher in patients with the V/V genotype than in patients with the A/A or A/V genotype, especially those with low plasma folate levels. The V allele of the MTHFR gene was significantly associated with cerebral infarction in an elderly Japanese population in a co-dominant manner. The V/V genotype may contribute to risk for ischemic stroke through a predisposition to increased plasma homocysteine levels, and dietary folate supplementation may be of benefit, particularly to patients with this genotype.

Attitudes Toward a Hypothetical Major Stroke

Patient beliefs, values, and preferences are crucial to decisions involving health care. In a large sample of persons at increased risk for stroke, Samsa and associates[12] from Durham and Winston Salem, North Carolina; Lawrence, Kansas; Rochester, New York; Minneapolis, Minnesota; and Indianapolis, Indiana, examined attitudes toward hypothetical major stroke. Respondents were obtained from the Academic Medical Center Consortium (n = 621), the Cardiovascular Health Study (n = 321), and United Health Care (n = 319). Preferences were primarily assessed by using the time trade off. Although major stroke is generally considered an undesirable event, responses were varied: although

45% of respondents considered major stroke to be a worse outcome than death, 15% were willing to trade off little or no survival to avoid a major stroke. Providers should speak directly with patients about beliefs, values, and preferences. Stroke-related interventions, even those with a high price or less than dramatic clinical benefits, are likely to be cost-effective if they prevent an outcome (major stroke) that is so undesirable.

Frequency of Stroke in Patients with Mitral Annular Calcium

Aronow and associates[13] from New York, New York, and Houston, Texas, investigated the frequency of thromboembolic strokes among 2,148 patients aged 60 years or older (mean age 81) in persons with mitral annular calcium (MAC) with associated AF, MS, and/or MR (Table 7-1). They found that persons with MAC had a 2.8 times higher prevalence of AF than persons without MAC. In persons with AF, MAC increased the incidence of new thromboembolic stroke 2.1 times if MS was associated with MAC, 1.7 times if 2 to 4+ MR was associated with MAC, and 1.4 times if 0 to 1+ MR was present. In persons with sinus rhythm, MAC increased the incidence of new thromboembolic stroke 3.6 times if MS was associated with MAC, 3.1 times if 2 to 4+ MR was associated with MAC, and 2.7 times if 0 to 1+ MR was present. Independent risk factors for new thromboembolic stroke were prior stroke (risk ratio 2.4), MAC (risk ratio 2.6), AF (risk ratio 3.0), and male gender (risk ratio 1.6).

Usefulness of Transesophageal Echocardiography in Stroke Patients

O'Brien and associates[14] from Baltimore and Bethesda, Maryland, tested the hypothesis that stroke patients without a coronary source of embolism

TABLE 7-1
Association of Mitral Annular Calcium (MAC) With Mitral Stenosis or Mitral Regurgitation With New Thromboembolic Stroke at 44-Month Follow-Up in Older Persons With Atrial Fibrillation and With Sinus Rhythm

	Thromboembolic Stroke	
	No.	%
Atrial fibrillation, no MAC (1)	30/85	35
Atrial fibrillation with mitral stenosis due to MAC (2)	31/42	74
Atrial fibrillation with MAC and 2–4+ mitral regurgitation (3)	53/90	59
Atrial fibrillation with MAC and 0–1+ mitral regurgitation (4)	45/93	48
Sinus rhythm, no MAC (5)	95/1,035	9
Sinus rhythm with mitral stenosis due to MAC (6)	13/41	32
Sinus rhythm with MAC and 2–4+ mitral regurgitation (7)	38/134	28
Sinus rhythm with MAC and 0–1+ mitral regurgitation (8)	148/628	24

$p < 0.0001$ comparing 1 with 2; $p = 0.002$ comparing 1 with 3; $p = 0.077$ comparing 1 with 4; $p = 0.006$ comparing 2 with 4; $p = 0.097$ comparing 2 with 3; $p = 0.154$ comparing 3 with 4; $p < 0.0001$ comparing 5 with 6, 5 with 7, and 5 with 8; $p = 0.680$ comparing 6 with 7; $p = 0.237$ comparing 6 with 8; $p = 0.241$ comparing 7 with 8.
Reproduced with permission from Aronow et al.[13]

suspected by clinical examination can be risk stratified by transesophageal echocardiography. Forty ischemic stroke patients without AF, prosthetic or bioprosthetic valves, EF less than 20%, or recent AMI underwent multiplane transesophageal echocardiography: 24 (designated high risk) had one or more of the following: left heart thrombus, vegetation, mass or spontaneous echo contrast, mobile ascending aortic or arch debris, patent foramen ovale, atrial septal defect or aneurysm, mitral annular calcium, mitral valve thickening, prolapse, or mitral valve strands. Endpoints were death, recurrent stroke, transient ischemic attack, AMI, or peripheral embolism. Thirty-eight patients (95%) (23 high, 15 low risk) were followed for 14 ± 8 months: 9 (24%) died of vascular causes including 4 who had a cardiac cause of death and 5 who had fatal strokes. Eight had recurrent strokes (4 nonfatal) and 1 nonfatal AMI occurred. Cardiovascular survival was predicted by transesophageal echocardiography: survival rates were 92% (low risk) and 63% (high risk) at 24 months. LA enlargement was independently associated with death from stroke (fatal stroke occurred in 25% of those with atrial enlargement compared to 8% of those with normal atrial dimension, as was LA spontaneous echo contrast (50% died vs. 9% without contrast). LV hypertrophy and aortic atherosclerosis were both associated with the risk of recurrent stroke (30% of patients with ventricular hypertrophy had recurrent stroke compared to 10% with normal wall thickness; 30% with aortic atherosclerosis had a recurrent stroke compared to none with a normal aorta. Thus, transesophageal echocardiography clearly identifies patients at high risk for cardiovascular mortality and morbidity after stroke despite an unsuspected source of embolism by clinical examination.

Global Utilization of Streptokinase and Tissue Plasminogen Activator for Occluded Coronary Arteries (GUSTO I) Trial Assessment of Nonhemorrhagic Stroke Risks

The GUSTO Investigators[15] studied 247 patients with nonhemorrhagic stroke who were randomly assigned to 1 of 4 thrombolytic regimens within 6 hours of symptom onset in the GUSTO I trial. They assessed the univariable and multivariable baseline risk factors for nonhemorrhagic stroke and created a scoring nomogram from the baseline multivariable modeling. They used time-dependent Cox modeling to determine multivariable in-hospital predictors of nonhemorrhagic stroke. Baseline and in-hospital predictors were then combined to determine the overall predictors of nonhemorrhagic stroke. Among 247 patients, 42 (17%) died and another 98 (40%) were disabled by 30-day follow-up. Older age was the most important baseline clinical predictor of nonhemorrhagic stroke, followed by higher heart rate, history of stroke or transient ischemic attack, diabetes, previous angina, and history of hypertension (Figure 7-6). These factors remained statistically significant predictors in a combined model, along with a worse Killip class, coronary angiography, bypass surgery, and atrial fibrillation/flutter. The authors conclude that the nomogram they have developed can predict the

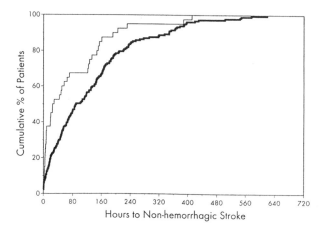

FIGURE 7-6. Cumulative frequency distribution of hours from enrollment to onset of nonhemorrhagic stroke in GUSTO I. Nonfatal nonhemorrhagic stroke is indicated by the heavy line, and fatal nonhemorrhagic stroke is indicated by the light line. Reproduced with permission from the GUSTO Investigators.[15]

1. Find Points For Each Risk Factor

Age, y		Heart rate, per min		Diabetes		Hypertension	
Age	Points	Rate	Points		Points		Points
20	10	0	0	Yes	11	Yes	7
30	20	20	5	No	0	No	0
40	30	40	11				
50	40	60	16				
60	50	80	21				
70	60	100	27				
80	70	120	32				
90	80	140	38	Previous CVD		Previous angina	
100	90	160	43		Points		Points
		180	48	Yes	20	Yes	9
		200	54	No	0	No	0
		220	59				
		240	64				
		260	70				

2. Sum Points For All Risk Factors

____ + ____ + ____ + ____ + ____ + ____ = ____
Age Heart rate Diabetes Hypertension Prev. CVD Prev. Angina Point Total

3. Look Up Risk Corresponding to Point Total

Points	Risk	Points	Risk	Points	Risk
67	0.5%	116	5%	153	25%
82	1%	132	10%	158	30%
97	2%	141	15%	162	35%
105	3%	148	20%		

FIGURE 7-7. Nomogram for the prediction of nonhemorrhagic stroke after thrombolysis for AMI. CVD = cerebrovascular disease. In 1, find the value most closely matching the patient's risk factors and circle the corresponding point assignment. In 2, sum the points of all predictive factors. In 3, determine the probability of in-hospital nonhemorrhagic stroke. For example, a 71-year-old nondiabetic patient with previous CVD, a history of hypertension, and previous angina who presents with a heart rate of 121 bpm would have a total score of 60 + 32 + 0 + 20 + 7 + 9 = 128. This score corresponds to a predicted probability of in-hospital nonhemorrhagic stroke of 10%. Reproduced with permission from the GUSTO Investigators.[15]

risk of nonhemorrhagic stroke on the basis of clinical characteristics (Figure 7-7).

Spiral Computed Tomography

Corti and colleagues[16] used spiral CT and duplex ultrasonography in 59 consecutive patients with a clinical suspicion of an obstructive lesion involving the carotid arteries. They analyzed a total of 354 segments from the extracranial carotid arteries, including the common, internal, and external carotid arteries. A total of 4 complete occlusions, 38 severe stenoses, and 32 moderate stenoses were identified by means of duplex ultrasonography and spiral CT. In 5 cases in which duplex ultrasonography did not allow sufficient evaluation of the carotid artery because of a poor ultrasonographic window or severe calcification, spiral CT allowed identification and correct measurement of the stenotic lesion. The comparison of the percentage of stenosis with both methods was good, r = 0.91. Thus, these data indicate that spiral CT of the extracranial cerebral arteries is a promising noninvasive complementary and nonoperator-dependent examination (Figure 7-8).

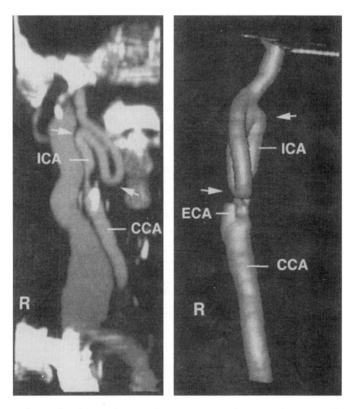

FIGURE 7-8. Kinking of right ICA by spiral CT in MIP and SSD techniques. Shown is severe kinking of right ICA describing a loop of 360° by MIP (left) and SSD reconstruction techniques with 90° clockwise rotation on its long axis (right). MIP reconstruction also shows a severe calcified stenosis (70%) at ICA origin. Arrows indicate knee of kinking loop. Reproduced with permission from Corti et al.[16]

Ischemic Limbs

Injection of Naked Plasmid DNA Promotes Collateral Vessel Development in Ischemic Limbs

Baumgartner and colleagues[17] wished to document the safety and feasibility of intramuscular gene transfer by use of naked plasmid DNA encoding and endothelial cell mitogen ($VEGF_{165}$) and to analyze potential therapeutic benefits in humans with critical limb ischemia. Gene transfer was performed in 10 limbs of 9 patients with nonhealing ischemic ulcers and/or rest pain (10 of 10) due to peripheral arterial disease. A total dose of 4,000 μg of naked plasmid DNA encoding the 165-amino-acid isoform of human vascular endothelial growth factor ($phVEGF_{165}$) was injected directly into the muscles of the ischemic limb. Gene expression was documented by a transient increase in serum levels of VEGF monitored by ELISA. The ankle-brachial index improved significantly (0.33 $\pm$ 0.05 to 0.48 $\pm$ 0.03, p$=$0.02) (Figure 7-9). Newly visible collateral blood vessels were directly documented by contrast angiography in 7 limbs and magnetic resonance angiography showed qualitative evidence of improved distal flow in 8 limbs (Figure 7-10). Ischemic ulcers healed or markedly improved in 4 of 7 limbs, including successful limb salvage in 3 patients who had been previously recommended to have below-knee amputations. Tissue specimens obtained from an amputee 10 weeks after gene therapy showed foci of proliferating endothelial cells by immunohistochemistry. PCR and Southern blot analyses indicated persistence of small amounts of plasmid DNA. Complications related to the procedure were primarily lower extremity edema in 6 patients, consistent with VEGF enhancement of vascular permeability.

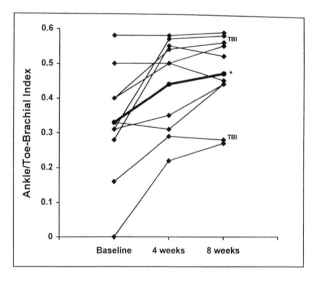

FIGURE 7-9. Gain in ABI and/or TBI in 10 limbs 4 and 8 weeks after intramuscular phVEGF$_{165}$ gene transfer. *Mean values, p = 0.02. Reproduced with permission from Baumgartner et al.[17]

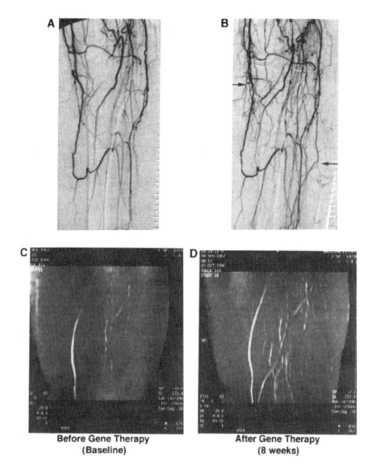

Before Gene Therapy
(Baseline)

After Gene Therapy
(8 weeks)

FIGURE 7-10. (A, B) Newly visible collateral vessels at calf level 8 weeks after phVEGF[165] gene transfer. Luminal diameter of newly visible vessels ranged from 200 to over 800 μm (arrow); most were closer to 200 μm, and these frequently appeared as a blush of innumerable collaterals. (C, D) MRA before and 8 weeks after gene therapy. After gene therapy, signal enhancement is clearly evident, consistent with improved flow in ischemic limb. Reproduced with permission from Baumgartner et al.[17]

Thus, these data suggest that intramuscular injection of naked plasmid DNA achieves constitutive overexpression of VEGF in amounts sufficient to cause angiogenesis in selected patients with critical limb ischemia.

Study of Leg Blood Flow Responses

Steinberg and associates[18] studied leg blood flow responses to graded intrafemoral artery infusions of the endothelium-dependent vasodilator, methacholine chloride, or the endothelium-independent vasodilator, sodium nitroprusside, in normal volunteers exhibiting a wide range of total cholesterol values within the normal range, lower than the 75th percentile. Leg blood flow

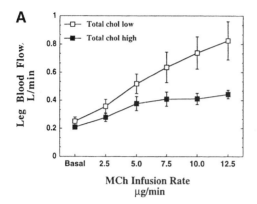

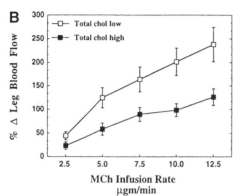

FIGURE 7-11. (A) Leg blood flow under basal conditions and in response to graded intra-femoral artery infusions of methacholine chloride (MCh) in the low (□) and high (■) normal cholesterol groups (p < 0.0001, ANOVA, low vs. high). (B) Percent incre-ments (%△) in leg blood flow above baseline in response to graded intrafemoral artery infu-sions of MCh in the low and high normal cho-lesterol groups (p < 0.0001, ANOVA, low vs. high). Reproduced with permission from Steinberg et al.[18]

increased in a dose-dependent fashion in response to the femoral artery infu-sion of both agonists. Leg blood flow responses to methacholine were signifi-cantly blunted in subjects with high normal cholesterol (195 ± 6 mg/dL, n = 13) compared with subjects with low normal cholesterol (146 ± 5 mg/dL, n = 20) (Figure 7-11). Maximal endothelium-dependent vasodilation in the high nor-mal group was decreased by nearly 50% compared with the low normal group. There was a negative correlation between total serum cholesterol and maximal endothelium-dependent vasodilation. Leg blood flow responses to nitroprus-side did not differ in the patients in the 2 different groups. Thus, these data suggest that patients with high serum cholesterols have endothelial dysfunc-tion, even when the serum cholesterols are in the "normal" range as presently defined.

Intermittent Claudication

Vitamin Supplementation and Intermittent Claudication

Tornwall and associates[19] in Helsinki, Finland, examined the primary pre-ventive effect of vitamin E (α-tocopherol) and β-carotene supplementation on intermittent claudication. The subjects, participants in the Alpha-Tocopherol, Beta-Carotene Cancer Prevention Study, were male smokers age 50–69 years who were randomly assigned to receive 50 mg α-tocopherol daily, 20 mg of β-carotene daily, both, or placebo. At baseline, there were 26,289 men with no history or symptoms of intermittent claudication. The Rose questionnaire on intermittent claudication was administered annually to discover incident cases. The investigators observed 2,704 cases of first occurrence of typical intermittent claudication during a median follow-up time of 4 years. Compared with placebo, the adjusted relative risks for typical intermittent claudication among those who received α-tocopherol was only 1.11; among those who received α-tocopherol and β-carotene, 1.02; and among those who received β-carotene only, 1.02. When investigators compared the α-tocopherol supplemented subjects with those that received no α-tocopherol, the adjusted relative risks for intermittent claudication was 1.05, and for β-carotene supplemented subjects compared with those who did not receive β-carotene, the relative risks were 0.96. In conclusion, no primary preventive effect on intermittent claudication was observed among middle-aged male smokers who were supplemented with α-tocopherol, β-carotene, or both.

Deep Venous Thrombosis

Streptokinase Versus Alteplase in Pulmonary Embolism

Various studies have compared different thrombolytic regimens in patients with massive pulmonary embolus. Meneveau and colleagues[20] from France sought to compare the efficacy of 2-hour regimens of alteplase and streptokinase in acute massive pulmonary embolism. The primary endpoint was immediate hemodynamic improvement and the secondary endpoints included early clinical efficacy and safety as well as 1-year clinical outcome. Sixty six patients with acute massive pulmonary embolism and mean PA pressure greater than 20 mm Hg were randomly assigned to receive either a 100 mg 2-hour infusion of alteplase or 1.5 million IU of streptokinase over 2 hours. In both groups, heparin infusion was started at the end of thrombolytic infusion and adapted thereafter. The results demonstrated that despite a faster fall of total pulmonary vascular resistance in the alteplase group, a similar hemodynamic effect was obtained at 2 hours when both thrombolytic regimens were completed. There was no significant difference in either pulmonary vascular obstruction at 36 to 48 hours or bleeding complication rates. One-year survival was similar in both groups as most events were related to concomitant disease. These authors conclude that a 2-hour regimen of streptokinase can be routinely used in patients with massive pulmonary embolism and cardiac output maintained without obviously compromising efficacy or safety.

Right Ventricular Function in Pulmonary Embolism

Inasmuch as the presence of RV overload in patients with pulmonary embolism is associated with a bad prognosis, evaluation of RV function in pulmonary embolism is of importance. This study by Ribeiro and associates[21] from Stockholm, Sweden, was done to establish if the degree of RV overload can be predicted from the extent of perfusion defects. One hundred twenty-one consecutive patients with pulmonary embolism diagnosed by lung scintigraphy were examined by Doppler echocardiography immediately after diagnosis. The extent of perfusion defects were graded visually in categories (lung scintigraphy score $1 = \leq 20\%$, $2 = \geq 20\%$ of total lung area) and on a continuous scale (normal perusion = 0, no perfusion = 1). The reproducibility of both methods was tested. RV wall motion was assessed on a 4-point scale (0 = normal to 3 = severely hypokinetic). The distance from the LV posterior wall to the RV anterior wall and dimensions of RV and LV were measured. PA systolic pressure was calculated by using the maximum velocity of TR. There were 51 patients with lung scintigraphy score 1 and 70 (58%) with score 2. In comparison with patients with lung scintigraphy score 1, those with score 2 more often had RV hypokinesis 2+ or 3+ (n=49 vs. n=16), larger RV (34 ± 6 mm [22 to 48] vs. 29 ± 5 [17 to 38] and higher PA systolic pressure (51 ± 13 mm Hg [21 to 83] vs. 42 ± 14 [20 to 81]). The variability in both groups was large. With continuous scaling, the extent of perfusion defects averaged 0.3. This was also the value that best discriminated RV hypokinesis 2+ or 3+ in a receiver operating characteristic curve. However, the variability for this scan scoring method was SD 0.073, giving a 95% confidence limit of ±0.15. There is a significant correlation between RV overload and extent of perfusion defects, but the variability is large; therefore, an estimate of the size of perfusion defects in lung scintigraphy cannot replace Doppler echocardiography in the assessment of PA systolic pressure and the degree of RV overload in pulmonary embolism.

Prevention of Venous Thromboembolism After Neurosurgery

In a multicenter, randomized, double-blind trial, Agnelli and colleagues[22] assessed the efficacy and safety of enoxaparin in conjunction with the use of compression stockings in the prevention of venous thromboembolism in patients undergoing elective neurosurgery. Enoxaparin (40 mg once daily) or placebo were given subcutaneously for not less than 7 days beginning within 24 hours after surgery. The primary endpoint was symptomatic, objectively confirmed venous thromboembolism or deep vein thrombosis assessed by bilateral venography, which was performed in all patients on day 8. Bleeding side effects were carefully evaluated. Among 307 patients assigned to treatment groups, 129 of the 154 patients receiving placebo (84%) and 130 of the 153 patients receiving enoxaparin (85%) had venographic studies adequate for analysis. An additional patient in the placebo group died before venography of autopsy-confirmed pulmonary embolism. In this analysis, 42 patients given placebo (32%) and 22 patients given enoxaparin (17%) had deep vein thrombosis, p=0.004. The rates of proximal deep vein thrombosis were 13% in patients receiving placebo and 5% in patients receiving enoxaparin, p=0.04. Two patients in the placebo group died of autopsy-confirmed pulmonary embolism on days 9 and 16. Major bleeding occurred in 4 patients receiving placebo (intracranial bleeding in all 4) and 4 patients receiving enoxaparin (intracranial bleeding in 3). Thus, enoxaparin combined with compression stockings is more effective than compression stockings alone for the prevention of venous thromboembolism after elective neurosurgery and does not cause excess bleeding.

Stenting

Neurological Complications with Carotid Stenting

Mathur and colleagues[23] from the University of Alabama at Birmingham, Alabama, analyzed the impact of various clinical, morphological, and procedural determinants on the development of procedural strokes in 231 patients who underwent elective (primary) stenting of 271 extracranial carotid arteries. The mean age of the patients was 68.7 years, and 165 were males; 139 of the patients had symptoms attributable to the lesion treated. One hundred sixty-four patients represented a high-risk subset (71%) having significant CAD. Ninety-one patients had bilateral carotid disease, and 28 had contralateral carotid occlusions. Among the untreated vessels, 59 (22%) had prior carotid endarterectomy, 66 (24%) had ulcerated plaques, and 87 (32%) had calcified lesions. Among 37 treated vessels 14% would have been eligible for inclusion in the North American Symptomatic Carotid Endarterectomy Trial. There were 17 (6%) minor and 2 (0.7%) major strokes during and within 30 days of the procedure. Multivariate analysis indicated that advanced age and the presence of long or multiple stenoses were independent predictors of procedural strokes (Table 7-2). Thus, neurological complications with carotid stenting are dependent on patient selection characteristics and advanced age and long or multiple stenoses are independent risks for procedural stroke.

Renal Vascular Disease

Renal Artery Stent Placement

Hypertension due to renal artery stenosis can be treated with balloon angioplasty. White and colleagues[24] from New Orleans, Louisiana, reported on

TABLE 7-2
Result of Multivariate Analysis for Predictors of Minor and Major Strokes After Carotid Stenting

Predictor	Coefficient	Odds Ratio	*P*	95% Confidence Limits
Age	0.117	1.1249	.0057	1.0348, 1.2228
Long/multiple stenoses	1.6376	5.1429	.0056	1.6145, 16.3824
Lesion severity	0.0464	1.0474	.0618	0.9977, 1.0996
Residual irregularity	0.9583	2.6073	.0852	0.8756, 7.7642

Reproduced with permission from Mathur et al.[23]

100 consecutive patients with hypertension and renal artery stenosis who also had stents placed. Angiographic success was obtained in 99% of 133 lesions. Early clinical success was achieved in 76% of the patients. Six months after stent placement, the systolic blood pressure was reduced from 173 to 147 and the diastolic pressure from 88 to 76. The mean number of antihypertensive medications per patient was reduced from 2.6 to 2.0. Angiographic follow-up at 9 months in 67 patients revealed stenosis in 19% of 80 stented vessels. These authors conclude that renal artery stenting is an effective treatment for renovascular hypertension with a low angiographic restenosis rate. Stent placement appears to be a very attractive therapy in patients with lesions difficult to treat with balloon angioplasty such as renal aorto-ostial lesions and restenotic lesions as well as after a suboptimal balloon angioplasty result.

Follow-Up of Renal Artery Stent Revascularization

Dorros and colleagues[25] in Phoenix, Arizona, successfully performed Palmaz-Schatz stent revascularization of renal artery stenosis in 163 consecutive patients with poorly controlled hypertension or preservation of renal function. Among these, 145 were eligible for 6 or more months of clinical follow-up of the effect of the procedure on renal function, BP control, number of antihypertensive medications, and survival. At 4 years, systolic and diastolic BPs significantly decreased and BP control was easier in approximately half of the patients. Creatinine decreased or remained stable in approximately two-thirds of the patients. The cumulative probability of survival was 74% ± 4% at 3 years with few deaths related to end-stage renal disease. Survival was good in patients with normal baseline renal function, fair in those with mildly impaired renal function, and poor in patients with elevated baseline creatinine levels of 2.0 or more mg/dL. The combination of impaired renal function and bilateral disease adversely affected survival. Thus, renal artery stent revascularization in the presence of normal or mildly impaired renal function had a beneficial effect on blood pressure control and a nondeleterious effect on renal function (Figure 7-12).

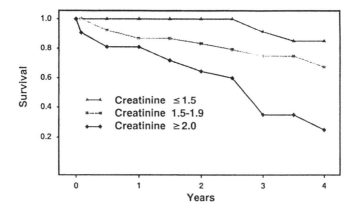

FIGURE 7-12. Actuarial analysis of renal artery stent revascularization patients as categorized by baseline serum creatinine at the time of procedure. Reproduced with permission from Dorros et al.[25]

1. Cohen A, Tzourio C, Bertrand B, Chauvel C, Bousser M-G, Amarenco P, on behalf of the FAPS Investigators: Aortic plaque morphology and vascular events: A follow-up study in patients with ischemic stroke. Circulation 1997 (December 2);96:3838–3841.
2. Ridker PM, Cushman M, Stampfer MJ, Tracy RP, Hennekens CH: Plasma concentration of C-reactive protein and risk of developing peripheral vascular disease. Circulation 1998 (February 10);97:425–428.
3. Sutton-Tyrrell K, Rihal C, Sellers MA, Burek K, Trudel J, Roubin G, Brooks MM, Grogan M, Sopko G, Keller N, Jandová R, for the BARI Investigators: Long-term prognostic value of clinically evident noncoronary vascular disease in patients undergoing coronary revascularization in the bypass angioplasty revascularization investigation (BARI). Am J Cardiol 1998 (February 15);81:375–381.
4. Mustonen P, Lepantalo M, Lassila R: Physical exertion induces thrombin formation and fibrin degradation in patients with peripheral atherosclerosis. Arterioscler Thromb Vasc Biol 1998 (February);18:244–249.
5. Meijer WT, Hoes AW, Rutgers D, Bots ML, Hofman A, Grobbee DE: Peripheral arterial disease in the elderly: The Rotterdam Study. Arterioscler Thromb Vasc Biol 1998 (February);18:185–192.
6. Schmidt H, Schmidt R, Niederkorn K, Horner S, Becsagh P, Reinhart B, Schumacher M, Weinrauch V, Kostner GM: Beta-fibrinogen gene polymorphism $((C_{148}{\rightarrow}T)$ is associated with carotid atherosclerosis: Results of the Austrian Stroke Prevention Study. Arterioscler Thromb Vasc Biol 1998 (March);18:487–492.
7. Khoury Z, Schwartz R, Gottlieb S, Chenzbraun A, Stern S, Keren A: Relation of coronary artery disease to atherosclerotic disease in the aorta, carotid, and femoral arteries evaluated by ultrasound. Am J Cardiol 1997 (December 1);80:1429–1433.
8. Barzilay JI, Kronmal RA, Bittner V, Eaker E, Foster ED: CAD in diabetic and nondiabetic patients with lower extremity arterial disease: A report from the Coronary Artery Surgery Study Registry. Am Heart J 1998 (June);35:1055–1062.
9. Rossi E, Citterio F, Vescio MF, Pennestri F, Lombardo A, Loperfido F, Maseri A: Risk stratification of patients undergoing peripheral vascular revascularization by combined resting and dipyridamole echocardiography. Am J Cardiol 1998 (August 1);82:306–310.
10. Tanne D, Yaari S, Goldbourt U: Risk profile and prediction of long-term ischemic stroke mortality: A 21-year follow-up in the Israeli ischemic heart disease (IIHD) project. Circulation 1998 (October 6);98:1365–1371.
11. Morita H, Kurihara H, Tsubaki S-I, Sugiyama T, Hamada C, Kurihara Y, Shindo T, Oh-hashi Y, Kitamura K, Yazaki Y: Methylenetetrahydrofolate reductase gene polymorphism and ischemic stroke in Japanese. Arterioscler Thromb Vasc Biol 1998 (September);18:1465–1469.
12. Samsa GP, Matchar DB, Goldstein L, Bonito A, Duncan PW, Lipscomb J, Enarson C, Witter D, Venus P, Paul JE, Weinberger M: Utilities for major stroke: Results from a survey of preferences among persons at increased risk for stroke. Am Heart J 1998 (October);136:703–713.
13. Aronow WS, Ahn C, Kronzon I, Gutstein H: Association of mitral annular calcium with new thromboembolic stroke at 44-month follow-up of 2,148 persons, mean age 81 years Am J Cardiol 1998 (January);81:105–106.
14. O'Brien PJ, Thiemann DR, McNamara RL, Roberts JW, Raska K, Oppenheimer SM, Lima JAC: Usefulness of transesophageal echocardiography in predicting mortality and morbidity in stroke patients without clinically known cardiac sources of embolus. Am J Cardiol 1998 (May 1);81:1144–1151.
15. Mahaffey KW, Granger CB, Sloan MA, Thompson TD, Gore JM, Weaver WD, White HD, Simoons ML, Barbash GI, Topol EJ, Califf RM, for the GUSTO-I Investigators: Risk factors for in-hospital nonhemorrhagic stroke in patients with acute myocardial infarction treated with thrombolysis. Results from GUSTO-I. Circulation 1998 (March 3);97:757–764.
16. Corti R, Ferrari C, Roberti M, Alerci M, Pedrazzi PL, Gallino A: Spiral computed tomography: A novel diagnostic approach for investigation of the extracranial cerebral arteries and its complementary role in duplex ultrasonography. Circulation 1998 (September 8);98:984–989.

17. Baumgartner I, Pieczek A, Manor O, Blair R, Kearney M, Walsh K, Isner JM: Constitutive expression of phVEGF$_{165}$ after intramuscular gene transfer promotes collateral vessel development in patients with critical limb ischemia. Circulation 1998 (March 31);97:1114–1123.
18. Steinberg HO, Bayazeed B, Hook G, Johnson A, Cronin J, Baron AD: Endothelial dysfunction is associated with cholesterol levels in the high normal range in humans. Circulation 1997 (November 18);96:3287–3293.
19. Tornwall ME, Virtamo J, Haukka JK, Aro A, Albanes D, Edwards BK, Huttunen JK: Effect of alpha-tocopherol (vitamin E) and beta-carotene supplementation on the incidence of intermittent claudication in male smokers. Arterioscler Thromb Vasc Biol 1997 (December);17:3475–3480.
20. Meneveau N, Schiele F, Metz D, Valette B, Attali P, Vuillemenot A, Grollier G, Elaerts J, Mossard J-M, Viel J-F, Bassand J-P: Comparative efficacy of a two-hour regimen of streptokinase versus alteplase in acute massive pulmonary embolism: Immediate clinical and hemodynamic outcome and one-year follow-up. JACC 1998 (April);31:1057–1063.
21. Ribeiro A, Juhlin-Dannfelt A, Brodin LA, Holmgren A, Jorfeldt L: Pulmonary embolism: Relation between the degree of RV overload and the extent of perfusion defects. Am Heart J 1998 (May);135:868–874.
22. Agnelli G, Piovella F, Buoncristiani P, Severi P, Pini M, D'Angelo A, Beltrametti C, Damiani M, Andrioli GC, Pugliese R, Iorio A, Brambilla G: Enoxaparin plus compression stockings compared with compression stockings alone in the prevention of venous thromboembolism after elective neurosurgery. N Engl J Med 1998 (July 9);339:80–85.
23. Mathur A, Roubin GS, Iyer SS, Piamsonboon C, Liu MW, Gomez CR, Yadav JS, Chastain HD, Fox LM, Dean LS, Vitek JJ: Predictors of stroke complicating carotid artery stenting. Circulation 1998 (April 7);97:1239–1245.
24. White CJ, Ramee SR, Collins TJ, Jenkins JS, Escobar A, Shaw D: Renal artery stent placement: Utility in lesions difficult to treat with balloon angioplasty. JACC 1997 (November 15);30:1445–1450.
25. Dorros G, Jaff M, Mathiak L, Dorros II, Lowe A, Murphy K, He T: Four-year follow-up of Palmaz-Schatz stent revascularization as treatment for atherosclerotic renal artery stenosis. Circulation 1998 (August 18);98:642–647.

8

Aortic Inflammation, Atherosclerosis, and Aneurysms

Aortic Obstruction

Aortic Atheromas and Systemic Emboli

The aorta is a source of thromboembolism. Studies using transesophageal echocardiography (TEE) have suggested an increased frequency of aortic atheroma in patients with systemic emboli. Dressler and colleagues[1] from St. Louis, Missouri, evaluated 31 patients who presented with a systemic embolic event who were found to have mobile aortic atheroma on TEE. They measured the dimensions of the mobile component. Patients not receiving warfarin had a higher incidence of vascular events (45% vs. 5%). Stroke occurred in 27% of these patients and in none of those treated with warfarin. The annual incidence of stroke in patients not taking warfarin was 0.32%. AMI occurred in 18% of patients in this group. Forty seven percent of patients with small mobile atheroma did not receive warfarin. Recurrent stroke occurred in 38% of these patients representing an annual incidence of 0.61. There were no strokes in patients with small mobile atheroma treated with warfarin. Likewise, none of the patients with intermediate or large mobile atheroma had a stroke during follow-up. Only 3 of these patients had not been taking warfarin. These authors conclude that patients presenting with systemic emboli and found to have mobile aortic atheroma on TEE have a high incidence of recurrent vascular events. Warfarin is efficacious in preventing stroke in this population. The dimensions of the mobile component of atheroma should not be used to determine the need for anticoagulation.

Beta-Blocker Therapy in Marfan Syndrome

It has been shown that β-adrenergic blocking agents may reduce the rate of aortic dilation and the development of aortic complications in patients with Marfan syndrome. This observation may be due to β-blocker-induced changes in aortic stiffness, of which distensibility and pulse wave velocity are *in vivo* measurable derivatives. Groenink and colleagues[2] from Leiden, The Netherlands, studied changes in distensibility at 4 levels of the aorta and pulse wave velocity along the entire aorta after 2 weeks of β-blocker therapy in 6 Marfan

505

syndrome patients and 6 healthy volunteers, using magnetic resonance imaging (MRI) combined with brachial artery BP measurements. In both groups, mean BP decreased significantly (Marfan: 86 ± 6 vs. 78 ± 5 mm Hg; control: 80 ± 8 vs. 73 ± 3 mm Hg) (all data expressed as mean ± 1 SD). At baseline, the Marfan syndrome patients exhibited decreased distensibility at the level of the ascending aorta (2 ± 1 vs. 6 ± 2 10^{-3} mm Hg^{-1} and increased pulse wave velocity (6.2 ± 0.4 vs. 3.9 ± 0.4 ms^{-1}) compared with control subjects. Only the Marfan syndrome patients had a significant increase in aortic distensibility at multiple levels and a significant decrease in pulse wave velocity after β-blocker therapy (ascending aorta distensibility: 2 ± 1 vs. 4 ± 1 10^{-3} mm Hg^{-1}; abdominal aorta distensibility: 5 ± 2 vs. 8 ± 3 10^{-3} mm Hg^{-1}; pulse wave velocity: 6.2 ± 0.4 vs. 5.0 ± 1.0 ms^{-1}). Thus, aortic stiffness in Marfan syndrome, together with mean BP, is reduced by β-blocker therapy, and MRI is well suited to detect these changes by measuring distensibility and pulse wave velocity.

Risk Factors for Abdominal Aortic Aneurysms

Degradation of Elastic Media in Abdominal Aortic Aneurysms

Degradation of the elastic media is a hallmark of abdominal aortic aneurysm (AAAs). Davis and coinvestigators[3] in Omaha, Nebraska, examined the expression of 2 elastolytic matrix metaloproteinases (MMPs), MMP-2 and MMP-9, in AAA aortic tissues compared with those from atherosclerotic occlusive disease (AOD) and nondiseased control tissues. Quantitative competitive reverse transcription polymerase chain reaction and gelatin zymography showed increased MMP-9 mRNA and protein in both AAA and AOD tissue compared with those in control tissues, but there was no significant difference between AAA and AOD. In contrast, MMP-2 mRNA and protein levels were significantly higher in AAA than in AOD or control tissues. Sequential extraction of the MMPs of the aortic tissue with a physiologic salt solution, 2% dimethylsulfoxide (DMSO), and 10 mol/L urea showed that large amounts of MMP-2 and MMP-9 were bound to the matrix. The most conspicuous finding was that the levels of MMP-2 were significantly elevated in the DMSO fraction and in AAA tissues compared with AOD and control tissue. In addition, a large portion of MMP-2 found in the DMSO and urea fractions was in the active 62-kDa form, indicating that precursor of MMP-2 in AAA is largely activated locally and binds to the tissue matrix tightly. By immunolocalization, MMP-9 was found to be produced primarily by macrophages and MMP-2 by mesenchymal cells. The production of MMP-2 was prominent when mesenchymal cells were surrounded by inflammatory cells, suggesting paracrine modulation of MMP-2 expression in AAAs (Figure 8-1). These observations emphasize that MMP-2 participates in the progression of AAAs by degrading aortic tissue matrix components.

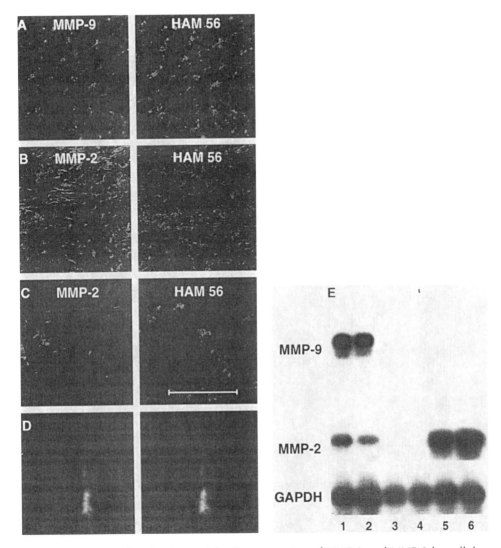

FIGURE 8-1. Immunolocalization and *in vitro* expression of MMP-2 and MMP-9 by cellular components of aorta. Sections of AAA tissue were double-immunolabeled with antibodies to MMP-2 or MMP-9 and anti-HAM 56 (macrophages). Primary antibody was visualized with secondary antibody conjugated to FITC (MMP-2, MMP-9) or TRITC (HAM-56). MMP-9 collocalized with HAM-56-staining cells (**A,** original magnification, ×200). MMP-2 localized to spindle-shaped cells in outer media and adventitia and rarely to macrophages (**B**). MMP-2 expression was distinctly decreased in areas with little inflammation (**C**). Sections treated with IgG alone served as immunohistochemical control (**D**). Bar = 30 μm. MMP-2 and MMP-9 mRNA expression was determined by RT-PCR (E) in unactivated macrophages (lane 1), LPS-activated macrophages (lane 2), unactivated T lymphocytes (lane 3), PHA-activated T lymphocytes (lane 4), aortic SMCs (lane 5), and adventitial fibroblasts (lane 6). Equal levels of GAPDH amplification product for each cell type indicate equivalence of total RNA for RT-PCR. Reproduced with permission from Davis et al.[3]

In-Hospital Cost of Repair of Abdominal Aortic Aneurysms

Surgical repair of abdominal aortic aneurysms (AAA) is increasingly being performed, but little is known about the correlates of in-hospital cost associated with this procedure. Baseline clinical characteristics, in-hospital outcomes, and total in-hospital costs were examined by Benzaquen and associates[4] from Cleveland, Ohio, and Montreal, Canada, among a retrospective cohort of 71 patients who underwent AAA repair. Median age was 68 years, and 75% of the patients were men. High-risk characteristics for perioperative complications were common and included hypertension (73%), documented CAD (66%), smoking (60%), previous myocardial infarction (47%), history of CHF (12%), urgent or emergent AAA repair (16%), and diabetes mellitus (11%). Perioperative complications included CHF (13%), myocardial infarction (11%), and death (1%). Median length of stay in the surgical intensive care unit (SICU) was 2 days (range 0 to 28), and median in-hospital stay was 9 days (range 5 to 39). In-hospital cost for the 71 patients ranged from $13,766 to $82,435 (mean $25,931). Univariate and multiple linear regression analyses demonstrated that among the potential correlates investigated, number of SICU days and total length of stay were the most closely associated with in-hospital cost. Among patients undergoing AAA repair, the major correlates of in-hospital cost are the number of days spent in the SICU and the total number of days spent in the hospital. These results suggest that any intervention that reduces length of stay may significantly reduce the total in-hospital cost associated with AAA repair.

Thoracic Aortic Aneurysms

Autosomal dominant inheritance of thoracic aortic aneurysms and dissections occurs in patients with Marfan syndrome, which results from mutations in the FBN1 gene on chromosome 15. A second chromosomal locus on 3p24-25 has been identified for a Marfan-like condition with thoracic aortic aneurysms. Milewicz and colleagues[5] from multiple USA medical systems described 6 families with multiple members with thoracic aortic aneurysms and dissections in the absence of the ocular and skeletal manifestations of Marfan syndrome (Figure 8-2). The authors reviewed medical records and autopsy reports on affected subjects in families with multiple members with thoracic aortic aneurysms and dissections. Subjects in these families at risk for developing aortic disease underwent echocardiography to evaluate the aorta. The pattern of inheritance of thoracic aortic aneurysms and dissections was autosomal dominant in these families. Most affected subjects presented with aortic root dilatation or acute type 1 dissection, but the age of onset of disease was variable and there was decreased penetrance of the disorder. In 2 of the families, the syndrome was not linked to FBN1 or 3p24-25. Familial thoracic aortic aneurysm and dissection is an autosomal dominant condition with marked variability in the age of onset of aortic disease and decreased penetrance, making identification of affected subjects difficult. This condition is not due to mutations in the FBN1 gene or the unidentified gene on 3p24-25.

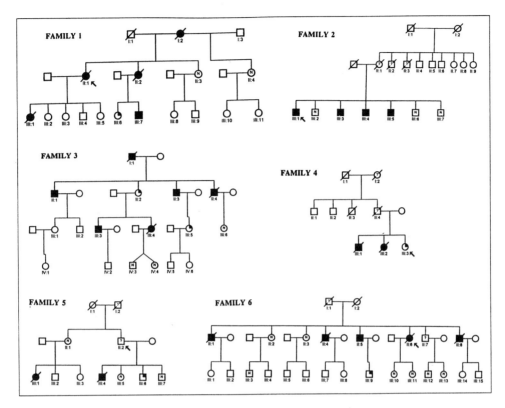

FIGURE 8-2. Pedigrees of the 6 families with thoracic aortic aneurysms/dissections. Blackened circles or squares indicate affected subjects who either died of aortic rupture or dissection, underwent surgical repair of an aortic aneurysm or dissection, or have aortic root dilatation. Circles or squares with the upper right corner blackened indicate subjects whose aortic root is at the upper limits of normal, based on their body surface area. Circles or squares with question marks indicate subjects who died suddenly of unknown causes, under circumstances suggestive of dissection or rupture of an aneurysm. Reproduced with permission from Milewicz et al.[5]

Pathogenesis of Abdominal Aortic Aneurysms

The basic feature in the pathogenesis of abdominal aortic aneurysm is the degradation of extracellular matrix components. This process is induced partly by cytokines secreted from inflammatory and mesenchymal cells. Circulating levels of inflammatory cytokines were studied by Juvonen and coinvestigators[6] in Oulu, Finland, in abdominal aortic aneurysm patients and compared with subjects suffering from atherosclerotic disease only. Furthermore, the predictive value of cytokine concentrations was evaluated for aneurysm expansion rate. Circulating levels of interleukin 1β, interleukin 6, tumor necrosis factor-α, and interferon-γ were measured in 50 abdominal aortic aneurysm patients (40 men, 10 women), in 42 patients with CAD (23 men, 19 women), and in 38 controls whose angiograms were normal (17 men, 21 women) (Figure 8-3). No differences in cytokine concentrations were found between the CAD patients

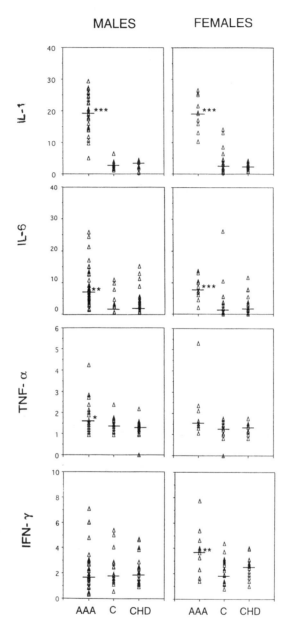

FIGURE 8-3. Cytokine concentrations (pmol/L) in the serum of male and female abdominal aortic aneurysm (AAA), coronary heart disease (CHD), and control (C) patients. The distributions of circulating cytokine concentrations in the AAA patients and the controls were compared using the Mann-Whitney U test. ***p < 0.001, **p < 0.005, and *p < 0.05. Reproduced with permission from Juvonen et al.[6]

and the controls. Abdominal aortic aneurysm disease was found to be associated with significantly higher interleukin 1β and interleukin 6 concentrations in both male and female patients than in either the CAD patients or the controls. Tumor necrosis factor-α levels were slightly higher in the abdominal aortic aneurysm patients than in the other groups. Interferon-γ levels were elevated significantly in the female abdominal aortic aneurysm patients compared with levels found in the other female or male patient groups. The measured cytokine concentrations were not related to the size of the aneurysm or the maximal thickness of the thrombus within the aneurysm. Interferon-γ concentrations showed a significant positive correlation to the aneurysm expansion and negative correlation to the concentration of aminoterminal propeptide of type 3 procollagen during 6 month follow-up. The results show that circulating levels of inflammatory cytokines are elevated in patients with abdominal aortic aneurysm disease, suggesting that the production of these cytokines is increased in these patients compared with CAD patients and controls. Elevated interferon-γ concentrations seem to predict an increased rate of expansion in abdominal aortic aneurysm.

1. Dressler FA, Craig WR, Castell R, Labovitz AJ: Mobile aortic atheroma and systemic emboli: Efficacy of anticoagulation and influence of plaque morphology on recurrent stroke. JACC 1998 (January);31:134–138.
2. Groenink M, de Roos A, Mulder BJM, Spaan JAE, van der Wall EE: Changes in the aortic distensibility and pulse wave velocity assessed with magnetic resonance imaging following beta-blocker therapy in the Marfan syndrome. Am J Cardiol 1998 (July 15);82:203–208.
3. Davis V, Persidskaia R, Baca-Regen L, Itoh Y, Nagase H, Persidsky Y, Ghorpade A, Baxter BT: Matrix metalloproteinase-2 production and its binding to the matrix are increased in abdominal aortic aneurysms. Arterioscler Thromb Vasc Biol 1998 (October);18:1625–1633.
4. Benzaquen BS, Eisenberg MJ, Challapalli RC, Nguyen T, Brown KJ, Topol EJ: Correlates of in-hospital cost among patients undergoing abdominal aortic aneurysm repair. Am Heart J 1998 (October);136:696–702.
5. Milewicz DM, Chen H, Park E-S, Petty EM, Zaghi H, Pai GS, Willing M, Patel V: Reduced penetrance and variable expressivity of familial thoracic aortic aneurysms/dissections. Am J Cardiol 1998 (August 15);82:474–479.
6. Juvonen J, Surcel H-M, Satta J, Teppo A-M, Bloigu A, Syrjala H, Ariaksinen J, Leinonen M, Saikku P, Juvonen T: Elevated circulating levels of inflammatory cytokines in patients with abdominal aortic aneurysm. Arterioscler Thromb Vasc Biol 1997 (November);17:2843–2847.

9
Cardiovascular Disease in the Young

Kawasaki Disease

Silent Myocardial Ischemia in Kawasaki Disease

Ogawa and colleagues[1] in Japan studied the effectiveness of PTCA in patients with silent myocardial ischemia (MI) detected by dobutamine stress scintigraphy, body surface mapping, and signal-averaged electrocardiograms in 76 asymptomatic patients with Kawasaki disease and coronary stenosis greater than 25%. Patients with coronary stenosis greater than 25% and a positive dobutamine stress test were considered to have silent MI. Eight patients had greater than 95% stenoses demonstrated by coronary angiography just prior to PTCA. After PTCA, coronary angiography showed that all of the coronary stenoses had been reduced to less than 50%. Intravascular ultrasonography performed in 5 patients before and after PTCA demonstrated adequate dilatation of the coronary stenosis. All 8 patients who had PTCA underwent dobutamine stress studies 3 months after PTCA, which demonstrated no regions of MI. Approximately 6 months later, the coronary arteriography was repeated and only 1 patient had developed restenosis. Thus, PTCA effectively dilates stenotic arteries in children with Kawasaki disease. Dobutamine stress myocardial scintigraphy studies are useful for detecting silent MI and estimating the effectiveness of PTCA in these patients.

Coronary Aneurysms in Kawasaki Disease

Beiser and associates[2] from Boston, Massachusetts, and Los Angeles, California, reviewed a multicenter database of 212 patients with acute Kawasaki disease in an attempt to construct a predictive instrument for the development of coronary artery abnormalities. The instrument was then validated in 3 test data sets of 192, 264, and 92 patients, respectively. Risk factors used in the sequential classification instrument included baseline neutrophil and band counts, hemoglobin concentration, platelet count, and temperature on the day after infusion of intravenous gamma globulin. In the developmental data set, the instrument classified 123 of 212 patients or 58% as low risk, and none developed coronary artery abnormalities. Among 89 patients classified as high risk, 3 of 36 females (8.3%) and 9 of 53 males (17.0%) developed coronary artery abnormalities. The instrument performed similarly in the 3 test data

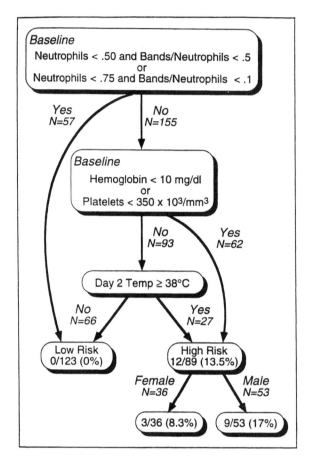

FIGURE 9-1. Diagram depicting the performance of the sequential classification scheme in the development data set. Reproduced with permission from Beiser et al.[2]

sets; no patient in any data set classified as low risk developed coronary artery abnormalities. This simple instrument (Figure 9-1) allows the clinician to identify within 1 day of treatment low-risk children in whom extensive and frequent cardiac testing may be unnecessary, as well as high-risk children who require closer monitoring and may be candidates for additional treatment. The authors warn that the instrument may not be accurate in patients who present after the tenth day of illness or who have atypical disease or in patients treated with a lower dose of intravenous globulin than 1.6 or 2 grams.

Coarctation of the Aorta

Recurrent Coarctation

Sakopoulos and associates[3] from Indianapolis, Indiana, reviewed a 27-year experience with surgical repair of recurrent aortic coarctation in 56 patients. The majority of recoarctations were repaired with a prosthetic patch technique with a greater than 96% success rate. There was a bimodal distribution of recurrence with roughly 1/3 of all patients undergoing a second operation within 2 years of the first operation and 50% undergoing a second operation from 7 to 15 years after the first operation. Follow-up was available in 71% of these 56 patients and ranged from 1 to 11 years. Medically controlled hypertension was present in 18%, and 5 patients had echocardiographic evidence of a gradient across the coarctation repair site. There was only 1 aneurysm following prosthetic patch repair of recurrent coarctation. These data were compared to previous data from other institutions regarding balloon aortoplasty. The wide range of residual or recurrent coarctation after balloon dilatation and post-dilatation aortic aneurysm makes comparison with surgery difficult. This series demonstrates that surgical reoperation can be performed with good success and low morbidity. The current use of stents for aortic recoarctation may prove a useful alternative.

Coarctation in Pregnancy

Saidi and associates[4] from Houston, Texas, reviewed female patients with coarctation born before 1980 who had undergone balloon angioplasty or surgery. Patients with Turner's syndrome and cyanotic congenital heart disease were excluded. There were 74 patients who met criteria and 52 were contacted. There were 36 pregnancies in 18 patients with 3 spontaneous and 4 elective abortions. Preeclampsia complicated 4 pregnancies in 3 woman and 1 patient had systemic hypertension. Delivery by cesarean section was performed in 11 infants. There were 29 births with an average weight of 3 kg with 5 preterm births, 4 to a teenage mother. Only 1 child (3%) had a congenital heart defect. In women with an arm-to-leg blood pressure gradient of less than 20 mm Hg after coarctation repair, pregnancy is successful. Preeclampsia incidence was similar to that in the general population. There continues to be concern about pregnancy in women with coarctation whether surgically repaired or treated with balloon dilatation because of previous reports of aortic complications in such patients. This small series shows pregnancy well tolerated, but a larger study is needed to determine the risk of pregnancy in this group.

Use of Stents for Coarctation

Ebeid and associates[5] from Cleveland, Ohio, report 9 patients younger than 10 years of age with coarctation in whom balloon dilation alone was thought to be ineffective and who underwent stent implantation. A previous operation, balloon dilation, or both had been performed in 7 of the patients and recurrent obstruction was present. At the time of implantation, the peak systolic and mean gradients decreased from a mean of 37 ± 7 and 14 ± 3 mm Hg to 4 ± 1 and $2 \pm .6$ mm Hg. The coarctation diameter increased from a mean of 9 ± 1 to 15 ± 1 mm. The patients have been followed for up to 42 months with no complications; the stents remain in position without fractures.

There was 1 successful redilation 3 years after implantation because of an exercise-induced gradient. The systolic gradient at the latest follow-up is 7 ± 2 mm Hg. The use of stents in coarctation is a feasible alternative to surgical repair or balloon angioplasty in selected patients. No patients have had significant neointimal growth resulting in significant restenosis.

Transposition of the Great Arteries

Arterial Switch Operation

Karl and associates[6] from Melbourne, Australia, review results of the arterial switch operation for both simple and complex transposition of the great arteries (TGA). Various anatomical factors that have been noted to increase risk for this operation, including intact septum beyond 21 days of age, intramural coronary arteries, other coronary artery patterns, aortic arch obstruction, the Taussig-Bing anomaly, congenitally corrected transposition, transposition with LV outflow obstruction, and univentricular heart with TGA and subaortic stenosis were considered in regard to current results. The coronary anatomy in TGA is clearly demonstrated in Figure 9-2 and the classic arterial switch operation depicted in Figure 9-3. In addition, the results of the double switch operation of congenitally corrected transposition is shown very elegantly in Figure 9-4. These authors show outstanding results for arterial switch in all patterns of coronary artery anatomy, including intramural coronary arteries. In addition, results for the Taussig-Bing operation and corrected transposition or tricuspid atresia are outstanding, although the number of patients in these latter 3 groups are small. These authors make a strong case for the more widespread use of the arterial switch operation for patients who were previously considered at additional risk for this operation.

Outflow Obstruction After Arterial Switch

Williams and associates[7] from New York, New York; Toronto, Ontario, Canada; and Birmingham, Alabama, presented data from the Congenital Heart Surgeons Society regarding outflow obstruction after the arterial switch for TGA. Percutaneous or surgical reintervention for obstruction after operation was selected as an endpoint for obstruction. Risk factors for obstruction were identified by time-related multivariable analyses of yearly follow-up data from 514 neonates with simple transposition or TGA with VSD. Patients were from 23 institutions and were entered into the study before 15 days of age. There were 62 patients undergoing 86 reinterventions for right-sided obstruction (83% free of obstruction at 10 years) and 6 for left-sided obstruction. (98% obstruction free at 10 years). After 2 years, right-sided obstruction occurred at a rate of about 1%/year and left-sided at a rate of about 0.1%/year. RV infundibular or valvular obstruction were associated with the aorta and pulmonary trunk positioned side-by-side, coexisting coarctation, use of prosthetic material

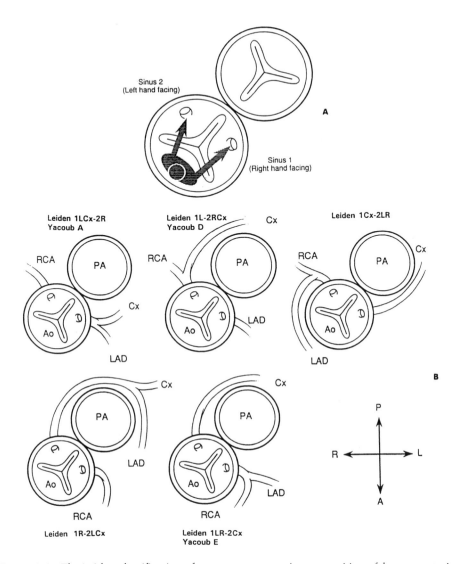

FIGURE 9-2. The Leiden classification of coronary anatomy in transposition of the great arteries. The right hand of an observer standing in the noncoronary sinus (facing the coronary ostia) points to sinus 1, the left hand to sinus 2. The most common pattern is 1 left, circumflex, 2 right. Ao = aorta; Cx = circumflex coronary artery; L = left; LAD = left anterior descending coronary artery; PA = pulmonary artery; R = right; RCA = right coronary artery. Reproduced with permission from Karl et al.[6]

in sinus reconstruction, one institution, and earlier institutional experience. Pulmonary trunk or PA obstruction were associated with lower birth weight, left coronary artery arising from sinus 2, coronary explantation away from the transection site, 3 institutions, and earlier institutional experience. The risk-adjusted base incidence of 0.5%/year for reintervention for right-sided obstruction continues late after operation. It is due in part to congenital variability or abnormality of RV outflow structures and to experience and surgeon variability resulting in suboptimal pulmonary trunk reconstruction. Obstruction to aortic

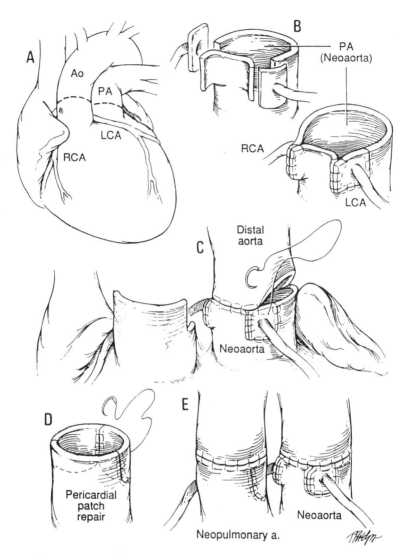

FIGURE 9-3. The arterial switch operation technique used at Royal Children's Hospital. Medially based rectangular flaps were used in the neoaortic sinuses for coronary translocation. The flaps decrease the arc of rotation and prevent tension on the anastomosis. Ao = aorta; LCA = left coronary artery; PA = pulmonary artery; RCA = right coronary artery. Reproduced with permission from Karl et al.[6]

outflow after switch operation fortunately is very rare and the suture line appears to show normal growth. Obstruction on the right side continues to be a problem although results continue to improve. Percutaneous intervention is helpful in some patients, but many will require reoperation.

Arterial Switch for Older Infants

Foran and associates[8] from London, United Kingdom, assessed the surgical outcome of 37 patients 3 weeks to 2 months old and 156 patients less than

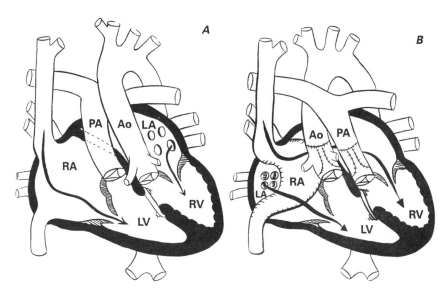

Figure 9-4. (A) "Classic" septation of a heart with discordant transposition of the great arteries, leaving the right ventricle and tricuspid valve in the systemic circuit. **(B)** The Senning technique plus an arterial switch operation restores concordant atrioventricular and ventriculoatrial connections, avoiding late problems attributable to a right ventricle in the systemic circuit. Ao = aorta; LA = left atrium; LV = left ventricle; PA = pulmonary artery; RA = right atrium; RV = right ventricle. Reproduced with permission from Karl et al.[6]

3 weeks old who underwent primary arterial switch with transposition with intact septum. There was 1 operative death in the late switch group, 13 deaths in the early switch group, and 1 late death in each group. Postoperative mechanical LV support was required in 1 of 37 late switch patients and 6 of 156 early switch patients. Neither death nor the need for mechanical LV support in the late switch group patients could be attributed to LV failure. In the late group, neither age, LV geometry, LV mass index, LV posterior wall thickness index, LV volume index, LV mass/volume, PDA, or pattern of coronary anatomy were predictive of death, duration of postoperative ventilation, inotropic support, or time in intensive care. Primary arterial switch operation may be appropriate treatment for infants with transposition as old as 2 months of age regardless of preoperative echocardiographic variables. The upper age limit for which primary switch operation is indicated is not yet defined.

Treadmill Test After Arterial Switch Operation

Massin and associates[9] from Aachen, Germany, present data from 50 asymptomatic children ages 4 to 9 years who underwent Bruce treadmill protocols after having an arterial switch operation for simple TGA in the neonatal age. They were compared with age-matched normal children. There were 47 of 50 patients who had normal exercise capacity and electrocardiographic parameters. There was 1 patient whose coronary angiogram showed occlusion of the left main coronary artery, who developed signs of myocardial ischemia during exercise. In 1 patient with a single right coronary artery and another who underwent a neonatal internal mammary bypass graft for obstruction of the right coronary artery, the resting electrocardiogram showed ventricular premature complexes and exercise stress-induced salvos of VT. Most children who underwent the neonatal arterial switch operation have a normal exercise capacity and no evidence for ischemia by Bruce treadmill protocol. These data suggest that treadmill exercise data may be useful in these patients during their late follow-up.

Mortality in Transposition of the Great Arteries

Soongswang and associates[10] from Toronto, Ontario, Canada, reviewed factors contributing to or causing death before surgery in neonates despite anatomy suitable for the arterial switch operation. Twelve out of 295 infants with TGA had anatomy suitable for the arterial switch operation but died prior to surgery. All had TGA with intact ventricular septum and presented with a severely restrictive ASD. In 11 of 12 cases, the cause of death was attributed to the profound hypoxemia from inadequate mixing. Contributing factors were prematurity in 42%, severe respiratory distress syndrome in 25%, and persistent pulmonary hypertension in 17%. All patients received PGE1 infusion, and urgent balloon septostomy was performed in 67% with improved oxygenation. Patients with an ASD less than or equal to 2 mm and/or a birth weight less than 2 kg were also reviewed. All patients with a small patent foramen who survived arterial switch had a significantly better response to PGE1 than the nonsurvivors. The operation was accomplished without mortality in 4 of 9 infants with a weight less than 2 kg. Although this group represents a small percentage of neonates with TGA, the consequences of inadequate atrial mixing due to a small ASD are extremely difficult to treat unless the patient is born at a high-risk unit where balloon atrial septostomy can be performed urgently.

Aortic Allograft

Metras and associates[11] from Marseilles, France, report the use of a tubular segment of an aortic autograft to connect the PA to the right ventricle for patients with TGA, VSD, and LV outflow obstruction. This method was used in 10 consecutive patients aged 2 months to 11 years. No valvular device was used for the RV outflow tract repair. There were no early or late deaths and only 1 patient with multiple VSDs needed an early reoperation for a residual VSD. All patients are asymptomatic without medications at a mean follow-up of 30 months. There have been no calcifications on the chest x-rays and a most recent echocardiogram showed RV pressures from 25 to 40 mm Hg with a mean of 33 mm Hg and no significant gradient between the right ventricle and PAs. The operation avoids the use of homograft material and apparently pulmonary insufficiency is tolerated well. Further follow-up is needed in terms of growth of the RV outflow and the autograft.

Repair of Transposition of Great Arteries with Other Abnormalities

Metras and associates[12] from Marseilles, France, report 12 patients with TGA, VSD, and severe LV outflow obstruction. Patients ranged in age from 2 months to 11 years with a mean of 32 months. Ten had severe PS and 2 had pulmonary atresia. In addition, 4 had a restrictive VSD and 2 had multiple VSDs. All patients underwent total repair with LV-aortic intraventricular connection with 4 needing VSD enlargement. Connection between the right ventricle and pulmonary arteries was established with a tubular segment of autograft aorta, without the anterior location of the bifurcation of the pulmonary arteries. No valvular device was used for the RV outflow tract (Figure 9-5). No early

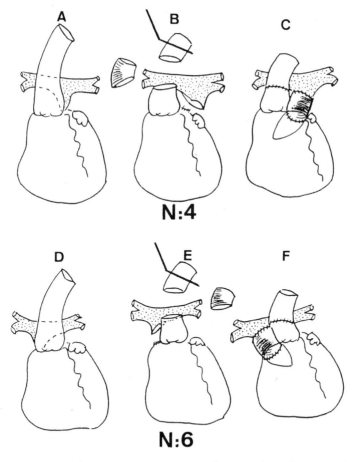

FIGURE 9-5. Operative technique: (A) Appearance of the transposed aorta with PA located toward the left. (B) Resection of a tubular segment of ascending aorta division, suture of proximal end of PA, and opening of main PA. (C) Autograft reconstruction on the left side of the aorta (4 patients). (D) Aspect of the transposed aorta with the PA located to the right. (E) Same as part B. (F) Autograft reconstruction on the right side of the aorta (6 patients). Reproduced with permission from Metras et al.[12]

or late deaths occurred and 1 patient with multiple VSDs needed an early reoperation for a residual VSD. All patients are asymptomatic without modification at a mean follow-up of 30 months. The most recent echocardiogram showed RV pressure ranging from 25 to 40 mm Hg and no significant gradient was found between the RV and the pulmonary artery. This modification of the Rastelli procedure avoids any tension on the RV–PA anastomosis, leaves the pulmonary arteries posterior to avoid anterior compression by the sternum, and can be used as a primary corrective operation even in infants. The autograft is living tissue and should grow with time. The disadvantage is that there is no pulmonary valve and late pulmonary regurgitation is a potential problem. Pulmonary regurgitation has not been a problem in early follow-up of these patients, and all patients were able to have primary sternal closure even after a prolonged cardiopulmonary bypass time.

Evaluation of Systemic Atrioventricular Valve Regurgitation in Congenitally Corrected Transposition

Lynch and associates[13] from Atlanta, Georgia, evaluated systemic AV valve regurgitation of the morphological tricuspid valve using serial echocardiography in 25 children with congenitally corrected TGA, both with and without surgery. Patient age was 6 months to 19 years and follow-up was from 5 months to 15 years with a median of 4. Initial assessment was at a median 65 days of age; only 9/25 (36%) had TR. At follow-up, 16/25 (64%) had TR with 2 requiring valve replacement. The tricuspid valve was abnormal in 16/25 (64%) of patients and in 11 of 16 (69%). TR worsened compared with 1 of 9 with "normal" morphologic tricuspid valve. Ebstein's anomaly was present in 9 of 25 (36%) and 3 of 9 (33%) had new TR develop. Of 17 patients who underwent cardiac surgery, 10 (59%) had new or increased TR compared with 3 of 8 (37%) of nonoperative patients. After intracardiac repair 8 of 11 (73%) had increased TR compared with 6 patients after extracardiac surgery. These authors shed more light on the progressive development of TR in patients with congenitally corrected TGA. It appears to develop in the majority of patients and frequently progresses after intracardiac repair.

Patent Ductus Arteriosus

Comparison of Coil Occlusion and Surgical Closure of Patent Ductus Arteriosus

Prieto and associates[14] from Cleveland, Ohio, compared the cost and clinical effectiveness of transcatheter coil occlusion and surgical PDA closure in 36 patients with a median age of 8.8 years for the coil patients and 7.3 years for the surgical patients. There were 24 patients who underwent coil occlusion and 12 who underwent surgical closure. Median procedural duration was 150 minutes for the coil group and 165 minutes for the surgical group. The total cost to the institution for coil occlusion was significantly lower than that of surgical closure ($5,273 vs. $8,509). The greatest difference was in the cost of hospital stay ($398 vs. $2,566) and in the professional costs ($1,506 vs. $2,782). Technical costs were similar ($2,156 for coil, and $2,151 for surgery), although use of the catheterization laboratory per unit of time was more expensive than use of the operating room ($800 vs. $400/hour). Additional technical costs of the surgical procedure related to general anesthesia and postoperative care made up the difference. No patient in either group had a residual PDA murmur at hospital discharge or thereafter. Follow-up echocardiography was performed in all coil occlusion patients, and tiny residual leaks were detected in 17%. Only 42% of the surgical patients had postoperative echocardiography and none had residual leaks. There were no deaths or major complications in either group. The difference in cost here of over $3,000 might be expected. Obvious differences in cost will relate to hospital charges and professional charges for these particular services. Coil closure of the PDA has now been shown to be very safe and cost effective in the majority of patients.

Reopening of Patent Ductus Arteriosus

Daniels and associates[15] from Columbus, Ohio, studied 22 patients after attempted coil occlusion of PDA. Clinical success was achieved in 20 patients and Doppler echocardiography was negative for PDA shunting in 19 patients or 90%. At follow-up, at a mean time of 6 months, 5 patients demonstrated reopening. The PDA minimal diameter was 1.4 mm for the reopened group and 1.2 mm for the other patients. The PDA length was 2.9 mm for the reopened group and 7.1 for all other patients. All 3 patients with type B PDA (conical with a shortened ductal ampulla) were in the reopened group. When independent variables were compared between groups, only PDA length and type B PDA predicted reopening. PDA reopening may occur after successful coil occlusion and warrants follow-up by clinical exam and echo Doppler in these patients. Short length PDAs may need variations of the coil technique to achieve complete and permanent closure.

Catheter Closure of Patent Ductus Arteriosus

Masura and associates[16] from the Slovak Republic, the United Kingdom, Greece, Jordan, and the United States report results in 24 patients who underwent attempted transcatheter closure of a PDA using the new self-expandable, repositionable Amplatzer ductal occluder device. Patients were a median age of 3.8 years and a median weight of 15.5 kg, with the smallest patient being 0.4 years and 6 kg. The mean PDA diameter at its narrowest segment was 3.7 mm and a 6 French long sheath was used for delivery of the device. Successful device placement was achieved in 24 patients and angiography showed that 7 patients had complete immediate closure, 14 had a trace residual shunt, and 4 had a small residual shunt. Within 24 hours, color Doppler revealed complete closure in all patients. The median fluoroscopy time was 13.5 minutes. All patients were discharged home the next day. The 1-month follow-up study was completed in 21 to 23 patients and all had continued complete closure. At 3 months, 18 of 23 patients completed the study and all had complete closure. This device can be used to close ductuses up to a diameter of 6 mm and hopefully will represent a new clinically useful method for patients with large PDAs.

Hypoplastic Left Heart

Fenestration Closure in Hypoplastic Left Heart

Lloyd and associates[17] from Ann Arbor, Michigan, studied hemodynamic responses to fenestration closure during catheterization in 40 consecutive patients who had a prior Fontan procedure performed. Hypoplastic left heart syndrome was present in 20 and other forms of univentricular hearts in 20. Hemodynamics before fenestration closure were nearly identical between the 2 groups. Significant changes after closure included increases in arterial saturation of 9%, mean arterial pressure of 3 mm Hg, baffle pressure increase of 1 mm Hg, and increase in arteriovenous oxygen content difference by 18 mL/L, with near elimination of right-to-left shunting. Cardiac output decreased by 21% and systemic oxygen transport by 13% with no differences between the 2 patient groups. Mean baffle pressures were lower than 17 mm Hg in 32 of 40 patients. The hypoplastic left heart syndrome patients responded in a similar fashion to other univentricular hearts to fenestration closure. Although oxygen transport fell, these patients improve symptomatically after this intervention.

Ventricular Septal Defect

Multiple Ventricular Septal Defects

Kitagawa and associates[18] from Ann Arbor, Michigan, reviewed the records of all 33 patients with multiple VSDs undergoing repair between January 1988 and October 1996. PA hypertension was present in 21 patients (group 1), and PS in the remaining 12 (group 2). Closure was accomplished from a right atriotomy alone in most patients, although an apical left ventriculotomy was used for apical defects. Among group 1 patients, the mean age of repair was 6 months and major associated anomalies included coarctation in 6, straddling tricuspid valve in 1, and critical AS in 1. Reoperation was performed in 2 patients for residual VSDs. Among group 2 patients, the mean age at repair was 6.6 years and major anomalies included TF in 2, PS in 4, double outlet right ventricle with hypoplastic LV in 1 and isolated LV hypoplasia in 1. There were 3 reoperations for residual VSDs. There were no early or late deaths and no episodes of heart block and no significant residual VSDs among group 1 patients. All these patients remain free of significant residual complications at a mean of 23 ± 5 months. Among group 2 patients, there was 1 early death in a patient with a small left ventricle. Complete heart block occurred in 2 patients and 1 required late mitral valve replacement. There were no late deaths; 7 remain alive without significant defects at a mean of 36 ± 8 months, and 2 required retransplantation for LV failure. Primary repair of multiple VSDs is associated with good late outcomes and the RA approach is satisfactory for most muscular defects, although limited apical left ventriculotomy was used for apical defects. These authors feel that pulmonary banding with the consequence of severe RV and septal hypertrophy make this operation harder, and they would favor primary repair unless one is dealing with a very small premature infant who is ventilator dependent. These investigators also feel that the limited left ventriculotomy was not associated with significant morbidity or mortality. The small number of patients with significant follow-up makes this an unproven hypothesis at present.

Atrioventricular Septal Defect Repair in Infancy

Reddy and associates[19] from San Francisco, California, report 72 infants who underwent primary repair of complete AV septal defect at the median age of 3.9 months with 40% younger than 3 months. A single-patch technique was used in all and the cleft was closed completely in 61 patients, partially in 10, and not at all in 1. Left AV valve annuloplasty was performed in 18 patients. On the basis of transesophageal echocardiography, 10 patients were returned to bypass for revision of the valve repair. There was 1 early death in a patient with a single left papillary muscle, no early reoperations, and no new permanent arrhythmias. Only 3 patients had moderate left AV regurgitation at discharge. During a median follow-up of 24 months, there was 1 late death and 5 reoperations for left AV valve regurgitation in 2 and/or systemic outflow obstruction in 4. Follow-up left AV valve regurgitation was moderate in 3 patients, mild in 14, and none or trace in 54. Age had no relation to postoperative AV valve regurgitation, death, or reoperation. These authors recommend elective operation between 4 to 8 weeks of age. Reoperation for moderate or severe left AV valve regurgitation usually reveals a broken suture that can be repaired effectively.

Aortic Atresia and Subaortic Obstruction

Aortic Atresia Survival

Jacobs and associates[20] from Browns Mill, New Jersey; Birmingham, Alabama; Loma Linda, California, and the Congenital Heart Surgeons Society present data from a total of 323 neonates with aortic atresia who were entered into a 21-institution prospective, nonrandomized study. There were 3 protocols that were used nonexclusively in many institutions: staged reconstructive surgery with initial palliation by a Norwood procedure and eventual Fontan operation, heart transplantation as initial definitive therapy, and nonsurgical management. Analysis was based on initial protocol assignment: staged reconstructive surgery in 253, heart transplantation in 49, and nonsurgical management in 21. For all patients initially entered into the 2 surgical treatment protocol, survival at 1, 3, 12, 24, and 36 months after entry was 67%, 59%, 52%, 51%, and 50%, respectively. A multivariable analysis found incremental risk factors for death at any time after entry to be lower birth weight, associated noncardiac anomaly, and entry into the nonsurgical or the staged reconstructive surgery protocol. There were 4 institutions with higher survival statistics; 2 used a heart transplantation protocol and 2 used a staged reconstructive surgery protocol. For the 113 patients treated at these 4 institutions, survival at 1, 3, 12, 24, and 36 months after entry were 77%, 70%, 64%, 62%, and 61%, respectively. Survival among these 4 institutions was similar. Among patients with aortic atresia, other features of cardiac structure including aortic size, degree of LV hypoplasia, and degree of mitral hypoplasia or atresia were not predictive of survival from 2 surgical protocols. The highest survival was achieved with either treatment strategy at institutions strongly committed to the use of 1 or the other surgical management strategies.

Subaortic Stenosis and Arch Obstruction

McElhinney and associates[21] from San Francisco, California, report the use of a modified Damus-Kaye-Stansel procedure in 14 neonates and 7 infants with single ventricle and subaortic stenosis, including 15 with arch obstruction. Diagnoses included double inlet left ventricle in 12, tricuspid atresia in 2, and other forms of hypoplastic ventricle in 7. Concurrent bidirectional Glenn shunt was performed in 3 patients. In the most recent 7 patients with arch obstruction, arch repair was achieved with an end-to-side anastomosis of the descending aorta to the ascending aorta with continuous upper body perfusion (Figure 9-6). There was 1 early death among 14 neonates and 3 deaths among infants for an early mortality of 19%. At a median follow-up of 33 months, there were no late deaths or neurological complications. Nine patients underwent subsequent bidirectional Glenn anastomosis, including 3 who had Fontan completion. No patients have required recurrent arch obstruction relief. The permanent relief of subaortic stenosis in infants with single ventricle remains difficult to achieve. This modified procedure may prove useful in patients with complex intraventricular anatomy and arch obstruction.

Pulmonary Atresia

Repair of Pulmonary Atresia

Tchervenkov and associates[22] from Montreal, Canada, report experience with single stage unifocalization and repair of infants with pulmonary atresia and VSD. Since 1989, 11 of 12 patients with pulmonary atresia, VSD, and major aortopulmonary collateral arteries have undergone complete surgical

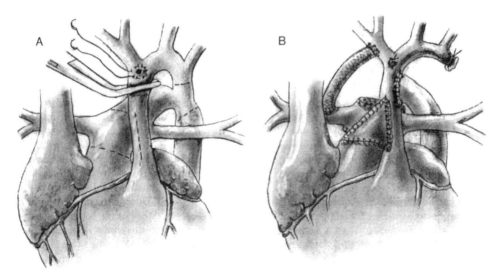

FIGURE 9-6. Modified technique for performing the Damus-Kaye-Stansel (DKS) procedure in a patient with coarctation of the aorta. The aortic inflow cannula is inserted at the base of the innominate artery, immediately distal to the aortic crossclamp. After institution of bypass, the patent ductus arteriosus is doubly ligated and divided. The pulmonary artery is transected above the sinotubular junction (dashed lines in the left frame indicate incisions) and at the origin of the ductus. Both defects in the central pulmonary artery are patched with either allograft or pericardium. The ascending aortotomy is performed with an L-shaped incision, and the flap of aortic tissue is retracted posteriorly as a flap for reconstruction of the posterior wall of the main pulmonary artery–ascending aorta anastomosis. The DKS anastomosis is completed anteriorly with a hood of allograft tissue. A longitudinal aortotomy is then made in the opposite side of the ascending aorta (left side in this example), all ductal tissue is resected, and arch repair is performed by advancing the descending aorta to the ascending aorta and performing an end-to-side anastomosis. In this manner, circulatory arrest to the brain is avoided. A modified Blalock-Taussig shunt is then placed. Reproduced with permission from McElhinney et al.[21]

correction. The first 7 patients were subject to staged bilateral unifocalization, with repair being achieved in 6. The last 5 patients have undergone 1 stage midline unifocalization and repair via a sternotomy. All patients in the first group had TF, whereas in the second group, 3 patients had TF, 1 had double outlet right ventricle, and 1 had complete AV septal defect and TGA. The operation was performed at a median age of 43 weeks in group 1 with complete repair at a median age of 4 years, and a mean of 3 operations required. In the single stage group, only 1 operation was needed to achieve complete repair at a median age of 28 weeks. The postoperative RV/LV pressure ratio was 0.49 in group 1 and .45 in group 2. There was 1 intraoperative death and 1 late death in the multistaged group, but no early or late deaths in the single stage group. The specific details of the surgical anatomy are illustrated for both groups in Figures 9-7 and 9-8. There continues to be considerable interest in the feasibility of doing 1 stage repair in infants with this complex condition. It is hoped that more patients are amenable to this approach. The multistage unifocalization is frequently associated with loss of flow to various bronchopulmonary segments due to progressive stenosis.

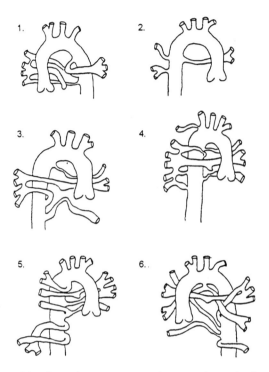

FIGURE 9-7. Pulmonary blood supply in patients undergoing the multiple-stage unifocalization followed by repair (group 1). Reproduced with permission from Tchervenkov et al.[22]

Right Ventricular Growth After Pulmonary Atresia Therapy

Ovaert and associates[23] from London, United Kingdom, report results with laser or radiofrequency-assisted balloon valvotomy in 12 neonates and infants with pulmonary atresia and intact ventricular septum. The atretic pulmonary valve was successfully perforated and dilated in 9 of 12 patients; 5 of 9 required additional transcatheter surgical procedures to augment pulmonary blood flow. Of 6 survivors, 5 are regularly followed-up with a median follow-up of 60 months (range 37 to 68 months). All 5 have 2-ventricle circulations; 2 of 5 required surgical enlargement of the RV outflow tract with or without closure of the ASD. Tricuspid valve dimensions and Z-values before transcatheter valvotomy tended to be smaller in the patients who died than in the survivors. In the survivors, the absolute tricuspid valve dimensions increased after valvotomy, but the Z-values tended to decrease or stayed constant. Of the 6 long-term survivors, tricuspid annulus at the time of presentation ranged from 8 to 12 mm with the Z-value within normal limits ranging from −1.3 to −0.4. Tricuspid valve/mitral valve ratio was 0.56–0.80. The tricuspid valve did grow in all of these patients, although the Z-value remained less than normal with a value of −2.3 at latest follow-up. Despite these borderline small tricuspid valves, these patients achieved biventricular repair and significant RV growth was achieved.

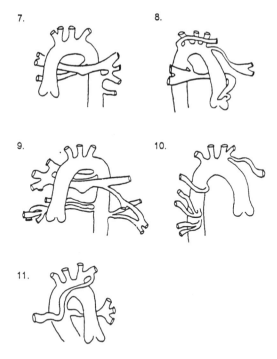

FIGURE 9-8. Pulmonary blood supply in patients undergoing single-stage midline unifocalization and repair (group 2). Reproduced with permission from Tchervenkov et al.[22]

Pulmonary Atresia with Intact Septum

Daubeney and associates[24] from Southampton, and London, United Kingdom, studied the impact of fetal echocardiography on the incidence of pulmonary atresia with intact septum at birth and postnatal outcome. All infants born with this diagnosis and all fetal diagnoses in the United Kingdom and Eire were studied. There were 183 live births with an incidence of 4.5/100,000 live births with the higher incidence in Eire and Northern Ireland. There were 86 fetal diagnoses made at a mean age of 22 weeks' gestation, leading to 53 terminations of pregnancy or 61%, 4 intrauterine deaths, and 29 live births. An initial diagnosis of critical pulmonary stenosis was made in 6 cases at a mean age of 22 weeks' gestation with progression to pulmonary atresia by 31 weeks. Probability of survival at 1 year was 65% and was the same for all live-born infants whether or not a fetal diagnosis was made. This condition remains difficult to treat. although 65% survival at 1 year probably represents a significant improvement in the last 10 to 20 years. Termination of pregnancy has resulted in a significant reduction in live-born incidence in mainland Britain. The fact that fetal diagnosis makes no difference in survival probably indicates that early postnatal diagnosis and prostaglandin treatment is almost universal, whether or not a prenatal diagnosis is made.

Tetralogy of Fallot

Obstruction Development After Tetralogy of Fallot Repair

Moran and associates[25] from Boston, Massachusetts, and Toronto, Ontario, Canada, report 552 children under 2 years of age who underwent primary TF repair at a median age of 6.7 months with long-term follow-up in 308 children. Of these, 17 children subsequently developed double-chambered right ventricle requiring reoperation. The median age at initial operation for this group was 7.9 months. During a median follow-up interval of 43 months, murmur intensity increased in all patients, and the average subpulmonary gradient at catheterization increased from 24 to 80 mm Hg in 7 children, and at Doppler echocardiography, from 14 to 89 mm Hg in 5 children. Before operation, 6 of 17 children were symptomatic. At a median age of 55 months, obstruction was relieved by incision of hypertrophied anomalous muscle bundles in all 17 patients, with prominent fibrosis noted in 8 patients. No new transannular patches were required and recurrent obstruction has occurred in 3 of these 17 children. Double chambered right ventricle is a medium-term complication of TF repair in infants, with a minimal incidence of 3%. The condition is progressive and is due to anomalous muscle bundle hypertrophy or fibrosis, or both, which may represent displaced insertion of a moderator band. Diagnoses can be made with echo and/or angiography as indicated in Figures 9-9–9-11. Because reobstruction can occur, continued follow-up is necessary.

Survival in Patients with Tetralogy of Fallot

Nollert and associates[26] from Munich, Germany, reviewed 658 patients who underwent correction of TF and were analyzed for survival. Of this patient group, 40% had previous palliation; operative and 1-year deaths were excluded for long-term calculations, resulting in a study group of 490 patients. Actuarial 10-, 20-, 30-, and 36-year survival rates were 97%, 94%, 89%, and 85%, respectively. Mortality increased 25 years postoperatively from 0.24%/year to 0.94%/year. The most common cause of death was sudden in 13 followed by CHF in 6. Multivariate correlates of impaired long-term survival were date of operation before 1970, preoperative erythrocytosis, and use of an RV outflow patch. Patients without preoperative erythrocytosis and RV outflow patch had a 36-year actuarial survival of 96% and normal life expectancy. Although these investigators showed a very high early mortality, late mortality is quite low. These patients were mostly operated on at an older age and data on infant repair are not available. Sudden cardiac death occurred in approximately 3% of long-term survivors and data on previous arrhythmias or residual hemodynamic abnormalities for these patients were not available.

Right Ventricular Function After Tetralogy of Fallot Repair

Singh and associates[27] from St. Louis, Missouri; Philadelphia, Pennsylvania; and South Hampton, United Kingdom, studied 10 of 19 consecutive pa-

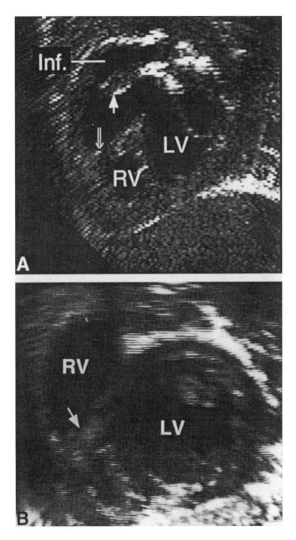

Figure 9-9. The subxyphoid short-axis view from a patient with tetralogy of Fallot revealed (**A**) a displaced moderator band (open arrow) with more rightward and superior insertion into the interventricular septum; anterior displacement of the conal septum is also shown (solid arrow). This has a similar appearance to the typical position of the moderator band in double chambered RV associated with a membranous VSD (**B**) Inf. = infundibulum; LV = left ventricle; RV = right ventricle. Reproduced with permission from Moran et al.[25]

tients with chronic pulmonary regurgitation age 14 ± 2 years (range 11 to 17 years) after surgery for primary repair of TF in infancy at a mean age of 7 ± 4 months. Patients were selected on the basis of freedom from reoperation, raised jugular venous pressure, residual intracardiac shunt, TR and RV outflow tract obstruction. There were no symptoms in 7 and mild symptoms in 3. Operations were performed with deep hypothermic circulatory rest with a mean arrest time of 58 ± 4 minutes. The RV outflow tract was reconstructed with a transannular patch to achieve a post-bypass systolic RV–LV pressure ratio less than 0.75. There were 7 age- and gender-matched controls. Cine magnetic

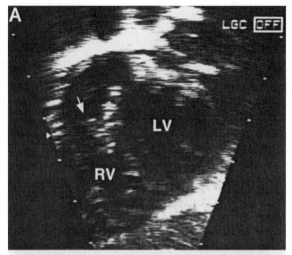

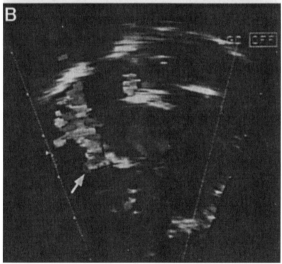

FIGURE 9-10. (A) The subxyphoid view in a patient after repair of tetralogy of Fallot. The prominent muscle bundle is shown (arrow) with a typical double chambered RV appearance. (B) Color Doppler interrogation illustrates the midcavity obstruction. LV = left ventricle; RV = right ventricle. Reproduced with permission from Moran et al.[25]

resonance imaging was performed to determine ventricular volume and time–volume curves of a complete RV cycle. RV volume was virtually twice normal and RVEF was 35% versus a normal value of 55%. In addition, the filling fraction during the first third of diastole was lower in patients than controls and RV peak filling rate also was significantly lower. Finally, the maximum work capacity and maximal heart rate achieved during modified Bruce protocol were both reduced in the patient group. This study demonstrates in a small group of patients with minimal or no symptoms that the current surgical trend of early primary repair of tetralogy in infants does not prevent late

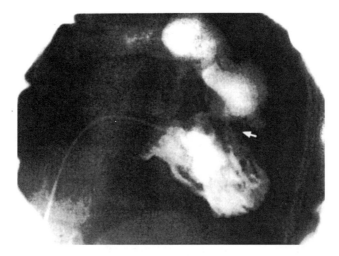

FIGURE 9-11. The anteroposterior projection after repair of tetralogy of Fallot, with an appearance typical of double chambered RV with midcavity obstruction at the level of the displaced moderator band (arrow). Reproduced with permission from Moran et al.[25]

RV systolic and diastolic dysfunction and diminished exercise performance if chronic pulmonary regurgitation results from RV outflow tract reconstruction.

Tetralogy Repair in Infancy

Munkhammar and associates[28] from Lund, Sweden, and London, England, United Kingdom, studied diastolic RV physiology after tetralogy repair in infancy. There were 47 patients from Lund and London investigated with a median age at repair of 0.78 years and median follow-up of 3 years. Restrictive RV physiology was assessed by Doppler echocardiography. There were 13 patients, or 28%, who had restrictive RV physiology at follow-up, 3 of 29 patients (16%) with transatrial repair, and 10 of 28 patients (32%) with transventricular repair, respectively. Restrictive physiology was present in 10% of patients repaired before 6 months of age, increasing to 38% with repair after 9 months. Transannular patch repair was performed in 55% of patients, including 8 of 10 with repair before 6 months of age, and restrictive physiology was present in 31% of all patients in this group. Restrictive patients had more severe preoperative pulmonary stenosis, were older at repair, and had a shorter duration of pulmonary regurgitation at follow-up. Restrictive RV physiology in inversely related to age at repair and is independent of type of outflow tract repair. Since transannular repair is more common in early repair and restriction seems to be less frequent, long-term follow-up to assess adverse effects of pulmonary regurgitation is needed. Predictors of postoperative restrictive RV physiology are unclear, but inadequate myocardial protection at the time of surgery, severe fibrosis prior to surgery, and the size of the RV and transannular incision are probably all related. It is still unclear whether patients with restrictive RV physiology will have a more favorable long-term outcome, since some data suggest that it will prevent severe pulmonary regurgitation.

Conotruncal Repair

Kurosawa and associates[29] from Tokyo, Japan, presented their conotruncal repair methodology for TF in 233 patients ages 2 months to 53 years with a mean of 5 years. The specific methodology used in this repair is illustrated by Figures 9-12 and 9-13; a monocusp was used to prevent severe pulmonary regurgitation. There were no early deaths, and only 2 late deaths occurred over a mean follow-up of 7 years. The actuarial survival was 99% and there were only 2 reoperations for residual anomalously connecting pulmonary veins. The mobility of the monocusp was detected in 85% and pulmonary regurgitation was less than mild in 82% at the late phase. The late right and left ventricular pressure ratio was 0.40 ± 0.14 and the late central venous pressure was 6 ± 2. Conotruncal repair has provided excellent midterm functional results with low central venous pressure and outstanding hemodynamics.

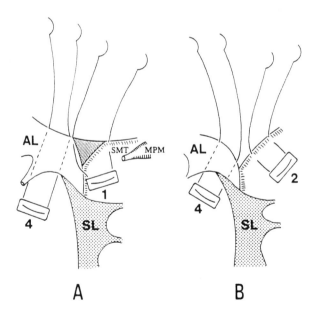

FIGURE 9-12. Two types of perimembranous outlet VSD in tetralogy of Fallot. The number of the sutures correspond to the number in Figure 9-13. (A) An "interventricular" membranous flap (shaded triangle) exists at the posteroinferior border of the VSD. Suture number 1 is stitched through the fibrous tissue of the septal leaflet at the junction with the membranous flap and through the muscular margin of the posterior extension of the septomarginal trabeculation (SMT) at the junction with the membranous flap. The membranous flap is indirectly used and is reinforced by a pledget. Suture number 4 is placed through the annulus of the anterior leaflet of the tricuspid valve corresponding to the fibrous continuity with the aortic noncoronary cusp. The medial papillary muscle (MPM) is divided for convenience. (B) The membranous flap is absent. Suture number 1 is simply skipped. Reproduced with permission from Kurosawa et al.[29]

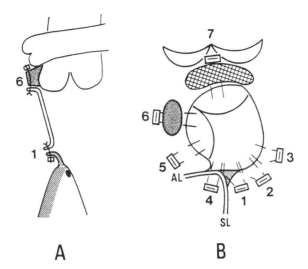

A   B

FIGURE 9-13. Sutures for patching the VSD: 1, at the membranous flap; 2, in the posterior extension of septomarginal trabeculation; 3, in the anterior limb of septomarginal trabeculation; 4, through the anterior "annulus" of the tricuspid valve, corresponding to the fibrous continuity with the aortic noncoronary cusp; 5, in the nonresected ventriculoinfundibular fold; 6, in the muscle stump after resection of hypertrophied muscle bundles; 7, in the subtotally resected infundibular septum. AL and SL = the annuli of the anterior and septal leaflets of the tricuspid valve, respectively. Reproduced with permission from Kurosawa et al.[29]

Ventricular Tachycardia After Tetralogy of Fallot Repair

Harrison and associates[30] from Toronto, Ontario, Canada, sought to determine features associated with sustained VT in adult patients late after repair of TF. In a retrospective review, 18 adult patients with VT were identified and compared with 192 with repaired TF free of sustained arrhythmia. There was no significant difference in age at repair, age at follow-up, or operative history. Patients with VT had frequent ventricular ectopic beats, low cardiac index, and more structural abnormalities of the right ventricle including outflow tract aneurysms and pulmonary regurgitation or tricuspid regurgitation than control patients. Electrophysiologic map-guided operation was performed in 10 of 14 patients; VT reoccurred in 3 of 10. Operation was not undertaken in 4 patients, 3 of whom received amiodarone and 1 received defibrillator implantation. Severe heart failure was present in 2 patients with VT and these patients died. Most patients with VT late after repair of TF have outflow tract aneurysms or pulmonary regurgitation or both. A combined approach of correcting significant structural abnormalities with intraoperative electrophysiologic-guided ablation may reduce the potential risk of deterioration of ventricular function and enable arrhythmia management to be optimized. An alternate strategy for these patients might be attempted preoperative ablation in the catheterization lab in order to decrease the operative time and to make them better candidates for their surgery.

Aortic and Pulmonic Valvular Stenosis

Repair for Discrete Aortic Stenosis

Brauner and associates[31] from Los Angeles, California, report follow-up for 75 of 83 consecutive patients operated on for discrete subaortic stenosis with an average duration of follow-up of 7 years. The lesion was discrete in 68 patients (91%) and of a tunnel type in 7, with associated VSD in 28 (37%). All underwent transaortic resection and there were no deaths. There were 18 recurrences in 15 patients (20%). Reoperation for recurrence of aortic valve disease was carried out in 13 patients (17%) who underwent 17 reoperations. The cumulative hazard of recurrence was 9%, 16%, and 29% and the hazard events including recurrence and reoperation were 9%, 18%, and 35% at 2, 5, and 10 years, respectively. Residual end-operative LV outflow obstruction gradient higher than 10 mm Hg and tunnel lesions were univariate predictors of recurrence; multivariate predictors included higher preoperative gradient and younger patients. There were only 2 recurrences in patients with a preoperative peak gradient of 40 mm Hg or less, whereas higher gradients were associated with a greater than sevenfold recurrence rate. The aortic valve required concomitant repair in 17 cases in the high gradient group and in only 8 in the low gradient group. Despite relief of the obstruction, progressive AR was noted at follow-up after 14 procedures in the high gradient group and after only 5 procedures in the low gradient group. Recurrent subaortic stenosis continues to be a significant problem despite multiple efforts to modify the operation. Although these authors show better results when operating on a lower gradient, this may be because these patients had milder disease and were more amenable to surgical relief.

Aorto-Arteriopathy in Childhood

D'Souza and associates[32] from Ontario, Canada, reviewed the experience with 14 pediatric patients with acquired stenotic aorto-arteriopathy who presented over a 16-year period. Most patients presented with a mid-thoracoabdominal coarctation and were diagnosed with Takayasu arteriitis. Differentiating between this diagnosis and fibromuscular dysplasia was difficult on clinical grounds or by angiography. Medical management of renovascular hypertension and selective percutaneous transluminal balloon angioplasty of the stenotic renal arteries met with minimal success. Renal autotransplantation had slightly better success. Dilation of stenosed aortic segments with balloon-expandable stents and subsequent renal autotransplantation proved the most useful treatment (Figure 9-14). Therapy should focus on interventions to minimize the end-organ damage caused by the vaso-occlusive manifestations of these disorders.

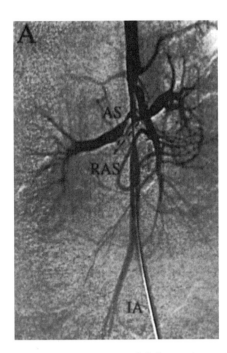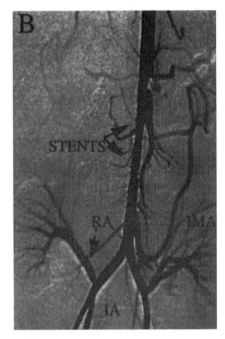

FIGURE 9-14. Angiograms of abdominal aorta in patient K. **(A)** before, and **(B)** after endovascular stent placement and bilateral renal autotransplantation. **(A)** Note small caliber of iliac arteries (IA) and aorta distal to stenotic segment (AS) before placement of stents. Renal artery stenosis (RAS) was limited to ostia bilaterally with marked post-stenotic dilation. Contrast this with **(B)** caliber of vessels after stents were placed. After renal transplantation, there was a mild, clinically insignificant narrowing at site of anastomosis of renal arteries (RA) to iliac arteries. Reproduced with permission from D'Souza et al.[32]

Discrete Subaortic Stenosis

Bezold and associates[33] from Boston, Massachusetts, and Houston, Texas, studied echocardiographic characteristics and clinical course of 100 patients with discrete sub-AS. In phase I, a prediction model was developed based on multivariant analysis of morphometric and Doppler variables in 52 children. In phase II, the performance characteristics of the model were tested in 48 patients. Patients were divided into 3 outcome groups: nonprogressive, progressive, and intermediate progression. In phase I, multivariant analysis identified 3 independent predictors of progressive disease: indexed aortic valve to subaortic membrane distance, anterior mitral leaflet involvement, and initial Doppler gradient. The characteristics associated with lack of regression were thin mobile folds near the aortic valve and low profile lesions along the lower margin of VSDs (Figure 9-15). Progressive lesions are most often thick, nonmobile, and echogenic, consistent with a fibrous or fibromuscular ridge located a short distance below the aortic valve with involvement of the anterior mitral leaflet. Accessory mitral tissue chordal attachments to the ventricular septum are more common in the intermediate group. These studies can be useful in trying to determine time for follow-up and indications for intervention. Determining optimal timing operation remains a difficult task in this patient group.

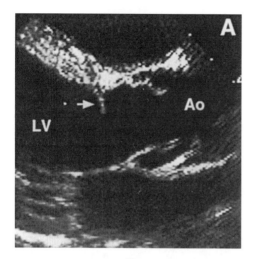

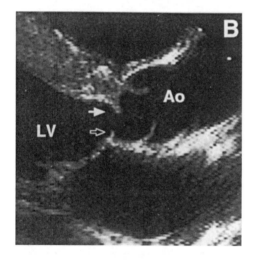

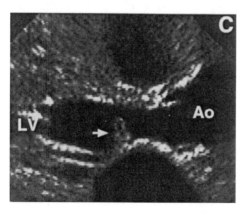

FIGURE 9-15. Representative examples of subaortic membrane and left ventricular outflow tract morphology in the 3 study groups as seen from the parasternal long-axis view. (A) Nonprogressive group: low profile membrane at the crest of the ventricular septum (arrow) in a patient with a small membranous ventricular septal defect (not seen in this plane). Notice that the membrane is thin and is located 8 mm below the aortic valve. (B) Progressive group: thick protrusive membrane located 2 mm below the aortic valve (solid arrow) with involvement of the anterior mitral leaflet (open arrow). (C) Intermediate group: mild subaortic stenosis produced by accessory mitral valve tissue (arrow) attaching to the subaortic septum. Ao = aorta; LV = left ventricle. Reproduced with permission from Bezold et al.[33]

Survival After Repair of Aortic Stenosis

Kovalchin and associates[34] from Houston, Texas, and San Francisco, California, studied 28 infants with a mean age of 1 day and a mean weight of 3.6 kg with critical AS to evaluate echocardiographic, hemodynamic, and morphometric factors that would predict which infants could undergo a biventricular repair as opposed to a Norwood, single ventricle operative procedure. A 2-ventricle repair was initially attempted in 19 of 28, and 9 of 28 had a Norwood operation. Among patients with a 2-ventricle repair, the hemodynamic factors associated with survival included predominant or total antegrade flow in the ascending and transverse aorta. Aortic valve gradient, mitral valve inflow, and direction of flow in the ductus arteriosus and descending aorta were unrelated to outcome. The morphometric factors associated with survival after 2-ventricle repair included the indexed aortic annulus, aortic root, ascending aorta, and LV long-axis length. LV volume, mass, ejection fraction, and mitral valve area were not related to outcome after 2-ventricle repair. The search for definitive measurements to choose between 1 and 2 ventricular repairs in infants with critical AS continuous LV size, mitral valve size, LV annulus, and subaortic size have all been used to help in the selection process. This article adds further data, but the number of patients is small. Further data on applying these and other measurements to a larger patient group could be useful in providing the best operation for those patients with a borderline size left ventricle.

Ross Procedure in Children

Reddy and associates[35] studied the geometric mismatch of pulmonary and aortic annuli in children undergoing the Ross procedure with implications for surgical management and autograft malfunction. Forty-one children who have undergone the Ross procedure were analyzed to determine risk factors predictive of autograft regurgitation. The diameter of the pulmonary valve was greater than that of the aortic valve by at least 3 mm in 20 cases, equal to or within 2 mm in 12 cases, and less by at least 3 mm in 9 cases, with differences ranging from $+10$ to -12 mm. In 12 patients with a larger pulmonary annulus, aorto-ventriculoplasty was used to correct the mismatch. In patients with a larger aortic annulus, the mismatch was corrected by gradual adjustment along the circumference of the autograft, rather than by tailoring of the native aortic annulus. At a follow-up (median 31 months), 2 patients had undergone reoperation on the neoaortic valve for moderate regurgitation, but in the remainder, regurgitation was none or trivial in 30, mild in 7, and moderate in 1. There was no correlation between regurgitation and age, geometric mismatch, or previous or concurrent procedures. These authors conclude that technical factors that may result in distortion of the valve complex are more important as determinants of autograft regurgitation than are indications for repair, geometric mismatch, or previous or concomitant outflow tract procedures.

Subpulmonary Homografts

Stark and associates[36] from London, United Kingdom, reviewed data on 656 conduits placed in the subpulmonary position between 1971 and 1993. Patients receiving heterografts or valveless conduits and patients dying within 90 days of insertion were excluded; thus 405 homograft conduits were studied. There were 293 aortic homografts, 94 pulmonary, and 18 of unknown type. The endpoint of conduit failure was defined by conduit replacement for whatever reason, balloon dilation of the conduit, or death of the patient with the conduit in place. Initial conduits and conduits inserted earlier in the series appeared to last longer than second and subsequent conduits and those inserted later in the series. Overall survival of conduits at 5, 10, and 15 years was 84%, 58%, and 31%, respectively. The longest surviving homograft conduit in this series lasted 23 years. Regarding univariate analysis, reoperation, recent operation, pulmonary versus aortic graft, cryopreserved rather than antibiotic preserved, and older age at operation are associated with poor outcome. In multivariant analysis, however, only reoperation and order number had significant predictive power. When patient survival was considered, patients operated on more recently survived longer despite the fact that their conduits were being replaced earlier. Overall, survival of patients at 5 and 15 years was 95% and 85%, respectively. The search for an optimal conduit or homograft continues. There may well be immunological factors that lead to graft failure in some patients, although it could not be proven in this study. Despite gradual deterioration of homograft or conduits, they remain essential for correction of many complex lesions with excellent 15-year patient survival.

Familial Atrial Septal Defects

Benson and associates[37] from Boston, Massachusetts, and Saint Louis, Missouri, identified 3 families with ASD and multiple generations. The lesion was transmitted as an autosomal dominant trait in each family and ASD was the most common anomaly, but other heart defects occurred alone or in association with ASD in individuals from each kindred. Linkage studies in 1 kindred localized a familial ASD disease gene to chromosome 5p. Assessment of 20 family members with the disease haplotype revealed that 9 had ASD, 8 were clinically unaffected, and 3 had other cardiac defects including AS, atrial septal aneurysm, and persistent left superior vena cava. Familial ASD did not map to chromosome 5p in the 2 other families. Familial ASD is a genetically heterogeneous disorder; 1 disease gene maps to chromosome 5p. Recognition of the heritable basis of familial ASD is complicated by low disease penetrance and variable expressivity. Identification of ASD or other congenital heart defects in more than 1 family member should prompt clinical evaluation of all relatives. The genetic base of congenital heart disease continues to broaden. Further studies such as this will hopefully continue to shed new light on cardiac embryogenesis and genetic abnormality.

Atrioventricular Septal Defect Repair

Najm and associates[38] from Toronto, Ontario, Canada, report 363 children who underwent repair of complete AV septal defect at a median age of 8.3 months and a mean age of 17 months. TF was present in 21 patients, double outlet RV in 4, sub-AS in 8, ventricular hypoplasia in 8, coarctation in 5, atrial isomerism in 2, and other congenital anomalies in 9. Down syndrome was present in 65%. A 1-patch technique was applied in 99, and a 2-patch technique in 243. Left AV valve cleft was closed partially in 181 and completely in 112. Early mortality was 10.5% with 10-year survival at 83%. At 10 years, freedom from reoperation for left AV valve repair was 86%, left AV valve replacement was 90%, sub-AS was 95%, residual VSD was 97%, permanent pacemaker insertion was 98%, and other types of reoperation was 95%. At the time of operation, older age, shorter ischemic time, absence of a double orifice left AV valve, and cleft closure were found to be significant independent predictors of survival. The rare patient with double orifice left AV valve remains difficult to treat surgically; hopefully, new surgical methods will be developed for this anomaly.

Atrioventricular Defect Repair

Michielon and associates[39] from Padova, Italy, report 100 patients, median age 6.1 months, who underwent repair of complete AV septal defect. Surgery was performed in 37% at less than 1 month of age (group 1) and in 63 patients more than 4 months of age (group 2). Double patch reconstruction was used in all and trifoliate reconstruction of the left AV valve was selected in 93%. Parametric time-related survival was 93% at 14 years in group 1 and 76% at 15 years in group 2. Multivariate analysis showed early repair as a negative risk factor for death. Freedom from reoperation was 83% at 15 years. Down syndrome was a negative risk factor for reoperation, whereas annular dilation increased the risk for this event. Early correction of complete AV septal defect is safe and beneficial not only in controlling heart failure but also in preventing annular dilation secondary to excessive pulmonary flow, which is a potential mechanism for left AV valve regurgitation.

Computed Tomography in Heterotaxy Syndrome

Chen and associates,[40] Taipei, Taiwan, performed computed tomography on 32 patients with clinical impression of heterotaxy syndrome. Interpretation of cardiac anomalies was performed by sequential analysis based on these cross-sectional images. There were 28 patients with bilateral trifurcated bronchi, and most of these (24 of 28) did not have a spleen. There were 4 patients with bilateral bifurcated bronchi, and 2 patients had polysplenia and the other 2 had a lobulated single spleen. This modality allowed the identification of laterality in all patients. In comparison to echocardiography and catheterization, this modality appeared superior in demonstration of pulmonary venous

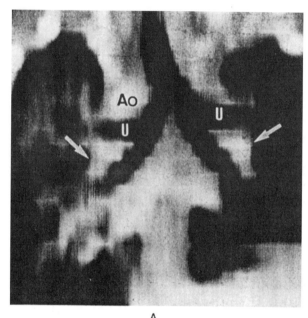

A

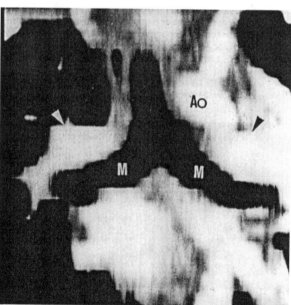

B

FIGURE 9-16. Coronal reconstructive computed tomographic image of airway. **(A)** Case 12: a 2-month-old girl with no spleen. Bilateral bronchi are symmetric with early branching and narrow subcarinal angle. Both pulmonary arteries (arrows) are below bilateral upper lobe bronchi (U). **(B)** Case 29: a 2-year-old girl with multiple splenules. Bilateral bronchi are symmetrical with wide subcarinal angle. Both pulmonary arteries (arrowheads) are straddling the bilateral main stem bronchi (M) before branching. Ao = aortic arch. Reproduced with permission from Chen et al.[40]

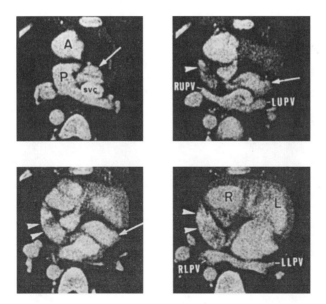

FIGURE 9-17. Case 17: a 5-year-old girl with no spleen. Her bilateral atrial appendages are rather symmetrical, wide-based, and triangular, but their axes are arranged in different orientation. The right-sided atrial appendage (arrowheads) is in dorsal-ventral orientation, whereas the left-sided appendage (arrows) is in caudal–cephalic orientation. Pulmonary veins connect to the junction between the SVC and the roof of the left-sided atrium. A = aorta; L = left ventricle; LLPV = left lower pulmonary vein; LUPV = left upper pulmonary vein; P = main pulmonary artery; R = right ventricle; RLPV = right lower pulmonary vein; RUPV = right upper pulmonary vein; SVC = superior vena cavae. Reproduced with permission from Chen et al.[40]

anatomy and presence of a very small rudimentary ventricle. In addition, associated visceral, bronchopulmonary, mediastinal, and intracardiac anomalies could be clearly delineated by computed tomography. A clear demonstration of bronchi is shown in (Figure 9-16). In addition, abnormalities of pulmonary venous anomalies may be clearly demonstrated (Figure 9-17). This technique may be useful in delineating some of the complex anatomy in these patients. We have a number of different modalities to use in these patients, and echocardiography with or without catheterization can delineate the anatomy in most cases. Most of the data that are needed to care for these patients are needed in the neonatal and young infant, and thus it is unclear as to how useful this new modality will be for this age group.

Antithrombotic Therapy in Children

Andrew and associates[41] from Hamilton and Toronto, Ontario, Canada; Worcester Massachusetts; and Burlington, Vermont, reviewed predisposing factors and management options for pediatric patients with thrombotic disease. The high incidence of venous thrombosis in patients with indwelling

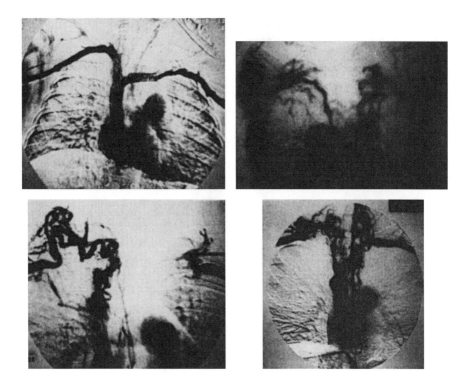

FIGURE 9-18. The top left panel is an example of a normal venogram in a child. The other 3 panels show the venograms of 3 patients receiving home total parenteral nutrition. There is venous occlusion with collateral circulation in all 3 cases. Reproduced with permission from Andrew et al.[41]

catheters is highlighted (Figure 9-18). Guidelines are given for the use of systemic heparin, warfarin therapy, and thrombolytic therapy for pediatric patients. With increasing success for operative intervention for complex congenital heart disease, more patients are spending prolonged recovery time in ICUs with indwelling catheters. As a consequence, thrombotic disease has become more prevalent. Many of these patients develop semi-effective collateral channels, diagnosis is frequently delayed, and the ability to intervene successfully can be compromised by such delay. This article provides excellent management guidelines for potential prevention and treatment of thrombotic disease in pediatric patients.

Arrhythmias

Congenital Long-QT Syndrome

Locati and associates[42] from Milan, Italy; Pavia, Italy; Salt Lake City, Utah; and Detroit, Michigan, studied age- and gender-related differences in clinical manifestations in patients with congenital long-QT syndrome (LQTS). Age-

and gender-related occurrence of events were analyzed in 479 probands of which 70% were females, as well as 1,041 affected family members with a Qtc greater than 440 ms. LQTS gene mutations were identified in 162 patients. Females predominated among 366 probands and 230 symptomatic family members. Male probands were younger than females at first event (8 ± 7 vs. 14 ± 10 years) and had a higher event rate by age 15 years than females (74% vs. 51%). Affected family members had similar findings. The event rate was higher in male than female LQT 1 carriers, but no age or gender difference in event rate was detected in LQT 2 or LQT 3 carriers. Among LQTS patients, the risk of cardiac events was higher in males until puberty and higher in females during adulthood. The same pattern was evident among long QT 1 gene carriers. Unknown sex factors modulate QT duration and arrhythmic events with preliminary evidence of gene-specific differences in age-gender modulation.

Atrial Pacing

Ragonese and associates[43] from Rome, Italy, studied the post-pacing clinical course in 18 patients with recurrent atrial reentry tachycardias unresponsive to conventional therapy who had an implanted atrial pacemaker. All patients had previous operations for complex congenital heart disease. The pacemaker was programmed at a pacing rate 20% faster than spontaneous mean daily rate previously determined with 24-hour monitoring. Monitoring after pacing documented greater than 80% paced rhythm during the daily hours in all patients during the follow-up. Antiarrhythmic medications were discontinued after 6 months if the patient remained arrhythmia free while on pacing. At the end of the follow-up, 83% were arrhythmia-free and only 2 were still on antiarrhythmic drugs. These investigators indicate that permanent atrial pacemaking may be an important adjunct to therapy for these patients with complex heart disease and difficult-to-manage atrial arrhythmias. Radiofrequency ablation may also be useful in selected patients in whom other modalities are unsuccessful.

Propafenone Use in Children

Janousek and associates[44] from Prague, Czech Republic, and Hannover, Germany, reviewed retrospective data from 27 European centers covering 772 patients treated with propafenone for reentrant SVT in 381, atrial ectopic tachycardia in 66, junctional ectopic tachycardia in 39, atrial flutter in 21, ventricular premature complexes in 140, VT in 78, and other arrhythmias in 39 patients. Structural heart disease was present in 32%. Significant electrophysiologic side effects for arrhythmia were found in 15 of 772 patients (1.9%) including sinus node dysfunction in 4, complete AV block in 2, aggravation of SVT in 2, acceleration of ventricular rate during atrial flutter in 1, ventricular proarrhythmia in 5, and unexplained syncope in 1. Cardiac arrest or sudden death occurred in 5 of 772 (0.6%). Of the patients who died, 2 had SVT due to WPW and a normal heart; the remaining 3 had structural heart disease.

Overall, adverse cardiac effects were more common in the presence than in the absence of structural heart disease 4.8% versus 1.5%. Propafenone is a relatively safe drug for the treatment of several pediatric arrhythmias and is 1 of the most frequently used antiarrhythmic drugs in infants, children, and adolescents in Europe.

Radiofrequency Catheter Ablation in Pediatric Patients

Tanel and associates[45] from Boston, Massachusetts, reviewed the results of the first 5 years of radiofrequency catheter ablation with a retrospective review of 410 consecutive procedures in 346 patients who underwent at least 1 application of radiofrequency energy for the treatment of recurrent SVT or VT. The overall final success rate for all diagnoses was 90%, with a higher success rate for patients with an accessory pathway (96%). The incidence of serious complications was only 1.2% with 1 late death, 1 ventricular dysfunction, 1 complete heart block, 1 cardiac perforation, and 1 cerebrovascular accident. Congenital heart disease was present in more than 20% of the patients, markedly increasing the complexity of the catheter ablation procedure. These authors consider ablation for infants younger than 1 year only after all medical options have been exhausted. Generally from 1 to 2 years, patients must have moderate symptoms that are not well controlled by medical therapy or drug-induced side effects to warrant ablation. From 2 to 5 years of age, freedom from symptoms must be dependent on continuous medical therapy before an ablation procedure is considered. There have been major advances in this form of therapy with outstanding results and only minimum morbidity and mortality. This mode of therapy is now one of the mainstays of treatment for pediatric and young adult patients with arrhythmias with or without associated congenital heart disease.

Congenital Heart Disease

Ultrafiltration and Myocardial Performance

Rivera and associates[46] from Cincinnati, Ohio, studied the effects of veno-venous ultrafiltration on myocardial contractility in children undergoing cardiopulmonary bypass for repair of congenital heart defects. There were 23 patients ages 2 months to 9 years who underwent ultrafiltration for 10 minutes after cardiopulmonary bypass. There were 12 patients who underwent ultrafiltration immediately after bypass (group A) and were studied before and after bypass, after ultrafiltration, and 10 minutes after ultrafiltration. There were 11 patients who underwent ultrafiltration 10 minutes after bypass (group B) and were studied before bypass, after bypass, and after a 10-minute delay before ultrafiltration, and finally after ultrafiltration. Contractility was estimated by the difference of the observed and predicted velocity of circumferential fiber shortening for measured wall stress, using transesophageal echocardiography.

There were significant improvements in contractility after ultrafiltration in both groups. In addition, myocardial thickness to cavity dimension decreased in both groups following ultrafiltration. Ultrafiltration improves hemodynamics by improving contractility and possibly by reducing myocardial edema in children early following cardiac surgery. This may be particularly important in patients with borderline ventricular function or who have prolonged ischemic times required for repair of their defect.

Pediatric Therapeutic Cardiac Catheterization

Allen and associates[47] from the Council on Cardiovascular Disease in the Young of the American Heart Association have provided a document on current status of pediatric therapeutic cardiac catheterization. This has been a field of rapid advancement, and the indications for use of these procedures, as well as some of the data regarding availability, is of wide interest to the cardiologist. These studies need to be performed by pediatric experts in interventional catheterization who have had special training and experience in these complex procedures. These therapeutic modalities have provided important new advancements in assuring optimal care for patients with congenital heart disease.

Reoxygenation Injury in Cyanotic Infants

Allen and associates[48] from Chicago, Illinois, studied 7 acyanotic and 21 cyanotic infants who were operated on for congenital heart disease using cardiopulmonary bypass. RA biopsies were performed to determine antioxidant reserve capacity. Of the cyanotic infants, 7 had bypass initiated at an Fio_2 of 1.0, 6 at an Fio_2 of 0.21, and 8 had undergone cardiopulmonary bypass using leukocyte filtration. There was a marked increase in malondialdehyde levels in cyanotic versus acyanotic patients, indicating a depletion of antioxidants. In addition, antioxidants were depleted less when bypass was initiated at an Fio_2 of 0.21. There was only a minimal increase in malondialdehyde induction in 8 of 21 infants in whom white blood cells were effectively filtered. These studies clearly show increased amounts of oxygen free radicals generated in cyanotic infants with initiation of cardiopulmonary bypass, and this production is reduced by initiating bypass at an Fio_2 of 0.21 or by effectively filtering white blood cells. White blood counts were effectively back to normal by the time the infants reached the intensive care unit, despite this filtration process. Although no direct studies on clinical outcome were available, the authors feel that the white blood cell-filtered patients had improved oxygenation, pulmonary compliance, fewer problems with postoperative hypertension, and lower requirements for inotropic support. There is a real need for hard data on these observations.

Intravascular Stents in Congenital Heart Disease

Shaffer and associates[49] from Houston, Texas, report long-term results from stent implantation from a single center in 200 patients. These include stents for treatment of arterial and venous stenosis. At stent implantation, pressure gradients decreased significantly from 46 ± 25 to 10 ± 13 in postoperative PA stenosis, from 71 ± 45 to 15 ± 21 in congenital PA stenosis, and from 7 ± 6 to 1 ± 2 in stenosis of systemic veins and venous anastomoses. Vessel diameters markedly increased from 6 ± 3 to 12 ± 3 in postoperative PA stenosis, from 3 ± 1 to 9 ± 1 in congenital PA stenosis, and from 3 ± 4 to 12 ± 4 in stenosis of systemic veins and venous anastomoses. In the postoperative and congenital PA stenosis groups, RV pressure indexed for femoral artery pressure and reported as a ratio decreased from 0.63 ± 0.2 to 0.41 ± 0.02 and from 0.71 ± 0.3 to 0.55 ± 0.35, respectively. Perfusion to a single affected lung increased from 31% ± 17% to 46% ± 14%. On recatheterization at a mean of 14 months, post-implantation results varied minimally. Repeat angioplasty of residual stent stenosis was safe and effective. Complications included 4 early patients with stent migration, 3 with stent thrombosis, and 2 deaths. There were no late complications. There was significant restenosis in only 3 patients. Intravascular stents for the treatment of vascular stenosis in congenital heart disease is an important aspect of care for patients with complex congenital heart disease. These studies must be performed by well-trained, experienced pediatric interventionalists and should be available in all centers that deal with large numbers of patients with congenital heart disease.

Coronary Perfusion Abnormalities

Donnelly and associates[50] from Ann Arbor, Michigan, used positron emission tomography to measure myocardial perfusion at rest and with adenosine in 5 infants after anatomic repair of congenital heart disease and in 5 infants after Norwood palliation for hypoplastic left heart syndrome. Infants with repaired heart disease had higher resting flow and less coronary flow reserve than previously reported for adults. After Norwood palliation, infants have less perfusion and oxygen delivery to the systemic ventricle than do infants with a repaired lesion. These results may in part explain why the outcome for Norwood palliation is less favorable than for patients with other conditions. Coronary perfusion abnormalities may contribute to myocardial dysfunction and arrhythmias despite what appears to be a good surgical result.

Abnormalities of Coronary Perfusion

Singh and associates[51] from Detroit, Michigan, evaluated myocardial flow reserve, LV function, and exercise performance in 11 patients at baseline and during maximal coronary dilation by adenosine using positron emission tomographic imaging in 11 patients at a median age of 17 years who had previously had repair of anomalous origin of the left coronary from the PA. Patients' median age at surgical repair was 7 months. All patients were asymptomatic and had normal ventricular function by echocardiography. Three patients were known to have occluded grafts. Basal myocardial blood flow was mildly reduced in the left coronary territories versus the control region. During hyperemia, flow in the left coronary territories was significantly lower than in the control region and as a result myocardial flow reserve was lower overall in the left coronary territories than in the control region. In addition, exercise performance was impaired in patients when compared with age-matched controls. Long-term survivors of anomalous left coronary artery surgery demonstrate regional impairment of myocardial flow reserve which may contribute to impaired exercise performance by limiting cardiac output reserve. Ventricular function usually improves dramatically in patients with anomalous left coronary who have establishment of a 2-coronary system. As might be expected, abnormalities of coronary perfusion can persist and need further evaluation by long-term follow-up.

Defects of Proteins Can Cause Dilated Cardiomyopathy

Deficiency of the sarcolemmal protein dystrophin has been linked to dilated cardiomyopathy. Some children with congenital muscular dystrophy have a deficiency of the laminin α_2 chain of merosin, an extracellular matrix protein linked to dystrophin through a group of glycoproteins. It has been shown that deficiency in one of these glycoproteins is responsible for muscular dystrophy and dilated cardiomyopathy. Children with laminin α_2 deficiency may be at risk for development of cardiomyopathy. Spyrou and associates[52] from London, United Kingdom, studied the cardiac function of a cohort of 16 children with congenital muscular dystrophy by using 2-dimensional echocardiography. The expression of the laminin α_2 of merosin in the patients was determined on a skin or muscle biopsy. Two of 6 merosin-deficient children had an EF less than 40%. The average EF of the merosin-deficient children was 43% ± 11%, which was significantly lower than the merosin-positive children (53% ± 5%). This study suggests that a deficiency of laminin α_2 can give rise to dilated cardiomyopathy, supporting the idea that defects of dystrophin, or of associated proteins, can cause dilated cardiomyopathy in addition to muscular dystrophy.

22q11 Deletions with Conotruncal Defects

Goldmuntz and associates[53] from Philadelphia, Pennsylvania, enrolled 251 patients with conotruncal defects and screened for the presence of 22q11 deletion. Deletions were found in 50% with interrupted aortic arch, 35% with truncus arteriosus, and 16% with TF. Only 2 of 6 patients with a posterior malalignment VSD and only 1 of 20 with double outlet right ventricle were found to have deletions. None of the 45 patients with TGA had a deletion. The frequency of deletions was higher in patients with anomalies of the pulmonary arteries, aortic arch, or its major branches compared to patients with a normal left aortic arch regardless of intracardiac anatomy. This study is helpful in drawing attention to those conotruncal anomalies with a high likelihood of having a 22q11 deletion. The authors are performing additional studies to include diagnoses such as thymic aplasia, palatal abnormalities, or symptomatic hypocalcemia in the neonate. In addition, it is unclear how many patients with known cardiac features will develop learning disabilities, hypernasal speech, neuro-psychiatric disorders, or facial dysmorphia, and whether these noncardiac abnormalities are directly related to certain aspects of the deletion.

Partial Biventricular Repair

Reddy and associates[54] from San Francisco, California, report 23 patients with a median age of 5.2 years who underwent partial biventricular repair. In 15 of these 23 patients, the entire repair including bidirectional cavopulmonary anastamosis, intracardiac repair, and RV outflow reconstruction, was performed as a planned procedure. The other 8 had previously been placed on Fontan track, but their circulations were converted to a partial biventricular circulation because of RV hypoplasia. There were no early deaths; complete AV block developed in 2 patients with straddling tricuspid valve. At a median follow-up of 17 months, there were no late deaths, but 3 patients had undergone reintervention, including partitioning of the PA to a classic Glenn anastamosis with antegrade flow to the left lung atrial septectomy, and revision of tricuspid valve repair. Partial biventricular repair is a versatile strategy that can be used to manage a variety of forms of complex congenital heart disease. In patients who have a bidirectional Glenn shunt, potential problems with forward pulmonary flow can arise when the RV output is substantial or when there is significant pulmonary insufficiency.

Right Ventricular Overload and Small Left Ventricle

Phoon and Silverman[55] from New York, New York, and San Francisco, California, studied 22 patients with RV overload lesions perioperatively to determine whether they had true LV hypoplasia or simply a compressed left ventricle due to underfilling. Preoperative LV volume was 15 ± 7 mL/m^2 and 59% of patients had a volume of less than 15 mL/m^2. Potential volume was calculated for given endocardial circumference by calculating from the maximal potential cross-sectional area (Figures 9-19 and 9-20). Potential volume was 20 ± 10 mL/m^2 and postoperative volume increased to 28 ± 9 mL/m^2. Preoperative potential volume correlated well with, but generally underestimated, postoperative volume, and postoperative increases in both LV circumference and length contributed to this discrepancy. In RV overload lesions, LV hypoplasia is primarily due to compression and underfilling. Many ventricles that appear hypoplastic can achieve an adequate cavity volume after operation with more optimal loading conditions.

Moyamoya Syndrome and Congenital Heart Disease

Lutterman and associates[56] from Boston, Massachusetts, report 5 patients with moyamoya syndrome and structural congenital heart disease. Associated

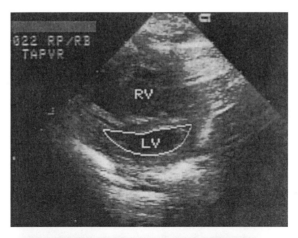

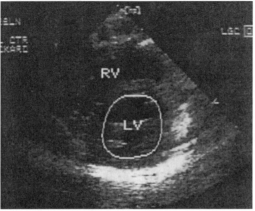

Figure 9-19. Echocardiographic short-axis views of the RV and LV in TAPVC. **Top:** A small LV compressed by right-to-left bowing of the interventricular septum due to RV volume overload. **Bottom:** The same patient after surgical repair shows normalization of the septal position and a normal, circular, cross-sectional LV geometry. Reproduced with permission from Phoon and Silverman.[55]

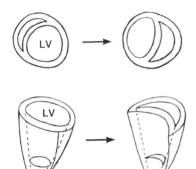

Figure 9-20. Schematic diagram of normal LV geometry **(left)** and geometry during RV overload conditions **(right).** In our model, RV overload causes right to left bowing of the interventricular septum. However, neither the endocardial circumference in the short-axis **(top)** nor the LV length **(bottom)** changes. Reproduced with permission from Phoon and Silverman.[55]

heart defects included: coarctation of the aorta, VSD, AS, MS, and TF. Surgical repair of the congenital heart disease was performed in 4 patients in the first year of life and 1 patient had balloon dilation of aortic coarctation at 5 years of age. In all patients, moyamoya syndrome was diagnosed after surgical intervention for congenital heart disease at 6 months of age in 1 patient, at 2 years of age in 3 patients, and at 6 years of age in 1 patient. Strokes were the most common presenting sign followed by seizures. By the age of 33 months, 4 of 5 patients had undergone cerebral revascularization surgery to halt the clinical progression of moyamoya syndrome. Moyamoya syndrome should be considered in the differential diagnosis of seizures and stroke in patients with structural congenital heart disease because prompt diagnosis and surgical management of the occlusive cerebral angiopathy could lead to improved neurological outcome.

Neonatal Heart Block in Maternal Lupus

Buyon and associates[57] from New York, Connecticut, Colorado, Maryland, and Oklahoma studied the demographics, mortality, morbidity and recurrence rates of autoimmune-associated congenital heart block using information from the Research Registry for Neonatal Lupus. The cohort included 105 mothers whose sera contain anti-SSA/Ro or anti-SSB/La antibodies, or both, and their 113 infants diagnosed with congenital heart block between 1970 and 1997. There were 87 pregnancies in which sufficient medical records were available, and bradyarrhythmia confirmed to be congenital heart block was initially detected before 30 weeks of gestation in 71 (82%) (median time 23 weeks). There were no cases in which major congenital cardiac defects were considered causal for the development of heart block; in 14 there were minor abnormalities. There were 22 of 113 children who died or 19%, and 73% of these 19 died within 3 months after birth. Cumulative probability of 3-year survival was 79%. Of 107 live-born children, 63% required pacemakers, 35 within 2 days of life, 15 within 1 year, and 17 after 1 year. There were subsequent pregnancies in 49 mothers and 16% had another infant with complete heart block. This series substantiates that autoantibody-associated heart block is not coincident with major structural abnormalities, is most often identified in the late second trimester, carries a substantial mortality in the neonatal period, and frequently requires pacing. The recurrence rate is at least 2 to 3 times higher than the rate for a mother with lupus and anti-Ro and anti-La antibodies who never had an affected child. These data support close echocardiographic monitoring in all subsequent pregnancies, with heightened surveillance between 18 and 24 weeks of gestation.

Myocardial Hypertrophy

Banerjee and associates[58] from Cincinnati, Ohio, studied systolic and diastolic properties of the left ventricle in children with myocardial hypertrophy. There were 10 children with congenital AS or coarctation of aorta and 9 control patients. Systolic properties were assessed by shortening fraction, end-systolic fiber elastance measured at resting heart rates, and force-frequency relationships measured at heart rates increasing from 110 to 160 beats/minute. Diastolic properties were estimated from the time constant of relaxation at matched heart rates, chamber stiffness constant, myocardial stiffness constant, and relaxation-frequency relationships measured at gradually increasing heart rates. Elastance remained unchanged by myocardial hypertrophy, however, and the time constant of relaxation was prolonged. Both chamber and myocardial stiffness constants remained unchanged. Incremental increases in heart rate produced incremental improvement in both contraction and relaxation. Slopes of force-frequency and relaxation-frequency relationships remained unchanged in the experimental group. This prolongation of relaxation in children with myocardial hypertrophy may play a role in diastolic dysfunction, which can be extremely detrimental to patients with complex heart disease undergoing surgery such as the bidirectional Glenn or Fontan operations. Further studies will be useful to determine diastolic properties in this group of patients who remain difficult to manage in the early postoperative period.

Cyanotic Ebstein's Anomaly

Yetman and associates[59] from Toronto, Ontario, Canada, reviewed clinical, angiographic, radiographic, and echocardiographic data on 46 neonates with Ebstein's anomaly presenting with cyanosis to determine possible risk factors for death. Mean systemic oxygen saturation was 62% and an ASD of 4 or more mm was noted in 20 patients (44%). A patent RV to PA connection was present in 10 (22%) and pulmonary atresia was functional in 25 (54%) and anatomic in 11 (24%). Surgical interventions were undertaken in 15 patients (35%). Total mortality was 70% versus 14% in acyanotic Ebstein's anomaly patients diagnosed during the same time. Death was related to low cardiac output and hypoxia in 62%, postoperative complications in 25%, and sudden death in 13%. Survival estimates were 61% at age 1 week, 48% at age 1 month, and 36% at both 1 and 5 years of age. Survival improved from 19% in 1954–1985 to 53% in 1986–1996. Significant independent predictors of mortality include an ASD of 4 mm or more, reduced LV function, and functional or anatomical pulmonary atresia. An echocardiographic ratio of the combined RA and atrialized RV area to the area of the functional right ventricle and left heart more than 1.0 was 100% predictive of mortality. Infants with Ebstein's anomaly, cyanosis, and a very large heart presenting as a neonate continue to present a difficult management problem. These authors document the correlation of cyanosis and a very large RA and atrialized right ventricle as very prominent risk factors for poor survival.

Repair of Ebstein's Anomaly

Hetzer and associates[60] from Berlin, Germany, report a modified technique for tricuspid valve repair in Ebstein's anomaly. The technique restructures the valve mechanism at the level of the true tricuspid annulus by using the most mobile leaflet for valve closure without plication of the atrialized chamber. Nineteen patients ages 2 to 54 years with a mean of 21 years were repaired with this technique. The indication for operation was CHF of various degrees in all patients. TR was grade II in 2 patients, grade III in 14, and grade

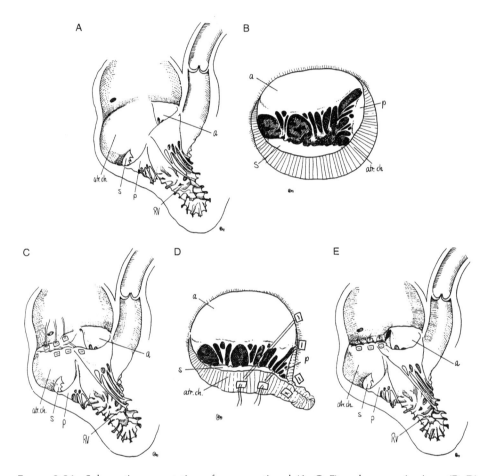

FIGURE 9-21. Schematic presentation of cross-sectional **(A, C, E)** and surgeon's views **(B, D)** of the intraoperative findings and the surgical technique applied in patients 2, 3, 4, 11, and 13 through 19. **(A, B)** The pathologic finding corresponds to Ebstein's anomaly of Carpentier type B, with the displaced septal (s) and posterior (p) leaflets toward the apex of the right ventricle (RV). Leaflet displacement creates an atrialized chamber (atr. ch.) below the anatomic tricuspid annulus. There is a large, mobile anterior leaflet (a). **(C, D, E)** The anterior part of the anterior leaflet was chosen for the valve-closing structure. A mattress suture of 3-0 polypropylene pledgeted with autologous pericardium is passed from the anterior leaflet annulus to the atrialized septum just below the natural tricuspid annulus. A row of these sutures is added toward the posterior annulus. These pledgeted stitches can also be placed through the septal anatomic annulus. After the sutures are placed, they are tied, resulting in obliteration of the posterior half of the anatomic tricuspid orifice. Thus the anterior annulus is approximated to the septum. When valve competence is tested by filling the ventricular cavity with saline solution, the anterior part of the anterior leaflet now coapts with the atrialized septum. The "atrialized chamber" is now incorporated into contracting right ventricular cavity. Reproduced with permission from Hetzer et al.[60]

IV in 3. Associated malformations were simultaneously repaired, including ASD in 18, VSD in 2, PS in 2, and MVP in 1. Follow-up ranged from 10 to 103 months with a median of 28 months and was complete for all patients. There were no operative deaths, but 1 patient with active endocarditis and pulmonary abscess died 2 months after operation. There were no late deaths. Functional classification improved from New York Heart Association functional class 2.8 before the operation to 1.9 without recurrent cyanosis, and TR decreased from a mean grade of 3.1 to 0.9, without any echocardiographic deterioration of the tricuspid valve function or RV dilation. This is an interesting technique whereby the atrialized chamber continues as part of the right ventricle in all patients. There were no instances of aneurysmal dilation of this part of the chamber and excellent results were obtained on midterm follow-up. This technique should be studied by all physicians who deal with complex congenital heart disease (Figures 9-21–9-24).

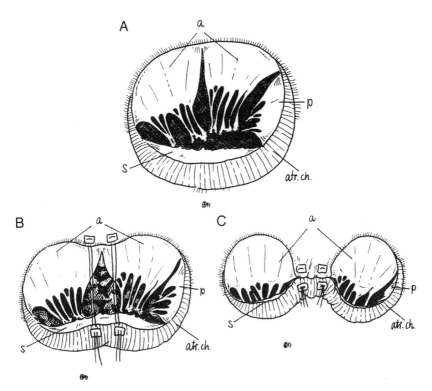

FIGURE 9-22. A view of the tricuspid valve in case 1 from the surgeon's side. **(A)** The anterior leaflet (a) is split by a cleft and shows deep fissures. There are some chordal adhesions of the leaflet to the right ventricular wall, which are dissected. **(B)** Two 3-0 polypropylene mattress sutures supported with autologous pericardium pledgets are passed through the middle portions of the anterior annulus and the atrialized septum just below the septal annulus. **(C)** When the sutures are tied, the anterior annulus is approximated to the septum, dividing the valve into 2 orifices and enabling valve closure by the solid part of the leaflets, which can now meet the atrialized septum and afford valve competence. p = Posterior leaflet; s = septal leaflet; atr.ch. = atrialized chamber. Reproduced with permission from Hetzer et al.[60]

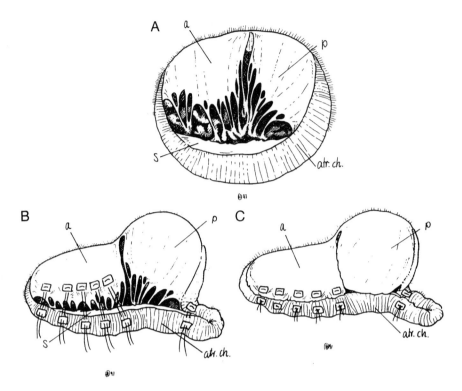

FIGURE 9-23. Schematic presentation of the valve repair technique used in cases 5, 8, and 10. **(A)** Anterior (a) and posterior (p) leaflets are almost equal in size. In case 10, there were additional chordal adhesions between the anterior leaflet and the right ventricular wall. The large posterior leaflet was selected for valve function. **(B)** The anterior leaflet was translocated to the atrialized septum by a row of 3-0 polypropylene pledgeted sutures. Furthermore, the posteroseptal angle of the anatomic annulus was plicated for closer approximation of the anterior annulus to the septum. The anterior half of the orifice is now closed with the anterior leaflet, and the posterior leaflet moves freely. **(C)** Testing of valve competence reveals appropriate valve closure achieved by good coaptation of the posterior leaflet with the septum. s = Septal leaflet. Reproduced with permission from Hetzer et al.[60]

Molecular Diagnosis for Genetic Cardiovascular Disease

Maron and associates[61] from the American Heart Association Scientific Councils reviewed the impact of laboratory molecular diagnosis on contemporary diagnostic criteria for the genetically transmitted cardiovascular diseases: hypertrophic cardiomyopathy, long QT syndrome (LQTS), and Marfan syndrome. This comprehensive, well-written article reviews these syndromes that are associated with autosomal dominant inheritance and demonstrate variable penetrance and expressivity. Although these syndromes are relatively uncommon in the general population, each confers a risk for unexpected sudden cardiac death in the young. Over the past 8 to 10 years, the application of molecular biology and DNA-based technology to the study of genetically transmitted cardiovascular disease has provided a measure of diagnostic clarifica-

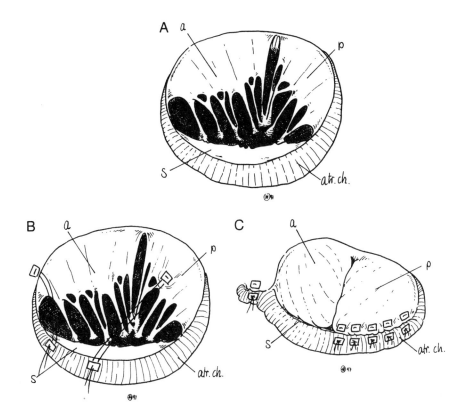

Figure 9-24. Schematic drawings of pathologic findings and applied surgical technique in cases 6 and 9. **(A)** The anterior (a) and the posterior (p) leaflets are of almost equal sizes. The anterior leaflet is mobile, but too small to close the orifice by itself. **(B)** The posterior leaflet is transposed with its septal free edge to the atrialized septum below the anatomic annulus. In addition, the anteroseptal commissure is plicated by a pledgeted suture. **(C)** On valve closure, the anterior leaflet plays the main closing part, which coapts with the fixed posterior leaflet and the atrialized septum. s = Septal leaflet; atr. ch. = atrialized chamber. Reproduced with permission from Hetzer et al.[60]

tion. Nevertheless, at present, most patients with these conditions can still be identified reliably by standard clinical diagnostic techniques (Figure 9-25; Tables 9-1 and 9-2). At present, the clinical utility of genetic testing for hypertrophic cardiomyopathy, LQTS, and Marfan syndrome is hampered by their substantial allelic heterogeneity and the time-intensive and costly nature of laboratory genotyping. Future initiatives directed toward molecular diagnosis will likely result from improved technology, gene sequencing, and the development of automatic screening methods for more rapid identification of mutations. At present, laboratory genetic analysis for these syndromes may be useful in selected patients in certain ambiguous areas, particularly those in which family history is suggestive of a high risk status. However, given the large number of genes and mutations already evident in these syndromes (and the realistic expectation for additional diversity), the future design of comprehensive molecular screening tests and therapy for these genetic cardiovascular diseases will continue to be a challenge.

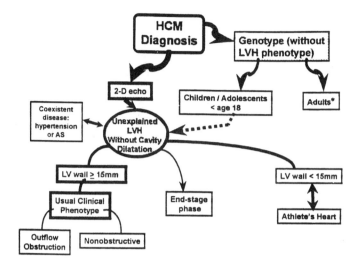

FIGURE 9-25. Diagram summarizing the clinical and laboratory diagnosis of hypertrophic cardiomyopathy (HCM). Although it is possible to establish this diagnosis in the laboratory setting by mutational analysis, in the vast majority of instances, HCM is identified clinically with 2-dimensional echocardiographic imaging (by virtue of a hypertrophied but nondilated left ventricle). Clinical diagnosis by this criterion can be confounded by associated cardiovascular diseases such as systemic hypertension or aortic valve stenosis, by evolution to the end-stage (or dilated) phase of HCM in which left ventricular wall thinning occurs, or if the subject is a highly trained athlete in selected sporting disciplines. LV = left ventricle; LVH = left ventricular hypertrophy; 2-D echo = 2-dimensional echocardiographic imaging; AS = aortic valve stenosis. * Genotype-positive, phenotype-negative adults are uncommon but appear to be more frequently associated with certain genetic defects, such as mutations in the gene for myosin-binding protein-C. Reproduced with permission from Maron et al.[61]

Cardiomyopathy

Use of Beta-Blocker Treatment in Children

Shaddy[62] from Salt Lake City, Utah, used β-blocker therapy in 4 children with cardiomyopathy who were referred for consideration of heart transplantation because of severe heart failure. Conventional therapy received prior to β-blockade included digoxin, diuretics, and angiotensin-converting enzyme inhibitors for a period of 3 ± 1.5 months without echocardiographic or symptomatic improvement on maximum tolerated doses of these medications. Over a follow-up period of 13 months with β-blocker treatment, LV fractional shortening increased from 14% to 26%, EF from 20% to 41%, and 2 children became asymptomatic (Figure 9-26). β-blockade may be effective in improving EF symptoms in some young children with cardiomyopathy and CHF unresponsive to standard therapy.

Use of Beta-Blocker Treatment in Infants

Buckhorn and associates[63] from Gottingen, Germany, report 6 consecutive infants with CHF due to large left-to-right shunt who were treated with pro-

TABLE 9-1
LQTS Diagnostic Criteria

	Points
ECG findings†	
A. QTc	
$\geq$480 ms$^{1/2}$	3
460–470 ms$^{1/2}$	2
450 ms$^{1/2}$ (in males)	1
B. Torsades de pointes	2
C. T-wave alternans	1
D. Notched T wave in 3 leads	1
E. Low heart rate for age‡	0.5
Clinical history	
A. Syncope	
With stress	2
Without stress	1
B. Congenital deafness	0.5
Family history	
A. Family members with definite LQTS§	1
B. Unexplained sudden cardiac death <30 years among immediate family members	0.5

Scoring: $\leq$1 point, low probability of LQTS; 2 to 3 points, intermediate probability of LQTS; $\geq$4 points, high probability of LQTS.

† In the absence of medications or disorders known to affect these electrocardiographic features.

‡ Resting heart rate below the second percentile for age.

§ Definite LQTS is defined by an LQTS score $\geq$4.

Reproduced with permission from Maron et al.[61]

pranolol after conventional therapy had proven unsuccessful in relieving their symptoms. Diagnoses were tricuspid atresia in 2, double outlet right ventricle with mitral atresia in 1, and complete AV septal defect in 3. Before beginning propranolol therapy, all infants had received digoxin and diuretics for at least 4 weeks. All infants had clinical signs of severe CHF with mean respiratory rates of 75/minute, diaphoresis at rest, and a decrease in weight over at least 4 weeks. There were all fed by nasogastric tube. Therapy was begun with a 1 mg dose, and if tolerated, continued with 1 mg/kg/day given in 3 divided doses and increased as tolerated up to 3 mg/kg/day. There was a significant decrease in respiratory rate averaging 11 breaths/minute, heart rate averaging 22 bpm, and mean arterial pressure of 4 mg Hg with no change in oxygen saturation. Mean plasma renin decreased from 124 to 20 ng/mL/hr and aldosterone levels decreased from 3,170 to 1,159 pg/L. After titration therapy for 2 to 3 weeks, the infants had a mean propranolol dosage of 1.8 mg/kg/day. The clinical course of these infants suggests a clear beneficial effect when adding propranolol therapy. No data were obtained on ACE inhibitor therapy that might also be useful prior to using the β-blockade. The fear of a decrease in cardiac index and worsening CHF was not realized in this small group of patients. These limited data suggest that this therapy may be useful in selected patients with severe CHF in infancy despite usual maximal medical therapy.

Table 9-2

Requirements for Diagnosis of Marfan Syndrome (Ghent Criteria)

For the index case:
- If the family/genetic history is not contributory, major criteria in ≥2 different organ systems and involvement of a third organ system.
- If a mutation known to cause Marfan syndrome in others is detected, 1 major criterion in an organ system and involvement of a second organ system.

For a relative of an index case:
- Presence of a major criterion in the family history, 1 major criterion in an organ system, and involvement of a second organ system.

Skeletal System

Major Criterion (Presence of ≥4 of the following manifestations is necessary to satisfy a major criterion):
- Pectus carinatum
- Pectus excavatum requiring surgery
- Reduced upper- to lower-segment ratio or arm span-to-height ratio >1.05
- Wrist and thumb signs
- Scoliosis of >20° or spondylolisthesis
- Reduced extension at the elbows (<170°)
- Medial displacement of the medial malleolus causing pes planus
- Protrusio acetabulae of any degree (ascertained on radiographs)

Minor Criteria
- Pectus excavatum of moderate severity
- Joint hypermobility
- Highly arched palate with crowding of teeth
- Facial appearance (dolichocephaly, malar hypoplasia, enophthalmos, retrognathia, down-slanting palpebral fissures)

For the skeletal system to be considered involved, at least 2 of the components comprising the major criterion or 1 component comprising the major criterion plus 2 of the minor criteria must be present.

Ocular System

Major Criterion
- Ectopia lentis

Minor Criteria
- Abnormally flat cornea
- Increased axial length of globe
- Hypoplastic iris or hypoplastic ciliary muscle causing decreased miosis

For the ocular system to be involved, at least 2 of the minor criteria must be present.

Cardiovascular System

Major Criteria
- Dilation of the ascending aorta with or without aortic regurgitation and involving at least the sinuses of Valsalva; or
- Dissection of the ascending aorta

Minor Criteria
- Mitral valve prolapse with or without mitral valve regurgitation;
- Dilatation of the main pulmonary artery, in the absence of valvular or peripheral pulmonic stenosis or any other obvious cause, younger than age 40;
- Calcification of the mitral annulus younger than age 40; or
- Dilatation or dissection of the descending thoracic or abdominal aorta younger than age 50.

For the cardiovascular system to be involved, 1 major criterion or only 1 of the minor criteria must be present.

(continued)

Table 9-2 *(continued)*

Pulmonary System
  Major Criteria
  • None
  Minor Criteria
  • Spontaneous pneumothorax; or
  • Apical blebs
  For the pulmonary system to be involved, 1 of the minor criteria must be present.
Skin and Integument
  Major Criteria
  • None
  Minor Criteria
  • Striae atrophicae (stretch marks) not associated with marked weight gain, pregnancy, or repetitive stress; or
  • Recurrent or incisional herniae
  For the skin and integument to be involved, 1 of the minor criteria must be present.
Dura
  Major Criterion
  • Lumbosacral dural ectasia by CT or MRI
  Minor Criteria
  • None
  For the dura to be involved, the major criterion must be present.
Family/Genetic History
  Major Criteria
  • Having a parent, child, or sibling who meets these diagnostic criteria independently;
  • Presence of a mutation in *FBN-1* known to cause MFS; or
  • Presence of a haplotype around *FBN-1,* inherited by descent, known to be associated with unequivocally diagnosed MFS in the family.
  Minor Criteria
  • None
  For the family/genetic history to be contributory, 1 of the major criteria must be present.

Reproduced with permission from Maron et al.[61]

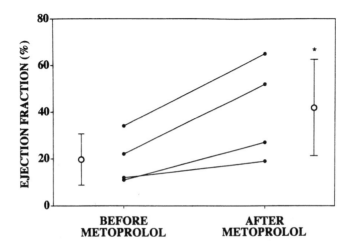

FIGURE 9-26. Increase in EF in patients after metoprolol therapy when compared with before initiation of metoprolol (*p < 0.05). Reproduced with permission from Shaddy.[62]

Hypertrophic Cardiomyopathy

Charron and associates[64] from Paris, Boulogne, and Nantes, France, studied 76 genetically affected subjects from 9 families with hypertrophic cardiomyopathy with 7 recently identified mutations in the cardiac myosin-binding protein C (MYBPC3) gene. Detailed clinical, electrocardiographic, and echocardiographic parameters were analyzed. An intergene analysis was performed by comparing the MYBPC3 group to 7 mutations in the β myosin heavy-chain gene (β-MHC). There were no significant phenotypic differences among the different mutations in the MYBPC3 gene. However, in the MYBPC3 group compared with the β-MHC group, prognosis was significantly better, no deaths occurred before the age of 40 years, the age of onset of symptoms was delayed, and before 30 years of age, the phenotype was particularly mild because penetrance was low, maximal wall thickness lower, and abnormal T waves less frequent. The survival probability for the 2 different gene groups is shown in Figure 9-27. These results are consistent with specific clinical features related to the MYBPC3 gene which appear to show a later onset of disease and significantly better prognosis than with the β-MHC gene. Hopefully, these findings will be useful for clinical management and more genotypes will be discovered with appropriate phenotypic differences that will allow better personalized management and genetic counseling in hypertrophic cardiomyopathy.

Screening for Hypertrophic Cardiomyopathy

Corrado[65] and associates from Padua, Italy, report results from screening of athletes from 1979 to 1996. The causes of sudden death in athletes and

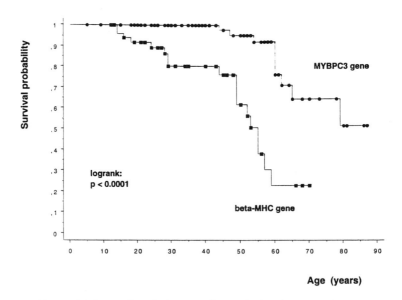

FIGURE 9-27. Kaplan-Meier product-limit curves for survival in the MYBPC3 group (7 mutations in this gene) compared with β-MHC group (7 mutations in this gene). Disease-related deaths and cardiac transplantations were considered events. Product-limit survival functions were significantly different between the 2 groups (p < 0.0001) by the log-rank test. Reproduced with permission from Charron et al.[64]

nonathletes were compared, and the pathological findings in the athletes were related to their clinical histories and electrocardiograms. Of 269 sudden deaths in young people, 49 occurred in competitive athletes. The most common cause of sudden death was RV cardiomyopathy in 22%, atherosclerosis in 18%, and anomalous origin of coronary artery in 12%. Hypertrophic cardiomyopathy caused only 1 sudden death among the athletes or 2% but caused 16 sudden deaths in nonathletes or 7%. Hypertrophic cardiomyopathy was detected in 22 athletes at preparticipation screening and accounted for 3.5% of the cardiovascular reasons for disqualification. None of the disqualified athletes with hypertrophic cardiomyopathy died during a mean follow-up of 8 ± 5 years. These authors report a strategy for cardiovascular screening which includes general clinical history taking, physical examination, and electrocardiogram for these competitive athletes. The data suggest that it has been successful in preventing death in hypertrophic cardiomyopathy patients by eliminating competitive sports. The numbers are small and the comprehensive evaluation and electrocardiogram may be prohibitive for many countries. Further follow-up with type of screening would be extremely useful in order to set appropriate guidelines for preparticipation screening.

Complications After Surgery

Duration of Heart Block After Surgery

Weindling and associates[66] from Boston, Massachusetts, prospectively studied all patients undergoing cardiac surgery between January 1991 and January 1994 who had complete heart block lasting longer than 4 hours postoperatively. Patients with preexisting second and third degree AV block or a history of transient AV block at prior operation were excluded. The timing of permanent pacing system implantation was left to the discretion of the surgeon. There were 54 operations that were complicated by complete heart block, representing 2% of total cardiac operations and 3% of those requiring cardiopulmonary bypass. The greatest risk for heart block occurred with surgery for LV outflow obstruction (8 of 46, 17%) and corrected transposition of the great arteries occurring (5 in 44, 11%). The incidence was less but still significant after VSD closure (18 of 474, 4%) and TF (6 of 206, 3%). Patients were divided into 2 groups for analysis with group 1 patients recovering AV conduction the first 30 days following surgery. Group 2 patients did not recover conduction or did so more than 30 days following surgery. Recovery of AV conduction after surgically induced complete heart block occurs in more than 95% of patients by postoperative day 9. In summary, heart block after surgery for congenital heart disease resolves in 2 of 3 patients, usually by the ninth postoperative day. It is important that even patients who appear to recover from heart block early have the potential for late development of AV conduction abnormalities such as Mobitz type II AV block, which was seen in 3 patients or 9% of those with transient complete heart block.

Effect of Surgical Volume on Mortality

Hannan and associates[67] from Albany, Syracuse, and New York, New York, and Chapel Hill, North Carolina, examined the relationship between hospital and surgeon volume on in-hospital mortality for pediatric cardiac surgery. All children undergoing congenital heart surgery in New York from 1992 to 1995 at 16 acute care hospitals were studied. The certificates of need to perform pediatric cardiac surgery were included in the analysis, and a total of 7,169 cases were analyzed. After controlling for severity of preprocedural illness using clinical risk factors, hospitals with annual pediatric cardiac surgery volumes of fewer than 100 had significantly higher mortality (8.3%) than hospitals with volumes of 100 or more (5.5%), and surgeons with annual volumes of fewer than 75 had significantly higher mortality rates (8.8%) than surgeons with annual volumes of 75 or more (5.9%). These data show the annual hospital volume and annual surgeon volume were both significantly related to inpatient mortality rate even after controlling for patient age, several clinical risk factors, and procedure complexity. The maximal difference in mortality rate between high and low volume providers was at 100 procedures annually for hospitals and 75 procedures annually for surgeons. In general, higher hospital volumes and higher surgeon volumes were associated with lower risk-adjusted mortality rates across all procedure volumes.

Cause of Death After Norwood Procedure

Bartram and associates[68] from Boston, Massachusetts, reviewed postmortem studies in 122 patients to determine probable cause of death after the Norwood procedure. The most important causes were found to be impairment of coronary perfusion in 27%, excessive pulmonary blood flow in 19%, obstruction of pulmonary arterial blood flow in 17%, neoaortic obstruction in 14%, RV failure in 13%, bleeding in 7%, infection in 5%, AV valve insufficiency in 6%, sudden death from arrhythmias in 5%, and necrotizing enterocolitis in 3%. In 21%, more than 1 factor appeared responsible for death. There continues to be significant morbidity and mortality associated with surgical treatment of patients with hypoplastic left hearts. A number of centers continue to show improvement in outcome as surgical methodology has evolved with attempts to optimize coronary perfusion, prevent excessive pulmonary blood flow, and aggressively treat neoaortic obstruction and AV valve insufficiency.

Aortopulmonary Defects

McElhinney and associates[69] from San Francisco, California, reviewed 24 patients with aortopulmonary defects who underwent repair at ages ranging from 2 to 172 days with a median of 34 days. There were complex associated anomalies in 12 patients including interrupted or hypoplastic arch in 9, TF in 1, pulmonary atresia in 1, and TGA in 1. The most recent 7 patients were diagnosed by echocardiography without catheterization. There were no early or late deaths among the 12 patients with simple defects; 4 patients with complex associated lesions died in the early postoperative period and another died 4 months after surgery. Long-term survival has been good, but repair of recurrent obstruction of the arch repair site has been needed in the majority of patients with interrupted or hypoplastic arch.

Conotruncal Anomalies with Aortic Arch Obstruction

Lacour-Gayet and associates[70] from Paris, France, report biventricular repair of conotruncal anomalies associated with aortic arch obstruction in 103 patients. The conotruncal anomalies included TGA in 59 with 44 having VSD, double outlet RV in 32, truncus arteriosus in 10, double outlet left ventricle in 1, and TF in 1. The aortic obstruction included 88 coarctation and 15 interrupted arch anomalies. One-stage repair has been the favored technique since 1990 and was performed in 58 neonates, including 38 with TGA or double outlet right ventricle and VSD, 10 TGAs with intact ventricular septum, and all of the infants with truncus arteriosus. The repair included 89 arterial switch operations, 2 Kawashima reroutings, 10 truncus arteriosus repairs, 1 double outlet left ventricle repair, and 1 TF repair. The aortic arch was reconstructed by direct anastomosis in 85 patients with a Gore-Tex conduit in 3 and more recently by an ascending aortic patch augmentation in 15 patients. The hospital mortality was 12% for the 1-stage repair and 20% for the 2-stage repair. There were 6 late deaths. Reoperations or angioplasties were mandatory in 12 RV outflow tract obstructions after arterial switch, involving 10 patients with double outlet right ventricle. In addition, there were 10 recurrent arch obstructions and 6 miscellaneous lesions. One-stage biventricular repair of conotruncal anomalies associated with arch obstruction can be achieved in selected patients with an 83% survival rate at 7 years. This is a very complex group of patients who are at high risk for mortality and morbidity with this challenging repair. These authors have gotten outstanding results, and hopefully, long-term follow-up will show that these results are enduring.

Echocardiographic Predictors of Left Ventricular Outflow Obstruction

Apfel and associates[71] from New York, New York, reviewed the preoperative echocardiograms and the postoperative clinical course and echocardiograms of 23 consecutive patients who underwent primary repair of interrupted aortic arch without widening of the subaortic region. Significant LV outflow obstruction occurred in 9 patients (39%) with a pressure gradient greater than 40 mm Hg. Obstruction was noted postoperatively in 7 of 9 patients by 1 month, 8 of 9 by 2 months, and 9 of 9 by 1 year. On retrospective analysis of the preoperative echocardiograms, indexed cross-sectional area of the LV outflow tract, the subaortic diameter index, and the subaortic diameter Z score were all significantly smaller in those requiring reintervention. Of these, indexed cross-sectional area had the least reproducibility and subaortic diameter index had the most. In conclusion, most patients who develop significant LV outflow obstruction after repair of interrupted arch do so within 1 month of operation, and several different measurements of subaortic diameter may provide the best method for predicting significant postoperative subaortic obstruction postoperatively. These patients frequently present difficult management decisions; i.e., when should one proceed with a Norwood I type repair versus conventional operation? There is still controversy on the proper use of preoperative echocardiographic data to make this decision.

Fontan Procedure

Protein-Losing Enteropathy After Fontan

Mertens[72] and associates from Leuven, Belgium; Rochester, Minnesota; Munchen, Germany; and London, United Kingdom, report a multicenter study that retrospectively analyzes the data on 114 patients with protein-losing enteropathy after Fontan-type surgery. In 35 participating centers, 3,029 Fontan operations were performed and protein-losing enteropathy was found in 114 patients (3.7%). The median age at Fontan-type surgery was 8 years (range 0.6 to 33 years). Median age at diagnosis of protein-losing enteropathy was 12 years with a median time interval between surgery and diagnosis of 3 years (range of 0.1 to 16 years). Edema was present in 79% and effusions in 75%. Hemodynamic data revealed a mean RA pressure of 17 with a cardiac index of 2.4. Medical treatment in 52 resulted in a complete resolution of symptoms in 25%, no improvement in 29%, and death in 46%. Surgical treatment in 52 was associated with relief of protein-losing enteropathy in 19%, no improvement in 19%, and death in 62%. In 13 patients, 16 percutaneous interventions were performed, resulting in symptomatic improvement after 12 interventions and no improvement after 4 interventions. This is an important paper indicating the fortunately rare occurrence of protein-losing enteropathy in a large number of Fontan patients. Unfortunately, treatment is frequently not successful. Complete hemodynamic evaluation and treatment of any lesions that could cause high central venous pressure should be undertaken in all patients. Creating or enlarging an atrial fenestration should be considered if there are no residual lesions to treat. Some patients may improve with high-dose steroid treatment or subcutaneous high molecular weight heparin. Heart transplantation should be considered in patients unresponsive to these strategies.

Nonfenestrated Fontan

Hsu and associates[73] from New York, New York, report postoperative course and preoperative risk factors in 61 consecutive patients with a median age of 3.3 years undergoing a single stage nonfenestrated Fontan operation with follow-up of 4 ± 2 years. Preoperative risk factors assessed included age younger than 2 years, branch PS, elevated mean PA pressure greater than 15 mm Hg, AV valve regurgitation, and decreased ventricular function. Total caval pulmonary anastomosis was performed in 53 patients and additional surgery was required at the time of the Fontan in 25 patients. The median duration of the mechanical ventilation was 1 day and median chest tube drainage was 5.5 days with a range of 1 to 35. Oxygen saturation rose from 83% to 95% and early mortality was 4.9%; 1 patient died from pacemaker failure in 9 months postoperatively, and 1 patient underwent heart transplant 4 months post-Fontan. One- and 5-year actuarial survival was 93%. No preoperative risk factor was associated with a failed Fontan or significant effusions. These authors report excellent results in this group of consecutive operations without using the fenestrated Fontan or the preoperative superior vena cava PA anastomosis as a preliminary procedure. The debate continues regarding the use of a 1-stage versus a 2-stage approach for these patients and the need for fenestration with Fontan repair. Certainly patients with good preoperative risk factors and older age can get excellent results with the 1-stage procedure. If one could eliminate the fenestration in a significant number of patients, this should decrease the incidence of postoperative thromboembolic phenomena with systemic embolization.

Thromboembolism After the Fontan Procedure

Monagle and associates[74] from Hamilton, Ontario; Melbourne, Australia; and Toronto, Canada, reviewed the current data regarding thromboembolic complications after the Fontan procedure and the role of prophylactic anticoagulation. Central venous and intracardiac thrombosis are major causes of morbidity and mortality after the Fontan procedure. Prophylactic anticoagulation with warfarin or antiplatelet agents after the procedure is frequently recommended. However, no consensus was found in the literature or in routine clinical practice regarding the efficacy of or the optimal type or duration of anticoagulation. The data viewed indicated a wide variation in thromboembolic complications reported, which may be related to differences in the methods used to detect these problems. Physicians who deal with these patients will find this report of interest. There is no definitive answer to the question of what is optimal prophylaxis for prevention of thromboembolism after the Fontan procedure. A multicenter, randomized controlled trial is needed to solve this dilemma.

Fontan Conversion and Cryoablation

Mavroudis and associates[75] from Chicago, Illinois, reviewed their experience with patients who had atriopulmonary Fontan connections and obstructive or arrhythmic indications for conversion to total cavopulmonary connection, arrhythmia circuit cryoablation, and placement of an atrial antitachcardia pacemaker. There were 14 patients with a mean age of 14 years who had conversion to total cavopulmonary connection 8 ± 3 years after the original operation primarily for atrial arrhythmias in 11, obstructive lesions in 2, and bradycardia with cyanosis in 1. Arrhythmia circuit ablation was performed on 11 patients and 10 had atrial antitachycardia pacemakers inserted. One patient had brain death presumably caused by resternotomy complications despite an excellent hemodynamic result. Another required reoperation for a maldeployed clamshell device after attempted fenestration closure. Average length of stay was 10 days and there were no long-term deaths with a mean follow-up of 1.7 years and a range of 5 months to 5 years. Postoperative arrhythmias occurred in 5 patients, 3 of whom had successful termination by antitachycardia pacemaker and 2 had pharmacological control of their respective junctional ectopic and slow atrial tachycardias. All patients have improved symptomatically. This operation, as depicted in Figures 9-28 and 9-29 has theoretical merit in improving the hemodynamics of the Fontan connection. In addition, decreasing the size of the atrium may decrease the potential for arrhythmias. In this series of patients, there were a number of strategies to improve control of life-threatening arrhythmias, and it is unclear whether hemodynamic improvement, cryoablation, or atrial antitachycardia pacemaker therapy had the most profound effect on outcome. It is probable that all contributed to symptomatic improvement.

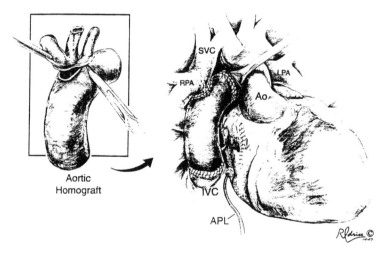

FIGURE 9-28. Diagrammatic representation of a total cavopulmonary artery extracardiac conversion in a patient with an established classic right Glenn/right atrium-to-left pulmonary artery Fontan connection. An aortic homograft was used to connect the left pulmonary artery with the inferior vena cava using the favorable curve of the ascending and transverse arch of the homograft. The Glenn anastomosis was connected side-to-side to the homograft to complete the reconstruction. A transmural bipolar steroid-eluting atrial lead (Medtronic, Inc., Minneapolis, MN) is placed in the left atrial appendage for antitachycardia pacemaker placement. Ao = aorta; APL = antitachycardia pacemaker lead; IVC = inferior vena cava; SVC = superior vena cava; LPA = left pulmonary artery; RPA = right pulmonary artery. Reproduced with permission from Mavroudis et al.[75]

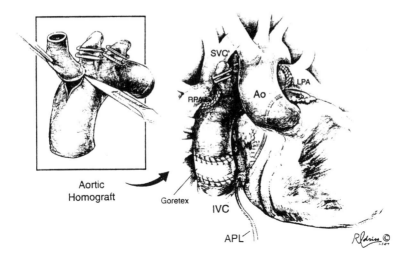

FIGURE 9-29. Total cavopulmonary artery extracardiac Fontan conversion (see Figure 9-28). Occasionally, the aortic homograft may require a PTFE graft extension (composite graft) to connect the left pulmonary artery with the inferior vena cava. The Glenn anastomosis can be connected to the homograft as appropriate. Abbreviations as in Figure 9-28. Reproduced with permission from Mavroudis et al.[75]

Valvular Disease in Children

Beneficial Therapy in Children with Chronic Aortic Regurgitation

A prospective study by Alehan and Ozkutlu[76] from Ankara, Turkey, was performed to assess the effects of 1 year of angiotensin-converting enzyme inhibition with captopril in 20 children (mean age 14 ± 2.3 years) with asymptomatic chronic AR. At 12 months, patients receiving captopril had a significant reduction in LV end-diastolic and end-systolic dimensions (57 ± 9.3 vs. 51 ± 9.5 mm; 35 ± 6.1 vs. 32 ± 6.8 mm), end-diastolic and end-systolic volume indexes (111 ± 36 vs. 94 ± 29 ml/m^2; 35 ± 13 vs. 30 ± 12 ml/m^2), and mass index (138 ± 37 vs. 109 ± 32 gm/m^2) determined by 2-dimensional echocardiography. Meridian and circumferential wall stresses also decreased significantly with therapy. Significant reduction (28%) was achieved in regurgitant fraction with captopril. These data show that long-term therapy with angiotensin-converting enzyme inhibitors is able to reverse LV dilation and hypertrophy and suggest that such therapy has the potential to favorably influence the natural history of the disease in children.

Rejection of Homograft Valves in Infants

Rajani and associates[77] from Cleveland, Ohio, reviewed 11 cryopreserved homograft valves removed at reoperation and 1 at autopsy. There were 6 valves from adults, 5 from infants, and 1 from a 13-year-old child. The failed homo-grafts from the adults and the 13-year-old child showed leaflet calcification, fibrosis, and degeneration, but no inflammation. The valves from the infants all failed in less than 8 months and showed valve thickening with evidence of multiple foci of inflammation consisting of T lymphocytes in all 5 infant cardiac valves and B lymphocytes in 3 of 5 infant valves. These observations are consistent with other reports of rapid failure of homograft valves in this age group. The issue of rejection of homografts needs to be further investigated. Despite the initial belief that homografts would provide excellent long-term palliation, this has not been the case in many patients.

Tricuspid Valve Repair

Reyes and associates[78] from Ann Arbor, Michigan, reviewed clinical and echocardiographic data on 59 consecutive patients with hypoplastic left heart. Patients with a moderate or severe degree of TR demonstrated by color flow Doppler before the hemi-Fontan or Fontan operation who underwent tricuspid valve repair were included. Patients with hypoplastic left heart and coexisting AV septal defect were excluded from the study. There were 8 patients (14%) who were found to have a minimum of 2 + or moderate TR before operation. In 5 of 8 patients, the valve was found to be myxomatous, thickened, and redundant. There were multiple regurgitant jets in 3 of 5 patients in this group. In the remaining 3 of 8 patients, the valve had a normal appearance and regurgitation was the result of lack of complete leaflet coaptation. All 8 patients underwent tricuspid valvuloplasty, and all experienced a decrease in regurgitation. In 5 of 8 patients, there was a reduction in insufficiency of 2 grades of severity, and in 3 of 8 there was a 1 grade improvement. Tricuspid valve stenosis was not documented after operation. In 7 of 8 patients, RV function was assessed as fair before repair and improved to good in 5 of 7 after the procedure. The remaining patient had good function both at baseline and after repair. Moderate to severe TR is a common finding in hypoplastic left heart patients. Tricuspid valvuloplasty carried a high success rate in this group and was associated with improved function. Although this represents only a small number of patients, the results are impressive. TR assessment by echo Doppler assessment remains a semiquanitative measure at best. By decreasing ventricular size with the Fontan or hemi-Fontan operation, TR is usually reduced without tricuspid valvuloplasty. Hopefully, other centers will report their data regarding TR before and after repair in these patients and appropriate guidelines can be developed as to which patients will benefit from valvuloplasty at the time of repair.

Congenital Mitral Valve Insufficiency

Chauvaud and associates[79] from Paris, France, report 145 patients who were operated on for congenital mitral valve regurgitation by means of the Carpentier's technique in a single center. These patients were younger than 12 years of age with a mean age of 6 years ranging from 0.17 to 12 years. Mitral

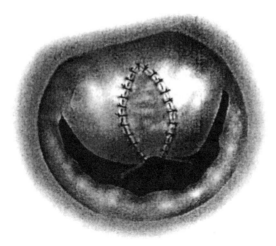

FIGURE 9-30. Cleft leaflet closed with a pericardial patch. Reproduced with permission from Chauvaud et al.[79]

regurgitation associated with AV septal defect, AV discordance, straddling mitral valve, acquired disease, Marfan syndrome, and degenerative disease were excluded from this study. According to the Carpentier classification, 31 patients had normal leaflet motion, 79 patients had leaflet prolapse, and 35 had restricted leaflet motion, with 15 having normal papillary muscles and 20 abnormal papillary muscles. There were associated lesions in 35%. A conservative operation was possible in 138 patients (95%) and among them, 70 patients required a prosthetic annuloplasty and 21 patients required valve extension with a pericardial patch (Figures 9-30–9-32). In-hospital mortality was 5% and mean follow-up was 9 ± 7 years with a range of 1 to 26 years. There were 10 late deaths, and actuarial survival at 10 years was 88% of patients who underwent valve repair and 51% of patients who underwent valve replacement. Late reoperation was required in 15% of patients who had undergone valve repair

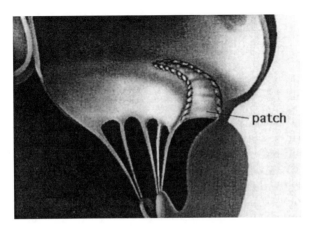

FIGURE 9-31. Hammock mitral valve. Posterior leaflet extension with pericardial patch. Reproduced with permission from Chauvaud et al.[79]

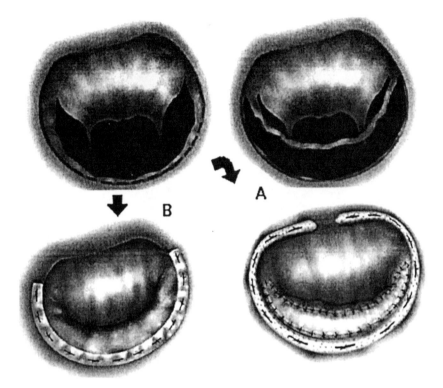

FIGURE 9-32. Restricted leaflet motion resulting from short chordae, associated with annular dilatation. Pericardial patch enlargement and prosthetic ring **(A)** compared with semicircular plication **(B).** Reproduced with permission from Chauvaud et al.[79]

and in 28% of patients with valve replacement. Causes of reoperation were recurrent LV failure in 1, residual or recurrent MR in 17, MS in 3, and calcification of bioprosthesis in 2. Actuarial freedom from reoperation was 68% at 15 years and there were no thromboembolic events in any group. Conservative surgery with Carpentier's technique is feasible in the majority of cases with congenital mitral insufficiency of these particular types. These techniques are extremely useful to avoid the problems associated with valve replacement anticoagulation in the young patient.

Cryopreserved Homografts

Mitchell and associates[80] from Boston, Massachusetts, studied 33 explanted left-sided or right-sided cryopreserved human allograft heart valves several hours to 9 years after operation, 14 nonimplanted allografts, and 16 aortic valves removed from transplanted allograft hearts 2 days to 4 years after operation. Cryopreserved valves had no viable cells, distorted but preserved collagen, and no evidence for immunological reactions. Valves from transplanted hearts showed remarkable structural preservation and evidence for inflammation. These results are in marked contrast to the findings by Rajani et al. (*J Thorac Cardiovasc Surg* 1997;115:111–117) of rejection of cryopreserved homograft cardiac valves in infants. The question of possible graft rejection of cryopreserved homografts is clinically important since immunotherapy might be considered in certain patients if there were more data to suggest immunological problems. This continues to be an active area of investigation.

Miscellaneous

Neonatal Vascular Thrombosis

Farnoux and associates[81] from Paris, France, report 16 patients with neonatal vascular thrombosis treated with recombinant tissue plasminogen activator (RTPA). Flow restoration was complete in 7 patients, partial in 7, and absent in 2. The safety of this technique was satisfactory provided contraindications were respected. Thrombosis continues to be a major problem in postoperative complex congenital heart disease patients. Frequently it is associated with indwelling catheters and prolonged intensive care. Rapid diagnosis and treatment are necessary in these patients to optimize survival. This study and the succeeding one (J Pediatr 1998;133:133–136) indicate that RTPA can be useful in this setting.

Markers of Adverse Events in Children

Duke and associates[82] from Victoria, Australia, attempted to determine physiological variables that predict major adverse events in children in the intensive care unit after cardiac operations. There were 90 patients undergoing open heart surgery for simple and complex congenital cardiac defects. The median age was 2.65 months with a range of 0.5 to 5.7 months. The median duration of cardiopulmonary bypass was 103 minutes and the median cross-clamp time was 51 minutes (range 40–71 minutes). Circulatory arrest was used in 21% of the operations. Major adverse events were prospectively identified as cardiac arrest, need for emergency chest opening, development of multiple organ failure, and death. There were 12 major adverse events and 4 deaths. Only blood lactate level, mean arterial pressure, and duration of cardiopulmonary bypass were significant independent predictors of major adverse events when measured at the time of admission to the intensive care unit. Independent significant predictors of major adverse events were lactate and carbon dioxide difference 4 hours after admission and lactate and base deficit 8 hours after admission. The odds ratios for major adverse events if the blood lactate level was greater than 4 mmol/L at 4 and 8 hours were 8.3 and 9.3, respectively. At no time in the first 24 hours were cardiac output, oxygen delivery, mixed venous oxygen saturation, toe-core temperature gradient, or heart rate significant predictors of major adverse events. These data suggest that routine determination of blood lactate level may add to the ability to prospectively identify patients at high risk for major adverse events and hopefully intervene to prevent these complications.

Right Atrial Isomerism

Hashmi and associates[83] from Toronto, Ontario, Canada, studied outcome of over 26 years of 91 consecutive patients with asplenia and RA isomerism. Most patients (89%) presented within the first month of life—62% at birth. Cardiac abnormalities included common AV valve in 81%, ventricular hypoplasia or single ventricle in 73%, abnormal ventriculoarterial connections in 96%, pulmonary outflow obstruction in 84%, anomalous pulmonary venous drainage in 87%, and pulmonary venous obstruction in 30%. The overall mortality was 69%. No interventions were planned or performed in 24%, and 95% of these died. The mortality rate for patients requiring their first operation in the neonatal period was 75% versus 51% for those with later first operations. The surgical mortality for patients undergoing pulmonary vein repair was 95%. Overall survival estimates were 71% at 1 month, 49% at 1 year, and 35% at 5 years. Independent risk factors for early death include the absence of pulmonary outflow obstruction, presence of major AV valve anomaly, and obstructed pulmonary veins. Despite the high mortality/morbidity rates in this patient group with complex anatomy, Fontan procedures can be successful for those patients who can be palliated successfully in early infancy. Only 3 patients were identified as having sepsis as the primary cause of death, although accurate records for cause of death were not always available. Successful transplantation has been performed in patients with heterotaxy syndrome with reported 5 years survival rates of 65% by the Loma Linda group. (*J Am Cardiol* 1997; 29A:105).

Pediatric Primary Benign Cardiac Tumors

An increase in the frequency of primary cardiac tumors has been reported since the development or enhancement of noninvasive imaging modalities. Beghetti and associates[84] from Toronto, Canada, identified 56 children with primary cardiac tumors. Forty-four (78%) children had rhabdomyomas, 6 (11%) had fibromas, 1 (2%) had pericardial teratoma, 1 (2%) had epicardial lipoma, 1 (2%) had multicystic hamartoma, and 3 (5%) had unspecified tumors. The mean age at diagnosis was 19 ± 35 months (median 4.7 months, range 0.03 to 204 months), excluding 12 patients who were given the diagnosis before birth. Among 27,640 patients assessed for cardiac disease, the frequency of tumors was 0.06% (1980–1984), 0.22% (1985–1989), and 0.32% (1990–1995). Diagnosis was made in 55 of 56 patients by echocardiography. Catheterization was performed in 5 patients and magnetic resonance imaging in 9. No tumor-related deaths occurred. Nine patients had surgery because of hemodynamically significant obstruction or arrhythmias. Partial or complete regression occurred in 25 (54%) of 44 patients with rhabdomyomas. Overall, the prognosis was excellent. Individualized surgery allowed early safe treatment of symptomatic tumors.

1. Ogawa S, Fukazawa R, Ohkubo T, Zhang J, Takechi N, Kuramochi Y, Hino Y, Jimbo O, Katsube Y, Kamisago M, Genma Y, Yamamoto M: Silent myocardial ischemia in Kawasaki disease. Circulation 1997 (November 18);96:3384–3389.
2. Beiser AS, Takahashi M, Baker AL, Sundel RP, Newburger JW, for the US multicenter Kawasaki Disease Study Group: A predictive instrument for coronary artery aneurysms in Kawasaki disease. Am J Cardiol 1998 (May 1);81:1116–1120.
3. Sakopoulos AG, Hahn TL, Turrentine M, Brown JW: Surgery for congenital heart disease: Recurrent aortic coarctation: Is surgical repair still the gold standard? J Thorac Cardiovasc Surg 1998 (October);116:560–565.
4. Saidi AS, Bezold LI, Altman CA, Ayres NA, Bricker JT: Outcome of pregnancy following intervention for coarctation of the aorta. Am J Cardiol 1998 (September 15);82:786–788.
5. Ebeid MR, Prieto LR, Latson LA: Use of balloon-expandable stents for coarctation of the aorta: Initial results and intermediate-term follow-up. J Am Coll Cardiol 1997 (December);30:1847–1852.
6. Karl TR, Cochrane A, Brizard CPR: Arterial switch operations: surgical solutions to complex problems. Tex Heart Inst J 1997 (November);24:322–333.
7. Williams WG, Quaegebeur JM, Kirklin JW, Blackstone EH: Outflow obstruction after the arterial switch operation: A multiinstitutional study. J Thorac Cardiovasc Surg 1997 (December);114:975–990.
8. Foran JP, Sullivan ID, Elliott MJ, DeLeval MR: Primary arterial switch operation for transposition of the great arteries with intact ventricular septum in infants older than 21 days. J Am Coll Cardiol 1998 (March);31:883–889.
9. Massin M, Hovels-Gurich H, Dabritz S, Messmer B, Bernuth GV: Results of the Bruce treadmill test in children after arterial switch operation for simple transposition of the great arteries. Am J Cardiol 1998 (January 1);81:56–60.
10. Soongswang J, Adatia I, Newman C, Smallhorn JF, Williams WG, Freedom RM: Mortality in potential arterial switch candidates with transposition of the great arteries. J Am Coll Cardiol 1998 (September);32:753–757.
11. Metras D, Kreitmann B, Riberi A, Yao JG, El-Khoury E, Wernert F, Pannetier-Mille A: Extending the concept of the autograft for complete repair of transposition of the great arteries with ventricular septal defect and left ventricular outflow tract obstruction: A report of ten cases of a modified procedure. J Thorac Cardiovasc Surg 1997 (November);114:746–754.
12. Metras D, Kreitmann B, Riberi A, Yao JG, El-Khoury E, Wernert F, Pannetier-Mille A: Extending the concept of the autograft for complete repair of transposition of the great arteries with ventricular septal defect and left ventricular outflow tract obstruction: A report of ten cases of a modified procedure. J Thorac Cardiovasc Surg 1997 (November);114:746–754.
13. Lynch KP, Da'Cheng BA, Sharma S, Dhar PK, Fyfe DA: Serial echocardiographic assessment of left atrioventricular valve function in young children with ventricular inversion. Am Heart J 1998 (July);136:94–98.
14. Prieto LR, DeCamillo DM, Konrad DJ, Scalet-Longworth L, Latson LA: Comparison of cost and clinical outcome between transcatheter coil occlusion and surgical closure of isolated patent ductus arteriosus. Pediatrics 1998 (June);101:1020–1024.
15. Daniels CJ, Cassidy SC, Teske DW, Wheller JJ, Allen HD: Reopening after successful coil occlusion for patent ductus arteriosus. J Am Coll Cardiol 1998 (February);31:444–450.
16. Masura J, Walsh KP, Thanopoulous B, Chan C, Bass J, Goussous Y, Gavora P, Hijazi ZM: Catheter closure of moderate-to large-sized patent ductus arteriosus using the new Amplatzer duct occluder: immediate and short-term results. J Am Coll Cardiol 1998 (March 15);31:878–882.
17. Lloyd TR, Rydberg A, Ludomirsky A, Teien DE, Shim D, Beekman RH, Mosca

RS, Bove EL: Late fenestration closure in the hypoplastic left heart syndrome: Comparison of hemodynamic changes. Am Heart J 1998 (August);136:302–306.

18. Kitagawa T, Durham III LA, Mosca RS, Bove EL: Techniques and results in the management of multiple ventricular septal defects. J Thorac Cardiovasc Surg 1998 (April);115:848–856.

19. Reddy VM, McElhinney DB, Brook MM, Parry AJ, Hanley FL: Atrioventricular valve function after single patch repair of complete atrioventricular septal defect in infancy: How early should repair be attempted? J Thorac Cardiovasc Surg 1998 (May);115:1032–1040.

20. Jacobs ML, Blackstone EH, Bailey LL, The Congenital Heart Surgeons Society: Intermediate survival in neonates with aortic atresia: A multi-institutional study. J Thorac Cardiovasc Surg 1998 (September);116:417–431.

21. McElhinney DB, Reddy VM, Silverman NH, Hanley FL: Modified Damus-Kaye-Stansel procedure for single ventricle, subaortic stenosis, and arch obstruction in neonates and infants: Midterm results and techniques for avoiding circulatory arrest. J Thorac Cardiovasc Surg 1997 (November);114:718–726.

22. Tchervenkov CI, Salasidis G, Cecere R, Beland MJ, Jutras L, Paquet M, Dobell ARC: One-stage midline unifocalization and complete repair in infancy versus multiple-stage unifocalization followed by repair for complex heart disease with major aorto-pulmonary collaterals. J Thorac Cardiovasc Surg 1997 (November);114:727–737.

23. Ovaert C, Oureshi SA, Rosenthal E, Baker EJ, Tynan M: Growth of the right ventricle after successful transcatheter pulmonary valvotomy in neonates and infants with pulmonary atresia and intact ventricular septum. J Thorac Cardiovasc Surg 1998 (May);115:1055–1062.

24. Daubeney PEF, Sharland GK, Cook AC, Keeton BR, Anderson RH, Webber SA: Pulmonary atresia with intact ventricular septum: Impact of fetal echocardiography on incidence at birth and postnatal outcome. Circulation 1998 (August 11);98: 562–566.

25. Moran AM, Hornberger LK, Jonas RA, Keane JF: Development of a double chambered right ventricle after repair of tetralogy of Fallot. J Am Coll Cardiol 1998 (April);31:1127–1133.

26. Nollert G, Fischlein T, Bouterwek S, Bohmer C, Klinner W, Reichart B: Long-term survival in patients with repair of tetralogy of Fallot: 36-year follow-up of 490 survivors of the first year after surgical repair. J Am Coll Cardiol 1997 (November 1);30:1374–1383.

27. Singh GK, Greenbert SB, Yap YS, Delany DP, Keeton BR, Monro JL: Right ventricular function and exercise performance late after primary repair of tetralogy of Fallot with the transannular patch in infancy. Am J Cardiol 1998 (June 1);1378–1382.

28. Munkhammar P, Cullen SH, Jogi P, De Leval M, Elliott M, Norgard G: Early age at repair prevents restrictive right ventricular physiology after surgery for tetralogy of Fallot, diastolic RV function after TOF repair in infancy. J Am Coll Cardiol 1998 (October);32:1083–1087.

29. Kurosawa H, Morita K, Yamagishi M, Shimizu S, Becker AE, Anderson RH: Conotruncal repair for tetralogy of Fallot: Midterm results. J Thorac Cardiovasc Surg 1998 (February);115:351–360.

30. Harrison DA, Harris L, Siu SC, MacLoghlin CJ, Connelly MS, Webb GD, Downar E, McLaughlin PR, Williams WG: Sustained ventricular tachycardia in adult patients late after repair of tetralogy of Fallot. J Am Coll Cardiol 1997 (November); 30:1368–1373.

31. Brauner R, Laks H, Drinkwater DC, Shvarts O, Eghbali K, Galindo A: Benefits of early surgical repair in fixed subaortic stenosis. J Am Coll Cardiol 1997 (December); 30:1835–1842.

32. D'Souza SJA, Tsai WK, Silver MM, Chait P, Benson LN, Silverman E, Hebert D, Balfe JW: Diagnosis and management of stenotic aorto-arteriopathy in childhood. J Pediatr 1998 (June);132:1016–1022.

33. Bezold LI, Smith EO, Kelly K, Colan SD, Gauvreau K, Geva T: Development and validation of an echocardiographic model for predicting progression of discrete subaortic stenosis in children. Am J Cardiol 1998 (February 1);81:314–320.

34. Kovalchin JP, Brook MM, Rosenthal GL, Suda K, Hoffman JIE, Silverman NH: Echocardiographic hemodynamic and morphometric predictors of survival after two-ventricle repair in infants with critical aortic stenosis. J Am Coll Cardiol 1998 (July);32:237–244.

35. Reddy VM, McElhinney DB, Phoon CK, Brook MM, Hanley FL: Geometric mismatch of pulmonary and aortic annuli in children undergoing the Ross procedure: Implications for surgical management and autograft valve function. J Thorac Cardiovasc Surg 1998 (June);115:1255–1263.

36. Stark J, Bull C, Stajevic M, Jothi M, Elliott M, de Leval M: Fate of subpulmonary homograft conduits: Determinants of late homograft failure. J Thorac Cardiovasc Surg 1998 (March);115:506–516.

37. Benson DW, Sharkey A, Fatkin D, Lang P, Basson CT, McDonough B, Strauss AW, Seidman JG, Seidman CE: Reduced penetrance, variable expressivity, and genetic heterogeneity of familial atrial septal defects. Circulation 1998 (May 26);97:2043–2048.

38. Najm HK, Coles JG, Endo M, Stephens D, Rebeyka IM, Williams WG, Freedom RM: Complete atrioventricular septal defects: Results of repair, risk factors and freedom from reoperation. Circulation 1997 (November 4);96(Suppl II):II-311–II-315.

39. Michielon G, Stellin G, Rizzoli G, Casarotto DC: Repair of complete common atrioventricular canal defects in patients younger than four months of age. Circulation 1997 (November 4);96(Suppl II):II-316–II-322.

40. Chen SJ, Li YW, Wang JK, Wu MH, Chiu IS, Chang CI, Hsieh SC, Su CT, Hsu JCY, Lue HC: Usefulness of electron beam computed tomography in children with heterotaxy syndrome. Am J Cardiol 1998 (January 15);81:188–194.

41. Andrew M, Michelson AD, Bovill E, Leaker M, Massicotte MP: Guidelines for antithrombotic therapy in pediatric patients. J Pediatr 1998 (April);132:575–588.

42. Locati EH, Zareba W, Moss AJ, Schwartz PJ, Vincent M, Lehmann MH, Towbin JA, Priori SG, Napolitano C, Rovinson JL, Andrews M, Timothy K, Hall WJ: Age- and sex-related differences in clinical manifestations in patients with congenital long QT syndrome findings from the international LQTS registry. Circulation 1998 (June 9);97:2237–2244.

43. Ragonese P, Drago F, Guccione P, Santilli A, Silvetti MS, Agostino DA: Permanent overdrive atrial pacing in the chronic management of recurrent postoperative atrial reentrant tachycardia in patients with complex congenital heart disease. PACE 1997 (December);20(Pt. I):2917–2923.

44. Janousek J, Paul T, for the Working Group on Pediatric Arrhythmias and Electrophysiology of the Association of European Pediatric Cardiologists: Safety of oral propafenone in the treatment of arrhythmias in infants and children (European Retrospective Multicenter Study). Am J Cardiol 1998 (May 1);81:1121–1124.

45. Tanel RE, Walsh EP, Triedman JK, Epstein MR, Bergau DM, Saul JP: Five-year experience with radiofrequency catheter ablation: Implications for management of arrhythmias in pediatric and young adult patients. J Pediatr 1998 (December);131:878–887.

46. Rivera ES, Kimball TR, Bailey WW, Witt SA, Khoury PR, Daniels SR: Effect of veno-venous ultrafiltration on myocardial performance immediately after cardiac surgery in children. J Am Coll Cardiol 1998 (September);32:766–772.

47. Allen HD, Beekman III RH, Garson Jr. A, Hijazi ZM, Mullins C, O'Laughlin MP, Taubert KA: Pediatric therapeutic cardiac catheterization: A statement for healthcare professionals from the Council on Cardiovascular Disease in the Young. Circulation 1998 (February);97:609–625.

48. Allen BS, Rahman S, Ilbawi MN, Kronon M, Bolling KS, Halldorsson AO, Feinberg H: Detrimental effects of cardiopulmonary bypass in cyanotic infants: Preventing the reoxygentation injury. Ann Thorac Surg 1997 (November);64:1381–1388.

49. Shaffer KM, Mullins CE, Grifka RG, O'Laughlin MP, McMahon W, Ing FF, Nihill MR: Intravascular stents in congenital heart disease: Short- and long-term results from a large single-center experience. J Am Coll Cardiol 1998 (March 1);31:661–667.

50. Donnelly JP, Raffel DM, Shulkin BL, Corbett JR, Bove EL, Mosca RS, Kulik TJ:

Resting coronary flow and coronary flow reserve in human infants after repair or palliation of congenital heart defects as measured by positron emission tomography. J Thorac Cardiovasc Surg 1998 (January);115:103–110.

51. Singh TP, DiCarli MF, Sullivan NM, Leonen MF, Morrow WR: Myocardial flow reserve in long-term survivors of repair of anomalous left coronary artery from pulmonary artery. J Am Coll Cardiol 1998 (February);31:437–443.

52. Spyrou N, Philpot J, Foale R, Camici PG, Muntoni F: Evidence of LV dysfunction in children with merosin-deficient congenital muscular dystrophy. Am Heart J 1998 (September);136:474–476.

53. Goldmuntz E, Clark BJ, Mitchell LE, Jawad AF, Cuneo BF, Reed L, McDonald-McGinn D, Chien P, Feuer J, Zackai EH, Emanuel BS, Driscoll DA: Frequency of 22q11 deletions in patients with conotruncal defects. J Am Coll Cardiol 1998 (August);32:492–498.

54. Reddy VM, McElhinney DB, Silverman NH, Marianeschi SM, Hanley FL: Partial biventricular repair for complex congenital heart defects: An intermediate option for complicated anatomy or functionally borderline right complex heart. J Thorac Cardiovasc Surg 1998 (July);116:21–27.

55. Phoon CKL, Silverman NH: Conditions with right ventricular pressure and volume overload, and a small left ventricle: "Hypoplastic" left ventricle or simply a squashed ventricle? J Am Coll Cardiol 1997 (November 15);30:1547–1553.

56. Lutterman J, Scott M, Nass R, Geva T: Moyamoya syndrome associated with congenital heart disease. Pediatrics 1998 (January);101:57–60.

57. Buyon JP, Hiebert R, Copel J, Craft J, Friedman D, Katholi M, Lee LA, Provost TT, Reichlin M, Rider L, Rupel A, Saleeb S, Weston WL, Skovron ML: Autoimmune-associated congenital heart block: Demographics, mortality, morbidity and recurrence rates obtained from a national neonatal lupus registry. J Am Coll Cardiol 1998 (June);31:1658–1666.

58. Banerjee A, Mendelsohn AM, Knilans TK, Meyer RA, Schwartz DC: Effect of myocardial hypertrophy on systolic and diastolic function in children: Insights from the force-frequency and relaxation-frequency relationships. J Am Coll Cardiol 1998 (October);32:1088–1095.

59. Yetman AT, Freedom RB, McCrindle BW: Outcome in cyanotic neonates with Ebstein's anomaly. Am J Cardiol 1998 (March 15);81:749–754.

60. Hetzer R, Nagdyman N, Ewert P, Weng YG, Alexi-Meskhisvili V, Berger F, Pasic M, Lange PE: A modified repair technique for tricuspid incompetence in Ebstein's anomaly. J Thorac Cardiovasc Surg 1998 (April);115:857–868.

61. Maron BJ, Moller JH, Seidman CE, Vincent GM, Dietz HC, Moss AJ, Towbin JA, Sondheimer HM, Pyeritz RE, McGee G, Epstein AE: Impact of laboratory molecular diagnosis on contemporary diagnostic criteria for genetically transmitted cardiovascular diseases: Hypertrophic cardiomyopathy, long-QT syndrome, and Marfan syndrome. A statement for healthcare professionals from the councils on clinical cardiology, cardiovascular disease in the young, and basic science. Circulation 1998 (October 6);98:1460–1471.

62. Shaddy RE: β-Blocker therapy in young children with congestive heart failure under consideration for heart transplantation. Am Heart J 1998 (July);136:19–21.

63. Buckhorn R, Bartmus D, Siekmeyer W, Hulpke-Wette M, Schulz R, Bursch J: Beta-blocker therapy of severe congestive heart failure in infants with left to right shunts. Am J Cardiol 1998 (June 1);81:1366–1368.

64. Charron P, Dubourg O, Desnos M, Bennaceur M, Carrier L, Camproux AC, Isnard R, Hagege A, Langlard JM, Bonne G, Richard P, Haique B, Bouhour JB, Schwartz K, Komajda M: Clinical features and prognostic implications of familial hypertrophic cardiomyopathy related to the cardiac myosin-binding protein c gene. Circulation 1998 (June 9);97:2230–2236.

65. Corrado D, Basso C, Schiavon M, Thiene G: Screening for hypertrophic cardiomyopathy in young athletes. N Engl J Med 1998 (August 6);339:364–369.

66. Weindling SN, Saul JP, Gamble WJ, Mayer JE, Wessel D, Walsh EP: Duration of complete atrioventricular block after congenital heart disease surgery. Am J Cardiol 1998 (August 15);82:525–527.

67. Hannan EL, Racz M, Kavey RE, Quaegebeur JM, Williams R: Pediatric cardiac surgery: The effect of hospital and surgeon volume on in-hospital mortality. Pediatrics 1998 (June);101:963–969.
68. Bartram U, Grunenfelder J, Praagh RV: Causes of death after the modified Norwood procedure: A study of 122 postmortem cases. Ann Thorac Surg 1997 (December); 64:1795–1802.
69. McElhinney DB, Reddy VM, Tworetzky W, Silverman NH, Hanley FL: Early and late results after repair of aortopulmonary septal defect and associated anomalies in infants less than 6 months of age. Am J Cardiol 1998 (January 15);81:195–201.
70. Lacour-Gayet F, Serraf A, Galletti L, Bruniaux J, Belli E, Piot D, Touchot A, Petit J, Houyel L, Planche C: Biventricular repair of conotruncal anomalies associated with aortic arch obstruction 103 patients. Circulation 1997 (November 4);96(Suppl II):II-328–II-334.
71. Apfel HD, Levenbraun J, Quaegebeur JM, Allan LD: Usefulness of preoperative echocardiography in predicting left ventricular outflow obstruction after primary repair of interrupted aortic arch with ventricular septal defect. Am J Cardiol 1998 (August 15);82:470–473.
72. Mertens L, Hagler DJ, Sauer U, Somerville J, Gewillig M: Protein-losing enteropathy after the Fontan operation: An international multicenter study. J Thorac Cardiovasc Surg 1998 (May);115:1063–1073.
73. Hsu DT, Quaegebeur JM, Ing FF, Selber EJ, Lamour JM, Gersony WM: Outcome after the single-stage, nonfenestrated Fontan procedure. Circulation 1997 (November 4);96(Suppl II) II-335–II-340.
74. Monagle P, Cochrane A, McCrindle B, Benson L, Williams W, Andrew M: Thromboembolic complications after Fontan procedures: The role of prophylactic anticoagulation. J Thorac Cardiovasc Surg 1998 (March);115:493–498.
75. Mavroudis C, Backer CL, Deal BJ, Johnsrude CL: Fontan conversion to cavopulmonary connection and arrhythmia circuit cryoablation. J Thorac Cardiovasc Surg 1998 (March);115:547–556.
76. Alehan D, Ozkutlu S: Beneficial effects of 1-year captopril therapy in children with chronic AR who have no symptoms. Am Heart J 1998 (April);135:598–603.
77. Rajani B, Mee RB, Ratliff NB: Evidence for rejection of homograft cardiac valves in infants. J Thorac Cardiovasc Surg 1998 (January);115:111–117.
78. Reyes A, Bove EL, Mosca RS, Kulik TJ, Ludomirsky A: Tricuspid valve repair in children with hypoplastic left heart syndrome during staged surgical reconstruction. Circulation 1997 (November 4);96(Suppl II) II-341–II-345.
79. Chauvaud S, Fuzellier JF, Houel R, Berrebi A, Mihaileanu S, Carpentier A: Reconstructive surgery in congenital mitral valve insufficiency (Carpentier's techniques): Long-term results. J Thorac Cardiovasc Surg 1998 (January);115:84–93.
80. Mitchell RN, Jonas RA, Schoen Frederick J: Pathology of explanted cryopreserved allograft heart valves: Comparison with aortic valves from orthotopic heart transplants. J Thorac Cardiovasc Surg 1998 (January);115:118–127.
81. Farnoux C, Camard O, Pinquier D, Hurtaud-Roux MF, Sebag G, Schlegel N, Beaufils F: Recombinant tissue-type plasminogen activator therapy of thrombosis in 16 neonates. J Pediatr 1998 (July);133:137–140.
82. Duke T, Butt W, South M, Karl TR: Early markers of major adverse events in children after cardiac operations. J Thorac Cardiovasc Surg 1997 (December);114:1042–1052.
83. Hashmi A, Abu-Sulaiman RA, McCrindle BW, Smallhorn JF, Williams WG, Freedom RM: Management and outcomes of right atrial isomerism: A 26-year experience. J Am Coll Cardiol 1998 (April);31:1120–1126.
84. Beghetti M, Gow RM, Haney I, Mawson J, Williams WG, Freed S: Pediatric primary benign cardiac tumors during 15 years. Am Heart J 1997 (December);134:1107–1114.

10

Transplantation

Transplantation (General Topics)

L-Type Calcium Channels in Failing and Nonfailing Hearts in Transplant Recipients

Schröder and colleagues[1] in Hamburg, Germany, investigated the properties of L-type calcium channels in LV myocytes isolated from nonfailing donor hearts (n = 16 cells) or failing hearts of transplant recipients with dilated (n = 9) or ischemic (n = 7) cardiomyopathy. The single-channel recording technique was used. Peak average currents were significantly enhanced in CHF versus non-CHF control hearts because of an elevation of channel availability and open probability within active sweeps. These differences closely resembled the effects of a cAMP-dependent stimulation with 8-Br-cAMP. Kinetic analysis of the slow gating showed that channels from CHF hearts remained available for a longer time, suggesting a defect in the dephosphorylation. The phosphatase inhibitor, okadaic acid, was unable to stimulate channel activity in myocytes from hearts with CHF. Expression of calcium channel subunits was measured by Northern blot analysis. Expression of the α_{1C}- and β-subunits was unaltered. Whole-cell current measurements did not reveal an increase of current density with CHF. Thus, individual L-type calcium channels are fundamentally affected in severe human CHF. This may be important in the known impairment of cardiac excitation-contraction coupling.

Plasma Levels of Oxidized Low Density Lipoprotein

Holvoet and coinvestigators[2] in Leuven, Belgium, used the monoclonal antibody 4E6-based ELISA to quantify levels of oxidized LDL in plasma of 65 control subjects, 47 patients transplanted for dilated cardiomyopathy, and 60 patients transplanted for CAD. Levels of oxidized LDL were 0.68 mg/dL, 1.27 mL/dL, and 1.73 mL/dL, respectively. Levels of oxidized LDL were significantly lower in transplanted patients with angiographically normal coronary arteries than in patients with mild or severe coronary artery stenosis (Figure 10-1). Logistic regression analysis identified 3 parameters that were significantly and independently correlated with post-transplant CAD: plasma levels of oxidized LDL, length of follow-up, and donor age. Thus, the study demonstrates that plasma levels of oxidized LDL correlate with the extent of CAD in transplant patients and suggests that elevated levels of oxidized LDL may be a marker for CAD.

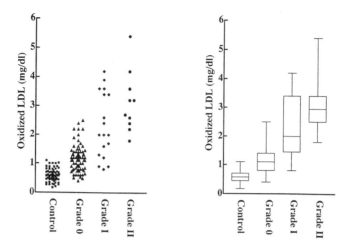

FIGURE 10-1. Scatter **(left)** and box-and-whisker **(right)** graphs illustrating individual oxidized LDL values and the distribution of oxidized LDL levels in control subjects and patients with grade 0, grade 1, and grade 2 post-transplant coronary artery stenosis. Whiskers extend from minimum to maximum values. Reproduced with permission from Holvoet et al.[2]

Comparison of Clinical and Morphological Cardiac Findings

Waller and colleagues[3] from Dallas, Texas, compared intergroup and intragroup clinical and morphological findings in patients with ischemic cardiomyopathy (IC), idiopathic dilated cardiomyopathy (IDC), and dilated hypertrophic cardiomyopathy (HC) undergoing cardiac transplantation (Table 10-1). Few previous publications have described findings in native hearts explanted at the time of CT. The explanted hearts in 92 patients undergoing cardiac transplantation were examined in uniform manner with particular attention to the sizes of the ventricular cavities and the presence of and extent of ventricular scarring. Of the 92 hearts examined, 47 had IC, 35 had IDC, and 10 had dilated HC. Although considerable degrees of intragroup variation occurred, the mean degree of LV dilatation was similar among the patients with IC, IDC, and dilated HC. All patients with IC had LV free wall scarring that was more extensive than that involving the ventricular septum, but the intragroup variation in the amounts of scarring was considerable. Nine of the 10 patients with dilated HC also had ventricular wall scarring, but it was more extensive in the ventricular septum than in the LV free wall and involvement of the RV wall also was present. Eight (23%) of the 35 IDC patients also had grossly visible ventricular scars, but they were small and only 1 of the 8 had coronary narrowing and that was not in the distribution of the scarring. Narrowing of 1 or more epicardial coronary arteries more than 75% in cross-sectional area by plaque was present in all 47 IC patients, in 8 of the 35 IDC patients (7 had no ventricular scars), and in none of the 10 dilated HC patients. Coronary angiography was the major clinical tool allowing separation of the IC, IDC, and HC patients. Coronary angiography did not detect narrowing in any of the 8 patients with IDC who were found to have coronary narrowing on anatomic study. Thus, among patients with IC, IDC, and dilated HC having cardiac transplantation, distinctive

TABLE 10-1
Clinical and Morphological Findings in the 47 Patients With Ischemic Cardiomyopathy

Pt. No.	Age (yr)	Sex	Interval (mo) S→CT	HW (g)	BW (kg)	T	CABG (grafts)	CA >75%↓	LVMD (cm)	H (%)	TC (mg/dL)	TG (mg/dL)	LVEDD (cm)	LVESD (cm)
							Morphology				**Laboratory**		**Echocardiogram**	
1	42	M	12	325	70	0	0	4	5.5	44	308	138	—	—
2	43	M	5	380	64	0	0	3	7.0	23	241	286	—	—
3	43	M	60	450	—	+(LV)	0	1	5.5	—	308	—	—	—
4	43	M	6	—	—	0	0	2	—	—	—	—	—	—
5	45	M	8	475	76	0	0	1	6.5	30	135	50	7.4	6.4
6	45	M	—	305	—	0	+(4)	4	4.0	—	—	—	—	—
7	46	F	4	365	73	0	+(4)	3	—	41	126	243	5.0	4.0
8	46	M	14	—	74	0	+(1)	3	—	50	168	—	—	—
9	49	M	8	351	58	0	+(3)	4	5.0	38	252	74	6.2	5.5
10	49	M	24	490	72	0	0	3	6.5	39	167	188	8.0	—
11	50	M	15	345	91	0	0	1	5.0	43	162	316	6.2	4.8
12	50	M	84	570	89	0	+(1)	3	6.0	42	125	115	6.5	5.8
13	50	M	30	395	78	0	0	3	6.5	30	180	97	5.5	4.8
14	51	M	11	440	73	0	+(2)	4	—	34	247	278	6.9	6.3
15	51	M	30	565	71	+(LV)	0	3	5.0	40	242	115	—	—
16	51	M	36	503	72	0	+(3)	3	5.0	46	155	54	7.0	6.0
17	51	M	7	450	70	0	0	2	5.5	32	194	90	—	—
18	52	M	41	510	75	0	+(2)	3	4.0	32	334	296	8.0	7.0
19	52	M	24	565	—	0	+(3)	3	5.0	—	240	—	—	—
20	53	M	6	260	—	0	0	3	—	33	260	658	4.3	2.9
21	53	M	11	535	96	0	+(4)	3	6.3	42	264	—	—	—
22	54	M	1	500	—	0	0	3	—	—	226	—	—	—
23	55	M	108	490	74	0	+(3)	4	5.5	37	158	156	6.0	5.5
24	55	M	—	430	—	0	+(3)	3	—	—	—	—	—	—
25	56	M	240	520	85	0	+(3)	2	6.0	43	204	180	6.5	—
26	56	M	15	430	82	0	0	4	6.0	39	280	501	—	—
27	56	F	60	385	50	0	0	3	6.0	30	219	168	6.2	5.7
28	56	M	33	720	103	0	0	2	7.9	31	240	123	7.4	6.2
29	56	M	36	—	—	0	+(4)	4	—	—	—	—	—	—
30	57	M	24	415	77	0	0	3	5.5	37	183	96	6.5	5.0
31	57	M	144	535	90	0	+(2)	3	6.5	34	227	147	8.0	—
32	57	M	4	—	—	0	+(4)	3	—	31	174	—	—	—
33	57	M	1	—	—	0	0	1	—	—	—	—	—	—
34	58	M	11	352	75	0	+(4)	4	—	35	281	147	4.3	3.8
35	58	M	56	580	99	0	+(4)	1	3.5	38	267	170	—	—
36	58	M	12	590	70	0	+(4)	4	6.6	37	132	—	—	—
37	59	M	8	390	—	0	0	1	5.5	—	—	—	7.0	6.5
38	59	M	13	490	88	0	+(3)	3	5.3	35	105	65	6.5	5.1
39	60	M	21	365	72	+(LV)	0	2	6.0	42	146	69	7.5	6.0
40	60	M	31	610	74	0	0	2	6.0	30	131	106	6.0	—
41	61	M	12	690	94	0	+(4)	3	6.5	39	198	147	5.7	4.2
42	61	M	47	385	77	0	+(4)	3	6.7	36	202	73	6.4	6.1
43	62	F	120	480	66	0	0	3	6.5	35	161	232	7.8	7.1
44	62	M	24	503	68	0	0	2	6.5	40	217	—	8.8	7.2
45	63	M	13	450	84	0	+(3)	3	4.5	33	209	83	6.0	4.8
46	63	M	36	750	80	0	0	3	6.3	42	—	—	—	—
47	65	M	1	280	—	0	0	3	5.0	—	—	—	—	—

* When not in atrial fibrillation.

AF = atrial librillation; BBB = bundle branch block; BW = body weight; CABG = coronary artery bypass graft; CHB = complete heart block; CI = cardiac index; CT = cardiac transplantation; H = hemotocrit; HW = heart weight; L = left; LAD = left atrial diameter; LV = left ventricle; LVEDD = left ventricular end-diastolic diameter; LVEF = left ventricular ejection fraction; LVESD = left ventricular and systolic diameter; LVFW = left ventricular free wall; LVMD = left ventricular maximum diameter; MR = mitral regurgitation; PAW = pulmonary artery wedge; R = right; RA = right otrium; RV = right ventricle; S = symptoms; SA = systemic arterial; s/d = peak systole/end diastole; T = thrombus; TC = total cholesterol; TG = triglyceride; TR = tricuspid regurgitation; VSW = ventricular septal width; VT = ventricular tachycardia; + = positive or present; 0 = negative or absent; — = no information available.

Reproduced with permission from Waller et al.[3]

anatomic features allow separation of patients with IC, IDC, and dilated HC, but within each group considerable variation in LV cavity size and extent of ventricular scarring occurs.

Low Lymphocyte Count in Advanced Heart Failure

Ommen and colleagues[4] in Rochester, Minnesota, evaluated the prognostic significance of a very low lymphocyte count in patients with advanced heart failure. Patients evaluated in the Mayo Clinic cardiac transplantation program between April 1988 and July 1995 were retrospectively reviewed. There were 263 patients; 52 patients were excluded because they had trauma, infection, surgery, MI, corticosteroid use, or history of malignancy. In the remaining 211 patients, they used the Cox proportional hazard analysis to examine the association between survival and transplant-free survival with baseline variables. Univariate analysis showed a significant association between time to death and the percentage of lymphocytes, New York Heart Association functional class, and maximal oxygen uptake. Univariate analysis of the endpoint of survival free from transplantation provided similar results. One- and 4-year survival rates for patients with a low lymphocyte percentage, i.e., less than 20%, were 78% and 34% compared with 90% and 73% for those with a normal percentage of lymphocytes. Multivariate analysis showed New York Heart Association functional class and percent lymphocyte count to be independent predictors of survival and survival free from cardiac transplantation (Figure 10-2). The authors conclude that a relative lymphocyte concentration is an

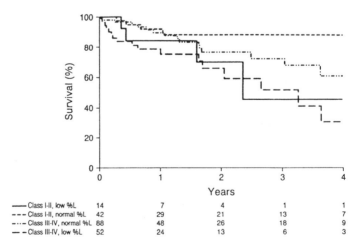

FIGURE 10-2. Survival curves for endpoint of death (with censoring at the time of transplantation) based on NYHA class and lymphocyte count. Survival rates for patients with NYHA class I to II symptoms with normal versus low lymphocyte count, respectively, were 92% versus 85% at 1 year and 89% versus 47% at 4 years. Survival rates for patients with NYHA class III to IV symptoms with normal versus low lymphocyte count, respectively, were 90% versus 76% at 1 year and 62% versus 32% at 4 years ($p = 0.003$ by log-rank test). %L indicates percentage of lymphocytes. Reproduced with permission from Ommen et al.[4]

inexpensive, readily available, simple prognostic marker in patients with symptomatic CHF who do not have a history of recent trauma, infection, surgery, MI, corticosteroid therapy, or malignancy. They further suggest that it should be incorporated in clinical protocols to predict patient outcome and to aid in the selection of patients for heart transplantation.

Progression of Chronic Cardiac Transplant Rejection

Hornick and colleagues[5] in London, United Kingdom, determined whether donor-specific tolerance could be detected in T cells with direct anti-donor allospecificity in human heart transplant recipients after prolonged graft residence. Two populations of T cells contribute to allograft rejection. T cells with direct allospecificity are activated after recognition of intact MHC alloantigens displayed at the surface of donor passage leukocytes carried within the graft. T cells with indirect allospecificity recognize donor alloantigens as processed peptides associated with self (recipient)-MHC class II molecules. In small animal models of transplantation, direct pathway T cells dominate the acute rejection process and are rendered tolerant to the graft after loss of donor passage leukocytes. Indirect pathway T cells contribute substantially to continual graft damage after passenger cell loss. Alloreactive helper and cytotoxic T cells were enumerated by use of limiting dilution analyses. These assay systems were refined to make them specific for the direct pathway of allorecognition and more sensitive in the case of the alloreactive helper cell assay. Recipient:anti-donor frequencies were generated in 10 long-term recipients of heart grafts with progressive chronic rejection and compared with those against equivalent HLA mismatched recipient:third-party controls. Alloreactive helper tolerant direct pathway donor-specific hyporesponsiveness was detected in 5 to 10 recipients. Among these 5 recipients, 4 also had low anti-donor cytotoxic T cells. In the 5th recipient, the cytotoxic T cells were greater than 1:100,000, significantly lower than that estimated against the third-party control. Donor-specific hyporesponsiveness was demonstrated in 50% of recipients in both the helper and cytotoxic T cell compartments of the direct alloresponse. Direct allorecognition, therefore, appears unlikely to be responsible for the progression of chronic rejection, thereby implicating indirect allorecognition as the primary immunological driving force.

Use of Photopheresis for Prevention of Rejection in Transplantation

Barr and colleagues[6] performed a preliminary study to assess the safety and efficacy of photopheresis in the prevention of acute rejection of cardiac allografts. Photopheresis is an immunoregulatory technique in which lymphocytes are reinfused after exposure to a photoactive compound (methoxsalen) and ultraviolet A light. A total of 60 consecutive eligible patients who were recipients of primary cardiac transplants were randomly assigned to standard triple-drug immunosuppression therapy of cyclosporine, azathioprine, and prednisone alone or in conjunction with photopheresis. The photopheresis group received a total of 24 photopheresis treatments, each pair of treatments given on 2 consecutive days, during the first 6 months after transplantation. The regimen for maintenance immunosuppression, the definition of treatment of rejection episodes, the use of prophylactic antibiotics, and the schedule for cardiac biopsies were standardized among the study centers. All the cardiac biopsy samples were graded in a blinded manner at a central pathology laboratory. Plasma from the subgroup of 34 patients who were enrolled at the 9 US centers were analyzed by polymerase chain reaction amplification for cytomegalovirus DNA. After 6 months of treatment, the mean number of episodes of acute rejection per patient was 1.44 in the standard therapy group and 0.91 in the photopheresis group ($p = 0.04$). Significantly more patients in the photopheresis group than in the standard therapy group had 1 or no rejection episode and significantly fewer patients in the photopheresis group had 2 or more rejection episodes than in the standard therapy group ($p = 0.02$). There was no significant difference in the time to a first episode of rejection, the incidence of rejection associated with hemodynamic compromise, or survival at 6 and 12 months. There were no significant differences in the rates or types of infection. Cytomegalovirus DNA was detected significantly less frequently in the photopheresis group than in the standard therapy group ($p = 0.04$). Thus, the addition of photopheresis to triple-drug immunosuppression therapy significantly decreased the risk of cardiac rejection without increasing the incidence of infection.

Endothelial Function of Internal Mammary Artery

The objective of this study by Berkenboom and associates[7] from Brussels, Belgium, was to examine the endothelial function of the internal mammary artery in patients with CAD and in heart transplant recipients. Therefore, the response of this artery to increasing concentrations of acetylcholine (1, 10, 20 μg/min for 2.5 min each) was assessed in 6 patients in a control group, in 16 patients with CAD (CAD group) matched for risk factors with 16 heart graft recipients (who underwent transplantation for nonischemic heart failure), and in 12 patients with CAD and peripheral vascular disease (PVD group). Diameters of proximal and middle segments of internal mammary artery were measured by quantitative angiography. The responses to the first concentration of acetylcholine were attenuated in these 3 groups compared with the control group. At the highest concentration of acetylcholine, the diameter increase was similar in the control and CAD groups, whereas the responses remained significantly impaired in the transplant and PVD groups. However, after selective infusion of L-arginine (30 mg/min for 11 min), the precursor of endothelium-derived nitric oxide, was performed, the responses to acetylcholine were restored in these 2 latter groups. Endothelin plasma levels were significantly enhanced in the PVD group, which exhibited the most severe impairment in acetylcholine-induced vasodilatation. Thus, some patients with CAD, mainly those with advanced atherosclerosis and cardiac transplant recipients, exhibit internal mammary artery endothelial dysfunction, and this abnormality may be reversible.

Allograft Coronary Artery Disease

Allograft CAD is a major cause of heart transplant failure. There is a need to identify patients who are at risk for the development of angiographic CAD early after transplantation since target therapy may be helpful. Akosah and colleagues[8] from Richmond, Virginia, and LaCrosse, Wisconsin, sought to determine the prognostic significance of serial dobutamine stress echocardiography in new heart transplant recipients. Twenty two such patients underwent dobutamine stress echocardiography at the time of their regularly scheduled endomyocardial biopsy. Seven patients had normal serial stress echo studies, 4 had transient inducible wall motion abnormalities, and 11 developed persistent wall motion abnormalities. During a mean follow-up time of 32 months, 8 of the 11 patients in the latter group developed angiographic coronary disease, myocardial infarction, or died. These results suggest that dobutamine-induced wall motion abnormalities, which are persistent in new heart transplant recipients, are predictive of the development of angiographic CAD, AMI, or death.

Luminal Narrowing in Cardiac Allograft Vasculopathy

Despite increasing knowledge about degree and distribution patterns of intimal hyperplasia in cardiac allograft vasculopathy, coronary artery remodeling is poorly understood in this disease. To evaluate vascular geometry, intravascular ultrasound was used by Pethig and associates[9] from Hannover, Germany, to characterize 57 advanced lesions in 35 consecutive transplant recipients. Lumen, plaque, and vessel area in these target lesions were compared with proximal and distal reference sites. Vascular remodeling by compensatory local vessel enlargement (positive remodeling) and circumscript vascular constriction (negative remodeling) could be demonstrated. Plaque area in stenotic lesions was significantly increased compared with the mean reference site (5.6 ± 3.0 mm^2 vs. 2.8 ± 1.5 mm^2); however, inadequate compensatory enlargement rather than intimal hyperplasia was shown to be the most important predictor of luminal obstruction.

Early Detection of Allograft Coronary Vasculopathy

Following heart transplantation, allograft vasculopathy is the most common cause of death. Anecdotal studies have suggested the efficacy of augmented immunosuppressive therapy after early detection of vascular involvement. In order to evaluate this concept further, Lamich and colleagues[10] from Barcelona, Spain, and Boston, Massachusetts, prospectively evaluated 76 cardiac allograft recipients and followed them for a period of 8 years. Angiography was performed at 1 month and every year after transplantation, and thallium-201 scintigraphy was performed 1, 3, 6, and 12 months after transplantation and twice a year thereafter. Eighteen of the patients developed either angiographic or scintigraphic evidence of coronary vasculopathy and were treated with 3-day methylprednisolone pulse and antithymocyte globulin. Of the 22 episodes of vasculopathy in 18 patients, 2 were detected only by angiography, 7 by angiography and scintigraphy, 4 by scintigraphy and histologic evidence of vasculitis, and 9 episodes only by thallium-201 scintigraphy. Angiographic and/or scintigraphic resolution was observed in 15 of the 22 episodes (68%) with augmented immunosuppression. The likelihood of regression was higher when treatment was instituted within the first year of transplantation (92%) than after the first year (40%). These authors conclude that early detection of allograft coronary vasculopathy is feasible with surveillance myocardial perfusion or coronary angiographic studies. When identified early after transplantation, immunosuppressive treatment may result in regression of coronary disease. These data are important since they provide the first prospective evidence that one may intervene appropriately to reduce this risk following heart transplantation.

1. Schröder F, Handrock R, Beuckelmann DJ, Hirt S, Hullin R, Priebe L, Schwinger RHG, Weil J, Herzig S: Increased availability and open probability of single L-type calcium channels from failing compared with nonfailing human ventricle. Circulation 1998 (September 8);98:969–976.
2. Holvoet P, Stassen J-M, Cleemput JV, Collen D, Vanhaecke J: Oxidized low density lipoproteins in patients with transplant-associated coronary artery disease. Arterioscler Thromb Vasc Biol 1998 (January);18:100–107.
3. Waller TA, Hiser WL, Capehart JE, Roberts WC: Comparison of clinical and morphologic cardiac findings in patients having cardiac transplantation for ischemic cardiomyopathy, idiopathic dilated cardiomyopathy, and dilated hypertrophic cardiomyopathy. Am J Cardiol 1998 (April 1);81:884–894.
4. Ommen SR, Hodge DO, Rodeheffer RJ, McGregor CGA, Thomson SP, Gibbons RJ: Predictive power of the relative lymphocyte concentration in patients with advanced heart failure. Circulation 1998 (January 6/13);97:19–22.
5. Hornick PI, Mason PD, Yacoub MH, Rose ML, Batchelor R, Lechler RI: Assessment of the contribution that direct allorecognition makes to the progression of chronic cardiac transplant rejection in humans. Circulation 1998 (April 7);97:1257–1263.
6. Barr ML, Meiser BM, Eisen HJ, Roberts RF, Livi U, Dall'Amico R, Dorent R, Rogers JG, Radovančević B, Taylor DO, Jeevanandam V, Marboe CC, for the Photophoresis Transplantation Study Group: Photopheresis for the prevention of rejection in cardiac transplantation. N Engl J Med 1998 (December 10);339:1744–1751.
7. Berkenboom G, Crasset V, Giot C, Unger P, Vachiery JL, LeClerc JL: Endothelial function of internal mammary artery in patients with CAD and in cardiac transplant recipients. Am Heart J 1998 (March);135:488–494.
8. Akosah KO, McDaniel S, Hanrahan JS, Mohanty PK: Dobutamine stress echocardiography early after heart transplantation predicts development of allograft coronary artery disease and outcome. JACC 1998 (June);31:1607–1614.
9. Pethig K, Heublein B, Wahlers T, Haverich A, for the Working Group on Cardiac Allograft Vasculopathy: Mechanism of luminal narrowing in cardiac allograft vasculopathy: Inadequate vascular remodeling rather than intimal hyperplasia is the major predictor of coronary artery stenosis. Am Heart J 1998 (April);135:628–633.
10. Lamich R, Ballester M, Marti V, Brossa V, Aymat R, Carrio I, Berna L, Camprecios M, Puig M, Estorch M, Flotats A, Bordes R, Garcia J, Auge JM, Padro JM, Caralps JM, Narula J: Efficacy of augmented immunosuppressive therapy for early vasculopathy in heart transplantation. JACC 1998 (August);32:413–419.

Appendix

Interviews with Selected Leaders of Cardiovascular Medicine/Surgery

Please note that the following interviews were originally published in the *American Journal of Cardiology* and are reproduced here with kind permission from Elsevier Medica.

JESSE EFREM EDWARDS, MD:
A Conversation With the Editor*

The first time I heard the name Jesse Edwards was in July 1959 shortly after I had come to the National Institutes of Health (NIH) in Bethesda, Maryland. Dr. Louis Thomas, who was in the Laboratory of Pathology of the National Cancer Institute and had trained in anatomic pathology at the Mayo Clinic, recommended that I read some of Dr. Edwards' writings. I was new at the NIH and within a few weeks of arriving found myself doing virtually all of the autopsies on patients from the National Heart Institute. At the time, most cases were either congenital heart disease or valvular heart disease. The Pathology Department of the Clinical Center of the NIH was actually located at that time in the National Cancer Institute, and, therefore, the faculty pathologists focused primarily on cancer, not heart disease. I was interested in the latter. Fortunately, I found the writings by Jesse Edwards to be enormously useful. Before 1959 was out, I had read virtually every one of his publications on cardiovascular disease and also his 1954 *Atlas of Congenital Anomalies of the Heart and Great Vessels* which had been introduced to me by Dr. Andrew Glenn Morrow, who was head of the Surgery Branch of the National Heart Institute and later the person who gave me my first permanent position at NIH. Jesse Edwards had also written the section on congenital heart disease in Gould's *Pathology of the Heart*, which was the most used book on morphologic aspects of heart disease at the time. Dr. Edwards' portion of that book on heart disease occupied nearly 300 pages and it soon became my Bible. Every time I did an autopsy on a patient with tetralogy of Fallot, for example, I reread Jesse Edwards' chapter on tetralogy of Fallot. It was not long before I had most of his chapters nearly memorized. Every cardiovascular subject I encountered for the next several years I first sought Jesse Edwards' writing on the topic before I went elsewhere. Thus, Jesse Edwards became my morphologic tutor in cardiovascular disease. I always found his writings to be logical, straightforward, and well illustrated. He had a wonderful capacity to simplify complicated subjects.

In June 1962, a week or so before leaving the NIH for a year at The Johns Hopkins Hospital, I visited Dr. Edwards at the Miller Hospital in St. Paul, Minnesota, where he had moved 2 years earlier. I was enormously impressed with the efficiency of his cardiovascular registry, with the love and respect that his fellows engendered toward him, and for the kindness he showed me during the visit. Jesse Edwards has trained well over 500 physicians and students. Unfortunately, I was not one among that number in St. Paul or Rochester, but I think no one has studied his publications quite as consistently and thoroughly as I have.

I consider Jesse Edwards a great man. Had he chosen surgery, internal medicine, or pediatrics or a non-medical career he also would have been superb. He has always been good with both his hands and his head. His contributions to our knowledge on virtually every cardiovascular disease is enormous. There are very few cardiovascular conditions that he has not written about. His publications in medical journals number over 700, his chapters in other physicians' books number over 70, and books which he has authored or co-authored number 12. In addition to his contributions to our fund of cardiovascular knowledge, his influence on his students has been widespread. Jesse Edwards is such a good human being, a good family man, a man of high principles. His influence will remain for decades after he is gone. It has been one of the pleasures in my life to know him and to study his contributions.

I am speaking with Dr. Edwards in his home in St. Paul, Minnesota, on October 17, 1997.

William Clifford Roberts, MD[†] (hereafter, WCR): *Dr. Edwards, I would like to discuss your career and try to find out what was it that instilled that desire in you to be such a leader in your profession. Let me start by asking you what was it like growing up in Hyde Park, Massachusetts? What did your parents do? How many siblings did you have? Just discuss your early family life, your early development.*

Jesse Efrem Edwards, MD[‡] (hereafter, JEE): I was born in Hyde Park, Massachusetts, but raised in eastern Connecticut. I grew up on a 150-acre farm and went to school through the eighth grade in a 1-room school. During that time I learned a lot about listening, because when we were in the first grade, we listened to the second grade. When you got to the second grade you knew all about it. In those days, sometimes we skipped a grade, and I skipped grade 6. I went the first year to high school in New London, Connecticut, and here I had a classical experience. Latin was a required subject in those days. I still recall Latin as being very important to me—sentence structure, vocabulary. This has stuck with me. That year was a sad time in my upbringing. My mother died and the family then moved to Boston where I completed high school.

WCR: *Your mother died when you were 13?*

JEE: Yes. She left a memory with me. I have hardly gone through a day without thinking of her even though she died almost 75 years ago. My father never remarried, and he was a great guide to me. One of the things he emphasized to me was never waste anything: "Don't waste things, don't waste time." This advice has stayed with me forever. When I see a specimen, a

*This interview is part of a series of interviews of prominent cardiovascular specialists, and the series is underwritten by an unrestricted grant from Bristol-Myers Squibb.
†Baylor Cardiovascular Institute, Baylor University Medical Center, Dallas, Texas 75248.
‡From the Jesse E. Edwards, Cardiovascular Registry.

0002-9149/98/$19.00
PII S0002-9149(98)00009-5

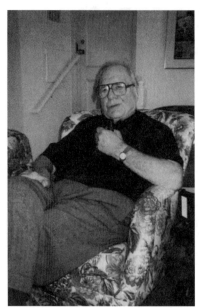
FIGURE 1. JEE during the interview in his home on 17 October 1997.

particular condition, I want to see who else I can interest in it to teach, so I constantly think of the days of being taught not to waste anything. If there is something that has teaching value I try to find a student and teach with it. That was maybe the reason eventually why I was put in a position where I collected hearts, first congenital and then acquired conditions, as a symbol that I was taught early not to waste.

WCR: *What did your father do?*

JEE: Basically he was a farmer, with poultry and gardening. He was self-educated. He had a very strong desire for his 3 kids to get educated. Everyone of us went to graduate school.

WCR: *Were your father and mother born in the USA or did they come from Europe? When did your family come to the USA?*

JEE: About 110 years ago. My father was born in the Ukrane. My mother was born in Poland.

WCR: *What year was your father born?*

JEE: In 1875. My mother was born in 1882.

WCR: *Did your father go to college?*

JEE: No, he never went to college, but he had great respect for education. He saw to it that each of his kids had the opportunity for an education.

WCR: *What did your mother die from?*

JEE: She had cancer of the stomach. As the years go by, I wonder, because she did not have an autopsy, if she did not have ovarian cancer.

WCR: *What was her age?*

JEE: She was 42 years old.

WCR: *How old was your father when he died?*

JEE: He was 70.

WCR: *So there were 3 children?*

JEE: I was the youngest, the baby. My sister, the eldest, became a teacher, and my brother became a surgeon at the Harvard Medical School.

WCR: *Your oldest sibling was how much older than you?*

JEE: Seven years.

WCR: *Your brother, who became a surgeon, was 5 years older than you. After high school, you went to Tufts in Boston. What did you major in at Tufts? As you look back over your college career what were the things that influenced you as you think about it now?*

JEE: I had my sights set for medicine. I majored in biology at Tufts. After 3 years, I entered the Tufts Medical School, and after 1 year of medical school, I then graduated from Tufts with a BS degree and had 3 more years of medical school.

WCR: *Because you skipped the sixth grade and then went to only 3 years of college, rather than 4, you entered medical school at age 20.*

JEE: Yes.

WCR: *You graduated from medical school in 1935?*

JEE: Yes.

WCR: *So you graduated from college in 1932, the heart of the depression, and then from medical school in 1935. Were you able to go through college and medical school financially okay?*

JEE: My father and sister helped. During the summers for several years I worked at the postal office to help toward tuition. Then my fourth year, I, along with 2 other classmates, was selected to be an instructor in anatomy for the first-year class, so I had free tuition from medical school that last year. The first half of the year I taught anatomy to the first-year students. This had a great impact on me: one thing was the teaching, which I enjoyed, and the other thing was that you had to love gross anatomy, which I still enjoy, and which plays a part in my day-to-day work.

WCR: *So you were a very good medical student, one of the select chosen during your senior year. You made AOA as a medical student. I presume you did quite well in your studies in college. Is that correct?*

JEE: So-So.

WCR: *Who do you remember in medical school that had an influence on you?*

JEE: The anatomy and physiology professors had great influence on me. The one I remember most was the Professor of Pathology. I got my lowest grade in medical school in pathology! The pathology teacher was Dr. Harold McMann who was superb. He was a young man, only in his second year as a professor. He was a great teacher and covered medicine with pathology. I think that had a great influence on me in my career to correlate pathology with medicine.

WCR: *When you were growing up, your mother had died, there were 3 of you; what was it like sitting around the dinner table at night? Your father must have been working very hard trying to support you 3. What do you recall? Were there active discussions around the dinner table at night? What was the atmosphere like?*

JEE: Not out of the ordinary. We had things to do. First we had to prepare the dinner and do the dishes.

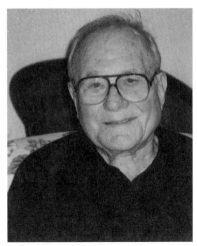
FIGURE 2. JEE during the interview.

WCR: *Each of you had your chores to do. Did you and your brother and sister get along well?*

JEE: Yes, we did. They treated me like a baby. They looked after me. I had no mother, but they participated in mothering me.

WCR: *So you enjoyed medical school a bit more than you enjoyed college. From a scholastic standpoint, you did better in medical school than you did in college. Is that correct?*

JEE: Yes.

WCR: *Why did you choose Tufts for both college and medical school?*

JEE: Tufts was simple. I could get there from home by streetcar.

WCR: *So when you went to college and medical school you lived at home? That saved a lot of money. How many students were in your medical school class?*

JEE: I think 110. We graduated with about 100.

WCR: *Did any of your colleagues in medical school have an illustrous career, even approaching yours?*

JEE: It would be ill-mannered of me to answer the question directly. When the Tufts Medical School celebrated its 100th anniversary the President picked out 7 graduates from the 100 classes and he chose me as one of them.

WCR: *In 100 years, you and 6 others were picked out as the most illustrious to graduate from Tufts Medical School?*

JEE: According to that President.

WCR: *When you graduated from medical school in 1935 you were only 24 years old. You decided to train in pathology and went to the Mallory Institute of Pathology at Boston City Hospital right there in Boston. What was that like? Did you enjoy your training?*

JEE: Yes, it was wonderful. That year we had a lot of deaths from lobar pneumonia. Five or 6 of us did autopsies and each 1 of us did about 20 or 30 cases of lobar pneumonia that year. This was before antibiotics. We all saw the multiple complications of lobar

pneumonia. Also, the histology of lobar pneumonia was very graphic and it got to be an experience of very major proportions. Also, in the general hospital we saw all kinds of things at other autopsies and the surgicals.

WCR: *I noticed that during your training at the Mallory Institute of Pathology you wrote the classic articles with your older brother on morphologic features of varicose veins in the legs. Was your brother training at Boston City Hospital also? How did that come about?*

JEE: At that time he was in practice in Boston. He maintained a connection with the medical examiner where he did some pathology to broaden his surgical experience. We had the opportunity to examine material in the medical examiner's office. From that material we described the pathology of the valves in varicose veins and in deep vein thrombosis in the legs.

WCR: *You are an enormously personable human being, you are easy with people, you are superb with your hands, you could have easily gone into a clinical field, internal medicine, surgery, and you elected to go into pathology. Was that decision easy for you in medical school or did you tustle with that decision a great deal?*

JEE: My first year out of school was pathology. This was intended to be an experience to precede training in medicine or surgery. My first year in pathology, maybe the experience with lobar pneumonia and the experience of teaching students, left me feeling that a career in pathology was very good for me. So during my first year of pathology I began to think that I should stay in pathology and, for that reason, I sought 1 year of clinical medicine my second year out of school. I was very anxious to get into pathology because to me it seemed a natural.

WCR: *At that time, 1935 until about 1940, the Mallory Institute of Pathology was one of the finest centers in the world in that particular specialty. Is that correct?*

JEE: Yes.

WCR: *How did you get interested in cardiovascular disease. I am aware that during that period of your training, roughly 1935 to 1940, you did do that work with your brother on varicose veins, and I consider those papers that you did with him the classic papers on the morphologic aspects of varicose veins and deep vein thrombosis. I am also aware that during the period of your training, that your Chief, Dr. Frederic Parker, wrote a paper on histologic findings in the lungs in patients with mitral stenosis. Did that background, in retrospect, have an impact on you?*

JEE: Yes, it did. Some years later when I was at the Mayo Clinic, I got the assignment of doing cardiac pathology. The experience at that time with congenital heart disease and the background I had had in Boston with the lungs in mitral stenosis led me to continue my interest in the vessels of the lung. Study of the pulmonary vessels turned into an everyday situation in congenital heart disease particularly.

WCR: *Dr. Edwards, I am not sure that everybody is aware of the fact that you were an outstanding re-*

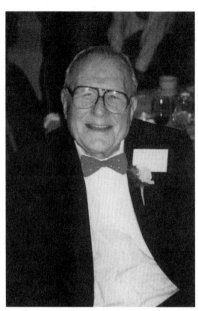

FIGURE 3. JEE at dinner banquet on the evening after his interview.

searcher in cancer. When I was at the National Institutes of Health, Dr. Harold Stewart was the Chief of the Laboratory of Pathology of the National Cancer Institutes. He could not have been more complimentary of you and your cancer work. How did you migrate to the National Institutes of Health in 1940 to do research in cancer?

JEE: In 1940, I had completed my formal training in pathology at Boston. I was interested in doing some work other than day-to-day pathology, so I sought the National Cancer Institute in Bethesda, Maryland. That was fairly new at that time, and I received an appointment as a Research Fellow where I continued for 2 years and then I went into the Army because of World War II.

WCR: I gather you went into the Army in 1942 when you were 31 years of age. It seems to me that your 4 years in the Army was quite an interesting experience for you. I gather that you were the commanding officer of the Central Laboratory for the U.S. Army in Europe and the European theater. Can you describe your activities during that period and what impact they had on your future career?

JEE: After having served in a U.S. general hospital and in England, I had a period during 1945, after World War II in Europe had ended, where I was in Europe serving as a pathologist on war crimes. During the summer of 1945 I was doing autopsies in Germany on American and British soldiers and there was the possibility that crimes had been experienced against these people. After the summer of 1945 doing that work, I was given the function of being the Chief Pathologist at the Central Laboratories in the United States theater in Europe. With that I was consultant to the Surgeon General in Europe for laboratory matters.

WCR: After you got out of the Army in 1946, you went directly to the Mayo Clinic. How did that come about? Here you had spent your entire civilian life in Massachusetts, Connecticut, Maryland; now all of a sudden you are in Rochester, Minnesota.

JEE: It came about when the Mayo Clinic was looking for a pathologist. The Mayo Clinic in 1946 made contact with the Army asking for potential people coming out of the Army who might be useful to them to fill the vacancy. At that time in Washington the Army knew about me because I had worked as Chief Officer in the laboratories in the European theater. Apparently, I had a good reputation because they offered my name. That is how the Mayo Clinic got interested in me.

WCR: Do you know who it was at the Mayo Clinic who contacted the Army?

JEE: Yes. The contact man was Dr. Bryl R. Kirklin, who was in charge of diagnostic radiology at the Mayo Clinic and he was in the Army at that time. His son, John, later became the prominent cardiovascular surgeon at the Mayo Clinic, and I worked closely with him.

WCR: Rochester, Minnesota, was quite a bit smaller than Boston, Massachusetts, where you had lived for a long time. You were used to farming country since your father was a farmer. How did Rochester, Minnesota, hit you, and how did you get into cardiovascular disease there?

JEE: I liked Rochester. At that time Rochester had a population of 40,000 people. It was a nice small town. The job I went to fill was in pathology. Quickly, I found I became a cardiovascular pathologist.

WCR: When you went there, you knew that that was the area of pathology you were going to focus on, or did that not come about until you got there?

JEE: It did not come about until I got there.

WCR: You wanted that?

JEE: No, they said the field was open and I had not done a tour in cardiac work and I had no great preference in one or another field. I was interested in doing human pathology; what field it was did not matter.

WCR: When you went to the Mayo Clinic you did recognize that the cardiovascular area was open and the Chief of the Department asked you at that time whether you would handle that. That's the way it was?

JEE: Yes.

WCR: What was the atmosphere like? Here you are at the Mayo Clinic in 1946, open heart surgery had not started yet. The only cardiac surgery at the time, I gather, included closure of or creation of a patent ductus arteriosus. How did cardiovascular disease develop there?

JEE: Gradually. When I came there they had operated on patients with patent ductus and constrictive pericarditis. Coarctation of the aorta had not yet been done. I came there in May 1946, and the first coarctation operation at the Mayo Clinic was in November 1946. Catheterization had not been done yet. Catheterization at the Mayo Clinic started a year later. It has been 50 years since the first catheterization was per-

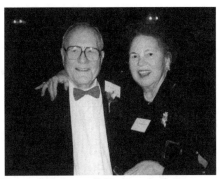

FIGURE 4. At the banquet with his devoted wife Marge.

formed at the Mayo Clinic. They celebrated the occasion this year.

WCR: *Fifty years of cardiac catheterization at the Mayo Clinic was celebrated in 1997. There have been an array of fantastic heart specialists at the Mayo Clinic, Jesse Edwards, Howard Burchell, Earl Wood, John Kirklin, Dwight McGoon, Jim DuShane. How did Burchell come to the clinic? How were these other figures attracted to the Mayo Clinic?*

JEE: Burchell came ahead of me. He was trained in internal medicine but also had experience in pathology and physiology. He was one of the young Mayo Clinic cardiologists when I met him. Wood had been trained at the University of Minnesota by Visiher, a physiologist. He was at the Mayo Clinic during World War II doing work developing and improving a decelerating machine for devices for flying. He was a physiologist but had not done any catheterizations yet. Kirklin came after I did. His fellowship in surgery was interrupted by service in the Army where he worked as a neurosurgeon. When he came back to the Clinic he was told he would be in cardiovascular surgery which developed with time. McGoon had trained at the Hopkins. By the time he came, the field was already established.

WCR: *Could you describe what the atmosphere was like at the Mayo Clinic in the late 1940s? The number of articles you published, almost from the moment you hit the Mayo Clinic, was incredible. What was your day like? What were your day-to-day activities?*

JEE: I had my regular work, along with 4 or 5 other pathologists. I took my turn with the next case, whatever it was, cancer of ovaries, cancer of the stomach, colon, all sorts of things. I participated in the autopsy in all of the congenital heart cases whether or not I was assigned that case. I got to see every congenital heart, even though I was not on duty. In the early days, we had a close connection between pathology and the other fields. We had no turf problems. We did not have the problem of the pathologist only talking about pathology. We could talk about physiology. The physiologist could talk about pathology. In the early days, we had a lot of interplay between the various fields. I would not hesitate in a surgical conference to make a suggestion for the shape of a patch to prevent reste-

nosis. The surgeon did not mind saying something about the autopsy. We had a free play of interest, crossing fields. I think that is what represented the gist of the development of the Mayo Clinic team.

WCR: *How did it work that you would see Burchell and DuShane periodically. Were there one or more adult and pediatric cardiology conferences a week? How did you interact with John Kirklin? When did you do it? How did it work out on a day-to-day basis?*

JEE: We had a lot of conferences. The autopsy conference would deal with all operative cardiac deaths. The surgeons were there, the cardiologists were there, the physiologists were there. When the physiologist held a conference the same people were there. We learned. We thought closely.

WCR: *So you, in essence, became a pretty good physiologist. Burchell became a pretty good cardiac morphologist, etc.*

JEE: Yes.

WCR: *What were your time commitments like in those early days? As a farm boy, so to speak, I gather you always arose early or what time would you get to the Mayo Clinic, what time would you leave home, what time would you wake up in the morning in those days, what time would you leave the Mayo Clinic at night? I gather you were single at the time. Were you working into the night? Can you give me an idea of what your activities were really like?*

JEE: I used to spend a lot of time in the library in the early days, searching the publications way back to the Civil War and beyond, so we could see the development of the field. We could see new developments, and also we could see deficiencies. We did a lot of work on classification of the diseases, for example, the so-called endocardial cushion defect. Burchell and I classified the various types of tricuspid atresia. Some cases have transposition of the great vessels with and without pulmonary stenosis. We also classified truncus arteriosis and even today our classification is used. In those days, every case we saw was something new. For example, I had seen one case of left-sided Ebstein's malformation—a 32-year-old person who had died of a brain abscess. Now with that case I suddenly became a expert on Ebstein's malformation. After that, an 8-year-old boy with Ebstein's had cardiac catheterization. Unfortunately, the patient died and I got on the telephone to Earl Wood and Earl said, "What did you find"? and I said, "Ebstein's", and he said, "What the hell is an Ebstein's?" That is how early it was and exciting.

WCR: *Tell me about your work habits then. You didn't have any specific training in heart disease, you trained yourself, and all of your colleagues were sort of learning together at that period of time, I gather, since cardiac catheterization was new, cardiac surgery was new, etc. What time did you get to the Mayo Clinic? What time did you leave home? What were your weekends like?*

JEE: I did most of my extra work at night, at the library or at my desk. I worked very frequently going to bed about 1:00 A.M. and I got up about 6:30 A.M., except when I wrote a 3-volume book, which took me

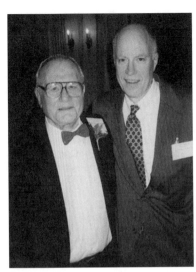
FIGURE 5. JEE at the banquet with WCR.

18 months, and during that period I worked on it from 6:30 until 8:00 each morning. At 8:00 A.M. the day started.

WCR: *You would go to bed at 1:00 A.M. and you would get up about 6:30 A.M. and that continued for many years? Where did you live in Rochester when you were single. I understand from Larry Elliott that you used to throw some nice parties and have a good number of people over. People liked to come to your house. What were your social activities like? What happened on the weekend?*

JEE: I had normal contacts. Sometimes I would have a group of young fellows over for dinner. It was mixed company. Sometime I would have a date and we would go out.

WCR: *When did you meet Marge and when did you get married?*

JEE: I met Marge 2 years before we were married. We had dates on weekends mostly and we married in 1952. I wish now that we had married earlier. We are proud of our children. One is a newspaper editor and the other is a cardiologist.

WCR: *You were 41 years of age? You had waited a bit long to get married. William Osler was 42 when he got married. I suspect it was quite hard for you to leave the Mayo Clinic. You built up a lot of friends there, you were enormously productive. How did it come about that you moved to St. Paul in 1960?*

JEE: It was hard for me to leave the Mayo Clinic, but the people at the University of Minnesota in Minneapolis were very good about making the cardiac material available to me. My primary hospital was the Miller Hospital in St. Paul, now called United. I wouldn't leave the Mayo Clinic for an ordinary job in pathology. Cardiac material had to be available. When the University said I could have all the cardiac material and the hospital supplied enough people to help me in general pathology, then I moved. I have had a great time working with people who were training at

the university. Sometimes we had as many as 12 fellows and graduate students at one time.

WCR: *Your moving to St. Paul was in actuality bringing a university to United Hospital, namely you. Nevertheless, I am sure you must have had some trepidation. That was a bit risky from a professional standpoint. Here you are at the Mayo Clinic. You've published an enormous number of articles in 14 years. You've written a number of books by that time. Your name was associated with the Mayo Clinic. You were one of the big 4, so to speak, and yet you made the St. Paul operation a magnificent success. You acquired a lot of money from NIH grants. As you say, you had a lot of fellows. How do you now look back on those first few years in St. Paul compared to the Mayo Clinic? Did it work out just as you had hoped it would work out?*

JEE: As it turned out, it was a good move. Had I stayed at the Mayo Clinic I am afraid I would have gotten old in the same job. By making the move I had to wake up and make my life here, and I think it worked out very well, but it was a risk.

WCR: *Dr. Edwards, you have published well over 700 articles in medical journals, you have published 12 books, 70 chapters in other people's books. Your name was first among your 726 articles in medical journals only about 100 times, and yet, I gather, you essentially wrote all or virtually all of those articles. In other words, you seem to me to have been an enormously unselfish person. People clammered to work with you. How did you write all these papers? Did you dictate them or did you write with pencil and paper? How did you do your writing work, particularly after you came to St. Paul?*

JEE: Mostly, pencil and paper. The fellows who worked with me usually would write the first draft, and then together we developed many drafts. Many have said to me, ''you've taught us a lot more than pathology.'' I spent a lot of time writing with the young people.

WCR: *As you look back over your illustrious last 40 years (from 1946 to now 1997) what accomplishments are you most proud of?*

JEE: My family and my friends.

WCR: *It seems your capacity for friendship is great. All of your fellows, it seems to me, are still your friends. You stay in touch with your many fellows. How many fellows have you had through the years?*

JEE: Counting medical students, over 500.

WCR: *You have a collection, as I understand it, of approximately 15,000 hearts. These are hearts with heart disease, either acquired or congenital. Autopsies in this country are continually getting fewer and fewer. This material is getting rarer and rarer. Here you can collect 146 cases studied at autopsy with the polysplenia syndrome, or nearly 50 cases of parachute mitral valve syndrome. Nowhere else in the world can anybody come up with this type of collection to study. How can this collection be preserved. Where can the money come from to keep it going?*

JEE: That's tough. We have some funds from the endowment but that is small. We probably have to seek more funds from people who are interested in this collection.

WCR: *You were President of the American Heart Association for 1 year. That was 1969 or something like that. What do you remember about that experience? Was that a good experience?*

JEE: It was a good experience. It's like owning a boat. It's great when you buy it and it's great when you sell it.

WCR: *You enjoyed having the opportunity of being president of the American Heart Association but when it was over you were glad it was over. I have admired you through the years by your ability not to travel too much. You seem to have stuck to your job and you must have had a lot of opportunities to go here and yon, but you seemed to have kept travel down. Could you talk about that a bit?*

JEE: My family was close and my in-laws (who are gone now) lived with us for about 17 years. My wife is an only child and she was very close to her family, and she was not very enthusiastic about travel, so I more or less did it her way. I think the family had a lot to do with it. The kids were raised in part by their grandparents. They had a great influence on the kids. I am happy the way it worked out.

WCR: *I asked you sometime ago to look over your publications and mark those that you thought were the most significant. You have 726 publications in medical journals and you only marked 18 of them. Now I can tell you that you passed over some classic papers. You did not mark enough! I realize you are a modest man but as you look back what are some of your professional accomplishments you are most proud of?*

JEE: First of all, I like young people and I like to help them develop into adults.

WCR: *Do you have any regrets? Were there some things professionally that you wanted to do that you did not do?*

JEE: Not really.

WCR: *As mentioned earlier, you are an extremely personable person. I am sure people have mentioned to you through the years that, "gosh, I wish you had been my doctor." Do you regret at all that you did not have that interpatient contact on a day-to-day basis? Obviously, you would have been very good at that.*

JEE: No, I am happy with the experience I had.

WCR: *It seems to me that you could not have accomplished what you did had you not had good hands. In other words, you were smart, clever, creative, but you also knew how to open the heart and how to illustrate it and how to make it understandable to those who didn't do that every day. Your diagrams have been reproduced by numerous people all over the world. You would have been a superb surgeon. Do you ever regret that you did not go into surgery like your brother did?*

JEE: I sometimes think if I had done something else that I would have prospered. I don't know. I am not dissatisfied with my experience.

WCR: *You have reviewed for cardiology editors and editors for other journals, literally hundreds of manuscripts through the years. You have done that*

very efficiently, quickly, and promptly. You have always made it a priority if someone asked you to write a chapter or review a manuscript that you got it in by the due date. I guess you get annoyed when people say they are going to do something and yet they don't do it. You seem to always deliver. Can you comment on that?*

JEE: A promise is a promise.

WCR: *Have other physicians or investigators influenced you considerably?*

JEE: I will mention *Bradley Patton*. When I started working at the Mayo Clinic on congenital heart disease, I contacted him and spent some time with him, both at work and some time at home. He taught me some basics of embryology. He gave me some insights that were helpful to me. I would also like to mention *Robert Benassi*. He is a medical illustrator with whom I have worked for the last 30 years or so and he has done most of the illustrations that I have developed. He was a great help to me. If I had a chance to illustrate something, he had the talent to do it. He has made about 5,000 illustrations for me. He worked freelance when I came to St. Paul. I worked with him for quite a few years and one day the Mayo Clinic called me and wanted to know about Bob Benassi. They wanted to give him a job and they did, but he assisted me and to this day he is still available to me.

WCR: *I always thought that you knew a lot about embryology but that you did not mix embryological terms with descriptive terms of congenital heart disease. In other words, you kept the nomenclature simple. You made your nomenclature readily understandable. One of your many contributions was making the nomenclature of corrected transposition of the great arteries reasonable, bringing together the concept of situs, simplifying the concept of detroversion and dextrocardia. I wonder if you could comment on that? I remember when I was a resident in anatomic pathology, one of the first cases that I encountered was a patient who had a large ventricular septal defect, and, in retrospect, both great arteries arose from the right ventricle. I remember keeping that heart in a basin in my office and I looked at it nearly everyday for a couple of months trying to figure it out. During that time, your classic article on the origin of both great arteries from the right ventricle appeared and you had 10 or 12 cases in that first paper. Then I knew exactly what it was, but I had not figured it out myself. Do you want to comment on your relative simplification of nomenclature, particularly in congenital heart failure?*

JEE: Basically I believe in simplicity, call it the way you see it, and I think if you do that people in other fields can understand. Of course, some people with congenital heart disease like to feel that they know it all and no other person can know what they think.

WCR: *Do you have hobbies, Dr. Edwards? What do you do when you are not doing medical things?*

JEE: Before I had my stroke I worked in the garden, and also I love to fish. Once I had my stroke, my son, Brooks, got me a rod and reel that is made for the handicapped. I cast out and then reel it in by pushing a button. The last time I fished, my wife and I caught a 4-pound Northern Pike.

WCR: *Your gardening, I presume, was a continuation of your farming as a youngster. Do you read a good bit? Do you read a lot other than medicine?*

JEE: No, I don't.

WCR: *Time factor, mainly, I presume?*

JEE: I think that also may be my schooling, when you could listen to the second grade when you were in the first grade.

WCR: *I wanted to tell you that I was not one of your 500 or more fellows, but you never had a fellow who read more of your publications than I did. If anybody ever asks me who was my instructor, I say, Jesse Edwards. When I have had fellows through the years, I always tell them, find out what Jess Edwards had to say about this before we go too much further.*

JEE: You are very kind, Bill, thanks.

WCR: *Thank you, Dr. Edwards. It is a real pleasure to see you. I appreciate your spending this time with me. You have a lovely home and it is a pleasure to be here.*

JEE's most important 149 publications selected by JEE among his 721 articles published in journals

1. Edwards EA, Edwards JE. The effect of thrombophlebitis on the venous valve. *SG & O* 1937;65:310–320.
3. Edwards JE, Edwards EA. The saphenous valves in varicose veins. *Am Heart J* 1940;19:338–351.
12. Edwards JE. Hepatomas in mice induced with carbon tetrachloride. *J National Cancer Inst* 1941;2:197–199.
28. Edwards EA, Edwards JE. The venous valves in thromboangiitis obliterans. *Arch Path* 1943;35:242–252.
31. Bartel CM, Edwards JE, Lamb ME. Mycotic and dissecting aneurysms of aorta complicating bacterial endocarditis. *Arch Pathol* 1943;35:285–291.
39. Gates RM, Rogers HM, Edwards JE. The syndrome of cerebral abscess and congenital cardiac disease. *Mayo Clin Proc* 1947;22:401–412.
42. Edwards JE. Retro-esophageal segment of the left aortic arch, right ligamentum arteriosum and right descending aorta causing a congenital vascular ring about the trachea and esophagus. *Mayo Clin Proc* 1948;23:108–116.
47. Rogers HM, Edwards JE. Incomplete division of the atrioventricular canal with patent interatrial foramen primum (persistent common cardioventricular ostium). Report of 5 cases and review of the literature. *Am Heart J* 1948;36:28–54.
48. Edwards JE. Anomalies of the derivatives of the aortic arch system. *Med Clin North Amr* 1948(July):925–949.
50. Edwards JE, Christensen NA, Clagett OT, McDonald JR. Pathologic consideration in coarctation of the aorta. *Mayo Clin Proc* 1948;23:324–332.
51. Edwards JE, Clagett OT, Drake RL, Christensen NA. The collateral circulation in coarctation of the aorta. *Mayo Clin Proc* 1948;23:333–339.
52. Edwards JE. "Vascular rings" related to anomalies of the aortic arches. *Mod Concepts Cardiovasc Dis* 1948 (August);17:1–3.
56. Dahlin DC, Edwards JE. Amyloid localized in the heart. *Mayo Clin Proc* 1949;24:89–98.
58. Ludden TE, Edwards JE. Carditis in poliomyelitis: an anatomic investigation of 35 cases and review of the literature. *Am J Pathol* 1949;25:357–381.
59. Larrabee WF, Parker RL, Edwards JE. Pathology of intrapulmonary arteries and arterioles in mitral stenosis. *Mayo Clin Proc* 1949;24:316–326.
61. Edwards JE, Burchell HB. Congenital tricuspid atresia: a classification. *Med Clin North Am* 1949 (July):1177–1196.
62. Collett RW, Edwards JE. Persistent truncus: a classification according to anatomic types. *Med Clin North Am* (Mayo Clin No) 1949 (August):1245–1270.
68. Edwards JE, DuShane JW. Thoracic venous anomalies. I. Vascular connection of the left atrium and the left innominate vein (levoatriocardinal vein) associated with mitral atresia and premature closure of the foramen ovale. II. Pulmonary veins draining wholly into the ductus venosus. *Arch Pathol* 1950;49:517–537.
75. Civin WH, Edwards JE. Pathology of the pulmonary vascular tree. I. A comparison of the intrapulmonary arteries in the Eisenmenger complex and in stenosis of the ostium infundibuli associated with biventricular origin of the aorta. *Circulation* 1950;2:545–552.
79. Becker DL, Burchell HB, Edwards JE. Pathology of the pulmonary vascular

tree. II. The occurrence in mitral insufficiency of occlusive pulmonary vascular lesions. *Circulation* 1951;3:230–238.
80. Civin WH, Edwards JE. The postnatal structural changes in the intrapulmonary arteries and arterioles. *Arch Pathol* 1951;51:192–200.
84. Edwards JE, Chamberlin WB Jr. Pathology of the pulmonary vascular tree. III. The structure of the intrapulmonary arteries in cor triloculare biatriatum with subaortic stenosis. *Circulation* 1951;3:524–530.
85. Edwards JE, DuShane JW, Alcott DL, Burchell HB. Thoracic venous anomalies. III. Atresia of the common pulmonary vein, the pulmonary veins draining wholly into the superior vena cava. IV. Stenosis of the common pulmonary vein (cor triatriatum). *Arch Pathol* 1951;51:446–460.
93. Bahn RC, Edwards JE, DuShane JW. Coarctation of the aorta as a cause of death in early infancy. *Pediatrics* 1951;8:192–203.
96. Williams RR, Kent GB Jr, Edwards JE. Anomalous cardiac blood vessel communicating with the right ventricle. Observations in a case of pulmonary atresia with an intact ventricular septum. *Arch Pathol* 1951;52:480–487.
106. Jordan RA, Miller RD, Edwards JE, Parker RL. Thrombo-embolism in acute and in healed myocardial infarction. I. Intracardiac mural thrombosis. *Circulation* 1952;6:1–6.
107. Miller RD, Jordan RA, Parker RL, Edwards JE. Thrombo-embolism in acute and in healed myocardial infarction. II. Systemic and pulmonary arterial occlusion. *Circulation* 1952;6:7–15.
115. Edwards JE. Malformations of the aortic arch system manifested as "vascular rings." *Lab Invest* 1953;2:56–75.
118. Kelsey JR, Gilmore CE, Edwards JE. Bilateral ductus arteriosus representing persistence of each sixth aortic arch. Report of a case. *Arch Pathol* 1953;55:154–161.
130. Clagett OT, Kirklin JW, Edwards JE. Anatomic variations and pathologic changes in 124 cases of coarctation of the aorta. *Surgery* 1954;36:72–83.
137. Barger JD, Creasman RW, Edwards JE. Bilateral ductus arteriosus associated with interruption of the aortic arch. *Am J Clin Pathol* 1954;24:441–444.
150. Becu LM, Swan HJC, DuShane JW, Edwards JE. Ebstein malformation of the left atrioventricular valve in corrected transposition of the great vessels with ventricular septal defect. *Mayo Clin Proc* 1955;30:483–490.
151. Rogers HM, Waldon BR, Murphey DFH, Edwards JE. Supravalvular stenosing ring of left atrium in association with endocardial sclerosis (endocardial fibroelastosis) and mitral insufficiency. *Am Heart J* 1955;50:777–781.
152. Becu LM, Tauxe WN, DuShane JW, Edwards JE. A complex of congenital cardiac anomalies: ventricular septal defect, biventricular origin of the pulmonary trunk, and subaortic stenosis. *Am Heart J* 1955;50:901–911.
157. Edwards JE, Burchell HB, Christensen NA. Specimen exhibiting the essential lesion in aneurysm of the aortic sinus. *Proc Mayo Clin* 1956;31:407–412, 464.
165. Barger JD, Bregmann EH, Edwards JE. Bilateral ductus arteriosus with right aortic arch and right-sided descending aorta. Report of a case. *Am J Roentgenol* 1956;76:758–761.
169. Kirklin JW, Harshbarger HG, Donald DE, Edwards JE. Surgical correction of ventricular septal defect: anatomic and technical considerations. *J Thorac Surg* 1957;33:45–59.
174. Edwards JE. The Lewis A. Conner Memorial Lecture. Functional pathology of the pulmonary vascular tree in congenital cardiac disease. *Circulation* 1957;15:164–196.
176. Lyons WS, Hanlon DG, Helmholz HF Jr, DuShane JW, Edwards JE. Congenital cardiac disease and asplenia: report of 7 cases. *Mayo Clin Proc* 1957;32:277–286.
177. Edwards JE, Burchell HB. Pathologic anatomy of deficiencies between the aortic root and the heart, including aortic sinus aneurysms. *Thorax* 1957;12:125–139.
183. Dines DE, Edwards JE, Burchell HB. Myocardial atrophy in constrictive pericarditis. *Mayo Clin Proc* 1958;33:93–99.
206. Edwards JE, Burchell HB. Endocardial and intimal lesions (jet impact) as possible sites or origin of murmurs. *Circulation* 1958;18:946–960.
219. Heath D, Wood EH, DuShane JW, Edwards JE. The structure of the pulmonary trunk at different ages and in cases of pulmonary hypertension and pulmonary stenosis. *J Path Bact* 1959;77:443–456.
223. Sommerville RL, Allen EV, Edwards JE. Bland and infected arteriosclerotic abdominal aortic aneurysms: a clinicopathologic study. *Medicine* 1959;38:207–221.
228. Edwards JE. Congenital stenosis of pulmonary veins. Pathologic and developmental considerations. *Lab Invest* 1960;9:46–66.
238. Edwards JE. The problem of mitral insufficiency caused by accessory chordae tendineae in persistent common atrioventricular canal. *Mayo Clin Proc* 1960;35:299–305.
240. Burroughs JT, Edwards JE. Total anomalous pulmonary venous connection. *Am Heart J* 1960;59:913–931.
250. Neufeld HN, DuShane JW, Wood EH, Kirklin JW, Edwards JE. Origin of both great vessels from the right ventricle. I. Without pulmonary stenosis. *Circulation* 1961;23:399–412.
253. Edwards JE. The congenital bicuspid aortic valve. *Circulation* 1961;23:485–488.
254. Neufeld HN, DuShane JW, Edwards JE. Origin of both great vessels from the right ventricle. II. With pulmonary stenosis. *Circulation* 1961;23:603–612.
256. Wagenvoort CA, Neufeld HN, DuShane JW, Edwards JE. The pulmonary arterial tree in ventricular septal defect. A quantitative study of anatomic features in fetuses, infants and children. *Circulation* 1961;23:740–748.

260. Edwards JE. Calcific aortic stenosis: pathologic features. *Mayo Clin Proc* 1961;36:444–451.

266. Lucas RV Jr, Adams P Jr, Anderson RC, Varco RL, Edwards JE, Lester RG. Total anomalous pulmonary venous connection to the portal venous system: a cause of pulmonary venous obstruction. *Am J Roentgenol* 1961;86:561–575.

268. Davignon AL, Greenwold WE, DuShane JW, Edwards JE. Congenital pulmonary atresia with intact ventricular septum: clinicopathologic correlation of two anatomic types. *Am Heart J* 1961;62:591–602.

271. Lucas RV Jr, Lund GW, Edwards JE. Direct communication of a pulmonary artery with the left atrium. An unusual variant of pulmonary arteriovenous fistula. *Circulation* 1961;24:1409–1414.

273. Spiekerman RE, Brandenburg JT, Achor RWP, Edwards JE. The spectrum of coronary heart disease in a community of 30,000. A clinicopathologic study. *Circulation* 1962;25:57–65.

281. Lucas RV Jr, Woolfrey BF, Anderson RC, Lester RG, Edwards JE. Atresia of the common pulmonary vein. *Pediatrics* 1962;29:729–739.

282. Elliott LP, Edwards JE. The problem of pulmonary venous obstruction in total anomalous pulmonary venous connection to the left innominate vein. *Circulation* 1962;25:913–915.

283. Lucas RV Jr, Neufeld HN, Lester RG, Edwards JE. The symmetrical liver as a roentgen sign of asplenia. *Circulation* 1962;25:973–975.

290. Edwards JE. On the etiology of calcific aortic stenosis. *Circulation* 1962; 26:817–818.

300. Shone JD, Sellers RD, Anderson RC, Adams P Jr, Lillehei CW, Edwards JE. The developmental complex of "parachute mitral valve," supravalvular ring of left atrium, subaortic stenosis, and coarctation of aorta. *Am J Cardiol* 1963;11: 714–725.

306. Titus JL, Daugherty GW, Edwards JE. Anatomy of the atrioventricular conduction system in ventricular septal defect. *Circulation* 1963;28:72–81.

311. Eliot RS, Wolbrink A, Edwards JE. Congenital aneurysm of the left aortic sinus. A rare lesion and a rare cause of coronary insufficiency. *Circulation* 1963;28:951–956.

316. Edwards JE. The direction of blood flow in coronary arteries arising from the pulmonary trunk. *Circulation* 1964;29:163–166.

321. Ruttenberg HD, Neufeld HN, Lucas RV Jr, Carey LS, Adams P Jr, Anderson RC, Edwards JE. Syndrome of congenital cardiac disease with asplenia. Distinction from other forms of congenital cyanotic cardiac diseases. *Am J Cardiol* 1964;13:387–406.

333. Noren GH, Raghib G, Moller JH, Amplatz K, Adams P Jr, Edwards JE. Anomalous origin of the left coronary artery from the pulmonary trunk with special reference to the occurrence of mitral insufficiency. *Circulation* 1964;30: 171–179.

335. Eliot RS, Kanjuh VI, Edwards JE. Atheromatous embolism. *Circulation* 1964;30:611–618.

338. Moller JH, Lucas RV Jr, Adams P Jr, Anderson RC, Jorgens J, Edwards JE. Endocardial fibroelastosis. A clinical and anatomic study of 47 patients with emphasis on its relationship to mitral insufficiency. *Circulation* 1964;30:759–782.

341. Eliot RS, Woodburn RL, Edwards JE. Conditions of the ascending aorta simulating aortic valvular incompetence. *Am J Cardiol* 1964;14:679–694.

349. Speckhals RC, Winchell P, Amplatz K, Edwards JE, From AHL. Idiopathic myocardiopathy with endocardial fibroelastosis occurring during pregnancy. *Am Heart J* 1965;69:551–558.

357. Todd DB, Anderson RC, Edwards JE. Inverted malformations in corrected transposition of the great vessels. *Circulation* 1965;32:298–300.

358. Ongley PA, Titus JL, Khoury GH, Rahimtoola SH, Marshall HJ, Edwards JE. Anomalous connection of pulmonary veins to right atrium associated with anomalous inferior vena cava, situs inversus and multiple spleens. A developmental complex. *Mayo Clin Proc* 1965;40:609–624.

361. Raghib G, Bloemendaal RD, Kanjuh VI, Edwards JE. Aortic atresia and premature closure of foramen ovale. Myocardial sinusoids and coronary arteriovenous fistula serving as outflow channel. *Am Heart J* 1965;70:476–480.

362. Jue KL, Raghib G, Amplatz K, Adams P Jr, Edwards JE. Anomalous origin of the left pulmonary artery from the right pulmonary artery. Report of 2 cases and review of the literature. *Am J Roentgenol* 1965;95:598–610.

363. Moller JH, Edwards JE. Interruption of aortic arch. Anatomic patterns and associated cardiac malformations. *Am J Roentgenol* 1965;95:557–572.

364. Peterson TA, Todd DB, Edwards JE. Supravalvular aortic stenosis. *J Thorac Cardiovasc Surg* 1965;50:734–741.

371. Jue KL, Noren G, Edwards JE. Pulmonary atresia with left ventricular-right atrial communication: basis for "circular shunt." *Thorax* 1966;21:83–90.

372. Mantini E, Grondin CM, Lillehei CW, Edwards JE. Congenital anomalies involving the coronary sinus. *Circulation* 1966;33:317–327.

375. Jue KL, Adams P Jr, Pryor R, Blount SG Jr, Edwards JE. Complete transposition of the great vessels in total situs inversus. Anatomic, electrocardiographic and radiologic observations. *Am J Cardiol* 1966;17:389–394.

379. Jue KL, Lockman LA, Edwards JE. Anomalous origins of pulmonary arteries from pulmonary trunk ("crossed pulmonary arteries"). Observation in a case with 18 trisomy syndrome. *Am Heart J* 1966;71:807–812.

380. Moller JH, Nakib A, Edwards JE. Infarction of papillary muscles and mitral insufficiency associated with congenital aortic stenosis. *Circulation* 1966;34:87–91.

381. Simmons RL, Moller JH, Edwards JE. Anatomic evidence for spontaneous closure of ventricular septal defect. *Circulation* 1966;34:38–45.

384. Moller JH, Nakib A, Eliot RS, Edwards JE. Symptomatic congenital aortic stenosis in the first year of life. *J Pediatr* 1966;69:728–734.

386. Moller JH, Noren GR, David PR, Amplatz K, Kanjuh VI, Edwards JE. Congenital stenosis of individual pulmonary veins without intracardiac anomalies. *Am Heart J* 1966;72:530–537.

394. Layman TE, Edwards JE. Anomalous mitral arcade. A type of congenital mitral insufficiency. *Circulation* 1967;35:389–395.

396. Levine MA, Moller JH, Amplatz K, Edwards JE. Atresia of the common pulmonary vein: case report and differential diagnosis. *Am J Roentgenol* 1967; 100:322–327.

405. Moller JH, Nakib A, Anderson RC, Edwards JE. Congenital cardiac disease associated with polysplenia. A developmental complex of bilateral "left-sidedness." *Circulation* 1967;36:789–799.

413. Stanger P, Benassi RC, Korns ME, Jue KL, Edwards JE. Diagrammatic portrayal of variations in cardiac structure. Reference to transposition, dextrocardia and the concept of four normal hearts. *Circulation* 1968;37,38(suppl IV):IV-1–IV-16.

421. Goor D, Edwards JE. Friction lesions of the right ventricular endocardium. Related to tricuspid chordae in cardiac hypertrophy. *Arch Pathol* 1969;87:100–109.

431. Stanger P, Lucas RV Jr, Edwards JE. Anatomic factors causing respiratory distress in acyanotic congenital cardiac disease: special reference to bronchial obstruction. *Pediatrics* 1969;43:760–769.

435. Koretzky ED, Moller JH, Korns ME, Schwartz CJ, Edwards JE. Congenital pulmonary stenosis resulting from dysplasia of valve. *Circulation* 1969;40:43–53.

458. Becker AE, Becker MJ, Edwards JE. Malposition of pulmonary arteries (crossed pulmonary arteries) in persistent truncus arteriosus. *Am J Roentgenol* 1970;110:509–514.

462. Becker AE, Becker MJ, Edwards JE. Pathologic spectrum of dysplasia of the tricuspid valve. Features in common with Ebstein's malformation. *Arch Pathol* 1971;91:167–178.

476. Vlodaver Z, Edwards JE. Pathologic changes in aortic-coronary arterial saphenous vein grafts. *Circulation* 1971;44:719–728.

477. Schroeckenstein RF, Wasenda GJ, Edwards JE. Valvular competent patent foramen ovale in adults. *Minn Med* 1972;55:11–13.

479. Van Tassel RA, Edwards JE. Rupture of heart complicating myocardial infarction. Analysis of 40 cases including nine examples of left ventricular false aneurysm. *Chest* 1972;61:104–116.

481. Claudon DG, Claudon DB, Edwards JE. Primary dissecting aneurysm of coronary artery. A cause of acute myocardial ischemia. *Circulation* 1972;45: 259–266.

500. Edwards JE, McGoon DC. Absence of anatomic origin from heart of pulmonary arterial supply. *Circulation* 1973;47:393–398.

503. Charuzi Y, Spanos PK, Amplatz K, Edwards JE. Juxtaposition of the atrial appendages. *Circulation* 1973;47:620–627.

513. Tandon R, Moller JH, Edwards JE. Communication of mitral valve with both ventricles associated with double outlet right ventricle. *Circulation* 1973; 48:904–908.

519. Waller BF, Carter JB, Williams HJ Jr, Wang K, Edwards JE. Bicuspid aortic valve. Comparison of congenital and acquired types. *Circulation* 1973;48:1140–1150.

521. Blieden LC, Randall PA, Castaneda AR, Lucas RV Jr, Edwards JE. The "goose neck" of the endocardial cushion defect: anatomic basis. *Chest* 1974;65: 13–17.

526. Marin-Garcia J, Tandon R, Moller JH, Edwards JE. Common (single) ventricle with normally related great vessels. *Circulation* 1974;49:565–573.

529. Tandon R, Edwards JE. Tricuspid atresia. A re-evaluation and classification. *J Thorac Cardiovasc Surg* 1974;67:530–542.

532. Rose AG, Beckman CB, Edwards JE. Communication between coronary sinus and left atrium. *Br Heart J* 1974;36:182–185.

542. Tandon R, Sterns LP, Edwards JE. Thoracopagus twins. Report of a case. *Arch Pathol* 1974;98:248–251.

544. Tandon R, Becker AE, Moller JH, Edwards JE. Double inlet left ventricle. Straddling tricuspid valve. *Br Heart J* 1974;36:747–759.

547. Knight L, Edwards JE. Right aortic arch. Types and associated cardiac anomalies. *Circulation* 1974;50:1047–1051.

561. Vlodaver Z, Edwards JE. Occlusion of coronary grafts-result of injury? *Ann Thorac Surg* 1975;20:719–720.

566. Baldwin JJ, Edwards JE. Rupture of right ventricle complicating closed chest cardiac massage. *Circulation* 1976;53:562–564.

571. Knight L, Neal WA, Williams HJ, Huseby TL, Edwards JE. Congenital left ventricular diverticulum. Part of a syndrome of cardiac anomalies and midline defects. *Minn Med* 1976;59:372–375.

572. Shrivastava S, Tadavarthy SM, Fukuda T, Edwards JE. Anatomic causes of pulmonary stenosis in complete transposition. *Circulation* 1976;54:154–159.

576. Guthrie RB, Edwards JE. Pathology of the myxomatous mitral valve. Nature, secondary changes and complications. *Minn Med* 1976;59:637–647.

581. Arom KV, Edwards JE. Relationship between right ventricular muscle bundles and pulmonary valve. Significance in pulmonary atresia with intact ventricular septum. *Circulation* 1976;54(suppl III):III-79–III-83.

592. Stanger P, Rudolph AM, Edwards JE. Cardiac malpositions. An overview based on study of sixty-five necropsy specimens. *Circulation* 1977;56:159–172.

596. Sotomora RF, Edwards JE. Anatomic identification of so-called absent pulmonary artery. *Circulation* 1978;57:624–633.

600. Edwards WD, Edwards JE. Hypertensive pulmonary vascular disease in d-transposition of the great arteries. *Am J Cardiol* 1978;41:921–924.

603. Sridaromont S, Ritter DG, Feldt RH, Davis GD, Edwards JE. Double-outlet right ventricle. Anatomic and angiocardiographic correlations. *Mayo Clin Proc* 1978;53:555–557.

606. Anderson JL, Durnin RE, Ledbetter MK, Angevine JM, Gilbert EF, Edwards JE. Pulmonary veno-occlusive disease. *Am Heart J* 1979;97:233–240.

615. Zollikofer CL, Vlodaver Z, Nath HP, Castaneda-Zuniga W, Valdez-Davila O, Amplatz K, Edwards JE. Angiographic findings in recanalization of coronary arterial thrombi. *Radiology* 1980;134:303–307.

620. Castaneda-Zuniga WR, Formanek A, Tadavarthy M, Vlodaver Z, Edwards JE, Zollikofer C, Amplatz K. The mechanism of balloon angioplasty. *Radiology* 1980;135:565–571.

622. Scholz DG, Lynch JA, Willerschneidt AB, Sharma RK, Edwards JE. Coronary arterial dominance associated with congenital bicuspid aortic valve. *Arch Pathol Lab Med* 1980;104:417–418.

624. Pritzker MR, Ernst JD, Caudill C, Wilson CS, Weaver WF, Edwards JE. Acquired aortic stenosis in systemic lupus erythematosus. *Ann Intern Med* 1980; 93:434–436.

628. Bramlet DA, Edwards JE. Congenital aneurysm of left atrial appendage. *Br Heart J* 1981;45:97–100.

632. Nath PH, Castaneda-Zuniga W, Zollikofer C, Delany DJ, Fulton RE, Amplatz K, Edwards JE. Isolation of a subclavian artery. *Am J Roentgenol* 1981;137:683–688.

633. Edwards BS, Edwards WD, Edwards JE. Aortic origin of conus coronary artery. Evidence of postnatal coronary development. *Br Heart J* 1981;45:555–558.

644. Castaneda-Zuniga W, Nath HP, Moller JH, Edwards JE. Left-sided anomalies in Ebstein's malformation of the tricuspid valve. *Pediatr Cardiol* 1982;3:181–185.

647. Braunlin E, Peoples WM, Freedom RM, Flyer DC, Goldblatt A, Edwards JE. Interruption of the aortic arch with aorticopulmonary septal defect. An anatomic review. *Pediatr Cardiol* 1982;3:329–335.

649. Chesler E, King RA, Edwards JE. The myxomatous mitral valve and sudden death. *Circulation* 1983;67:632–639.

653. Peoples WM, Moller JH, Edwards JE. Polysplenia: a review of 146 cases. *Pediatr Cardiol* 1983;4:129–137.

660. Edwards BS, Edwards WD, Connolly DC, Edwards JE. Arterial-esophageal fistulae developing in patients with anomalies of the aortic arch system. *Chest* 1984;86:732–735.

663. Edwards BS, Edwards WD, Edwards JE. Ventricular septal rupture complicating acute myocardial infarction: identification of simple and complex types in 53 autopsied hearts. *Am J Cardiol* 1985;54:1201–1205.

665. Edwards BS, Lucas RV Jr, Lock JE, Edwards JE. Morphologic changes in the pulmonary arteries after percutaneous balloon angioplasty for pulmonary arterial stenosis. *Circulation* 1985;71:195–201.

667. Topaz O, Edwards JE. Pathologic features of sudden death in children, adolescents and young adults. *Chest* 1985;87:476–482.

670. Peterson MD, Roach RM, Edwards JE. Types of aortic stenosis in surgically removed valves. *Arch Pathol Lab Med* 1985;109:829–832.

672. Hanson TP, Edwards BS, Edwards JE. Pathology of surgically excised mitral valves. One hundred consecutive cases. *Arch Pathol Lab Med* 1985;109:823–828.

674. Feigl D, Feigl A, Sweetman KM, Lobo FV, Moller JH, Edwards JE. Accessory tissue of the tricuspid valve protruding into the left ventricle through a septal defect. *Arch Pathol Lab Med* 1986;110:144–147.

680. Braunlin EA, Moller JH, Patton C, Lucas RV Jr, Lillehei CW, Edwards JE.

Predictive value of lung biopsy in ventricular septal defect: long-term follow-up. *J Am Coll Cardiol* 1986;8:1113–1118.

691. Blatchford JW III, Franciosi RA, Singh A, Edwards JE. Vascular ring in interruption of the aortic arch with bilateral patent ductus arteriosi. *J Thorac Cardiovasc Surg* 1987;94:596–599.

692. Edwards BS, Weir EK, Edwards WD, Ludwig J, Dykoski RK, Edwards JE. Coexistent pulmonary and portal hypertension: morphologic and clinical features. *J Am Coll Cardiol* 1987;10:1233–1238.

694. Tuna IC, Edwards JE. Aortico-left ventricular tunnel and aortic insufficiency. *Ann Thorac Surg* 1988;45:5–6.

696. Pierpont MEM, Gobel JW, Moller JH, Edwards JE. Cardiac malformations in relatives of children with truncus arteriosus or interruption of the aortic arch. *Am J Cardiol* 1988;61:423–427.

700. Tveter KJ, Edwards JE. Calcified aortic sinotubular ridge: a source of coronary ostial stenosis or embolism. *J Am Coll Cardiol* 1988;12:1510–1514.

703. Tuna IC, Bessinger FB, Ophoven JP, Edwards JE. Acute angular origin of left coronary artery from aorta: an unusual cause of left ventricular failure in infancy. *Pediatr Cardiol* 1989;10:39–43.

704. Silberbach M, Castro WL, Goldstein MA, Lucas RV Jr, Edwards JE. Comparison of types of pulmonary stenosis with the state of the ventricular septum in complete transposition of the great arteries. *Pediatr Cardiol* 1989;10:11–15.

708. Gikonyo BM, Jue KL, Edwards JE. Pulmonary vascular sling: report of 7 cases and review of literature. *Pediatr Cardiol* 1989;10:81–89.

709. Kanjuh VI, Katkov H, Singh A, Franciosi RA, Helseth HK, Edwards JE. Atypical total anomalous pulmonary venous connection: two channels leading to infracardiac terminations. *Pediatr Cardiol* 1989;10:115–120.

712. Yomtovian RA, Walley VM, Bollinger DJ, Edwards JE. Isolated valvular amyloid. *Am J Cardiovasc Pathol* 1989;2:365–370.

714. Lobo FV, Heggtveit HA, Butany J, Silver MD, Edwards JE. Right ventricular dysplasia: morphological findings in 13 cases. *Can J Cardiol* 1992;8:261–268.

Books authored or coauthored by JEE

1. Edwards JE, Dry TJ, Parker RL, Burchell HB, Wood EH, Bulbulian AH. *An Atlas of Congenital Anomalies of the Heart and Great Vessels.* Springfield, ILL: Charles C Thomas, 1954:202.

2. Edwards JE. *An Atlas of Acquired Diseases of the Heart and Great Vessels.* Vol. 1–3. Philadelphia: WB Saunders, 1961:1401.

3. Fontana RS, Edwards JE. *Congenital Cardiac Disease: A Review of 357 Cases Studied Pathologically.* Philadelphia: WB Saunders, 1962:291.

4. Wagenvoort CA, Heath D, Edwards JE. *The Pathology of the Pulmonary Vasculature.* Springfield, Ill: Charles C Thomas, 1964:494.

5. Stewart JR, Kincaid OW, Edwards JE. *An Atlas of Vascular Rings and Related Malformations of the Aortic Arch System.* Springfield, Ill: Charles C Thomas, 1964:171.

6. Edwards JE, Carey LS, Neufeld HN, Lester RG. *Congenital Heart Disease. Correlation of Pathologic Anatomy and Angiocardiography.* Vol. 1 and 2. Philadelphia: WB Saunders, 1965:890.

7. Edwards JE, Goot B. *The Illustrated Coronary Fact Book.* New York: Arco, 1973:101.

8. Voldaver Z, Neufeld HN, Edwards JE. *Coronary Arterial Variations in the Normal Heart and in Congenital Heart Disease.* New York: Academic Press 1975:171.

JOHN WEBSTER KIRKLIN, MD:
A Conversation With the Editor*

I first met John Kirklin in 1969 when he was 52 years old. The occasion was a committee which had been formed to unify the nomenclature and coding of cardiovascular disease in children. That committee met on several occasions, and thus, I had an opportunity in a small room to witness John Kirklin in action. I remember being enormously impressed with the quiet precision with which he stated his views. There was never any doubt what his views were on a particular topic, but his manner was gentlemanly and persuasive without being overbearing. Of course, I had been fascinated by his rapid rise to fame at such a young age at the Mayo Clinic, and his essentially capturing cardiac surgery at that famous institution in his early 30s, and then within about 10 years becoming the first Chairman of Surgery there. His move to Alabama in 1966 when he was 49 years old was both a surprise to me and a fascination for me. I wondered why a man at the peak of his influence at a world famous institution would leave to move to a relatively impoverished state and to a medical center that was anything but the Mayo Clinic at the time. It was not long, however, before patients from all over the world were coming to Birmingham and young physicians were knocking on his door to train in his department. His high volume of publications continued after his coming to Birmingham, and it was not long before the Medical Center at the University of Alabama in Birmingham was well known all over the world.

Then in February 1978 I had another encounter with John Kirklin, and it had a lasting impact on me. A year earlier The American College of Cardiology had asked me to direct a course at their newly built Heart House, and I suggested one on the multidisciplinary approach to congenital heart disease. Jesse Edwards, Mary Ellen Engle, Sam Kaplan, and John Kirklin participated. During the 3 days of the meeting, 21 specific congenital cardiovascular malformations were discussed with either Jesse Edwards or myself describing morphologic features, either Mary Ellen Engle or Sam Kaplan describing the clinical, roentgenographic, electrocardiographic, and echocardiographic features, and John Kirklin discussing operative treatment and results. The malformations reviewed in this course included such topics as atrial septal defect, ventricular septal defect, aorticopulmonary defects, isolated pulmonic stenosis, tetralogy of Fallot, aortic isthmic coarctation and interruption, aortic valve stenosis, aortic valve atresia and other hypoplastic left heart syndromes, discreet and tunnel subaortic stenosis, supravalvular aortic stenosis, cardiac malpositions, transposition complexes, origin of both great arteries from the right ventricle, asplenia and polysplenia syndromes, pulmonic valve atresia with intact ventricular septum, tricuspid valve atresia, congenital mitral regurgitation and mitral valve prolapse, anomalous origin of one or both major coronary arteries, left ventricular inflow obstruction, the Epstein malformation, persistent truncus arteriosus, vascular rings, and congenital aortic regurgitation. John Kirklin presented his data with numbers and results for each of these specific anomalies. The science and precision of his presentations were overwhelming. Any observer at that conference could appreciate the desire for precision and quantitation sought in every aspect of his life by John Kirklin. I thought that 3-day conference personified the essence of this man. He brought that precision and conciseness to the operating room, to the intensive care unit, and to life in general. John Kirklin is the greatest scientific cardiac surgeon of this century and his contributions will continue to be influential many decades after he is gone.

William Clifford Roberts, MD[†] (hereinafter, WCR): *Dr. Kirklin, what I would like to try to learn from you is what gave you that desire to excel far above the pack. I wonder if you could start by talking about your parents. What it was like growing up in Muncie, Indiana? Did you have brothers and sisters? What do you remember from very youngest times?*

John Webster Kirklin, MD[‡] (hereinafter, JWK): Well, what drove me, I suppose, is *the lure of the unknown*. Maybe that is what everybody says, but that is a very conscious appeal to me. What is not known has always made me curious, challenged me. As far as growing up, I don't remember very much about Muncie, Indiana, because my family left there when I was about 8 years old and my father accepted a position as a radiologist at the Mayo Clinic. I really grew up in Rochester, Minnesota. I don't have any outstanding memories of that era, at least related to medicine, except that when I left to go to college at the University of Minnesota the one thing I was pretty sure of was that I did not want to be a doctor. At the University of Minnesota, those 4 years were very formative to me in a lot of ways. I don't know exactly why, maybe just my age, or whatever it was, but I came under the influence of a biochemist named, Gortner, a great guy, not very well-known today, probably long ago dead, but he taught biochemistry at the University of Minnesota out on what was called "the farm" campus, not really part of the main university. He was a great man and had a reputation with all great chemists. The people in the Department of Chemistry and also in the Department of Physics at the University of

* This series of interviews are underwritten by an unrestricted grant from Bristol Myers Squibb.

† Baylor Cardiovascular Institute, Baylor University Medical Center, Dallas, Texas 75246.

‡ Department of Surgery, Division of Cardiovascular Surgery, University of Alabama School of Medicine, Birmingham, Alabama 35294-0007.

0002-9149/98/$19.00 **1027**
PII S0002-9149(98)00068-X

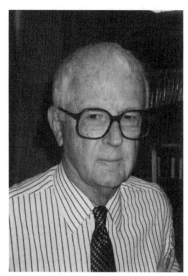

FIGURE 1. Photograph of JWK during the interview (by WCR).

Minnesota really attracted me. I liked what they did and what they taught. I suppose those years shaped me as much as anything else. Plus, the first year at Harvard Medical School, there was a guy named, A. Baird Hastings, teaching biochemistry. I spent the summer between the first and second years of medical school in Boston working in the laboratories of that department with Logan. I stayed with a couple of friends of mine, Bill Christiansen, and another from Michigan, Bill Vandorlaan, who became a well-known endocrinologist on the West coast. No doubt I was enormously enamored by those sciences and I suppose I developed a little bit of snootiness, intellectual arrogance, if you will, just a little, not a lot but a little, just enough to make me want to be different than most physicians. That is probably what started it.

WCR: *Did you have brothers and sisters?*

JWK: I had one sister, 4 years younger than me, and she is now dead. No brothers.

WCR: *You were the only boy and you were the older of the 2 siblings. Was there medicine in your family other than your father?*

JWK: No, there wasn't, and my father did not bring his work home. There was not much talk about medicine around the house. By the time I was beginning to finish at the university and was interested in medicine, I spent a lot of time with my father and watched him work, watched the operations and all that. Before that I had not particularly paid much attention to the Mayo Clinic.

WCR: *What was home life like in Minnesota. When your father came home, I presume his hours were relatively regular, did you'll sit around the dining table at night and have discussions on this or that topic? Was it an intellectual environs that you grew up in?*

JWK: Not particularly. I have a little trouble separating that period from later periods, but I don't think it was a particularly intellectual environment. I always was great in school. It was very easy for me. I got great grades and they all liked that, but there really wasn't much intellectual format.

WCR: *When you were in high school, did you play sports?*

JWK: Not competitively. I played the usual stuff kids play, tennis, basketball, a little bit of baseball, but never competitively.

WCR: *You were sort of a small guy.*

JWK: Yes, I was a small guy and still am. In college I weighed only 130 pounds.

WCR: *Why did you decide to go to the University of Minnesota to college? What were you planning to major in when you went off to college?*

JWK: I went to the University of Minnesota because a lot of my friends were going to Dartmouth, Harvard, Yale, and all of that, and I decided I wouldn't try, I would go to the university. I don't think any of my friends from Rochester went to the University of Minnesota when I did. It was a big school, much bigger now, but it was even then a huge university—easy to get lost in the mob. I figured if I made it there, I could make it anyplace.

WCR: *So you enjoyed the challenge of a big environs. You must have liked your home to want to go only 100 miles or so away to college.*

JWK: I am not sure that had much to do with it. I didn't go home very much.

WCR: *You were born in 1917. You went off to college in 1934?*

JWK: Yes, and I graduated from Harvard Medical School in 1942. I spent 4 years in college and 4 years in medical school. I graduated from the University of Minnesota in 1938.

WCR: *So that was in the midst of the depression. Were you conscious of the depression going on in the USA in Minnesota as a youngster?*

JWK: I was conscious of it, but I think one of the many things my father did for me was to shield me from it. He never talked about money, never complained about money, never said he had to borrow money to help me go to school, all of which he did, but he never discussed it with me. He just shielded me from that world.

WCR: *So you sort of took it for granted that you could go wherever you wanted and your family was supportive of that.*

JWK: Absolutely. My father played no role in where I went. He said, "That is up to you."

WCR: *What do you remember about college? Did you enjoy it? Did you have a good time?*

JWK: I had a wonderful time. I was the student manager of the football team for 4 years. At that time, the University of Minnesota football team was the greatest in the country, national champions for 3 years. I traveled with the team, and I adored every second of that football job. It is perhaps my fondest memory of the university. I also graduated with a lot of degrees, along with Phi Beta Kappa, and I liked that, but that was easy for me. I spent long hours on that dumb football manager's job.

WCR: *What did you do? What did "student manager" mean?*

JWK: As the freshman and sophomore manager, you were just an equipment "scuff pup." You picked up the footballs and shoulder pads after the players were done and put them away. In the junior and senior years, it was a white collar job and a very nice job, because you got to know the players, the coaches, you traveled with the team. It was fun.

WCR: *So you learned something about management during that period of time.*

JWK: The team had a great coach, a fellow named Bernie Berman. Nowadays most people do not remember him, but he was great by any standard. I enjoyed knowing him a lot.

WCR: *Have you kept up with some of the football players and coaches?*

JWK: Only, Bud Wilkinson. He was also in the same fraternity. He was one year ahead of me in school, and of course, he was a great football player. I knew him quite well.

WCR: *What did you major in in college?*

JWK: I think I majored in psychology because I could get to all those classes and still be the manager of the football team. I think I had 2 minors: 1 in biochemistry and 1 in abnormal psychology.

WCR: *So you went to the University of Minnesota without the intention of going to medical school. What made you switch to medicine?*

JWK: I don't know Bill. I suppose deep in my heart I always wanted to but would not let it surface. I don't know, just all of a sudden I wanted to go to medical school, and I wanted to go to Harvard Medical School.

WCR: *Why did you choose Harvard?*

JWK: I don't know. It was said to be hard to get into. Perhaps that was one reason. I don't really know. It had a great reputation. I asked around in Rochester, and everybody thought Harvard was a pretty good school.

WCR: *So you went off to Boston in 1938, having lived in a relatively small town (Rochester) and in a relatively large town (Minneapolis). Was Boston agreeable to you once arriving as a 21 year old?*

JWK: Yes.

WCR: *In medical school, did you find the teaching good? Was it better than it was at the University of Minnesota? Were you impressed with the way they taught or were you a bit disappointed?*

JWK: Neither. I was impressed with the people primarily.

WCR: *Your student colleagues or the faculty?*

JWK: I really meant the faculty, but the student colleagues were outstanding also. Many of them were my best friends for many, many years after that. The faculty was highly impressive. For example, in our freshman years, there were Saturday morning courses and one morning early in the year there was a course in wound healing given by Robert E. Gross, and when he walked in the room and had talked for a few minutes, there were 100 cardiac surgeons in the audience. A lot of people like that had a profound impression on all of us.

WCR: *So you eventually went up and trained with him?*

JWK: Yes, right after I got out of the Army.

WCR: *Who had the biggest impact on you in medical school?*

JWK: Robert Gross, no question about it.

WCR: *How long was it after you entered medical school that you decided that "by golly, I am going to be a surgeon"?*

JWK: I don't know. I suppose I always wanted to be a surgeon. Maybe the glamour of it.

WCR: *Did you always like to work with your hands? Did you like to build things when you were a youngster.*

JWK: A little bit but I don't think anymore than anybody else. Not particularly.

WCR: *When you were in medical school, did you do any research?*

JWK: Yes, I spent one summer in the biochemistry laboratories.

WCR: *You enjoyed that?*

JWK: I did.

WCR: *You went 4 years to medical school, although the war had started in your senior year.*

JWK: The accelerated programs had not quite begun. The 999 internship program was in effect at that time.

WCR: *Who were some of your classmates in medical school that have done very well?*

JWK: There are so many, and one was Hans Zinsser. I can't think but there were a bunch of them. John Merrill, perhaps, was one of the best known. Some of them were surgeons. A few of them were heart surgeons.

WCR: *How many were in your class at Harvard?*

JWK: I think 110.

WCR: *Were you number 1 in your graduating class?*

JWK: I think so.

WCR: *Were you number 1 when you graduated from the University of Minnesota as far as you could tell.*

JWK: I was in a very small top percent.

WCR: *Did you have to study hard to make those grades or did they seem to come easy for you.*

JWK: Easy, I think.

WCR: *Here you were in Boston, you had the Brigham Hospital, the Massachusetts General, and you in 1942 decided to intern at the University of Pennsylvania. What was behind that decision?*

JWK: Sitting here thinking back, I suppose I was just sort of contrary. I did not want to follow the herd. Everybody said, "You've got to intern in Boston. It is the only place in the world." I knew it was not the only place in the world so I decided to go somewhere else.

WCR: *How did you like the University of Pennsylvania Hospital? Was that what you wanted after you got there?*

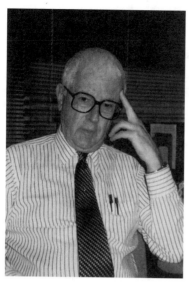

FIGURE 2. Photograph of JWK during the interview (by WCR).

JWK: It was a rotating internship. The Boston internships were all straight internships. I was interested in a rotating internship. I don't know why, but I was.

WCR: *During your year in Philadelphia, was there anybody who really had an impact on you?*

JWK: Perhaps 2 people, Jonathan Rhodes was there. Remember now that this was during World War II and a lot of those people were off to the war. Dr. Rhodes was there. Then there was a guy who was an assistant resident in medicine named Franklin Murphy. I don't know if you ever knew him, but he became a very famous person. He went to the University of Kansas as the Dean and then maybe as the vice-president. Then he went to California to the new school in Los Angeles, UCLA, built around a fancy new hospital. He went out there where he became the Chancellor. Then he went to become the CEO of the Times/Mirror Corporation. He was a high-school all-state halfback. A very unusual guy who I got to know pretty well, and who I enjoyed a lot. He had a big impact on me.

WCR: *Even though you decided to take a rotating internship, you always knew you wanted to go into surgery.*

JWK: Absolutely.

WCR: *In retrospect, were you glad you did the rotating internship?*

JWK: Surely.

WCR: *Most of your classmates took a straight medicine or straight surgical internship? So you were sort of a rebel in your choice? In other words, not many people from Harvard Medical School went for rotating internships.*

JWK: No, no one had for a long time.

WCR: *What did your colleagues, your classmates, and the faculty at Harvard think about this, the top fellow in the class taking a rotating internship?*

JWK: I don't know and I didn't care.

WCR: *Why did you decide to leave Philadelphia after 1 year to go to the Mayo Clinic?*

JWK: It was the 999 era, and you took a 9-month internship, then you had to commit to another 9 months or be willing to be drafted. I just decided to go back to Rochester for 9 more months, rather than staying in Pennsylvania. I did not think it was all that great, and I was anxious to get started with a surgical career, so I decided to go back to Rochester to do a surgical residency.

WCR: *Had you known a good number of the surgery faculty at the Mayo Clinic through your father? Would they come over to your house?*

JWK: No, not so much. I knew most of them, a little, not very well.

WCR: *When you got back there you liked it right away? You were pleased you made the change?*

JWK: Fairly pleased. I was disappointed in having to spend so much time on the medical service, but other than that I was pleased. I was happy.

WCR: *Did you get to do enough operating yourself right away or not?*

JWK: No, the Mayo Clinic does not work that way or it didn't then. It does now. I was just learning and excited about everything. I met my wife.

WCR: *You met your wife there? Your wife is a physician? At what stage was she?*

JWK: She came there as a resident in medicine at the same time I came as a resident in surgery.

WCR: *That was April 1943. When did you get married?*

JWK: In December 1943.

WCR: *You met and 6 months later you were married? Has your wife practiced while you have been married or not?*

JWK: Don't forget this was World War II. I went off to the service, knew I was going to go to a U.S. place for awhile so she decided she would go with me. She was pregnant at the time, and our child was born in an Army Hospital. Then, when I finished the service, we went back to Rochester. We had 2 children by then so she was pretty busy. She never finished her training, but when we came to Birmingham she began to work again, not as a practicing physician but in various clinics.

WCR: *So at age 26 in December 1943, you got married. Where did you go in the Army? What did you do those 27 months?*

JWK: I was a neurosurgeon!

WCR: *Where were you?*

JWK: The reason is that I had enough general surgical training to get a B medical occupational specialty in surgery but not an A. When I went in the service it was just at the time of the landing on the Normandy beaches, the Spring of 1944. The Army had a massive number of head injuries, peripheral nerve injuries, so they took some of us who had some general surgical training, not enough to be qualified general surgeons, sent us to neurosurgical school, sent me back to Philadelphia for 5 weeks, then we were neurosurgeons. For $2\frac{1}{2}$ years I practiced neurosurgery in the U.S. Army.

WCR: *Where were you?*

JWK: I was in Springfield, Missouri, at a place called O'Reilly General Hospital.

WCR: *You spent your full time there other than the 5 weeks or so in Philadelphia.*

JWK: I had just joined one of those auxiliary surgical teams as the war came to a close. I had just been assigned to go to the Pacific as the war ended.

WCR: *That must have been an exciting experience to learn a new specialty.*

JWK: I operated day and night, every day of the week practically. Worked under a wonderful man named Francis Murphy who was a neurosurgeon in Memphis. He is now dead. I got a lot of experience. It was a wonderful experience.

WCR: *You were the prime operator in no time flat. You were doing craniotomies, etc.*

JWK: Mostly peripheral nerve injuries, some sympathectomies, a few craniotomies, not many. Those people usually did not live to get there.

WCR: *Your period in the Army was in actuality a period of surgical training for you?*

JWK: Absolutely.

WCR: *So when you went back to the Mayo Clinic, it was almost like you had had a continual surgical residency since you began essentially in July 1943? You went back to the Mayo Clinic after the Army in October 1946. As a resident you only had 2 more years of training in surgery officially there at the Mayo Clinic. Is that correct?*

JWK: I went back to the Mayo Clinic primarily to spend a little time before I could go back to Boston to work with Dr. Gross for 6 months, which I did in 1948.

WCR: *The first 2 years back at the Mayo Clinic you were doing essentially general surgery. Did you do much chest surgery in that period? When you finished the Mayo Clinic did you feel comfortable in chest surgery?*

JWK: I felt comfortable with surgery in general. I had fantastic experience in the Army so I knew my way around the extremities, the neck, and then with my subsequent training at the Mayo Clinic, I was really a general surgeon. I did hysterectomies and so on.

WCR: *So during the 2 years of residency at the Mayo Clinic you were operating all you wanted to? Then in 1948 you went to the Children's Hospital for 6 months? What was that like.*

JWK: It was a great, great experience, primarily, I suppose, because of Dr. Gross, who was a fabulous surgeon, even in retrospect.

WCR: *When you say fabulous, do you mean technically, exquisitely, precise or what?*

JWK: Technically, an exquisite surgeon with a good mind, and just a great man.

WCR: *Was he the best surgeon technically you had encountered?*

JWK: I think so. We used to sit around at night with notebooks (I wished I had saved them), drawing all the things we could do if we could ever get inside the heart. In 1948, I had tons of drawings about fixing ventricular septal defects and repairing tetralogies, fixing mitral valves, all ready once we could get into the heart. It was interesting.

WCR: *Were these discussions with Gross?*

JWK: No, with colleagues, other residents.

WCR: *You were sort of off on your own in many of these many mental exercises before the pump came along.*

JWK: After I got back to Rochester, a fellow named Jesse Edwards was there and he was a very important component in that sort of internal operating. I learned about cardiac pathology from Jesse.

WCR: *When you went to work for Robert Gross for these 6 months, were you the only fellow with him?*

JWK: No, I was the junior resident technically. I had to wait for a spot, because, of course, everybody wanted to work with him. So I was a junior resident and the first rotation I was on was neurosurgery for I think 2 months, but the rest of the 6 months I spent scrubbing with Dr. Gross and doing a few hernias.

WCR: *In actuality you would have taken the 6 months with Robert Gross anytime during that 3-year period after you went back to the Mayo Clinic, when the slot opened up?*

JWK: I arranged that when I was still in the Army. It was very hard to get a job with him.

WCR: *When you worked with Gross, you were the first assistant? Did he let you do any cases as primary operator?*

JWK: I don't think I did any with him. I did a lot of cases at Children's as the primary operator, but I don't think I did with Gross.

WCR: *You enjoyed operating with him? How was he in the operating room? Did he talk or chat or was he totally focused on the job he was doing?*

JWK: The answer to that question is best answered by the following: I would pass him in the halls frequently, of course, and sometimes he would see me coming down the hall and he never said a word, so I did not say anything to him either. Sometimes I would pass him and he would stop and chat, so I got along great with him, because I think I knew how to get along with him. If he did not want to talk, I wouldn't. It was the same in the operating room. He would sometimes talk about the election of the Mayor of Boston, how lousy he was. Other times he would go 2 or 3 cases and not say a word, so I did not say anything either.

WCR: *So you figured out when to keep you mouth shut and when to converse with him. You felt parallel or in communication with him.*

JWK: I felt totally comfortable with him.

WCR: *Did he invite you to his house? Did you become friends with his wife and 2 daughters?*

JWK: Not close friends, but friends.

WCR: *When you left after those 6 months, did you consider him the best you had thus far encountered?*

JWK: Yes, and I was lucky enough to somehow keep crossing his path and seeing him. I sort of thought I had a special relationship with the guy.

WCR: *What were his work habits like? What time did he get to the hospital?*

JWK: Bill, I don't know. It just seems to me he was always there. I think he must have come early, but he was not a slave to the business by any means. He enjoyed living a lot. He was just a great guy to me, but not for everybody. A lot of people did not like him.

WCR: *You felt very comfortable that when he operated on people they were getting the best at that time. Was he an arrogant man?*

JWK: Many people would say so. He was not my definition of arrogance.

WCR: *He was still a pretty young fellow at that time. How did he rise so quickly up there.*

JWK: He closed a ductus while, his boss, Dr. William E. Ladd, was out of town. He became famous overnight. Dr. Gross was a senior resident. Gross did the ductus, the kid survived, and Gross was famous.

WCR: *From that point on people came directly to see Gross? How did Ladd react to all of that?*

JWK: Dr. Ladd was quite an old man by then. He was still fully active, but he retired within a few years. I think he had retired by 1948 when I was there. Dr. Gross was the Professor. There was not much time for Dr. Ladd to react. People said he did not like it very well, and he raised hell when he got back to work after the famous ductus, but what could he do. When you have a famous pupil, what can you do?

WCR: *Then, you went back to the Mayo Clinic and you had another year. Were you still in training for another year?*

JWK: Yes, I interrupted my training there to be with Dr. Gross.

WCR: *In actuality when you went back to the Mayo Clinic you were doing the same thing you were doing before, continuing your residency in general surgery.*

JWK: Yes. It was not until January 1950 that I became a member of the staff with full operating privileges.

WCR: *You knew they were going to ask you to join the staff, but you did not know that when you went back for that final year?*

JWK: No.

WCR: *So at age 31 years old, you are a member of the surgical staff of the Mayo Clinic. At that time were there boards in thoracic surgery?*

JWK: In thoracic surgery, yes, but not in cardiac surgery.

WCR: *You took your boards in general and then in thoracic surgery? Once you went on the faculty, you were doing more thoracic than you were doing general or not?*

JWK: Fifty/fifty perhaps. That was sort of the manner of living at that time. That is what everybody did.

WCR: *Up until that point, you had not published any articles in medical journals?*

JWK: I had published 1 article the summer in medical school while working in biochemistry. I published 2 or 3 articles while doing neurosurgery in the Army.

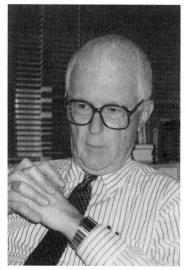

FIGURE 3. Photograph of JWK during the interview (by WCR).

WCR: *Here you are the 31-year-old new faculty person. Was anybody smothering you or looking over your shoulder or were you sort of on your own?*

JWK: I was for sure on my own, but I had a guy named Jim Clagett, and his predecessor, Dr. Harrington, who were senior thoracic surgeons at the Mayo Clinic, who were very good to me, totally supportive, very helpful, could not have been better.

WCR: *Clagett was how old then?*

JWK: I would guess 40.

WCR: *You mentioned when we started this discussion that what drove you was your curiosity, your desire to figure things out, to learn new things, to make innovations. Did you know Gibbon in Philadelphia when you were in that city?*

JWK: No, he was away with the U.S. Army or Navy. Also, he worked at Jefferson, a different hospital.

WCR: *So, when did you get wind of Gibbon's working on a heart/lung machine?*

JWK: I am not sure, Bill. All I can remember is that in 1952, at the Surgical Forums of the American College of Surgeons, Dr. Gross was presiding, and Dr. Gibbons gave a paper about his experience with dogs, and he said, "I think we are soon going to use this on people." That is when I suppose I really became conscious of it. Up until that time, I did mainly 2 operations at the Mayo Clinic: lymph node biopsies and mitral commissurotomies. That is what I did most everyday. Once in a while a gastric resection or colon resection, mitral commissurotomies, a new exciting operation, and sometimes a hernia.

WCR: *So you were the Mayo Clinic mitral commissurotomy person. How did you capture that? That was an exciting thing. Clagett did not want to do that?*

JWK: No, he didn't. Bob Glover had been trained at the Mayo Clinic. I knew him quite well, and somehow or another things were much easier being that I knew Dr. Bailey quite well. I knew Dwight Harken, of course. I had known him in Boston. We used to remark about his working in the dog lab doing this stuff. Mitral commissurotomy was sort of like the back of my hand to me. Before I had ever done one I had learned a lot about it, heard about it, lived and breathed it. It was exciting. There were only a few places in the world doing this. Mayo Clinic had plenty of cases so I did them.

WCR: *You enjoyed being in the heart?*

JWK: Sure. Absolutely.

WCR: *What was the first creative, innovative thing you did at the Mayo Clinic?*

JWK: I don't know the answer to that. I right away found myself in the middle of probably the most exciting group of people I had ever worked with, Howard Burchell, Earl Wood, Jesse Edwards, David Donald, and less well-known, but an experimental surgeon, Jim DuShane, and with that group of people, life was just terribly exciting. I think together we did a hell of a lot of innovative things. It is hard to take them apart, but we published tons of papers, and everyday was something new and exciting.

WCR: *Gibbon closed an atrial septal defect in 1953?*

JWK: Yes, it was in 1953. I can remember very well the period when that was done. My life in that era began when I was sitting talking to Earl Wood, who had just come back from an autopsy done by Jesse Edwards on a patient of Howard Burchell's who I had operated on by the closed method, a patient with pulmonary stenosis and a severe subvalvular (infundibular) obstruction. Earl Wood said: "You know, you are never going to do any better until you get inside that heart and look at it." I said, "Yes, I guess so." I was depressed, of course, about losing somebody. I think we decided that day to move ahead. "Okay, that is what we are going to do," we said. That was 1952, and Gibbon did not do his first successful case until 1953. We made a trip around the country then. Howard didn't go, Jesse didn't go, Earl went part of the time. I went all the time. Dave Donald went. We visited Gibbon's place. We visited Dewey Dodderal in Detroit and Bill Mustard in Toronto. Dodderal's pump looked like a car engine. He was a well-known thoracic surgeon, well-known for working experimentally with a machine built by General Motors. Gibbon was working with his machine which looked like an IBM computer because it had been built by IBM. Bill Mustard was working with monkey lungs as an oxygenator. Nobody was doing any clinical work. I suppose if I have any great, good luck it is that I am very impatient with people talking vaguely and promising, "We are fixing to get ready to do that." So, I decided to hell with it, we needed to do it, not just sit around talking about it or doing it on dogs. I had already had about a year and one-half in the dog lab with a simple pump oxygenator. We got permission from Gibbon and IBM to build essentially their machine. It was different from the General Motors one, but a little similar, quite a bit better. When we had it, we used it.

WCR: *When did you first use it?*

JWK: March 1955, and every year on that day I still get a letter from Howard Burchell, including 1996, 1997, and I'm sure I will get one in 1998. He is a special guy.

WCR: *Did you see Howard Burchell, Jesse Edwards, Earl Wood, a lot?*

JWK: Everyday practically.

WCR: *When you were at the Mayo Clinic, it is my understanding you operated every other day. So 1 week you operated 3 days, the next week 2 days.*

JWK: That came into effect while I was there, but it was not that way initially. You operated every other day including Saturday.

WCR: *So it became 3 days a week. Did you like that?*

JWK: It was okay. It was all I knew.

WCR: *The days you were not operating, you were seeing patients you were going to operate on the next day?*

JWK: Plus, working in the experimental laboratory.

WCR: *After the first pump operation, I gather that open heart surgery by you just absolutely took off, and each year the number of cases increased.*

JWK: So did the length of the waiting period. It became over a year sometimes. I will tell you a little story about that period, about Russell Brock, because you probably knew him and know that he was a very difficult, tough guy. I forget what day we did the first operation, let's say it was a Tuesday, and Tuesday night Dr. Varco called me from Minneapolis (We all knew each other quite well.) so, among other things, he said, "We have a visitor who would like to come down and talk to you." I said "That is fine, who is it?," and he said, "Russell Brock." He wanted to know if we were going to do another case, and I said, "Yes, we are going to do one Thursday." Russell came down Wednesday from Minneapolis and said, "Now, I guess you are going to do a case tomorrow." I said, "We are." He said, "I won't come to the operation." I said, "You have to, you are most welcome." He said, "No, I think there will be concern over a famous visitor." I said, "You will be most welcome." He said, "I want to sit in the gallery someplace where I won't be conspicuous, I don't want to bother you." He came and sat and did not open his mouth, just sat there. Absolutely the most consideration to a young surgeon that you can imagine. Most people don't think that about Russell Brock, but that is the way he was. That was a great period and, of course, it was a period when nobody knew the indications and so on. I saw a lot of patients that nobody knew whether they should be operated on or not. That is the reason I saw Howard Burchell, Jim DuShane and all those people quite a lot.

WCR: *So most of the conditions of the patients having cardiac operations using cardiopulmonary bypass had never been operated on before. You could not read about these conditions in the library because no one had operated on them before. You were oper-*

ating so much you could not put all the new innovations together at once.

JWK: We published them pretty much as they occurred.

WCR: *What was life like on a day-to-day basis. Your bibliography, no question, just sky rocketed during that period of time.*

JWK: The work ethic in southern Minnesota is enormous. Everybody works very hard. You don't survive through the winter if you don't work hard and plan ahead. We sort of reflected the area. You had to plan, work hard, "no rest for the wicked." We all worked very hard. We would get to work at 5:30 in the morning. It was an exciting, terribly busy, wonderful time.

WCR: *What time would you leave the hospital at night as a rule?*

JWK: As a rule, I don't know, but often it was 10:00 or 11:00 P.M.

WCR: *You were living at that hospital during that period. How did you write your manuscripts? Did you dictate, did you write them in pencil?*

JWK: I wrote them in pencil.

WCR: *When would you do most of your writing?*

JWK: Probably on the weekends and nonoperative days. I don't remember exactly, but I am almost sure that is when it was.

WCR: *It must have been a loss when Jesse Edwards left in 1960.*

JWK: It was a big loss. Actually, however, he never really left. Even to this day he goes back pretty frequently.

WCR: *At least you did not see him on a day-to-day basis. You found him very helpful, particularly early on, in your getting familiar with the inside of the heart?*

JWK: Extremely helpful. One day I asked Jess, "Where is the bundle of His?" He said, "I am not sure, but I'll tell you a person who does know and that is Maurice Lev and you should go see him." The next day I got on an airplane and went down to Miami to see him. I cannot say too much positive about Jess Edwards' influence on all of us. He was just a very important member of a small group.

WCR: *You were the first and I gather the only one to use the pump there early on, 1955 or 1956. Did anybody else at the Mayo Clinic do cases using cardiopulmonary bypass early on. I gather that Dwight McGoon did not come until later?*

JWK: Dwight came in 1958. A fellow named Bunky Ellis, who went to Boston about a year after I left, came and he did some of the cases.

WCR: *In 1964 you became Chairman of the Department of Surgery at the Mayo Clinic. How did that work out?*

JWK: I wanted it badly. There had never been a Chairman of a Department before. Everybody was equal among kings.

WCR: *Really. You were the first Chairman of Surgery at the Mayo Clinic.*

JWK: I think that is true. It became more and more obvious to me that the Surgery Department needed a Chairman. That was a very important period for me. I totally changed the residency system, became a member of the Board of Governors, so I had some voice in the overall clinic policy. It was an added challenge.

WCR: *But it was good preparation for what came later, I presume, or did you already know what you wanted to do?*

JWK: No, I didn't. I was too busy to know what I wanted to do the next year. I was just too busy, too happy, too faced with problems needing solutions which required a lot of thought and effort. I had no idea of leaving the Mayo Clinic until about 1965 when I began to get invitations to various places who wanted a Professor of Surgery. I thought about it. I had a second son, Jim, who was a state champion springboard diver, and he did not want to leave until after his senior year. For one reason or another, I stayed there, even after I began to be bitten by that bug, until 1966.

WCR: *Why did you get bitten? Here you were on the Board of Governors, the Chairman of the Department of Surgery. Were those things going to run out? I mean, you weren't going to be on the Board of Governors forever?*

JWK: No, but they were not about to run out. "What else could I do?" I asked myself.

WCR: *How did the University of Alabama come about? I am sure you had plenty of offers to a lot of different places. At the time you received an offer from the University of Alabama at Birmingham (UAB), I guess cardiology was quite good at the UAB.*

JWK: It was pretty good. The main thing about the UAB was that there was not much here.

WCR: *So that just aroused your competitive spirit?*

JWK: Not quite exactly. Even though I had been terribly busy, operating, and thinking about things, doing special studies, all the time in my mind, I suppose, I was formulating a lot of opinions about how things should be done, what should determine the number of residents that a hospital takes, how a surgical program really should be run, should the residents just be turned free to operate willy-nilly or should they never operate or something in between. What were the appropriate arrangements between people, financial arrangements, everything, and it was time for me to do an experiment, so I came to the UAB. I have never said it that way before but that is really it.

WCR: *So you wanted to see if you could pull off what you had formulated in your mind as an ideal Department of Surgery?*

JWK: My interests were not strictly in the Department of Surgery. They were in the UAB. It was the entire medical center.

WCR: *So you thought you would have an institutional impact as well as a departmental impact?*

JWK: I was sure I would. At least, I hoped I would.

WCR: *How did it actually come about. Did you receive a letter from the Dean or President or Provost from UAB? What were the details?*

JWK: Do you remember a man named Joe Reeves? Joe was there. He called me, and that is the way I first knew about it. They had invited Frannie Moore (Boston) to be their external advisor and he called me. That is the way I got started.

WCR: *Joe Reeves called you and said "come on down here and visit us."*

JWK: He said, "We need a new Professor of Surgery." Dr. Lyons had died of a brain tumor, suddenly, unexpectedly. So they suddenly needed a new chairman.

WCR: *Here you were, having grown up in and now living in Rochester, Minnesota, with relatively brief spans in Minneapolis and Boston, and suddenly you are looking at a spot in the deep South. When you came down to Birmingham to look things over, what happened? How did you react? All these buildings that I see here now were not here then.*

JWK: No, they weren't here. I knew what I was getting into. I came down here a few times. I knew it would be really tough, very difficult. All of my friends in Rochester said, "How in the world can you go down there with their attitude about the blacks?" Nobody in Rochester knew anything about blacks. A big surprise is that I was able to continue my cardiac surgical life at the same pace as in Rochester, found new colleagues, good colleagues. The patients came.

WCR: *When you came down here the first time, did you say "no, I don't want to get into this" or did you keep investigating?*

JWK: I said to them and to myself, "I need to know more about this." I think I came down 3 times.

WCR: *When you decided to come here, you came not only as Chairman of the Department of Surgery with yourself being Director of the Division of Cardiovascular Surgery, you also came as Chief of the Medical Staff. You must have come down here with the authority to carry out all the objectives that you had formulated in your mind that you wanted to do if you had a department you could make your own. In other words, did you have hiring and firing rights of people in the intensive care unit? Did you have control over the nursing service in surgery?*

JWK: Bill, I did not organize any of that ahead of time. I figured if I couldn't hack it by being there, I couldn't. I figured I could get the authority just because I have always been successful in getting it when I wanted it, and when I wanted it I went after it and got it. I ended up with a whole lot of authority, but no more than I had had at the Mayo Clinic.

WCR: *It sounds to me like you just wanted a fresh challenge. You had conquered about all there was to conquer at the Mayo Clinic. You were now still at a young age, 47, Chairman of the Department of Surgery, already full Professor for 7 years, on the Board of Governors at the Mayo Clinic. Is Jim your oldest or middle child?*

JWK: Middle, we have 3 children.

WCR: *Is the third one a boy or girl?*

JWK: Girl.

WCR: *So you have boy, boy, girl. So your third one was a junior in high school when you left Roch-*

ester. So 1 more year and they are gone to college. The kids were soon to be gone.

JWK: My wife was perhaps a little restless in Rochester, because she is a very bright person, was AOA in medical school, and I think she never urged me to stay or leave, but she was favorable to moving.

WCR: *Where was your wife from? Where did she grow up?*

JWK: The state of Washington.

WCR: *So she is a Northwesterner. Where did she go to medical school?*

JWK: Buffalo.

WCR: *She came to Buffalo to go to medical school. Where did she go to college?*

JWK: She went to college at Washington State for her first year and then the University of Oregon.

WCR: *When you came to the UAB, I presume, you changed faculty a good bit, you changed house staff a good bit, relatively rapidly. All of a sudden a flock of patients were coming from all over the world to the UAB. Overnight the whole medical center changes. So everybody was happy. Now what did you find your biggest challenge? Here you are studying patients after operations. When did you get into evaluating who should be operated on, when, timing the procedures, the statistical analyses that you brought into the evaluation. How did this evolve?*

JWK: I think the way everything evolves. You attract colleagues dependent on the environment you build. I was very lucky. I think it must have been 1969 or 1970 when a young man named Gene Blackstone walked into my office and wanted an internship. He has been here ever since and he is a genius, literally.

WCR: *He wanted a surgery internship? Where had he gone to medical school?*

JWK: The University of Chicago.

WCR: *So he walked into your office. I figured you had recruited him. How did you know he was a genius?*

JWK: He walked into my office and said, "I want an internship." I said, "Well, you have to apply through the internship committee, the national mechanism was operating then." He said, "I am not eligible for that." I thought, "Oh God, here is another guy that flunked out of medical school." I said, "Why aren't you eligible?" He said, "Well, I graduated 2 years ago." I said, "What have you been doing since?" He said he had been working with . . . He named off the famous people at the University of Chicago. I said, "Have you been getting a Ph.D.?" He said, "No, I didn't have time." So Gene was already a very exceptional person, and as he worked as an intern, it was really obvious he was an exceptional person. He owed the Army/Air Force some time which he then gave to them, came back here, and has been here ever since. He is right next door, and we work very closely together and have for 25 years.

WCR: *Does he operate?*

JWK: No, he is not a surgeon. He is an investigator. He told me, "I don't want to be a surgeon. I want to be an investigator, and I figure the place to do that

is in the Department of Surgery where the action is.''
I figured he was right.

WCR: *He learned statistics on his own.*

JWK: No, at the University of Chicago he worked under Paul Meier for a year or 2.

WCR: *You were no slouch in the stuff at that time yourself.*

JWK: We pooled our efforts and there happens to be a statistician here who is very special, very unique. I am of the opinion that you will go any place and you will find a few special people. There were a few special people here and that made it possible.

WCR: *When you came to the UAB, rather than operating every other day, you started operating every day. Is that right?*

JWK: That is true.

WCR: *What was your typical day like after you had been here 2 or 3 years.*

JWK: I would get up at 4:30 in the morning, work for an hour at home on something, a book, a paper, or something like that, come to work, operate maybe until 1:00 or 2:00.

WCR: *You would get to the hospital at what time?*

JWK: Seven o'clock.

WCR: *But you had been up since 4:30 more or less. What time would you walk into the operating room.*

JWK: Seven-thirty. I never liked walking in when someone else was preparing the patient.

WCR: *Did you do the thoracotomy?*

JWK: Yes, on the first case. Not necessarily on the next one. We had a lot of wonderful residents.

WCR: *Why did you want to do that? Not many Chairman of Departments that are cardiac surgeons do thoracotomies anymore, do they?*

JWK: No, not many people accomplish what I have done either. Maybe there is a correlation. It is just that I suppose I am at the same time both confident and fearful. I just want to remember how to pound in the nails and saw the lumber, and I don't want to be in a position where I can't survive by myself, requiring an entourage around me. I never wanted to be in that position.

WCR: *So on your typical day, you would arrive at the hospital at 7:00 A.M. You had been up for a couple of hours before that. First case at 7:30. So how many patients were you operating on each day at UAB?*

JWK: Not so many a day, maybe 3.

WCR: *So your operations were finished as a rule by 1 or 2:00 P.M.*

JWK: Usually, but, you know, there is always the exception that goes until 7:00 or 8:00 P.M.

WCR: *Most days you had some time to take care of certain administrative tasks later in the afternoon.*

JWK: Administrative, research, data analysis, things like that.

WCR: *What time would you leave the hospital as a rule?*

JWK: Usually after dark 7:30, 8:00 o'clock.

WCR: *Were you any good after you got home?*

JWK: No.

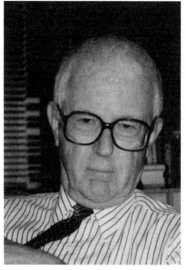

FIGURE 4. Photograph of JWK during the interview (by WCR).

WCR: *Did you have a cocktail when you got home?*

JWK: Usually.

WCR: *Would you do something else or would you go to bed early?*

JWK: Go to bed early. Both my wife and I enjoy music a lot so we usually sit down in the living room and put on a CD or record and have a drink and talk for a while, eat dinner, not do much after that.

WCR: *You were pretty good when you woke up in the mornings, but not once you got home at night.*

JWK: I almost never worked at home at night.

WCR: *Now when your kids were young you did not get home until 10:00 or 11:00 P.M.*

JWK: Too often.

WCR: *What kind of Daddy were you, are you?*

JWK: Probably not very good.

WCR: *When your son Jim was in the diving meets, you were there?*

JWK: Always.

WCR: *What do your other 2 children do?*

JWK: My oldest son was interested in track. He ran the 440 in high school. I would always go to that. Our daughter Helen did the usual things young girls do, ballet schools. She plays the violin. My wife is a pianist, not a concert pianist but a serious one. Helen has fulfilled her desires in that regard. Helen lives in Gainesville, Florida, where her husband is a professor of English. She plays in the Jacksonville Symphony. She is a very talented gal.

WCR: *What does your older son do?*

JWK: He went to Dartmouth College, graduated with all the honors, went to Harvard Law School where he lost a little interest in excelling. Then he was offered a position in a prestigious law firm in New York which he took, but after about 6 or 8 years, he became disenchanted with work, very introspective, tried to commit suicide at one point, ultimately divorced his wife (they have 2 kids), married another woman, still lives in New York. I think he has gotten his act somewhat together now, not at a high level. Maybe he didn't like it there in some way. I don't totally understand. He is different and perhaps when you asked if I was a good father probably not. If I had been, that probably should not have happened to young John. But life unfolds in strange directions.

WCR: *You stepped down as Chairman of the Department of Surgery in 1982, and as Director of the Cardiothoracic Division in 1985. You kept operating. When did you stop operating?*

JWK: I am not sure. Anne, my secretary could tell us, but it must have been about 1990.

WCR: *Why did you stop operating. You look healthy, vigorous.*

JWK: I always knew I would sometime. I have always known that. You may remember Professor E. J. Zerbini, who was a great surgeon in Sal Paulo, Brazil. We all watched him operate long after he should have stopped. I never wanted that to happen to me. I thought the Mayo Clinic plan at that time was a bit too rigorous, no reason to stop at 65 or something just because you reached that age if you were still fit. But I began to wonder if I was doing as good a job as someone else could have done, and you can only live with that so long and then you quit.

WCR: *Did you feel a difference. You are 79 and will be 80 this year. You didn't stop operating until you were 71?*

JWK: Probably.

WCR: *Did you feel at 70 that you were as good as at 40?*

JWK: I probably was better at 70 because I knew more, had more good sense, more experience. Technically, I don't think there is much deterioration. I thought I still did a good job and I always promised myself (I am not sure I hit it exactly) that I would quit before people began to think I needed to.

WCR: *So you were operating and all of a sudden, boom. You said, "This is it."*

JWK: One day I walked out and I have never been back.

WCR: *Are you glad you did that?*

JWK: Yes, I am glad I did it. I am sorry the time came, but I am glad I did it.

WCR: *How many operations do you figure you have done in your life?*

JWK: 10,000, something like that.

WCR: *You mentioned in your book your group did 50,000 operations. How did the book,* Cardiac Surgery, *come about?*

JWK: You remember what you wrote about that, that it would never have a second edition? That is the reason we brought out a second edition! I don't know exactly when I began thinking about a book, but whenever it was, I was in South America at a meeting where Brian Barratt-Boyes was and somehow we found out that each of us was thinking about writing a book. I said to Brian "why don't we do it together?"

He was never in love with the idea, still isn't, but we did it, and I think it was better for having done so.

WCR: *The first edition was 1988. You said in all of the chapters that both of you contributed to each chapter. If you initiated one, you sent it to him and vice versa. You both participated in each of those chapters. Each chapter is really an in-depth discussion of the topic of that particular chapter. You not only provide your own experiences but those that you considered worthwhile. How did you do all that literature work?*

JWK: I suppose we had a little bit of help but mostly we did it ourselves. Besides, Bill, it may be difficult today, but we knew everybody, we talked to everybody, we visited everybody, so, therefore, we remembered their articles very well because you could see the guy in the paper. I think we just knew the field terribly well. We lived in it.

WCR: *How long did it take to do the book?*

JWK: Three or four years.

WCR: *What was your work pattern like? Would you work on that book in the mornings? You were still operating then.*

JWK: I did the first book primarily at home in the mornings. The second edition was done mostly at the university, because that is where I had some help and the whole thing to look at.

WCR: *You wrote out your first draft in pencil? You did not dictate?*

JWK: Very little. I must say I can always tell when someone has dictated a paper.

WCR: *I actually like your reference way with the alphabet, then the number, and, as you say, if you want to later on, you can plug a reference in without having to change every lousy number in the whole shebang. Now that system has not taken off very well. Has anybody else copied you there? I think it is very reasonable. I admire your innovation here.*

How did you like being Editor of the Journal of Thoracic and Cardiovascular Surgery?

JWK: As one editor to another, I actually enjoyed it. I resented to some extent the time it took. As you well know, it takes a huge amount of time, but it was made worthwhile, I thought, by the 5% or 10% of papers that I positively, very favorably improved by being editor, by the people we sent them to, by the decisions we made when they came back, by the suggestions we made to the authors. I think we did a worthwhile job. You must feel that way.

WCR: *How much time did you spend on it?*

JWK: A lot. As I recall, it bridged the period between when I was operating and when I wasn't. So in a way, it was a refuge for using the time that was set free by not operating. I spent a lot of time on it.

WCR: *In retrospect, are you glad you waited to do that magnificent book until you were 71 years of age? So many people do books at age 40. You could not have had as many original contributions, it seems to me, if you had done that way back.*

JWK: I could not have for sure. It seemed a natural time.

WCR: *I think Dwight McGoon's foreword was the*

most beautiful I have ever read in a book. When you were operating, what was your favorite operation? If you could do just 3 operations and that was it, which ones would they have been?

JWK: I suppose the tetrology because it was so varied and so much of it. We lived to create a lot of that stuff. The knowledge maybe as much as the technique.

WCR: *Did you do a lot of switch operations for complete transposition or not?*

JWK: I don't think I ever did that. I was beginning to back away when the arterial switch came along. I am very familiar with it, however.

WCR: *Do you think there will ever be another surgeon that will do the whole gamut like you have done?*

JWK: No. I don't know why, but partly because it is not the fashion. But Dr. Gibbon once said to me, "Kirklin, I am not interested in fashion."

WCR: *It must have been very exciting to see your operative schedule and have these exciting cases lined up one after the other: tetralogy with varying degrees of right ventricular outflow obstruction, then pulmonic valve atresia with ventricular septal defect, then mitral valve replacement, then a coronary bypass for example. Did you like doing the coronary bypass operation?*

JWK: Yes. I think it is very exciting. It is not an easy operation. Everybody does so many of them, I guess they are good, but yes, I thought it was an interesting operation.

WCR: *Can you describe the atmosphere of your operating room? What was it like to be in your operating room when you were doing a tetralogy case, for example?*

JWK: Well, I didn't like the music on, never did, never will. I think it is a distraction to everybody, anytime during the procedure. If I were the patient I wouldn't want anybody, the circulating nurse, or anybody else distracted. This is very serious business, all compacted into a short period of time. At the same moment, people don't perform well if their tension gets too high so you have to break it a little bit. I think it is a very exciting orchestra to be able to conduct. That is the way I tried to play it. Everyone was responsible for everything else. The anesthesiologist was responsible for the "rib spreader" being in properly, and I was held responsible for the endotracheal tube, in a way shared responsibility, a very exciting experience, much more exciting than to be a solo. It is great to forge a group that really acts as one, all for the same purpose.

WCR: *Did you talk much during the operations?*

JWK: I was not silent like Robert Gross. It is not my nature, but I am not terribly talkative. Some people talk every second. I think I talked a fair amount especially once the critical part was over.

WCR: *How did you relax your help, so to speak?*

JWK: Very important maneuver. I think I did it by knowing them quite well, by being sure I knew their names, always, I didn't forget them, and by some little joke or brief report of some sort, half-kidding, half-

serious. One has to do that. The people have to like working if they are going to give that extra little bit that once in a while is required.

WCR: *If one of your patients, lets say, bled postoperatively and you had gone home, did you come back?*

JWK: Usually. Almost always.

WCR: *Did you follow your patients postoperatively? You saw them everyday?*

JWK: Well, I wouldn't say I saw them everyday by the 5th, 6th, or 7th day, but early on I always saw them daily and I saw them before they went home.

WCR: *How were you able to get such good follow-up on all the patients you operated on? You couldn't see them.*

JWK: Just like everybody, plain hard work. We organized a whole bunch of people out there. We spent our money that way instead of taking it home.

WCR: *Do we have too many cardiac surgeons? How is the number going to be cut down?*

JWK: Well, one of the things I am very proud of is that when I came down here eons ago, I set about talking to people, getting information, to see how many new surgeons we needed rather than deciding how many residents we took by the amount of work to be done at the hospital. I figured the state of Alabama needed about 1 new cardiac surgeon every 5 to 8 years, something like that. I was not popular for my thinking and talking that way, but that is what needed to be done. We just overproduced ourselves. I believe it was because the hospital needed to dictate the number of residents rather than society.

WCR: *It seems to me that surgeons today don't get the kind of experience that you had. You grew up on the aorta and esophagus and all the rest of it. You mastered the congenital challenges, valve replacements, the whole gamut. Ninety percent of cardiac operations today are bypasses. Now the congenital heart surgeons are not doing any of the other stuff.*

JWK: That is why I didn't go to the Boston Children's Hospital when I had a chance to go. You never did that yourself. You moved freely through the field of cardiac pathology. It must have been the same reason.

WCR: *More fun that way.*

JWK: It is more fun that way. Absolutely more fun. More exciting, more stimulating.

WCR: *As you look back, did you make any mistakes.*

JWK: Sure, 100's. I think I always tried to identify them and prevent them in the future, but sure I made mistakes.

WCR: *You always analyzed what you were doing? How do you relax?*

JWK: My wife and I had been married about 3 or 4 years and it was very apparent what lay ahead and we would grow further and further apart. I was working all the time. She had the kids to worry about. So we decided we had to find something we could do together that was outside, that was a little dangerous, a little exciting, so we bought a couple of horses. She and I have been riding ever since. Her horse got unruly and she was dislodged from the saddle and broke her hip about 5 or 6 years ago. I still ride 3 times a week.

WCR: *Where do you live here?*

JWK: We built a house outside of town 30 years ago, and we still live there.

WCR: *Do you have acreage to ride on your property?*

JWK: No, I keep the horses boarded out.

WCR: *So, where you board them is where you ride? How long does it take you to get into work from where you live?*

JWK: Not very long. That was a prime consideration. I had to be able to get into work in 10 or 15 minutes. Somebody's bleeding, I need to get there. Now it takes a little longer because it has all built up around us, but where we lived originally south of town, it was in the booneys.

WCR: *Did you play a musical instrument when you were a boy?*

JWK: I used to play the piano some.

WCR: *What are you most proud of that you have been able to accomplish in your professional and personal careers?*

JWK: I think there must be a missing part in me somewhere because I never feel very proud of anything, happy with it, but not particularly proud of it. There is something inside me that makes me take it apart and say I could have done that a little better. I am relatively proud of my contributions to the cardiothoracic world. I am relatively proud of that. I would be disappointed if it had not included clinicians and pathologists. I think we contributed a little but we learned a lot from you. I think I am pleased, maybe not proud of the fact that I have been able to continue to concentrate on details, not be satisfied with just a broad picture. I am proud of the work we have done, but I wish we could have done more and better.

WCR: *The precision.*

JWK: The precision, I think, is the key to everything—in your head, you hands, and everything.

WCR: *Did you do much teaching of medical students when you came to the UAB?*

JWK: I did. Early on every afternoon for an hour I went down to one of the surgical wards where the students were. I was interested in that because I found out very early that the caliber was just as good here as it was where I had come from, but that their early education wasn't, and I found it quite interesting to inquire as to why. It was because of the desperate economic conditions in Alabama between World War I and World War II. It was just pitifully poor. I could only learn all that by really working with the students. Then, I had been here for 6 or 8 years when this epidemic came through of students grading the faculty. I spent zero time after that teaching medical students. Not because they graded me poorly, but I didn't like the idea.

WCR: *How many medical students are there at the UAB.*

JWK: I am not sure—100 I am tempted to think about in every class.

WCR: *The surgery housestaff and fellows in car-*

diothoracic surgery have been reduced. You need to start cutting down the numbers of medical students.

JWK: It is a difficult problem. The world today is full of enormous problems. You must think so too. You are thoughtful about things and much of the world today is not very thoughtful. It seems to react more than anything.

WCR: *In the 50 years you have been in medicine and surgery, what surgeons do you really admire?*

JWK: Stanley Crawford. Maybe his is the first name that comes to mind. I had an enormous amount of respect, admiration and love for this man, all those things for Stanley Crawford. He was a great surgeon. Stanley stayed a generalist although he was the world's best when it came to the aorta, and he was also a superb abdominal surgeon. He was probably my greatest hero.

WCR: *You never worked with him?*

JWK: Never, but I somehow got to know him very well, spent a fair amount of time watching him operate. He would come up to Rochester ever so often. There are a lot of great surgeons. I shouldn't really single him out, but that is the name that comes to my mind when one asks about great surgeons.

WCR: *Do you think operating on some portions of the aorta, like the descending thoracic, is a bit more difficult than say aortic valve replacement or a mitral valve replacement?*

JWK: Absolutely. Very difficult.

WCR: *You can't make any mistakes in the aorta.*

JWK: No, and everything is more difficult. The exposure is more difficult, control of the bleeding is more difficult, the diseases are more difficult. There is nothing like an aortic dissection to challenge a surgeon. I think it is a tough, tough area and Stanley was just a master.

WCR: *You must be enormously pleased to have your son follow in your footsteps.*

JWK: I don't know Bill. I never felt particularly pleased, I liked it. The thing I like best is the story about it. He went to Ohio State because they had a great diving coach for college. In his third year, he called me to say, "I think I want to go to medical school." I said, "What?" He said, "Now, I even want to go to Harvard." I said, "That is nice, but you have to be more than wanting to. Why did you call." He said, "Well, I wanted a piece of advice." This was a first. He said, "Should I continue to dive next year? If I continue to dive I am risking not getting into Harvard. I think I will get into medical school some place, but I want to go to Harvard." I said, "Why?" He said, "It is supposed to be the best. If I can't dive, I think I probably can." I told him to go ahead and dive, and he nevertheless got into Harvard. He never dived again after beginning medical school because he was busy studying. Yes, I am proud of him. He has picked a very tough area, cardiac transplantation. I like it better than if he were doing something else, being a lawyer or business man or something.

WCR: *What is on the horizon out there in cardiac surgery? Jim is how old now?*

JWK: Fifty. Does not seem possible.

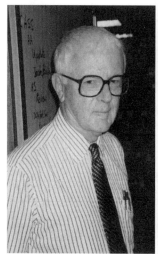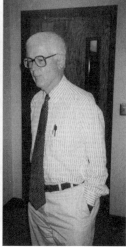

FIGURE 5. Photograph of JWK during the interview (by WCR).

WCR: *So he has 20 years more of operating.*

JWK: Fifteen, he says.

WCR: *Let's pick a 30-year-old surgeon. What is a 30-year-old cardiovascular surgeon today going to be doing at 55?*

JWK: I am sure things we have not thought about. I am afraid the world around him will limit his repertoire. I am afraid it will, and the reason I think that's bad is that he wants to do as well as he could on whatever he is doing as if he had a little more broad continuing experience. It is no good to be broadly trained and then thereafter do some little deal. People are still people and patients with heart trouble sometimes have trouble with their feet and so forth. I don't know. I think "where is medicine as a whole going to be?" It is very hard to see. I am guessing you and I have lived through the best years.

WCR: *You have interviewed a lot of people through the years, you have picked people to surround you that have obviously done very well on their own. When you pick a person to be a surgery resident or staff person, this is your person, what are you looking for? What characteristics are absolutely essential for you to find out about?*

JWK: I don't agree with the statement I am about tell you completely, but it is a little close. There was a surgeon at the Mayo Clinic called John Waugh, a great surgeon. John used to say, "I can tell you who is going to be a good surgeon by walking down the hall with him." I think there is a little truth to that. In other words, it is a very intuitive plus an analytical thing. I don't think there is any correct answer to the question, and I am not sure I have followed a consistent path. I was disappointed ever so often, but in general I think you just have to pay close attention to details, especially concentrating on the whole person. I can't answer that any other way.

WCR: *How do you handle a person you interview, looks like this person comes with a good record in*

medical school or further back than that, and low and behold you take him on your service and his hands are atrocious. You just know you don't want this person operating on anybody. How do you handle that type situation?

JWK: It is difficult. I think the worst solution maybe is to tell him/her that. The best solution is if one can somehow find things that not only he is good at, but he likes, that are outside the operating room, gradually pushing him in that direction so he seems to have made the decisions himself. Often these people are aware of that after a while. They are not ignorant. So I think you just do your best to steer them, encourage them in other directions, for which they have more influence.

WCR: *When you were making the intensive care unit very technologically sophisticated, was that happening elsewhere around the country? You were ahead of the game there by a long shot. Is that not correct?*

JWK: As a matter of fact when we presented a paper at The American Surgical Association a long time ago, Jim Maloney from Los Angeles got up and showed a picture of a distressed child in the intensive care unit, and said "now that picture tells you more than all of this analytical approach could possibly have." I guess I could not have possibly disagreed with anything more. I think we were the first people to automate an intensive care unit, to bring computers into it. We were the first people ever to even have an intensive care unit. Cardiac surgery units were the first intensive care units. I am proud of that. I don't know if I am pleased with it. I think it was a good and correct thing to do. It does not mean you have to forget to smell things, feel things, does not mean that at all. It does not mean you are not a good clinician. It just means you are better if you have some information.

WCR: *It puts science and precision into it. Would you say that the desire to put precision and science* into everything you do has been maybe your outstanding contribution?

JWK: I hope so. I sincerely hope so.

WCR: *How would you state that?*

JWK: Just the way you did.

WCR: *You mentioned analyzing the minutia, the details, and when you started measuring pressure in pulmonary arteries, nobody else was measuring this. This is 1 simple example, so to speak.*

JWK: Probably congenitally I was lucky. I just always had a desire to have quantitative information. Information, wherever possible, rather than vagueness. Somehow it was just the way I came. I think the results kept getting better and better because of it.

WCR: *Were there some days in the operating room you were just a lot better than others?*

JWK: I am sure that is true.

WCR: *You had 2 cups of coffee before you walked into the operating room or you had zero?*

JWK: Never. I drank a cup of coffee at breakfast. I never drank coffee before I went in or between cases, not because it makes me jittery but because it just puts you a little bit on edge. You loose the serenity that is necessary for good decision making.

WCR: *May I ask what your life is like socially? Do you have a lot of friends here?*

JWK: I suppose many people think of us as loners, my wife and I. We have friends. She has friends that I don't know that she plays tennis with. I think we each have friends but we are not great socializers.

WCR: *You enjoy the quietness of the home when you are away from the hustle/bustle. Do you take off much?*

JWK: Probably less than most people.

WCR: *When you were operating so much, did you go on vacations?*

JWK: Always. We usually went for several relatively short times rather than 1 long time. We did not go on round-the-world cruises. We would go for a week or so, some place with the kids or later on by ourselves.

WCR: *You felt that a very useful thing to do?*

JWK: Absolutely. For a lot of reasons.

WCR: *You obviously get a lot of invitations to give talks and so on. You must have had to limit that a great deal.*

JWK: I did. I always felt that people who were talking a lot ended up without much to talk about. I did try to limit it.

WCR: *Is there anything that you would like to put in the record, so to speak, Dr. Kirklin, or discuss anything that we have not touched on?*

JWK: Gee, I think we have talked about most everything. I can't think of anything we have left out.

WCR: *Sir, it was a pleasure.*

JWK's best publications selected by JWK among his 750 articles in medical journals

12. Kirklin JW, McDonald JR, Harrington SW, New GB. Parotid tumors: histopathology, clinical behavior, and end results. *Surg Gynecol Obstet* 1951;92: 721–733.

22. Kirklin JW. Surgical treatment of mitral stenosis. *Proc Staff Meet Mayo Clin* 1952;27:357–360.

23. Kirklin JW, Burchell HB, Pugh DG, Burke EC, Mills SD. Surgical treatment of coarctation of the aorta in a ten week old infant: report of a case. *Circulation* 1952;6:411–414.

25. Knight CD, Kirklin JW. Abdominal incisions in infants. *Surgery* 1952;32: 689–695.

26. Kirklin JW, Openshaw CR, Tompkins RG. Surgical treatment of infundibular stenosis with intact ventricular septum: report of a case. *Ann Surg* 1953;137: 228–231.

27. Connolly DC, Lev R, Kirklin JW, Wood EH. The problem of isolated valvular versus infundibular pulmonic stenosis with particular reference to cardiac catheterization data and records obtained at the time of operation. *Proc Staff Meet Mayo Clin* 1953;28:65–71.

31. Kirklin JW, Jampolis RW. Intrapericardial dissection in left pneumonectomy for bronchiogenic carcinoma. *J Thorac Surg* 1953;25:280–285.

38. Kirklin JW. Surgical treatment of anomalous pulmonary venous connection (partial anomalous pulmonary venous drainage). *Proc Staff Meet Mayo Clin* 1953;28:476–479.

41. Kirklin JW, Connolly DC, Ellis FH Jr, Burchell HB, Edwards JE, Wood EH. Problems in the diagnosis and surgical treatment of pulmonic stenosis with intact ventricular septum. *Circulation* 1953;8:849–863.

45. Clagett OT, Kirklin JW, Edwards JE. Anatomic variations and pathologic changes in coarctation of the aorta: a study of 124 cases. *Surg Gynecol Obstet* 1954;98:103–114.

49. Silver AW, Swan HJC, Kirklin JW. Demonstration by dye dilution techniques of preferential flow across atrial septal defects from right pulmonary veins and inferior vena cava. *Fed Proc* 1954;13:138.

50. Lev R, Connolly DC, Kirklin JW, Wood EH. The immediate hemodynamic effects of mitral commissurotomy during surgery. *Surg Forum* 4:13–17.

52. Mears TW, Kirklin JW, Woolner LB. The fate of patients with alveolar-cell tumor of the lungs. *J Thorac Surg* 1954;27:420–424.

55. Fletcher G, DuShane JW, Kirklin JW, Wood EH. Aortic-pulmonary septal defect: report of a case with surgical division along with successful resuscitation from ventricular fibrillation. *Proc Staff Meet Mayo Clin* 1954;29:285–293.

62. Connolly DC, Kirklin JW, Wood EH. The relationship between pulmonary artery wedge pressure and left atrial pressure in man. *Circ Res* 1954;2:434–440.

68. Kirklin JW, Swan HJC, Wood EH, Burchell HB. Anatomic, physiologic, and surgical considerations in repair of interatrial communications in man. *J Thorac Surg* 1955;29:37–49.

70. Jones RE, Donald DE, Swan HJC, Harshbarger HG, Kirklin JW, Wood EH. Apparatus of the Gibbon type for mechanical bypass of the heart and lungs: preliminary report. *Proc Staff Meet Mayo Clin* 1955;30:105–113.

71. Donald DE, Harshbarger HG, Hetzel PS, Patrick RT, Wood EH, Kirklin JW. Experiences with a heart-lung bypass (Gibbon type) in the experimental laboratory: preliminary report. *Proc Staff Meet Mayo Clin* 1955;30:113–115.

72. Kirklin JW, McDonald JR, Clagett OT, Moersch JH, Gage RP. Bronchogenic carcinoma: cell type and other factors relating to prognosis. *Surg Gynecol Obstet* 1955;100:429–438.

76. Kirklin JW, Allen EV, Odel HM, Shick RM. Atherosclerosis and thrombosis of the distal part of the abdominal aorta: clinical and surgical considerations. *Circulation* 1955;11:799–805.

77. Kirklin JW, DuShane JW, Patrick RT, Donald DE, Hetzel PS, Harshbarger HG, Wood EH. Intracardiac surgery with the aid of a mechanical pump-oxygenator system (Gibbon type): report of 8 cases. *Proc Staff Meet Mayo Clin* 1955;30:201–206.

83. Clagett OT, Kirklin JW, Ellis FH Jr. Surgical treatment of coarctation of the aorta. *Surg Clin North Am* 1955;35:937–946.

90. Ellis FH Jr, Kirklin JW. Anomalous pulmonary venous connection. *Surg Clin North Am* 1955;35:997–1004.

97. Shepherd JR, Callahan JA, DuShane JW, Kirklin JW, Wood EH. Coarctation of the aorta with patent ductus arteriosus opening at the coarctation. *Am Heart J* 1955;50:225–236.

102. Kirklin JW, Daugherty GW, Burchell HB, Wood EH. Repair of the partial form of persistent common atrioventricular canal: so-called ostium primum type of atrial septal defect with interventricular communication. *Ann Surg* 1955;142: 858–862.

105. Ellis FH Jr, Kirklin JW, Callahan JA, Wood EH. Patent ductus arteriosus with pulmonary hypertension. *J Thorac Surg* 1956;31:268–282.

106. Kirklin JW, Ellis FH Jr, Wood EH. Treatment of anomalous pulmonary venous connections in association with interatrial communications. *Surgery* 1956; 39:389–398.

109. DuShane JW, Kirklin JW, Patrick RT, Donald DE, Terry HR Jr, Burchell HB, Wood EH. Ventricular septal defects with pulmonary hypertension: surgical treatment by means of a mechanical pump-oxygenator. *JAMA* 1956;160:950–953.

114. Kirklin JW, Weidman WH, Burroughs JT, Burchell HB, Wood EH. The hemodynamic results of surgical correction of atrial septal defects: a report of 33 cases. *Circulation* 1956;13:825–833.

118. Fuquay MC, Carey LS, Dahl EV, Kirklin JW, Grindlay JH. Myocardial revascularization: a comparison between internal mammary and subclavian-artery implantation in the dog. *Surg Forum* 1956;6:211–215.

120. Silver AW, Kirklin JW, Wood EH. Demonstration of preferential flow of blood from inferior vena cava and from right pulmonary veins through experimental atrial septal defects in dogs. *Circ Res* 1956;14:413–418.

121. Kirklin JW, Donald DE, Harshbarger HG, Hetzel PS, Patrick RT, Swan HJC, Wood EH. Studies in extracorporeal circulation. 1. Applicability of Gibbon-type pump-oxygenator to human intracardiac surgery: 40 cases. *Ann Surg* 1956; 144:2–8.

122. Donald DE, Harshbarger HG, Kirklin JW. Studies in extracorporeal circulation. II. A method for the recovery and use of blood from the open heart during extracorporeal circulation in man. *Ann Surg* 1956;144:223–227.

123. Becu LM, Fontana RS, DuShane JW, Kirklin JW, Burchell HB, Edwards JE. Anatomic and pathologic studies in ventricular septal defect. *Circulation* 1956; 14:349–364.

124. Cooley JC, Kirklin JW. The surgical treatment of persistent common atrioventricular canal: report of 12 cases. *Proc Staff Meet Mayo Clin* 1956;31: 523–527.

127. Kirklin JW, Ellis FH Jr, Barratt-Boyes BG. Technique for repair of atrial septal defect using the atrial well. *Surg Gynecol Obstet* 1956;103:646–649.

132. Kirklin JW, Harshbarger HG, Donald DE, Edwards JE. Surgical correction of ventricular septal defect: anatomic and technical considerations. *J Thorac Surg* 1957;33:45 47.

138. Kirklin JW, Patrick RT, Theye RA. Theory and practice in the use of a pump-oxygenator for open intracardiac surgery. *Thorax* 1957;12:93–98.

147. Berkson J, Harrington SW, Clagett OT, Kirklin JW, Dockerty MB, McDonald DJ. Mortality and survival in surgically treated cancer of the breast: a statistical summary of some experiences of the Mayo Clinic. *Proc Staff Meet Mayo Clin* 1957;32:645 670.

148. Theye RA, Patrick RT, Kirklin JW. The electro-encephalogram in patients undergoing open intracardiac operations with the aid of extracorporeal circulation. *J Thorac Surg* 1957;34:709–716.

149. Sturtz GS, Kirklin JW, Burke EC, Power MH. Water metabolism after cardiac operations involving a Gibbon-type pump-oxygenator. 1. Daily water metabolism, obligatory water losses, and requirements. *Circulation* 1957;16: 988–999.

150. Sturtz GS, Kirklin JW, Burke EC, Power MH. Water metabolism after cardiac operations involving a Gibbon-type pump-oxygenator. II. Benign forms of water loss. *Circulation* 1957;16:1000–1003.

152. Harshbarger HG, Kirklin JW, Donald DE. Studies in extracorporeal circulation. IV. Surgical techniques. *Surg Gynecol Obstet* 1958;106:111–118.

159. Kirklin JW, McGoon DC. Surgical technique for repair of high ventricular septal defects. *J Thorac Surg* 1958;35:584–590.

161. Kirklin JW, Silver AW. Technic of exposing the ductus arteriosus prior to establishing extracorporeal circulation. *Proc Staff Meet Mayo Clin* 1958;33:423–425.

163. Berkson J, Clagett OT, Dockerty MB, Harrington SW, Kirklin JW, McDonald JR. Treatment of breast cancer: the question of "selection." *Lancet* 1958;2:516–518.

165. Heath D, Helmholz HF Jr, Burchell HB, DuShane JW, Kirklin JW, Edwards JE. Relation between structural changes in the small pulmonary arteries and the immediate reversibility of pulmonary hypertension following closure of ventricular and atrial septal defects. *Circulation* 1958;18:1167–1174.

168. Kirklin JW, Ellis FH Jr, McGoon DC, DuShane JW, Swan JHC. Surgical treatment for the tetralogy of Fallot by open intracardiac repair. *J Thorac Surg* 1959;37:22–46.

169. McGoon DC, Swan JHC, Brandenburg RO, Connolly DC, Kirklin JW. Atrial septal defect: factors affecting the surgical mortality rate. *Circulation* 1959;19:195–200.

177. DuShane JW, Kirklin JW. Selection for surgery of patients with ventricular septal defect and pulmonary hypertension. *Circulation* 1960;21:13–20.

179. Kirklin JW. Surgical treatment of ventricular septal defects. *Am J Cardiol* 1960;5:234–238.

181. McGoon DC, Miff EA, Theye RA, Kirklin JW. Physiologic studies during high flow, normothermic, whole body perfusion. *J Thorac Cardiovasc Surg* 1960;39:275–287.

182. DuShane JW, Weidman WH, Brandenburg RO, Kirklin JW. Differentiation of interatrial communications by clinical methods: ostium secundum, ostium primum, common atrium, and total anomalous pulmonary venous connection. *Circulation* 1960;21:363 371.

185. Kirklin JW, Payne WS. Surgical treatment of tetralogy of Fallot after previous anastomosis of systemic to pulmonary artery. *Surg Gynecol Obstet* 1960;110:707–713.

186. Lyons HA, DuShane JW, Kirklin JW. Postoperative care after whole-body perfusion and open intracardiac operations: use of Mayo-Gibbon pump-oxygenator and Browns-Emmons heat exchanger. *JAMA* 1960;173:625–630.

189. Savard M, Swan HJC, Kirklin JW, Wood EH. Hemodynamic alterations associated with ventricular septal defects. In: Congenital Heart Disease. Washington: American Association for the Advance of Science, 1960:141–164.

190. Levin MB, Theye RA, Fowler WS, Kirklin JW. Performance of the stationary vertical-screen oxygenator (Mayo-Gibbon). *J Thorac Cardiovasc Surg* 1960;39:417–426.

194. Uihlein A, Theye RA, Dawson B, Terry HR Jr, McGoon DC, Daw EF, Kirklin JW. The use of profound hypothermia, extracorporeal circulation and total circulatory arrest for an intracranial aneurysm: preliminary report with reports of cases. *Proc Staff Meet Mayo Clin* 1960;35:567–578.

196. Kirklin JW, Payne WS, Theye RA, DuShane JW. Factors affecting survival after open operation for tetralogy of Fallot. *Ann Surg* 1960;152:485–493.

198. Beck W, Swan JHC, Burchell HB, Kirklin JW. Pulmonary vascular resistance after repair of atrial septal defects in patients with pulmonary hypertension. *Circulation* 1960;22:938–946.

199. Kirklin JW, McGoon DC, DuShane JW. Surgical treatment of ventricular septal defect. *J Thorac Cardiovasc Surg* 1960;40:763–775.

201. Kirklin JW, Devloo RA. Hypothermic perfusion and circulatory arrest for surgical correction of tetralogy of Fallot with previously constructed Potts-anastomosis. *Dis Chest* 1961;39:87–91.

205. Kirklin JW, DuShane JW. Repair of ventricular septal defect in infancy. *Pediatrics* 1961;27:961–966.

207. Kirklin JW, Devloo RA, Weidman WH. Open intracardiac repair for transposition of the great vessels: 11 cases. *Surgery* 1961;50:58–66.

209. Kirklin JW, Dawson B, Devloo RA, Theye RA. Open intracardiac operations: use of circulatory arrest during hypothermia induced by blood cooling. *Ann Surg* 1961;154:769–776.

213. Taylor LM, Theye RA, Devloo RA, Kirklin JW. Patterns of acid-base changes during surgical convalescence. *Surg Gynecol Obstet* 1962;114:97–101.

216. Theye RA, Kirklin JW, Fowler WS. Performance and film volume of sheet and screen vertical-film oxygenators. *J Thorac Cardiovasc Surg* 1962;43:481–488.

218. Moffitt EA, Kirklin JW, Theye RA. Physiologic studies during whole-body perfusion in tetralogy of Fallot. *J Thorac Cardiovasc Surg* 1962;44:180–188.

219. Kirklin JW, Payne WS. Tetralogy of Fallot. In: Benson CO, Mustard WT, Ravitch MA, Synder WH Jr, Welch KJ, eds. Pediatric Surgery. Chicago: Yearbook Medical Publishers, 1962:462–471.

220. Kirklin JW, Theye RA. Whole-body perfusion from a pump oxygenator for open intracardiac surgery. In: Gibbon JH Jr, ed. Surgery of the Chest. Philadelphia: WB Saunders, 1962:694–707.

224. Rehder K, Kirklin JW, Theye RA. Physiologic studies following surgical correction of atrial septal defect and similar lesions. *Circulation* 1962;26:1302–1311.

228. Payne WF, Theye RA, Kirklin JW. Effect of carbon dioxide on rate of brain cooling during induction of hypothermia by direct blood cooling. *J Surg Res* 1963;3:54–57.

233. Theye RA, Kirklin JW. Physiologic studies following surgical correction of ventricular septal defect. *Circulation* 1963;27:530–540.

235. Theye RA, Kirklin JW. Physiologic studies early after repair of tetralogy of Fallot. *Circulation* 1963;28:42–52.

241. Theye RA, Kirklin JW. Vertical film oxygenator performance at 30°C and oxygen levels during rewarming. *Surgery* 1963;54:569–572.

242. Kirklin JW, Theye RA. Cardiac performance after open intracardiac surgery. *Circulation* 1963;28:1061–1070.

243. Michenfelder JD, Kirklin JW, Uihlein A, Svien HJ, MacCarty CS. Clinical experience with a closed-chest method of producing profound hypothermia and total circulatory arrest in neurosurgery. *Ann Surg* 1964;159:125–131.

244. Sturridge MF, Theye RA, Fowler WS, Kirklin JW. Basal metabolic rate after cardiovascular surgery. *J Thorac Cardiovasc Surg* 1964;47:298–307.

247. Albertal G, Swan HJC, Kirklin JW. Hemodynamic studies two weeks to six years after repair of tetralogy of Fallot. *Circulation* 1964;29:583–592.

252. Kirklin JW, Harp RA, McGoon DC. Surgical treatment of origin of both vessels from right ventricle including cases of pulmonary stenosis. *J Thorac Cardiovasc Surg* 1964;48:1026–1036.

254. Rastelli GC, Weidman WH, Kirklin JW. Surgical repair of the partial form of persistent common atrioventricular canal, with special reference to the problem of mitral valve incompetence. *Circulation* 1965;31,32:I-31–I-35.

257. Rastelli GC, Ongley PA, Davis GD, Kirklin JW. Surgical repair for pulmonary valve atresia with coronary-pulmonary artery fistula: report of case. *Mayo Clin Proc* 1965;40:521 527.

258. Rastelli GC, Ongley PA, Kirklin JW. Surgical correction of common atrium with anomalously connected persistent left superior vena cava: report of case. *Mayo Clin Proc* 1965;40:528–532.

260. Frye RL, Kincaid OW, Swan HJC, Kirklin JW. Results of surgical treatment of patients with diffuse subvalvular aortic stenosis. *Circulation* 1965;32:52–57.

263. Kirklin JW, Wallace RB, McGoon DC, DuShane JW. Early and late results after intracardiac repair of tetralogy of Fallot: 5-year review of 337 patients. *Ann Surg* 1965;162:578–589.

273. Rastelli GC, McGoon DC, Ongley PA, Mankin HT, Kirklin JW. Surgical treatment of supravalvular aortic stenosis. *J Thorac Cardiovasc Surg* 1966;51: 873–882.

276. Mielke JE, Hunt JC, Maher FT, Kirklin JW. Renal performance during clinical cardiopulmonary bypass with and without hemodilution. *J Thorac Cardiovasc Surg* 1966;52:229–237.

278. Rastelli GC, Kirklin JW, Titus JL. Anatomic observations on complete form of persistent common atrioventricular canal with special reference to atrioventricular valves. *Mayo Clin Proc* 1966;41:296–308.

280. Hooksema TD, Wallace RB, Kirklin JW. Closed mitral commissurotomy: recent results in 291 cases. *Am J Cardiol* 1966;17:825–828.

286. Cartmill TB, DuShane JW, McGoon DC, Kirklin JW. Results of repair of ventricular septal defect. *J Thorac Cardiovasc Surg* 1966;52:486–499.

296. Daicoff GR, Brandenburg RO, Kirklin JW. Results of operation for atrial septal defect in patients 45 years of age and older. *Circulation* 1967;35,36(suppl I):1-143–I-147.

297. Woods JE, Taswell HF, Kirklin JW, Owen CA Jr. The transfusion of platelet concentrates in patients undergoing heart surgery. *Mayo Clin Proc* 1967;42:318–325.

298. Rastelli GC, Kirklin JW. Hemodynamic state early after replacement of aortic valve with ball-valve prosthesis. *Surgery* 1967;61:965–971.

303. Reid DJ, Digerness S, Kirklin JW. Intracellular fluid volume in surgical patients measured by simultaneous determination of total body water and extracellular fluid. *Surg Forum* 1967;18:29–30.

305. Woods JE, Kirklin JW, Owen CA Jr, Thompson JH Jr, Taswell HF. Effect of bypass surgery on coagulation-sensitive clotting factors. *Mayo Clin Proc* 1967;42:724–735.

307. Reid DJ, Digerness S, Kirklin JW. Changes in whole body venous tone in surgical patients. *Surg Gynecol Obstet* 1967;125:1212–1216.

309. Kiser JC, Ongley PA, Kirklin JW, Clarkson PM, McGoon DC. Surgical treatment of dextrocardia with inversion of ventricles and double-outlet right ventricle. *J Thorac Cardiovasc Surg* 1968;55:6–15.

311. Kirklin JW. The tetralogy of Fallot, Caldwell Lecture, 1967. *Am J Roentgenol Radium Ther Nucl Med* 1968;103:253–266.

317. Sheppard LC, Kouchoukos NT, Kurtts MA, Kirklin JW. Automated treatment of critically ill patients following operation. *Ann Surg* 1968;168:596–604.

318. Reid DJ, Digerness SB, Kirklin JW. Changes in whole body venous tone and distribution of blood after open intracardiac surgery. *Am J Cardiol* 1968;22:621–623.

322. Hightower BM, Barcia A, Bargeron LM Jr, Kirklin JW. Double-outlet right ventricle with transposed great arteries and sub-pulmonary ventricular septal defect: the Taussing-Bing malformation. *Circulation* 1969;49,50(suppl I):I-207–I-213.

325. Breckenridge IM, Digerness SB, Kirklin JW. Validity of concept of increased extracellular fluid after open heart surgery. *Surg Forum* 1969;20:169–171.

327. Shepard RB, Kirklin JW. Relation of pulsatile flow to oxygen consumption and other variables during cardiopulmonary bypass. *J Thorac Cardiovasc Surg* 1969;58:694–702, 718–720.

333. Breckenridge IM, Digerness SB, Kirklin JW. Distribution volume, equilibration time, and exponential analysis of 82Br after open intracardiac operations. *Ann Surg* 1970;171:583–589.

337. Breckenridge IM, Digerness SB, Kirklin JW. Increased extracellular fluid after open intracardiac operation. *Surg Gynecol Obstet* 1970;131:53–56.

341. Kirklin JW. Systems analysis in surgical patients with particular attention to the cardiac and pulmonary subsystems (Macewen Memorial Lecture). Glasgow: University of Glasgow Press, 1970.

345. English TAH, Digerness SB, Kirklin JW. Karp RB. Pulmonary capillary blood volume and lung water in pulmonary edema. *Surg Gynecol Obstet* 1971;132:93–100.

347. Kouchoukos NT, Barcia A, Bargeron LM, Kirklin JW. Surgical treatment of congenital pulmonary atresia with ventricular septal defect. *J Thorac Cardiovasc Surg* 1971;61:70–84.

359. Kouchoukos NT, Kirklin JW, Sheppard LC, Roe PA. Effect of elevation of left atrial pressure by blood infusion on stroke volume early after cardiac operations. *Surg Forum* 1971;22:126–127.

362. Kirklin JW. A university department of surgery. *Am Surg* 1971;37:706–712.

368. Kouchoukos NT, Doty DB, Buettner LE, Kirklin JW. Treatment of postinfarction cardiac failure by myocardial excision and revascularization. *Circulation* 1972;45,46(suppl I):I-72–I-78.

372. Bargeron LM Jr, Karp RB, Barcia A, Kirklin JW, Hunt D, Deverall PB. Late deterioration of patients after superior vena cava to right pulmonary artery anastomosis. *Am J Cardiol* 1972;30:211–216.

377. Kirklin JW. Replacement of the mitral valve for mitral incompetence. *Surgery* 1972;72:827–836.

378. Stewart S III, Edmunds LH Jr, Kirklin JW, Allarde RR. Spontaneous breathing with continuous positive airway pressure after open intracardiac operations in infants. *J Thorac Cardiovas Surg* 1973;65:37–44.

379. Kirklin JW, Pacifico AD. Surgery for acquired valvular heart disease. *N Engl J Med* 1973;288:133–140, 194–199.

385. Ceballos R, Kirklin JW. Long-term anatomical results of intracardiac repair of tetralogy of Fallot. *Ann Thorac Surg* 1973;15:371–377.

388. Pacifico AD, Kirklin JW. Surgical repair of complete atrioventricular canal with anterior common leaflet attached to an anomalous right ventricular papillary muscle. *J Thorac Cardiovasc Surg* 1973;65:727–730.

392. Kirklin JW. Evaluating the results of cardiac surgery (Lewis A. Conner Memorial Lecture). *Circulation* 1973;48:232–238.

393. Archie JP, Kirklin JW. Effect of hypothermic perfusion on myocardial oxygen consumption and coronary resistance. *Surg Forum* 1973;24:186–188.

394. Pacifico AD, Bargeron LM Jr, Kirklin JW. Primary total correction of tetralogy of Fallot in children less than 4 years of age. *Circulation* 1973;48:1085–1091.

397. DuShane JW, Kirklin JW. Late results of the repair of ventricular septal defect on pulmonary vascular disease. In: Kirklin JW, ed. Advances in Cardiovascular Surgery. New York: Grune & Stratton, 1973:9–16.

407. Wisheart JD, Archie JP, Kirklin JW, Tracy WG. Myocardial blood flow and oxygen consumption in man early after valve replacement. *Circulation* 1974;49:933–942.

408. Sapsford RN, Blackstone EH, Kirklin JW, Karp RB, Kouchoukos NT, Pacifico AD, Roe CR, Bradley EL. Coronary perfusion versus cold ischemic arrest during aortic valve surgery. A randomized study. *Circulation* 1974;49:1190–1199.

409. Parr GVS, Kirklin JW, Pacifico AD, Blackstone EH, Lauridsen P. Cardiac performance in infants after repair of total anomalous pulmonary venous connection. *Ann Thorac Surg* 1974;17:561–573.

411. Kouchoukos NT, Kirklin JW, Oberman A. An appraisal of coronary bypass grafting (presented by Dr. Kirklin as Sixth Annual George C. Griffith Lecture). *Circulation* 1974;50:11–16.

414. Pacifico AD, Kirklin JW, Bargeron LM Jr, Soto B. Surgical treatment of common arterial trunk with pseudotruncus arteriosus. *Circulation* 1974;49,50(suppl II):II-20–II-25.

419. Parr GVS, Blackstone EH, Kirklin JW. Cardiac performance and mortality early after intracardiac surgery in infants and young children. *Circulation* 1975;51:867–874.

430. Fox LS, Kirklin JW, Pacifico AD, Waldo AI, Bargeron LM Jr. Intracardiac repair of cardiac malformations with atrioventricular discordance. *Circulation* 1976;54:123–127.

432. Blackstone EH, Kirklin JW, Bradley EL, Dushane JW, Appelbaum A. Optimal age and results in repair of large ventricular septal defects. *J Thorac Cardiovasc Surg* 1976;72:661–679.

439. Parr GVS, Kirklin JW, Blackstone EH. The early risks of re-replacement of aortic valves. *Ann Thorac Surg* 1977;23:319–322.

440. Stephenson LW, Kouchoukos NT, Kirklin JW. Triple-valve replacement: an analysis of 8 year's experience. *Ann Thorac Surg* 1977;23:327–332.

446. Pacifico AD, Kirklin JW, Blackstone EH. Surgical management of pulmonary stenosis in tetralogy of Fallot. *J Thorac Cardiovasc Surg* 1977;74:382–395.

447. Castaneda AR, Kirklin JW. Tetralogy of Fallot with aorticopulmonary window. Report of 2 surgical cases. *J Thorac Cardiovasc Surg* 1977;74:467–468.

452. Kirklin JW, Bargeron LM Jr, Pacifico AD. The enlargement of small pulmonary arteries by preliminary palliative operations. *Circulation* 1977;56:612–617.

458. Laws HL, Kirklin MK, Diethelm AG, Hall J, Kirklin JW. Training and use of surgeon's assistants. *Surgery* 1978;83:445–450.

460. Berger TJ, Kirklin JW, Blackstone EH. Pacifico AD, Kouchoukos NT. Primary repair of complete atrioventricular canal in patients less than 2 years old. *Am J Cardiol* 1978;41:906–913.

461. Katz NM, Kirklin JW, Pacifico AD. Concepts and practices in surgery for total anomalous pulmonary venous connection. *Ann Thorac Surg* 1978;25:479–487.

464. Alfieri O, Blackstone EH, Kirklin JW, Pacifico AD, Bargeron LM Jr. Surgical treatment of tetralogy of Fallot with pulmonary atresia. *J Thorac Cardiovasc Surg* 1978;76:321–335.

473. Gale AW, Arciniegas E, Green EW, Blackstone EH, Kirklin JW. Growth of the pulmonary anulus and pulmonary arteries after the Blalock-Taussig shunt. *J Thorac Cardiovasc Surg* 1979;77:459–465.

474. Blackstone EH, Kirklin JW, Pacifico AD. Decision-making in repair of tetralogy of Fallot based on intraoperative measurements of pulmonary arterial outflow tract. *J Thorac Cardiovasc Surg* 1979;77:526–532.

479. Kirklin JW, Conti VR, Blackstone EH. Prevention of myocardial damage during cardiac operations. *N Engl J Med* 1979;301:135–141.

480. Kirklin JW, Blackstone EH, Pacifico AD, Brown RN, Bargeron LM Jr. Routine primary repair vs two-stage repair of tetralogy of Fallot. *Circulation* 1979;60:373–386.

482. Blackstone EH, Kirklin JW, Bertranou EG, Labrosse CJ, Soto B, Bargeron LM Jr. Preoperative prediction from cineangiograms of postrepair right ventricular pressure in tetralogy of Fallot. *J Thorac Cardiovasc Surg* 1979;78:542–552.

483. Kirklin JW. A letter to Helen. *J Thorac Cardiovasc Surg* 1979;78:643–654.

493. Bharati S, Kirklin JW, McAllister HA Jr, Lev M. The surgical anatomy of common atrioventricular orifice associated with tetralogy of Fallot, double outlet right ventricle and complete regular transposition. *Circulation* 1980;61:1142–1149.

500. Kouchoukos NT, Oberman A, Kirklin JW, Russell RO Jr, Karp RB, Pacifico AD, Zorn GL. Coronary bypass surgery: analysis of factors affecting hospital mortality. *Circulation* 1980;61(suppl I):I-84–I-89.

504. Rizzoli G, Blackstone EH, Kirklin JW, Pacifico AD, Bargeron LM Jr. Incremental risk factors in hospital mortality rate after repair of ventricular septal defect. *J Thorac Cardiovasc Surg* 1980;80:494–505.

506. Fuster V, McGoon DC, Kennedy MA, Ritter DG, Kirklin JW. Long-term evaluation (12 to 22 years) of open heart surgery for tetralogy of Fallot. *Am J Cardiol* 1980;46:635–642.

508. Kirklin JW. The replacement of cardiac valves. *N Engl J Med* 1981;304:291–292.

509. Chenoweth DE, Cooper SW, Hugli TE, Stewart RW, Blackstone EH, Kirklin JW. Complement activation during cardiopulmonary bypass: evidence for generation of C3a and C5a anaphylatoxins. *N Engl J Med* 1981;304:497–503.

513. Kirklin JK, Blackstone EH, Kirklin JW, Stewart RW, Pacifico AD, Bargeron LM Jr. Management of the cardiac subsystem after cardiac surgery. In: Parenzan L, Crupi G, Graham G, eds. Congenital Heart Disease in the first 3 months of life. Medical and Surgical Aspects. Bologna, Italy: Patron Editore, 1981:33–41.

519. Kirklin JK, Blackstone EH, Kirklin JW, McKay R, Pacifico AD, Bargeron LM Jr. Intracardiac surgery in infants under age 3 months: incremental risk factors for hospital mortality. *Am J Cardiol* 1981;48:500–506.

520. Kirklin JK, Blackstone EH, Kirklin JW, McKay R, Pacifico AD, Bargeron LM Jr. Intracardiac surgery in infants under age 3 months: predictors of postoperative in-hospital cardiac death. *Am J Cardiol* 1981;48:507–512.

537. Katz NM, Blackstone EH, Kirklin JW, Pacifico AD, Bargeron LM Jr. Late survival and symptoms after repair of tetralogy of Fallot. *Circulation* 1982;65:403–410.

538. Fox LS, Blackstone EH, Kirklin JW, Stewart RW, Samuelson PN. Relationship of whole body oxygen consumption to perfusion flow rate during hypothermic cardiopulmonary bypass. *J Thorac Cardiovasc Surg* 1982;83:239–248.

540. Bergdahl LAL, Blackstone EH, Kirklin JW, Pacifico AD, Bargeron LM Jr. Determinants of early success in repair of aortic coarctation in infants. *J Thorac Cardiovasc Surg* 1982;83:736–742.

541. Blackstone EH, Kirklin JW, Stewart RW, Chenoweth DE. Damaging effects of cardiopulmonary bypass. In: Wu KK, Rossi ED, eds. Prostaglandins in Clinical Medicine. Cardiovascular and Thrombotic Disorders. Chicago: Year Book Medical Publishers, 1983:355–369.

558. Ceballos R, Soto B, Kirklin JW, Bargeron LM Jr. Truncus arteriosus. An anatomical-angiographic study. *Br Heart J* 1983;49:589–599.

563. Kirklin JW, Blackstone EH, Kirklin JK, Pacifico AD, Aramendi J, Bargeron LM Jr. Surgical results and protocols in the spectrum of tetralogy of Fallot. *Ann Surg* 1983;198:251–265.

564. Treasure T, Naftel DC, Conger KA, Garcia JH, Kirklin JW, Blackstone EH. The effect of hypothermic circulatory arrest time on cerebral function, morphology, and biochemistry. An experimental study. *J Thorac Cardiovasc Surg* 1983; 86:761–770.

566. Kirklin JK, Westaby S, Blackstone EH, Kirklin JW, Chenoweth DE, Pacifico AD. Complement and the damaging effects of cardiopulmonary bypass. *J Thorac Cardiovasc Surg* 1983;86:845–857.

572. Fox LS, Blackstone EH, Kirklin JW, Bishop SP, Bergdahl LAL, Bradley EL. Relationship of brain blood flow and oxygen consumption to perfusion flow rate during profoundly hypothermic cardiopulmonary bypass. An experimental study. *J Thorac Cardiovasc Surg* 1984;87:658–664.

575. Kirklin JW, Blackstone EH, Pacifico AD, Kirklin JK, Bargeron LM Jr. Risk factors for early and late failure after repair of tetralogy of Fallot, and their neutralization. *J Thorac Cardiovasc Surg* 1984;32:208–214.

577. Stefanelli G, Kirklin JW, Naftel DC, Blackstone EH, Pacifico AD, Kirklin JK, Soto B, Bargeron LM Jr. Early and intermediate-term (10 year) results of surgery for univentricular atrioventricular connection ("single ventricle"). *Am J Cardiol* 1984;54:811–821.

578. Cleveland DC, Kirklin JK, Naftel DC, Kirklin JW, Blackstone EH, Pacifico AD, Bargeron LM Jr. Surgical treatment of tricuspid atresia. *Ann Thorac Surg* 1984;38:447–457.

590. Pacifico AD, Naftel DC, Kirklin JW, Blackstone EH, Kirklin JK. Ventricular septation within the spectrum of surgery for double inlet ventricles. *J Jpn Assoc Thorac Surg* 1985;33:593–601.

591. Kirklin JK, Kirklin JW, Pacifico AD. Homograft replacement of the aortic valve. *Cardiol Clin* 1985;3:329–341.

593. Blackstone EH, Kirklin JW. Death and other time-related events after valve replacement. *Circulation* 1985;72:753–767.

597. Kirklin JK, Blackstone EH, Zorn GL Jr, Pacifico AD, Kirklin JW, Karp RB, Rogers WJ. Intermediate-term results of coronary artery bypass grafting for acute myocardial infraction. *Circulation* 1985;72(suppl II):II-175–II-178.

602. Kirklin JK, Chenoweth DE, Naftel DC, Blackstone EH, Kirklin JW, Bitran DD, Curd JG, Reves JG, Samuelson PN. Effects of protamine administration after cardiopulmonary bypass on complement, blood elements, and the hemodynamic state. *Ann Thorac Surg* 1986;41:193–199.

610. Ferrazzi P, McGiffin DC, Kirklin JW, Blackstone EH, Bourge RC. Have the results of mitral valve replacement improved? *J Thorac Cardiovasc Surg* 1986; 92:186–197.

612. Quagebeur JM, Rohmer J, Ottenkamp J, Tuis T, Kirklin JW, Blackstone EH, Brom AG. The arterial switch operation. An eight-year experience. *J Thorac Cardiovasc Surg* 1986;92:361–384.

614. Kirklin JW, Pacifico AD, Blackstone EH, Kirklin JK, Bargeron LM Jr. Current risks and protocols for operations for double-outlet right ventricle. *J Thorac Cardiovasc Surg* 1986;92:913–930.

618. Kirklin JK, Blackstone EH, Kirklin JW, Pacifico AD, Bargeron LM Jr. The Fontan operation: ventricular hypertrophy, age, and date of operation as risk factors. *J Thorac Cardiovasc Surg* 1986;92:1049–1064.

622. Kirklin JK, Pacifico AD, Kirklin JW. Intraventricular tunnel repair of double outlet right ventricle. *J Cardiac Surg* 1987;2:231–245.

623. Sand ME, Naftel DC, Blackstone EH, Kirklin JW, Karp RB. A comparison of repair and replacement for mitral valve incompetence. *J Thorac Cardiovasc Surg* 1987;94:208–219.

631. Coles JG, Kirklin JW, Pacifico AD, Kirklin JK, Blackstone EH. The relief of pulmonary stenosis by a transatrial versus a transventricular approach to the repair of tetralogy of Fallot. *Ann Thorac Surg* 1988;45:7–10.

632. Castaneda AR, Trusler GA, Paul MH, Blackstone EH, Kirklin JW, and the Congenital Heart Surgeons Society. The early results of treatment of simple transposition in the current era. *J Thorac Cardiovasc Surg* 1988;95:14–27.

644. Shimazaki Y, Maehara T, Blackstone EH, Kirklin JW, Bargeron LM Jr. The structure of the pulmonary circulation in tetralogy of Fallot with pulmonary atresia. *J Thorac Cardiovasc Surg* 1988;95:1048–1058.

645. Kirklin JW, Blackstone EH, Shimazaki Y, Maehara T, Pacifico AD, Kirklin JK, Bargeron LM Jr. Survival, functional status, and reoperations after repair of tetralogy of Fallot with pulmonary atresia. *J Thorac Cardiovasc Surg* 1988;96: 102–116.

647. Blackstone EH, Shimazaki Y, Maehara T, Kirklin JW, Bargeron LM Jr. Prediction of severe obstruction to right ventricular outflow after repair of tetralogy of Fallot and pulmonary atresia. *J Thorac Cardiovasc Surg* 1988;96: 288–293.

659. Kirklin JW. Reply to the editor on early primary repair of tetralogy of Fallot. *Ann Thorac Surg* 1988;46:711.

663. Kirklin JW, Naftel DC, Blackstone EH, Pohost GM. Summary of a consensus concerning death and ischemic events after coronary artery bypass grafting. *Circulation* 1989;79(suppl I):I-81–I-91.

671. Fernandez G, Costa F, Fontan F, Naftel DC, Blackstone EH, Kirklin JW. Prevalence of reoperation for pathway obstruction after Fontan operation. *Ann Thorac Surg* 1989;48:654–659.

678. Fontan F, Fernandez G, Costa F, Naftel DC, Tritto F, Blackstone EH, Kirklin JW. The size of the pulmonary arteries and the results of the Fontan operation. *J Thorac Cardiovasc Surg* 1989;98:711–724.

681. Kirklin JK, Naftel DC, Blackstone EH, Kirklin JW, Brown RC. Risk factors for mortality after primary combined valvular and coronary artery surgery. *Circulation* 1989;79(suppl I):I-185–I-190.

682. Kirklin JK, Pacifico AD, Kirklin JW. Surgical treatment of prosthetic valve endocarditis with homograft aortic valve replacement. *J Cardiac Surg* 1989;4: 340–347.

686. Kirklin JW, Fernandez G, Fontan F, Naftel DC, Ener A, Blackstone EH. Therapeutic use of right atrial pressures early after the Fontan operation. *Eur J Cardiothorac Surg* 1990;4:2–7.

688. Kirklin JW, Blackstone EH, Kirklin JK, Pacifico AD. Predicting the degree of relief of the pulmonary stenosis of atresia after the repair of tetralogy of Fallot. *Semin Thorac Cardiovasc Surg* 1990;2:55–60.

693. Fontan F, Kirklin JW, Fernandez G, Costa F, Naftel DC, Tritto F, Blackstone EH. Outcome after a "perfect" Fontan operation. *Circulation* 1990;81: 1520–1536.

705. Kirklin JW, and the ACC/AHA Task Force Subcommittee on Coronary Artery Bypass Graft Surgery. Guidelines and Indications for the coronary artery bypass graft operation. *Circulation* 1991;83:543–589, 1125–1173.

712. Kirklin JW, Blackstone EH, Shimazaki Y, Kirklin JK, Mayer JE Jr, Pacifico AD, Castaneda AR. Morphologic and surgical determinants of outcome events after repair of tetralogy of Fallot and pulmonary stenosis. A two-institution study. *J Thorac Cardiovasc Surg* 1992;103:706–723.

713. Shimazaki Y, Blackstone EH, Kirklin JW, Jonas RA, Mandell V, Colvin EV. The dimensions of the right ventricular outflow tract and pulmonary arteries in tetralogy of Fallot and pulmonary stenosis. *J Thorac Cardiovasc Surg* 1992; 103:692–705.

720. Crawford ES, Kirklin JW, Naftel DC, Svensson LG, Coselli JS, Safi HJ, Hess KR. Surgery for acute ascending aortic dissection: should the arch be included? *J Thorac Cardiovasc Surg* 1992;104:46–59.

722. Kirklin JW, Blackstone EH, Tchervenkov CI, Castaneda AR, and the Congenital Heart Surgeons Society. Clinical outcomes after the arterial switch operation for transposition. Patient, support, procedural, and institutional risk factors. *Circulation* 1992;86:1501–1515.

723. Walters HL, Digerness SB, Naftel DC, Waggoner JR, Blackstone EH, Kirklin JW. The response to ischemia in blood perfused vs. crystalloid perfused isolated rat heart preparations. *J Mol Cell Cardiol* 1992;24:1063–1077.

618

HOWARD BERTRAM BURCHELL, MD:
A Conversation With the Editor*

Howard Burchell was born in Canada in November 1907 and came to live in the United States 26 years later when he went to Pittsburgh to continue his training in medicine. He never returned to Canada thereafter on a permanent basis. A fellowship at the Mayo Clinic in 1936 eventually led to his permanent position at the Clinic in Rochester in 1946. In 1968, he moved to the Minneapolis/St. Paul area where he headed the Section of Cardiology for several years at the University of Minnesota.

Dr. Burchell is a scholar and a lover of medicine. He was a major force in cardiology in the early years at the Mayo Clinic immediately following World War II. He has always been a student of cardiovascular information and a splendid teacher of medicine. His scholarship, creativity, and teaching abilities have brought him many honors, including the Gold Heart Award and the James B. Herrick Award of the American Heart Association, The Gifted Teacher Award of the American College of Cardiology, and the Outstanding Achievement Award of the University of Minnesota. Dr. Burchell was Editor-in-Chief of *Circulation* from 1965 to 1970. At age 90, he still is an avid reader of cardiovascular publications and attendee of cardiovascular conferences. His scholarship goes beyond medical writings, and his medical writings extend to historical vignettes and biographical sketches. Dr. Burchell has great capacity for friendship. His friends cherish his many handwritten letters. He remains the epitome of what a cardiologist or any physician should strive to be.

I spoke with Dr. Burchell in his home in St. Paul, Minnesota, on October 18, 1997.

William C. Roberts, MD‡ (hereafter, WCR): *Dr. Burchell, what I would like to try to do here is to learn more about you. I gather you were born in Ontario, Canada. Could you tell a bit about your upbringing, who your parents were, what they did, your siblings, and what your growing up was like?*

Howard B. Burchell, MD‡ (hereafter, HBB): Both of my parents came from an agricultural background from farms on either side of the St. Lawrence River. They had come over as immigrants from Ireland in the 18th century. My father left the farm very early, became a school teacher, and then principal of a high school. I had 4 brothers and 1 sister. My father was very interested in our athletic development in school as well as pushing us in our education. We were kind of "proud poor" at that time. After high school, I had doubts that I could get into medical

school and finance it, but my father said, "oh, we can do that." I had been interested in being a physician since a grade school child. I remember wanting to be a medical missionary. I ended up going to the University of Toronto, where I graduated in 1932. My 65th reunion was just last year, and I received a videotape for being one of the survivors of our class.

WCR: *You said you had 4 brothers and 1 sister. Where are you in the hierarchy?*

HBB: My sister was the oldest and she was kind of a second mother. I was right in the middle. My first brother became an actuary and my second brother, a school teacher. Then there was me. My next brother became an engineer. My youngest brother went into the British Navy where he became somewhat of a hero in World War II as Radar Officer to Admiral Cunningham in the Mediterranean fleet.

WCR: *Where is Athens, Ontario, located?*

HBB: If one can visualize the St. Lawrence River going out of Lake Ontario into the gulf, it is about half way along. Maybe some people remember Kingston, which is the place where Lake Ontario empties into the St. Lawrence, and then about 100 miles further along there is a little town by the name of Brockville, then Gananoque, and then Athens is just 10 miles north of Brockville.

WCR: *Neither your mother nor father went to college, and all of your siblings did?*

HBB: My mother never went to college. My father went for 1 year to what was called "normal school" before receiving his teaching certificate. Then, over the next 10 years he finally got a college degree by going intermittently in the summers to Queens University.

WCR: *You were the only one who became a physician? Do you remember what turned you onto medicine? You mentioned that even in grade school you thought about medicine.*

HBB: It always seemed interesting. I had no particular idol at that time as a physician.

WCR: *Were there any particular teachers in high school or junior high school that had a particular influence on you? Did you have any particular mentors who took a particular interest in you and that influenced you a good bit?*

HBB: Actually, my father did, though I was not cognizant of it at the time. He taught science in high school where he was principal, and I was there. I was kind of a "nerd," a good little boy, and did not misbehave.

WCR: *Did you play sports?*

HBB: I was very active in hockey, in particular, and this was supported by the whole community. I remember at the time we were winners in our little local area. The team was scouted by the New York

*This series of interviews are underwritten by an unrestricted grant from Bristol-Myers Squibb.

‡Baylor Cardiovascular Institute, Baylor University Medical Center, Dallas, Texas 75246.

†Division of Cardiology, Department of Medicine, University of Minnesota, Minneapolis, Minnesota 55417.

0002-9149/98/$19.00 **1187**
PII S0002-9149(98)00187-8

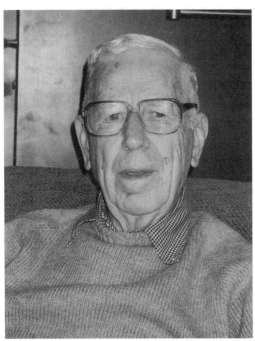

FIGURE 1. Photograph of H.B. Burchell taken by W.C. Roberts during the interview.

Rangers and I was terribly disappointed that I was not offered a job on one of their farm teams.

WCR: *Where did you go to college?*

HBB: The University of Toronto.

WCR: *What was college like? What do you remember about college?*

HBB: I found it very pleasant. There were no ups or downs at that time. I was particularly interested in the opening up of the tremendous vastness, you might say, of the knowledge that might be attained. Even at that time, I was an avid library patron.

WCR: *You stayed at the University of Toronto for medical school? How was medical school? Did you enjoy it?*

HBB: I did indeed. It was a lot of work, but I liked it. Perhaps, in medical school the person who influenced me the most was *Dr. Charles Best.* When I was in medical school he was made a Professor of Physiology and he was the youngest professor ever appointed. I think he was only 28 or 29. For some reason, he became interested in me and gave me an encouraging word once in a while.

WCR: *This was the* Best *of insulin fame?*

HBB: Yes.

WCR: *When it came time to pick an internship, did you have a hard time deciding what you wanted, medicine or surgery or something else?*

HBB: I think it was a general aspiration of most medical students at the University of Toronto Medical School to apply for a general medicine internship. I applied for that and was accepted. In this particular

track, a person after the first year often went into the laboratory for awhile. I suppose this is partly the pattern of Sir William Osler, though I didn't recognize it at the time. I applied for an internship in pathology for a year and did that at the Toronto General Hospital in the Department of Pathology and Bacteriology. The next step would ordinarily be to go to a senior internship in the same institution, but the Professor of Pathology, *Dr. Oskar Klotz,* had a friend at the University of Pittsburgh who wanted someone to continue work on what I had been doing at the University Toronto. So I went to Pittsburgh. I was expecting to stay there a year, but I stayed 2 years. They wanted me to continue, but after 3 years in the laboratory I wanted to go back into clinical medicine. *Dr. Maclacklan,* my mentor, along with the people at the Mellon Institute, who were producing various types of chemotherapeutic reagents which I had been testing, suggested that if I wanted to be in clinical medicine I should go to Rochester, Minnesota. I applied to the Mayo Clinic and was accepted. The curious thing about that was that as soon as I arrived there my particular mentor was *Dr. Arlie Barnes* who looked at my background and said, "well, I think you should go up to the institute," so I went back into the laboratory and worked on coronary flow with *Dr. Hiram Essex* for a year.

WCR: *You had a rotating internship which included both medicine and surgery. Then you had a year in pathology. Then, for the next 2 years you were really doing research.*

HBB: Right. I also had clinical teaching duties at the University of Pittsburgh at the Mercy Hospital, where there was a ward which was dedicated to the study of patients with pneumonia. At that time, the coal miners in the Pittsburgh area had practically epidemic pneumonia in the winter. There was a ward with 8 to 10 patients in it. The mortality rate of pneumococcal pneumonia at that time was about 25%. I introduced the typing of the pneumococcus. The mortality rate of type I pneumonia was around 20%, and type II, almost 40%.

WCR: *So you did spend 3 years at the Mayo Clinic?*

HBB: That started a long period at the Mayo Clinic. That was when I was I oriented toward cardiology with Dr. Arlie Barnes.

WCR: *He was considered a cardiologist at that time?*

HBB: Yes. All the people at the Mayo Clinic at that time kept their basic interest in internal medicine, but he spent most of his time in cardiology. He had one landmark article on the electrocardiographic localization of myocardial infarcts. He was very interested in getting people to work in the laboratory.

WCR: *A cardiologist in 1939 to 1949 really meant that you knew something about electrocardiography?*

HBB: That is right. I thought, if I were going to be a cardiologist that I should work with other cardiologists at the time, and obtained a position at the University of Minnesota, Minneapolis, campus to work with *Dr. Maurice Visscher.* I was there for about 6 months. Then I went to England for 6 months.

WCR: *What was it like studying in England?*

HBB: The English system of graduate teaching at that time was interesting because you could go to various open clinics, such as the Heart Hospital and the London Hospital and see patients. There would be a discussion of them afterwards. *Dr. John Parkinson* was particularly helpful. He was a gentleman and a cardiologist right on the top of the pedestal. I also studied with *Dr. Bedford* who was interested in the history of cardiology. I suppose that he was an authority on the development of cardiology in France. He became a close friend of mine. Later in life, when I became editor of *Circulation* (many years afterwards), he contributed articles on the history of cardiology.

WCR: *What did Dr. Parkinson have to say about Sir James MacKenzie?*

HBB: He was an admirer of MacKenzie, and MacKenzie's first assistant in London.

WCR: *When you went to London for those 6 months, was it understood that you would come back to the Mayo Clinic and join the faculty there?*

HBB: Not definitely. I told Dr. Barnes that I wanted to go to England, and at that time I had no idea where I was going to be afterwards. Being unmarried, I did not feel any particular responsibility, but after I was over there for about 3 months, Dr. Barnes wrote me and asked when I was going to come back, indicating I had a place at the Mayo Clinic.

WCR: *You joined the Mayo Clinic as a full time faculty person in 1940?*

HBB: It was kind of understood that I would be soon. Initially, I was a first assistant. Even before the Pearl Harbor bombing, I had indicated to the people in Canada that I might go back to its army services, but they said they did not need doctors in 1940. So then I became an American citizen. Right after Pearl Harbor, I volunteered and entered the US Army. Since I had been working at that time at the Mayo Clinic with the low-pressure chamber with *Randy Lovelace* and *Walter Booth,* it was apparent that where I might be most useful, which was at Randolph Field, Texas.

WCR: *How long were you at Randolph Field?*

HBB: Two years. Then I was in the European theater for 2 years.

WCR: *What did you learn in your investigations?*

HBB: I was teaching physiology. We had a course for the flight surgeons, and I started a course for aviation physiologists. I just taught that for the one session. There were people in that first group who were much more knowledgeable than I was. The new trainees were then scattered all over the world to run the low-pressure chambers.

WCR: *What did you do in Europe for the 2 other years you were in the Armed Services?*

HBB: I went to the Central Medical Establishment, which was just a temporary organization formed by the Headquarters of the 8th Air Force for the study of people with various medical problems. My duties over there were threefold: (1) working with individuals

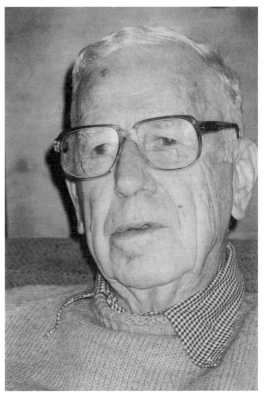

FIGURE 2. Photograph of H.B. Burchell taken by W.C. Roberts during the interview.

who had physiological problems, disorientation, psychological stresses, and combat fatigue; (2) consulting in the surrounding hospitals where the Air Force personnel might have been hospitalized; and (3) working on the criteria for injuries, psychological and physical, that might require the soldier's being discharged from duty.

WCR: *Did you enjoy your tour over there?*

HBB: Yes, very much.

WCR: *It sounds to me like your 4 years in the Air Force really furthered your medical career a good bit.*

HBB: It forwarded my medical career from the understanding of people with general problems. It did not forward my career very much from the point of view of cardiology, though at Randolph Field, I was closely associated with *Dr. Charles Kossmann,* a cardiologist from New York who had trained with Dr. Wilson at Ann Arbor, Michigan, and we talked quite a bit about cardiology. We were the referring center for individuals where there would be a question of a cardiac disability or a murmur.

WCR: *After World War II you returned to the Mayo Clinic? That was 1946?*

HBB: Yes, January 1946.

WCR: *What was it like on a day-to-day basis at the Mayo Clinic in 1946?*

HBB: One worked in a section which took all

types of medical cases, but the cardiac cases were concentrated in 2 sections.

WCR: *At that time were you seeing patients in both mornings and afternoons 5 days a week?*

HBB: The system there was that you had a period in the hospital and during that time you were full time in the hospital. That was somewhat more enjoyable than working in what would be the equivalent of the outpatient clinic. Full time in the hospital then was for about 3 months of the year.

WCR: *It was not long before most of the patients you were seeing had cardiac conditions?*

HBB: I always had a continued interest in diagnosis of general medical problems. Even in the last years I had many referrals and consultations, I was probably seeing 20% of people with problems which were not cardiac.

WCR: *How did you develop your relationships with Earl Wood, John Kirklin, Jesse Edwards, Jim DuShane? Here, they are, these magnificent magnets for attracting patients with heart disease. How did you folks interact? Did you have a lot of conferences? Were you seeing a lot of patients with heart disease that had not been properly diagnosed or someone had given up on? How did it go?*

HBB: My interest in electrocardiography continued. In England during the last year of the war, I used to drop by various English hospitals. I saw a cardiac catheterization done by Sharpey-Schafer and thought that this was the coming thing, relatively easy, relatively safe, and it opens the window to understanding. One of my first objectives when I got back to the Mayo Clinic was to initiate cardiac catheterizations. When I got back in January 1946, the first thing was to sell the idea. The background I had had in the metabolic laboratory gave me the knowledge to get someone to do the oxygen intakes. At that time, there was *Dr. John Pender* in anesthesiology who was putting catheters in veins to introduce an anesthetic in a more efficient way. He had established a reputation of being able to get into any vein. The first group was John Pender, myself, and a technician from what was called the metabolic laboratory, and we did the first catheterization at the Mayo Clinic. In a way, it was a demonstration case to indicate its feasibility within a large institution as well as a diagnostic procedure. A patient came along with an atrial septal defect. At the time, we were pretty certain of our diagnosis from the point of view of the auscultatory findings and the chest x-ray. This patient of *Dr. Charles Mayo* also had gallstones. I suggested that we might catheterize this patient before surgery, indicating it might give me an even better ability to appraise the cardiac risk. I was exaggerating a little bit. It was done and it went very smoothly. We established the fact that there was a big shunt at the atrial level, and that helped to convince my colleagues that the procedure was feasible, safe, and diagnostic. At that time, it so happened that *Dr. Earl Wood,* who had been very busy during the war years on research of the physiology of ''blackout'' on the human centrifuge at the Mayo Clinic, was beginning to look for something else to do. When I suggested that he might take on the cardiac catheterization laboratory, he did. He revolutionized the way cardiac catheterization was done by the development of oximeters so that the blood oxygen content could be determined without having to send a sample to the laboratory. Then he improved techniques to measure the intravascular pressures.

At the time, *Raymond Pruitt,* a medical fellow about 8 years my junior, had developed an interest in electrocardiography and I suggested he might go to study electrocardiography under Frank Wilson, which he did. When he came back, he and I worked together on recording intracardiac electrograms.

Jesse Edwards was recruited in early 1946 when he got out of the Army. He came to the clinic with the idea that he might do cancer research, but somehow Dr. Arlie Barnes, in concert with *Dr. Kernohan* of the Department of Pathology, got him interested in the collection of congenital hearts that were there.

WCR: *You actually got the cardiac catheterization laboratory up and running after you came back to the Mayo Clinic in January 1946?*

HBB: That gives me a little bit too much credit. I arranged the first catheterization and got it running on a regular schedule.

WCR: *Where was the catheterization laboratory first located?*

HBB: In the Medical Science Building, which was connected by a tunnel to the downtown hospital. It was in a nonclinical building. You had to bring the patient from the hospital, perhaps from the Clinic, and then back. It had some disadvantages, particularly when we were doing very young children. The second laboratory was established later in the St. Mary's Hospital and *Dr. Jim DuShane* and others were responsible for that.

WCR: *When was the first cardiac catheterization at the Mayo Clinic?*

HBB: It was the first week of November 1946.

WCR: *So it took awhile to get this going? You left the Mayo Clinic in 1969? How many cardiac catheterization laboratories were present at the Mayo Clinic when you left?*

HBB: There were 2. When I left, the one in the Medical Science Building was still running for adult catheterizations and the one at St. Mary's Hospital was largely, if not entirely, for pediatric cases. *Jeremy Swan* was instrumental in expanding St. Mary's hospital catheterization activities. *Kincaid* and *George Davis* added intracardiac angiocardiography, and *Robert Frye* expanded the coronary arteriography. Many others including *Sabu Rahimtoola* and *Ben McCallister* were wonderful collaborators.

WCR: *When you came back to the Mayo Clinic in 1946, the only intrathoracic cardiovascular operations being done at that time, I gather, were closure of patient ductus arteriosus, resection of coarctation of aorta, pericardial resection, and mitral valvulotomy? Rapid developments occurred. What happened early on?*

HBB: Dr. Wood and Dr. Code had their PhD's from the University of Minnesota, and even in 1939 we were dreaming of direct-vision intracardiac repair. One of the projects I did with Dr. Visscher before the war was to look at a new type of oxygenator and he said, "what can you do here to make this work better?" I worked with it for awhile, but I was not very successful. The main problem was to prevent blood frothing. Even in the mid 1940s cardiopulmonary bypass was kind of a dream, and when I was in the service, people I met from Sweden, France, and Belgium were thinking along the same lines. At the forefront were the surgeons at the University of Minnesota. The cross circulation procedure pioneered by *Dr. Walton Lillehei* was a tremendous advance. The development of the bubble oxygenator thereafter was good, too. There was some competition between who might do the first cardiopulmonary bypass operation with an artificial heart–lung machine, either Rochester, Minnesota, or Minneapolis, Minnesota. Interest in doing this existed also in Detroit, Stockholm, and Paris and probably in other centers.

WCR: *But the first one was actually done in Philadelphia?*

HBB: Yes.

WCR: *But it spread immediately. The Mayo Clinic pump was simultaneously being developed?*

HBB: Right, it was patterned after the Gibbon machine. This is where *Dr. John Kirklin* came prominently into the picture. An engineer who came from Minneapolis, *Richard Jones,* contributed tremendously to the project. The first open heart operation with the heart–lung apparatus in Rochester, I remember very well, on March 22, 1955. That was over 2 years after the first one was performed in Philadelphia.

WCR: *What cardiac condition did that first patient have?*

HBB: It think it was a ventricular septal defect.

WCR: *What was it like on a day-to-day basis by 1950 at the Mayo Clinic? What were your activities like? Were you seeing patients primarily? How many conferences did you have a week?*

HBB: I was seeing patients primarily. We had a number of conferences. I had an informal electrocardiographic conference during the noon hour several times a week. I would be reading electrocardiograms and people who were interested would drop in and we would discuss them. We had a weekly clinicopathological conference with Dr. Jesse Edwards. Then, I had a review of catheterizations with Earl Wood once a week.

WCR: *Those were taking place primarily at noon time?*

HBB: Yes. We also had one cardiac conference that started at 8:00 A.M.

WCR: *What was your actual schedule with patients? When did you see patients, 9 to 12, 1 to 5? How did it actually work?*

HBB: The people at the desk would arrange for patients to come in at certain hours, but it was a very loose schedule. There would be some patients that would be put in a room for a consultation and the signal was right there and those lights indicated that that patient was waiting for you.

WCR: *So it was a very efficient system of seeing patients?*

HBB: The patients might not say that because there were often quite long waiting periods, but it was efficient from the point of view of the fact that the patient was satisfied because when they were seen, they were not hurried.

WCR: *How many cardiologists were at the Mayo Clinic in the early 1950s? You mentioned Ray Pruitt.*

HBB: There were 2 sections. I think there were 5 physicians in each section. Then, there was also a section in hypertension which was headed by *Ed Allen, Nelson Barker,* and *Edgar Hines.* There were 5 in that section also. They took care of those patients who had special problems in high blood pressure. I regarded them as circulation specialists, even though they were not specialists in hearing the heart sounds and murmurs.

WCR: *After surgery on patients with cardiopulmonary bypass was begun in 1955, I assume the number of patients coming to the Mayo Clinic with cardiovascular disease must have skyrocketed. Was that the situation?*

HBB: I don't know if it would be equivalent to the influx of patients with congenital heart disease that occurred at The Johns Hopkins Hospital, for instance, after the Blalock-Taussig shunt, but certainly there were more and more patients coming for a diagnosis. The numbers increased rapidly; "skyrocketed," would be an exaggeration.

WCR: *In 1965, you became editor of* Circulation *and were editor for 5 years? You were required to step down after 5 years. As you look back over your editorship, did you enjoy it, was it a pleasant experience?*

HBB: Very much so. One reason it was acceptable, you might say, "to step down" was the fact that for me it was a 7-day business. When offered the editorship, I discussed it with administration at the Clinic. I told them that I would like to continue doing clinical work, but wished that to be half time. Thus, I had the mornings for *Circulation* and the afternoons for patients. It turned out that I was working evenings and weekends rather constantly with *Circulation* affairs, but that was enjoyable. I developed contacts with many physicians around the country. When I went to the University of Minnesota in 1968, I asked an epidemiologist (*Henry Blackburn*) and a pediatric cardiologist (*Ray Anderson*) to join me as Associate Editors.

WCR: *You left the Mayo Clinic in 1968 for the University of Minnesota in Minneapolis?*

HBB: After early retirement from the Mayo Clinic in 1968 at age 60, I went to the Department of Medicine to work with *Richard Ebert.* At that time, there was no separation of specialties in the Department of Medicine. There were people in the department, of course, in various subspecialties, but there were no administrative sections. After I came, Dr. Ebert instituted the separation of sections. I was there about a year when sections were established in the subspecialties. Then I became Head of the Cardiac Section in the

Department of Medicine. During this time I had some periods of study abroad—sabbaticals. I had one in Scotland and one in Holland. In Holland, in particular, I became very close to *Dr. Dirk Durrer*. He established a heart institute in Amsterdam.

WCR: *What did you do in Scotland?*

HBB: Teaching and research conferences.

WCR: *Where was that?*

HBB: That was at St. Andrews University. The clinical work was done across the river in the city of Dundee.

WCR: *Why did you decide to take early retirement from the Mayo Clinic and move to Minneapolis?*

HBB: I was interested in undergraduate education and just curious. I thought people in Rochester did not need me particularly.

WCR: *How did it work out?*

HBB: It worked out well. I was very lucky in 2 ways: first, in respect to my health and also my family. I wondered what might happen if I became sick or disabled. I took some financial loss coming to Minneapolis.

WCR: *Both you and John Kirklin left the Mayo Clinic about the same time?*

HBB: Yes. He was tempted to go to Birmingham because it was going to be "the Harvard of the South," and I understood that he was offered practically anything he wanted. He established an outstanding cardiac surgery program there.

WCR: *Jesse Edwards had left the Mayo Clinic in 1960?*

HBB: Yes.

WCR: *After you resigned as Chief of the Section of Cardiology at the University of Minnesota, you remained active in teaching and writing?*

HBB: At the time I accepted the position, it was not a division, it was a section. Initially, I thought someone else would be coming soon. The one who finally came was *Jay Cohn*. He really made the group a division instead of a section. He developed a terrific program.

WCR: *How do you now compare the atmosphere at the University of Minnesota with the atmosphere at the Mayo Clinic?*

HBB: They are certainly different. At the time I was leaving the Clinic, a visitor came and when he had learned I was going he said "why are you leaving here? It's like taking off from a beautiful cruise ship into a large working freighter," indicating that I would find things different. Things at the University were not as well organized, perhaps did not go so smoothly in regard to patients. The emphasis at the University of Minnesota was on laboratory research; at the Mayo Clinic the emphasis was on the care of the patients. I was comfortable, however, in both places. I liked them both; they were just different.

WCR: *As you look back over your career, what activities brought the greatest pleasure to you? What are you most pleased with in what you have done professionally?*

HBB: I suppose it is my associations and perhaps making some minor contributions to new approaches.

I have been long interested in electrocardiography. I think maybe I made some little contributions in the diagnosis of arrhythmias and myocardial injuries. When I was in Amsterdam in about 1960, Dick Durrer and I were particularly interested in the Wolff-Parkinson-White syndrome which, as you know, is a type of electrocardiographic abnormality associated with arrhythmias, and caused by "bypass" across the atrioventricular groove or some area close to the bundle. We were thinking at that time of ablation techniques. We theorized that we could do this with an ablation by recording simultaneously from the atrial side and the ventricular side, and ablated where we had identified the location of the bypass tract.

WCR: *I presume that you always were on salary both at the Mayo Clinic and at the University of Minnesota? What is your view about cardiologists and cardiac surgeons being on fee-for-service compensation? In other words, when you can charge x-dollars to do a cardiac catheterization and you get paid a good bit for that, there might be an added incentive to do the catheterization, whereas if you are on salary, whether you do a cardiac catheterization or not, you are going to get the same salary. Do you think money is too influential now in cardiovascular judgments?*

HBB: That is a difficult question to answer "yes" or "no." I believe in a fee-for-service system, as a philosophy, but I really think it would be better if physicians were on salary. I have a daughter now who is in internal medicine and she is on a fee-for-service. She does all right. Actually, she has a business head, which probably I never had. I have always thought myself very, very lucky because I was doing the things I wanted to do and did not have to worry about how I was getting my living. I liked being on a salary. I was looked at benevolently, you might say, by the people who were paying my salary.

WCR: *When did you marry?*

HBB: In 1941. When I went into the Army, I more or less said goodbye to my girlfriend, the person who was closest to me. I told Margaret: "Well, I am going into the Army and therefore you had better put off any ideas of getting married until after this confrontation is over." She had different ideas and said she would like to get married and came down to visit me in Texas. We were married in the chapel at Randolph Field.

WCR: *You had how many children?*

HBB: Four.

WCR: *What do your children do?*

HBB: Of the 4 girls, the oldest went to Radcliffe and studied genetics. As a senior, she was married, graduated from Barnard. She had 2 children, and then she went to medical school and is practicing internal medicine in New Jersey. The second one went to Smith College in Massachusetts and left in her senior year. That was a time of the Vietnam war problems. She became a potter, an artist, and is doing very well, but different. The third one went to Stanford University. Her husband, Richard Patterson, is a Professor of Philosophy at Emory University, and she also teaches history there. They both have tenure at Emory. The last one went to Stanford University also, studied botany, and ended up at the University of Virginia, where she is now. She is not teaching, but she has a family and is married to a biologist, Henry Wilbur.

WCR: *So you have very scholarly offspring?*

HBB: Yes.

WCR: *How did you meet your wife?*

HBB: A blind date in Rochester, Minnesota.

WCR: *Is she a scholarly person?*

HBB: Yes, I think so. She went to Smith and majored in sociology and then became a nursery school teacher. She established a nursery school in Rochester.

WCR: *I have always thought of you as a very scholarly physician and one who enjoyed medicine for the enjoyment of it, in addition to what you do for people. You have written a number of articles on important figures in medicine. You have been interested in the history of medicine for many years. How did that come about?*

HBB: I guess I just drifted into it. I remember in medical school going to one class where the Professor of Pathology had said that King George II had syphilitic aortitis and then went into another class where the professor said he had ruptured his heart. That was my first case study in history. I found that King George II did indeed rupture his heart, his right ventricle, and he also had a dissecting aneurysm. At that time, *Mr. Thomas Keys* worked in the History of Medicine Department at the Mayo Clinic, and we reported that story together. I became very interested in eponyms and wondered who the person was from whom a disease might have been named.

WCR: *I noticed that you wrote a piece on William Ernest Henley. Who was he?*

HBB: He wrote the poem about the problems of having a disability, probably a tuberculous infection of his foot and ankle. He was in the Edinburgh Infirmary for a long time as a patient of Dr. Lister. Henley then became a poet, a literary man at the time of Sir Walter Scott.

WCR: *The piece entitled, "The Other Wise Man." What is that about?*

HBB: It was a story by Henry Van Dyke about an individual who started out to find Christ by following the stars. But during his search he had many diversions and those diversions were caused by his doing his duty to his fellow man. He was delayed in his search for Christ, arriving only at the crucifixion ending. I compared that story to the general practitioner who often did not get to the medical meetings and things like that because he was looking after patients at home.

WCR: *What about the piece on "Hedgehog and Foxes"?*

HBB: This caught my attention because of a little book Isach Berlin had written by that title, based on Tolstoy, a story of war and peace. This was an attempt to sort out individuals with a different approach to life. It goes something like this: the fox knows many things, the hedgehog but one. Which would be better, the one who had many little approaches to things or an individual who is motivated by a single principle.

WCR: *Which side did you come down on?*

HBB: I couldn't decide.

WCR: *You wrote a piece on "Osler: In Quest of the Gnostic Grail in Morbid Anatomy"? What does that mean?*

HBB: What was it that "drove" Osler in his professional life? Pathology was the prime basis of Osler's knowledge. As you and probably everyone else knows, after Osler graduated from medical school, he studied pathology and did literally hundreds of postmortems. It was from this source of information I think that he became so knowledgeable in disease processes and the clinical manifestations of those diseases.

WCR: *You wrote a piece on Sir Thomas Lewis. Do you consider Sir Thomas Lewis a great man?*

HBB: Oh, I do indeed. I went to some of his clinics when I was in England in 1939. Lewis was a tremendous individual and he said of himself, "I am not a clinician primarily," though he said he could do that, but he was "a clinical investigator." The very first clinic of Lewis' that I went to, he had actually discussed cases. He picked me out for some reason. I think it was the fashion of many of the top medical teachers in England to try "to pick on" Americans, maybe because Americans were thought of as not being real scholars. He said, "Well, Burchell, as an American, what do you know about this?" I answered, "not much." He was talking about the auscultatory findings in mitral stenosis, that old story. Lewis said, "People really can't say this person has a presystolic murmur. It *is* a presystolic murmur, but they don't know that. All they know is that they hear that noise complex of the first sound and they know from phonocardiographic records that it is presystolic; however, when they listen to the patient they don't know that is a presystolic from listening."

WCR: *You have encountered a number of important figures in cardiovascular disease in the past 60 years. You must have met most of them. Who strikes you in these last 60 years of men and women that you have encountered as way above the pack?*

HBB: There are a number, of people, of course, who were exceptionally good. With my early laboratory background, I was initially more active in the American Physiological Society than the American Heart Association. I got to know *Paul White* pretty well because he and I were on the Heart Council together. I never met or got to know *Samuel Levine*. Many people from Boston say that Dr. Levine was the greatest cardiologist, but I never knew him. I liked and admired *Howard Spraque* and *"Coke" Andrus*. An individual who stands out from Philadelphia, who I thought was exceptionally good from a clinical point of view, was *Francis Wood*. Then, from serving on various research committees, I was privileged to get to know *Louis Katz*. I had a tremendous respect for him. There were so many who were leaders. I suppose Paul White would the person in this country who stands out predominantly in my mind. *Arlie Barnes* from the Mayo Clinic was an individual with tremendous insight and a great supporter of research. They were all Presidents of the American Heart Association.

WCR: *What characteristics of Paul Dudley White made him stand out so much in your mind now?*

HBB: He was one of the first persons who said as a young man, "I am going to be a heart specialist." Early in his career, White did basic research work as a student with Sir Thomas Lewis. Many of his articles were case reports with unusual things enlightening the physiological and pathological background of those conditions. He was very public-health oriented. That particular activity may have stemmed from his knowledge of the work of the New York Heart Association. That Association started cardiac clinics for the poor, and then from those clinics, particularly those focusing on rheumatic fever, the concept emerged that certain cardiac diseases could be prevented. Paul White gave great support to *Ancel Keyes* at the beginning of the now famous 7 country study. *Frank Wilson* in Ann Arbor was outstanding in electrocardiography.

WCR: *What do you do most of the time now?*

HBB: You can see I am surrounded by books. I read a great deal. I cannot keep up with the cardiological literature, of course. I go to the History of Medicine Library a couple of times a week, look for various things, and I still go to grand rounds if it is on a cardiac subject. I go to the clinicopathologic correlation conferences. I am as addicted to clinicopathological conferences as some people are to opera, because one can really see life played out there.

WCR: *Did you enjoy the year you spent entirely in pathology?*

HBB: Yes.

WCR: *What did you do mainly? Autopsies?*

HBB: I spent most of the time doing autopsies.

WCR: *That background made working with Jesse Edwards a given, almost.*

HBB: You could say that. I could recognize which was the right and left ventricle. I mentioned that because with the more or less complete disappearance of postmortems, I don't think students know what the heart is like, and this came up in relation to what the candidates knew when they came for the accreditation examination for cardiology. When I took that accreditation cardiovascular discourse in 1939, pathology was something you could choose to do. You were able to coast through it pretty well. When I later came on the accreditation board, we really established a thorough examination with 2 cases and 2 examiners, one of whom was just a "standby" and supporter of the students to a certain extent when the other man was quizzing. Then there were short tests of about 15 minutes each in separate rooms. Routine electrocardiograms were passed out. Then heart specimens were shown. Then there were radiographs, pharmacology, and cardiac catheterization data. Some candidates would not be able to tell anything about the heart specimen. Most knew how the heart worked but most did not know what it looked like.

WCR: *As you look back is there anything professionally you would have liked to have done that you were not able to do?*

HBB: Of course, I would have liked to have done things better. Maybe developed better electrocardiographic equipment for the study of arrhythmias at the time of surgery. The people at Duke really did this so well, and they had the equipment and knowledge that surpassed my abilities back in the 1960s.

WCR: *Do you have hobbies other than medicine? I presume the history of medicine is a hobby to you.*

HBB: That is right.

WCR: *Do you have other hobbies?*

HBB: I used to care about fishing and hunting. Earl Wood is a great hunter. I never went deer hunting with him, but many times we went game hunting and duck hunting together. I had a dog ordinarily. In fact, one time I had one of the outstanding retrievers in Minnesota. I used to go to hunting trials.

WCR: *How much time off did you take off, as a rule, when you were at the Mayo Clinic? Did you get a month a year off?*

HBB: It depended upon the length of service. I think you started when you went on staff, getting 3 weeks' vacation, and 2 weeks travel time for meetings. Then, after a certain period of time, maybe it was 10 years on the staff, you got a month off. After 20 years, I think you got 6 weeks off. I was extremely fortunate. When I got up to having 4 to 6 weeks off a year, I used to go back to the laboratory for about half of that time. For 2 or 3 weeks, Ray Pruitt and I would get clinical experiments done in relation to excitation patterns.

WCR: *Did your whole family go on family vacations when your kids were growing up?*

HBB: Yes, we used go on skiing vacations as a family practically every year. One year we saved up to go to a ranch for a couple of weeks one summer.

WCR: *You have had a happy life?*

HBB: Yes. I have been very fortunate.

WCR: *You see your daughters very much now?*

HBB: No, not very much. They have their own things to do and they shouldn't come to see me. They have too many things to do.

WCR: *How many grandchildren do you have?*

HBB: Nine. Three have graduated from college and 2 have just begun.

WCR: *Is your wife healthy?*

HBB: Yes.

WCR: *So you are 90?*

HBB: I will be 90 in November 1997.

WCR: *What is your wife's age?*

HBB: She is 80, so a 9- to 10-year difference depending on the time of year.

WCR: *Do you ever go south in the wintertime to get warm?*

HBB: I was again fortunate in being offered opportunities to take a period at Stanford and for 7 years I went out there for the winter quarter. Donald Harrison invited me. What I did out there was have open-room discussions with the cardiac fellows. Occasionally, I made rounds. For 2 years I went to the University of Arizona for a period, so that was nice also.

WCR: *You must have gotten many invitations to go here and there to speak. I gather you had to limit* *that a good bit, particularly when you were at the Mayo Clinic. Is that right?*

HBB: I did not have to limit it a great deal. I made choices of course. I was able to go where I really wished to go.

WCR: *Do you enjoy traveling?*

HBB: I did. I don't enjoy it any more. I am happy at home with a familiar environment. I have a hearing problem and it is so much easier being at home.

WCR: *Dr. Burchell, it has been a pleasure. I have been privileged to have this opportunity to talk with you.*

HBB'S BEST PUBLICATIONS AS SELECTED BY HBB

2. Burchell HB, Barnes AR, Mann FC. The electrocardiographic picture of experimental localized pericarditis. *Am Heart J* 1939;18:133–144.

3. Burchell HB. Adjustments in coronary circulation after experimental coronary occlusion with particular reference to vascularization of pericardial adhesions. *Arch Int Med* 1940;65:240–262.

8. Barnes AR, Burchell HB. Acute pericarditis simulating acute coronary occlusion, a report of fourteen cases. *Am Heart J* 1942;23:247–268.

12. Burchell HB. Observations on additional instances of a supernormal phase in the human heart. *J Lab Clin Med* 1942;28:7–11.

17. Pruitt RD, Burchell HB, Barnes AR. The anoxia test in the diagnosis of coronary insufficiency, a study of 289 cases. *JAMA* 1945;128:839–845.

21. Burchell HB, Glagett OT. The clinical syndrome associated with pulmonary arteriovenous fistulas, including a case report of a surgical cure. *Am Heart J* 1947;34:151–162.

22. Burchell HB. Cardiac manifestations of anxiety. *Proc Staff Meet, Mayo Clin* 1947;22:433.

32. Burchell HB, Pritt RD, Barnes AR. The stress and the electrocardiogram in the induced hypoxemia test for coronary insufficiency. *Am Heart J* 1948;36:373–389.

42. Burchell HB. An evaluation of esophageal electrocardiograms in the diagnosis of healed posterior myocardial infarction. *Am J Med Sc* 1948;216:492–500.

57. Burchell HB. Sino-auricular block, interference dissociation, and different recovery rates of excitation in the bundle branches. *Br Heart J* 1949;11:230–236.

67. Burchell HB, Taylor BE, Knutson JRB, Wood EH. Circulatory adjustments to the hypoxemia of congenital heart disease of the cyanotic type. *Circulation* 1950;1:404–414.

70. Burchell HB, Taylor BE, Knutson JRB, Wakim KG. Coarctation of the aorta with hypotension in the left arm. Physiologic observations on direct intra-arterial pressures and flow of blood. *M Clin N Am* 1950:1177–1185.

101. Bartholomew LG, Burchell HB. Wolff-Parkinson-White syndrome associated with situs inversus, report of case simulating myocardial infarction electrocardiographically. *Proc Staff Meet, Mayo Clin* 1952;27:98–104.

107. Burchell HB, Essex HE, Pruitt RD. Studies on the spread of excitation through the ventricular myocardium II. The ventricular septum. *Circulation* 1952;6:161–171.

120. Burchell HB, Essex HE, Lambert EH. Action potentials supporting the presence of specialized conduction pathways in the dogs ventricle. *Circulation Res* 1953;1:186–188.

129. Burchell HB, Swan JHC, Wood EH. Demonstration of differential effects on pulmonary and systemic arterial pressure by variation in oxygen content of inspired air in patients with patent ductus arteriosus and pulmonary hypertension. *Circulation* 1953;8:681–694.

300. Atwood RM, Burchell HB, Tauxe WN. Pulmonary scans achieved with macroaggregated radioiodinated albumin, use in diagnosis of pulmonary artery agenesis. *Amer J Med Sci* 1966;252:84–88.

313. Burchell HB, Frye RL, Anderson MW, McGoon DC. Atrio-ventricular and ventriculoatrial excitation in Wolff-Parkinson-White syndrome (type B): temporary ablation at surgery. *Circulation* 1967;36:663–672.

321. Burchell HB. A cardiologist's view of modern cardiovascular surgery. *Dis Chest* 1969;55:323.

323. Burchell HB, Merideth J. Management of cardiac tachyarrhythmias with cardiac pacemakers. *Ann New York Acad Sci* 1969;167:546.

366. Burchell HB, Tuna N. The interpretation of gross left axis deviation in the electrocardiogram. *Eur J Cardiol* 1979;10:259–277.

368. Burchell HB. Potassium and the cardiologist—1980 close encounters. *Cardiovasc Rev Rep* 1980;1:316–324.

Historical Pieces

9. Burchell HB, Keys TE. The heart of George II of England. *Bull Med Libr Assn* 1942;30:198–202.

249. Burchell HB. Stephen Hales, September 17, 1677–January 4, 1761, (editorial). *Circulation* 1961;23:1–6.

259. Burchell HB. William Ernest Henley (1849–1903), medical frame of reference for the poem invictus. *Ad Med* 1961;30:510–515.

269. Burchell HB. Henry Van Dyke and his angina pectoris, a note on the story of the other wise man and an analogy to the practitioner. *JAMA* 1962;182:1029–1030.

286. Burchell HB. The other wise man. *New Physician* 1964;13:459–470.

297. Burchell HB. Hedgehog and foxes, renascent reflections of a tyro editor. *JAMA* 1966;195:285–286.

349. Burchell HB. Osler: In quest of the gnostic grail in morbid anatomy. *J Hist Med* 1975;30:235–249.

351. Burchell HB. Hutchinson's "Don'ts" for diagnosticians. His principles of diagnosis revisited. *Geriatrics* 1975;30:105–111.

WILLIAM HOWARD FRISHMAN, MD:
A Conversation With the Editor*

Dr. Bill Frishman is Professor of Medicine and Pharmacology and Chairman of the Department of Medicine of New York Medical College in Valhalla, New York, and also Chief of Medicine at Westchester County Medical Center in Valhalla, which is located in the northern suburbs of New York City. He was born in the Bronx, grew up in the Bronx, and except for his 6 years in Boston, he has always lived in the Bronx. His father's premature death convinced him that he wanted to be a physician and cardiologist and to work in his beloved Bronx. His career at Albert Einstein stretched from 1976 until 1997 and during this period he published approximately 180 original communications in medical journals; 391 monographs, reviews, and book chapters, and 14 books. His work has involved primarily evaluation of drugs to decrease myocardial ischemia, heart failure, blood pressure, and various arrhythmias. He has been involved in the evaluation of 50 drugs beginning with propranolol in 1973. Bill Frishman is a self-made man devoted to his family, community, country, and medical center. He is also a good guy with a good sense of humor and a good capacity for friendship.

William Clifford Roberts, MD† (hereafter WCR): *I am speaking with Dr. Bill Frishman on December 15, 1997, in my office at Baylor University Medical Center. Dr. Frishman has just presented at our Medical Grand Rounds. Dr. Frishman, I would like to find out what it was in you that made it possible for you to stand "above the herd," so to speak. Maybe we could start with your childhood. How was it growing up in the Bronx? Who were your mother and father? Did you have siblings? What do you remember of your young years?*

William Howard Frishman, MD‡ (hereafter WHF): I was born in the southeast Bronx, a lower middle-class community of New York City, where many first- and second-generation European Americans had settled after moving from crowded neighborhoods in Manhattan to seek greater living space. My great grandparents and grandparents had emigrated from eastern Europe at the turn of the century, and they all worked in the garment industry which was located in lower Manhattan. My father was born in Hoboken, New Jersey, just across the Hudson River from New York City, and my mother was born on the lower east side of Manhattan. Their families moved to the Bronx after World War I.

As a child, I was fortunate to have 2 loving parents

and large extended family, all who lived in the same community. My father owned a men's and boys clothing store in the neighborhood, and my mother worked as a bookkeeper for a ceramics factory located in the community. We lived in a small apartment; few people in the neighborhood owned automobiles.

I developed a love of learning from my parents. My father and mother were high school graduates and were reading constantly in their limited spare time. I would go to the local public library every week to borrow books, and I developed from my book browsing a love of history, especially historical biographies.

I attended a local public elementary and junior high school. They were not the easiest places to learn in, with large classes of 35 to 40 students. However, I had many wonderful teachers who were devoted to their work. It was from these experiences, I sought a career as an educator. I was impressed with the impact a teacher can make on a youngster, even in the formative years. The instructor who had the greatest influence on me during these years was a junior high school General Science teacher, Eugene Smolar. I have modeled my teaching style after Mr. Smolar. He made difficult scientific concepts easy to learn, with a sense of humor mixed with firmness. He also had great respect for his students, and I developed a real appreciation for science from him. In subsequent years, I was fortunate to attend the Bronx High School of Science (Figure 1), one of the first specialty science schools in the country. Entry to Bronx Science was based on a competitive examination and grade performance in junior high school. At Bronx Science the student body included young men and women from all over the city, most coming from inner city homes with families struggling to succeed. It was the most competitive school environment I would ever work in, however, an extremely stimulating atmosphere for learning, with the best teachers in the city. Bronx Science has had more Nobel Prize winners than any high school in the U.S., and many alumni would go on to future careers in the physical and biological sciences, medicine, and mathematics. Jimmy Carter's Secretary of Defense, Harold Brown, was a Bronx Science graduate. Some graduates did go on to nonscience careers, such as Stokeley Carmichael, William Safire, and Bobby Darin (Walden Cassatto Jr.) who would eventually die from rheumatic heart disease.

My high school years were clouded by the sudden death of my father from an acute myocardial infarction, a great catastrophe for our family, which would ultimately lead to my becoming a cardiologist. My father was a vibrant, active man who worked very hard, 6 days a week from morning until night; unfortunately he had been a heavy cigarette smoker since his teenage years. My mother had also smoked but quit the habit because of migraine headaches. One

*This series of interviews are underwritten by an unrestricted grant from Bristol-Myers Squibb.
†Baylor Cardiovascular Institute, Baylor University Medical Center, Dallas, Texas 75246.
‡Department of Medicine, New York Medical College, Valhalla, New York 10598.

0002-9149/98/$19.00 **1323**
PII S0002-9149(98)00224-0

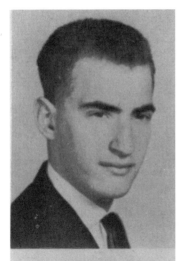

WILLIAM FRISHMAN   SY 2-3115
1366 White Plains Rd., Bx. 62
Ed.-in-Chief of Observatory,
Science Editor Journal of Bio.,
Physical Science Journal, Math
Bulletin, Arista Tutor, Track
Team, ARISTA.

FIGURE 1. Graduation from Bronx High School of Science at the age of 16.

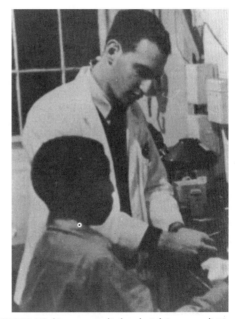

FIGURE 2. Working as a medical student doing my pediatrics rotation at Boston City Hospital, 1967.

childhood remembrance I have is being sent by my parents to buy them cigarettes which in the 1950s sold for 24 cents a pack. A youngster could buy cigarettes during those years without any question from the merchant. My father first suffered myocardial infarction in his 30s and had been warned to stop smoking, but continued after his recovery, right until his death at age 46. My father's death was a tremendous loss, and I learned from this tragedy that an individual with modifiable risk factors for coronary artery disease bears a responsibility not just for his/her own well being, but the well being of their family. Children should not be orphaned by the premature death of a parent from preventable conditions. My father's death occurred just before final exams during my junior year of high school, and I made an immediate decision to become a heart doctor who would work to see that what happened to my family would not happen to other families. I became extremely focused and goal oriented.

I also had more pleasant experiences during my high school years that would influence my future work. First, I was appointed Editor-in-Chief of my high school year book. From my year book work, I learned how to organize a detailed compendium within a defined time limit, since your classmates are counting on the year book being printed before graduation. Second, I worked after classes at a local pharmacy as a stock and delivery boy. I would read the labels on all the medicine bottles. From this experience I developed both a love of pharmacology and an

appreciation of the work of pharmacists. Finally, I was awarded a National Science Foundation grant at Cornell Medical School during one of my summer vacations. I worked on my own research project entitled "Cardiac Manifestations of Hyperthyroidism" under the direction of a Cornell physician-biometrician, Dr. Melvin Schwartz. I used the books at the Cornell Medical Library to try to teach myself electrocardiography of the white Wistar rat, a clinical skill I still have not yet mastered.

Following high school, I attended the Boston University 6-year medical program, one of the first such accelerated programs in the U.S. After high school, one was guaranteed admission to medical school after passing all the course work during the 2-year undergraduate portion of the program. For many individuals, this is not the best route for a medical education, but in my eagerness to become a physician, it was just right for me. It was a wonderful experience being a college and medical student in Boston during the 1960s (Figure 2). I had wonderful professors in medical school, and since the class size was relatively small, I was able to know many of the faculty very well, including Stanley Robbins, the editor of the Pathology Text. My chiefs of medicine at Boston University were Franz Ingelfinger and Arnold Relman, who subsequently became editors-in-chief of the *New England Journal of Medicine*, Dr. Norman Levinsky, who would become Chair of Medicine at BU for 25 years, Aram Chobanian, who is now the Dean at Boston University, and John Harrington, who is the Dean at Tufts. An upper classmate at Boston University, Marcia Angell, is now the executive editor of *The New England Journal of Medicine*. The research thrust at Boston University during these years was hypertension and atherosclerosis, a tradition that continues today under Apstein, Gavras, and Loscalzo. Cardiology was beginning to blossom as a scientific discipline during the 1960s, and my experiences at Boston University reinforced my desire to be an academic cardiologist. One experience at BU that had a great impact on my future work as a teacher was the opportunity to work one-on-one with a faculty member in preparation of a required doctoral thesis. This project had to be of such quality that it could stand the light of day if submitted to a peer-reviewed journal. This provided an opportunity to know a faculty member well, something that is lost now in large medical school classes.

WCR: *Dr. Frishman, let me go back just a bit, and put some dates on things. You were born in what year?*

WHF: I was born on November 9, 1946.

WCR: *Your father died in what year?*

WHF: 1961.

WCR: *So you were 15 when your father died. Did you have siblings?*

WHF: Yes, I have a sister who is 2 years younger than I. I picked up other stepsiblings later when my mother remarried, but that was many years later when I was already in medical school. I also had grandparents, many uncles, aunts, and cousins. My entire family was very close and we all lived in the same community.

WCR: *What was your living like? Did you live in an apartment? What was day-to-day situation like? When your father was alive, did you have a lot of discussions at the dinner table at night? Was he home at night? How did that work out on a day-to-day basis?*

WHF: We always lived in an apartment. I shared a bedroom with my sister, while my parents slept in the living room. They never had their own bedroom. That was how we lived until I went away to college and medical school.

My father worked 6 days a week, and came home early only on Tuesday evenings for dinner. Because he had a retail clothing business, he worked Monday thru Saturday and was off only on Sunday. I remember my father, with the little time he had, always reading a book, even during spare moments at work. I had the good fortune to spend time with my father at his business which was close to our home. My mother was one of the first women in the community to go to work, and that was to help the financial situation of the family. Many times during my school vacations, I stayed with my father at his place of work where I had a chance to know him very well. Despite his long work hours, I could always count on his help if I had difficulty in school, where he could always point me in the right direction. My father had also been a great athlete in his youth; a champion handball player. However, because of his work schedule in the later years, he could not get involved in athletic activities, except for playing ball with my sister and me.

WCR: *What did you do in your spare time when you were a youngster in high school? You mentioned working in your father's place of work? Was that close? Could you just walk there or ride your bicycle?*

WHF: I use to go with my father to his place of work either by bus or car. The Bronx also provided wonderful diversions for a young boy growing up in the 50s and early 60s. Those were the "glory days" of the New York Yankees, the Bronx Bombers. From 1949 to 1964, the Yanks won the American League Pennant 14 times. I used to go to the games with my dad and uncles, usually on Tuesday night. The games we were involved with as children were the New York "street sports." There were few playing fields available, so we spent time playing ball games on the sidewalk and even in the middle of the street, having to dodge oncoming traffic. I was also active in the Boy Scouts. Until my dad's passing, for an inner city youngster, I think I had an idyllic childhood.

WCR: *So you were a happy youngster?*

WHF: Yes

WCR: *How did you get into the Bronx School of Science?*

WHF: The Bronx School of Science was a New York City magnet school that was started in 1938, and the students came from all over New York City. It was a highly competitive school, where admission was based on grades, specifically performance in math and science in elementary and junior high school. We also had to take a competitive entry exam. I entered the school in 1960 in a newly remodeled building in the west Bronx which had a planetarium and other laboratory facilities that few high schools could provide, either public or private. It was a wonderful environment for learning, with very dedicated teachers.

WCR: *Was that close to home? Could you walk to school?*

WHF: My daily commute involved taking 2 subway trains each way. The high school was in the West Bronx, and I lived in the East Bronx. The transportation in the Bronx is only good north to south, not east to west. I had to take a train to Manhattan, and then another uptown to the West Bronx.

WCR: *How long did it take to get to school?*

WHF: An hour by train, each way.

WCR: *You spent 2 hours a day just getting to school and back?*

WHF: Yes. And the train stop was also 5 to 6 blocks from school.

WCR: *Did you think safety when walking around in the Bronx?*

WHF: New York is actually a relatively safe city. However, from the popular press there was always a fear of crime. I think when you live in the inner city you learn how to avoid trouble. At least in the 1950s and 60s young people were not armed with guns. Of course there were a lot of street encounters, most of which were fist fights, but rarely did anyone get seriously hurt. At Bronx Science we did have pressures on us from other neighborhood high schools. They had some tough kids and one always had to defend oneself or learn to run fast. However, I was never fearful for my safety in those situations. You avoided walking alone, especially in a neighborhood you were not familiar with.

WCR: *What floor did you live on in your apartment house?*

WHF: We lived on the 2nd floor and then we moved to a slightly larger apartment on the 1st floor.

WCR: *When you father was not at home, what was it like at dinner time? Your mother was working. When you came home, you came into an empty apartment.*

WHF: I had many relatives in the community, including my grandparents who lived close by. My mother would come home from work around 6 o'clock, and until then my sister and I were on our own. Mom would always prepare dinner, and she did whatever was necessary to get us ready for school the next day. I absorbed a tremendous work ethic from both my mother and father. My mother just kept going, even after my father's death. Although at times with her busy schedule, I think it became a bit overwhelming for her. When my father was alive, he would come home very late on work days. Most often dinner would include just my sister, my mother, and me. My mother would make dinner again for my father when he came home from work.

WCR: *You mentioned your father's reading. Was your mother intellectually inclined?*

WHF: My mother was a bookkeeper. She was a high school graduate and read as much as she could. On Saturday afternoons when my father was at work, my mother would go to the public library. Our entire family always had a reverence for books. Even today in her retirement, my mother can always be found at the public library.

WCR: *Did you have many books in your house?*

WHF: We didn't have space for a library. I would use the encyclopedia in the public library which was located a few blocks from our home. Sometimes I would study there because it was quiet.

WCR: *Did you always feel a bit crowded in the house?*

WHF: Yes, in fact our apartment was really just a place to sleep and eat. I would spend free time on the street with friends. During inclement weather, we congregated in the hallways of our building, went to the movies or to the local bowling alley.

WCR: *You were a reasonable athlete in junior high school and high school?*

WHF: Yes and no. I was a fair athlete but more accomplished in my knowledge of sports trivia.

WCR: *You were always playing some sport, chasing some ball?*

WHF: We played baseball, handball, and stickball during the warm months and basketball and touch football in the winter. If we played with a tennis ball, it was not on a regulation court, but against the outside wall of our apartment building. I also competed on the track team in high school.

WCR: *What did you do?*

WHF: I was a quarter miler.

WCR: *I gather neither your mother nor father went to college.*

WHF: My dad attended the City University as a part-time student for 2 years. My mother would attend college at the City University many years later.

WCR: *You mentioned your grandparents were in the Bronx. You had aunts and uncles. I presume most of them did not go to college either.*

WHF: No, in fact one of my grandmothers could not read or write English; however, she did read the Yiddish newspapers.

WCR: *Where did your mother and father actually come from?*

WHF: My great grandparents and grandparents were born in eastern Europe. My maternal grandmother was from Hungary, my paternal grandmother from Austria, and my two grandfathers were from Russia. My grandparents all married in the U.S. Both my parents were born in the U.S., and I am a second-generation American.

WCR: *Your father was how old when he died?*

WHF: He was 46. He had suffered a previous heart attack while he was in his mid-30s.

WCR: *Your mother is now how old?*

WHF: 79

WCR: *What was the age difference between your mother and father?*

WHF: 3 years

WCR: *You went to Boston University for that 6-year combined liberal arts/medical school program. You came from a family without a lot of financial resources. Did you have a scholarship to Boston University? How did that work out? How did you choose Boston University?*

WHF: I was attracted to the program because of the ability to accelerate in pursuit of a medical degree. I had a partial scholarship and had student loans. I always worked at after-school jobs in college and in medical school. As an undergraduate I worked for room and board as a telephone switchboard operator and as a food server in the dormitory cafeteria.

WCR: *How many hours did you work a week?*

WHF: 10 to 15 hours.

WCR: *You were how old when you went off to college?*

WHF: 16

WCR: *Therefore, you graduated from college and medical school at age 22?*

WHF: Yes. I was in a hurry to get on with a medical career.

WCR: *Your mother and relatives in the Bronx must have been enormously proud of you to have one of theirs go off to college and medical school when they did not have that opportunity to do so themselves.*

WHF: Yes, I was really the first one in my family who went to an out-of-town school. My sister and cousins attended the local public colleges.

WCR: *What about your sister?*

WHF: My sister attended the City University of New York, and she is now a physical education and math teacher in the New York City public school system.

WCR: *Is she back in the Bronx?*

WHF: She teaches in Queens, but she lives on Long Island now.

WCR: *What do you remember about your 2-year liberal arts education at Boston University?*

WHF: The liberal arts program was quite rigorous. We essentially completed 3 years of college by also attending classes through 2 summers. Although we had to take the regular premedical courses, organic chemistry, physics, physical chemistry and biology, there was also time for the humanities. The curriculum was not just concentrated on science. We had very short vacations, 3 weeks at the end of each summer. We eventually received a Bachelor of Arts degree at the time we graduated from medical school.

WCR: *Did any teachers in the liberal arts program have a major impact on you?*

WHF: My physical chemistry professor, Alfred Prock, was an outstanding instructor, and he still teaches in the current 7-year program at Boston University. Physical chemistry was a difficult course for a college freshman, but Dr. Prock made it both enjoyable and easy to understand. In fact, he's another individual whose teaching style I would adopt later. My Western Civilization teacher (I always liked history) also had a great influence on me. I was impressed how teachers could make subject matter come to life through the enthusiasm and dedication they have for their jobs. I consider teaching to be one of the noblest professions.

The 1960s was an interesting time to go to school. John F. Kennedy was assassinated in November of my freshman year of college. In fact he had just visited Boston with his family the week before he went to Dallas. I think individuals growing up at that time (Kennedy was elected when I was in high school) were greatly affected by his assassination, and I don't think the U.S. has ever been the same. I think a lot of the drive and enthusiasm the country had was lost for many years, and of course would be affected more so by the Vietnam War. Many of my former high school classmates at Bronx Science, some of the brightest people I had ever met, were swallowed up by the war. I say "swallowed up" not by being involved in combat, but by the antiwar protests on the college campuses. Many of my friends never pursued their planned scientific careers. I myself was affected greatly by what was going on at the time.

WCR: *You started college in the combined program in September 1963 and Kennedy was shot in November 1963.*

WHF: Most of us looked to Kennedy as the patriarch of the country. He was on television and had a great influence on young people. He was a pro-science, pro-intellectual, pro-athletic type president.

WCR: *I gather from your growing up in the Bronx, you and your family did not go on vacations in the summer time. You didn't travel much outside of New York City.*

WHF: In fact we did. One of the things about living in the New York City in the 1950s was the lack of air conditioners since most of the apartment buildings were not properly wired. The only air conditioners were found in the movie theaters. It was terribly hot and humid during the summer in the 1950s, and our entire family would go to the public beach at Rockaway Peninsula in Queens. In the 1960s our family would go to the Catskill Mountains for the summer, about 100 miles north of the city. I was always in the care of relatives as my parents continued to work through the summer in the city. My family could not afford to send me to camp.

WCR: *Your parents essentially never vacationed?*

WHF: I remember my father having only one weekend off during my early years.

WCR: *When you went to Boston you were, in a way, upgrading your living standards?*

WHF: Well I had my own room for the first time.

WCR: *How did that affect you?*

WHF: It was a wonderful change. I shared a suite of rooms in the dormitory with a group of roommates who today remain my close friends. We were all in the 6-year program together. My 4 roommates were from different parts of the northeast, and we were very supportive and respectful of one another. One became a cardiothoracic surgeon, one became a general surgeon, 2 of us became cardiologists, and one became a psychoanalyst.

WCR: *So you all roomed together the entire 6 years?*

WHF: Yes. We were assigned together at random and not by our choosing. It really worked out well. In fact, George Hines who is now a cardiothoracic surgeon on the faculty of Stony Brook Medical School remains one of my best friends. He and I always sat next to each other during college and medical school final exams for good luck. Even now, when we go out together with our wives, the two of us will sit next to each other. Whoever gets to the restaurant first, saves the place for the other one.

WCR: *What other broadening experiences in college and medical school opened up to you in Boston? After 6 years how did you see yourself compared to when you left the Bronx 6 years earlier?*

WHF: I was a completely different person (Figure 3). Being away from home really helped me in my overall development. First of all, it allowed me to meet people from other parts of the country, particularly other parts of the Northeast. It was also an exciting time to be in Boston, which is a wonderful place to go to school, and a great college town. Overall, it was a mind-expanding experience, but I also worked very hard during these years. Because of the jobs I had and the attention I had to give my studies, I probably had less spare time than most of my peers. However, I still found time to get involved in some athletic activities.

WCR: *Were you a pretty good track man in high school?*

WHF: In the Bronx you learn to run fast.

WCR: *In medical school what kind of jobs did you have? You mentioned those in college.*

WHF: In medical school I worked as a medical technician at the Joslin Clinic because there were no house officers working there at the time. It was a good

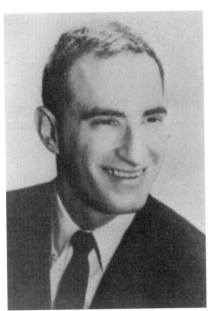

FIGURE 3. Graduation from the Boston University 6-Year Liberal Arts-Medicine Program, 1969.

job except I worked through the night. I worked in all the clinical labs—chemistry, blood banking, hematology and bacteriology—and I did this once or twice a week. I also had a job as an attendant in the Boston Garden, where we covered the first aid room during all the sporting events. That was a time when the Boston Celtics were in their "glory days." I also worked during the Boston Bruins hockey games and all the professional wrestling matches.

WCR: *You actually saw the events and you were just called if someone needed you?*

WHF: It was just a wonderful job for someone who enjoyed team athletics as much as I do, and it was a real thrill to be so close to the players, such as Bill Russell and John Havlicek. I was able to go to many games and actually found the time to study during some of the less exciting competitions.

WCR: *Did learning always come easy for you or did you have to bear down a great deal?*

WHF: Learning came easy but I still studied very hard. I always felt it was not enough to study just to pass an exam. I wanted to learn in such a manner that I would retain the information indefinitely. I was never a good note taker in school and relied a great deal on book reading. I was fortunate in that I had a good memory. In those years, especially in medical school, a good memory was important. I was able to perform well because of that, and I could recall facts later on which I would have forgotten if I had only studied to pass examinations.

WCR: *What do you mean you were not a good note taker?*

WHF: I have a bad handwriting. When I got home I often could not read my notes. To take good notes, I

had to write slowly. As a consequence, I would often miss points in the lecture. I attended lectures faithfully but I needed to do more supplementary reading than my peers.

WCR: *While in college and medical school, were you always worried that you did not have enough money?*

WHF: I had real concerns about how I would perform in school because of my outside jobs. Sometimes I would work through the entire night and then have to go to class the next day. However, working did not affect my academic performance. I was able, in those years, as I am today, to balance many different activities. I don't think my medical school instructors realized that I was involved in so much outside work.

WCR: *Did you sleep much? What was your sleeping life like?*

WHF: I slept whenever I could, but even today I can always get around without much sleep. In those years I could get by on 4 to 5 hours of sleep a night.

WCR: *After completing medical school did you return to the Bronx?*

WHF: Yes. That was part of my life plan. I had made a promise to myself that I was going to be a cardiologist and practice in the community where I was raised. I returned to the Bronx to do just that.

WCR: *I gather you had no problem deciding what specialty you wanted to pursue in medical school?*

WHF: I knew I wanted to be a cardiologist in high school. I was so focused. What was still needed to be decided finally was the type of cardiologist. When I finished medical school I was not sure whether I would be a private practitioner or an academician. Because of the wonderful experiences I had in medical school, I was leaning towards an academic career.

WCR: *Although you returned to the Bronx you had not known medicine in the Bronx when you left 6 years earlier. How did you find medicine in the Bronx after having experienced it at Boston University Medical Center, Boston City Hospital, the Boston Veterans Administration Hospital, and some other Boston institutions?*

WHF: One of the interesting things about the Bronx is that it has many similarities to Boston. The Bronx and Boston are the same size, and the types of patients I was caring for in the Bronx really did not differ much from those I cared for in medical school. Because I was used to a rigorous schedule in medical school, I was able to function well working every other night or every third night.

WCR: *What was your living like when you became an intern? Did you live at the hospital?*

WHF: I lived at the hospital in an attached apartment building.

WCR: *You did a year of internship and your first year of residency at Montefiore Hospital. Who influenced you there?*

WHF: Montefiore is an institution with a long and distinguished history. It had initially been an affiliate of Columbia University Medical School during the years that it functioned as a chronic disease hospital. Since so many cardiac diseases were chronic because they could not be treated years ago, Montefiore always had a strong reputation in cardiology. The hospital changed its mission to encompass more acute care in the 1960s, and developed a strong academic affiliation with the newly formed Albert Einstein Medical School. Montefiore would ultimately became the university hospital for the Einstein Medical School and it provided a very good environment for medical training. The faculty included many excellent teachers in both internal medicine and cardiology; the cardiology faculty included Doris Escher and Seymour Furman who had put in the first transvenous pacemaker. Indeed, there was a lot of cardiology history at Montefiore. My Chief of Medicine was David Hamerman who was a gifted teacher and basic scientist in rheumatology. I got to know him quite well. The hospital had a large housestaff that included 48 interns. The Montefiore training program included working at the private hospital and also at an affiliated public hospital in the south Bronx, which was located in an indigent community. The experiences there complimented what we had in the private voluntary hospital. We were exposed to all types of patients one might see in a busy city practice.

WCR: *What do you mean by a "voluntary hospital"?*

WHF: In New York there is a large public hospital system. The voluntary hospitals were private, "not for profit" institutions.

WCR: *How much time did you spend at the south Bronx hospital?*

WHF: Two-thirds of the time were spent at Montefiore Hospital, one-third at the public hospital. One of the bonuses that came with working at Montefiore Hospital was the opportunity I had to meet a very attractive ward nurse who I eventually married.

WCR: *What made you decide to take your final year of medical residency at the Bronx Municipal Hospital?*

WHF: The Bronx Municipal Hospital had an extremely competitive housestaff program, which was located on the Einstein Medical School campus. It was actually closer to my home of origin in the Bronx. In those days physicians in training rarely completed an internal medicine program at one institution and it was not uncommon for people in the middle of internal medicine training to go to another hospital to complete their residency. I was not unhappy at Montefiore; I simply wanted to expand my experiences at another institution.

WCR: *Who influenced you a great deal at the Bronx Municipal Hospital?*

WHF: The Bronx Municipal Hospital is Einstein Medical School's oldest affiliated institution. The clinical faculty at the hospital have a strong research tradition. Many staff physicians who taught on the wards also had basic research laboratories at the medical school. There was more of a focus on research at the Bronx Municipal Hospital than at Montefiore. I was impressed by how many of the staff physicians were able to bring their work from the laboratory directly to the bedside.

WCR: *What made you decide to go to Cornell-New York Hospital to do your cardiology fellowship?*

WHF: Again, it was to get a different experience. Cornell had a superb Chief of Cardiology, Thomas Killip III, and the institution was one of the national leaders in coronary disease research. Cornell had one of the early NIH-sponsored Myocardial Infarction Research Units (MIRU) and had established one of the first coronary care units in the country. The MIRU program was involved in the development of the Swan-Ganz catheter and had pioneered bedside hemodynamic monitoring of myocardial infarction patients. I had the opportunity through the meetings of the various MIRU center faculties to interact with some of the leadership and future leadership of academic cardiology: Charles Rackley (University of Alabama at Birmingham); Jeremy Swan, William Ganz, William Parmley, and James Forrester (Cedars of Sinai); Eugene Braunwald, John Ross, Robert O'Rourke, and Bert Sobel (University of California-San Diego); Richard Ross, Bernadine Healy, Myron Weisfeldt, J. O'Neal Humphries, C. Richard Conti, and Bertram Pitt (Johns Hopkins), and Paul Yu (University of Rochester). This was one of the most exciting times in academic cardiology.

WCR: *Before you started your cardiology fellowship, you had no medical publications? Is that correct?*

WHF: I had written a thesis in medical school but it was not published.

WCR: *In your cardiology fellowship you had several publications during that 2-year span.*

WHF: I had 2 interesting opportunities at New York Hospital. It was a time when the beta blockers were first being introduced in the U.S. for the management of various cardiovascular disorders. I always had an interest in pharmacology. Tom Killip had spoken to some of the senior fellows first to see if they wanted to be involved in an angina project using propranolol as a treatment. I was the third one he spoke with and he did not have to convince me. My research career in cardiovascular pharmacotherapy began with propranolol. Also in the basic laboratory at that time, there was a lot of work being done examining platelet function and its relationship to both acute and chronic coronary disease syndromes. Cornell had a major platelet research effort under Ralpha Nachman, now the Chairman of Medicine at Cornell, and Babette Weksler. I worked with Babette on projects to examine whether or not platelets were activated in chronic or acute coronary syndromes.

WCR: *So your first publication in a medical journal was 1973?*

WHF: I had a case report published in 1973, and an original investigation published in *Circulation* in 1974.

WCR: *How did publishing hit you? I gather that investigation leading to publication, writing up, putting a ribbon around it, turned you on right away?*

WHF: It goes back to my yearbook work in high school, college, and medical school. I really enjoyed taking a research project from the early hypothesis stage and seeing it through to the end: making sure the study is carried out and analyzed properly, being able to do the necessary background research, putting together a manuscript, and seeing it through to publication, being able to present data at national forums. My fellowship experiences had really inspired me to a life in academic cardiology.

WCR: *How did you like New York Hospital? Here is quite a sophisticated hospital in downtown Manhattan, with a lot of private patients who were well off. How did all that phase you at the time?*

WHF: It was a little bit of culture shock at first. I did not live in Manhattan while I trained at Cornell, but continued to reside in the Bronx with my family because it was less expensive and had more living space. Cornell provided me a complimentary experience from what I had encountered from inner city hospitals. New York Hospital was in a very special central academic region of New York, across the street from Memorial Sloan Kettering Hospital and next to the Rockefeller Institute. The intellectual environment was incredible.

WCR: *How long did it take you to get back and forth to the Bronx?*

WHF: About an hour.

WCR: *So you were use to that from high school? I gather you used that time for reading?*

WHF: I would drive and occasionally get stuck in a New York City traffic jam and regret having taken the car. Then I would take the subway and go back to driving. It depended on how I felt each day. Once while trapped in a traffic jam only 2 blocks from the hospital, I had to leave my car to help carry a patient from an ambulance that was directly behind me. The patient was having an acute myocardial infarction. After delivering the patient to the emergency room, I returned to find my car and the ambulance in the same place in the traffic jam.

WCR: *After the fellowship in cardiology, which I gather you completed in June 1974, you went into the service for a couple of years.*

WHF: Because I was so young when I graduated from medical school, I was a prime target for being drafted into the service. I joined the Berry Plan as a way of trying to postpone my military duty, and I was luckily deferred so that I could finish all my internal medicine and cardiology training. In 1974 I entered the military for 2 years.

WCR: *Being in the Berry Plan prevented you from going to the NIH?*

WHF: I had to join the Berry Plan relatively early because I was fearful of being drafted, having been recently married.

WCR: *I gather your 2 years in the armed services actually turned out to be a useful endeavor for you. Could you describe that?*

WHF: I was assigned to a 500-bed military hospital, U.S. Walson Army Hospital in Fort Dix, New Jersey, which was located 1-3/4 hours from where my wife and I lived in the Bronx. I was also able to keep a faculty appointment at Cornell. I was able to balance going to New York Hospital where I was completing

some of my research studies, while maintaining a full-time job at Fort Dix where I served as Chief of Cardiology at the hospital. The previous chiefs of Cardiology at Fort Dix included Carlos deCastro and Melvin Marcus who had just preceded me. At Fort Dix there were about 120 physicians like myself, trained in excellent academic programs from different parts of the country. My active duty military experience turned out to be a real opportunity for me.

WCR: *What made it so?*

WHF: First of all, there was great camaraderie in the medical corp and I was always patriotic. My father and uncles had served in the military during World War II. I felt that the soldiers involved in the Vietnam War and their families had made a great personal sacrifice, and the military physician had an obligation to them. I felt privileged to be in the Army, and grateful to the service for allowing me the time to go back to New York Hospital to complete my research studies.

WCR: *Did you enjoy being Chief of Cardiology at Fort Dix?*

WHF: It was a wonderful experience and a unique opportunity. Fort Dix is located in Burlington County, New Jersey, in a rural area close to Philadelphia and Trenton. Surrounding the military camp was a large, retired military population whom we cared for. What was also remarkable about being stationed there for military duty was that outside the gates of the fort, within walking distance, was the Deborah Heart/Lung Institute, one of the leading cardiology specialty hospitals in the U.S. at that time, and an affiliate of Temple Medical School. I was able to present many of our problem military patients at Deborah. Working with the Deborah faculty was comparable to having 2 more years of fellowship, since I had the opportunity to participate in their conferences and other academic functions. There were 3 historical events also that affected me during my military service. First, I entered the Army in July 1974, and in August 1974 President Nixon resigned. That event had a great impact on me with the war winding down and the terrible morale hovering over the military because of feelings of defeatism, especially with the president being brought to his knees. Second, the war officially ended in Vietnam in April 1975 with the evacuation of the U.S. embassy in Saigon. Subsequently many Vietnamese refugees were brought to the U.S. I was pulled out of my unit at Fort Dix for a month and sent to Fort Bragg, North Carolina, to work in a combat hospital during extensive military maneuvers (Figure 4). Although I left the Army in July 1976, I was still on active duty in the military on July 4th when the U.S. Bicentennial was celebrated. This was a very memorable experience for me. I very much enjoyed working with the people in the military, and I was blessed to be able to contribute something to my country.

WCR: *That 2-year experience did indeed have an impact on you?*

WHF: Yes, and I do not think I would have been the same without it.

WCR: *Can you expand on that a little bit?*

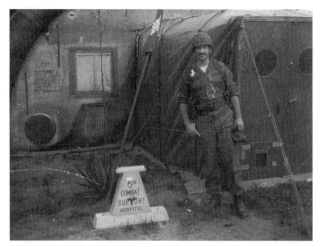

FIGURE 4. At combined Armed Forces war games with the 82nd Airborne Division Medical Corp., Fort Bragg, North Carolina, 1975, just after the end of the Vietnam War.

WHF: I learned to appreciate the many sacrifices the dependents of military personnel actually make. It was not only the soldier and sailor, but their dependents who were making a sacrifice. I felt that what I was doing in the military at that time as a physician actually paled compared to what they were going through. Because of my good experiences in the Army, I joined the Reserves afterwards. Overall, it was a very positive experience for me, and it completed my training as a physician.

WCR: *Are you still in?*

WHF: Not since 1990.

WCR: *Did you actually live in the Bronx when in the Army.*

WHF: Yes, I drove home at night. However, I would stay over when I was on hospital call. My wife would come down to visit at times. We had a small house on the base, but we kept our apartment in the Bronx.

WCR: *How did it come about that you went back to the Bronx?*

WHF: It fulfilled my promise that I would come back as a heart doctor to my community.

WCR: *Did you ever tell your father that, or did you ever have the chance?*

WHF: No I never had the chance, but that was my promise to honor his memory. There was also a great opportunity available at Einstein. Ed Sonnenblick had just come from Harvard and Peter Bent Brigham to be Chief of Cardiology at Einstein. I had the opportunity to work with him.

WCR: *When you joined the faculty, where was your office?*

WHF: I went to work at the Bronx Municipal Hospital and the Einstein College Hospital which was physically attached to the Einstein College of Medicine. I always wanted to be near the medical school. Bronx Municipal Hospital was the public hospital for

the Albert Einstein College of Medicine, and the college hospital was affiliated with Montefiore Hospital.

WCR: *Was Dr. Sonnenblick the one who actually hired you?*

WHF: Right. He recruited me. I also had the opportunity to continue on the faculty at New York Hospital, but my commitment was really to the community where I was raised.

WCR: *When you first went back, what happened? How did you start off when you got back?*

WHF: I started off as Director of the Non-Invasive Cardiac Labs and ultimately became the Chief of Medicine at the hospital and Associate Chairman and Professor of Medicine at the medical school. I also restarted my clinical drug trials. There was a very strong tradition in basic research already at the medical school. Einstein was always a national leader in receiving extramural NIH funding for basic research. What I was able to do was to get the clinical research programs started. Ed Sonnenblick was a basic researcher and had a strong basic cardiac laboratory presence. I realized the possibilities in clinical research with a population that was well-known to me and at the same time was medically underserved. There were not enough physicians in that area of the city. I had the opportunity to carry out the types of trials I had started at Cornell, and I went right to work in this direction.

WCR: *What were the initial trials?*

WHF: They involved the second-generation β blockers. Propranolol was already out, and there was a whole new generation of β blockers that were being introduced, followed later by the calcium blockers, and the ACE inhibitors. It was a gradual progression. I was able to do a great deal of the clinical investigations involving all the new drug breakthroughs that were occurring. In fact, until propranolol appeared, the cardiology pharmacopeia was similar to that in 1930—nitroglycerin, digitalis, isosorbide, and quinidine. The revolution that occurred in human cardiovascular pharmacotherapy began in the early 1970s and is continuing today. I was fortunate to be there at the beginning.

WCR: *You obtained a large number of grants, both from the NIH and from industry. Since you proved yourself rapidly that you could take one of these agents and evaluate it carefully, whether myocardial infarction or congestive heart failure, whether systemic hypertension or arrhythmia, after awhile the pharmaceutical companies must have started coming to you rather than your going to them.*

WHF: Yes, and I also had a very good population of patients to work with, and a wonderful research staff. The patients were individuals I knew from the neighborhood where I grew up. I was very close to them and supportive of their needs. Many of the patients were able to walk to the medical school and hospital. We always had a large cadre of patients that were very reliable and who we could follow carefully in studies.

WCR: *From 1976 to the time you left in 1997, you had 21 years of investigative efforts. You became full professor in 1985?*

WHF: Yes.

WCR: *When did you move to Montefiore Hospital?*

WHF: I always stayed at Montefiore. What happened was that Montefiore had taken over the administrative functions for the Hospital of the Albert Einstein College of Medicine. So technically, I was working at a Montefiore affiliate all the time. I never left the medical school campus.

WCR: *Where you went in 1976 is where you stayed until you left in 1997? What was your life like on a day-to-day basis? Here you were enormously productive. From 1974 until 1997 you published 571 papers in medical journals and 14 books. You were raising a family of 3 children. What was your day-to-day activity like? What time did you wake up in the morning? What time did you get to the hospital? What time did you leave home in the morning? What time did you get home from work? What time did you go to bed? How much sleep were you obtaining during that period? Can you give a flavor of your day-to-day activities?*

WHF: My days were very full. I still wake up early. I do my best work between 4:30 and 7:00 A.M.

WCR: *So you wake up about what time?*

WHF: 4:30 or 5:00.

WCR: *Everyday?*

WHF: For the most part except if I'm on vacation. I work at home in the early morning, and then we always have breakfast as a family. I do not go to work until after the children go to school, which is about 8 A.M. I would get to work about 8:15 or 8:30 after a 20-minute auto commute. We moved out of the Bronx in 1978 to the northern suburb of Westchester, to a town called Scarsdale where we still live.

WCR: *So you moved to a house?*

WHF: Yes, we bought a house.

WCR: *So that was 1978 and you were born in 1946, you were 32.*

WHF: The house was initially too quiet for me. I had trouble sleeping because I was used to the noise of the city. Probably, if it were not for my wife who had grown up in a house, I would have stayed in an apartment in the Bronx.

WCR: *So you would leave home at 8 A.M.? What did you do mainly at work?*

WHF: My work involved a very full day because I combined both my clinical research with clinical practice and large teaching load. I really work nonstop and rarely eat lunch. I always found that by not eating lunch I had an extra hour to get some important work done while other people were eating lunch. I found that was an important hour to have for myself. I work a full day, usually until 6 or 7 o'clock.

WCR: *When you go home, does your family eat together?*

WHF: Yes, we tried. My wife would try to wait until I arrived home. If I cam home really late, she would feed the children first, and we would have dinner together, just as my parents did.

WCR: *Did you try to make your dinners intellectual?*

WHF: We would review what each of us did during the day. We also discussed current events and other things with the children.

WCR: *What then did you do?*

WHF: My wife and I would help the kids with their homework, I would try to read journals or textbooks, and something nonmedical, before I would go to sleep.

WCR: *What time did you go to bed?*

WHF: Usually around midnight.

WCR: *You would wake about around 4:30 or 5 A.M.? What about the weekends?*

WHF: I had to go to the hospital for part of the weekend to care for patients. But mostly I involved myself with the childrens' activities. I was very active in all their team sports. My children say I never missed a game they were involved with or a musical performance. I could not be a full-time coach because of the time commitment, but I would always help out. All my children participated actively in sports throughout the school year.

WCR: *So you and your wife made parenting a major priority?*

WHF: Yes.

WCR: *How old are your kids now?*

WHF: My oldest daughter Sheryl is 26, my daughter Amy is 21, and my son Michael is 16 (Figure 5).

WCR: *What does your older daughter do?*

WHF: She's an attorney that specializes in problems of the elderly. She has always been socially responsive to the needs of people. In fact, she worked with me when she was in college on some of the geriatric research that I was involved with, and that is how she became interested in working with older people. She ultimately married a classmate who is also an attorney. They currently live in Manhattan, but will soon move into a house close to us.

WCR: *Your second daughter?*

WHF: My second daughter is a senior in New York University and she is studying to be a special education teacher, and will be attending graduate school at NYU following completion of her undergraduate studies.

WCR: *And your son?*

WHF: My son is 16 and is a junior in high school. He is a very good student, a class officer, a musician and an athlete, participating in football, baseball, and basketball. He is learning how to balance a very busy work and sports schedule.

WCR: *What do you think he will do?*

WHF: My son is just crossing the line now realizing that he may not make it as a professional football player, to thinking about medicine.

WCR: *Do you keep up well with all your cousins, aunts, and uncles living in the Bronx? Is this still a close-knit family?*

WHF: Yes. I think one of the advantages, or maybe a slight disadvantage, of living around my entire fam-

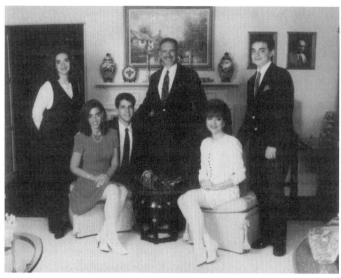

FIGURE 5. My greatest sources of inspiration: from *left*, my daughter Amy, my daughter Sheryl (seated), and my son-in-law Rob, my wife Esther (seated), and my son Michael, in our living room in Scarsdale, New York.

this course, and received both the Teaching Scholar Award of the American Heart Association and the Preventive Cardiology Academic Award from the NIH for my efforts in this area. I was also involved in the development of an independent scholars program at Einstein where all the students have to prepare a scholarly thesis for graduation. I would mentor 10% to 15% of the class in this activity which involved having a one-to-one relationship with students that provided an experience for them that was similar to mine as a student in Boston. One of the things I am most proud of from all my teaching activities was my ability to mentor hundreds of Einstein students as a thesis advisor. As a result of my efforts in medical education, I was nominated by the medical school to receive the AAMC Distinguished Teacher Award (Figure 6).

WCR: *The only other cardiologist who ever won this national teachers award is W. Proctor Harvey of Georgetown.*

WHF: Yes, and I think that was at the time the award was first presented.

WCR: *Why did you decide to leave the Albert Einstein College of Medicine in 1997 to become Chairman of Medicine at New York Medical College in Valhalla, New York, and Chief of Medicine at the Westchester Medical Center? Was that a difficult decision for you?*

WHF: Yes and no. I have had a wonderful career at Einstein. I had been a hospital Chief and really done all the jobs in the department of medicine, having served as clerkship leader, subinternship leader, and course leader. I was looking for an opportunity to be departmental chairman and make an even greater impact. New York Medical College happens to be located close to where I live. When the Chairman's job became available there, I thought that was an opportunity I could not refuse. The health care mission at New York Medical College, in a way is comparable to Einstein's and New York City's other medical schools. The school has a large hospital network that extends from Staten Island in the southern part of New York City, to just south of Albany, covering almost a 200 mile distance. I was really looking at the chairmanship as an opportunity to grow something new. Although I felt very comfortable at Einstein, I felt I had accomplished what I wanted to do there. I wanted to leave like Jerry Seinfeld, at the top of my form. New York Medical College has particularly great strength in basic cardiology research, which was attractive to me, as well as great expertise in pharmacology, physiology, and medicine. The Open Heart Surgery Program and Interventional Cardiology Program are well known in the region. The medical

ily is that when they have medical problems, I am the first one they call. I am involved with every medical issue that goes on with my aunts and uncles and cousins.

WCR: *Where is your wife from?*

WHF: My wife was born in Israel but was raised in the West Bronx. She is a research coordinator who works with me in the federally funded Women's Health Initiative trial. She is my best friend and a source of great strength for our family. We are extremely devoted to each other and to our children.

WCR: *You have won a number of teaching awards at Einstein School of Medicine. You recently received the Association of American Colleges Distinguished Teacher Award as the nation's outstanding medical educator. That sounds impressive to me. Tell me about it.*

WHF: Because of how I was influenced by my teachers and coming from a family where learning was very important, I always wanted to impart knowledge to students. In almost every activity I was involved with, whether through practice or through research, I always had students with me. I was also involved in teaching at the medical school on all levels, from the first through the fourth year. I have taught basic science, including physiology, epidemiology, pathophysiology, and pharmacology. I always teach on the wards and in the clinics. I also was involved in some innovative course design. We had a course Einstein called the "Return to Basic Science" where students, after being on the ward for a year in their third year of medical school, went back to the classroom for a brief basic science course where we would reinforce a lot of the basic science principles that may not have been appreciated during the first years of medical school. I was involved in directing

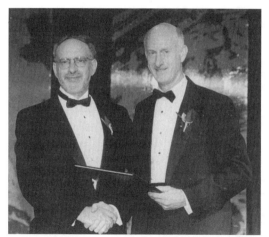

FIGURE 6. Receiving the national Distinguished Teacher Award at the 1997 Association of American Medical Colleges, Washington, DC from Dr. David Dale, President of Alpha Omega Alpha and the former Dean of the University of Washington School of Medicine.

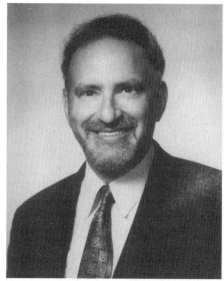

FIGURE 8. Bill Frishman (1997), currently the Professor of Medicine and Pharmacology and Chairman of the Department of Medicine, New York Medical College, and Director of Medicine at Westchester University Medical Center, Valhalla, New York.

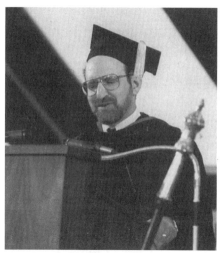

FIGURE 7. Giving the 1989 Commencement Address at the Albert Einstein College of Medicine.

school is the third largest in the U.S., and sponsors a large graduate medicine program. I felt well qualified for the task, having worked closely with 3 distinguished chairmen of medicine at Einstein, Milford Fulop, Louis Sherwood, and James Scheuer, from whom I learned a great deal.

WCR: *Where is the medical center that you will be working at?*

WHF: Westchester Medical Center, where I am also the Chief of Medicine (Figure 8). This was also an opportunity to become involved in planning health care delivery for a large region. I am very interested in maximizing health care delivery, while trying to make the health care system work better both for patients and their physicians. Again, I was very happy to make

a move, although sad to leave a place where I have had such wonderful memories. However, there is a saying: "You can never really get out of the Bronx." Indeed, I have a visiting faculty appointment at Einstein and continue to participate in collaborative research projects there. I am a co-principal investigator of the national Women's Health Initiative trial in New York City, and will still be working in that capacity while in my new school role.

WCR: *For someone like you who has investigated so many drugs, you will not be able to continue in the investigative arena quite to the same extent that you were before taking on the chairmanship of this large department of medicine medical school. Does that bother you?*

WHF: I may not be able to do all the "hands on work" that I did before, but I will have the opportunity to have a greater impact in helping to train a whole new generation of clinical scientists who will be able to continue the work.

WCR: *It must be a great source of satisfaction to you to receive the Distinguished Alumni Award from Boston University School of Medicine where you went to college and medical school, and an Honorary Alumnus Award from the Albert Einstein College of Medicine where you worked for so many years. You are now 51. What are your goals now?*

WHF: I think there are great opportunities in medicine. I want to rejuvenate the enthusiasm in young people for a career in medicine. I have always enjoyed doing that. Although physicians work hard, there is a tremendous amount of personal gratification that comes from a career in science and health care. There is also an exciting era just beginning in clinical research where many of the discoveries in the basic

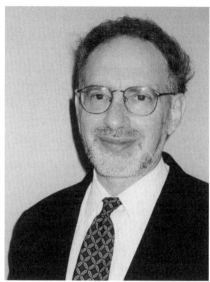

FIGURE 9. Photograph of WHF taken by WCR during the interview.

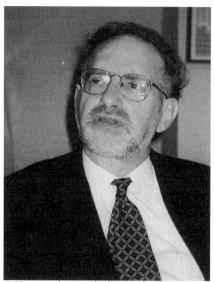

FIGURE 10. Photograph of WHF taken by WCR during the interview.

laboratory are now coming to the clinic. There are new agents being looked at for angiogenesis, and a whole new group of biological agents are being used that potentially could replace the traditional pharmacological approaches that I had investigated in years past. The thrombolytics are a product of that. I see a great opportunity in this area and I always want to remain a part of the drug discovery mission.

WCR: *How have you handled travel through the years? You have been visiting professor at many medical centers around the country. How does traveling fit into your scheme?*

WHF: When traveling, I try to get work done that I cannot do at home. Very often I'm writing a manuscript, correcting, or reviewing a paper. When I come home from a trip, I am able to spend more time with my family rather than less. One of the things I was cautious about all these years, even with my travels, was the time I spent home with my family. I always try to be there for them. Therefore I actually use the time away to get a lot of paperwork done that would not bog me down when I return home. The travel, in a way, complimented my hospital work.

WCR: *What about your vacations in these 22 years with your family? Have you regularly gone away for a period of time?*

WHF: Whenever I was at a meeting, I tried to bring the whole family along, which was an opportunity for them to see what kind of work I was involved with. When our children got older and my wife could not come with me, I would take at least one of the children with me on a trip so we could have a one-on-one experience together. Our family takes 2 one-week vacations during the winter in Florida where we have a home. I always liked being at the beach, since it reminds me of my youth when we frequented the public beach. Our Florida home is in Hallendale, an area north of Miami, where we have a beachfront view. We have true family vacations. I try to do a lot of my pleasure reading when I am away. I still try to squeeze in, even during a busy day, some reading unrelated to medicine.

WCR: *What are you reading right now?*

WHF: I am reading a new biography of John Quincy Adams. During this past year, I read for the second time, all of Shakespeare's histories. I appreciated these plays a lot more the second time around. Most of my reading is either biography or historical fiction.

WCR: *You do some nonmedical reading every day?*

WHF: Yes. Right before I go to bed. I often wake up with the book open next to me. This was always a very relaxing thing for me to do.

WCR: *So you live by Osler's recommendation of reading the masters the last 30 minutes of each day?*

WHF: I always felt I was a better physician because I did clinical research and therefore had a much better understanding of disease processes and how best to treat them. But also because of my nonmedical reading, I was also able to communicate more effectively with my patients. Knowledge of sports and current events helps you interact closely with patients, relieving the stress they may be under. I also think the lessons of literature help you to become more sensitive and caring when you are at the bedside.

WCR: *Tell me about your private practice. You have always seen a lot of patients. How much time a week, when you were at Einstein, were you spending seeing patients?*

WHF: I would spend a portion of my day teaching and participating in clinical research. My internal medicine and cardiology practice allowed me to take care of many patients in a holistic way. Even though a patient may have come to me with a cardiac problem, I would manage all other medical problems they had on a chronic basis. I have always worked one full day in the office as a practitioner. In actuality, I was practicing 7 days a week while involved in clinical research because I would have to become directly involved with problems that developed in the studies. As a clinical researcher and a principal investigator, you are always "on call." You cannot sign out to a colleague when you are involved in double-blind studies with a sick population; you always have to be available. I have to say that even though I go on vacation, my staff always knows where to get me if there is a problem. Again, I have always enjoyed practice, and would never give it up. In fact at the end of my career, what I would like best to be doing is seeing patients.

WCR: *If you were offered the head of the FDA, would you take that?*

WHF: If I cannot have the opportunity to be involved in direct patient care, I would have problems with such a position.

WCR: *Is there anything you would like to discuss that we have not discussed?*

WHF: The other areas I wanted to discuss relate to my ongoing research work in other disciplines like geriatrics and womens health. One advantage I always had in working in my old neighborhood was I was able to be involved in many large, community-based studies, such as the Bronx Aging Study and the Womens Health Initiative. I am hoping to continue this work, even in my new chairman's role, since my new medical school is also affiliated with many hospitals both in New York City and the surrounding suburbs. I have even begun to enter into new collaborations with my old and my new schools.

WCR: *Of the various activities you do, which do you enjoy the most or do you like the variety?*

WHF: I like the variety and I enjoy all the roles that I'm involved with. I enjoy being a good son, a good brother, trying to be a good parent, a good husband, a good friend, a good teacher, a caring physician for my patients, a good researcher, and a fair-minded administrator. I feel all these roles have been important in rounding me off as a person (Figure 10).

WCR: *You have worked hard at all these various roles. Do you think you will continue to go on 4½ hours sleep from here on?*

WHF: From the way my schedule looks now, maybe 3½. Even during this visit I awoke early this morning to write.

WCR: *Your plane did not arrive until after 11 P.M., so you must not have gotten to the hotel until around midnight?*

WHF: I had my 4½ hours of sleep, and was up at 4:30 this morning.

WCR: *You looked fresh when I picked you up at 7:15 A.M. It has been a pleasure. I appreciate your honoring us with your presence here at Baylor University Medical Center. Speaking for the AJC readers, I appreciate your opening up your life to us so we can all learn from it. Thank you.*

WHF: Thank you Dr. Roberts.

Best Publications of WHF Selected by WHF

2. Frishman WH, Epstein A, Kulick S, Killip T. Heart failure sixty-three years following traumatic arteriovenous fistula. *Am J Cardiol* 1974;34:733–736.

3. Frishman W, Weksler B, Christodoulou J, Smithen C, Killip T. Reversal of abnormal platelet aggregability and change in exercise tolerance in patients with angina pectoris following oral propranolol. *Circulation* 1974;50:887.

4. Frishman W, Smithen C, Befler B, Kligfield P, Killip T. Non-invasive assessment of clinical response to oral propranolol. *Am J Cardiol* 1975;35:635–644.

7. Frishman W, Christodoulou J, Weksler B, Smithen C, Killip T, Scheidt S. Aspirin therapy in angina pectoris: effects on platelet aggregation, exercise tolerance and electrocardiographic manifestations of ischemia. *Am Heart J* 1976; 92:3–10.

9. Frishman WH, Christodoulou J, Weksler B, Smithen C, Killip T, Scheidt S. Abrupt propranolol withdrawal in angina pectoris. Effects on platelet aggregation and exercise tolerance. *Am Heart J* 1978;95:169.

12. Sonnenblick EH, Frishman WH, LeJemtel TH. Dobutamine: a new synthetic cardioactive sympathetic amine. *N Engl J Med* 1979;300:17–22.

13. Frishman WH, Ribner H. Anticoagulation in myocardial infarction: a modern approach to an old problem. *Am J Cardiol* 1979;43:1207.

15. Frishman WH, Kostis J, Strom J, Hosler M, Elkayam U, Davis R, Weinstein J, Sonnenblick EH. Clinical pharmacology of the new beta blocking drugs. Part 6. A comparison of prindolol and propranolol in treatment of patients with angina pectoris. The role of intrinsic sympathomimetic activity. *Am Heart J* 1979;98: 526–535.

19. Frishman WH, Factor S, Jordan A, et al. Right atrial myxoma: unusual clinical presentation and glandular histology. *Circulation* 1979;59:1070.

24. Elkayam U, LeJemtel T, Mathur M, Frishman W, Ribner H, Strom J, Sonnenblick EH. Prazosin therapy in congestive heart failure: importance of prolonged hemodynamic evaluation of vasodilator agents. *Am J Cardiol* 1979; 441:540–545.

25. Becker R, Frishman W, Frater RWM. Surgical management of mitral valve endocarditis: a review of 26 patients. *Chest* 1979;75:314.

31. Davis R, Strom J, Frishman W. Echographic findings of vegetations in bacterial endocarditis: an indication for urgent valvular replacement. *Am J Med* 1980;69:57–63.

35. Matsumoto M, Oka Y, Strom J, Frishman W, Kadish A, Becker RM, Frater RWM, Sonnenblick EH. Application of transesophageal echocardiography to continuous intraoperative monitoring of left ventricular performance. *Am J Cardiol* 1980;46:95–105.

36. Strom J, Frishman W, Davis R, Matsumoto M, Becker R, Frater RWM. Echocardiographic and surgical correlations in bacterial endocarditis. *Circulation* 1980;62:1–164.

38. Frishman W. β-adrenoceptor antagonists. New drugs and new indications. *N Engl J Med* 1981;305:505–506.

39. Frishman W. Nadolol: a new beta-adrenoceptor blocking drug. *N Engl J Med* 1981;305:678.

40. Frishman WH, Strom J, Kirschner M, Poland M, Klein N, Halprin S, LeJemtel T, Kram M, Sonnenblick EH. Labetalol therapy in patients with systemic hypertension and angina pectoris: effects of combined alpha and beta-adrenoceptor blockade. *Am J Cardiol* 1981;48:917–928.

42. Klein N, Siskind S, Frishman W, Sonnenblick E, LeJemtel T. Hemodynamic comparisons of intravenous amrinone and dobutamine in patients with severe congestive heart failure. *Am J Cardiol* 1981;48:170–175.

44. Fein S, Klein N, Frishman W. Exercise testing soon after uncomplicated myocardial infarction. *JAMA* 1981;245:1863.

47. LeJemtel TH, Keung E, Frishman WH, Ribner HS, Sonnenblick EH. Hemodynamic effects of captopril in patients with severe chronic heart failure. *Am J Cardiol* 1982;49:1484–1488.

48. Frishman WH, Klein NA, Strom JA, Willens H, LeJemtel TH, Jentzer J, Siegel L, Klein P, Kirschen N, Silverman R, Doyle R, Kirsten E, Sonnenblick EH. Superiority of verapamil to propranolol in stable angina pectoris: a double-blind randomized crossover trial (abstr). *Circulation* 1982;65 (suppl I):I-51–59.

49. Frishman WH. Atenolol and timolol: two new systemic β-adrenoceptor antagonists. *N Engl J Med* 1982;306:1456–1462.

52. Packer M, Frishman WH. Verapamil therapy for stable and unstable angina pectoris: calcium channel antagonists in perspective. *Am J Cardiol* 1982;50:881.

53. Frishman WH, Klein N, Klein P, Strom JA, Tawil R, Strair R, Wong B, Roth S, LeJemtel T, Pollack S, Sonnenblick EH. Comparison of oral propranolol and verapamil for combined systemic hypertension and angina pectoris: a placebo-controlled, double-blind, randomized, crossover trial. *Am J Cardiol* 1982;50: 1164–1172.

54. Frishman WH, Klein N, Strom J, Cohen MN, Shamoon H, Willens H, et al. Comparative effects of abrupt withdrawal of propranolol and verapamil in angina pectoris. *Am J Cardiol* 1982;50:1991–1195.

55. Frishman WH, Kirsten E, Kates R. Clinical relevance of verapamil plasma levels in stable angina pectoris. *Am J Cardiol* 1982;50:1180.

57. Kostis JB, Frishman WH, Hosler M, et al. The treatment of angina pectoris with pindolol. The significance of intrinsic sympathomimetic activity of β-blockers. *Am Heart J* 1982;104:496.

58. Kugler J, Maskin C, Laragh J, Sealy J, Frishman WH, Sonnenblick EH, LeJemtel T. Regional and systemic metabolic effects of angiotensin converting enzyme inhibition during exercise in patients with severe heart failure. *Circulation* 1982;66:1256–1261.

59. Maskin, C, Forman R, Frishman W, Sonnenblick E, LeJemtel TH. Failure of dobutamine to increase exercise capacity despite hemodynamic improvement in severe chronic heart failure. *Am J Cardiol* 1983;51:177–182.

61. Frishman WH. Multifactorial actions of β-adrenergic blocking drugs in ischemic heart disease. *Circulation* 1983;67(Suppl 1):I-11–18.

62. Frishman WH. Pindolol: a new β-adrenoceptor antagonist with partial agonist activity. *N Engl J Med* 1983;308:940–944.

63. Michelson EL, Frishman WH, Lewis JE, et al. Multicenter clinical evaluation of the long-term efficacy and safety of labetalol in the treatment of hypertension. *Am J Med* 1983;75(4A):68.

64. Jacob H, Brandt L, Farkas P, Frishman WH. Beta-adrenergic blockade and the gastrointestinal system. *Am J Med* 1983;74:1042–1051.

69. Frishman WH, Weinberg P, Peled HB, Kimmel B, Charlap S, Beer N. Calcium-entry blockers for the treatment of severe hypertension and hypertensive crisis. *Am J Med* 1984;77(2B):35.

70. Frishman WH, Furbert CD, Friedewalk WT. β-Adrenergic blockade in survivors of acute myocardial infarction. *N Engl J Med* 1984;310:830–837.

72. Frishman WH, Crawford MH, DiBianco R, Farnham DJ, Katz RJ, Kostis JB, Mohiuddin SM, Sawin HS, Thadani U, Zellner S. Combination propranolol and bepridil therapy in angina pectoris. *Am J Cardiol* 1985;55:43C–49C.

77. Frishman WH, Kirkendall W, McCarron D, et al. Diuretics versus calcium entry blockers in systemic hypertension: a preliminary multicenter experience with hydrochlorothiazide and sustained-release diltiazem. *Am J Cardiol* 1985;56:92H–96H.

79. Frishman WH, Kimmel B, Charlap S, Saltzberg S, Stroh J, Weinberg P, Moniszko E, Wiezner J, Dorsa F, Pollack S, Strom J. Twice daily administration of oral verapamil in the treatment of essential hypertension. *Arch Intern Med* 1986;146:561–565.

81. Robbins MJ, Frater RWM, Soeiro R, Frishman WH, Strom JA. Influence of vegetation size on the clinical outcome of right-sided infective endocarditis. (Recipient of Grand Prize Award ACP Associates Competition). *Am J Med* 1986;80:165.

84. Goldberger J, Stroh J, Peled H, Cohen M, Frishman WH. The natural history and prognosis of acute pulmonary edema. *Arch Intern Med* 1986;146:489.

87. Frishman WH, Zawada ET, Smith LK, Sowers J, Swartz SL, Kirkendall W, Lunn J, McCarron D, Moser M, Schnaper H. A comparative study of diltiazem and hydrochlorothiazide as initial medical therapy for mild to moderate hypertension. *Am J Cardiol* 1987;59:615.

93. Frishman WH, Garofalo JL, Rothschild A, Rothschild M, Greenberg SM, Soberman J. Multicenter comparison of the nifedipine gastrointestinal system and long-acting propranolol in patients with mild to moderate systemic hypertension receiving diuretics: a preliminary experience. *Am J Med* 1987;83(6B):15–19.

94. Frishman WH, Charlap S, Kimmel B, Teicher M, Cinnamon J, Allen L, et al. Diltiazem compared to nifedipine and combination treatment in patients with stable angina: effects on angina, exercise tolerance and the ambulatory ECG. *Circulation* 1988;77:774–786.

96. Frishman WH, Charlap S. Calcium-channel blockers for combined systemic hypertension and myocardial ischemia (abstr). *Circulation* 1988;75(suppl V):V-154.

103. Frishman WH, Glasser SP, Strom JA, Schoenberger J, Liebson P, Poland M. Effects of dilevalol on left ventricular mass and function in non-elderly and elderly hypertensive patients: double-blind comparisons with atenolol and metoprolol. *Am J Cardiol* 1989;63:69I–74I.

104. Frishman WH, Flamenbaum W, Schoenberger J, Schwartz GL, Vidt DG, Neri GS, Greenberg S, Lazar E, Godrey JC, Stevenson A, Lamon KD, Chang Y, Magner DJ. Celiprolol in systemic hypertension: results of a placebo-controlled double-blind titration study. *Am J Cardiol* 1989;63:839–842.

109. Frishman WH, Giles T, Greenberg S, Heiman M, Raffidal L, Soberman J, Laifer L, Nadelmann J, Lazar E, Strom J. Sustained high-dose nitroglycerin transcutaneous patch therapy in angina pectoris: evidence of attenuation of effect over time. *J Clin Pharmacol* 1989;29:1097–1105.

112. Aronson MK, Ooi WL, Morgenstern PH, Hafner A, Masur D, Crystal H, Frishman W, Fisher D, Katzman R. Women, myocardial infarction and dementia in the very old. *Neurology* 1990;40:1102–1106.

115. Nadelmann J, Frishman WH, Ooi WL, Tepper D, Greenberg S, Guzik H, Lazar EJ, Heiman M, Aronson M. Prevalence, incidence and prognosis of recognized and unrecognized myocardial infarction in persons aged 75 years or older: The Bronx Aging Study. *Am J Cardiol* 1990;66:533–537.

116. Frishman WH, Lazar EJ. Reduction in mortality, sudden death, and nonfatal reinfarction with beta-adrenergic blockers in survivors of acute myocardial infarction: a new hypothesis regarding the cardioprotective action of beta-adrenergic blockade. *Am J Cardiol* 1990;66:66G–70G.

119. Frishman WH, Heiman M, Soberman J, Greenberg S, Eff J, for the Celiprolol International Angina Study Group. Comparison of deliprolol and propranolol in stable angina pectoris. *Am J Cardiol* 1991;67:665–670.

123. Aronson MK, Ooi WL, Geva D, Masur D, Blau A, Frishman WH. Dementia: age-dependent incidence, prevalence and mortality in the old. *Arch Intern Med* 1991;151:989–992.

125. Frishman WH, Heiman M, for the Nisoldipine Multicenter Angina Study Group. Usefulness of nisoldipine for stable angina pectoris. *Am J Cardiol* 1991;68:1004–1009.

126. The SHEP Cooperative Research Group. Prevention of stroke by antihypertensive drug treatment in older persons with isolated systolic hypertension: final results of Systolic Hypertension in the Elderly Program (SHEP). *JAMA* 1991;265:3255–3264.

129. SOLVD Investigators. Effects of angiotensin converting enzyme inhibition with enalapril on survival in patients with reduced left ventricular ejection fraction and congestive heart failure. *N Engl J Med* 1991;325:293–302.

132. Zimetbaum P, Frishman WH, Ooi WL, Derman MP, Aronson M, Gidez LI, Eder HA. Plasma lipid and lipoproteins and the incidence of cardiovascular disease in the old: The Bronx Longitudinal Aging Study. *Arterioscler Thromb* 1992;12:416–425.

133. Guzik H, Ooi WL, Frishman WH, Greenberg S, Aronson MK. Hypertension: Cardiovascular implications in a cohort of old old. *J Am Geriatr Soc* 1992;40:348–353.

135. Frishman WH, Nadelmann J, Ooi WL, Greenberg S, Heiman M, Kahn S, Guzik H, Lazar E, Aronson M. Cardiomegaly on chest x-ray: prognostic implications in a 10 year study of an old old cohort. A report from the BAS. *Am Heart J* 1992;124:1026–1030.

136. Frishman WH. Comparative efficacy and concomitant use of bepridil and beta blockers in the management of angina pectoris. *Am J Cardiol* 1992;69:50D–60D.

137. Gradman AH, Frishman WH, Kaihlanen PM, Wong SC, Friday KJ. Comparison of sustained-release formulations of nicardipine and verapamil for mild to moderate systemic hypertension. *Am J Cardiol* 1992;70:1571–1575.

138. SOLVD Investigators. Effect of enalapril on mortality and the development of heart failure in asymptomatic patients with reduce left ventricular ejection fractions. *N Engl J Med* 1992;327:685–691.

142. Conigliaro J, Frishman WH, Lazar EJ, Croen L. Internal medicine housestaff and attending physician perceptions of the impact of New York State 405 regulations on working conditions and supervision of residents in two training programs. *J Gen Med* 1993;8:502–507.

146. Landau A, Frishman WH, Alturk N, Adjei-Poku M, Fornasier-Bongo M, Furia S. Improvement in exercise tolerance and immediate β-adrenergic blockade with intranasal propranolol in patients with angina pectoris. *Am J Cardiol* 1993;72:995–998.

147. Frishman WH, Bryzinski BS, Coulson LR, DeQuattro VL, Vlachakis ND, Mroczek WJ, Dukart G, Alemaychu D, Koury K. A multifactorial trial design to assess combination therapy in hypertension: treatment with bisoprolol and hydrochlorothiazide. *Arch Intern Med* 1994;154:1461–1468.

150. Frishman WH, Brobyn W, Brown RD, Johnson BF, Reeves RL, Wombolt DG. Amlodipine versus atenolol in essential hypertension. *Am J Cardiol* 1994; 73:50A–54A.

151. Crystal HA, Ortof E, Frishman WH, Gruber A, Hershman D, Aronson M. Serum vitamin B12 levels and incidence of dementia in a healthy elderly population: a report from the Bronx Longitudinal Aging Study. *J Am Geriatr Soc* 1994;42:933–936.

161. Hershman DL, Simonoff PA, Frishman WH, Paston F, Aronson MK. Drug utilization in the old old, and how it relates to self-perceived health and all cause mortality. Results from The Bronx Aging Study. *J Am Geriatr Soc* 1995;43:356–360.

162. Feinfeld DA, Guzik H, Carvounis CP, Lynn RI, Somer B, Aronson M, Frishman WH. Sequential changes in renal function tests in the old old: results from The Bronx Longitudinal Aging Study. *J Am Geriatr Soc* 1995;43:412–414.

163. Frishman W, Pepine CJ, Weiss R, Baiker WM, for the Zatebradine Study Group. Addition of zatebradine, a direct sinus node inhibitor, provides no greater exercise tolerance benefit in patients with angina pectoris taking extended-release nifedipine: results of a multicenter, randomized, double-blind, placebo-controlled, parallel group study. *J Am Coll Cardiol* 1995;26:305–312.

168. Frishman WH, Ram CVS, McMahon FG, Chrysant SG, Graff A, Kupiec JW, Hsu H, for the Benazepril/Amlodipine Study Group. Comparison of amlodipine and benazepril monotherapy to combination therapy in patients with systemic hypertension: a randomized, double-blind, placebo-controlled parallel group study. *J Clin Pharmacol* 1995;35:1060–1066.

169. Pratt CVM, McMahon RP, Goldstein S, Pepine CJ, Andrews TC, Dyrda I, Frishman WH, Geller NL, Hill JA, Morgan NA, Stone PH, Knatterud GL, Sopko G, Conti CR, for the ACIP Investigators. Comparison of subgroups assigned to medical regimens used to suppress cardiac ischemia (The Asymptomatic Cardiac Ischemia Pilot (ACIP) Study. *Am J Cardiol* 1996;77:1302–1309.

170. Kahn S, Frishman WH, Weissman S, Ooi WL, Aronson M. Left ventricular hypertrophy on electrocardiogram: prognostic implications from a 10 year cohort study of older subjects. A report from the Bronx Longitudinal Aging Study. *J Am Geriatr Soc* 1996;44:524–529.

171. Stone PH, Chaitman B, McMahon RP, Andrews TC, MacCallum G, Sharaf B, Frishman W, Deanfield JE, Sopko G, Pratt C, Goldberg AD, Rogerts WJ, Hill J, Proschan M, Pepine CJ, Bourassa MG, Conti CR, for the ACIP Investigators. Relationship between exercise-induced and ambulatory ischemia in patients with stable coronary disease. The Asymptomatic Cardiac Ischemia Pilot (ACIP) Study. *Circulation* 1996;94:1537–1544.

174. Frishman WH, Heiman M, Karpenos A, Ooi WL, Mitzner A, Goldkorn R, Greenberg S. Twenty-four hour ambulatory electrocardiography in elderly subjects: prevalence of various arrhythmias and prognostic indications. A report from the Bronx Longitudinal Aging Study. *Am Heart J* 1996;132:297–302.

176. Bernstein JM, Frishman WH, Chang CJ. Value of ECG PR and QTc interval prolongation and heart rate variability for predicting cardiovascular morbidity and mortality in the elderly: the Bronx Aging Study. *Cardiol in Elderly* 1997;5:31–41.

178. Frishman WH. Mibefradil: a new selective T-channel calcium antagonist for hypertension and angina pectoris. *J Cardiovasc Pharmacol Ther* 1997;2:321–330.

181. Frishman WH, Gomberg-Maitland M, Hirsch H, et al. Differences between male and female patients with regard to baseline demographics and clinical outcome in the Asymptomatic Cardiac Ischemia Pilot (ACIP) Trial. *Clin Cardiol* 1998;21:184–190.

Books

6. Frishman WH. Current Cardiovascular Drugs, 2nd ed. Philadelphia: Current Science, North American edition, 1995.

7. Goldberg DE, Frishman WH. Beta3 Adrenergic Agonism: A New Concept in Human Pharmacotherapy. New York: Futura Publishing, 1995.

10. Frishman WH, Sonnenblick EH (eds). Cardiovascular Pharmacotherapeutics. New York: McGraw Hill, 1997.

13. Frishman WH, Sonnenblick EH (eds). Cardiovascular Pharmacotherapeutics Companion Handbook. New York: McGraw Hill 1998, in press.

14. Frishman WH (co-editor). Yearbook of Medicine 1998. St. Louis: Mosby 1998, in press.

Monographs, Chapters in Books

6. Frishman WH. Clinical pharmacology of the new beta-adrenergic blocking agents. part I: Pharmacodynamic and pharmacokinetic properties. *Am Heart J* 1979;97:663–670.

49. Spivack C, Ocken S, Frishman WH. Calcium antagonists: clinical use in treatment of systemic hypertension. *Drugs* 1983;25:154–177.

50. Frishman WH, Charlap S. Verapamil in the treatment of chronic stable angina. *Arch Intern Med* 1983;143:1407.

56. Michelson EL, Frishman WH. Labetalol: an alpha-beta adrenergic blocker. *Ann Intern Med* 1983;99:553.

70. Frishman WH, Furberg CD, Friedewald WT. The use of β-adrenergic blocking drugs in patients with myocardial infarction. *Curr Probl Cardiol* 1984; 9:3–70.

111. Frishman WH. Beta-adrenergic blocker withdrawal. *Am J Cardiol* 1987;59: 26F–32F.

114. Maza SR, Frishman WH. Therapeutic options to minimize free radical damage and thrombogenicity in ischemic/reperfused myocardium. *Am Heart J* 1987;114:1206–1215.

118. Kralstein J, Frishman WH. Malignant pericardial disease: diagnosis and treatment. *Am Heart J* 1987;113:785.

133. Schoen RE, Frishman WH, Shamoon H. Hormonal and metabolic effects of calcium-channel antagonists in man. *Am J Med* 1988;84:492–504.

146. Hachamovitch R, Strom JA, Sonnenblick EH, Frishman WH. Left ventricular hypertrophy in hypertension and the effects of antihypertensive drug therapy. *Curr Probl Cardiol* 1988;13:371–421.

153. Frishman WH, Skolnick AE, Strom JA. Effects of calcium-entry blockade on hypertension-induced left ventricular hypertrophy. *Circulation* 1989;80(suppl IV):IV-151–IV-161.

169. Skolnick AE, Frishman WH. Calcium channel blockers in myocardial infarction. *Arch Intern Med* 1989;149:1669–1677.

170. Charlap S, Lichstein E, Frishman WH. Electromechanical disassociation: diagnosis, pathophysiology, and management. *Am Heart J* 1989;118.

177. Frishman WH, Garofalo JL, Rothschild A, Rothschild M, Greenberg SM, Soberman J. The nifedipine gastrointestinal therapeutic system in the treatment of hypertension. *Am J Cardiol* 1989;64:65F–69F.

182. Frishman WH, Sokol S, Aronson MK, Wassertheil-Smoller S, Katzman R. Risk factors for cardiovascular and cerebrovascular diseases and dementia in the elderly (monograph). *Curr Probl Cardiol* 1998;23:1–68.

188. Frishman WH, Charlap S. The alpha- and beta-adrenergic blocking drugs. In: Parmley WW, ed. Cardiology. Philadelphia: Lippincott, 1990;1–18.

192. Frishman WH. "Something Special". Valedictory Address to the 1989 Graduating Classes of the Albert Einstein College of Medicine and the Sue Golding Graduate Division of Yeshiva University. *Einstein Uart J Biol Med* 1990;8:31–33.

205. Nadelmann J, Frishman WH. Clinical use of β-adrenoceptor blockade in systemic hypertension. *Drugs* 1990;39:862–876.

217. Zimetbaum P, Frishman W, Aronson M. Hyperlipidemia, vascular diseases, and dementia with advancing age: epidemiologic considerations. *Arch Intern Med* 1991;151:240–244.

219. Frishman WH, Lazar EJ, Gorodokin G. Pharmacokinetic optimization of therapy with beta-adrenergic blocking agents. *Clin Pharmacokin* 1991;20:311–318.

222. Frishman WH, Skolnick AE, Miller KP. Secondary prevention post infarction: the role of β-adrenergic blockers, calcium-channel blockers and aspirin. In: Gersh BJ, Rahimtoola SH, eds. Management of Myocardial Infarction. New York: Elsevier Science, 1991:469–492.

234. Dustan HP, Caplan LR, Curry CL, DeLeon AC, Douglas FL, Frishman W, Hill MN, Washington RL, Steigerwalt S, Shulman N, Taubert K, Champagne B. Report of the Task Force on the Availability of Cardiovascular Drugs to the Medically Indigent. *Circulation* 1992;85:849–860.

237. Frishman WH. Comparative pharmacokinetic and clinical profiles of angiotensin converting enzyme inhibitors and calcium antagonists in systemic hypertension. *Am J Cardiol* 1992;69:17C–25C.

253. Frishman WH. Tolerance, rebound and time-zero effect of nitrate therapy. *Am J Cardiol* 1992;70:43G–48G.

261. Frishman WH. β-Adrenergic blockers. In: Izzo JL, Jr, Black HR, eds. Hypertension Primer of the American Heart Assn. 1993;297–300.

273. Frishman WH, Sonnenblick EH. β-adrenergic blocking drugs and calcium blockers. In: Alexander RW, Schlant RC, Fuster V, eds. The Heart, 9th ed. New York: McGraw Hill 1998:1583–1618.

279. Landau AJ, Gentilucci M, Cavusoglu E, Frishman WH. Calcium antagonists for the treatment of congestive heart failure. *Coron Artery Dis* 1994;5:37–50.

291. Kang PM, Landau AJ, Eberhardt RT, Frishman WH. Angiotensin II receptor antagonists: a new approach to blockade of the renin-angiotensin system. *Am Heart J* 1994;127:1388–1401.

296. Loskove J, Frishman WH. Nitric oxide donors in the treatment of cardiovascular and pulmonary diseases. *Am Heart J* 1995;129:604–613.

298. Schwartz J, Freeman R, Frishman W. Clinical pharmacology of estrogens: focus on their cardiovascular actions and cardioprotective benefits of replacement therapy in postmenopausal women. *J Clin Pharmacol* 1995;35:314–329.

299. Frishman WH, Huberfeld S, Okin S, Wang Y-H, Kumar A, Shareef B. Serotonin and serotonin antagonism in cardiovascular and non-cardiovascular disease. *J Clin Pharmacol* 1995;35:541–572.

301. Katz B, Rosenberg A, Frishman WH. Controlled release drug delivery systems in cardiovascular medicine. *Am Heart J* 1995;19:359–368.

302. Frishman WH, Cavusoglu E. β-Adrenergic blockers and their role in the therapy of arrhythmias. In: Podrid PJ, Kowey PR, eds. Cardiac Arrhythmias—Mechanisms, Diagnosis and Management. Baltimore: Williams & Wilkins, 1995: 421–433.

304. Opie LH, Frishman WH. Lipid-lowering and antiatherosclerotic drugs. In: Opie LH, et al, eds. Drugs for the Heart, 4th ed. Philadelphia: WB Saunders, 1995:288–307.

305. Opie LH, Sonnenblick EH, Frishman WH, Thadani U. β-Blocking drugs. In: Opie LH, et al, eds. Drugs for the Heart, 4th ed. Philadelphia: WB Saunders 1995:1–30.

306. Opie LH, Frishman WH, Thadani U. Calcium channel antagonists. In: Opie LH, et al, eds. Drugs for the Heart, 4th ed. Philadelphia: WB Saunders 1995: 50–82.

309. Patel RC, Frishman WH. Aids and the Heart: Clinicopathologic assessment. *Cardiovasc Pathol* 1995;4:173–183.

310. Cavusoglu E, Frishman WH. Sotalol: a new β-adrenergic blocker for ventricular arrhythmias. *Prog Cardiovasc Dis* 1995;37:423–440.

312. Tamirisa P, Frishman WH, Kumar A. Endothelin and endothelin antagonism: roles in cardiovascular disease and health. *Am Heart J* 1995;130:601–610.

313. Frishman WH, Burns B, Atac B, Alturk N, Altajar B, Lerrick K. Novel antiplatelet therapies for treatment of patients with ischemic heart disease. Inhibitors of platelet glycoprotein IIb/IIa integrin receptor. *Am Heart J* 1995;130:877–892.

317. Frishman WH. Postinfarction survival: role of β-adrenergic blockade. In: Fuster V, Ross R, Topol EJ, eds. Atherosclerosis and Coronary Artery Disease. Philadelphia: Lippincott-Raven, 1996:1205–1214.

321. Frishman WH, Sung HM, Yee HCM, Liu LL, Keefe D, Einzig A, Dutcher J. Cardiovascular toxicity with cancer chemotherapy. *Curr Probl Cardiol* 1996; 21:225–288.

329. Frishman WH, Hotchkiss H. Selective and non-selective dopamine receptor agonists: an innovative approach to cardiovascular disease treatment. *Am Heart J* 1996;132:861–870.

335. Gomberg-Maitland M, Frishman WH. Recombinant growth hormone: a new cardiovascular drug therapy. *Am Heart J* 1996;132:1244–1262.

339. Frishman WH. Faculty practice plan governance and management. Faculty Practice Plans. Florida: Am Coll Phys Exec, 1997.

341. Landzberg BR, Frishman WH, Lerrick K. Pathophysiology and pharmacological approaches for prevention of coronary artery restenosis following coronary artery balloon angioplasty and related procedures. *Prog Cardiovasc Dis* 1997;34:361–398.

ROBERT McKINNON CALIFF, MD:
A Conversation With the Editor*

D r. Rob Califf is Professor of Medicine, Associate Vice-Chancellor for Clinical Affairs, and Director of the Clinical Research Institute of Duke University Medical Center in Durham, North Carolina. He was born in Anderson, South Carolina, in 1951. He graduated from Duke University in 1973, having been elected to Phi Beta Kappa, and from Duke University School of Medicine in 1978, having been elected to Alpha Omega Alpha. He was president of his senior class in medical school. His internship and residency in internal medicine were at the University of California, San Francisco, from 1978 to 1980, and his fellowship in cardiology was at Duke University Medical Center from 1980 to 1983. As a resident he received the Distinguished Resident Teaching Award from the University of California Medical School. His first publication was in 1978 as a medical student and since that time he has had over 400 publications in various peer-reviewed medical journals. Nearly all of his publications have focused on coronary artery disease. Along with Dr. Eric Topol, Rob Califf has been the world's leader of multicenter cardiologic studies during the past 15 years. He has established the world's finest databank in cardiovascular disease and the data generated has had a major impact on management of patients with heart disease. I believe it fair to say that Dr. Califf, along with Dr. Topol, are the fathers of evidence-based information for cardiovascular decision making.

William Clifford Roberts, MD[†](Hereafter, WCR): *I am talking with Rob Califf in my office at Baylor University Medical Center on April 7, 1998. Dr. Califf just gave a beautiful presentation at our medical grand rounds. Dr. Califf, I would like to talk to you primarily about your upbringing, where you were born, where you grew up, what your home life was like, what your parents and siblings were like.*

Robert McKinnon Califf, MD[‡] (Hereafter, RMC): I was born in Anderson, South Carolina, at a hospital that is still standing and does a great job with clinical trials. My dad was a teacher in the architecture school at Clemson University at the time. Anderson was the closest hospital. Both my parents are native South Carolinians. They grew up in the low country, Charleston and St. George, South Carolina, which is steeped in historical tradition. I lived in Clemson until I was 5. I don't remember much about it except for going to football games and being very happy. We moved to Columbia, South Carolina, when I was 5 and I went to grammar school, junior high school, and

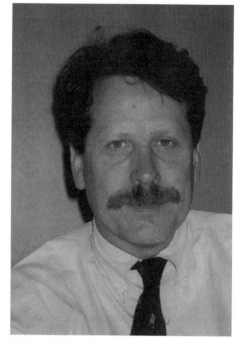

FIGURE 1. RMC during the interview.

high school there. That was also a very pleasant experience.

I had the distinction in 1960, while in junior high school, of being one of only a few students to vote for Kennedy in a mock election in my class of 300 or 400. We lived in an area of Columbia known as Republican Hills. Those following politics in the South since recognize that it was an omen of things to come. I felt fortunate to have a remarkable group of people to go to high school with. Many of them went on to political careers and did things related to those activities. Lee Atwater, who went on to become a famous Republican political campaign manager, was a classmate. Whether one agrees with the politics or not, it certainly was interesting to be so close to a colorful part of American history.

WCR: *How big was Columbia, South Carolina, when you were growing up there?*

RMC: I believe about 100,000. It was the State capital. It was dominated by 3 things: (1) the state government; (2) the University of South Carolina; and (3) Fort Jackson. Fort Jackson was one of the early training grounds for soldiers who were headed to Vietnam. We lived on the side of town with Fort Jackson so I could hear the guns at night.

Columbia was an interesting place to grow up. It was big enough that there was a fair amount of intel-

---

*This series of interviews are underwritten by an unrestricted grant from Bristol-Myers Squibb.

†Baylor Cardiovascular Institute, Baylor University Medical Center, Dallas, Texas 75246.

‡Duke Clinical Research Institute, Duke University Medical Center, Durham, North Carolina 27710.

0002-9149/98/$19.00 **639**
PII S0002-9149(98)00482-2

lectual activity, but it was also very much at the cross roads of what was happening in the South; not so much as Atlanta, but certainly many changes occurred during the time I was in junior high and high school.

WCR: *When your father left Clemson University, he went into the private practice of architecture in Columbia?*

RMC: He taught me many things in a very quiet sort of way. One of the main things he taught me was integrity—the importance of trying to do what is right, even if it is not popular. I think that is a quality we could use a little more today. Watching him deal with the world of architecture, which is very dependent on contracts and wheeling and dealing to get the big jobs, was a growing up lesson for me. Also, he used to take me on Saturdays to the buildings that were being built after he designed them. It was interesting to watch how subcontractors and architects try to get things done together. That was formative for me in some ways.

My father is a man who does not say a lot. His real focus is on architectural design and history. He had been the editor of the yearbook at Clemson when a student there, and had a lot of interesting experiences related to that. During his student days, Clemson was a military school. His class was called to war and arrived in Europe just in time to be at the Battle of the Bulge, which was a major disaster for the American troops. I think that left a permanent impression on him.

WCR: *You have 3 siblings?*

RMC: Yes.

WCR: *Where are you in the hierarchy?*

RMC: I am the second. I have an older brother who is also a Duke graduate and has spent time working in historical architectural work and computer programming. He is currently spending his time with computer programming. My younger brother is an orthopedic surgeon and a graduate of Duke Medical School. He is Chief of Staff at Alamance Regional Medical Center in Burlington, North Carolina, this year. I have a younger sister who lives in Houston. We have quite a family! Our parents' 50th anniversary is coming up this summer. We are all going to congregate at Myrtle Beach and try to get along together.

WCR: *What is your mother like? Did she have a lot of impact on you when you were growing up?*

RMC: Mothers usually do. My mother was a school teacher. At first she stayed home, then she did substitute teaching, and then full-time teaching. She looked out for us and saw that we did what we were supposed to do. She had a big impression that way. She taught us a lot about persistence. I remember not making it on the Little League team the first year I tried out, her making a phone call, and the next thing I knew I was on the team. It was not a political favor. It was probably the coach saying, "If I don't put this kid on the team, I will never hear the end of it." Sometimes you do find in life if you make it easier for people to do what they should do (or harder to do what they shouldn't do), that they will be more likely to do what you want them to do.

WCR: *You mentioned that you enjoyed school? Did you enjoy your studies in high school? Were they easy for you?*

RMC: For the most part, I enjoyed the reading and thinking part of my studies, but I didn't focus on test taking. I was fortunate to have great teachers. I had classmates who were very intellectually active. Of course, it was an interesting time because as we hit high school the Vietnam War was unfolding. Anybody in that class of 1969 in the USA has distinct memories of political speeches and decisions being made in the face of great uncertainty about what was going to happen in life. It was not as if the problem of war was unique to our generation, but 1969 was perhaps the peak of that kind of concern.

We had a tightly bonded class. Probably the most meaningful social thing I did was to play on the basketball team. Another interesting lesson—I had been on the second team in junior high school and there were a group of us who were really good friends who were on the first and second team in junior high school. Some of us on the second team thought we should be on the first team, but we never got the break. When we got to the 10th grade we were on the Junior Varsity team together and the varsity team was having a rough go of it. The coach got frustrated early into the season and said, "Okay, I am just going to call it quits and we are going to have tryouts including all the Junior Varsity and Varsity players, and whoever plays the best will be on the varsity team." One other guy and I got picked for the varsity team and we both started. I went from second team Junior Varsity to starting on the varsity team in 1 day and got 12 points in my first varsity game. We did not have a great year that year but I learned that if you persist in working towards your goal, sometimes unexpected pleasant surprises do happen. The next year we finished second in the state, and in my senior year we won the AAAA state championship in South Carolina, a tremendous team achievement. It was a group of kids who had been together for several years plus a team flavored by the initial integration of secondary schools in South Carolina. Integration in our schools sort of started with basketball. We had kids who had played together since the 7th grade and 3 minority players who came in and made a big impact.

WCR: *You went to public junior high and high school?*

RMC: Yes, public schools.

WCR: *What did you play in basketball?*

RMC: I was too slow to be a guard and too short to be a forward, so I sort of played in between guard and forward. We were blessed with a real big guy center and really good shooting guards. We had a mixture of about 8 or 9 kids who played well together and got along well.

WCR: *How tall are you?*

RMC: Six foot 1 inch.

WCR: *Did you play other sports in high school?*

RMC: Just for fun I played tennis and golf. My grandfather played golf and I got exposed to that at a young age and really enjoyed it as a 12- and 13-year old. Then I gave it up after high school and picked it up again about 8 years ago.

WCR: *When your family had dinner at night when you were a teenager did you discuss US or world topics? Were there intellectual discussions at the dinner table or how did that go?*

RMC: I think it is fair to say that we had a mixture of the usual family chaos with a fairly intellectual flavor. My parents were both interested in events in the world. They are both very bright. There was always a big emphasis in our family on the importance of education. My maternal grandfather had been a Baptist minister so there was a flavor of religion and doing the right thing in the family was very strong. My paternal grandfather had been in the military as an engineer and had been all around the world, so we had the world influence. We had a lot of intellectual discussions. But we also had the usual squabbling and sibling rivalries that most families go through.

One thing I did not learn that I should have was that we *did* have family meals together. I did not understand the importance of this until a little later with my own wife and children. It is something I really try to emphasize with trainees and junior faculty now. I think it is a missing ingredient in many medical families.

WCR: *To be home before dinner?*

RMC: Yes, even if you come back to work later. The discussion time together is important to kids, even if they don't realize it until later on.

WCR: *Did your family go on vacations in the summer time?*

RMC: Yes, but we were not a well-traveled family. We had a lot of relatives in the state so we would gather at the beach. I have fond memories of crabs being thrown in a pot on the beaches in South Carolina. If you have read Pat Conroy, you know that the low country of South Carolina is an unbelievably culturally rich environment and it is mostly oriented towards outdoor family activities. It was a great place to grow up, but we did not travel far. We went to the mountains of Tennessee and we went to the coast of South Carolina and that was pretty much it. I was never on an airplane until I was out of college.

WCR: *Did you have jobs in the summers?*

RMC: I worked most summers. I did bag-boy grocery jobs, and then made prefabricated siding for apartments in a lumber yard. The first summer after college was probably one of the most intense summers of discussion and reflection I ever had. I worked in a rock quarry with 4 or 5 of my friends, including Lee Atwater. Our job was to service the trussels that the big machines dropped the rocks into. Lee had gone to Newberry College (he had barely made it through high school) and gotten involved in Republican politics, and I had been at Duke and gotten very involved in anti-Vietnam War activities. We spent the summer in fairly intense political discourse about the future. He went on, of course, to run campaigns for Republicans, including George Bush's successful run for the Presidency, and I went on into medicine. The discussions we had then were quite formative in terms of thinking

about our future conduct. Not that we were all that wise at the time, but we were listening to a lot of people, reading, discussing, and coming to different conclusions about things.

WCR: *In junior high and high school were there teachers who had a major impact on you?*

RMC: There were in different kinds of ways. In the eighth grade, I had a science teacher who made us do presentations and I was a fairly shy kid. I liked to do things by myself. I had friends but I was fairly shy. She made us give presentations and encouraged me and I learned that I actually liked to talk about things that I knew something about, and that I could do it. That really made a lasting impression on me. Beyond that there was no individual teacher in high school, but it was a great environment where there was always something to do in our high school. When I look at high schools now in our community and others, I often wish the kind of environment we had could be recreated. It was relatively open and stimulating. People got along. We had our problems, but there were no significant physical threats and we had a pretty good time in high school.

WCR: *Were you valedictorian of your class?*

RMC: No. Nowhere near it. We ended up with about a dozen kids going to Ivy League schools. I did not study to make grades. I was sort of interested in certain things and worked on those and did not work as hard on others. I was very interested in sports.

WCR: *How many in your graduating high school class?*

RMC: Around 550.

WCR: *Where were you among those 550?*

RMC: I might have been 40th.

WCR: *How did you decide to go to Duke University?*

RMC: My brother had gone there and I thought it was kind of a neat place. I wanted to get away from home but not too far from home. I had never traveled much. The other college I really thought about was Clemson, because I still loved the town of Clemson and I think it is a great school. I decided to give Duke a shot. It was an interesting experience. I learned a lot. We have our 25th reunion coming up this year.

WCR: *What did you major in in college?*

RMC: Last night I was talking to Joe Mitchell, one of my old roommates who lives here in Dallas and is an attorney, about how we came along at a time where to show your outrage about the Vietnam War you signed a paper saying you were not going to take exams and they still nevertheless passed you. It was an odd time for academics. There were a lot of other issues on campus at the same time—fairness to racial minorities in the workforce, and wages.

I ended up majoring in psychology. My goal was to work in the prison system and try to improve it. I basically took courses I thought were interesting, which was an advantage I had. The thing about the university that was most important to me was that I met a lot of people from places I had never been. They came from different backgrounds with different expe-

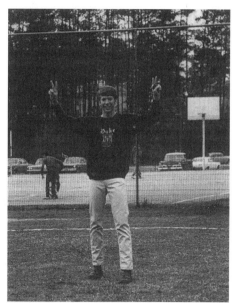

FIGURE 2. RMC as a senior in high school. His beloved car (the "Savoy") is in the background just to the left of the basketball hoop.

riences and I learned a heck of a lot from that. It was a great experience. I enjoyed just about all of it.

WCR: *Who had a significant influence on you in college? Was it primarily your classmates? Did any teachers stand out?*

RMC: As opposed to high school where my classmates dominate my memory (we were a pretty self-directed high school group) with modifying influences by teachers, I would say in college I had a lot of intense relationships with professors. One of the things I joke about with my kids now is that at the time I started the freshman year they actually had Saturday morning English tutorials where you had to bring in your writings and sit there with the professor and have your writing critiqued.

I am sure you see the same problems I see with writing, Bill. In editing a cardiology journal right now, I find it amazing how many bright people cannot write. Having to expose your writing and thoughts to a teacher in a one-on-one session was a tremendous experience. There was a psychology professor named Richard Kramer who had a way of teaching about the human brain that was fascinating. He had an influence on me, not that I admire some of the things that were done with psychotropic experimentation at that time, but it was fascinating to see people begin to understand better the capacity of the human mind and how it can be changed, sometimes for the worse.

WCR: *How did you decide to major in psychology in college?*

RMC: I thought I wanted to do something that was socially meaningful. I came from a Baptist sort of mentality that you need to do something that improves the world. My mother made me take all these achieve-ment and vocational tests. They kept saying I should be a lawyer, and I did not want to be a lawyer. The psychologist position came up high on the list. I was not particularly interested in biological science at that time. It seemed dealing with the human mind would be a good thing to do.

WCR: *When did you decide that you wanted to be a physician?*

RMC: It was very specific. I got a job in the State prison in South Carolina during college one summer. That was a phenomenal experience. They put me in the work-release program. I worked at a facility over in West Columbia. There were 30 to 40 inmates who had done well enough that they were nearing release, and they got jobs out in the communities but had to live in the facility. My job was to help them and make sure they stayed on the premises. We had a basketball team, which I coached. I did not have a gun or anything like that. If there was a problem, I just had to make a phone call and things would be taken care of. I found it to be frustrating, and although I admire people who can work in that environment and struggle with it, it almost seemed like by the time people had gotten into prison there was very little one could do to change behavior.

My ultimate moment of frustration came during one of the Friday nights when I escorted them to the speedway or to the bowling alley (the allowed recreation). A couple of fellows on work release were guys I had played high school ball against. This particular night at the bowling alley, they picked my pocket! Here I was helping these guys and they took my wallet right out of my pants. I didn't even know it was gone until I got back. No one would say who did it. At that point, I thought, this field is not far enough along for me to do what I want to do to improve it. I probably needed some more tangible rewards. I thought maybe I should go into something more physical, like medicine. I had taken no science courses until the summer of my junior year.

WCR: *So you took all your premedical science courses during the summer after your junior year and during your senior year in college?*

RMC: Yes, but also during the summer after my senior year. I had to wait out a year to apply to medical school because I did not get to take organic chemistry in time.

WCR: *That is why you had 5 years between the beginning of college and medical school? What did you do during the rest of the year?*

RMC: Lydia and I got married right after my graduation from Duke in May. (Our 25th wedding anniversary is coming up this year.) We had been high school sweethearts, so we have been together a long time. She was in nursing school at the University of North Carolina at Greensboro and had one more year to go, so I had a fabulous year. We lived in Columbia in a little apartment for the summer. I took organic chemistry and she worked in a hospital as sort of a practicum for her nursing training. We had no money, so we were living off her wages with a little help from our parents. We then went up to Greensboro and she finished her undergraduate degree while I worked as an orderly in a local hospital for 9 months.

It was a great experience. I worked 8 hours a day, 5 days a week. I got to know, at a very fundamental level, what happens to people in a hospital. I had a lot of very personal experiences with patients when putting in a Foley catheter and emptying the bed pans. I did a lot of work in the emergency department and got fascinated by defibrillation. I saw some people resuscitated. When I was not working, I was reading books and playing basketball and cooking. We had a great time, probably the most relaxed time ever. After about 6 months of that, I was ready to do something with a broader purpose and was happy to be headed to medical school.

WCR: *You graduated from college Phi Beta Kappa so you had no problem getting into medical school?*

RMC: I wanted to go to the University of Virginia because they had a program where you could design your own curriculum, and I thought that would be the best thing for me. I still to this day cannot stand sitting in classroom sessions. They did not think enough of me to admit me, however. I got into Duke and Tulane. I did not think I would want to go back to Durham. I thought I had spent enough time there. I started to go to Tulane and then at the last minute—I am still not sure why actually—I decided to go to Duke. Tulane still claims 300 precious dollars of ours that we could not get back because we decided too late to attend Duke.

WCR: *Had anybody in your family ever been a physician?*

RMC: I have a picture of a relative on my father's side who practiced as a horse and buggy physician in the low country of South Carolina. My great-great grandfather graduated from the Medical University of South Carolina in Charleston, and I have his diploma hanging on my wall. There is a family tradition of physicians, but it skipped a couple of generations. That was not a main motivating factor for me. I had seen something that I thought I could do and would enjoy doing.

WCR: *When you picked the medical profession, you really had not known what doctors do every day?*

RMC: Only in that one of my best friends growing up, *Ken Graham,* had a father who was a family doctor. We basketball groupees spent much time at his house because he had a nice court outside his garage, and over his garage he had a pool table in a separate room where we could hang out. I spent enough time to know about the personal interactions of a doctor, but I did not have a good feel for the procedural stuff until I did that year as an orderly. Then, I got a good understanding. I did everything from help out with some autopsies to emptying bed pans to setting up defibrillators and doing some cardiopulmonary resuscitation.

WCR: *So when you entered medical school in 1974 you had a pretty good sense what medicine was all about?*

RMC: I had a good sense for that time about what

doctors did in the real world. I had very little sense of what medical school was all about.

WCR: *How did you enjoy medical school?*

RMC: Duke is an interesting place for medical school, because it has a very tough, intense first year where you cram 2 years of work into one. In return you get a third year where you can pretty much do what you want to do. I would say that the first year was very colorful and I learned a heck of a lot, but it was incredibly stressful in every way. The payback was phenomenal though. I had an outstanding third year and actually set my career based on that experience.

I was going to be a pediatrician until I got involved more in the cardiovascular research world. I started out the second year just doing a job working with the Duke Cardiology Databank to make some money and ended up spending the whole third year putting Holter monitors on patients and measuring who had sudden death. That really got me excited about developing evidence and understanding whether what we do actually works.

WCR: *When you got a job in the Duke Databank as a sophomore in medical school had you had any previous experience with computers?*

RMC: Absolutely none.

WCR: *What happened that year?*

RMC: My job was to assist in the clinic. Data would be marked down on sheets and somebody would enter it into a computer. I saw that going on, but as I got involved in the third year, where I actually spent a lot of time with *Kerry Lee,* a senior statistician, who has been a very influential person in my career, it was evident that doctors have a hard time remembering or synthesizing all the information that they experience. It did not take a lot of work to see that the computer would come out with answers about the natural history of disease that were far superior to what the individual doctor could recognize from his/her own experience.

WCR: *You have been on a computer ever since?*

RMC: I would not say on a computer. I am actually not very good with computers myself. I am a computer user, but I don't do any of my own programming. I just use what computers can bring and depend on other people to do the things they like to do. I am more of an interface person. I like to try to interface what computers can do with the world of clinical practice.

WCR: *So your junior year in medical school was essentially spent in the Databank?*

RMC: That brings up the question, "What is medical school for, after all?" I went to medical school when most medical schools didn't do a very good job of education. They offered didactic courses, which I don't consider to be the way you really learn. I was unprepared for what medical school was like, and I continue to think much of medical school is wasted the way it is done presently.

WCR: *If you were a Dean of a medical school right now, how would you set up the medical school?*

RMC: If I were a Dean with unlimited authority?

I believe in the university without walls. If you ask the question, "Why do we have medical schools?" the answer probably is "to train doctors." Then you would ask the question, "What do doctors need to know?" It is at least my contention that we have far too much emphasis on rote learning and basic science constructs that doctors will never use and not enough about what they actually need to know to deal with the world they are going into. That has to do with how health systems work, how to supervise people, how to negotiate, how to interact effectively with other human beings, and how to understand evidence, both clinical and financial. There is very little about that in medical school today. Yet, if you look at what doctors are going to be doing, that is what they need to know.

I would say let's make a self-learning curriculum available for the basic sciences that one could pass or be certified in at any point along the way. Let's get rid of all these classrooms of people sitting through dry lectures. Let's make that kind of learning more interactive, based on computer interaction, one-on-one tutorials, or small tutorials for concepts and feedback. Let's really build in a curriculum that teaches people how to evaluate what needs to be done with other human beings in the practice of medicine. I would see more of a blend of what is currently done in business school and what we try to teach housestaff now. I think the time medical students are not seeing patients should be shortened in the medical school curriculum, with a fair amount of infiltration of what is taught in public health school.

WCR: *You would expose medical students to patients right away?*

RMC: Yes, and I think a lot of schools are doing that. But I think the lecture time is not all that well spent. If medical education stops when you graduate, it is not going to work because the jobs that doctors do are going to change substantially, and the things they need to know, looking at the pace that information is increasing, will change enormously. We should be focused on the skills of self-instruction.

WCR: *Who had the most impact on you in medical school?*

RMC: The most impact all together was by my wife, Lydia. She has kept me humble and aware that the small things in life really are important.

In terms of people at the medical school with the most impact on me, *Eugene Stead*, far and away. I think a lot of people who studied the history of modern medicine know that Dr. Stead is someone who has had a profound influence. He sees the world differently than most other people. He tends to see things other people don't see. The kinds of things that he would do would lead you to learn from them. Often you would initially have no earthly idea what it was you had learned; it would slowly come to you later on.

WCR: *What is an example of that?*

RMC: A concrete example is the first time I gave a talk to a group of doctors where he was in the audience. He walked up to me, took my slide carousel, took the top of it off and turned it upside down on the floor. He said, "Pick them back up, don't think about

what order they are in, and give the talk." Obviously, at the time, I did not think that was a very nice thing to do and I did not see how that would teach me anything, but by going through a number of exercises like that I learned how to give a talk, whether or not I had the slides or the projector broke or whatever. It was a great lesson. Half the time he would say things that sounded odd, and he would disregard things that we took as fundamental. After we would think about it, we would realize that he was just ahead of his time. The concept of "outcomes-research"—measuring, quantifying the natural history of disease using computers—seems so straightforward now, but when he was proposing it and writing about it in the 1960s he was considered way out in left field.

WCR: *Did Dr. Stead know anything about computers?*

RMC: No.

WCR: *Did he ever use one as far as you know?*

RMC: Not as far as I know.

WCR: *How much contact did you have with him in medical school?*

RMC: A fair amount. He had retired as Chief of Medicine at a young age and he basically did what he wanted to do, which was mostly to get money to support good ideas with grants and contracts and develop this database. He would come by and talk.

WCR: *This was when you were a junior spending the entire year in the databank?*

RMC: Yes, at that time the world was kind of divided into "Stead disciples" and "non-Stead disciples." He had a way of saying things that would make you scratch your head. Some people would say, "This guy is crazy." Other people would say, "There is something here I need to figure out." They would go off and figure it out and generally do better because they had.

Another person, who was hired by Dr. Stead, was *Kerry Lee*, who is still the senior statistician in our group. He was hired from the University of North Carolina at a time when there was no place for a statistician in Duke Medical Center. In fact, no department except Community and Family Medicine would offer Kerry a position. He ended up with a position in the Department of Community and Family Medicine, but he worked on the cardiology database.

I think a lot of people in medical school are taught a view of medical research that when you construct a hypothesis you pretty much rig the experiment to make the answer come out the way you want. You go into the whole experiment with a bias about what the answer will be. I remember taking my first data set to Kerry Lee, and he said, "Okay, let's do a regression model." I said, "What is a regression model?" He had all these computer cards and he punched out some stuff. The result was different from what we expected. I was unhappy with it because we wanted to show that ventricular premature complexes were really the root cause of sudden death. That was our hypothesis, yet every way we analyzed the data it turned out that left ventricular ejection fraction, not ventricular premature complexes, was the key factor. Kerry kept saying,

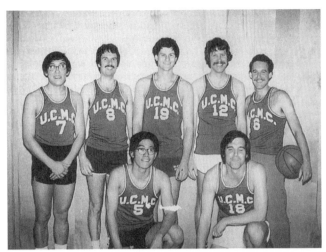

FIGURE 3. RMC (top row, second from right) with the University of California-San Francisco houseofficer basketball team.

"You don't need to tell the experiment what the answer is. You need to look at the result and try to understand it and put it in perspective." In retrospect, of course, his advice was pretty good. We have learned since that trying to suppress the frequency of ventricular premature complexes is not necessarily a good thing to do. We all know that people with bad left ventricular function are at high risk of sudden death. Therapies that don't necessarily suppress ventricular premature complexes also prevent sudden death in patients.

WCR: *That was your first paper in 1978?*

RMC: Yes.

WCR: *This article was published while you were in medical school? It was the year you graduated that it was published?*

RMC: Right. There was a tremendous emphasis on publishing what you did at Duke, particularly in cardiology. Obviously, I took this to heart.

WCR: *When you were in medical school you got into the Cardiology Databank early as a sophomore, just to get a job. Then you were so fascinated you spent your entire junior year there. By that time, did you know you wanted to be a cardiologist?*

RMC: I spent a lot of time hanging out with the cardiology fellows. I got to work in the catheterization laboratory, in the noninvasive laboratory, in the exercise laboratory; I put Holter monitors on patients. I just found it fascinating. This was something I could intuitively understand and deal with. I think everybody's mind is a little bit different. I learned that I did have a grasp of data, being able to look at it, draw conclusions, and take action. It also seemed to just fit together extremely well.

When it came time for matching on internship, Lydia and I went around to look at internships all over the country. Neither of us previously had ever been out of the Southeast. I decided I wanted to go to the west coast. Lydia was interested but really wanted to

stay in the Southeast. She was pregnant for the first time when the match came out, and when I matched the University of San Francisco she was pretty upset. She was not too thrilled with that opportunity. I was obviously delighted because that was a tough place to get into, and I knew I would meet a lot of people who would be interesting. I guess I had done well enough in that third year that I was able to arrange a fellowship in cardiology to return to back at Duke before I went to California. That also was a time when there was a special deal with the American Board of Internal Medicine, where if you did enough research in your fellowship you could do 2 years of internal medicine and get credit for the third year. We arranged for 2 years in San Francisco and then came back to Duke to start the cardiology fellowship.

WCR: *So that saved you a year? You went to San Francisco for internship in 1978 and stayed for 1 year of residency.*

RMC: Right.

WCR: *How did you enjoy your time in San Francisco?*

RMC: It was a phenomenal experience. Just about every part of it was interesting. We loved it. We lived in Buena Vista Park, which is right in the Haight-Ashbury District, and saw a lot of kinds of people we had not spent time with previously. Culturally, it was an extremely diverse city and that was interesting.

The medical training was superb with *Holly Smith* as Chief of Medicine. He was someone you could easily look up to. Although he had lost his South Carolina accent, he was from Camden, South Carolina. I got to know him fairly well. For a place that had done so well in research, the environment for the housestaff was extraordinarily friendly and personal. The ability to go over to San Francisco General and spend a third of your time there with one of the busiest emergency departments in the country was a great opportunity. Although we had excellent attending physicians, there was more to do than they could do, so as a houseofficer you really got to run the show in the emergency department and that was a fantastic experience.

I could get on my bicycle from home and ride right through the Golden Gate Park and go to the prettiest piece of real estate in the world, the San Francisco Veterans' Administration Hospital, right at the Golden Gate. You can look out the window and see the boats going by. I think it was a great choice for me and I learned a lot. There were things going on at the time which, again, like other times in life, we did not understand at all. This was right in the middle of the gay influx into the San Francisco community. We took care of patients with AIDS and did not know what AIDS was. I distinctly remember several patients who had AIDS. We just did not know what it was.

WCR: *What did you call it?*

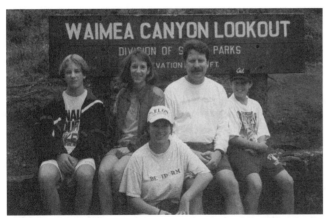

FIGURE 4. The Califf clan: left to right top row: Sam, Lydia, Rob, and Tom; kneeling: Sharon.

RMC: We called it whatever the manifestation was. If it was pneumonia, we called it "pneumonia." If they had weird skin lesions we called it "weird skin lesions" and tried to figure out what they were. It was a very rowdy political time, mostly related to the cultural clashes, the Harvey Milk assassination (a city council leader who was murdered in his office).

Also, the year I arrived, Proposition 13 had just been passed under the Reagan leadership and they had promised about $13,000 a year to interns. After arriving in San Francisco, I learned that they were only going to pay me $11,500. They breached their contract, but said there was nothing I could do about it. It was State law and if I didn't like it I could take it up with Ronald Reagan. I learned about the influence of government on medicine.

WCR: *You mentioned Holly Smith. Who had an impact on you during your internship and year of residency in San Francisco?*

RMC: There were a number of people, but the biggest impact was really from several people for different reasons. Although our daughter Sharon had been born in Durham, it was not until 3 weeks after we arrived in San Francisco that we learned she had congenital heart disease and the diagnosis of coarctation of the aorta, atrioventricular septal defect with a cleft mitral valve was made. We had no money, and were living from month to month on this small income. Sharon was in severe heart failure at the time of diagnosis. The surgeon, *Paul Ebert*, who earlier had been at Duke and was world renowned, had a system for taking care of these sick kids that was phenomenal. It was a system obviously built around his expertise, knowledge, and artistic capability in doing these heart operations. We saw him only a few times. All the other care was rendered by a variety of people who seemed to know exactly what they were supposed to do and when they were supposed to do it, ranging from the anesthesiologist, who resuscitated her after a postoperative cardiac arrest, to the pediatric cardiolo-

gist who took excellent personal care of her, to the nurses who were very tuned in to our needs.

Sharon spent a month in the hospital postoperatively, and I was a new intern. You can imagine the situation. She had a big operation where they tried to fix everything at one time, something her cardiologist told us could not be done. We learned later that that was a set up. This was a lesson I learned that I have employed in intensive care medicine ever since, which is when you initially meet a family and the situation is serious, it is probably better to tell them to expect the worst and you are going to do everything you can, than to tell them that everything is going to be all right. If things do turn out okay, it is a great sense of positivity, but if you expect everything to be all right and things turn out badly I think it is a worse situation for a family. It is realistic in those circumstances to expect the worst and that way you actually think about what you need to do.

Paul Ebert taught me that you certainly need to build your healthcare around technical competence, but the systematic approach to the management of illness, using a broad range of people with different talents, is something that makes a big difference. His system was in contrast to a lot of other systems at the University of California at San Francisco at the time, which were very good academically, from the point of view of traditional academic medicine, but were really not very efficient. To watch these children come from all over the world, have their families have a place to stay, see them get through the system, and have their needs taken care of, and have the technical competence too, was really something to watch. My daughter did well and she is now a bright and healthy college student.

Even in one of the best of systems, we had the experience of having a pediatric cardiologist who turned out not to be a pediatric cardiologist. This actually got to be a fairly well-known case. This gentleman was assigned to help in her care, and he ended up being her personal physician after surgery. He was a very nice guy, very attentive, but he turned out to be a fake doctor. He had taken his cousin's credentials and had gotten an internship and had risen through the ranks at University of California at San Francisco. When he came up to be head of the neonatal intensive care unit, which was a pretty big job at that time, his credential check flushed him out. We had the experience of hearing on the news that our child's doctor was not a doctor after all. These experiences reinforced a personal view that the physician has a special responsibility because of the trust of patients.

There was a guy named *Jim Naughton* who ran the housestaff program, and the personal attention that we got during this time of crisis, the little things he and his wife did meant so much to Lydia and me. We spent a month in the hospital just about 24 hours a day while Sharon was recovering. People brought us meals and he made accommodations to my responsibilities. I continued to work and we would make rounds on Sharon every day with the team. I was given some leeway to take care of this crisis in the middle of trying to be an intern. Those little things mean a lot to people when they come from those who are in a position of influence. This is probably something that I have not paid enough attention to, but something I think about fairly often and try to correct myself and do it more.

The other big influence was *Kanu Chatterjee*. Rounding with him on the coronary care unit was just a phenomenal experience because he thinks about human physiology in a way that is great to watch and to learn from. In a way, it was a luxury at the time. The hospital was not that busy a place in cardiology. It was not a high volume facility like many other places, so time was taken on rounds to listen to the heart, talk to the patients, and try to put everything together. I think that had an influence on a whole generation of us who went through the system.

WCR: *Were coronary care unit rounds with Dr. Chatterjee a long experience?*

RMC: They were not particularly long. They were sort of medium. We took time with each patient. He did not waste time on frivolous things. Another thing he did, which was a lesson I learned when I came to run my own coronary care unit and I think is a fundamental system, is that he had a rule that if you were on call at night as an intern or resident, and the nurses did not like what you were doing, they called him at home. He did not always agree with the nurses but he did render judgment on whether what you were doing met standards. His concept in medical care, that there should be a basic level of quality that can be recognizable and enforceable by people who are there as permanent employees, has been useful to me.

WCR: *Did anybody else during those 2 years have a significant impact on you?*

RMC: There were a lot of people, but I would not name anyone in particular. There is a lot of dedication in that institution to training.

WCR: *You said Holly Smith was a superb chairman. What were his qualities that made him so?*

RMC: First of all, he seemed to care about the people on his housestaff. He gave you a sense that he knew who you were and he was concerned that you should do well. Secondly, there was a sense of tradition that had developed there. There were certain things that were done. There were annual get togethers and ways of interacting that were comforting, considering you had a conglomeration of people from all over the country. Then lastly, his demeanor when he dealt with you was respectful and positive. He was a man of enough distinction he did not need to be that way, it was just the way he did things. I think when you saw the way he interacted with other people it set a tone that was great for the whole program. This was not an easy time in terms of society and how people

got along. There was a lot going on in San Francisco at that time, but he managed extraordinarily well.

WCR: *Did you have much contact with Bill Parmley?*

RMC: Actually, almost none, but I have since gotten to know Bill Parmley and he has had an influence on me the last couple of years in a very positive way. He is a paragon of integrity.

WCR: *What about your fellow housestaff? Who were some of your fellow housestaff and what kind of impact did they have on you?*

RMC: We had a great group of housestaff and the interactions were formative. The two housestaff with whom I have maintained a very close relationship, I was not particularly close to as house officers. We respected each other but just ended up not being on the same rotations together. They were *Eric Topol* and *Dean Kereiakes*. There were many bright people on the housestaff one could learn from and exchange ideas with. Sitting in the on-call room at San Francisco General Hospital at 4:00 A.M. trying to figure out what to do with a patient was a tremendous experience. The friendships made there are still carrying on. *Ralph Brendis*, who was a Chief Resident 2 years ahead of me and is now the head of the cardiac catheterization laboratory at Kaiser San Francisco, had a very positive influence on me in terms of maintaining enthusiasm and positivity. *Mike Clayman*, who went on to be a nephrologist and head of cardiovascular research at Eli Lilly, has remained a collaborator. Of course, I still have a relationship with Dean Kereiakes, who I work with every day in clinical trials and clinical research. Eric Topol and I have had a very close relationship over the years, and we have done a lot of things together and tend to think alike about how things should be done. *Jay Siegal* was a year ahead of me and is one of the leaders in the Bureau of Biologics at the Federal Food and Drug Administration. There were many people in that housestaff program who have gone on to be people I have interacted with on the national scene in the research that we have done.

WCR: *Did you and Lydia enjoy California?*

RMC: We really did. We laugh about it a lot now, because we did not have a lot of money. We rented a U-Haul truck and drove out to San Francisco with our daughter and our dog and cat. Lydia cried all the way to the Mississippi River on the way out there, and then when it came time to come back she did not want to come back and she cried all the way to the Mississippi River on the way back. We made a lot of friends there and had a great experience. Living in a city of such diversity and being able to go out to the Golden Gate Park on any given day and do interesting things or go across the Golden Gate Bridge and hike in Marin County or experience the California coast and the national parks was awesome. We learned a lot and had a great time. Oftentimes, I have wondered whether it would not have been better for me just to stay out there, but I think on balance we made the right move. On a sobering note, we lived in a predominantly gay community and many of the friends we made are now dead. I would say that most have died of HIV-related illnesses.

WCR: *What happened when you came back to Duke to do your cardiology fellowship? How did that work out?*

RMC: I came back and did the usual things that a fellow does the first year. I did research in the Databank and focused on natural history studies of coronary disease. It was a wonderful time because it was still in the era when there was enough money in the academic medical system that people saw patients for a certain number of hours in the day and then they had time to think. There was a guy named *Phil Harris*, who was a fellow who had come from Australia to spend a couple of years. Phil had a positive influence on an entire group of us. There was *Kerry Lee*, and there was *Frank Harrell*, another statistician; to this day Frank is the most creative thinker about data I have ever met. We all spent a lot of time looking at data and thinking about what it meant. It was a great time. I went on to do my clinical rotations and those were fun.

When I finished that second year of fellowship, *Jim Wyngaarden* was leaving to run the NIH. He had been the Chairman of Medicine, and *Andy Wallace*, who had been Chief of Cardiology, left the Division to run the hospital. They picked *Joe Greenfield* to run Cardiology and then eventually to be the Chair of Medicine. Joe called me and said, "We need someone to run the CCU. How would you like to do that instead of your third year of fellowship?" I ended up sort of being a fellow-faculty, which meant a year of being on call every other weekend and every week night for $35,000. It was a privilege to do it. I learned an incredible amount during that time dealing with acute coronary disease. It is hard for young people to understand this. We did not have thrombolytics or anything else to do to improve outcomes in acute MI. We did not even know about the benefits of aspirin.

WCR: *This was 1982?*

RMC: Yes. We basically put Swan-Ganz catheters in people and tried to modify the hemodynamics to try to make things better. We put in temporary pacemakers if someone went into heart block. We saw a lot of people go down the tubes that year, without being able to do a whole lot about it.

WCR: *I presume when Joe Greenfield asked you to take over the coronary care unit, your third year of fellowship, it was assumed you would stay on the faculty thereafter.*

RMC: There was a fair amount of uncertainty, because whenever you have a new Chief of Medicine you are not sure exactly what is going to happen, but that seemed reasonable and Joe had a very personable way of making you feel like if things did not work out he would help you find something that was to your benefit. That is a key quality in leaders that I see missing a lot today. The personal touch of reassuring those who work for you that even if it is not right for you, I will personally see to it that you get something that is right for you. He also never tried to take credit

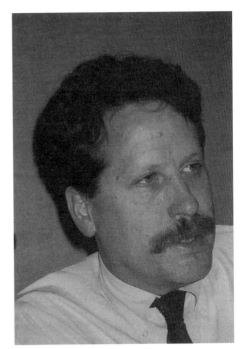

FIGURE 5. RMC during the interview.

for someone else's idea. Too many medical leaders today thrive on personal power and glory.

WCR: *Who in cardiology had an impact on you during your fellowship?*

RMC: *Bob Rosati*, who ran the Databank. He was a very bright person who had a lot of insight into how to look at data, but he had sort of gotten side tracked into looking at data before he had a chance to flex all his clinical muscles. He taught me a lot, but just as I finished the fellowship and the first year in the coronary care unit, he felt like he wanted to go back to clinical medicine so he decided not to run the Databank anymore. *Galen Wagner* also had a big influence. Galen had looked out for me during my third year of medical school. He is a person who has always had a different point of view about things and has persevered with the institution for many years. At the time, he was helping with the fellowship program.

WCR: *When Bob Rosati decided to go back into clinical medicine, you sort of captured the Cardiovascular Databank. Is that how that worked out?*

RMC: David Pryor was a colleague who was a year ahead of me, and we sort of split things up. David took over the leadership of the Databank and I took over the coronary care unit. The deal was that we would work together, that I would focus on the clinical enterprise and try to integrate that with the Databank, and he would do the more research-specific and administrative tasks, which he was very interested in. Joe Greenfield, when he called us into his office to talk about this, basically said, "This is an interesting idea of Dr. Stead's, but I don't think it is worth anything, and you have 5 years to prove it is worth something or I am turning it off." That stimulated us at a fairly young age to try to figure out how to make it a productive endeavor. Probably the most creative couple of months of my career in terms of thinking about how to do things was when David and I spent a few months on Saturday mornings trying to think about how to diversify the funding for the Databank.

WCR: *That is when you decided to get commercial support?*

RMC: Up until that time, most of the support for the Databank had come from the NIH to fund the computerization of medical records. People were beginning to realize that business was so far ahead of medicine in terms of computer programming and databases that it was pretty clear the funding was going to dry up for that aspect. We also were getting some grants from the National Center for Health Services Research, which was a very small agency at the time, to look at the observational treatment comparisons of bypass surgery and medical therapy. But, as Bob Rosati said when he decided to move on, "Bypass surgery has been around for awhile and I don't think we will make many advances with this comparison." Little did he know that *Gruentzig* was over there in his kitchen about that same time cooking up angioplasty, which cast a whole new light on the field. Basically, what David and I did was really believe in our hearts and minds that quantitation of medical phenomena was going to be important. This belief had been inspired to a large extent by Bob Rosati's influence. We developed a set of domains of funding that we thought would be worthwhile and useful. It included what became Agency for Health Care Policy and Research (AHCPR), which at the time was the NCHSR, and the NIH and the foundation and industry. We talked about clinical trials, but we did not know a whole heck of a lot about clinical trials at the time.

As it turned out, right about the same time, Eric Topol, who had been an intern when I was a resident at UCSF, had come to Duke to interview but had decided to go to Hopkins for his fellowship. I was disappointed by that, because I thought he really had a talent and a knack for thinking about data. We kept in touch through telephone conversations. As he was finishing his fellowship, thrombolytic therapy was just beginning to come on the scene, but none of us knew what it would amount to. I had given a fair amount of streptokinase to a dozen or so patients at Duke with *Richard Stack*, and Eric Topol had really focused on the science of plasminogen activators. We had a connection with Genentech, because the company had been formed by former University of California at San Francisco professors. *Bill O'Neill* and Richard Stack had been residents together and were good friends. Eric joined Bill at the University of Michigan. We thought it would be fun to see what this new recombinant molecule might do in terms of reperfusion of coronary arteries. In talking about it we said, "Why don't we get a group of friends together and do a clinical trial." I was able to leverage our computer facility, and with Eric's incredible energy and leadership, we did the Thrombolysis and Angioplasty in Myocardial Infarction (TAMI-1) study. I'm really proud of what Eric and I have accomplished. Over the years his creativity and insight into the interface between science and medicine have been incredible.

WCR: *That was the first clinical trial where data outside Duke came into your data center? That was the beginning of the huge number of clinical trials that you later managed?*

RMC: Right, and it was just a group of friends working together. Overall we lost money doing the research, but at the time we had core funding at Duke from NIH for statistics and computing. We were able to get the research done. We did 3 cardiac catheterizations on each of 386 patients for about $300 a patient. Times have obviously changed since then.

There was a great lesson in that trial because we thought doing an angioplasty immediately after thrombolytic therapy would be beneficial and it turned out not to be. We were just trying to demonstrate the benefit of a practice we were sure about, and it turned out we were doing the wrong thing in practice. Along with the Thrombolysis In Myocardial Infarction (TIMI)-2 study and the European Cooperative Group, it led to significant changes in the way people managed thrombolytic therapy.

WCR: *After that you saw that clinical trials were the way to go?*

RMC: I would not put it that way. I think what we saw was that randomization is a powerful tool. When it comes down to deciding if one treatment is better than another, a randomized trial is the best evidence one can get. Chances for bias are so great if you don't employ randomization. Besides that, trials were fun and, in those early days, we had meetings with people who enjoyed spending time with each other. We would all bring our cans of film from the cases we had done. We would see things nobody had ever seen before and try to figure out what to do about them in clinical practice. It was a very exciting time. Everyone wanted to do a series of TAMI studies all the way to TAMI-9.

WCR: *How many clinical trials are you now involved with?*

RMC: The word "involved" is a dangerous word in this regard, but today we have something like 40 clinical trials in which I have involvement on some aspect or another.

WCR: *That data is fed into your Databank?*

RMC: No. The ones we handle the data for are more in the order of 15 or 16, but we work as partners with collaborators on a number of other clinical trials.

WCR: *So you are involved in the design and in the carrying out of 15 to 40 clinical trials?*

RMC: Yes. Some involvement in the design of maybe 30 or 40. In some cases, I might be on a data and safety monitoring committee, and in other cases I may be on a steering committee but our center may not be handling the data.

WCR: *You remained head of the coronary care unit at Duke until when?*

RMC: Until about 2 years ago.

WCR: *When you were head of the coronary care unit, how much of your time was spent in that activity?*

RMC: Until about 4 years ago I was spending over 50% of my time there making rounds and caring for patients. We have a very busy clinical practice. We went through an exciting period before catheterization laboratories proliferated in the state of North Carolina, where we had a helicopter service and brought in a lot of patients who needed revascularization from small hospitals. We developed a lot of innovative approaches to providing care in the region, ranging from outreach clinics with cardiology fellows to catheterization laboratory trucks which brought an experienced crew of cardiologists to outlying hospitals to do the cases. *Harry Phillips* and I instituted the first "modern" group practice at Duke. Harry continues to amaze me with his attunement to the needs of the clinical practice. Those who provide first class patient care in academic centers don't get enough credit—Harry has contributed greatly to Duke over the years.

WCR: *Has that worked out well?*

RMC: Yes, very well. Over the years we have evolved to a practice of 18 cardiologists, and we have set up a clinical model to integrate evidence-based medicine into our practice. The practice that Harry developed has contributed huge amounts of money to the teaching and research mission of the institution.

WCR: *How many trucks do you have?*

RMC: We have 2 trucks and they are busy all the time.

WCR: *You have how many helicopters now?*

RMC: Two helicopters in service at a time, and we've developed a sophisticated ground transport system.

WCR: *They go all over the state?*

RMC: There is a network with other tertiary referral centers, and they pretty much cover the state. We did some interesting things. We were involved in the early digitalis toxicity studies at a time when there was a limited supply of the antibody to reverse the toxicity. We had some helicopter relays that were pretty exciting. At one point, we had a child in South Carolina who was in and out of sustained VT and really sick, and we met the helicopter from there halfway and handed off the Digibind and got the kid treated and the kid did fine from digitalis toxicity. We had a lot of high volume clinical experience.

During the last couple of years, I have spent less time seeing patients and more time with administrative responsibilities.

WCR: *How many people do you have in the Duke Clinical Research Institute?*

RMC: This is a little tricky because we have a lot of "parts" of people. There are many people who see patients or work as nurses and who handle clinical research work part time as well. The total would be 650. We also have people who don't live in Durham who monitor data in outlying regions.

Our hope is to serve as a training facility for those who will develop the evidence for better medical practice in addition to a center for performing research. The support of the Duke Health System leadership, *Bill Donelan* and *Ralph Snyderman*, has made a huge difference. The DCRI now includes faculty from 10 other areas of medicine including primary care, otolaryngology, and psychiatry.

WCR: *How big a budget do you have to run this operation?*

RMC: It is somewhere around $40 million a year.

WCR: *How much of that comes from NIH or foundations or pharmaceutical companies?*

RMC: About 20% from NIH or foundations and 80% from industry. The large clinical trials require extensive clinical research networks and that accounts for a fairly large portion of the funding that we get. We also now work with professional societies and managed care organizations in measurement of outcomes and quality improvement.

WCR: *Your activities have evolved since 1983 in just an incredible way. It has been 15 years since you took over the coronary care unit. What do you think you will be doing 15 years from now?*

RMC: I wish I knew the answer to that question. I think that probably what I am destined to do for the foreseeable future is push this concept of evidence-based medicine and try to help make that happen in the best way that I can. I hope I will continue to see patients. I still consider it a privilege to see patients, but I don't do it enough now to consider myself to be a real contributor to the patient-care enterprise the way I used to in those early years on the Duke CCU.

I really believe that given the advances of science and the societal issues concerning what we pay for and what we don't pay for and what is valuable and what is not, that we are going to need to take a quantum leap in terms of developing the evidence for evidence-based medicine.

WCR: *As I understand it, you were one of the finalists in 1995 to be Chairman of the Department of Medicine at Duke. It seems to me that being a Chairman of such a large department is not something that you need quite yet at age 46. With the tremendous amount of data you are generating and the contributions you are making to management of cardiovascular disease through that data, would you still be interested in a departmental chairmanship? Is that something on your horizon?*

RMC: I think there are people wiser than me who made that selection, but I think the path I am going down is something that I am better suited for than being a Chairman of a Department of Medicine. It is such a big job helping people to put together systems to generate the data we need that this endeavor is a better way for me to spend my time. In my institutional role, which has evolved, I feel like an intern. I am working with experts in the neurosciences and all different varieties of medicine, pediatrics, surgery, and trying to help the faculty set up programs that will develop the evidence to help them know how to treat patients more effectively.

WCR: *You are spreading out from coronary disease?*

RMC: I have been for a while.

655

dead. I would say that most have died of HIV-related illnesses.

WCR: *What happened when you came back to Duke to do your cardiology fellowship? How did that work out?*

RMC: I came back and did the usual things that a fellow does the first year. I did research in the Databank and focused on natural history studies of coronary disease. It was a wonderful time because it was still in the era when there was enough money in the academic medical system that people saw patients for a certain number of hours in the day and then they had time to think. There was a guy named *Phil Harris*, who was a fellow who had come from Australia to spend a couple of years. Phil had a positive influence on an entire group of us. There was *Kerry Lee*, and there was *Frank Harrell*, another statistician; to this day Frank is the most creative thinker about data I have ever met. We all spent a lot of time looking at data and thinking about what it meant. It was a great time. I went on to do my clinical rotations and those were fun.

When I finished that second year of fellowship, *Jim Wyngaarden* was leaving to run the NIH. He had been the Chairman of Medicine, and *Andy Wallace*, who had been Chief of Cardiology, left the Division to run the hospital. They picked *Joe Greenfield* to run Cardiology and then eventually to be the Chair of Medicine. Joe called me and said, "We need someone to run the CCU. How would you like to do that instead of your third year of fellowship?" I ended up sort of being a fellow-faculty, which meant a year of being on call every other weekend and every week night for $35,000. It was a privilege to do it. I learned an incredible amount during that time dealing with acute coronary disease. It is hard for young people to understand this. We did not have thrombolytics or anything else to do to improve outcomes in acute MI. We did not even know about the benefits of aspirin.

WCR: *This was 1982?*

RMC: Yes. We basically put Swan-Ganz catheters in people and tried to modify the hemodynamics to try to make things better. We put in temporary pacemakers if someone went into heart block. We saw a lot of people go down the tubes that year, without being able to do a whole lot about it.

WCR: *I presume when Joe Greenfield asked you to take over the coronary care unit, your third year of fellowship, it was assumed you would stay on the faculty thereafter.*

RMC: There was a fair amount of uncertainty, because whenever you have a new Chief of Medicine you are not sure exactly what is going to happen, but that seemed reasonable and Joe had a very personable way of making you feel like if things did not work out he would help you find something that was to your benefit. That is a key quality in leaders that I see missing a lot today. The personal touch of reassuring those who work for you that even if it is not right for you, I will personally see to it that you get something that is right for you. He also never tried to take credit

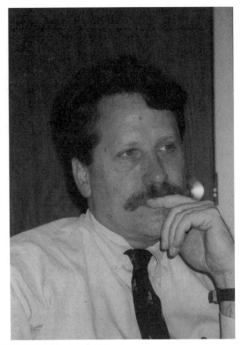

FIGURE 5. RMC during the interview.

for someone else's idea. Too many medical leaders today thrive on personal power and glory.

WCR: *Who in cardiology had an impact on you during your fellowship?*

RMC: *Bob Rosati*, who ran the Databank. He was a very bright person who had a lot of insight into how to look at data, but he had sort of gotten side tracked into looking at data before he had a chance to flex all his clinical muscles. He taught me a lot, but just as I finished the fellowship and the first year in the coronary care unit, he felt like he wanted to go back to clinical medicine so he decided not to run the Databank anymore. *Galen Wagner* also had a big influence. Galen had looked out for me during my third year of medical school. He is a person who has always had a different point of view about things and has persevered with the institution for many years. At the time, he was helping with the fellowship program.

WCR: *When Bob Rosati decided to go back into clinical medicine, you sort of captured the Cardiovascular Databank. Is that how that worked out?*

RMC: David Pryor was a colleague who was a year ahead of me, and we sort of split things up. David took over the leadership of the Databank and I took over the coronary care unit. The deal was that we would work together, that I would focus on the clinical enterprise and try to integrate that with the Databank, and he would do the more research-specific and administrative tasks, which he was very interested in. Joe Greenfield, when he called us into his office to talk about this, basically said, "This is an interesting idea of Dr. Stead's, but I don't think it is worth anything, ologists together in a cardiovascular center, and you would have oncology, which would include surgeons, internists, and radiation experts. You would have orthopedics and rheumatology working together. I think people function better when there is an alignment between what they do in their everyday lives and who their boss is. I would advocate more of a practice-oriented alignment for clinicians in medical schools. And that is beginning to happen at Duke and in a number of places, and I think that trend is going to continue and that is good.

Similarly, those who do basic research increasingly are not, or should not be, limited by departmental lines. If you are interested in a particular type of cellular signaling it should not matter whether you are a biochemist or a microbiologist by your initial training; this is really what you are interested in. Artificial departmental boundaries can be very restrictive. In clinical research, the methodology is common to all diseases, and I think there needs to be more of a focus on good methodology in clinical research. By the same token in a clinical practice plan, which is trying to stay alive in a very competitive world, if your salary is set by someone who is not primarily interested in the practice plan, for that part of your work that is clinical you have a misalignment, which can lead to a lot of difficulties. I think people who are primarily interested in clinical medicine have a lot in common and should hang together.

WCR: *You became editor of the* American Heart Journal *in July 1996? What are your plans for that journal? Are you enjoying it? How much time do you spend on it?*

RMC: I cannot say exactly how many hours I spend on it. *Dan Mark* has been a tremendous driving force and does much of the hands-on editorial work. He is very good at it. We have *Penny Hodgson* as managing editor; she has managed a lot of journals in the past. Our goal is to turn it into a journal devoted to clinical investigation. We are very interested in trying to stimulate research in clinical trials, health policy, and outcomes in cardiovascular disease. I don't think there is enough of that being done. I think we will begin to see some progress in that regard.

Although it is the *American Heart Journal*, we encourage non–US-based studies and are happy to give them the same priority as US-based studies. However, I believe that the potential in the USA to turn out good clinical research has not been met. We would like to be a stimulus to help make that happen.

WCR: *How much teaching do you do, Rob?*

RMC: When I was around the coronary care unit more, that was an everyday teaching experience. Now I spend only a month a year on that activity, and my teaching about individual patient care is less. I do a lot of teaching about clinical research. We have started a master's level course. We have had a course in biometry for over a decade, which has been very successful. We have recently reconfigured it to be very specifically oriented to clinical investigators. That has been an extremely good experience this year. In addition, we have a large number of fellows and junior faculty who spend time in the Clinical Research Institute. I spend a lot of time with them trying to help them sort through issues that they are dealing with as they do their research. Some of the most interesting teaching is continuing medical education. This is most fun when we are reviewing findings from a clinical study with the investigators who participated in the trial. The thirst for knowledge about how to improve practice is substantial in the practice community.

WCR: *You are involved in a lot of different professional activities? How do you do all this? Do you sleep? Maybe you could go through a typical day. What time do you wake up, what time do you get to the hospital, what time to you get home at night, what time do you go to bed?*

RMC: I usually get up around 6:00 A.M. or a little before, have a cup of coffee, read the paper. I go into work a little bit before 7:00 A.M. and start out the day by answering a bunch of e-mails I need to figure out what to do with. On a bad day, I will have meeting after meeting, talking about administrative issues or financial issues. On a good day, I will have a bunch of meetings where I am looking at data with people or going over a new study or thinking about an analysis. I am striving to have more of those good days and fewer of those bad days. I generally will have some kind of meeting or research conference during lunch. I will eat lunch on the fly and then work until between 6:00 and 7:00, usually closer to 7:00, and then head for home and have dinner with the family.

I have a very nice computer setup at home so I can sit at home and get my work done there. I used to have to go back to work at night, but I don't have to do that anymore unless I am on call for the coronary care unit.

WCR: *You finish dinner about 8:00? Are you much good to work after that now?*

RMC: It depends on the situation. There is always some kind of work I can do. That is a good time for me to review manuscripts or talk on the phone or answer e-mails. My best creative time is early in the morning, no doubt about that. If I want to work on something new, I will try to get up early in the morning and work on it, but early for me is 6:00 A.M. At night, by about 11:00, I have had it.

WCR: *What about weekends?*

RMC: I get most of my creative work done on weekends. I get up early in the mornings before the family does. I have a bunch of late sleepers in my family. I put on a pot of coffee, put on some classical music, and go to work. That is a very productive time for me. We are churchgoers on Sunday. We go to the Duke Chapel, which is a beautiful place for worship. It has a lot of traditions and a phenomenal choir and organ. Then the family will go out to lunch and review the situation for the week, whatever it may be.

WCR: *You have 3 children?*

RMC: Right.

WCR: *How old are they?*

RMC: Sharon will be 20 next week. She is at Elon College and doing great. She had her heart surgery at a young age and has done extremely well. I am really proud of her and she is enjoying college. Sam is 15.

He is a musician. He plays the electric guitar. He has a big concert tomorrow at school. He enjoys golf as I do. He is just a good guy to be around, and very bright. Tom, who is 13, is the athlete in the family. He plays on the basketball and soccer teams. He is very good with computers, much better than I am. I feel confident that each of the three will make a positive contribution to the world. It is fascinating how different each one is. We are enjoying the family life. My biggest regret is not spending more time at home when the children were little.

WCR: *You are trying to make up for that now?*

RMC: To some extent, as best I can. It is a struggle.

WCR: *Are you a pretty good daddy?*

RMC: You would have to ask them. I feel like I am. I think our children feel loved and cared for at home. Maybe that is something we don't see enough of these days.

WCR: *Do you take family vacations?*

RMC: We do. Lydia's parents have a beach house at Long Beach just south of Wilmington, North Carolina, and we go there every summer. We, at times, have gone to the mountains of North Carolina. We tend to spend a lot of time at home during the summer, even some vacation times just around the house.

WCR: *How much time do you take off a year, as a rule?*

RMC: Not enough. A couple of weeks.

WCR: *You obviously do a lot of traveling. These multicenter studies require meetings outside Durham; you go places to give talks, participate in educational meetings, visiting professorships. How much time are you gone?*

RMC: We just went over this on the homefront. I am gone about 60 days a year.

WCR: *So that is 60 nights away from home?*

RMC: If you average it out, it is probably a bit fewer than that because a lot of my trips these days are to Washington, and I can go back and forth in the same day. I am away probably about 40 nights a year (not including vacations). Face to face meetings are critical, and I really enjoy the relationships I have developed with clinicians and researchers around the world.

WCR: *For somebody who did not do any traveling when growing up you certainly have made up for it now. Are you going to be able to continue this pace for the next 20 years?*

RMC: I hope not. I hope that I will now settle into a lifestyle that is a little less frenetic but intellectually just as challenging. There are a lot of people in our research group now who are more skilled than I am at things I used to do myself. My goal is to have them develop even further, and I would like to focus on the background work to make the systems more effective.

WCR: *Do you have any ambitions to get other titles, seek other challenges? Would you look at opportunities outside of Duke?*

RMC: No, I think Duke is a great place to be right now. We are busy developing an integrated health system where we can actually try to use evidence as best we can to guide us to practice better medicine. This concept of evidence-based medicine is something people have talked about for a long time. We all know that much of managed care has failed because the financial pressures have been so great. Perhaps the time has come for academic health systems to step forward. The ability to have people who are cared for by your healthcare system over time, and to have information about how they are doing so that you can try to provide the best system of care is an exciting opportunity, and Duke is making an effort to be a leader in that category.

The support for the Clinical Research Institute has been great. The university built a new building that we are getting ready to move into. It will have the latest telecommunications and computer equipment. I might be able to cut out some more of my traveling just by being beamed out and talking with people that way. That would be greatly advantageous to me. I don't really enjoy sitting in airplanes and when I travel I generally don't get time to do things that would be fun. Travel for me is just a way to exchange knowledge and information.

The goal of the DCRI is to improve the practice of medicine and therefore the outcomes of patients through the use of quantitative principles. We hope to facilitate the chain of evidence from translational research to therapeutic trials to outcomes studies. I am grateful to our many collaborators and employees who have made the DCRI successful.

WCR: *Cardiology obviously has become a technology driven specialty. Do you think 12 years from now that there will be as many angioplasties and bypass operations done as there are today?*

RMC: If I had to bet, I would say there probably will be just as many, but it might not be much longer than 12 years that cardiology is going to be so technology driven. As we develop new ways to grow new blood vessels and use biological means to change pathophysiology, we may not need to do nearly as many invasive procedures as we are doing now. In 20 years, the procedures that we will be doing will be very different from today. I think they will be much more biologically oriented.

WCR: *Do we have too many physicians, too many medical schools? What should we be doing?*

RMC: I am not an expert on the number of medical schools, but it is my impression that we are probably training too many doctors right now. I don't think we are training too many healthcare providers. We need a somewhat different positioning of what people do. We are going to need an army of people to deal with the ravages of chronic disease and the aging population. It may not be that the technologically oriented physician is the right person to do that. If I had to bet, the best system would be one in which there is a physician who is trained not only in medicine, but also in management who is the leader of a squad of healthcare delivery people, including nurse practitioners, physician's assistants, and others, who provide most of the hands-on patient care. For example, in heart failure, we already know that you need a good diagnosis, and that needs to be done by someone who is highly trained, and serious effort needs to be put into the design of a treatment plan. But follow-up on that plan can be much more efficiently done by nurse practitioners and physician assistants than by physicians. We will need systems of calling people at home and interacting on the internet. A lot of patients come back once a month to the doctor's office for management of chronic medical problems and this could be done better by nonphysicians. I think the world will change substantially. The question of how many medical schools are needed may be supplanted by a question of how many places do we need for training and re-training of people who are providing medical care.

WCR: *Whether physicians or non-physicians?*

RMC: Right.

WCR: *It sounds to me like you and your wife Lydia have a very close relationship.*

RMC: We do and she has tolerated a lot over the years. She and I are sort of bookends. She frequently says I have no right brain and she doesn't like to use the left side of her brain as much. She really has an incredibly intuitive sense of what needs to be done, how to deal with people, how to notice small things and take care of them, and a tremendous sense of responsibility. I am burdened with often times thinking about the big picture, but missing really obvious things right in front of me that need to be dealt with, so she plays the key role in keeping me straight on those things. I'm often dealing with people who want to be important, and she keeps reminding me that most people are just trying to get through the day. She's been great for me. We are getting ready to celebrate 25 years of marriage and hopefully another 25 or so after that.

WCR: *Both of you were 21 when you got married?*

RMC: Right.

WCR: *Do you have hobbies?*

RMC: I like to play golf.

WCR: *Do you play much?*

RMC: I am playing a lot now. I am not getting any better, but I get out and hit maybe 3 or 4 times a week.

WCR: *Nine holes each time?*

RMC: I joined a golf club. It is not very crowded. I can walk 9 holes in an hour and a half. I can do that at the end of the day, particularly now that we have daylight savings time back. This year for the first time, I go to the driving range, which might improve my game. Both my boys play golf now.

WCR: *Do you have other hobbies?*

RMC: I like to listen to music, but I don't play an instrument. I love to watch basketball, but everybody in North Carolina loves to watch basketball. We've had season tickets to Cameron Indoor Stadium for Duke home games since 1982. I still like to get out and shoot baskets a little bit. I exercise. I finally got some equipment at home so I can ride the bicycle at home and watch television while doing it. I like to follow politics, which I find interesting.

WCR: *Do you do much reading outside of medicine?*

RMC: Not really at this point. I keep thinking I will go back to reading, but I am not doing a lot of reading outside of news magazines, newspapers, and medical stuff.

WCR: *It is pretty hard with your schedule. Who do you admire in cardiology or in medicine in general? You have mentioned Eugene Stead, Holly Smith. Who are medical heroes to you?*

RMC: I am not much of a hero worshiper. What I tend to see are attributes that people have that are admirable that are worth emulating. For example, Joe Greenfield had the personal touch of being able to meet with people and sort of know what they needed. One of our junior faculty once said he had calculated that working for Joe was worth $40,000 in salary. And most of us gave up more than that to work for Joe. Eric Topol's ability to see through data and draw a conclusion is tremendously effective. I aspire to be as good at that as he is. Gene Braunwald's ability to assimilate information and put it together in a way that can be explained to people is phenomenal. If you look at his career, the writing and lecturing he has done, it has transmitted a tremendous amount of information. I think Kanu Chatterjee's ability to see the patient and put things together has been great. If you asked me the one person who I just want to be like more than anybody else, I really would tend to see parts of people, but no single individual I would aspire to copy myself after.

WCR: *Do you think leadership is something neglected when committees get together to pick a chairman of this or that department in medical schools?*

RMC: I think leadership is hard to quantify, but it is something tangible when you look for it, and I don't think it is looked for enough. Of course, leadership, the ability to get people to follow, can be good or bad depending on what your underlying ideas are, but I think it is absolutely critical. We just saw *Primary Colors* over the weekend and that sort of quality that causes people to stop what they are doing and reorient themselves is an important attribute. I think that on balance, we need more emphasis on leadership because life is not a process. We need processes. We need methods of doing things, but the thing that draws the best out of people is when they figure out a way to do it differently and have the inspiration to accomplish a goal. We need more game plans—doing something for a purpose—not just processes. I think leaders bring out those qualities in people.

WCR: *When you are gone, when you cross the river, so to speak, what do you want to be remembered for?*

RMC: I don't really care if I am remembered, except by my family. I want my family to remember that I was a good person and that I had qualities that were passed on to them that they would want to emulate. Where I had qualities that were not admirable—like not coming home for dinner often enough or not paying attention to the little thing that a child did—I would hope to have recognized my deficiency and discussed it with the family so that they would try to do better than I did. I think that in the end these are the only things that really matter in terms of memory.

On a more general level, it is not important that I am remembered as a person, but I would hope to leave behind a better (I have gotten very focused on this issue) method of quantifying medicine so that we can know what we are doing when we treat people. I think if I can leave behind an improvement in the system of evidence-based medicine, I will feel I have done what I was intended to do. It really does not matter to me that I am the one who is remembered. But it does matter to me that the medical care system is better and that it works and that people are closer to getting what they need in the way of medical care. No matter what we do in medical care, if we get people to live longer or not be as ill, they can do something that is enjoyable and worthwhile in the time they have. The medical part is only a part of the equation. I think creating the circumstances to give others opportunity is very good use of one's time.

WCR: *Is there anything you would like to discuss that we haven't? Anything you would like to leave to your grandchildren to read about 25 years from now?*

RMC: I think probably that last part I said is what the grandchildren ought to listen to. You have pretty well exhausted me and I think I said pretty much what is on my mind.

WCR: *Rob, thank you. It has really been a treat. Thank you for sharing your thoughts and your career with the AJC readers.*

RMC PUBLICATIONS SELECTED BY HIM AS HIS BEST

1. Califf RM, Burks JM, Behar VS, Margolis JR, Wagner GS. Relationships among ventricular arrhythmias, coronary artery disease, and angiographic and electrocardiographic indicators of myocardial fibrosis. *Circulation* 1978;57:725–732.

3. Califf RM, McKinnis RA, Burks J, Lee KL, Harrell FE Jr, Behar VS, Pryor DB, Wagner GS, Rosati RA. Prognostic implications of ventricular arrhythmias during 24 hour ambulatory monitoring in patients undergoing cardiac catheterization for coronary artery disease. *Am J Cardiol* 1982;50:23–31.

7. Califf RM, McKinnis RA, McNeer JF, Harrell FE Jr, Lee KL, Pryor DB, Waugh RA, Harris PJ, Rosati RA, Wagner GS. Prognostic value of ventricular arrhythmias associated with treadmill exercise testing in patients studied with cardiac catheterization for suspected ischemic heart disease. *J Am Coll Cardiol* 1983;2:1060–1067.

8. Califf RM, Tomabechi Y, Lee KL, Phillips H, Pryor DB, Harrell FE Jr, Harris PJ, Peter RH, Behar VS, Kong Y, Rosati RA. Outcome in one-vessel coronary artery disease. *Circulation* 1983;67:283–290.

11. Pryor DB, Harrell FE Jr, Lee KL, Califf RM, Rosati RA. An improving prognosis over time in medically treated patients with coronary artery disease. *Am J Cardiol* 1983;52:444–448.

13. Roberts KB, Califf RM, Harrell FE Jr, Lee KL, Pryor DB, Rosati RA. The prognosis for patients with new-onset angina who have undergone cardiac catheterization. *Circulation* 1983;68:970–978.

19. Hlatky MA, Lee KL, Harrell FE Jr, Califf RM, Pryor DB, Mark DB, Rosati RA. Tying clinical research to patient care by use of an observational database. *Statistics in Medicine* 1984;3:375–384.

21. Komrad MS, Coffey CE, Coffey KS, McKinnis R, Massey EW, Califf RM. Myocardial infarction and stroke. *Neurology* 1984;34:1403–1409.

27. Califf RM, Hlatky MA, Mark DB, Lee KL, Harrell FE Jr, Rosati RA, Pryor DB. Randomized trials of coronary artery bypass surgery: impact on clinical practice at Duke University Medical Center. *Circulation* 1985;72:136–144.

28. Califf RM, Phillips HR III, Hindman MC, Mark DB, Lee KL, Behar VS, Johnson RA, Pryor DB, Rosati RA, Wagner GS, Harrell FE Jr. Prognostic value of a coronary artery jeopardy score. *J Am Coll Cardiol* 1985;5:1055–1063.

35. Hlatky MA, Haney T, Barefoot JC, Califf RM, Mark DB, Pryor DB, Williams RB. Medical, psychological and social correlates of work disability among men with coronary artery disease. *Am J Cardiol* 1986;58:911–915.

37. Lee KL, Pryor DB, Harrell FE Jr, Califf RM, Behar VS, Floyd WL, Morris JJ, Waugh RA, Whalen RE, Rosati RA. Predicting outcome in coronary disease: statistical models versus expert clinicians. *Am J Med* 1986;80:553–560.

38. Papanicolaou MN, Califf RM, Hlatky MA, McKinnis RA, Harrell FE Jr, Mark DB, McCants B, Rosati RA, Lee KL, Pryor DB. Prognostic implications of angiographically normal and insignificantly narrowed coronary arteries. *Am J Cardiol* 1986;58:1181–1187.

41. Blackshear JL, O'Callaghan WG, Califf RM. Medical approaches to prevention of restenosis after coronary angioplasty. *J Am Coll Cardiol* 1987;9:834–848.

44. Mark DB, Hlatky MA, Harrell FE Jr, Lee KL, Califf RM, Pryor DB. Exercise treadmill score for predicting prognosis in coronary artery disease. *Ann Intern Med* 1987;106:793–800.

46. Pryor DB, Harrell FE, Rankin JS, Lee KL, Muhlbaier LH, Oldham HN, Hlatky MA, Mark DB, Reves JG, Califf RM. The changing survival benefits of coronary revascularization over time. *Circulation* 1987;76:13–21.

48. Topol EJ, Califf RM, George BS, Kereiakes DJ, Abbottsmith CW, Candela RJ, Lee KL, Pitt B, Stack RS, O'Neill WW, and the Thrombolysis and Angioplasty in Myocardial Infarction Study Group. A randomized trial of immediate versus delayed elective angioplasty after intravenous tissue plasminogen activator in acute myocardial infarction. *N Engl J Med* 1987;317:581–588.

53. Bounous EP, Mark DB, Pollock BG, Hlatky MA, Harrell FE Jr, Lee KL, Rankin JS, Wechsler AS, Pryor DB, Califf RM. Surgical survival benefits for coronary disease in patients with left ventricular dysfunction. *Circulation* 1988;78:151–157.

54. Califf RM, Harrell FE Jr, Lee KL, Rankin JS, Mark DB, Hlatky MA, Muhlbaier LH, Wechsler AS, Jones RH, Oldham HN Jr, Pryor DB. Changing efficacy of coronary revascularization: implications for patient selection. *Circulation* 1988;78:185–191.

56. Califf RM, Mark DB, Harrell FE Jr, Hlatky MA, Lee KL, Rosati RA, Pryor DB. Importance of clinical measures of ischemia in the prognosis of patients with documented coronary artery disease. *J Am Coll Cardiol* 1988;11:20–26.

57. Califf RM, O'Neill W, Stack RS, Aronson L, Mark DB, Mantell S, George BS, Candela RJ, Kereiakes DJ, Abbottsmith C, Topol EJ, and TAMI Study Group. Failure of simple clinical measurements to predict perfusion status after intravenous thrombolysis. *Ann Intern Med* 1988;108:658–662.

58. Califf RM, Topol EJ, George BS, Boswick JM, Abbottsmith C, Sigmon KN, Candela R, Masek R, Kereiakes D, O'Neill WW, Stack RS, Stump D, and the TAMI Study Group. Hemorrhagic complications associated with the use of intravenous tissue plasminogen activator in treatment of acute myocardial infarction. *Am J Med* 1988;85:353–359.

59. Califf RM, Topol EJ, George BS, Boswick JM, Lee KL, Stump D, Dillon J, Abbottsmith C, Candela RJ, Kereiakes DJ, O'Neill WW, Stack RS, and the TAMI Study Group. Characteristics and outcome of patients in whom reperfusion with intravenous tissue-type plasminogen activator fails: results of the thrombolysis and angioplasty in myocardial infarction (TAMI) I trial. *Circulation* 1988; 77:1090–1099.

62. Hlatky MA, Califf RM, Harrell FE Jr, Lee KL, Mark DB, Pryor DB. Comparison of predictions based on observational data with the results of randomized controlled clinical trials of coronary artery bypass surgery. *J Am Coll Cardiol* 1988;11:237–245.

70. Stack RS, Califf RM, Phillips HR, Pryor DB, Quigley PJ, Bauman RP, Tcheng JE, Greenfield JC Jr. Interventional cardiac catheterization at Duke Medical Center. *Am J Cardiol* 1988;62:3F–24F.

71. Stack RS, O'Connor CM, Mark DB, Hinohara T, Phillips HR, Lee MM, Ramirez NM, O'Callaghan WG, Simonton CA, Carlson EB, Morris KG, Behar VS, Kong Y, Peter RH, Califf RM. Coronary perfusion during acute myocardial infarction with a combined therapy of coronary angioplasty and high-dose intravenous streptokinase. *Circulation* 1988;77:151–161.

78. Califf RM, Harrell FE Jr, Lee KL, Rankin JS, Hlatky MA, Mark DB, Jones RH, Muhlbaier LH, Oldham HN, Pryor DB. The evolution of medical and surgical therapy for coronary artery disease: a 15-year perspective. *JAMA* 1989; 261:2077–2086.

82. Gersh BJ, Califf RM, Loop FD, Akins CW, Pryor DB, Takaro TC. Coronary bypass surgery in chronic stable angina. *Circulation* 1989;79:46–59.

84. Hlatky MA, Boineau RE, Higginbotham MB, Lee KL, Mark DB, Califf RM, Cobb FR, Pryor DB. A brief self-administered questionnaire to determine functional capacity (the Duke Activity Status Index). *Am J Cardiol* 1989;64:651–654.

86. Kereiakes DJ, Topol EJ, George BS, Abbottsmith CW, Stack RS, Candela RJ, O'Neill WW, Anderson LC, Califf RM, and the TAMI Study Group. Favorable early and long-term prognosis following coronary bypass surgery therapy for myocardial infarction: results of a multicenter trial. *Am Heart J* 1989;118:199–207.

92. Stump DC, Califf RM, Topol EJ, Sigmon K, Thornton D, Masek R, Anderson L, Collen D, and the TAMI Study Group. Pharmacodynamics of thrombolysis with recombinant tissue-type plasminogen activator: correlation with characteristics of and clinical outcomes in patients with acute myocardial infarction. *Circulation* 1989;80:1222–1230.

94. Topol EJ, George BS, Kereiakes DJ, Stump DC, Candela RJ, Abbottsmith CW, Aronson L, Pickel A, Boswick JM, Lee KL, Ellis SG, Califf RM, and the TAMI Study Group. A randomized controlled trial of intravenous tissue plasminogen activator and early intravenous heparin in acute myocardial infarction. *Circulation* 1989;79:281–286.

97. Abbottsmith CW, Topol EJ, George BS, Stack RS, Kereiakes DJ, Candela RJ, Anderson LC, Harrelson L, Califf RM. Fate of patients with acute myocardial infarction with patency of the infarct-related vessel achieved with successful thrombolysis versus rescue angioplasty. *J Am Coll Cardiol* 1990;16:770–778.

99. Bengston JR, Mark DB, Honan MB, Rendall DS, Hinohara T, Stack RS, Hlatky MA, Califf RM, Lee KL, Pryor DB. Detection of restenosis after elective percutaneous transluminal coronary angioplasty using the exercise treadmill test. *Am J Cardiol* 1990;65:28–34.
103. Hlatky MA, Califf RM, Harrell FE Jr, Lee KL, Mark DB, Muhlbaier LH, Pryor DB. Clinical judgement and therapeutic decision making. *J Am Coll Cardiol* 1990;15:1–14.
104. Hlatky MA, Lipscomb J, Nelson C, Califf RM, Pryor D, Wallace AG, Mark DB. Resource use and cost of initial coronary revascularization: coronary angioplasty versus coronary bypass surgery. *Circulation* 1990;82:208–213.
105. Honan MB, Harrell FE Jr, Reimer KA, Califf RM, Mark DB, Pryor DB, Hlatky MA. Cardiac rupture, mortality, and the timing of thrombolytic therapy: a meta-analysis. *J Am Coll Cardiol* 1990;16:359–367.
112. Ohman EM, Califf RM, Topol EJ, Candela R, Abbottsmith C, Ellis S, Sigmon KN, Kereiakes D, George B, Stack R, and the TAMI Study Group. Consequences of reocclusion after successful reperfusion therapy in acute myocardial infarction. *Circulation* 1990;82:781–791.
117. Ohman EM, Califf RM, George BS, Quigley PJ, Kereiakes DJ, Harrelson-Woodlief L, Candela RJ, Flanagan C, Stack RS, Topol EJ. The use of intraaortic balloon pumping as an adjunct to reperfusion therapy in acute myocardial infarction. *Am Heart J* 1991;121:895–901.
118. Califf RM, Topol EJ, Stack RS, Ellis SG, George BS, Kereiakes DJ, Samaha JK, Worley SJ, Anderson JL, Harrelson-Woodlief L, Wall TC, Phillips HR, Abbottsmith CW, Candela RJ, Flanagan WH, Sasahara AA, Mantell SJ, Lee KL. Evaluation of combination thrombolytic therapy and timing of cardiac catheterization in acute myocardial infarction: results of thrombolysis and angioplasty in myocardial infarction-phase 5 randomized trial. *Circulation* 1991;83:1543–1556.
121. Kereiakes DJ, Topol EJ, George BS, Stack RS, Abbottsmith CW, Ellis S, Candela RJ, Harrelson L, Martin LH, Califf RM, and the TAMI Study Group. Myocardial infarction with minimal coronary atherosclerosis in the era of thrombolytic reperfusion. *J Am Coll Cardiol* 1991;17:304–312.
122. Kirklin JW, Akins CW, Blackstone EH, Booth DC, Califf RM, Cohen LS, Hall RJ, Harrell FE Jr, Kouchoukos NT, McCallister BD, Naftel DC, Parker JO, Shelden WC, Smith HC, Wechsler AS, Williams JF Jr. Guidelines and indications for coronary artery bypass graft surgery: a report of the American College of Cardiology/American Heart Association task force on assessment of diagnostic and therapeutic cardiovascular procedures (subcommittee on coronary artery bypass graft surgery). *J Am Coll Cardiol* 191;17:543–589.
123. Mark DB, Shaw L, Harrell FE Jr, Hlatky MA, Lee KL, Bengtson JR, McCants CB, Califf RM, Pryor DB. Prognostic value of a treadmill exercise score in outpatients with suspected coronary artery disease. *N Engl J Med* 1991;325: 849–853.
128. Sane DC, Stump DC, Topol EJ, Sigmon KN, Clair WK, Kereiakes DJ, George BS, Stoddard MF, Bates ER, Stack RS, Califf RM, and The Thrombolysis and Angioplasty in Myocardial Infarction Study Group. Racial differences in responses to thrombolytic therapy with recombinant tissue-type plasminogen activator, increased fibrin(ogen)olysis in blacks. *Circulation* 1991;83:170–175.
130. Smith LR, Harrell FE Jr, Rankin JS, Califf RM, Pryor DB, Muhlbaier LH, Lee KL, Mark DB, Jones RH, Oldham HN, Glower DD, Reves JG, Sabiston DC Jr. Determinants of early versus late cardiac death in patients undergoing coronary artery bypass graft surgery. *Circulation* 1991;84:245–253.
134. Bengtson JR, Kaplan AJ, Pieper KS, Wildermann NM, Mark DB, Pryor DB, Phillips HR III, Califf RM. Prognosis in cardiogenic shock after acute myocardial infarction in the interventional era. *J Am Coll Cardiol* 1992;20:1482–1489.
135. Bickell NA, Pieper KS, Lee KL, Mark DB, Glower DD, Pryor DB, Califf RM. Referral patterns for coronary artery disease treatment: gender bias or good clinical judgement? *Ann Intern Med* 1992;116:791–799.
138. Mark DB, Lam LC, Lee KL, Clapp-Channing NE, Williams RB, Pryor DB, Califf RM, Hlatky MA. Identification of patients with coronary disease at high risk for loss of employment: a prospective validation study. *Circulation* 1992; 86:1485–1494.
142. Pryor DB, Shaw L, McCants CB, Lee KL, Mark DB, Harrell FE, Muhlbaier LH, Califf RM. Value of the history and physical in identifying patient's at increased risk for coronary artery disease. *Ann Intern Med* 1993;118:81–90.
143. Topol EJ, Califf RM, Vandormael M, Grinds CL, George BS, Sanz ML, Wall TC, O'Brien M, Schwaiger M, Aguirre FV, Young S, Popma JJ, Sigmon KN, Lee KL, Ellis SG, and the Thrombolysis and Angioplasty in Myocardial Infarctions-6 Study Group. A randomized trial of late reperfusion therapy for acute myocardial infarction. *Circulation* 1992;85:2090–2099.
144. Williams RB, Barefoot JC, Califf RM, Saunders WB, Peterson BL, Haney TL, Pryor DB, Hlatky MA, Siegler IC, Mark DB. Prognostic importance of social and economic resources among medically treated patients with angiographically documented coronary artery disease. *JAMA* 1992;267:520–524.
145. Chapman GD, Ohman EM, Topol EJ, Candela RJ, Kereiakes DJ, Samaha J, Berrios E, Pieper KS, Young SY, Califf RM. Minimizing the risk of inappropriately administering thrombolytic therapy (thrombolysis and angioplasty in myocardial infarction [TAMI] study group). *Am J Cardiol* 1993;71:783–787.
148. Granger CB, Califf RM, Young S, Candela R, Samaha J, Worley S, Kereiakes DJ, Topol EJ, and the TAMI Study Group. Outcomes of patients with diabetes mellitus and acute myocardial infarction treated with thrombolytic therapy. *J Am Coll Cardiol* 1993;21:920–925.
155. O'Connor CM, Meese R, Carney R, Smith J, Conn E, Burks J, Hartman C, Roark S, Shadoff N, Heard M III, Mittler B, Collins G, Navetta F, Leimberger J, Lee K, Califf RM, for the DUCCS Group. A randomized trial of intravenous heparin in conjunction with anistreplase (Anisoylated Plasminogen Streptokinase Activator Complex) in acute myocardial infarction: The Duke University Clinical Cardiology Study (DUCCS) Group. *J Am Coll Cardiol* 1994;23:11–18.
160. Tenaglia AM, Fortin DF, Frid DJ, Nelson CL, Gardner L, Miller M, Navetta FI, Smith JE, Tcheng JE, Califf RM, Stack RS. Predicting the risk of abrupt vessel closure after angioplasty in an individual patient. *J Am Coll Cardiol* 1994;24:1004–1011.
165. Krucoff MW, Croll MA, Pope JE, Granger CB, O'Connor CM, Sigmon KN, Wagner BL, Ryan JA, Lee KL, Kereiakes DJ, Samaha JK, Worley SJ, Ellis SG, Wall TC, Topol EJ, Califf RM, for the TAMI 7 Study Group. Continuous 12-lead ST segment recovery analysis in the TAMI 7 Study: performance of a noninvasive method for real time detection of failed myocardial reperfusion. *Circulation* 1993;88:437–446.
167. Newby KL, Rutsch WR, Califf RM, Simoons ML, Aylward PE, Armstrong PW, Woodlief LH, Lee KL, Topol EJ, Van de Werf F, for the GUSTO-I Investigators. Time from symptom onset to treatment in the outcomes after thrombolytic therapy. *J Am Coll Cardiol* 1996;27:1646–1655.
168. Simoons ML, Maggioni AP, Knatterud G, Leimberger J, de Jaegere P, Van Domburg R, Boersma E, Grazia M, Califf RM, Schroder R, Braunwald E. Risk factors for intracranial hemorrhage during thrombolytic therapy. *Lancet* 1993; 342:1523–1528.
170. Tenaglia AN, Califf RM, Candela RJ, Kereiakes DJ, Berrios E, Young SY, Stack RD, Topol EJ. Thrombolytic therapy in patients requiring cardiopulmonary resuscitation. *Am J Cardiol* 1991;68:1015–1019.
172. Mark DB, Nelson CL, Califf RM, Harrell FE Jr, Lee KL, Jones RH, Fortin DF, Stack RS, Glower DD, Smith LR, DeLong ER, Smith PK, Reves JG, Jollis JG, Tcheng JE, Muhlbaier LH, Lower JE, Phillips HR, Pryor DB. Continuing evolution of therapy for coronary artery disease: initial results from the era of coronary angioplasty. *Circulation* 1994;89:2015–2025.
174. Ohman EM, Topol EJ, Califf RM, Bates ER, Ellis SG, Kereiakes DJ, George BS, Samaha JK, Kline E, Sigmon KN, Stack RS, and the Thrombolysis Angioplasty in Myocardial Infarction Study Group. An analysis of the cause of early mortality after administration of thrombolytic therapy. *Coron Art Dis* 1993;4:957–964.
176. Granger CB, Hirsh J, Califf RM, Col J, White HD, Betriu A, Woodlief LH, Lee KL, Bovill EG, Simes RJ, Topol EJ, for the GUSTO-I Trial. Activated partial thromboplastin time and outcome after thrombolytic therapy for acute myocardial infarction: results from the GUSTO-I Trial. *Circulation* 1996;93:870–878.
183. Gore JM, Granger CB, Sloan MA, Van de Werf F, Weaver WD, Califf RM, White HD, Barbash GI, Simoons ML, Aylward PE, Topol EJ, for the GUSTO Investigators. Stroke after thrombolysis: mortality and functional outcomes in the GUSTO-I Trial. *Circulation* 1995;92:2811–2818.
184. Knaus WA, Harrell FE, Lynn J, Goldman L, Phillips RS, Connors AF Jr, Dawson NV, Fulkerson WJ, Califf RM, Desbiens N, Layde P, Oye PK, Bellamy PE, Hakim RB, Wagner DP, for the SUPPORT Investigators. The SUPPORT prognostic model: objective estimates of survival for seriously ill hospitalized adults. *Ann Intern Med* 1995;122:191–203.
186. GUSTO IIa Investigators. Randomized trial of intravenous heparin versus recombinant hirudin for acute coronary syndromes. *Circulation* 1994;90:1631–1637.
191. Califf RM, Adams K, McKenna W, Gheorghiade M, Uretsky B, McNulty SE, Darius H, Schulman KA, Zannad F, Handberg-Thurmond E, Harrell FE Jr, Wheeler W, Soler-Soler J, Swedburg K. A randomized controlled trial of epoprostenol therapy for severe congestive heart failure: the Flolan international randomized survival trial (FIRST). *Am Heart J* 1997;134:44–54.
196. O'Neill WW, Brodie B, Ivanhoe R, Knopf W, Taylor G, O'Keefe J, Weintraub R, Sickinger B, Berdan LG, Tcheng JE, Woodlief LH, Strzelecki M, Hartzler G, Califf RM. Primary coronary angioplasty for acute myocardial infarction (the primary angioplasty registry). *Am J Cardiol* 1994;73:627–634.
201. Topol EJ, Califf RM, Weisman HF, Ellis SG, Tcheng JE, Worley S, Ivanhoe R, George BS, Fintel D, Weston M, Sigmon K, Anderson KM, Lee KL, Willerson JT, for the EPIC Investigators. Randomized trial of coronary intervention with antibody against platelet IIb/IIa integrin for reduction of clinical restenosis: results at 6 months. *Lancet* 1994;343:881–886.
204. Tcheng JE, Jackman JD, Nelson CL, Gardner LH, Smith LR, Rankin JS, Califf RM, Stack RS. Outcome of patients sustaining acute ischemic mitral regurgitation during myocardial infarction. *Ann Intern Med* 1992;117:18–24.
215. Granger CG, Miller JM, Bovill EG, Gruber A, Tracy RP, Krucoff MW, Green C, Berrios E, Harrington RA, Ohman EM, Califf RM. Rebound increase in thrombin generation and activity after cessation of intravenous heparin in patients with acute coronary syndromes. *Circulation* 1995;91:1929–1935.
219. Califf RM, Fortin DF, Frid DJ, Harlan WR, Bengston M Jr, Nelson CL, Tcheng JE, Mark DB, Stack RS. Restenosis after coronary angioplasty: an overview. *J Am Coll Cardiol* 1991;17:2B–13B.
220. Mark DB, Shaw L, DeLong ER, Califf RM, Pryor DB. Influence of gender on referral to cardiac catheterization: physician bias or appropriate management. *N Engl J Med* 1994;33:1101–1106.
221. Hillegass WB, Jollis JG, Granger CB, Ohman EM, Califf RM, Mark DB. Intracranial hemorrhage risk and new thrombolytic therapies in acute myocardial infarction. *Am J Cardiol* 1994;73:444–449.
225. The GUSTO Investigators. An international randomized trial comparing 4 thrombolytic regimens consisting of tissue plasminogen activator, streptokinase, or both for acute myocardial infarction. *N Engl J Med* 1993;329:673–682.
229. The EPIC Investigators. Use of a monoclonal antibody directed against the platelet-glycoprotein IIb/IIa receptor in high risk coronary angioplasty. *N Engl J Med* 1994;330:956–961.

235. The GUSTO Angiographic Investigators. The effects of tissue plasminogen activator, streptokinase, or both on coronary-artery patency, ventricular function, and survival after acute myocardial infarction. *N Engl J Med* 1993;329:1615–1622.

242. White HD, Barbash GI, Califf RM, Simes RJ, Granger CB, Weaver WD, Kleiman NS, Aylward PE, Gore JM, Vahanian A, Lee KL, Ross AM, Topol EJ, for the GUSTO-I Investigators. Age and outcome with contemporary thrombolytic therapy: results from the GUSTO-I Trial. *Circulation* 1996;94:1826–1833.

244. Mark DB, Talley JD, Topol EJ, Bowman L, Lam LC, Anderson KM, Jollis JG, Cleman MW, Lee KL, Aversano T, Untereker WJ, Davidson-Ray L, Califf RM, for the EPIC Investigators. Economic assessment of platelet glycoprotein IIb/IIa inhibition for prevention of ischemic complications of high-risk coronary angioplasty. *Circulation* 1996;94:629–635.

245. Wall TC, Califf RM, Blankenship J, Talley JD, Tannenbaum M, Schwaiger M, Gacioch G, Cohen MD, Sanz M, Leimberger JD, Topol EJ, and the TAMI-9 Research Group. Intravenous fluosol in the treatment of acute myocardial infarction: results of the thrombolysis and angioplasty in myocardial infarction 9 trial. *Circulation* 1994;90:114–120.

249. O'Connor CM, Meese RB, McNulty S, Lucas KD, Carney RJ, LeBoeuf RM, Maddox W, Bethea CF, Shadoff N, Trahey TF, Heinsimer JA, Burks JM, O'Donnell G, Krucoff MW, Califf RM, for the DUCCS-II Investigators. A randomized factorial trial of reperfusion strategies and aspirin dosing in acute myocardial infarction. *Am J Cardiol* 1996;77:791–797.

250. Mark DB, Naylor CD, Hlatky MA, Califf RM, Topol EJ, Granger CB, Knight JD, Nelson CL, Lee KL, Clapp-Channing NE, Sutherland W, Pilote L, Armstrong PW. Use of medical resources and quality of life outcomes after acute myocardial infarction in Canada versus the United States. *N Engl J Med* 1994; 331:1130–1135.

252. Granger CB, White HD, Bates ER, Ohman EM, Califf RM. A pooled analysis of coronary arterial patency and left ventricular function after intravenous thrombolysis for acute myocardial infarction. *Am J Cardiol* 1994;74:1220–1228.

256. Kleiman NS, White HD, Ohman M, Ross AM, Woodlief LH, Califf RM, Holmes DR Jr, Bates E, Pfisterer M, Vahanian A, Topol EJ, for the GUSTO Investigators. Mortality within 24 hours of thrombolysis for myocardial infarction: the importance of early reperfusion. *Circulation* 1994;90:2658–2665.

257. Tcheng JE, Harrington RA, Kottke-Marchant K, Kleiman NS, Ellis SG, Kereiakes DJ, Mick MJ, Navetta FI, Smith JE, Worley SJ, Miller JA, Joseph DM, Sigmon KN, Kitt MM, du Mée CP, Califf RM, Topol EJ, for the IMPACT Investigators. Multicenter, randomized, double-blind, placebo-controlled trial of the platelet integrin glycoprotein IIb/IIa blocker integrelin in elective coronary intervention. *Circulation* 1995;91:2151–2157.

261. Lee KL, Woodlief LH, Topol EJ, Weaver WD, Betriu A, Col J, Simoons M, Aylward P, Van de Werf F, Califf RM, for the GUSTO-I Investigators. Predictors of 30-day mortality in the era of reperfusion for acute myocardial infarction: results from an international trial of 41,021 patients. *Circulation* 1995;91:1659–1668.

266. Simes RJ, Holmes DR Jr, White HD, Rutsch WR, Vahanian A, Simoons ML, Morris D, Betriu A, Califf RM, Topol EJ, Ross AM, for the GUSTO Investigators. The link between the angiographic substudy and mortality outcomes in a large randomized trial of myocardial reperfusion: the importance of early and complete infarct vessel reperfusion. *Circulation* 1995;91:1923–1928.

270. Califf RM, Woodlief L, Harrell FE Jr, Lee KL, White HD, Guerci A, Barbash GI, Simes RJ, Wever WD, Simoons ML, Topol EJ, for the GUSTO-I Investigators. Selection of thrombolytic therapy for individual patients: development of a clinical model. *Am Heart J* 1997;133:630–639.

272. Holmes DR Jr, Topol EJ, Califf RM, Leya F, Berger PB, Talley JD III, Kellett MA Jr, Shani J, Gottlieb RS, Whitlow PL, Adelman AG, Pinderton CA, Lee KL, Pieper K, Keeler GP, Ellis SG, for the CAVEAT-II Investigators. A multicenter, randomized trial of coronary angioplasty versus directional atherectomy for patients with saphenous vein bypass graft lesions. *Circulation* 1995;91: 1966–1974.

280. Newby LK, Califf RM, Guerci A, Weaver WD, Col J, Horgan JH, Mark DB, Stebbins A, Van de Werf F, Gore JM, Topol EJ, for the GUSTO Investigators. Early discharge in the thrombolytic era: an analysis of criteria for uncomplicated infarction from the global utilization of streptokinase and t-PA for occluded coronary arteries (GUSTO) trial. *J Am Coll Cardiol* 1996;27:625–632.

284. Mark DB, Hlatky MA, Califf RM, Naylor CD, Lee KL, Armstrong PW, Barbash G, White H, Simoons ML, Nelson CL, Clapp-Channing N, Knight JD, Harrell FE Jr, Sims E, Topol EJ. Cost effectiveness of thrombolytic therapy with tissue plasminogen activator as compared with streptokinase for acute myocardial infarction. *N Engl J Med* 1995;332:1418–1424; erratum appears in *N Engl J Med* 1995;333:267.

285. Mahaffey KW, Granger CB, Collins R, O'Connor CM, Ohman EM, Bleich SD, Col JJ, Califf RM. Overview of randomized trials of intravenous heparin in patients with acute myocardial infarction treated with thrombolytic therapy. *Am J Cardiol* 1996;77:551–556.

291. Califf RM, Karnash Sl, Woodlief LH. Developing systems for cost-effective auditing of clinical trials. *Control Clin Trials* 1997;18:651–660.

292. Puma JA, Sketch MH Jr, Tcheng JE, Gardner LH, Nelson CL, Phillips HR, Stack RS, Califf RM. Percutaneous revascularization of chronic coronary occlusions, an overview. *J Am Coll Cardiol* 1995;26:1–11.

297. Betriu A, Califf RM, Bosch X, Guerci A, Stebbins AL, Barbagelata A, Aylward PE, Vahanian A, Van de Werf F, Topol EJ, for the GUSTO-I Investi-

gators. Recurrent ischemia after thrombolysis: importance of associated clinical findings. *J Am Coll Cardiol* 1998;31:94–102.

301. Selker HP, Griffith JL, Beshansky JR, Schmid CH, Califf RM, D'Agostino RB, Laks MM, Lee KL, Maynard C, Selvester RH, Wagner GS, Weaver WD. Patient-specific predictions of outcomes in myocardial infarction for real-time emergency use: the thrombolytic predictive instrument (TPI). *Ann Intern Med* 1997;127:538–556 with corresponding editorial.

304. The SUPPORT Investigators. A controlled trial to improve care for seriously ill hospitalized patients: the study to understand prognoses and preferences for outcomes and risks of treatments (SUPPORT). *JAMA* 1995;274:1591–1598.

306. Peterson ED, Shaw LK, DeLong ER, Pryor DB, Califf RM, Mark DB. Racial variation in the use of cardiac revascularization procedures: are the differences real? Do they matter? *N Engl J Med* 1997;336:480–486.

307. Puma JA, Sketch MH Jr, Tcheng JE, Gardner LH, Nelson CL, Phillips HR, Stack RS, Califf RM. The natural history of single-vessel chronic coronary occlusion: a 25 year perspective. *Am Heart J* 1997;133:393–399.

310. Pilote L, Sapp S, Miller DP, Mark DB, Weaver DB, Gore JM, Armstrong PW, Ohman EM, Califf RM, Topol EJ, for the GUSTO Investigators. Regional variation across the United States in the management of acute myocardial infarction. *N Engl J Med* 1995;333:565–572.

315. Ohman EM, Armstrong PW, Christenson RH, Granger CB, Katus HA, Hamm CW, O'Hanesian MA, Wagner GS, Kleiman NS, Harrell FE Jr, Califf RM, Topol EJ, for the GUSTO-IIa Investigators. Risk stratification with admission cardiac troponin T levels in acute myocardial infarction. *N Engl J Med* 1996;335:1333–1341.

316. Califf RM, White HD, Van de Werf F, Sadowski Z, Armstrong PW, Vahanian A, Simoons ML, Simes J, Lee KL, Topol EJ, for the GUSTO-I Investigators. One-year results from the global utilization of streptokinase and TPA for occluded coronary arteries (GUSTO-I) Trial. *Circulation* 1996;94:1233–1238.

322. Fuster V, Califf RM, Chesebro JH, Cohen M, Comp PC, Gheorghiade M, Hall J, Halperin J, Khan S, Kopecky S, and the Coumadin Aspirin Reinforcement Study (CARS) Investigators. Randomized double-blind trial of fixed low-dose warfarin with aspirin after myocardial infarction. *Lancet* 1997;350:389–396.

327. Connors AF Jr, Speroff T, Dawson NV, Thomas C, Harrell FE Jr, Wagner D, Desbiens N, Goldman L, Wu AW, Califf RM, Fulkerson WJ, Vidaillet H, Broste S, Bellamy P, Lynn J, Knaus WA, for the SUPPORT Investigators. The effectiveness of right heart catheterization in the initial care of critically ill patients. *JAMA* 1996;276:889–897.

329. Berkowitz SD, Granger CG, Pieper KS, Lee KL, Gore JM, Simoons M, Armstrong PW, Topol EJ, Califf RM, for the Global Utilization of Streptokinase and Tissue Plasminogen Activator for Occluded Coronary Arteries (GUSTO-I) Investigators. Incidence and predictors of bleeding after contemporary thrombolytic therapy for myocardial infarction. *Circulation* 1997;95:2508–2516.

331. Pilote L, Miller DP, Califf RM, Rao JS, Weaver WD, Topol EJ. Determinants of the use of coronary angiography and revascularization after thrombolysis for acute myocardial infarction in the United States. *N Engl J Med* 1996;335: 1198–1205.

335. Hathaway WR, Peterson ED, Wagner GS, Granger CB, Zabel KM, Pieper KS, Clark KA, Woodlief LH, Califf RM, for the GUSTO-I Investigators. Prognostic significance of the initial electrocardiogram in patients with acute myocardial infarction? *JAMA* 1998;279:387–391.

337. Topol EJ, Califf RM, de Werf F, Simoons M, Hampton J, Lee KL, White H, Simes J, Armstrong PW, for the Virtual Coordinating Center for Global Collaborative Cardiovascular Research (VIGOUR) Group. Perspectives on large-scale cardiovascular clinical trials in the new millennium. *Circulation* 1997;95: 1072–1082.

342. Jollis JG, DeLong ER, Peterson ED, Muhlbaier LH, Fortin DF, Califf RM, Mark DB. Outcome of acute myocardial infarction according to the specialty of admitting physician. *N Engl J Med* 1996;335:1880–1887.

353. Califf RM, Armstrong PW, Carver JR, D'Agostino RB, Strauss WE. Task Force 5, stratification of patients into high, medium, and low risk subgroups for purposes of risk factor management. *J Am Coll Cardiol* 1996;27:964–1047.

362. Ohman EM, Kleiman NS, Gacioch G, Worley SJ, Navetta FI, Talley JD, Anderson HV, Ellis SG, Cohen MD, Spriggs D, Miller M, Kereiakes D, Yakubov S, Kitt MM, Sigmon KN, Califf RM, Krucoff MW, Topol EJ, for the IMPACT-AMI Investigators. Combined accelerated tissue-plasminogen activator and platelet glycoprotein IIb/IIIa integrin receptor blockade with integrilin in acute myocardial infarction: results of a randomized, placebo-controlled, dose-ranging trial. *Circulation* 1997;95:846–854.

364. Barefoot JC, Helms MJ, Mark DB, Blumenthal JA, Califf RM, Haney TL, O'Connor CM, Siegler IC, Williams RB. Depression and long-term mortality risk in patients with coronary artery disease. *Am J Cardiol* 1996;78:613–617.

371. Tcheng JE, Lincoff AM, Sigmon KN, Lee KL, Kitt MM, Califf RM, Topol EJ, Juran N, Worley S, Tuzi J, et al, and the IMPACT II Investigators. Randomized placebo-controlled trial of effect of eptifibatide on complications of percutaneous coronary intervention—IMPACT II. *Lancet* 1997;349:1422–1428.

387. Topol EJ, Califf RM, Granger C, Van de Werf F, Aylward P, Simes J, Col J, Armstrong P, Vahanian A, Neuhaus K, et al, and the Global Use of Strategies to Open Occluded Coronary Arteries (GUSTO) IIb Investigators. A comparison of recombinant hirudin versus heparin for the treatment of acute coronary syndromes. *N Engl J Med* 1996;335:775–782.

392. Califf RM, Abdelmeguid AE, Kuntz R, Popma JJ, Davidson CJ, Cohen EA, Kleiman NS, Mahaffey KW, Topol EJ, Pepine CJ, Lipicky R, Granger CB, et al.

Myonecrosis after revascularization procedures. *J Am Coll Cardiol* 1998;31:241–251.

404. Peterson ED, Shaw LJ, Califf RM. Clinical guideline: Part II. Risk stratification after myocardial infarction. *Ann Intern Med* 1997;126:561–580.

410. Betriu A, Phillips H, Ellis S, Topol E, Califf RM, Van de Werf F, Ardissino D, Armstrong PW, Aylward P, Bates E, et al, and the GUSTO-IIb Angioplasty Substudy Investigators. A clinical trial comparing primary coronary angioplasty with tissue plasminogen activator for acute myocardial infarction. *N Engl J Med* 1997;336:1621–1628.

413. BARI (The Bypass Angioplasty Revascularization Investigators) Investigators. Comparison of coronary bypass surgery with angioplasty in patients with multivessel disease. *N Engl J Med* 1996;335:217-225.

414. Thel MC, Armstrong AL, McNulty SE, Califf RM, O'Connor CM, for the Duke Internal Medicine Housestaff. A randomized trial of magnesium in in-hospital cardiac arrest (MAGIC). *Lancet* 1997;350:1272–1276.

419. Topol EJ, Weisman HF, Tcheng JE, Ellis SG, Kleiman NS, Ivanhoe RJ, Wang AL, Miller DP, Anderson KM, Califf RM, for the EPIC Investigators Group. Protection from myocardial ischemic events in a randomized trial of brief integrin β3 blockage with percutaneous coronary intervention. (EPIC 3-year results). *JAMA* 1997;278:479–484.

420. Topol EJ, Califf RM, Lincoff AM, Tcheng JE, Cabot CF, Weisman HF, Kereiakes D, Lausten D, Runyon JP, Howard W, et al, and the EPILOG Investigators. Platelet glycoprotein IIb/IIIa receptor blockade and low-dose heparin during percutaneous coronary revascularization. *N Engl J Med* 1997;336:1689–1696.

429. Ross AM, Coyne K, Moreyra E, Reiner JS, Walker P, Simoons ML, Draoui Y, Califf RM, Topol EJ, Van de Werf F, Lundergan CF, for the GUSTO-I Angiographic Investigators. Impact of early reperfusion on long term survival after myocardial infarction. *Circulation* 1998;97:1549–1556.

431. Ryan TJ, Andreson JL, Antman EM, Braniff BA, Brooks NH, Califf RM, Hillis LD, Hiratzka LF, Rapaport E, Riegel BJ, Russell RO, Smith EE III, Weaver WD, and the ACC/AHA Task Force on Practice Guidelines (Committee on Management of Acute Myocardial Infarction). ACC/AHA Guidelines for the management of patients with acute myocardial infarction. A report of the American College of Cardiology/American Heart Association Task Force on Practice Guidelines (Committee on Management of Acute Myocardial Infarction). *J Am Coll Cardiol* 1996;28:1328–1428.

433. Cohen M, Demers C, Gurfinkel EP, Turpie AGG, Fromell GJ, Goodman S, Langer A, Califf RM, Fox KAA, Premmereur J, Bigonzi F, for the Efficacy and Safety of Subcutaneous Enoxaparin in Non-Q-Wave Coronary Events (ES-SENCE) Study Group. A comparison of low-molecular-weight heparin with unfractionated heparin for unstable coronary artery disease. *N Engl J Med* 1997;337:447–452.

454. The GUSTO III (The Global Use of Strategies to Open Occluded Coronary Arteries) Investigators. A comparison of reteplase with alteplase for acute myocardial infarction. *N Engl J Med* 1997;337:1118–1123.

REVIEWS

19. Califf RM. Why are large-scale trials needed? *Coron Art Dis* 1992;3:92–95.

39. Califf RM, Bengtson JR. Cardiogenic shock. *N Engl J Med* 1994;330:1724–1730.

EDITORIALS

1. Califf RM, Rosati RA. The doctor and the computer. *Western J Med* 1981;135:321–323.

2. Califf RM, Pryor DB, Greenfield JC Jr. Beyond randomized clinical trials: applying clinical experience in the treatment of patients with coronary artery disease. *Circulation* 1986;74:1191–1194.

10. Califf RM, Harrelson-Woodlief L, Topol EJ. Left ventricular ejection fraction may not be useful as an endpoint of thrombolytic therapy comparative trials. *Circulation* 1990;82:1847–1853.

12. Topol EF, Armstrong P, Van de Werf F, Kleiman N, Lee KL, Morris D, Simoons M, Barbash G, White H, Califf RM, on behalf of the Global Utilization of Streptokinase and Tissue Plasminogen Activator for Occluded Coronary Arteries (GUSTO) Steering Committee. Confronting the issues of patient safety and investigator conflict of interest in an international clinical trial of myocardial infarction. *J Am Coll Cardiol* 1991;19:1123–1128.

28. Califf RM, Jollis J, Peterson E. Operator-specific outcomes: a call to professional responsibility. *Circulation* 1996;93:403–406.

EUGENE BRAUNWALD, MD:
A Conversation With the Editor*

Eugene Braunwald is a name recognized by most physicians around the world. His first 9 years were spent in Vienna, Austria, and he and his family barely escaped the German Reich. Nine years after he and his family came to the states he graduated magna cum laude from New York University, and 3 years later he graduated first in his class from New York University School of Medicine. By the time he began his internship he was committed to a career in cardiology and beginning immediately after his internship, he was "full steam ahead" in cardiovascular research except for his medical residency at The Johns Hopkins Hospital. During his nearly 10 years as Chief of Cardiology at the National Heart Institute in Bethesda he published 370 articles in medical journals on numerous cardiovascular topics, and nearly all of them were major contributions to the particular field of investigation. From age 38 until age 66 he was chairman of a major department of internal medicine, the first 4 years at the University of California in San Diego and the next 24 years as the Hersey Professor of the Theory and Practice of Medicine and the Chairman of the Department of Medicine at Harvard Medical School; initially, at the Peter Bent Brigham Hospital and then at both the Brigham and Women's Hospital and the Beth-Israel Hospital. During his chairmanship in Boston, Barry Brenner, who headed his renal division, told me that Braunwald was the most productive member of the Department of Medicine. His publication list in medical journals now totals over 1,000. He has been co-editor of *Harrisons' Principles of Internal Medicine* (since 1967) and the founding author/editor of *Heart Disease, A Textbook of Cardiovascular Medicine* (since 1980). These 2 books, which are revised every 3 or 4 years, are the world's leading texts in both internal medicine and in cardiology. Nearly 40% of his *Heart Disease* is authored or co-authored by Braunwald.

He has served as President of the American Society for Clinical Investigation and the Association of Professors of Medicine. His honors and awards include the Research Achievement and Herrick Awards of the American Heart Association, the Distinguished Scientist Award of the American College of Cardiology, the Phillips Award of the American College of Physicians, the Williams Award of the Association of Professors of Medicine, and the Kober medal of the Association of American Physicians for 1998. He is

the recipient of 8 honorary degrees from distinguished universities throughout the world. In 1996 Harvard University created the Eugene Braunwald Professorship in Medicine as a permanently endowed chair.

Dr. Braunwald is the father of 3 daughters, one of whom is a physician, another a health lawyer, and a third a clinical psychologist, and he is the grandfather of 6 children. For almost 4 years he has been happily married to his second wife, Elaine. His late, first wife, Dr. Nina Braunwald, was the first female board-certified cardiothoracic surgeon in the USA and the first surgeon to replace a mitral valve. Dr. Braunwald recently honored his late wife by providing a $1.5 million gift to the Society of Thoracic Surgeons. For an internist/cardiologist to make such a gift to a surgical organization is remarkable, and such a cross-departmental occurrence has not occurred, to my knowledge, since Harvey Cushing, the great general surgeon/neurosurgeon, published in 1926 the Pulitzer Prize winning *A Life of William Osler* about the renowned internist.

I first met Dr. Braunwald in late 1959 when I began attending his cardiology ward rounds at NIH. Not long afterward he became the Chief of the newly formed Cardiology Branch in the National Heart Institute. Two years later Dr. Braunwald helped me obtain a medical residency on the Osler Medical Service at The Johns Hopkins Hospital, and in 1964, I had the privilege of spending 6 months in his cardiac catheterization laboratory. Thus, during an 8-year period I was able to observe Dr. Braunwald in action. I had never met a physician quite like him. From scratch he quickly built the best cardiology group in the world. He made ward rounds on the cardiology patients virtually every day and weekly he rounded on the postoperative cardiac surgical patients. Every Friday afternoon he presided over the cardiac catheterization conference where the data on every patient studied in cardiology that week were presented as well as the follow-up data in the postoperative patients. It was the best cardiac conference I've ever attended, and I rarely missed it. In addition to running a busy clinical service, Braunwald's research endeavors were astounding. Never previously had a cardiologist been so productive. Several nights a week one or more of his associates were called to his home to work on a manuscript. During his last 3 years at NIH he also was the Clinical Director of the National Heart Institute, and in this position his impact, particularly in teaching and learning, was felt in the entire institute.

Braunwald is an excellent teacher, a magnificent researcher, a superb clinician, and a giant leader. He was the most efficient user of time of anyone I had seen then or subsequently. During the 8 years in which I saw Gene usually several times a week, I never heard him speak about his upbringing in Vienna, the close

*This series of interviews are underwritten by an unrestricted grant from Bristol-Myers-Squibb.

†Baylor Cardiovascular Institute, Baylor University Medical Center, Dallas, Texas 75246.

‡Distinguished Hersey Professor of Medicine; Faculty Dean, Brigham and Women's Hospital and Massachusetts General Hospital, Harvard Medical School; Vice President for Academic Programs, Partners HealthCare System, Boston, Massachusetts 02115.

0002-9149/98/$19.00   **93**
PII S0002-9149(98)00283-5

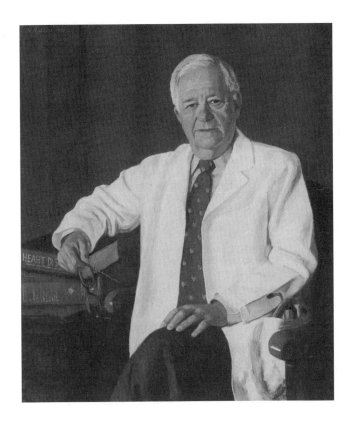

FIGURE 1. EB portrait in amphitheater at Brigham and Women's Hospital, with 5th edition of *Heart Disease* and 13th edition of *Harrison's Principles of Medicine.*

escape he and his family had from the German invaders, or his early period in New York City. He loved new ideas no matter where they came from. He required excellence from all those around him and his standards had to be met. I remember well during my early period in his cardiac catheterization laboratory that some of the presentations at one Friday conference were a bit "casual." Immediately after the conference, several of us were called into his office and in just a few minutes we all were aware of the high performance he expected from each of us. There was never any doubt what he thought on an issue. His decisiveness and ability to see and focus on the important or most important issue not only made him a superb investigator, teacher and writer, but it also made him a terrific consultant. I remember that Andrew Glenn Morrow, the cardiac surgeon in charge, sought Braunwald's opinions on many patients. Braunwald's recommendations usually were numbered: do this, this and this. No fussiness. There was never confusion about his recommendations. His questions at the monthly clinicopathologic conference, for which I was responsible, were predictably always the most perceptive and penetrating.

And he is a good guy with a good heart and a good sense of humor. Common sense abounds in him. His advice is usually right on. He rarely forgets a friend. Braunwald let my son Chuck work in his lab at Harvard for 2 summers, and he supported his endeavors enthusiastically. I am proud to have had the opportunity to study this great man who has been such an inspiration to so many of us in our profession.

William Clifford Roberts, MD† (hereafter, WCR): *I am speaking with Dr. Eugene Braunwald in my office at Baylor University Medical Center on January 27, 1998. Dr. Braunwald, thank you for coming to Baylor, for your splendid lecture at Medical Grand Rounds, and for your willingness to be interviewed for* The American Journal of Cardiology. *Could I start by asking about your memories of your first 9 years in Vienna? I gather you were born on August 15, 1929, and during those first 9 years lived in Austria.*

Eugene Braunwald, MD‡ (hereafter, EB): My memory of that period falls into 2 very distinct phases: before and after March 13, 1938. On that date the Nazis occupied Austria in the so-called *Anschluss.* My childhood was idyllic before that. We lived in one of the elegant areas of Vienna, I went to an excellent school and had private tutors in English and piano. My parents were very interested in opera, and by the time I was 6 they had begun taking me to the Vienna State Opera. Vienna was a gracious city in the 1930s, the cultural capital of central Europe. Then, suddenly, on March 13, 1938 everything changed. I recall vividly the enthusiastic crowds welcoming Hitler and his troops marching into Vienna. My father's and other Jews' businesses were taken over several days later and their liquidation was begun. We lived in constant terror from March until the end of July 1938, when we

665

escaped from Austria. Many people in our situation, of course, did not escape.

WCR: *Before March 13, 1938, you lived next to your father's business? What was your father like? Your mother like? What were your day-to-day activities, not only at school, but at home in those more pleasant moments?*

EB: Our apartment was just off the Schottenrink, Vienna's major thoroughfare, close to the University and to the State opera. I saw a good deal of my father because the proximity of our apartment to his business allowed him to have lunch with us quite frequently. In childhood, both of my parents had been too poor to receive an education beyond high school. My father was fifth generation Viennese, and my mother was born in a small town in the east of what was then the Austro-Hungarian empire. Her family fled to Vienna at the end of World War I because of an anti-Jewish pogrom in her town.

My father had built a successful wholesale clothing business by the time I was born, and we enjoyed a very pleasant life. The 3 most important things that I learned from those early years were: a central focus on the well being of the nuclear family; a reverence for learning; and an interest in classical music. As I just mentioned, we lived not far from the University of Vienna, and when I was 6 or 7 years old my mother took me for walks in the Stadtpark adjacent to the University. She would point to the University and say to me, "You will be a professor there someday." Because my parents had been deprived of an education themselves, they made my education their highest priority.

WCR: *Were there a lot of books around the house? Did you have intellectual discussions at the dinner table at night or at lunch time? How was learning pushed on you by both parents, neither of whom had the benefit of going to college themselves?*

EB: I remember discussions of history, economics and politics at the dinner table. My parents probably did emphasize such discussion because of their own lack of higher education. Of course, there was much talk about music. Actually, my parents had met in the standing room area at the Vienna State Opera!

WCR: *So they were poor initially, but your father was quite successful?*

EB: Yes. By the time of the *Anschluss* he had a prosperous business, but the Nazis quickly sent SS officers to liquidate all Jewish businesses. The officer who was assigned to my father's business had, I believe, been imprisoned for the assassination of Chancellor Dolfuss of Austria several years earlier. I got to know this SS officer because sometimes he came over to the apartment for lunch or coffee.

WCR: *What was he like?*

EB: He was cold and businesslike but always polite, as he went about destroying our livelihood. The liquidators themselves were able to make off with most everything, and therefore he wanted the process to be rapid and complete.

WCR: *How did it come about that your father was arrested by the Nazis within a couple of months of their invading Austria?*

EB: It was the proverbial knock on the door in the middle of a night in May 1938. I remember being awakened by my parents at about 3:00 A.M. My mother was hysterical, screaming, "They are taking your father away." He had 15 minutes to get dressed and to say goodbye to us. I now recall that he was remarkably stoic about it. Then my mother, my younger brother and I ran to the window and saw him herded into an open truck with 15 or 20 other men. they were then driven off to the railroad station.

WCR: *How did your mother get him back? I gather he came back the next day?*

EB: Yes. It is incredible what life can hinge on. When "our" S.S. officer came to the business the next morning, he asked for my father. My very upset mother said he had been taken away, presumably to a work camp. He shrugged his shoulders. (My mother and I subsequently talked about this event innumerable times.) Then came the pivotal moment. She said something along the following: "You need him back because you have liquidated only half of the business, and if you get him back you can liquidate the rest. Look how much richer you would be." He replied, "You might be right." He then phoned the depot to find that my father was about to board the train. My mother only overheard his side of this conversation in which he pulled rank on the officer at the depot, saying, "I don't care if you are a full colonel in the German army, I am a captain in the SS and I want this Jew returned!" So it ultimately became a matter of authority. By 11 A.M. my father was returned to us. He had been gone for only 8 hours, but is was a very close call. If my mother had not acted at that moment, none of our family would have survived, and of course, we wouldn't be having this interview.

WCR: *From that point it was about 2 months before you escaped? What happened in the interim?*

EB: My father had actually begun preparations for our escape in March immediately after the occupation, but he redoubled his efforts after his brief arrest. There were several opportunities for him to leave Vienna alone and to try to bring us along later, but he refused to allow the family to be separated. He insisted that we stay together even though that made escape more difficult. But he obviously calculated correctly. We left at the end of July 1938, in something that resembled the *Sound of Music* story, except that there was no music. We ended up in London, totally destitute, literally with only the shirts on our backs. We were taken care of by a relief agency. I spoke a little English because of the special tutoring I had received, but my parents did not then speak a word of English. (They later learned English in night school.)

WCR: *Could you, Dr. Braunwald, explain in a little more detail actually how you escaped from Vienna? Did you go by car, train? Did you take any possessions with you?*

EB: No. As a matter of fact, neither my brother, who is four years younger than I, nor I knew we were leaving. My parents did not want to risk our speaking about it to anyone. I was no longer attending school, and we were no longer allowed to play outdoors. On one Saturday morning, my parents told us we were going on a picnic. That seemed quite strange to me, given what our life had become. We took no belongings except what we carried on our persons, a few sandwiches and a thermos of tea. We started our trip by trolley, then took a taxi and then a train. We went through Switzerland to Paris and then on to London. Fortunately, everything went smoothly.

WCR: *You had no problem getting across the border?*

EB: This had been very carefully arranged by my father.

WCR: *Why did your parents decide to go to England?*

EB: It was the only place which would give us refuge. A business acquaintance of my father's in London was very helpful in making the arrangements. His help saved our lives.

WCR: *So you went through France by train?*

EB: Yes.

WCR: *When you got to London, what did you and your brother do? You were 9 and he was 5? I gather that he did not speak English.*

EB: No, but a 5-year-old learns very quickly. I was not fluent in English but also improved rapidly. I was sent by the refugee relief agency to a boarding school in Hove, near Brighton on the Channel coast of England, and stayed there from September 1938 to June 1939. In was hard for me to be separated from my family in a strange country. In September 1939, when World War II began and the London blitz started, the children living in London were evacuated to small towns, mostly in northern England. My parents felt that my brother was too young to be evacuated by himself, so we were shipped off together to a small village near Leeds. There we were accepted by a wonderful family with 6 children. I started to go to school there and then received a telegram from my father saying "Come back to London, we are going to America!" At the end of November 1939, we came to the United States on the *President Harding*. This was one of the last large American ships to make the trip to the States from England, because the German U-boats had already become quite active in the North Atlantic. We arrived in New York City on the day after Thanksgiving, 1939, and settled in Brooklyn.

WCR: *How did it work out that your father and mother decided to come to the USA? Did they have relatives in New York City?*

EB: Although England provided an emergency stop, it was not possible for Jewish refugees to stay there permanently. We knew that we had to leave or be interned in a camp for "enemy aliens." My parents began exploring opportunities to emigrate immediately upon our arrival there. To come to the United States, you needed a "sponsor" who would provide an affidavit that you would not be a burden to the state. At first, we had difficulty identifying a sponsor. My parents had actually already booked boat tickets to

Australia, which had much more liberal immigration laws than the U.S. Then, my mother's aunt, who lived in New York and whom she had never met, provided sponsorship for us and for many of our relatives who had also escaped from Vienna. So, we came to the United States through the enormous kindness of American relatives who had until then really been total strangers.

WCR: *How did you get the money for the tickets?*

EB: By that time my parents were working as shipping clerks at Selfridge's, a large department store in London. They saved every penny they could for the tickets.

WCR: *You came to Brooklyn. What do you remember about living in Brooklyn? You were now 10 years old?*

EB: I remember that it was not at all the image of the USA that I had from Vienna and London. I had imagined a land of skyscrapers, airplanes, helicopters and automobiles speeding on elevated freeways. That certainly was not what Brooklyn was like in 1939. Nevertheless, it was a tremendous relief to come to the USA. The events of my early childhood have given me a feeling of great loyalty to this country. I can never forget that we were rescued, and I will never take this country for granted. I think I have always been more tolerant of this country's faults than most native-born Americans.

WCR: *You arrived in Brooklyn. It's school time. You go to public school and you are in the fifth grade.*

EB: I didn't quite fit in. Curiously, we were again classified as "enemy aliens," and the other kids did not quite know what to make of me, but I did well in school. Three years after our arrival I graduated as valedictorian of my grade school class in 1943. It was the height of World War II, when electronics, mechanical engineering, and science were the rage. I gained admission to Brooklyn Technical High School, which required a very demanding entrance exam. Brooklyn Tech had an important influence on my subsequent interest in science, and ultimately in cardiology.

WCR: *How did it turn you toward science and medicine in particular?*

EB: It was a pre-engineering high school. I was introduced to the concepts of electrical circuits, electronics, and hydraulics. In 1945 I entered an accelerated program in which I completed both high school and college in 5 years. At the time there were many special accelerated programs for high school and college for veterans who had come back from the War and who had lost 4 or 5 years of their normal education time. I attended New York University (NYU) undergraduate school.

WCR: *You were 16 when you started NYU undergraduate school?*

EB: Yes. My parents could not afford to send me away to college, so I lived at home both during college and medical school and commuted by subway. I did not enjoy college much because I went through it too rapidly (2½ years) with classmates who were mostly much older than I. Anyway, I had set my sights on getting into medical school and focused on that almost exclusively. Because of the influx of veterans who properly were given preference for medical school admission, and the very strict "Jewish quotas" at the time, it was necessary for me to get almost straight "A"s to have a chance for admission.

WCR: *Essentially in college, you took the subway to NYU, went to your classes, came home, studied and went back the next day? There was not much of a social life. There was not extra money to do a lot of fun things that most college students do?*

EB: Yes. Living at home during those years, between ages 16 and 19, working under intense pressure with classmates who had had the war experience and who were passionately devoted to completing college and trying to catch up with their lives, made for a pretty disciplined time.

WCR: *Did you encounter at Brooklyn Technical High School or at NYU any particular teachers that really had an impact on you?*

EB: My professor of Biology at NYU, Malvina Schweiter, befriended me, excited my interest in Biology, and I maintained contact with her for 40 years! She subsequently moved to Washington and worked for Claude Lenfant (Director of the NHLBI), and we saw a fair amount of each other in Washington. There also was my Professor of Organic Chemistry, William MacTavish, who was influential in another way, as a "holy terror." I also took courses in my love: classical music. Being in New York City, with the New York Metropolitan Opera nearby also gave me the memorable chance to become an "extra" at the Met. For example, I was paid a dollar a night for being a spear carrier in a production of Aida! To be on the stage of the Metropolitan Opera in one of these grand productions was an unforgettable experience. I continued as an "extra" through medical school, but I had to quit during internship because I could not adjust my schedule to the Met's.

WCR: *That was your most pleasurable experience in college at any rate?*

EB: Yes, along with the Toscanini concerts. Arturo Toscanini conducted the NBC Symphony, and admission to their concerts was free because it was a radio broadcast. The NBC Symphony was one of the great orchestras of the time. I would get to the studio a couple of hours early and sit on the floor in the hall outside doing my homework, and that got me a seat in the first row. I must have attended nearly 100 Toscanini concerts over a 6-year period. He was the greatest conductor of the 20th century, perhaps of all time. Sitting in the first row, 10 feet away from this great man and getting caught up in the music is simply impossible to describe in words.

WCR: *You mentioned playing the piano when you were in Vienna. Did you continue that?*

EB: Yes, but I showed little talent. I do think playing helped my overall understanding of music.

WCR: *Did your mother and father play a musical instrument?*

EB: No, they didn't, but they wanted me to.

WCR: *In Austria, England, and the USA you always did well in school? Was it easy for you or did you have to work very hard at it?*

EB: I always did well scholastically, but I always worked hard at it also.

WCR: *It was a struggle because it was so intensely competitive or was it something more inside of you because of all these veterans trying to get into medical school, the quota systems limiting the numbers of Jews permitted in the schools of higher learning?*

EB: All of the above. I felt intense pressure and the need to excel scholastically.

WCR: *What was your apartment like in Brooklyn? Did you have a room of your own when you were coming home from college? Was your brother still there?*

EB: My brother and I shared a room when I attended college. When I was in medical school he had gone away to college. We had moved to Queens by then and I had my own room for the first time. I was still commuting by subway.

WCR: *How long did it take?*

EB: About 45 minutes each way and standing room only. As a freshman medical student, I would lug the box of anatomy bones, my microscope, and Gray's *Anatomy* on the subway.

WCR: *Getting into medical school must have been an enormous relief?*

EB: It was the most important day of my life. I'll always be grateful for that admission. I was the last one admitted to NYU's class of '52!

WCR: *How did you find that out?*

EB: At the time of graduation, I was told "Last in—first out."

WCR: *NYU was the only medical school you applied to?*

EB: No, I applied to and was admitted to several other schools. I had become friends with a classmate in college, who became my first wife, Nina. She had been admitted to NYU Medical School. I wanted to stay in New York City so that we could stay together.

WCR: *Nina, in actuality, determined where you went to medical school? Where else were you accepted?*

EB: Boston University.

WCR: *Your parents were working?*

EB: My father had re-established himself. He had become very successful in business a second time. It was inspiring for me to observe him.

WCR: *I gather your parents are not living?*

EB: My father died in 1977 at age 73, and my mother, in 1992 at 87.

WCR: *You are in medical school as a freshman, aged 19, and you finished medical school before your twenty second birthday in 1952. Describe your medical school experience.*

EB: I loved medical school. It was a privilege to go to NYU Medical School at that time. The faculty was spectacular and generally made themselves available to the students. The Chair of Physiology, Homer Smith, was the greatest renal physiologist of all time. We used to joke "He discovered the kidney." Colin

McCloud, the co-discoverer of DNA, was the Chair of Microbiology. Otto Leowi, a Noble Prize winner, was my laboratory instructor in pharmacology and Severo Ochoa, another Nobelist, was our Professor of Biochemistry! The quality of the basic science departments at NYU aroused my interest in science. Bellevue Hospital, NYU's teaching hospital, the first public hospital in the U.S., was then the flagship teaching hospital in the New York City system. The clinical training was very strong. The Chair of Medicine, William Tillett, was a member of the National Academy of Sciences. He had discovered streptokinase and was doing clinical investigation with streptokinase on the ward where I served my medical clerkship. I observed clinical research on streptokinase as a medical student in 1950!

WCR: *Did you do any research while in medical school?*

EB: Yes. I worked in the laboratory of Ludwig Eichna, who directed one of the first research cardiac catheterization laboratories in the country. Saul Farber, for many years Dean of NYU Medical School, was also my mentor. I took a 3-month elective with Eichna in my senior year in 1951 and studied the hemodynamics of heart failure. That aroused my lifelong interest in heart failure. This was also in the very early days of medical use of radioisotopes. One of the first papers I published was from work as a student on measuring the sodium concentration of sweat using isotopic methods. Our hypothesis was that sodium might be reduced in sweat in congestive heart failure. About 10 years before the discovery of aldosterone, it was thought that patients with heart failure might be under the influence of a sodium-retaining hormone, and that the action of such a hormone might be reflected in low sodium concentration of sweat.

WCR: *It must have been quite unusual in 1951 to take an elective while a medical student? Not many medical schools had that opportunity for their students at that time. Is that correct?*

EB: Yes, that was one of the wonderful things about NYU. It was one of the first schools to provide electives and to encourage student research. Medical curricula were pretty much in lock step at the time.

WCR: *Was it easy or difficult for you to decide which area of medicine you wanted to go into, whether you wanted to go into medicine or surgery or basic science, be a practitioner? How did you decide what you wanted to do?*

EB: Actually, it was easy. I made the decision very early on that I was interested in internal medicine. It was more cerebral than surgery, which I wanted to avoid because I didn't have much manual dexterity. The exposure to electronics and hydraulics which I had had in high school pointed me to cardiology. When I completed that 3-month elective in my senior year, my course was pretty much set for the rest of my professional life.

WCR: *Thus, that elective had a very powerful impact on you, not only from the research standpoint but on what type of research you would pursue the rest of your life. Let me go back one moment. Both you and*

your brother became physicians. Were there other physicians in your family? Did you know any doctors yourself, for example?

EB: No, we had no physicians in our family, but our parents were certainly in favor of our going into medicine and encouraged us.

WCR: *During your last year in medical school you decided to intern at Mt. Sinai Hospital in New York City. Why did you pick Mt. Sinai?*

EB: The strength of the cardiology faculty there—Charles Friedberg, Arthur Master, Simon Dack, among others, attracted me to Mt. Sinai.

WCR: *Did you continue to live in Brooklyn?*

EB: No, Nina and I were married the weekend after we graduated from medical school. We moved into an efficiency apartment on East 70th Street about halfway between Mt. Sinai and Bellevue, where she interned.

WCR: *You spent 2 years at Mt. Sinai?*

EB: Yes.

WCR: *Who had an impact on you at Mt. Sinai? Did you enjoy that 2-year experience?*

EB: Enormously. The Chief of Medicine, Isadore Snapper, a Dutchman, was a legendary clinician, a great Professor of Internal Medicine in the best preWar European tradition. I got to know Charles Friedberg reasonably well. I admired him and wanted to emulate him. As an intern I often ran into him in the hospital library at 11 P.M. working away at the first edition of his great textbook, even though he was in private practice. I got to do a fair amount of research at Mt. Sinai. My most important paper was one that reported the first measurement of the pressure gradient across a stenotic human heart valve. The paper was published in *Circulation* 1955;12:69–81 (Braunwald et al. The hemodynamics of the left side of the heart as studied by simultaneous left atrial, left ventricular, and aortic pressures: particular reference to mitral stenosis).

WCR: *How did that actually come about?*

EB: Cardiac surgery was in its infancy. I was assigned to the catheterization laboratory and the operating room. It was before left heart catheterization had been developed. It was exciting to make these first measurements of the pressure gradient with the cooperation of the cardiac surgeons.

WCR: *From there you went back to Bellevue Hospital to spend a year as a research fellow with Andre Cournand. How did you arrange that?*

EB: Dr. Cournand had described cardiac catheterization. He was about to win the Nobel Prize and was almost a deity. Ludwig Eichna's laboratory where I had taken my senior elective was 5 floors from Cournand's laboratory, and during that elective I attended some of his lectures and laboratory conferences. They were extremely stimulating, and I desperately wanted to continue my training in his laboratory.

WCR: *You really knew what you wanted to do early on. So immediately after internship you put yourself in a position where you could collect clinical data and publish it. I gather that experience "turned you on" right away?*

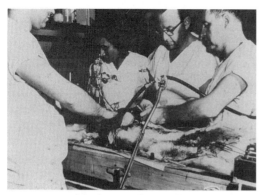

FIGURE 2. EB *(right)* with Dr. Stanley Sarnoff at NIH in 1955 when EB was 26 years old.

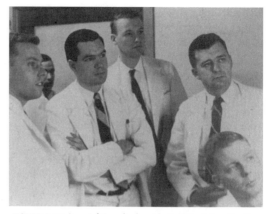

FIGURE 3. EB *(top right)* medical resident at The Johns Hopkins Hospital, 1957.

EB: I was committed to an academic career, and specifically to clinical research in cardiovascular disease. I knew pretty much what I wanted to do by the time I was 22.

WCR: *What happened in Dr. Cournand's laboratory during the period when you were there? Was that a year of more or less basic research? Did you see patients?*

EB: I did what we might now call basic human research, published in journals such as *Circulation Research* and the *American Journal of Physiology*. I had a couple of clinics, and I taught physical diagnosis to second year Columbia medical students. Cournand's laboratory was small; there were only 3 fellows. We would discuss data with him daily. Life in a top flight research laboratory was very different in those days. Dr. Cournand came to work every morning at 8:00 and left at 6:00 in the evening. He traveled very little. The laboratory group was like a very small, closely knit family.

WCR: *So you really got to know Dr. Cournand during that one year.*

EB: Yes. He introduced creativity in research to me. He was very supportive of me later in my career.

WCR: *How did it come about that you went to the National Institutes of Health (NIH) to work with Stanley Sarnoff?*

EB: I felt that to really learn cardiac physiology I had to devote extended time to work in an animal laboratory. The Clinical Center of the NIH had just opened in Bethesda, Maryland, and I had the opportunity to spend what was initially planned to be 2 years there. Stanley Sarnoff had come there from the Department of Physiology at Harvard. He was a charismatic, and exciting physiologist. He taught me a great deal.

WCR: *How did you hear about NIH? How did you hear about the availability of positions at NIH at that time? We are talking about 1955?*

EB: It was during the Korean War. I joined the U.S. Public Health Service as did many other young physicians aspiring to become scientists in those years.

WCR: *So you loved working in Sarnoff's laboratory?*

EB: Yes, but I also had the opportunity as a Clinical Associate in the National Heart Institute (now the National Heart, Lung, and Blood Institute) to see a lot of cardiac patients. I developed a close association with our mutual friend, the late Dr. Andrew Glenn Morrow, who was the new, dynamic young Chief of Cardiac Surgery. We developed a very productive relationship that extended from 1955 until 1968. My late wife, Nina, began her pioneering career as a cardiac surgeon in Morrow's group.

WCR: *After those 2 years at NIH I gather you felt that you had to have an additional year in internal medicine to become board qualified so you went to The Johns Hopkins Hospital in Baltimore, Maryland. Did that year have an influence on you?*

EB: A profound influence. The Hopkins tradition was one of learning medicine primarily by taking almost total responsibility for your patients. In that era residents on the Osler medical service had no scheduled time off all year except for a 2-week vacation. You were on call all the time including weekends, although you could sign out to a colleague. The year at Hopkins profoundly influenced my subsequent 28 years as Chairman of Medicine.

WCR: *Were there certain figures at Hopkins that had memorable influences on you?*

EB: A. McGehee Harvey, the Chief of Medicine, and E. Cowles Andrus, the Chief of Cardiology. I also got to know Helen Taussig. Even though I was a medical resident, I went to many of her conferences. Also, Richard Ross, who subsequently became Chief of Cardiology, was a wonderful teacher. I went to some of Alfred Blalock's clinics. I got to know some of the great young cardiac surgeons of that era: David Sabiston, Henry Bahnson, Frank Spencer. Although I was only a medical resident, since I had by that time spent 4 years of research in cardiology, the rich opportunities of the Johns Hopkins opened to me. After I returned to the NIH I maintained a part-time appointment at the Hopkins, as I think you did, Bill. This continued association provided rich experiences.

WCR: *Now it is July 1958, you're 29 and you return to NIH for 10 glorious years. Shortly after returning you became Chief of Cardiology, and recruited these extremely bright young people to work with you? As you look back on those 10 years how do they strike you now?*

EB: It was Camelot! I was fortunate to be in the right place at the right time. Resources were abundant, the patients were extremely interesting, my colleagues were extraordinarily talented, and it was a time when there were great things to be discovered in cardiology that mattered a great deal. It was like exploring the West in the days of Lewis and Clark! I recall coming home in the evening and telling Nina that I had worked on 5 exciting projects in the course of the day and had made some progress on each.

WCR: *You had a good deal of contact with Robert Berliner, who was Head of the Intramural Research Program in the National Heart Institute at the time. I gather he had some impact on you.*

EB: Yes. Robert Berliner is on of the strongest scientists I have ever encountered. Although he was not a cardiologist, he was my principal scientific mentor. Even as Chief of Cardiology, I had to clear every manuscript and every major project with him and that did me a lot of good. He brought an objective view to what I was doing from the perspective of a rigorous scientist. He also taught me how it is possible to have a large administrative job, in which you are responsible for many people and large programs, and at the same time maintain your personal scientific program. During the years that he was Director of Intramural Research at the Institute his own personal contributions to science were enormous.

WCR: *So it was an atmosphere of living one's work everyday, many new ideas, and resources to pursue them.*

EB: We really had the unique opportunity to bring cardiology together in a single unit for the first time. Today's cardiology divisions are large units, but that was not the case in 1960. In close physical proximity we had a floor of carefully selected cardiac patients, 2 superbly equipped cardiac catheterization laboratories and a row of basic science laboratories with people working on separate but interrelated projects: Ed Sonnenblick, studying the mechanics of isolated papillary muscle; John Ross and Jim Covell experimenting on the intact heart; Charles Chidsey, Burton Sobel, and Peter Pool working on the biochemical features of normal and failing cardiac muscle. The closeness of the unit allowed all of us to move rapidly from one area to another. We worked closely with an excellent cardiac surgery unit headed by Glenn Morrow, and of which my wife, Nina, was a member. You provided important insights into cardiac pathology. It was nirvana!

WCR: *It seems to me that you were the first cardiologist who ever worked intimately with a cardiac surgeon. The monograph on hypertrophic cardiomyopathy in 1964 is the epitome of cardiologic-surgical collaboration. So here you are at 38 years of age and you receive a call from the University of California at* San Diego *asking you to be the Professor and Founding Chairman of their Department of Medicine. That must have been a very difficult decision to go to California and to leave Bethesda. Here every day was glorious. You could not have been more productive. It seems to me that you accelerated the pace of cardiac research everywhere. You would have to start over completely if you went to California. How did you come to grips with that major decision?*

EB: I was getting restless, maybe a little jaded. I think of the following analogy. I love eating steak, but I had been "eating steak" 3 times a day 7 days a week for 12 years. I simply wanted to explore some other areas of medicine without giving up cardiology. There were 2 things that drove me in this direction. First, I wanted to be more involved in medical education and in general medicine. I had become an editor of *Harrison's Principles of Internal Medicine* in 1967. I had a Clinical Professorship at Georgetown University in Washington, DC, and made general medical rounds there for 5 years, so I knew there was something in medicine outside of cardiology. I sensed there were going to be profound changes in medical education and medical care and I wanted to be part of that process. It just seemed like a new frontier, going to the West, particularly to an area that was as beautiful as La Jolla was in those days, and to be given a clean slate to draw on, just like I had been given at the NIH 10 years earlier. It seemed like a great adventure and an awesome challenge.

There was a second reason. My research interest had switched to acute myocardial infarction. I knew that I could not study acute myocardial infarction at the NIH. I felt that if I was going to do credible research in the field that I had to be involved in the care of patients with this condition.

WCR: *How did it work out? You were in California for a total of 4 years?*

EB: It was an exhilarating experience. I was one of the 5 founding chairmen. We built a medical school from scratch. The creation was something like a MASH operation. When I first went out to San Diego, before my family joined me, I lived in a room in the University hospital for 6 weeks to get a "feel" for the hospital. I learned what it was like at 3:00 A.M. to go to the x-ray department and see whether or not you could retrieve a film. I became totally immersed in the University and the community. We had to get ourselves established as a medical center. It was not always glamorous. I remember going to the Tijuana Medical Society to give talks on high blood pressure and other general medical topics. At the time, the Society met in a basement; there were 15 members: 10 physicians, 1 dentist, 2 chiropractors, 1 nurse, and 1 faith healer!

We recruited about 75 faculty members to the Department of Medicine during those 4 years and developed a new medical residency. We developed a new curriculum in which the Department of Medicine taught not only medicine but also physiology, pharmacology, and microbiology. I stayed there through the graduation of the charter class. One measure of our success was that the charter class at the University of California San Diego Medical School came in first in the nation on the National Board Examinations! We had great students. Judy Swain, now Bloomfield Professor and Chair of Medicine at Stanford took an elective with me. Peter Libby, now Chief of Cardiology at the Brigham and Mallinckrodt Professor at Harvard worked in my dog laboratory. They were both in the second class. I was very proud of our students. Last year I returned to UCSD to address the 25th graduating class and see many members of the charter class again. Many of them have made important contributions to medicine.

WCR: *This medical school was quite different in the fact that the faculty of clinical specialties really taught the basic science courses.*

EB: It was quite "avant garde" for the time. Now this approach has been adopted in different forms by other medical schools, but the concept of faculty in clinical departments taking on the principal responsibility for education in the first 2 years was first tried at UCSD. The surgeons, for example, taught anatomy. The only truly separate pre-clinical department was pathology. It was both a thrill and a valuable learning experience for me to be involved in the creation of the school: to understand how an organization works, to help to develop the interaction between a new University and its medical school, and to learn about town-grown interactions, not all of which were pleasant. It opened a totally new world to me, and to my surprise it allowed me to start a new and exciting chapter in my research career.

WCR: *After a few months or maybe a year you got your laboratory going again in San Diego?*

EB: I did, at first on a very part-time basis. I did not feel that it was my job to do research, but I was like an alcoholic. I just couldn't stay away from it. We had gotten this idea of trying to salvage severely ischemic myocardium in Bethesda, and I wanted desperately to explore it.

WCR: *So you are in San Diego <4 years before you get a call from Harvard Medical School. Was that a difficult decision to move back East?*

EB: That decision was also an easy one. If you are in academic medicine you simply don't turn down that kind of opportunity. But I found the move back East to be more difficult than the earlier move to the West because our 3 children were older and had roots in school. The move to Boston also uprooted my own laboratory for the second time in 4 years, and this certainly disrupted my research.

WCR: *Do you think you would have been offered the Harvard position as Chairman of the Department of Medicine and the Hersey Professorship if you had not gone through the San Diego experience?*

EB: No, I don't think so. Even if I had, I would have been eaten alive if I had gone directly from the NIH to Harvard and the then Peter Bent Brigham Hospital.

WCR: *So you had really faced most of the problems that came subsequently during the 4-year San Diego period?*

EB: Developing a new medical school exposed me to every aspect of academic medicine. When I went to San Diego it was not with the intention of using it as a jumping off spot. I expected to stay there for the rest of my professional life. We bought a beautiful home on a bluff overlooking the Pacific which we thought was permanent and began to establish ourselves in the University community. The invitation to Harvard came out of the blue. Having said that, the experience of those 4 years of not only being a Chairman but being one of the founders of the school gave me an enormous advantage when coming to Harvard. I was able to bring outside views.

WCR: *The Peter Bent Brigham Hospital when you went there to be its Physician in Chief in 1972 was a small hospital—only 300 beds or so. Things changed a great deal during the 24 years that you were Chairman of Medicine. As you look back over your 24 years as Chairman of Medicine at the Brigham, what are the accomplishments you are most proud of?*

EB: I am most proud of the quality of the Internal Medicine Training Program that I developed with Marshall Wolf, my Associate Chief. We concentrated on its flexibility. "Special programs for special people!" We created the first research residency track, an idea that grew out of my NIH experience. The graduates of that track have become the most outstanding academic leaders, many now holding major chairs of internal medicine in this country. In 1973 we created one of the first primary care medical residencies in the country. Then we established an important educational association with the Harvard Community Health Plan, the first academically based HMO. In building the department at the Brigham, I emphasized basic sciences as they affect medicine, something I had learned in San Diego. The close relation that we developed between the Department of Medicine at the Brigham and the strong basic science departments on the Harvard quadrangle brings me much satisfaction.

WCR: *The Harvard School of Medicine is just next door to the Brigham?*

EB: Yes, but curiously when I came to Boston it was as if the Brigham Hospital and the Medical School were miles apart. We helped bring them closer together. It was largely by putting basic science chairs on the search committees for our division chiefs, recruiting some incredibly talented people and my helping them develop strong programs, trying to be supportive without micromanaging.

WCR: *By 1980, let's say, before the Beth Israel Hospital came into your life, how many full-time faculty did you have in your department at the Brigham Hospital?*

EB: About 180.

WCR: *What about when you left in 1996?*

EB: 523.

WCR: *How many fellows did you have in 1996?*

EB: About 800 in the Department of Medicine at the Brigham.

WCR: *How many house staff in 1996?*

EB: 125.

WCR: *How about secretaries and technicians in the Department of Medicine?*

EB: I don't know, but the annual research budget in the Department was about $80,000,000, and the clinical operation about $50,000,000.

WCR: *How many faculty did you have in 1972 when you arrived in Boston?*

EB: About 45. The 70s was a period of tremendous growth. During that time, the Peter Bent Brigham, the Robert Breck Brigham, and the Boston Hospital for Women merged into the Brigham and Women's Hospital. There were great people at the Brigham, great department and divisional chairs, outstanding hospital leadership under Dr. Richard Nesson. I enjoyed the support of Dean Robert Ebert, who had recruited me to Harvard, and then Dean Daniel Tosteson with whom I worked very closely for 20 years.

WCR: *How did it come about in 1980 that you also took on the Chairmanship of Medicine at the Beth Israel Hospital and became the Herrman Blumgart Professor of Medicine at that hospital?*

EB: The Dean and the President of the Beth Israel (BI) Hospital asked me to do this, i.e., attempt to unify the programs at the BI and the Brigham. Initially it was for 5 years, which grew into 9. As Physician-in-Chief, I took resident reports in both hospitals almost daily. I walked across Longwood Avenue twice a day for most of 9 years and wore out a lot of shoes. It is very interesting and gratifying that the new Dean of the Medical School, Dr. Joseph Martin, is now reenergizing the effort of integrating the Harvard hospitals.

WCR: *It sounds to me like your experience in trying to unify the medical programs between the Brigham and Women's Hospital and the Beth Israel Hospital is ideal for what you are now trying to do between the Brigham and Women's Hospital and the Massachusetts General Hospital. What are your goals now?*

EB: It is a very exciting period at Partners Health-Care System, the parent corporation formed by the merger of these 2 great hospitals. We are trying to make the transition from 2 tertiary-quaternary medical centers, ivory towers if you will, to an integrated healthcare system with a distributed network of physicians in the region and many other community hospitals and care organizations. In many ways this challenge is reminiscent of other things that I got into on the ground floor earlier, at NIH and at UCSD.

WCR: *Tell me about your editing.*

EB: Serving as an editor of *Harrison's Principles of Internal Medicine* has been a major and very rewarding part of my life since 1967. Harrison's is translated into 11 languages, and it is awesome, thrilling, and gratifying to think of teaching medicine to many hundreds of thousands of physicians and students with each edition. I started on the sixth edition, was Editor in Chief of the 11th edition, and will be Editor in Chief of the next edition (the 15th) now in the planning stages. We are also bringing out *Harrison's On-Line,* which should be available soon. I view the transition of this textbook to the Internet as a very important task. I am also beginning to think actively about the next (6th) edition of *Heart Disease.* Because much cardiac care is not delivered by cardiologists now but by primary care physicians, Lee Goldman and I have just completed the first edition of *Primary Cardiology* that takes a totally different approach to cardiology than does *Heart Disease.* I hope that it will assist generalists in dealing with patients who have cardiac diseases.

WCR: *Are you active in research now?*

EB: I chair the Thrombolysis In Myocardial Infarction (TIMI) trial group, an organization that is headquartered at the Brigham and Women's Hospital. We now have a network of 850 hospitals on 4 continents and we are conducting 6 trials right now. As cardiologists, we all take great pride in the reduction of mortality from myocardial infarction from about 35% to 8%, but we cannot be satisfied. Therefore, we are actively trying to test new drugs, especially platelet glycoprotein IIb/IIIa inhibitors, to try to further reduce this mortality.

WCR: *Gene, the quantity of work that you put out daily or weekly is really incredible. I wonder if you could share some of your work habits with us. For example, what time do you wake up in the mornings? What time do you get to the hospital? How much work do you do at night after you get home, etc.?*

EB: I wake up around 6:30 A.M., and am usually at one of my several work locations by 8:00 or 8:30 A.M. I usually get home for dinner by 7:30 P.M., and work after dinner until around 10:00 or 11:00 P.M. on weekdays. I also normally do about 14 hours of writing or editing each weekend.

For each edition of *Heart Disease,* I have gone on a semisabbatical. I can do *Harrison's* while doing my other jobs, but *Heart Disease* is another matter. I feel strongly that an editor should not be someone who just invites authors and transmits their work to the publisher. I write a lot of chapters in both books and spend much time editing those I don't write. I took a full year off to do the first edition of *Heart Disease* (from July 1, 1978, to June 30, 1979), and have taken 6- to 8-month sabbaticals for each subsequent edition.

WCR: *Do you write the books at home during these minisabbaticals?*

EB: Yes. A lot of it is done by fax between my staff at the office and me. A taxi takes a package from my house every morning and another comes back every evening.

WCR: *Everyday you have a certain amount written and you send it to your office to get it typed?*

EB: Yes or fax it to the office.

WCR: *I know that when you were at NIH you wrote your manuscripts out, paper and pencil. Do you do that now? How much do you dictate?*

EB: I mostly still write them by hand. Old habits die hard.

WCR: *Classical music is still a very important thing in your life?*

EB: As much as ever. I listen to classical music while I read, write, or edit. At this point I can't write or edit well without listening to classical music.

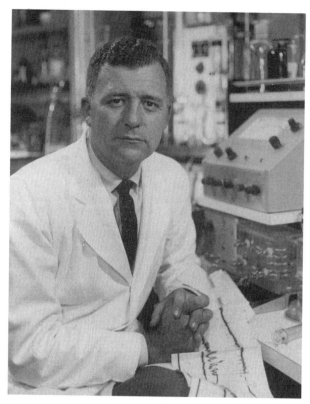

FIGURE 4. EB at time of appointment as Chief, Cardiology Branch, National Heart, Lung, and Blood Institute, in 1960 at age 31. By this young age, Braunwald had already had 7 years in cardiovascular research.

WCR: *You have 3 daughters? You have been extremely busy all your life and yet you appear to be a devoted father. The daughters have been very successful. Are you proud of your fathering?*

EB: I am proud of my daughters, but I think that I could have done better as a father. I was always very busy during the years in which they grew up, but we have stayed close. After their professional educations, they returned to the Boston area, and they and their families (6 grandchildren) live within 10 to 15 minutes of the home I share with my second wife, Elaine. We both enjoy the family tremendously, but again, I do not spend as much time with them as I would like to, although I see them almost every weekend.

WCR: *Is Sunday the day you relax a bit more?*
EB: Yes.

WCR: *Let's spend some time on your research accomplishments. You began in Ludwig Eichna's laboratory in Bellevue Hospital, did a number of left-sided hemodynamic studies at the Mt. Sinai Hospital and in Andre Cournand's laboratory at Bellevue Hospital. With Sarnoff at NIH you examined the determinants of myocardial oxygen consumption and continued that work, among others, later in your own laboratory at NIH. You also explored the roles of the adrenergic nervous system and the carotid sinus reflex in cardiovascular control. I gather that you had* learned *that stimulation of the carotid-sinus nerves reflex reduced all 3 major determinants of myocardial oxygen consumption that you had already defined, namely systemic arterial pressure, heart rate, and myocardial contractility. Can you discuss your work with carotid-sinus stimulation and how that led to your major work of limiting the size of an evolving acute myocardial infraction?*

EB: In 1966 Seymour Schwartz in the Department of Surgery at the University of Rochester, New York, was experimenting with an implanted electrical stimulator that provided continuous stimulation of the carotid sinus nerves and used this technique to reduce arterial pressure in conscious dogs with renovascular hypertension. When, on a visit to his laboratory in 1966, I observed this intriguing preparation it occurred to me that patient-controlled, transient electrical stimulation of these nerves might relieve angina pectoris by reducing myocardial oxygen consumption. Back in Bethesda, Stephen Epstein, Andrew Wechsler, Gerald Glick, my late wife Nina, and I developed a system whereby patients could self-activate a radiofrequency stimulator whenever they experienced severe angina pectoris. The device consisted of a stimulator with an external power source, not much larger than a pack of cigarettes, a transmitter taped to the surface of the chest, and an antenna inserted into the subcutaneous tissue that led to electrodes attached to the carotid sinus nerves. As we hoped, the stimulation reduced myocardial oxygen consumption and thereby relieved intractable angina. Having obtained considerable physiologic information from use of this device in patients, we had just begun a large clinical trial when Favoloro and Effler's landmark report on coronary artery bypass grafting made this approach to the treatment of angina pectoris obsolete.

However, this was not a wasted effort. A fortuitous event involving one of these patients with the implanted electrodes led to a watershed event in my professional life. We were concerned with the possible risk of excessive hypotension and bradycardia with carotid-sinus nerve stimulation if patients developed myocardial infarction. Therefore, we instructed our patients not to activate their stimulators if the ischemic discomfort was unusually severe or was not alleviated after a few minutes of stimulation. One patient who presented to us at the NIH with an evolving infarction left the carotid sinus stimulator activated, contrary to advice. Although when I first saw him I immediately turned it off, I noted on my return to the beside about 20 minutes later that he had reactivated it, and I deactivated it a second time. When we looked at the patient's ECG that evening, it was clear that during the periods when he had disregarded my instructions and activated the stimulator, the ST seg-

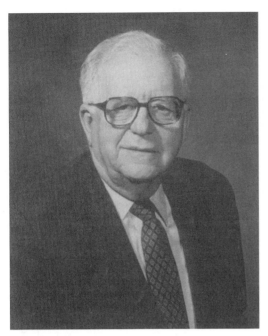

FIGURE 5. EB today.

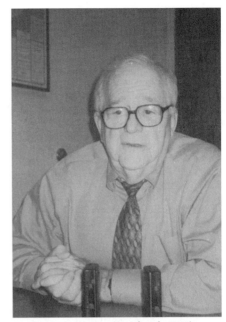

FIGURE 6. EB during the interview (photo by WCR).

ments on the electrocardiograms were almost isoelec-tric, while they were abnormally elevated when the stimulator was deactivated. At the time, the size of myocardial infarcts was thought to be irrevocably determined by the site of coronary artery occlusion and by the extent of the collateral circulation. But the finding that elevated ST segments in a patient under-going myocardial infarction could be normalized by an intervention that reduces myocardial oxygen con-sumption suggested that it might be possible to dimin-ish the extent of myocardial ischemic damage—i.e., to limit the size of an evolving infarction—by establish-ing a more favorable balance between myocardial oxygen supply and demand.

In 1968, when we moved to San Diego, I re-established my laboratory, albeit a much smaller one than I had at NIH. In addition to John Ross, Burton Sobel, Peter Poole, Bill Friedman, and James Covell, who had joined me, I also had an imaginative post-doctoral fellow, the late Peter Maroko. Peter and I studied anesthestized dogs with transient coronary oc-clusion. In an attempt to modify infarct size, we in-creased myocardial oxygen demand with beta-adren-ergic agonists and pacing-induced tachycardia and we reduced it with beta-adrenergic antagonists. At John Ross' suggestion, we determined the extent and se-verity of ischemia by recording epicardial ST seg-ments. We found that following coronary artery oc-clusion, the extent and severity of ischemia—which correlates closely with the size of the evolving infarc-tion—could be modified. Those interventions which simultaneously increased the delivery of oxygen to the myocardium and reduced myocardial demand for oxy-

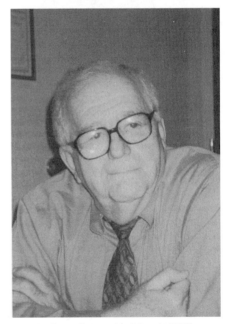

FIGURE 7. EB during the interview (photo by WCR).

gen, such as intraaortic balloon counterpulsation, were particularly effective in reducing infarct size. The infusion of glucose, insulin, and potassium to increase the generation of myocardial energy through anaero-bic metabolism was also helpful. Hypotension and beta-adrenergic agonists, on the other hand, increased ischemic injury, presumably by reducing perfusion of the ischemic area through collaterals and augmenting myocardial oxygen needs, respectively. Coronary reperfusion was particularly effective in limiting infarct size.

Initially in San Diego and later at Harvard, I continued my collaboration with Peter Maroko and later with James Muller and Robert Kloner. In trying to refine methods for assessing the severity and extent of ischemic injury in the dog, we turned to the anatomic measurement of infarct size and ultimately were able to relate necrosis to the quantity of myocardium within the area of distribution of the occluded artery—i.e., the area at risk. Our hope, of course, was to extend to patients the concept of limiting ischemic injury during an evolving infarction. We monitored the extent of ischemic injury in patients by measuring ST-segment elevations using a 35-lead precordial electrode system. In acute experiments, the use of beta blockade seemed helpful in limiting infarct size in patients.

The management of patients with acute myocardial infarction changed radically in 1979 when Rentrop and his collaborators showed that intracoronary thrombolytic therapy made it feasible to restore myocardial perfusion, improving the balance between myocardial oxygen supply and demand. By 1981, our group at the Beth Israel had shown that this intervention reduced infarct size in patients. In 1984, I was invited by the National Heart, Lung, and Blood Institute to chair the TIMI trials. In the first of these multicenter trials we demonstrated that the then-new thrombolytic agent, tissue plasminogen activator, was superior to the "reference" thrombolytic agent, streptokinase, in opening occluded, infarct-related arteries. This provided the exciting opportunity to administer one of the first pharmaceutical agents produced by recombinant technique and allowed us, after a struggle of almost 2 decades, finally to limit infarct size in patients with an approach that could easily be applied to patients in a variety of settings—the home, the ambulance, and the hospital emergency room.

At present, my research as chairman of the TIMI trials—with the TIMI 18 trial in the series now underway, and TIMI 19 and 20 on the drawing boards—continues to focus on attempts to reduce ischemic damage and thereby improve the outcome in patients with acute myocardial infarction and unstable angina. We are now studying newer antithrombotic and antiplatelet agents.

WCR: *What about your other efforts to study myocardial infarction?*

EB: In the course of experiments in the dog with experimentally induced myocardial ischemia, first carried out in the laboratory of Stephen Vatner (who had been one of my associates in San Diego) and subsequently in my laboratory with Bob Kloner, a previously unknown connection between myocardial ischemia and left ventricular dysfunction was identified. After relief of a brief (15 to 30 minutes) period of severe ischemia, not long enough to cause myocardial necrosis, myocardial dysfunction can persist for hours, or even for several days, before function recovers.

Bob Kloner and I termed this "myocardial stunning." Once we began to look for it we found that myocardial stunning was quite prevalent and could be identified in a wide variety of common clinical conditions including unstable angina, variant angina, in patients with acute myocardial infarction treated by reperfusion, and postcardiac surgery patients. In 1982 we suggested that prolonged stunning could develop with chronic, moderate ischemia. This condition, subsequently referred to as " myocardial hibernation," is quite widespread. It can be recognized by several imaging techniques, and the presence of chronically stunned (hibernating) myocardium is now a frequent indication for myocardial revascularization.

One closely related aspect of our work on limiting myocardial dysfunction in myocardial infarction dealt with attempts to reduce the impact of myocardial infarction on ventricular function and thereby to prevent later heart failure. In the late 1970s, Marc and Janice Pfeffer and I began to investigate the late consequences of myocardial infarction. In studies of coronary occlusion in the rat, Marc and Jan noted that late remodeling of the left ventricle was a consequence of large transmural infarction. In 1980 we obtained small quantities of captopril, the newly developed angiotensin-converting enzyme inhibitor, and found that this agent was enormously effective in preventing postinfarct ventricular remodeling and subsequent left ventricular failure in the rat. We then extended this concept to patients. In the Survival and Ventricular Enlargement (SAVE) trial, we observed that captopril reduced long-term total and cardiovascular mortality, as well as the development of heart failure and of recurrent infarction in patients who had experienced a myocardial infarction.

WCR: *Gene, you mentioned that had you not traveled to Rochester, New York, in 1966; your work on carotid-sinus stimulation in humans would probably not have come about and this work in turn led to your multiple landmark studies on limiting the size of acute myocardial infarcts. Thus, at least on this occasion, a single trip was enormously rewarding. You have had to travel a good bit in your career. How have you managed your traveling obligations? Do you recoup or deplete your energies during your travels? I know you do a good bit of work on your travels. How has traveling played with your other responsibilities?*

EB: I think, like most people in academic medicine, I travel too much. But you're right, the experience is often intellectually enriching, occasionally unexpectedly so.

WCR: *Do you take vacations?*

EB: My wife, Elaine, and I enjoy traveling together. We often add 4 or 5 days onto a cardiology meeting in an interesting location.

WCR: *How are your energy levels, your capacity for work, now compared to 30 years ago? It looks to me as if you have not changed at all. Do you feel it a bit more now?*

EB: I need a little more sleep. I sure have problems with "all nighters." On the other hand, I think that I

INTERVIEW: EUGENE BRAUNWALD **105**

676

work more efficiently now and I guess that's the tradeoff.

WCR: *I wonder if you could comment on your medical statesmanship. Here you have been departmental chairman for 28 years, you have taken on another responsibility now which is more challenging than your department. You have other medical school responsibilities as Faculty Dean at Harvard, you are on a number of advisory boards, presidential, etc. It is unending, but each of these brings a new experience I would presume?*

EB: To me these various facets of my professional life have been mutually reinforcing. I served for 2 nonconsecutive terms on the National Heart, Lung, and Blood Institute's Advisory Council, and I have had a number of other responsibilities of that nature including some at Harvard Medical School. I appreciate those opportunities. We live in the most exciting period in the history of medicine and biomedical science and it is challenging to attempt to influence the field in a positive way and a privilege sometimes to have the chance to do so. It is often very slow-going on these committees, and I tend to get very impatient, but every once in a long while you do get the chance influence matters in a positive way.

WCR: *Dr. Braunwald, thank you for sharing your thoughts, your past, and your desires for the future with the AJC readers.*

EB: Thank you, Bill. It's an honor to join the luminaries in your series.

Selected Publications of EB Selected by EB
Selected Books and Monographs

Braunwald E, Lambrew CT, Rockoff SD, Ross J Jr, Morrow AG. Idiopathic hypertrophic subaortic stenosis. *Circulation* 30: (suppl 4) 1964, 119 pp.

Braunwald E, Ross J Jr, Sonnenblick EH. Mechanisms of Contraction of the Normal and Failing Heart, 1st ed. Boston: Little, Brown & Co., (2nd ed. 1976).

Braunwald E (ed). The Myocardium: Failure and Infarction. New York: H.P. Publishing, Co., Inc., 1974.

Braunwald, E (ed). Beta-Adrenergic Blockade—A New Era in Cardiovascular Medicine. New York: Elsevier, 1978.

Braunwald, E (ed). Heart Disease: A Textbook of Cardiovascular Medicine, 1st ed. Philadelphia: WB Saunders, 1980. (Subsequent editions in 1984, 1988, 1992, and 1997).

Braunwald E, Mock MB, Watson JT (eds). Congestive Heart Failure: Current Research and Clinical Applications. New York: Grune & Stratton, 1982.

Braunwald E, Isselbacher KJ, Petersdorf RG, Wilson JD, Martin JB, Faucix AS (eds). Harrison's Principles of Internal Medicine. 11th ed. New York: McGraw Hill, 1987. (Other editions in 1970, 1974, 1977, 1980, 1983, 1991, 1994, and 1998).

Bleifeld W, Hamm CW, Braunwald E (eds). Unstable Angina. Berlin: Springer Verlag, 1990.

Haber E, Braunwald E (eds). Thrombolysis—Basic Contributions and Clinical Progess. St. Louis: Mosby Year Book, 1991.

Braunwald E (ed). Atlas of Heart Diseases, 14 volumes. Philadelphia: Current Medicine, 1995–1998.

Goldman L, Braunwald E (eds). Primary Cardiology. Philadelphia: WB Saunders, 1998.

Physiology, Pathophysiology, and Pharmacology*

5. Braunwald E, Moscovitz HL, Amram S, Lasser RP, Sapin SO, Himmelstein A, Rvaitch MM, Gordon AJ. The hemodynamics of the left side of the heart as studied by simultaneous left atrial, left ventricular, and aortic pressures; particular reference to mitral stenosis. *Circulation* 1955;12:69–81.

12. Braunwald E, Fishman AP, Cournand A. Time relationship of dynamic events in the cardiac chambers, pulmonary artery and aorta in man. *Circ Res* 1956;4:100–107.

---

*From EB's sequentially numbered bibliography.

26. Braunwald E, Welch, GH Jr, Sarnoff SJ. Hemodynamic effects of quantitatively varied experimental mitral regurgitation. *Circ Res* 1957;5:539–545.

33. Sarnoff SJ, Braunwald E, Welch GH Jr, Case RB, Stainsby WN, Marcruz R. Hemodynamic determinants of oxygen consumption of the heart with special reference to the tension-time index. *Am J Physiol* 1958;192:148–156.

34. Braunwald E, Sarnoff SJ, Case RB, Stainsby WN, Welch GH Jr. Hemodynamic determinants of coronary flow: effect of changes in aortic pressure and cardiac output on the relationship between myocardial oxygen consumption and coronary flow. *Am J Physiol* 1958;192:157–163.

72. Ross J Jr, Waldhausen JA, Braunwald E. Studies on digitalis. I. Direct effects on peripheral vascular resistance. *J Clin Invest* 1960;39:930–936.

168. Chidsey CA, Kaiser GA, Braunwald E. Biosynthesis of norepinephrine in isolated canine heart. *Science* 1963;139:828–829.

180. Braunwald E, Chidsey CA, Harrison DC, Gaffney TE, Kahler RL. Studies on the function of the adrenergic nerve endings in the heart. *Circulation* 1963; 28:958–969.

248. Epstein SE, Robinson BF, Kahler RL, Braunwald E. Effects of beta-adrenergic blockade on the cardiac response to maximal and submaximal exercise in man. *J Clin Invest* 1965;44:1745–1753.

250. Mason DT, Braunwald E. The effects of nitroglycerin and amyl nitrite on arteriolar and venous tone in the human forearm. *Circulation* 1965;32:755–766.

253. Sonnenblick EH, Ross J Jr, Covell JW, Kaiser GA, Braunwald E. Velocity of contraction as a determinant of myocardial oxygen consumption. *Am J Physiol* 1965;209:919–927.

418. Vatner SF, Franklin D, Van Citters RL, Braunwald E. Effects of carotid sinus nerve stimulation on the coronary circulation of the conscious dog. *Circ Res* 1970;27:11–21.

452. Eckberg DL, Brabinsky M, Braunwald E. Defective cardiac parasympathetic control in patients with heart disease. *N Engl J Med* 1971;285:877–883.

Diagnostic Methods and Clinical Cardiology

31. Braunwald E, Tanenbaum HL, Morrow AG. Localization of left-to-right cardiac shunts by dye-dilution curves following injection into the left side of the heart and into the aorta. *Am J Med* 1958;24:203–208.

87. Ross J Jr, Braunwald E, Morrow AG. Left heart catheterization by the transseptal route: a descrption of the technic and its applications. *Circulation* 1960;22:927–934.

96. Cornell WP, Braunwald E, Morrow AG. Precordial scanning: applications in the detection of left-to-right circulatory shunts. *Circulation* 1961;23:21–29.

108. Braunwald E, Brockenbrough EC, Frahm, CJ, Ross J Jr. Left atrial and left ventricular pressures in subjects without cardiovascular disease: observations in eighteen patients studied by transseptal left heart catheterization. *Circulation* 1961;24:267–269.

121. Folse R, Braunwald E. Determination of fraction of left ventricular volume ejected per beat and of ventricular end-diastolic and residual volumes. *Circulation* 1962;25:674–685.

128. Folse R, Braunwald E. Pulmonary vascular dilution curves recorded by external detection in the diagnosis of left-to-right shunts. *Br Heart J* 1962;24:166–172.

148. Braunwald NS, Braunwald E, Morrow AG. The effects of surgical abolition of left-to-right shunts on the pulmonary vascular dynamics of patients with pulmonary hypertension. *Circulation* 1962;26:1270–1278.

162. Braunwald E, Goldblatt A, Aygen MM, Rockoff SD, Morrow AG. Congenital aortic stenosis. Clinical and hemodynamic findings in 100 patients. *Circulation* 1963;27:426–450.

264. Roberts WC, Braunwald E, Morrow AG. Acute severe mitral regurgitation secondary to ruptured chordae tendineae. Clinical, hemodynamic and pathologic considerations. *Circulation* 1966;33:58–70.

386. Mason DT, Ashburn WL, Harbert JC, Cohen LS, Braunwald E. Rapid sequential visualization of the heart and great vessels in man using the wide-field anger scintillation camera: radioisotope-angiography following the injection of technetium-99m. *Circulation* 1969;39:19–28.

454. Ashburn WL, Braunwald E, Simon AL, Peterson KL, Gault JH. Myocardial perfusion imaging with radioactive-labeled particles injected directly into the coronary circulation of patients with coronary artery disease. *Circulation* 1971; 44:851–865.

Hypertrophic Cardiomyopathy

89. Braunwald E, Morrow AG, Cornell WP, Aygen MM, Hilbish TF. Idiopathic hypertrophic subaortic stenosis. Clinical, hemodynamic and angiographic manifestations. *Am J Med* 1960;29:924–945.

147. Braunwald E, Ebert PA. Hemodynamic alterations in idiopathic subaortic stenosis induced by sympathomimetic drugs. *Am J Cardiol* 1962;10:489–495.

216. Braunwald E, Lambrew CT, Rickoff SD, Ross J Jr, Morrow AG. Idiopathic hypertrophic subaortic stenosis. A description of the disease based upon an analysis of 64 patients. *Circulation* 1964;30 (suppl IV):3–119.

293. Ross J Jr, Braunwald E, Gault JH, Mason DT, Morrow AG. The mechanism of the intraventricular pressure gradient in idiopathic hypertrophic subaortic stenosis. *Circulation* 1966;34:558–578.

311. Cohen LS, Braunwald E. Amelioration of angina pectoris in idiopathic hypertrophic subaortic stenosis with beta-adrenergic blockade. *Circulation* 1967; 35:847–851.

Ventricular Function, Hypertrophy, and Failure

112. Braunwald E, Frahm CJ, Ross J Jr. Studies on Starling's law of the heart. V. Left ventricular function in man. *J Clin Invest* 1961;40:1882–1890.

141. Aygen MM, Braunwald E. Studies on Starling's law of the heart. VIII. Mechanical properties of human myocardium studied in vivo. *Circulation* 1962; 26:516–524.

144. Chidsey CA, Harrison DC, Braunwald E. Augmentation of the plasma norepinephrine response to exercise in patients with congestive heart failure. *N Engl J Med* 1962;267:650–654.

181. Chidsey CA, Braunwald E, Morrow AG, Mason DT. Myocardial norepinephrine concentration in man: effects of reserpine and of congestive heart failure. *N Engl J Med* 1963;269:653–658.

211. Ross J Jr, Braunwald E. Studies on Starling's law of the heart. IX. The effects of impeding venous return on performance of the normal and failing human left ventricle. *Circulation* 1964;30:719–727.

212. Chidsey CA, Kaiser GA, Sonnenblick EH, Spann JF, Braunwald E. Cardiac norepinephrine stores in experimental heart failure in the dog. *J Clin Invest* 1964;43:2386–2393.

234. Glick G, Sonnenblick EH, Braunwald E. Myocardial force-velocity relations studied in intact unanesthetized man. *J Clin Invest* 1965;44:978–988.

263. Chidsey CA, Sonnenblick EH, Morrow AG, Braunwald E. Norepinephrine stores and contractile force of papillary muscle from the failing human heart. *Circulation* 1966;33:43–51.

284. Covell JW, Chidsey CA, Braunwald E. Reduction of the cardiac response to postganglionic sympathetic nerve stimulation in experimental heart failure. *Circ Res* 1966;19:51–56.

321. Spann JF Jr, Buccino RA, Sonnenblick EH, Braunwald E. Contractile state of cardiac muscle obtained from cats with experimentally produced ventricular hypertrophy and heart failure. *Circ Res* 1967;21:341–354.

347. Gault JH, Ross J Jr, Braunwald E. Contractile state of the left ventricle in man. Instantaneous tension-velocity-length relations in patients with and without disease of the left ventricular myocardium. *Circ Res* 1968;22:451–463.

467. Higgins CB, Vatner SF, Eckberg DL, Braunwald E. Alterations in the baroreceptor reflex in conscious dogs with heart failure. *J Clin Invest* 1972;51: 715–724.

478. Higgins CB, Vatner SF, Franklin D, Braunwald E. Effects of experimentally produced heart failure on the peripheral vascular response to severe exercise in conscious dogs. *Circ Res* 1972;31:186–194.

658. Pfeffer JM, Pfeffer MA, Mirsky E, Braunwald E. Regression of left ventricular hypertrophy and prevention of left ventricular dysfunction by captopril in the spontaneously hypertensive rat. *Proc Natl Acad Sci* 1982;79:3310–3314.

744. Pfeffer JM, Pfeffer MA, Braunwald E. Influence of chronic captopril therapy on the infarcted left ventricle of the rat. *Circ Res* 1985;57:84–95.

812. Pfeffer MA, Lamas GA, Vaughan DE, Parisi AF, Braunwald E. Effects of captopril on progressive ventricular dilatation after anterior myocardial infarction. *N Engl J Med* 1988;319:80–86.

842. Pfeffer MA, Braunwald E. Ventricular remodeling following myocardial infarction: experimental observations and clinical implications. *Circulation* 1990; 81:1161–1172.

870. Pfeffer JM, Pfeffer MA, Fletcher PJ, Braunwald E. Progressive ventricular remodeling in rat with myocardial infarction. *Am J Physiol* 1991;260:H1406–H1414.

895. Pfeffer MA, Braunwald E, Moye LA, Basta L, Brown EJ Jr, Cuddy TE, Davis BR, Geltman EM, Goldman S, Flaker GC, Klein M, Lamas GA, Packer M, Rouleau J, Rouleau JL, Rutherford J, Wertheimer JH, Hawkins CM, on behalf of the SAVE Investigators. Effect of captopril on mortality and morbidity in patients with left ventricular dysfunction after myocardial infarction. Results of the Survival and Ventricular Enlargement Trial. *N Engl J Med* 1992;327:669–677.

926. Braunwald E (Chairman of Task Force). Report of the Task Force on Research in Heart Failure, National Heart, Lung, and Blood Institute 1994:1–108.

Myocardial Ischemia and Infarction

334. Braunwald E, Epstein SE, Glick G, Wechsler A, Braunwald NS. Relief of angina pectoris by electrical stimulation of the carotid sinus. *N Engl J Med* 1967;277:1278–1283.

432. Maroko PR, Kjekshus JK, Sobel BE, Watanabe T, Covell JW, Ross J Jr, Braunwald E. Factors influencing infarct size following experimental coronary artery occlusion. *Circulation* 1971;43:67–82.

474. Maroko PR, Libby P, Sobel BE, Bloor CM, Sybers HD, Shell WE, Covell JW, Braunwald E. Effect of glucose-insulin-potassium infusion on myocardial infarction following experimental coronary artery occlusion. *Circulation* 1972; 45:1160–1175.

491. Libby P, Maroko PR, Covell JW, Malloch CI, Ross J Jr, Braunwald E. Effect of practolol on the extent of myocardial ischemic injury after experimental coronary occlusion and its effects on ventricular function in the normal and ischemic heart. *Cardiovasc Res* 1973;7:167–173.

500. Maroko PR, Braunwald E. Modification of myocardial infarct size after coronary occlusion. *Ann Intern Med* 1973;79:720–733.

518. Braunwald E. Reduction of myocardial infarct size. *N Engl J Med* 1974; 291:525–526.

529. Muller JE, Maroko PR, Braunwald E. Evaluation of precordial electrocardiographic mapping as a means of assessing changes in myocardial ischemic injury. *Circulation* 1975;52:16–27.

544. Mudge GH Jr, Grossman W, Mills RM Jr, Lesch M, Braunwald E. Reflex coronary artery vasoconstriction in patients with ischemic heart disease. *N Engl J Med* 1976;295:1333–1336.

593. Pfeffer MA, Pfeffer JM, Fishbein MC, Fletcher PJ, Spadaro J, Kloner RA, Braunwald E. Myocardial infarct size and ventricular function in rats. *Circ Res* 1979;44:503–512.

613. Antman E, Muller J, Goldberg S, MacAlpin R, Rubenfire M, Tabatznik B, Liang E, Heupler F, Achuff S, Reicheck N, Geltman E, Kerin NS, Neff RK, Braunwald E. Nifedipine therapy for coronary artery spasm: experience in 127 patients. *N Engl J Med* 1980;302:1269–1273.

625. DeBoer LWV, Strauss HW, Kloner RA, Rude RE, David RF, Maroko PR, Braunwald E. Autoradiographic method for measuring the ischemic myocardium at risk: effects of verapamil on infarct size after experimental coronary artery occlusion. *Proc Natl Acad Sci* 1980;77:6119–6123.

648. Markis JE, Malagold M, Parker JA, SIlverman KJ, Barry WH, Als AV, Paulin S, Grossman W, Braunwald E. Myocardial salvage after intracoronary thrombolysis with streptokinase in acute myocardial infarction: assessment of intracoronary thallium-201. *N Engl J Med* 1981;305:777–782.

653. Ertl G, Kloner RA, Alexander RW, Braunwald E. Limitation of experimental infarct size by angiotensin-converting enzyme inhibitor. *Circulation* 1982;65: 40–48.

672. Braunwald E, Kloner RA. The stunned myocardium: prolonged, postischemic ventricular dysfunction. *Circulation* 1982;66:1146–1149.

682. Ellis SG, Henschke CI, Sandor T, Wynne J, Braunwald E, Kloner RA. Time course of functional and biochemical recovery of myocardium salvaged by reperfusion. *J Am Coll Cardiol* 1983;1:1047–1055.

690. Kloner RA, Ellis SG, Lange R, Braunwald E. Studies of experimental coronary artery reperfusion. Effects on infarct size, myocardial function, biochemistry, ultrastructure and microvascular damage. *Circulation* 1983;68 (suppl II):II-8–II-15.

694. DeBoer LWV, Rude RE, Kloner RA, Ingwall JS, Maroko PR, Davis MA, Braunwald E. A flow- and time-dependent index of ischemic injury after experimental coronary occlusion and reperfusion. *Proc Natl Acad Sci* 1983;80:5784–5788.

704. Ellis SG, Wynne J, Braunwald E, Henschke CI, Sandor T, Kloner R. Response of reperfusion-salvaged, stunned myocardium to inotropic stimulation. *Am Heart J* 1984;107:13–19.

711. Muller JE, Turi ZG, Pearle DL, Schneider JF, Serfas DH, Morrison J, Stone PH, Rude RE, Rosner B, Sobel BE, Tate C, Scheiner E, Roberts R, Hennekens CH, Braunwald E. Nifedipine and conventional therapy for unstable angina pectoris: a randomized, double-blind comparison. *Circulation* 1984;69:728–739.

718. Hammerman H, Kloner RA, Briggs LL, Braunwald E. Enhancement of salvage of reperfused myocardium by early beta-adrenergic blockade. *J Am Coll Cardiol* 1984;3:1438–1443.

725. Laffel GL, Braunwald E. Thrombolytic therapy: a new strategy for the treatment of acute myocardial infarction. *N Engl J Med* 1984;311:710–717;707–776.

755. Muller JE, Stone PH, Turi ZG, Rutherford JD, Czeisler CA, Parker C, Poole WK, Roberts R, Robertson T, Sobel BE, Willerson JT, Braunwald E, and the MILIS Study Group. Circadian variation in the frequency of onset of acute myocardial infarction. *N Engl J Med* 1985;313:1315–1322.

782. Braunwald E, Rutherford JD. Reversible ischemic left ventricular dysfunction: evidence for the "hibernating myocardium." *J Am Coll Cardiol* 1986;8: 1467–1470.

787. Sheehan FH, Braunwald E, Canner P, Dodge HT, Gore J, Van Netta P, Passamani ER, WIlliams DO, Zaret B, Co-Investigators. The effect of intravenous thrombolytic therapy of left ventricular function: a report on tissue-type plasminogen activator and streptokinase from the Thrombolysis in Myocardial Infarction (TIMI Phase I) trial. *Circulation* 1987;75:817–829.

792. The TIMI Study Group, Braunwald E (Chairman). The thrombolysis in myocardial infarction trial. *N Engl J Med* 1985;312:932.

829. The TIMI Study Group, Braunwald E (Chairman). Comparison of invasive and conservative strategies after treatment with intravenous tissue plasminogen activator in acute myocardial infarction. Results of the Thrombolysis in Myocardial Infarction (TIMI) Phase II trial. *N Engl J Med* 1989;320:618–627.

836. Braunwald E. Unstable angina—a classification. *Circulation* 1989;80:410–414.

837. Braunwald E Enhancing thrombolytic efficacy by means of "front-loaded" administration of tissue plasminogen activator. *J Am Coll Cardiol* 1989;14:1570–1571.

845. Rogers WJ, Baim DS, Gore JM, Brown BG, Roberts R, Williams DO, Chesebro JH, Babb JD, Sheehan FH, Wackers FJTh, Zaret BL, Robertson TL, Passamani ER, Ross R, Knatterud GL, Braunwald E. Comparison of immediate invasive, delayed invasive, and conservative strategies after tissue-type plasminogen activator—results of the Thrombolysis in Myocardial Infarction (TIMI) Phase II-A trial. *Circulation* 1990;81:1457–1476.

908. Kim CB, Braunwald E. Potential benefits of late reperfusion of infarcted myocardium: the open artery hypothesis. *Circulation* 1993;88:2426–2436.

918. The TIMI III B Investigators, Braunwald E (Chairman). Effects of tissue plasminogen activator and a comparison of early invasive and conservative strategies in unstable angina and non-Q-wave myocardial infarction. Results of the TIMI III B trial. *Circulation* 1994;89:1545–1556.

925. Braunwald E (Panel Chair). Unstable Angina: diagnosis and Management. Clinical Practice Guideline #10. Agency for Health Care Policy and Research, National Heart, Lung, and Blood Institute (publication no. 94-0602) 1994:1–154.
938. Kloner RA, Shook T, Prezyklenk K, Davis VG, Junio L, Matthews RV, Burstein S, Gibson CM, Poole WK, Cannon CP, McCabe Ch, Braunwald E, for the TIMI-4 Investigators. Previous angina alters in-hospital outcome in TIMI 4: a clinical correlate to preconditioning? *Circulation* 1995;91:37–45.
945. Cannon CP, Braunwald E, McCabe CH, Antman EM. The Thrombolysis in Myocardial Infarction (TIMI) trials: the first decade. *J Intervent Cardiol* 1995; 8:117–135.
950. Lamas GA, Flaker GC, Mitchell G, Smith SC, Gersh BJ, Wun C-C, Moyé L, Rouleau JL, Rutherford JD, Pfeffer MA, Braunwald E, for the Survival and Ventricular Enlargement (SAVE) Investigators. Effect of infarct artery patency on prognosis after acute myocardial infarction. *Circulation* 1995;92:1101–1109.
960. Gibson CM, Cannon CP, Daley WL, Dodge JT, Alexander B, Marble SJ, McCabe CH, Raymond L, Fortin T, Poole WK, Braunwald E. TIMI frame count: a quantitative method of assessing coronary artery flow. *Circulation* 1996;93: 879–888.
971. Antman EM, Tanasijevic MJ, Thompson B, Schactman M, McCabe CH, Cannon CP, Fischer GA, Fung AY, Thompson C, Wybenga D, Braunwald E. Cardiac-specific troponin I levels to predict the risk of mortality in patients with acute coronary syndromes. *N Engl J Med* 1996;335:1342–1349.
975. Cannon CP, McCabe CH, Gibson CM, Ghali M, Sequiera RF, McKendall GR, Breed J, Modi NB, Fox NL, Tracy RP, Love TW, Braunwald E, and the TIMI 10A Investigators. TNK-tissue plasminogen activator in acute myocardial infarction. *Circulation* 1997;95:351–356.
1012. Cannon CP, McCabe CH, Borzak S, Henry TD, Tischler MD, Mueller HS, Feldman R, Palmeri ST, Ault K, Hamilton SA, Rothman JM, Novothy WF, Braunwald E, for the TIMI 12 Investigators. Randomized trial of an oral platelet glycoprotein IIb/IIIa antagonist, sibrafiban, in patients after an acute coronary syndrome: results of the TIMI I2 trial. *Circulation* 1998;97:340–349.

Policy and Education

378. Braunwald E. The teaching of physiology. VI. A clinician's view of physiological training for the future physician. *J Med Ed* 1968;43:1161–1165.
419. Braunwald E, Grobstein E. The clinical department as a critical scientific mass. Implications for instruction in the preclinical disciplines. *J Med Ed* 1970; 45:525–530.
428. Braunwald E. The Loyal Opposition. Presidential Address, American Federation for Clinical Research. *Clin Res* 1970;18:555–559.

471. Braunwald E. Future shock in academic medicine. Presidential Address, Western Society of Clinical Research. *N Engl J Med* 1972;286:1031–1035.
523. Braunwald E. The training of manpower for biomedical research. *N Engl J Med* 1975;292:290–293.
530. Braunwald E. Can medical schools remain the optimal site for the conduct of clinical investigation? Presidential Address, American Society for Clinical Investigation. *J Clin Invest* 1975;56:i–vi.
662. Braunwald E. The present state and future of academic cardiology. The James B. Herrick Lecture. *Circulation* 1982;63:487–490.
729. Braunwald E. Thirty-five years of progress in cardiovascular research. *Circulation* 1984;70 (suppl III):III-8 –III-25.
762. Goldman L, Shea S, Wolf M, Braunwald E. Clinical and research training in parallel: the internal medicine research residency track at the Brigham and Women's Hospital. *Clin Res* 1986;34:1–5.
804. Braunwald E. On future directions for cardiology. The Paul D. White Lecture. *Circulation* 1988;77:13–32.
861. Braunwald E. Subspecialists and internal medicine: a perspective. *Ann Intern Med* 1991;114:76–78.
911. Braunwald E. Cardiology—division or department? *N Engl J Med* 1993; 329:1887–1890.
976. Braunwald E. The evolution of academic divisions of cardiology. *Circulation* 1997;95:545.
988. Braunwald E. Shattuck Lecture—cardiovascular medicine at the turn of the millennium: triumphs, concerns, and opportunities. *N Engl J Med* 1997;337: 1360–1369.

Other Subjects

779. Goldhaber SZ, Vaughan DE, Markis JE, Selwyn AP, Meyerovitz MF, Loscalzo J, Kim DS, Kessler CM, Dawley DL, Sharma GVRK, Sasahara A, Grossbard EB, Braunwald E. Acute pulmonary embolism treated with tissue plasminogen activator. *Lancet* 1986;2:886–889.
970. Sacks FM, Pfeffer MA, Moye LA, Rouleau JL, Rutherford JD, Cole TG, Brown L, Warnica JW, Arnold JM, Wun C-C, Davis BR, Braunwald E, for the CARE Investigators. The effect of pravastatin on coronary events after myocardial infarction in patients with average cholesterol levels: results of the Cholesterol and Recurrent Events (CARE) Trial. *N Engl J Med* 1996;335:1001–1009.
1016. Sacks FM, Moye LA, Davis BR, Cole TG, Rouleau JL, Nash DT, Pfeffer MA, Braunwald E. Relationship between plasma LDL concentrations during treatment with pravastatin and recurrent coronary events in the Cholesterol and Recurrent Events Trial. *Circulation* 1998;97:1446–1452.

ROBERT OGDEN BONOW, MD:
A Conversation With the Editor*

Bob Bonow was born in Camden, New Jersey, on 11 March 1947, and grew up in New Jersey in the suburbs of New York City. He graduated from Lehigh University magna cum laude in chemical engineering in 1969, and from the University of Pennsylvania School of Medicine in 1973. His medical internship and residency were at the Hospital of the University of Pennsylvania. In 1976 he went to the National Heart, Lung, and Blood Institute in Bethesda, Maryland, where he remained until 1992 when he moved to Chicago to be the Goldberg Distinguished Professor of Cardiology and Chief of the Division of Cardiology in the Department of Medicine of Northwestern University Medical School. Dr. Bonow is one of the world's outstanding cardiologists. He is a superb clinician, splendid clinical investigator, and marvelous teacher. He is also a nice guy and a good friend. I had the privilege of interviewing Dr. Bonow in his office at Northwestern University Medical Center in Chicago on 31 October 1997.

William Clifford Roberts, MD[†] (Hereafter, WCR): *Dr. Bonow, I would like to talk primarily about you as a person rather than about the work. I wonder if you could start by talking about your upbringing, where you were born, where you grew up, your family, your mother and father, your siblings.*

Robert Ogden Bonow, MD[‡] (Hereafter, ROB): I was born in New Jersey and grew up in the 1950s in a New York suburb. We originally lived in a little town called Wood Ridge, New Jersey. This same town produced several other cardiologists who have done quite well, including Raymond Gibbons at the Mayo Clinic. Ray and I played baseball in the same little league. My father was a chemical engineer and my mother was a homemaker. Both of them spent a lot of time with their kids and were very nurturing parents. There were a lot of things we did as a family. My father was very much involved in little league, Boy Scouts, and sports with his children. I have a brother, Tom, who is 2 years older and is now living in Dallas. I have a sister Kathryn who is 4 years younger and she lives in New Jersey. I came away from my childhood with the feeling from my parents that family is very important and spending time with children and nurturing them is a very important part of what being an adult is all about.

WCR: *What was it like around the dinner table at night when you would come home from school? Did you have a lot of discussions, was it an intellectual*

type of environs? What was it like on a day-to-day basis?

ROB: As youngsters, we dealt with the usual day-to-day things kids do and kids remember. I would not say it was terribly intellectual until perhaps when we were teenagers and could talk in a more adult style. We had a true family relationship, which I find very difficult to maintain in my own career. Sometimes I feel I am not giving to my family what I should, based upon what my parents gave me. My father traveled and had business obligations. He was not home every night, but when he was not traveling he was home for dinner. Even when he was traveling he somehow made it possible to be there when I had a baseball or basketball game. I played basketball in high school and college. He would travel sometimes hundreds of miles to get to the game, despite his own busy professional life. He was always there. I can't say our dinner conversations were always on the most intellectually fascinating things regarding finance, culture, politics or what was happening at that point in time in world history, but we were pretty much together as a family.

WCR: *You were an athlete. You played both basketball and baseball. What did you play in baseball?*

ROB: I played baseball (first baseman) up through high school and then dropped out when I was a junior. I was pretty good in the field, but not that good at batting. I stuck with basketball instead. As a high school student and college student I wound up practicing basketball almost every day of my life, maybe 6 or 7 years straight.

WCR: *Dr. Bonow, you went to Lehigh University in Bethlehem, Pennsylvania to college. Were you planning to be an engineer?*

ROB: Lehigh has a rich tradition in engineering. Initially, I was more or less following in the footsteps of my father. I did very well academically in science and math in high school, and engineering seemed like a rather natural and comfortable field for me to gravitate into. Three-quarters of the way through with my chemical engineering training I realized that I was not going to feel very gratified in that career. I had enough of the basic requisites through the engineering curriculum to be eligible to apply to medical school with a little extra biology and biochemistry in my senior year. Initially, I considered going into biomedical engineering, but with a little more experience in biomedical sciences, I realized that what I really wanted to be was a doctor.

WCR: *Did you go to college on a basketball scholarship?*

ROB: No, I was a walk-in candidate. Lehigh has a great tradition in wrestling, but it did not have much of a tradition in basketball. However, we competed among some of the better schools in the East, such as

*This series of interviews was underwritten by an unrestricted grant from Bristol-Myers Squibb.
[†]Executive Director, Baylor Cardiovascular Institute, Baylor University Medical Center, Dallas, Texas 75246.
[‡]Chief, Division of Cardiology; Goldberg Distinguished Professor, Northwestern University Medical School, Chicago, Illinois 60611.

0002-9149/98/$19.00
PII S0002-9149(98)00282-3

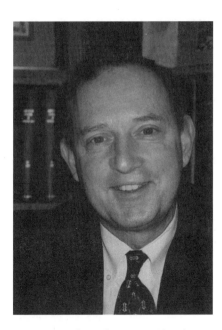

FIGURE 1. ROB during the interview (photo by WCR).

the Ivy League schools and the big 5 schools in Philadelphia. We played Army, and I played against Mike Krzyzewski when Bobby Knight was the coach at Army and against Jim Valvano when he played at Rutgers. Pete Carril was our coach at Lehigh before he went to Princeton, and so among many mentors there is one who is now in the basketball Hall of Fame. Coach Carril was like another father to me and instilled in me a sense of discipline, competitiveness, and goal orientation. He was only with us for a year at Lehigh before he went on to great success for 30 years at Princeton, but I remember many aspects of that year vividly, in almost minute-to-minute detail.

WCR: *You were on the varsity team all 4 years?*

ROB: Back then the NCAA had a freshman rule that permitted only 3 years of varsity eligibility. The same rule kept Lew Alcindor, who became Karem Abdul Jabbar, from playing 4 years of varsity ball at UCLA. They also had a rule about dunking. You could not dunk in college and you could only spend 3 years on the varsity team. The former rule affected Lew Alcindor more than me, but the latter rule affected both of us. I played on the freshmen team and then 3 years on the varsity. I was a co-captain my senior year.

WCR: *What position did you play on the basketball team?*

ROB: I was not big enough to play up front, so I was a shooting guard. I usually guarded someone a few inches taller than me. I could not handle the ball well enough to be the point man, but I had a pretty good outside shot. I would get out there in what is now 3-point territory. Unfortunately, the 3-point shot was not in effect at that time. If the 3-point shots were

credited as such at the time, I would have had a hefty increase in my total field goal scoring.

WCR: *You scored a lot of points?*

ROB: Of course, not as many as I would have liked to. I had a couple of 20-point games, but my average was in single figures. The 3-point shot would have been a big help.

WCR: *Were you first team all 3 years on the varsity?*

ROB: I started about 50% of the games. I probably was on the starting team in more games as a sophomore under Pete Carril. Then we started winning some games, and they began recruiting some talented underclassmen to better the team.

WCR: *You mentioned your basketball coach as a mentor. Was there anybody in your family who had been a physician? Were there other mentors in high school that had an influence on you?*

ROB: I am the first physician in the family, although my father had a major influence in helping me decide my ultimate career goals. I had several important mentors in high school. My basketball coach in high school, Bob Sanislow, is a wonderful guy, and he still keeps in contact. I went to high school in Westfield, New Jersey. Bob still lives in Westfield and we exchange notes around Christmas time. He was a true mentor on and off the court. He taught me enormously about how to get along with people in life, work as a team, work for common goals. He had great faith in me and in my potential and I hope I delivered. I remember many other teachers very fondly from high school—English, science, math—all of whom had a formative effect on me but are too numerous to mention here.

WCR: *You went to public high school?*

ROB: Yes.

WCR: *Who influenced you at Lehigh University?*

ROB: There were a number of people, most notably the basketball coaches, and my classmates. The Chairman of the Chemical Engineering Department, *Leonard Wenzel*, had a major influence on me. I remember having a meeting with him when I made the decision that engineering was not the field I wanted to pursue as a career. He was not disappointed in my decision and helped my plans to attend medical school. He was a very good advisor, very good at pointing me in the right direction. He recognized that I was setting my sights too low. I had done very well scholastically in the engineering curriculum, but as I was not in the premed curriculum, I did not believe that I would be a competitive applicant for the better schools. When I showed him my list of possible medical school applications, he quickly x'd out about 75%, because I was not shooting high enough.

WCR: *You played on the varsity basketball team in college as a walk-on, you made the team, and you made all A's in your studies. Was college a wonderful experience for you?*

ROB: I think most people look back at college as being a kind of wonderful time of life because this is a time when you have a lot of opportunities, a lot of time to think and dream, and not a whole lot of responsibility. Having said this, I should point out that I was an undergraduate during the era of the Vietnam War when there was tremendous turmoil and unrest on college campuses, enormous social changes, a large number of thought-provoking issues. I was caught up in all of it at that time, along with everyone else. The climate on the college campuses was unique during that era and shaped the lives of everyone in my generation.

WCR: *That was 1965 to 1969?*

ROB: That's right.

WCR: *Then you went to the University of Pennsylvania to medical school? That is the one you wanted to go to?*

ROB: Yes, Penn ended up being top on my list. Both of my parents were from Philadelphia. My mother's family had been there for generations going back to the Quaker settlement of Pennsylvania. My father had grown up there as well. Even though I grew up in the suburbs of New York City, most of my family roots were in Philadelphia. That was one of the reasons why I wanted to go to Penn, along with its terrific ranking among medical schools. I was delighted to be accepted there. I really enjoyed that experience.

WCR: *You were accepted there after a major in chemical engineering in college?*

ROB: That is correct.

WCR: *As you look back on medical school, how does that hit you now? Who had a major impact on you in medical school?*

ROB: I think more so than the professors I had as an undergraduate, the professors I had in medical school are the people I think of as the individuals who really shaped me. There were so many it is really hard to be fair in naming any, but I will name a few. I encountered *Darwin Prockop* on my first day of medical school when he gave a lecture that captivated me on the metabolic basis of inherited disease. I knew something about biochemistry before entering medical school, but he put some biochemical concepts in context with patients, and I was really captivated by the whole idea that learning on the scientific front could be directly translated to disease of patients. I spent 2 summers doing biochemical genetics in the laboratory of *William Mellman*, Chief of the Genetics Department. We developed a close relationship. Along the way, I encountered *Sam Thier* and *Arnold Relman*; Sam was the Associate Chairman and Arnold Relman was the Chairman of Medicine. They had recently come to Pennsylvania. I remember as a second-year medical student shaking in my boots because I had to present a case of mitral stenosis to Sam Thier who was legendary for being a great teacher, but also for being an intimidating figure. Somehow I survived the case presentation with Sam, learned a lot about one-on-one roundsmanship, and Sam, even though he is not a cardiologist, also taught me a lot about mitral stenosis. I remember to this day how that case presentation went. Drs. Relman and Thier were my Chairman and Associate Chairman during my residency in medicine before Dr. Relman went on to become Editor of *The New England Journal of Medicine* and Dr. Thier went

on to become Chairman of Medicine at Yale, President of the Institute of Medicine, President of Brandeis University, and, currently, Director of the Partners Hospitals in Boston.

In cardiology there were some notable figures also. *Stan Briller* was at Penn before he moved to Pittsburgh. I spent a summer in his laboratory with Gary Gerstenblith who is now a Professor of Medicine in the Cardiology Division at Johns Hopkins. *Richard Helfant*, I think, is a person who ultimately was the single most important individual in making me choose cardiology as a subspecialty career focus. Dick recently had come from the Peter Bent Brigham Hospital to the University of Pennsylvania and he was the Chief of Cardiology at Presbyterian Hospital. He and *Steve Miester* had at that point the premier cardiology rotation for the medical students. I went there to do 1 month with them and liked it so much I ended up doing 2 months. I saw in Dick Helfant the possibility of being a triple threat, taking care of patients and doing procedures, doing research and teaching. Until that point, I was uncertain regarding my career focus and whether I was going to be in practice or academics. Dick Helfant made it clear to me that cardiology was an exciting subspecialty and that an academic career could be rewarding; he also had the knack of making learning cardiology enjoyable and exciting. My fourth year, *Joe Perloff* came to Penn as the Chief of Cardiology and Joe, of course, is a master teacher. I already knew I was going to be a cardiologist, but Joe's arrival was wonderful for me; I spent hours listening to his lectures and making rounds with him. I stayed at Penn for my internship and residency and was able to continue learning from Joe and the faculty he brought to Penn, most notably *Doug Rosing*, *Nat Reichek*, and *John Hirshfeld*. I should not leave out *Jim Shelburne* and *Joel Manchester* who made the cath lab and the coronary care unit an exciting and entertaining environment.

WCR: *What about your classmates in medical school? Did they have much impact on you? Did some of your classmates go on to prestigious positions?*

ROB: I have several good friends from medical school, most of whom are currently in practice. I know they are still enjoying their medical careers even though they are under the same enormous pressures that are facing everyone right now. I have several good friends who have done quite well in academics as well. *Al Buxton*, a classmate, is now Professor of Medicine and Associate Chief of Cardiology at Temple University; *Jerome Strauss* is Professor of Obstetrics and Gynecology at the University of Pennsylvania; *Neil Goldman* is a Professor of Physiology at Penn; *Stephen Parnes* is Chief of Otolaryngology at the State University of New York at Albany; and *Frank James* is on the faculty in Cardiology at Temple. I think the individuals who had the biggest impact on me as colleagues were not so much my medical school classmates but the medical residents I trained with after medical school. As you know, residency is an intense experience and one develops close bonds with other residents in the middle of the night taking

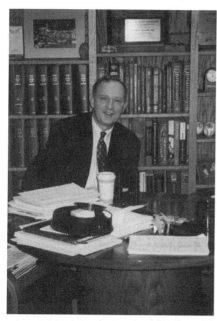

FIGURE 2. ROB during the interview (Photo by WCR).

care of sick patients. You also get to know who you can trust and whose judgment you can respect. I trained at a time when residents were on call every other night or every third night. I have a number of very close friends from my residency days. Again, many of them have wound up in practice settings but several are doing very well in academic circles also. *Irwin Klein*, a very close friend, is Professor of Medicine at New York University and Chief of Endocrinology at North Shore University Hospital, Long Island. Irwin's cutting edge research on hormonal regulation of myocyte growth makes him far more of a cardiologist than an endocrinologist. *Al Buxton*, already mentioned, was also a resident with me. Six or 7 members of our residency class went into cardiology. I keep in touch with them professionally and personally. These include *Eric Michelson* who was Chief of Cardiology at Hahnemann before assuming his current position as Vice-President of Astra Merck; *Arthur Riba*, who was the Chief of Cardiology at the West Haven Veterans Administration Hospital and a faculty member at Yale before taking his current practice position in Michigan; *Taylor Cope* and *Willie Lam*, practicing cardiologists here in Illinois; *Alan Speilman*, an electrophysiologist in Philadelphia; *John Coyle,* practicing cardiology in Tulsa, Oklahoma; and *Leonard Horowitz* was a year ahead of me and was a nationally recognized electrophysiologist at Penn before his untimely death, and *Bill Follansbee* was a year behind me in training and is now Professor of Medicine in the Cardiology Division at the University of Pittsburgh.

WCR: *In medical school you mentioned that cardiology appealed to you relatively early. Did you know you wanted to go into medicine pretty quickly?*

Did you have a problem deciding whether to go into medicine or into surgery? Was that decision relatively easy for you?

ROB: It was not easy. I was grappling with the usual uncertainties many students face. When I first went to medical school I thought I was going to be a pediatrician. I enjoyed the pediatric experience, but I determined I would go into internal medicine around the same time I determined I would go into cardiology.

WCR: *You began your internship in 1973 at the University of Pennsylvania. After the internship you did 2 years of residency in general medicine there.*

ROB: That is correct.

WCR: *Did you do any research in college?*

ROB: I did some research because it was expected as a chemical engineer student. To get my diploma I had to complete a research project. I studied crystal formation as liquid suspensions freeze on metal surfaces and the characteristics of the crystals that were deposited. This is about all I can tell you about it because it certainly did not stick with me. That was my research experience in college.

WCR: *Did that lead to a publication?*

ROB: It led to an in-house piece of work I wrote to pass the course. That research experience also occurred when I was practicing basketball daily and/or was on the road with the team. I can't say this was an intense research experience, because I was not able to devote sufficient time or mental energy to it. On the other hand, I don't want to minimize the importance of that experience, as it instilled the idea that there is a scientific process and there are suitable hypotheses that one can develop and test. It also lead me to understand that doing research was an important part of my education when I was in medical school.

WCR: *What did you do research in in medical school?*

ROB: The summer work with *Stan Briller* dealt with new methods of computerizing electrocardiograms. I spent that summer working with a wall-to-wall computer. That did not lead to a publication but it helped Stan Briller with his work and some of the publications he was preparing at that time. I was not a co-author there and did not deserve to be. The research in the early and midpart of my medical school career was with *Bill Mellman* in the genetics department there. We studied galactosemia and galactokinase deficiency and identified some new familial forms of galactokinase deficiency. That lead to 2 publications and also my first oral presentation at a national scientific meeting as a medical student. That experience paid off later when I applied for a position at the NIH.

WCR: *By the time you graduated from medical school you had how many publications?*

ROB: Two. Actually, both were published when I was a resident, but the work with Bill Mellman was done while in medical school.

WCR: *It seems to me that doing research in medical school is a key element to look at in somebody's*

CV because so many people who go on to successful academic careers have done research early on.

ROB: I agree entirely. That is a topic of discussion here among the faculty and I explore the issue when we are interviewing our fellowship candidates. It is important to capture people early in their careers. They have to get the bug early. A successful career in research requires discipline and extra effort. Research is fun, exciting, and worth the extra time, effort and frustration that is added on to an otherwise very busy complicated life in medicine. However, if you don't attract talented young people in the early stages of their careers, you risk loosing them to the other exciting opportunities medicine has to offer.

WCR: *After the 2 years of residency at the University of Pennsylvania, you went to the Cardiology Branch at the National Heart, Lung, and Blood Institute (NHLBI) of the National Institutes of Health in Bethesda, Maryland, in 1976. You had no cardiology fellowship training before that point?*

ROB: That's right.

WCR: *How did it come about that you went to NIH?*

ROB: I decided as a resident, given the backdrop of my cardiology experience in medical school, that I wanted an academic career in cardiology. I wanted to have a solid research experience. I had some friends in my residency program who had either been at NIH or were going to NIH, and it was apparent that this might be an excellent opportunity for a young person to spend a couple of years of completely protected research time, either in a basic or clinical laboratory and to really get a foothold in a research career. This was at a time right toward the end of the Vietnam War when positions at the NIH were very competitive to get into. I remember that there were 4 of us in my residency class who were applying for 1 of the 6 positions in the Clinical Associate program at the NHLBI. The NHLBI was not necessarily looking for residents interested in clinical cardiology training for, I think, legitimate reasons. The NHLBI was seeking individuals who either had a research background or clearcut research potential. Of the 4 of us, I was the 1 person who had done research in medical school and my research had been in genetics. I think that basic laboratory experience was quite helpful in making me a very competitive candidate for 1 of those 6 positions at the NIH. Of course, I don't know for certain what led to the decision to accept me, but I was accepted and was thrilled with the decision.

WCR: *You came to NIH as a Clinical Associate in the NHLBI. You were not automatically in the Cardiology Branch when you first came so how did it work out that you joined the Cardiology Branch?*

ROB: You know the system there since you were there for so long and had a very important leadership role. The 6 Clinical Associates rotated through all the clinical branches of the NHLBI including the Cardiology, Pulmonary, Hypertension, Hematology, and Metabolic Disease Branches. There were very prominent figures in all of those areas: *Robert Levy, Brian Brewer, Ronald Crystal, Art Neinhaus, Harry Keiser,*

and *Fred Bartter.* We had great opportunities in many areas but, again, I went there because I wanted to be involved in cardiovascular research, so on day one, I made it clear to *Steve Epstein,* the Cardiology Branch Chief, that his Branch was where I wanted to be. I did have several months of research time during my first year to begin work with the Cardiology Branch members, and, in my spare time, in the clinical rotation could continue that work. The person I hooked up with initially was *Walt Henry* who was, at that time, one of the leading figures in echocardiography. Walt and I did some work initially in patients with aortic valve disease. I credit Walter early on for stimulating my interest in valve disease and turning it into a more academic focus regarding left ventricular function, prognosis, and timing of aortic valve replacement. I am indebted to Walter Henry for guiding and mentoring me this entire area. However, it was Steve Epstein, who guided me later on in this area of investigation, and I credit Steve for mentoring me in developing deliberate, methodical, hypothesis-driven research pathways.

WCR: *After your 2 years as a Clinical Associate in the NHLBI you moved into the Cardiology Branch and that became very quickly a full time position.*

ROB: That's right. In fact, the Clinical Associateship was a 3-year position. It was a 1-year training position with the clinical rotations and then 2 years of research. The third year and part of the fourth year, *Dr. Lewis Lipson* and I shared the responsibilities of being chief fellow of the clinical cardiology service. In a way, this resulted in a 4-year training period.

WCR: *Then you became a full member of the staff of the Cardiology Branch. You never actually had a fellowship in cardiology?*

ROB: That is true, in a pure sense. However, fellowship requirements for board certification in the subspecialty of cardiology codified at a later point in time. It was around 1980 when I was completing my training and became Board-certified. In today's environment, I would probably do a year or 2 of research at the NIH and then be required to do 2 years of clinical fellowship training somewhere else, because the NHLBI program is not considered an accredited training program. However, the clinical training I received in 4 years at the NHLBI was equivalent to most fellowship programs in the 1970s and superior to many. This was the era before coronary angioplasty and thrombolytic therapy. The training I received from *Steve Epstein, Kenny Kent, Walt Henry,* and *Jeff Borer* occurred at the time the NIH was at the forefront of most areas in clinical cardiology including coronary, valvular, and myocardial diseases. The experience I obtained in echocardiography and nuclear cardiology, these new areas of noninvasive imaging, were clearly equivalent to the best training programs at the time. My experience in the cardiac catheterization laboratory included studies of patients with complex congenital heart disease, valvular disease, and cardiomyopathies. Every patient undergoing surgery at the NHLBI returned at 6 months for repeat cardiac catheterization. Hence, I did many transseptal punctures and percutaneous left ventricular punctures to obtain pressure measurements in patients who had prosthetic heart valves. This was routine. Kenny Kent was among the first cardiologists in this country to perform coronary angioplasty, at a time when I was an attending cardiologist in the cath lab. I don't have any problems regarding my clinical training in cardiology and regarding my ability to take care of patients with many forms of heart disease.

WCR: *Your training in cardiology actually was similar to that of people like Eugene Braunwald, John Ross, Ed Sonnenblick, Dean Mason, Donald Harrison. Those individuals never took official cardiology fellowships. They just learned cardiology along the way in their day-to-day work.*

ROB: That's right and obviously from very good mentors and teachers. I was not going to put it quite in those terms, but I am glad you did. There are many other cardiologists both in my generation and earlier generations who came through the process at the NIH. Cardiologists in many other programs in that era also did not sit through what is now considered the requirements for fellowship training and board eligibility.

WCR: *Dr. Bonow you were at NIH in the Cardiology Branch from 1976 until you came here to Chicago in 1992, a period of 16 years. As you look back at your period at NIH what accomplishments are you most pleased about? How do you fit your NIH experience into your present activities?*

ROB: That is a big question, so it is not possible to answer in a single word or two. There were several things. First, the mentorship I received there was from many individuals, among them *Steve Epstein*, *Kenny Kent*, *Walt Henry*, *Doug Rosing*, *Barry Maron*. It was very important, not only in developing me, but in allowing me to recognize the importance of mentorship and transmitting it to others. During my time at the NIH I was able to contribute to the development of other individuals who were in the program with me or a year or 2 behind me. *Marty Leon* and *Richard Cannon* were a year or 2 behind me. We became very good friends and, because of my being a few years ahead, I was able to provide some seniority and guidance in the early parts of their careers. *Jim Udelson*, who is now at Tufts-New England Medical Center, and a well known nuclear cardiologist, and *Vasken Dilsizian*, who now directs the nuclear cardiology program at the NIH, are other individuals in the next generation with whom I have a very strong personal connection. One of the values that grew out of the NIH experience is that mentorship is important, both on the receiving end and the giving end.

Second, the NIH, at that point in time and I hope beyond the current time, is a national treasure where young people can develop strong career foundations, where research opportunities are unique regarding protected time—the ability to develop and test hypotheses, and do what is considered high-risk research. I have certainly realized that creating this environment in Chicago or anywhere else in the world, for that matter, outside the NIH is very difficult. There are funding issues and clinical pressures. As a Chief of a

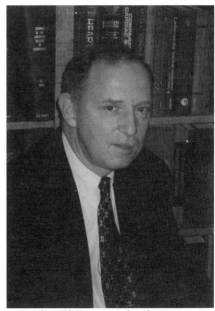

FIGURE 3. ROB during the interview (Photo by WCR).

Division of Cardiology in a major medical school, I also have a large number of other responsibilities that are administrative and academic, so my own ability to do research is limited. However, I can develop a research atmosphere, help to develop research themes, and work to develop funding mechanisms. In addition, I can impart how to ask the questions and how to go about answering those questions. The ability to transmit that information to others is very important. That is something else I owe to my experience at the NIH.

Also, the NIH was one of those rare places 15 or 20 years ago where basic research was done a hallway away from where patient care was provided. Although I can't say that we were as a group any more successful than others in taking basic concepts from the laboratory to the bedside, I think 15 years ago we had our share of success in that area. Steve Epstein was a master of taking ideas and concepts developed in the animal laboratory and thinking of ways of applying them to patients, either in practice or at least in theory. Examples include the use of nitroglycerin and aspirin in acute coronary syndromes and the use of calcium channel blockers in chronic coronary disease. Of course, this translational research is what we are all striving for in the current era of molecular biology and genetics. We obviously still have a long way to go in cardiovascular disease. This concept is nothing unusual or surprising in 1997, but in the 1970s there were very few places in the world equipped to think along these terms.

Finally, what is helping me the most in my current position is the fact that to do good clinical research, you have to be a good doctor. You have to know how to take care of patients and how to explain the details of diseases and the limitations of our current treatments with patients and their families. That has helped me tremendously in moving from 16 years in a scientific institution to what is much closer to the real world. Although a university medical school is not necessarily the real world, we are also part of a very successful and progressive hospital. Here in Chicago we compete with several other medical schools and a large number of community hospitals. We have to be very good clinically to grow our program and develop clinical services, which is the basis of our research and teaching programs. I believe strongly that my 16 years at the NIH have made me a much better physician. I am recognizable here as being a good doctor as much as I am for any other accomplishments I have achieved previously. In fact, I suspect most of the internists inside and outside my institution who refer patients to me don't know much about my research background. They know that I take care of their patients well, that I relate to them professionally as a physician should, and that the patients, hopefully, not only receive good care but are satisfied with me as their physician. The most important thing I learned at the NIH is that you have to be a skilled physician to do high quality clinical research. That is something that will never leave me.

WCR: *In the 16 years at NIH you obviously did a lot of investigations there. You became a world authority in nuclear cardiology. Your work of patients with certain types of valvular disease, particularly valvular regurgitation—when to operate, when not to operate on them—is masterful. As you look back on the work you did, what are you most pleased with now?*

ROB: There are a couple of things. I am certainly proud of the accomplishments in valvular heart disease, particularly aortic regurgitation and mitral regurgitation, and that has helped me as well in my current position. We have great expertise in valvular disease here at Northwestern, both in cardiology and cardiac surgery. I am also pleased with my studies of the impact of myocardial ischemia on left ventricular function, both in defining prognosis of patients with coronary artery disease and in identifying reversible left ventricular dysfunction, myocardial hibernation and stunning. I am pleased with the work I did with Vasken Dilsizian in my latter years at the NIH in the assessment of myocardial viability. Many of the original ideas were Vasken's, not mine, but I provided a great deal of help in formulating the questions and developing the protocols to address them. Together we created a great team. The viability issue is a big item here in the management of patients with coronary disease and impaired ventricular function and in selecting high-risk patients for revascularization to improve prognosis and also improve function. That is something we do essentially every day here both for clinical investigation and clinical care. The valve studies and the viability studies are probably the 2 most important areas in which the research I did has actually had a broad impact on patient care. The other areas of research I pursued at the NIH were fun, including assessment of left ventricular diastolic func-

tion and development of new radionuclide tests and procedures. The relationship I had at the NIH with nuclear medicine physicists and physicians was unique. *Steve Bacharach* and *Mike Green* are world class nuclear physicists. We worked closely together for 15 years. They taught me tremendously, and we remain close friends. I am trying to develop that kind of relationship between cardiology and nuclear medicine. I guess there are several reasons I am proud of my NIH days not only related to research productivity but also to the firm foundation provided for my subsequent career here in Chicago.

WCR: *Dr. Bonow, what was your day-to-day life like at NIH? Let's say 2 or 3 years before you left. How much time were you spending at NIH? Were you working at night on papers, weekends?*

ROB: The last couple of years there were quite different from my first 12 or 13 years. Again, those later years prepared me for my current position rather well. First of all, the cardiac surgery program was discontinued at the NIH, as you know. I won't discuss all the reasons for that because it is not pertinent here, but that had an impact on us as cardiologists both in terms of patient care and also in trying to recruit patients for clinical research protocols. Around the same point in time, Steve Epstein, who had already established himself as one of the nation's great teachers and clinical cardiologists, and whose research had touched patients all over the world, around 1990, determined that he wanted to embark on a new career path in molecular biology. He took a sabbatical for about 18 months during which time I was acting Chief of Cardiology. I took on many more administrative responsibilities in helping to run the program. This was at a time when the Surgery Branch had just been dismantled, and we needed to develop mechanisms to take care of our patients who required surgery. We developed a contracting process to provide care for our patients at 3 of the Washington, DC, area hospitals, each of which had great expertise in cardiac surgery: Georgetown University, the Washington Hospital Center, and Fairfax Hospital. That process, which was a new experience for me, was a difficult and laborious process, dealing with different hospital types, a university hospital on the one hand and 2 private hospitals on the other, dealing with the surgeons who worked in 3 hospitals, and at the same time dealing with the NIH and contracting officers. That experience, in retrospect, was not bad—learning how the world operates outside the NIH, which was helpful to me when I came to Chicago.

My daily life at NIH prior to those last 3 to 4 years was much different. Before that my professional life was busy but enjoyable. It actually was grueling work. We had to care for our patients and communicate with referring physicians regarding the care of their patients with complex heart disease. We had to recruit patients for research protocols, obtain informed consent from them, and discuss the implications of our research findings with them and their families. We had an enormous amount of data that was being generated for numerous ongoing protocols. We were understaffed in terms of nursing support, research nurses, research technicians, and fellows. Therefore, the attending physicians did a lot of the work themselves, work which in most academic institutions is routinely handled by nurses and technicians. This was an accepted part of the daily routine. Therefore, writing manuscripts was not done from 9:00 A.M. to 5:00 P.M. Even in the most austere research environment like the NIH, virtually all of the writing I did was on evenings and weekends. That sort of lifestyle was fine when I was single but created obvious conflict when I became a husband and a father. This went against the grain of what my parents had taught me when I was little about having quality time as a family. My wife, Pat, has been incredibly understanding and supportive and, of course, she has made most of the sacrifices because I would either get home late or, worse, get home and become preoccupied with professional things, trying to get my papers completed, trying to review manuscripts, trying to get my own manuscripts revised and sent back in for publication. Again, almost all of that was being done after hours and on weekends. This is also the way it is here for me now. My day-to-day life is tied up with either clinical issues or administrative issues. The last 4 years at NIH, when I had much more administrative responsibilities, slowed down my hands-on research. The publications, luckily, kept rolling since I had just terrific collaborative projects, proceeding with Vasken Dilsiziam, Richard Cannon, Arshed Quyyumi, and Barry Maron. Luckily, the research activity kept up and I was able to continue contributing. Although I missed the hands-on level of research, I realized that somebody had to mind the shop and provide leadership and administrative stability to keep the rest of the group productive.

WCR: *Dr. Bonow, in 1992, when you were 45 years of age, you had a major decision on your hands. I gather you were offered the Chiefship of the Division of Cardiology at Northwestern, one of the most prestigious medical schools in the world. You had only 4 years or so before you reached 20-year retirement in the Public Health Service at NIH which would be nice change in your pocket for the rest of your life. How did it come about that you came to Northwestern? Once you received the offer, was it easy to say "yes" or was it difficult for you?*

ROB: That is a good point. It is true that a number of people at the NIH worked with an eye on that 20-year clock because of the potential retirement package. That certainly was a factor for me to consider. I had looked at other positions over the course of many years, including some very good positions at very prestigious institutions. For one reason or another, I decided that what I was doing at the time in Bethesda was more important to me and my family, and I turned down the earlier opportunities. The Northwestern offer came at a time when there were changes going on in my life. I was already doing a lot of administrative work, and my own individual research productivity was not where it had been earlier. Although I had more of a leadership role in the Cardiology Branch by then, Steve Epstein had returned

from his sabbatical and resumed his role as Branch Chief. I was beginning to wonder where the tide would take from there on out. I certainly could have stayed there. I was still pretty happy there and my relationship with Steve Epstein was good and remains terrific to this day. When the opportunity in Chicago came along it was an opportunity that was only going to stay open for short time. I had to suddenly stop and look. Most of my colleagues over the years at the NIH had an inkling that they were not there forever, and sooner or later they had ventured out to a more real world environment. I had originally planned to spend 3 years at the NIH, but I stayed because it was fun, interesting, exciting, and productive. All along I kept my feelers out for the right situation at the right time to make a move such as the one I ultimately made. Steve Epstein counseled me early on that as long as I was productive in what I was doing, there is no reason to make a premature move, as greater productivity would bring bigger and better opportunities. That was good advice because through my tenure there the job market did not evaporate but only got better and more tantalizing. The Northwestern offer materialized as a great opportunity at the right time. Northwestern is a very interesting institution with enormous potential in a very big and great city, where it is easy to recruit physicians and scientists to work. We are located in one of the best parts of the city where patients are not concerned about the neighborhood. Northwestern Memorial Hospital is a very prestigious and successful institution. It has terrific experience and recognition and reputation in patient care. We are building a new hospital as we speak that will be open in 1999. The medical school is one of the major schools of Northwestern University. It is a very forward-thinking institution with new leadership. The new Chairman of Medicine, *Lewis Landsberg*, had arrived 2 years earlier from Beth-Israel Hospital in Boston and had initiated a search for a new Chief of Cardiology. *Francis Klocke* had arrived here a year earlier to run the Feinberg Cardiovascular Research Institute in the medical school. Fran and I had known each other for years and had similar research interests. It looked like an opportunity worth exploring. The more I developed a relationship with Dr. Landsberg and understood the potential here in cardiology it became apparent that this was an opportunity where, with a little bit of careful thought and maybe a little bit of good luck, one could do very well in terms of recruiting young faculty, developing clinical programs, and developing research programs. And so I decided to accept the Northwestern offer. I could have stayed where I was and might still be at the NIH, and I suspect if I was there my life would be a little easier. I knew I was ending one of the happiest periods of my life leaving Bethesda and venturing out to Chicago. On the other hand, my family and I live in a wonderful community north of Chicago where we love our home and neighbors and the town we live in.

The experience I have had here at Northwestern has actually been terrific. I have learned a tremendous amount about the way clinical programs develop and

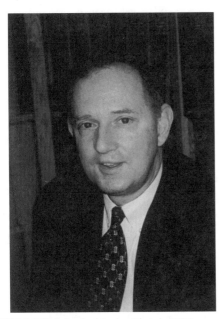

FIGURE 4. ROB during the interview (Photo by WCR).

the close relationship required between the faculty and the hospital to develop programs to provide services and attract patients. I think I have also become much more rounded as a clinical cardiologist. I have gotten up to speed with a number of aspects of heart failure, acute coronary care, and interventional cardiology, which were not part of my day-to-day life at the NIH. I am pretty conversant in these areas and have been successful at recruiting individuals who have helped balance out the program I inherited to create a program which is pretty solid in all aspects of the clinical components of cardiology. In addition to covering all the bases, we have considerable depth. We have 2 or 3 people in each aspect of the various subspecialties of cardiology, and this provides depth in terms of clinical care, teaching, and research. We do need greater development in basic science research. When I first arrived, given all the changes that were going on in terms of managed care and the enormous demands initially to turn around some aspects of the clinical programs, I was not able to concentrate on the development of basic research initiatives. Those pressures have not gone away, but at least we have been able to turn things around and be successful in terms of our clinical volume. Our patient volume has increased substantially in everything we do. This has fostered excellent clinical investigation, but it has taken a lot of work. I think now is an opportune time to develop our basic research program.

WCR: *Dr. Bonow, how many physicians do you have in the Division of Cardiology here at Northwestern? What size of division are you talking about?*

ROB: We have both full-time and voluntary faculty (private cardiologists who are part of the division). All cardiologists with hospital privileges at

Northwestern Memorial Hospital are members of the faculty at the medical school; so I am their Chief, whether they are full-time or private cardiologists. I try to do what is best for everybody on both sides, in terms of academic appointments and research as well as clinical privileges and activities. In the total we have 25 full-time cardiologists, in varying degrees devoted to research, teaching, and patient care. We have roughly 20 private cardiologists on the voluntary faculty. Both groups have grown since I have been here and I have done recruitment for both private and full-time cardiologists. I think that is a good balance. I think it is helpful for residents and fellows to see different approaches to patient care. It creates very interesting discussions at our cath conference or cardiology grand round series, just 2 of the many conferences we have every week. Our trainees receive a balance of different approaches for patient care. Our patients, many times, have a preference for a physician who is on the cutting edge of research and new developments in the field, while others prefer physicians taking care of patients in a private practice setting. I think we have a good balance here in terms of what our patients are looking for, and that balance has helped us be as successful as we have been. It is not a huge division. One could certainly find other larger divisions around Chicago, and elsewhere they may be larger.

WCR: *Now you have 25 full-time cardiologists and 20 volunteer cardiologists who are in private practice and they are all members of your faculty. How many full-timers did you have when you came in 1992?*

ROB: We had roughly the same number but there has been some transition and attrition in various areas. Several previous full-timers left to go into practice. Other physicians have left for movement up the ladder academically. One has become Chief of Cardiology at another medical school, and one has become director of an echocardiography laboratory at another medical school. Their career choices left us with important vacancies that needed to be filled. As difficult as it is to lose good people, the loss also represents an opportunity for it allows you to recruit good people to fill their ranks, people who can come in and grow academically. It is a challenge to keep things in balance. I may be missing the numbers by 1 or 2 physicians. I think in general we are about where I started, although it is true in most academic programs that one of the jobs of the Chief is constant recruitment. This year we will add more cardiologists because our clinical volume has risen to the point where we are really stretched thin in several areas.

WCR: *If you add secretaries and lab technicians to your 25 full-time faculty, how many people are you talking about in this division? How many cardiology fellows do you have?*

ROB: The answer to the fellowship issue is quite easy. We used to have 5 fellows per year but we have downsized from 5 to 4 to 3. This was our first year of bringing in only 3 first-year fellows. We have 5 in the third year, 4 in the second year, and 3 in the first. That gives a total of 12 fellows. We also have 2 fourth-year fellows in electrophysiology and interventional cardiology. We have a total of 14 fellows right now with 1 other research fellow. That will continue to get smaller as we continue to evolve into 3 per year for 3 years. At our tightest we will probably be down to 11 total. That has an impact, not so much on the fellows who continue to receive everything they have received in the past, but on the faculty who will have more to do with fewer fellows to support the clinical demands. There are some months in some of the clinical laboratories when an attending cardiologist cannot count on a fellow being present. We do make sure a fellow is always in a rotation where a fellow is necessary. You can't run a cardiac catherization laboratory or a large coronary care unit without a cardiology fellow.

In addition to the fellows, we have technicians, nurses, and secretaries, some of whom are hospital personnel, some of whom are employed by the medical school, and some of whom are employed by the faculty. Depending upon how you analyze this, we could be talking anywhere from 65 to 100 cardiologists and support personnel in the full-time components of the Division.

WCR: *The private practitioners are the volunteer faculty. They are not housed here in Northwestern Hospital quarters, are they? They have their own private offices?*

ROB: Yes, they are for the most part, practitioners who practice only here. Some of the practitioners also have privileges at other hospitals, but their offices are within the immediate area, either on campus or a few blocks away. Many of them have satellite activities going on or may have 2 offices, 1 downtown here, for example, near the university hospital or 1 in the suburbs, and they split their time. Their offices are not housed here in the hospital.

WCR: *Bob, you deal with a faculty of 45 physicians. It seems to me that 30 years ago that was how many people were on the entire faculty of the Department of Medicine. Today, you are equivalent to a Departmental Chairman as of several decades ago. How many physicians and PhDs are in the entire Department of Medicine here?*

ROB: I think it is roughly 120 to 140. It is true cardiology takes up a large percentage of the faculty in the Department of Medicine. Obviously, the things we do are very important for the department in terms of our teaching responsibilities and our clinical revenue. In return, we also receive support back from the department for our ongoing activities.

WCR: *Do you have much contact with the Chairman of the Department of Medicine?*

ROB: Yes, I have a very good, close, and collegial relationship with the department chairman. He has been very supportive. Again, he recruited me and I believe I was the first Division Chief he recruited after his arrival here. I have gone through a number of important agenda items since I have been here that have required his advice and support. He does have some firm ideas many times about the direction the department should be going and luckily most of the

time we see eye to eye. At the times we don't, we discuss our differences. Sometimes he wins, sometimes I win, but there has never been a clash of personalities. I can't think really of an incident in which I have not felt supported in moving forward, even in situations where we disagree. Around 1992 when I took this position, the Association of the Professors of Cardiology, APC, which is an organization for the division chiefs of the university-based cardiology programs nationwide, was going through a major revolutionary thought process regarding whether cardiology divisions should remove themselves from the departments of medicine and become their own free-standing departments, which would have altered some of the financial relationships between divisions of cardiology and departments of medicine. As a new recruit here, it would have been suicidal for me to consider doing that. I actually discussed this whole issue with the department chairman. He and I believe that in the current era of evolving managed care, this may not be the best thing for divisions of cardiology. At Northwestern, we are a part of a very large multispecialty practice group in which many of the issues about contracting and referrals from general specialists to subspecialists, capitation, etc., can be handled in a pretty efficient way. I think if our cardiology division was separated out, that would become more problematic. In addition, many of the current breakthroughs in cardiovascular research involve very tight collaboration with hematologists, immunologists, and other specialties. These collaborative interactions can occur interdepartmentally but are more natural and more easily fostered if they develop within the same department.

WCR: *Bob, you are responsible for a broad range of activities: patient care, teaching, research. Each of these activities are in and of themselves full-time activities. You are just one person, you have a family. What is your day-to-day life like? Let's start from the time you wake up in the morning. What time do you wake up? How long does it take you to get to the hospital? What time do you get out of the hospital at night? How long does it take you to get home? What do you do after you get home? Are you exhausted by that time so you don't do anymore professional work once you get home? What time do you go to bed? Can you discuss that in detail?*

ROB: I mentioned earlier that perhaps if I had stayed at the NIH, in some ways my life would be a lot simpler. That is related to your question. This is grueling. I actually enjoy what I am doing and I enjoy the responsibilities, but it is difficult to handle all these various aspects of the job and keep everybody happy, handle the balance of clinical care versus research, and also remain active in professional societies. Even if that balance can be achieved, it is at the expense of something else. This has been the major issue I have. Chicago is a big city. To have a nice home and a yard for your children to play in, good school systems, etc., most physicians live outside of the city, especially those with children. Our 2 boys are 13 and 9, and my wife, Pat, and I decided to move to our current home

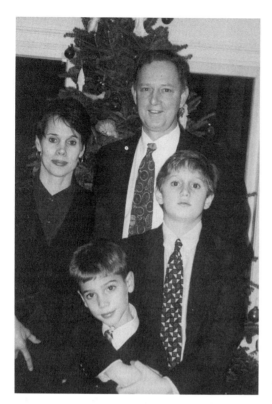

FIGURE 5. ROB and his wife Pat and their 2 boys.

because of the school system and the community. However, it is a long way from work. In Bethesda I commuted 1 mile to work and I could be there in 5 minutes. Here in Chicago it is a 30-minute drive when there is no traffic, but the rush hour is a big problem. I usually get up between 5:00 and 5:30 A.M. and hit the road about half an hour later. If I am going in that early I can usually be there in about half an hour. Any later, it may take me an hour. I just can't commit that kind of time to sitting in a car. The same is true about going home at night. I usually end up leaving after the rush hour and getting home around the time to get the kids to bed if I am lucky. Sometimes the children have not seen me for a couple days.

WCR: *So what time do you get home?*

ROB: Average time would be somewhere between 8:30 and 9:30 P.M., but there are times when I have set the record here at Northwestern for leaving late. There are some things, though, that I have built into my commitments. The boys participate in some sports. The last couple of years I have been a coach on the little league baseball team and now the basketball team. I am assistant scout master for the Boy Scout troop that my older son is involved in. I have spent a week camping with the Boy Scouts the last 2 summers, go to the weekly meeting at night, and participate in several weekend activities each year. The Boy Scouts is a great organization. I was an Eagle Scout as

a teenager and my older son is almost there. I try to get home when the boys' activities are going on. I can't say that I am doing this as well as my father did. I am not there for dinner most nights. I am not there to help the kids with their homework as much as I would like. All of this responsibility falls on my wife. Obviously, this creates a lot of struggle internally for me as to whether I am doing the right thing for my family and whether this is the kind of thing I can continue to do. On the other hand, I am not sure it would be much different if I were in a different location or even be in a different job these days in medicine. I know, although I often compare my life now to my life in Bethesda, times have changed. These are not really comparable points in time and most of my colleagues in medicine have very similar stories of the demands they are under, either in practice or in academics.

WCR: *So you wake up about 5:00 A.M. You get to the hospital about 6:30 or 7:00 A.M. You leave the hospital at night, that's variable, but 8:00 or 8:30 and you get home on the average at 9:00. What time do you go to bed?*

ROB: I never answered the earlier part of your question about what I do when I get home. I make sure the kids have not unraveled and have their school work done and try to help get them ready for bed. If I have not had dinner here at the hospital I have some dinner. I try to deal with any of the other home fires that are still burning. I cut the pumpkins last night for Halloween, for example, somewhere around 11:00 P.M. If I am just too burned out, I sit and talk to my wife for awhile and then go to bed, but more likely, that is the time when I have to pick up a manuscript that I am reviewing for the AJC or another journal or try to do some writing. I am still involved with what I think are important aspects of the American Heart Association (AHA) and the American College of Cardiology (ACC), so I have committee work to do there. I am Vice-Chairman of the Scientific Session Program Committee for the AHA and also Vice-Chair of the AHA Council on Clinical Cardiology. I am chairing the ACC/AHA committee to develop guidelines for management of valvular heart disease. I will soon become Chairman of the ACC Extramural Education Committee. I am also serving on the Subspecialty Board on Cardiovascular Disease of the American Board of Internal Medicine. That stuff, again, I am doing after hours for the most part. A lot of it is being done at home once I get home. Many times I go to bed at 12:00 or 1:00 A.M. Average sleep time here is 4 to 5 hours.

WCR: *What about weekends? Do you come into the hospital?*

ROB: I come in when I am on service. I do attend on the clinical cardiology service, but I don't do that as often as many of the other attendings do. I want to be visible and I enjoy seeing patients very much. I wish I could do more of that. When I am on the service I come in both Saturday and Sunday and make rounds. However, on the weekends when I am not involved clinically, I stay home. I take a couple of briefcases home. I usually have more than 1 briefcase full of papers that goes back and forth. I spend the weekends with a lot of hours of work, but I try as much as I can to put that off until the evening or the early morning hours so that during the key hours of Saturday and Sunday I am there with my wife and kids. We go to church every Sunday and we are active in some of the activities in the community, primarily those involved around children.

WCR: *Do you have a social life? Do you go out on Friday or Saturday evenings? Do you have friends over or go to their houses? Do you have time for that?*

ROB: Nothing scheduled. On Friday or Saturday we may go out, go to a ballgame or friend's house, go out to dinner, or have friends over for dinner. We probably do not do as much socializing as we should or would like. We are trying to balance the demands of the family versus the professional demands. My wife is now back at work. She received a master's degree in journalism here at Northwestern and is now working part time so her life has become much more complicated. Having people over can place a lot of extra demands on a situation that is already pretty demanding. We tend to go out more than we have people in, but we do socialize. We have several parties a year for the division members in cardiology in the summer and at Christmas time. We try to get to the symphony occasionally, to plays and museums. I wish we were doing more of that.

WCR: *Bob, what about vacations? How much time do you take off from work? Do you take off a month a year?*

ROB: We probably have a vacation in its truest sense, where I am devoid from work, not traveling because I am going to a meeting, a total of 2 weeks a year. I mentioned that I take a week out with the Boy Scouts. That is good for the 1 son that goes with me but not for the other one or my wife. This year we took a week at the beach. We are going for a week to Orlando next spring for the boys' school break. We usually go skiing for several days in the winter, not for a full week necessarily, and usually surrounding a ski meeting in which I give a lecture or 2. True vacations probably average about 2 weeks a year, not all at one time but spread out.

WCR: *You mentioned professional travels. How many trips do you go on? How many cities do you go to to give talk(s) or as a visiting professor or to committee meetings? Travel is a very tiring thing. I know you limit that some. How do you handle it?*

ROB: I try to limit it. You know how demanding that can be. However, when a good friend asks you up to do something you hate to say no. I enjoy teaching. I was a visiting professor at the Mayo Clinic last year where the fellows created a grueling schedule of rounds, conferences, and bedside teaching with the fellows, and I loved it. It was very tiring, but I really enjoyed it. That was 3 days away in a true professional visiting professor-type setting. I don't do that very often, perhaps once a year. That was kind of a unique and wonderful experience. Usually, as you know, travels consists of going away for 1 day and giving a lecture or participating in a committee meeting. I try

to limit that, but I still do it maybe once or twice a month. There are symposia where I am invited to speak, and I still do that. That probably averages once or twice a month as well. Unfortunately, many of these continuing education activities now occur on weekends, which cuts further into the family time. I go to 3 national scientific meetings each year. There are also a number of committee meetings, but luckily in Chicago a lot of those committee meetings occur at O'Hare Airport at the airport hotel so I don't have to travel as much. Still I am on the road a lot even though I try to keep it under control. Despite my best efforts, though, I tend to get myself over committed. Traveling has to be kept under control because there are not only the family pressures but also the pressures at work. Things have to get done for the medical school and the hospital. You have to be visible and be able to take care of your patients and be a role model for the other faculty. I am not the busiest doctor around, but I see a large number of outpatients, including many new patients. That is demanding also and places limits on traveling. I try to balance those things as best I can.

WCR: *What about trips abroad? Do you take 3 or 4 a year?*

ROB: Probably 2 to 4 a year. This year I was at the European meeting at Stockholm and 2 meetings in Italy. I will be going to Uruguay in December for their national meeting. I know I will be going to the World Congress next spring in Rio and a Congress on Valvular Heart Disease later in London. I try to limit those long trips, and I often do some crazy things like trying to go in overnight, give a lecture, and come back again without spending a lot of time to decompress and enjoy the location. I try to keep time away to a minimum. I may spend an extra day in a foreign city but usually I will not spend a week there.

WCR: *Bob, your schedule is obviously a grueling one, you are pulled in numerous directions by faculty, by fellows, by responsibilities in the medical center outside the division of cardiology, by the national committees you are on, and by the pressures to publish and review manuscripts. You review numerous manuscripts for various editors. You have been an unbelievably good reviewer for* The American Journal of Cardiology, *a very unselfish thing to do. You get very little credit for that. Your colleagues don't know that you are providing these splendid reviews all the time. Your family is pulling on you. You want to see your kids more. You want to see your wife more. You want to spend more time at home. I presume you want to read books other than medicine sometimes. I presume you would like to develop this hobby or that hobby a little better. Do you have hobbies?*

ROB: Photography remains my hobby. I am doing less of that than I used to do. Sports have always been fun and interesting and I can do that with the kids, but you are right, it is hard. I don't have very many other hobbies at the current time because I am caught up in the whirlwind of all you mentioned. The children do provide a nice outlet though because we get involved in their activities, namely sports, scouts, or things they do at school. We do some things together as a family, such as skiing, but I would like to be doing more of that.

WCR: *Did your athletic endeavors as a younger person in a way provide more stamina for you than if you had not been an athlete?*

ROB: Yes. They have given me more stamina so I had the physical energy to accomplish what I was doing, but also sports were very helpful in college in making me budget my time. I had limited time to study and that was it. I did not have time to goof off. I had basketball practice for several hours every afternoon from September until April. We traveled so I would either be reading on the bus to our game or would be getting back late from practice having only an hour or 2 to study. So I am pretty good at turning things off and focusing, which is very helpful at present with my time being very limited. That is the reason why I believe children should really be encouraged to participate in extracurricular activities. It really does heighten their ability to deal better with the other demands that develop later in life. Otherwise, they have all this time on their hands and run the risk of learning how to procrastinate.

WCR: *Are you going to be able to handle this grueling day-to-day schedule for 15 or 20 more years? You are 50 now? Do you have other goals or other things you might like to do for 5 or 10 years during the next 20 years?*

ROB: Yes. It may be just that I am not a good long-range planner, which is true. I think my short-term goals are to continue developing the program here, get the research program on a much more solid base. I do not have a major interest in moving up the ladder to become a Department Chairman. I have not been burned out enough yet. I can keep this going for awhile longer and for the most part I enjoy it and we have been successful. It is not like I have been hitting my head against the wall and not been able to produce. Our clinical and research activities are growing and that keeps me enthused to keep going. If this had been a loosing proposition here I would feel much different, but right now I am still enthusiastic and optimistic that my current position, and academic medicine in general, can still be fun, rewarding, and productive. I enjoy working with young people and developing their talents, and I can continue doing that for a while longer.

WCR: *It seems to me that you are an enormously diplomatic person. You rarely raise your voice. You are very kind to other people, very gracious. Do you think this is an absolute necessity in the environs we live in today, to make sure that we get along with everybody?*

ROB: That is a really good question. I don't know the answer. I think sometimes I might be better at what I do if I were tougher or meaner or raised my voice more. I think it is true that when I do get angry people do sit up and listen. It does not happen often. I think my personality has helped me as a person to be reasonably effective at accomplishing things. For other people it may not work as well. Diplomacy is one way of doing things, but I don't think it is an absolute necessity.

WCR: *You have very tough environs here in Chicago. Chiefs of Medicine, Chiefs of Cardiology don't last too long historically, and yet you seem to be thriving very well. Is there anything you would like to discuss that we haven't?*

ROB: No, I think you have asked some tough questions that I probably have not discussed in a public forum before. It is fun to think some of these things through with you. I cannot think of anything we have not discussed. You have covered a lot of bases already.

WCR: *Bob, it has been a pleasure. Thank you.*

BOOKS

Most Important Publications Selected by ROB from His 261 Publications

2. Tedesco TA, Bonow RO, Miller K, Mellman WJ. Galactokinase: evidence for a new racial polymorphism. *Science* 1972;178:176–177.

4. Henry WL, Bonow RO, Borer JS, Ware JH, Kent KM, Redwood DR, McIntosh CL, Morrow AG, Epstein SE. Observations on the optimal time for operation for aortic regurgitation. I. Evaluation of the results of aortic valve replacement in symptomatic patients. *Circulation* 1980;61:471–483.

5. Henry WL, Bonow RO, Rosing DR, Epstein SE. Observations on the optimal time for operative intervention for aortic regurgitation. II. Serial echocardiographic evaluation of asymptomatic patients. *Circulation* 1980;61:424–492.

6. Henry WL, Bonow RO, Borer JS, Kent KM, Ware JH, Glancy DL, Redwood DR, Itscoitz SB, McIntosh CL, Conkle DM, Morrow AG, Epstein SE. Evaluation of aortic valve replacement in patients with valvular aortic stenosis. *Circulation* 1980;61:814–825.

9. Bonow RO, Borer JS, Rosing DR, Henry WL, Pearlman AS, McIntosh CL, Morrow AG, Epstein SE. Preoperative exercise capacity in patients with aortic regurgitation as a predictor of postoperative left ventricular function and long-term prognosis. *Circulation* 1980;62:1280–1290.

15. Bonow RO, Lipson LC, Sheehan FH, Capurro NC, Isner JM, Roberts WC, Goldstein RE, Epstein SE. Lack of effect of aspirin on myocardial infarct size in the dog. *Am J Cardiol* 1981;47:258–264.

19. Bonow RO, Borer JS, Rosing DR, Green MV, Bacharach SL, Kent KM. Left ventricular functional reserve in adult patients with atrial septal defect: pre and postoperative studies. *Circulation* 1981;63:1315–1322.

20. Bonow RO, Bacharach SL, Green MV, Kent KM, Rosing DR, Lipson LC, Leon MB, Epstein SE. Impaired left ventricular diastolic filling in patients with coronary artery disease: assessment with radionuclide cineangiography. *Circulation* 1981;64:315–323.

21. Lipson LC, Kent KM, Rosing DR, Bonow RO, McIntosh CL, Condit JS, Epstein SE, Morrow AG. Long-term evaluation of porcine heterografts in the mitral position for more than five years. *Circulation* 1981;64:397–401.

24. Bonow RO, Rosing DR, Bacharach SL, Green MV, Kent KM, Lipson LC, Maron BJ, Leon MB, Epstein SE. Effects of verapamil on left ventricular systolic function and diastolic filling in patients with hypertrophic cardiomyopathy. *Circulation* 1981;64:787–795.

29. Kent KM, Bonow RO, Rosing DR, Lipson LC, McIntosh CL, Epstein SE. Improved myocardial function during exercise after successful percutaneous transluminal coronary angioplasty. *N Engl J Med* 1982;306:441–446.

30. Bonow RO, Leon MB, Rosing DR, Kent KM, Lipson LC, Bacharach SL, Green MV, Epstein SE. Effects of verapamil and propranolol on left ventricular systolic function and diastolic filling in patients with coronary artery disease: radionuclide angiographic studies at rest and during exercise. *Circulation* 1982; 65:1337–1350.

33. Maron BJ, Bonow RO, Seshagiri TN, Roberts WC, Epstein SE. Hypertrophic cardiomyopathy with ventricular septal hypertrophy localized to the apical region of the left ventricle ("apical hypertrophic cardiomyopathy"). *Am J Cardiol* 1982;49:1838–1848.

35. Bonow RO, Kent KM, Rosing DR, Epstein SE. Timing of operation for chronic aortic regurgitation. *Am J Cardiol* 1982;50:25–336.

38. Bonow RO, Kent KM, Rosing DR, Lipson LC, Bacharach SL, Green MV, Epstein SE. Improved left ventricular diastolic filling in patients with coronary artery disease after percutaneous transluminal coronary angioplasty. *Circulation* 1982;66:1159–1167.

47. Bonow RO, Frederick TM, Bacharach SL, Green MV, Goose PW, Maron BJ, Rosing DR. Atrial systole and left ventricular filling in patients with hypertrophic cardiomyopathy: effect of verapamil. *Am J Cardiol* 1983;51:1386–1391.

51. Bonow RO, Rosing DR, McIntosh CL, Jones M, Maron BJ, Lan KKJ, Lakatos E, Bacharach SL, Green MV, Epstein SE. The natural history of asymptomatic patients with aortic regurgitation and normal left ventricular function. *Circulation* 1983;68:509–517.

52. Bonow RO, Ostrow HG, Rosing DR, Lipson LC, Kent KM, Bacharach SL, Green MV. Verapamil effects on left ventricular systolic and diastolic function in patients with hypertrophic cardiomyopathy: pressure-volume analysis with a non-imaging scintillation probe. *Circulation* 1983;68:1062–1073.

61. Maron BJ, Bonow RO, Epstein SE, Wyngaarden MK, Hurley YE. Obstructive hypertrophic cardiomyopathy associated with minimal left ventricular hypertrophy. *Am J Cardiol* 1984;53:377–378.

64. Bonow RO, Rosing DR, Maron BJ, McIntosh CL, Jones M, Bacharach SL, Green MV, Clark RE, Epstein SE. Reversal of left ventricular dysfunction after aortic valve replacement for aortic regurgitation: influence of duration of left ventricular dysfunction. *Circulation* 1984;70:570–579.

65. Bonow RO, Kent KM, Rosing DR, Lan KKJ, Lakatos E, Borer JS, Bacharach SL, Green MV, Epstein SE. Exercise-induced ischemia in mildly symptomatic patients with coronary artery disease: identification of subgroups at risk of death during medical therapy. *N Engl J Med* 1984;311:1339–1345.

75. Cannon RO, Bonow RO, Bacharach SL, Green MV, Rosing DR, Leon MB, Watson RM, Epstein SE. Left ventricular dysfunction in patients with angina pectoris, normal epicardial coronary arteries and abnormal vasodilator reserve. *Circulation* 1985;71:218–226.

77. Bonow RO, Vitale DF, Bacharach SL, Frederick TM, Kent KM, Green MV. Asynchronous left ventricular regional function and impaired global diastolic filling in coronary artery disease: reversal after coronary angioplasty. *Circulation* 1985;71:297–307.

78. Bonow RO, Dilsizian V, Rosing DR, Maron BJ, Bacharach SL, Green MV. Verapamil-induced improvement in left ventricular diastolic filling and increased exercise tolerance in patients with hypertrophic cardiomyopathy: short- and long-term effects. *Circulation* 1985;72:853–864.

81. Bonow RO, Picone AL, McIntosh CL, Rosing DR, Maron BJ, Clark RE, Epstein SE. Survival and functional results after valve replacement for aortic regurgitation from 1976 to 1983: influence of preoperative left ventricular function. *Circulation* 1985;72:1244–1256.

83. Bonow RO, Epstein SE. Indications for coronary artery bypass surgery: implications of the multicenter randomized trials. *Circulation* 1985;72(suppl V):V-23–V-30.

91. Betocchi S, Bonow RO, Bacharach SL, Rosing DR, Maron BJ, Green MV. Isovolumic relaxation period in hypertrophic cardiomyopathy: assessment by radionuclide angiography. *J Am Coll Cardiol* 1986;7:74–81.

92. Cannon RO, Schenke WH, Bonow RO, Leon MB, Rosing DR. Left ventricular pulsus alternans in patients with hypertrophic cardiomyopathy and severe obstruction to left ventricular outflow. *Circulation* 1986;73:276–285.

94. Spirito P, Maron BJ, Bonow RO. Noninvasive assessment of left ventricular diastolic function: a comparative analysis of Doppler echocardiographic and radionuclide angiographic techniques. *J Am Coll Cardiol* 1986;7:518–526.

95. Palmeri ST, Bonow RO, Myers C, Sieppe CA, Jenkins J, Bacharach SL, Green MV, Rosenberg SA. Prospective evaluation of doxorubicin cardiotoxicity by serial rest and exercise radionuclide angiography. *Am J Cardiol* 1986;58:607–613.

105. Tracy CM, Winkler JA, Brittain E, Leon MB, Epstein SE, Bonow RO. Determinants of ventricular arrhythmias in mildly symptomatic patients with coronary artery disease and influence of inducible left ventricular dysfunction on arrhythmia frequency. *J Am Coll Cardiol* 1987;9:483–488.

106. Bonow RO, Vitale DF, Maron BJ, Bacharach SL, Frederick TM, Green MV. Regional systolic and diastolic asynchrony and impaired global left ventricular diastolic filling in hypertrophic cardiomyopathy: effect of verapamil. *J Am Coll Cardiol* 1987;9:1108–1116.

108. Spirito P, Maron BJ, Bonow RO, Epstein SE. Occurrence and significance of progressive left ventricular wall thinning and relative cavity dilatation in patients with hypertrophic cardiomyopathy. *Am J Cardiol* 1987;60:123–129.

109. O'Gara PT, Bonow RO, Maron BJ, Damske BA, Van Lingen A, Bacharach SL, Larson SM, Epstein SE. Myocardial perfusion abnormalities assessed by thallium-201 emission computed tomography in patients with hypertrophic cardiomyopathy. *Circulation* 1987;76:1214–1223.

111. Bonow RO, Bacharach SL, Green MV, Lafreniere RL, Epstein SE. Prognostic implications of symptomatic vs asymptomatic (silent) myocardial ischemia induced by exercise in mildly symptomatic and in asymptomatic patients with angiographically-documented coronary artery disease. *Am J Cardiol* 1987;60:778–783.

113. Maron BJ, Bonow RO, Cannon RO, Leon MB, Epstein SE. Hypertrophic cardiomyopathy: interrelation of pathophysiology, clinical manifestations and therapy. *N Engl J Med* 1987;316:780–789, 844–852.

116. Bonow RO, Epstein SE. Is preoperative left ventricular function predictive of survival and functional results after aortic valve replacement for chronic aortic regurgitation? *J Am Coll Cardiol* 1987;10:713–716.

119. Bonow RO, Vitale DF, Bacharach SL, Maron BJ, Green MV. Effects of aging on asynchronous left ventricular regional function and global ventricular filling in normal human subjects. *J Am Coll Cardiol* 1988;11:50–58.

122. Dilsizian V, Bonow RO, Cannon RO, Tracy CM, Vitale DF, McIntosh CL, Clark RE, Bacharach SL, Green MV. The effect of coronary artery bypass grafting on left ventricular systolic function at rest: evidence for preoperative subclinical myocardial ischemia. *Am J Cardiol* 1988;61:1248–1254.

124. Epstein SE, Quyyumi AA, Bonow RO. Myocardial ischemia: silent or symptomatic. *N Engl J Med* 1988;318:1038–1042.

127. Bonow RO. Prognostic implications of exercise radionuclide angiography in patients with coronary artery disease. *Mayo Clin Proc* 1988;63:630–634.

130. Bonow RO, Dodd JT, Maron BJ, O'Gara PT, White GG, McIntosh CL, Clark RE, Epstein SE. Long-term serial changes in left ventricular function and reversal of ventricular dilatation after valve replacement for chronic aortic regurgitation. *Circulation* 1988;78:1108–1120.

131. Brush JE, Cannon RO, Schenke WH, Bonow RO, Leon MB, Maron BJ, Epstein SE. Microvascular angina in patients with hypertension without left ventricular hypertrophy. *N Engl J Med* 1988;319:1302–1307.

135. Udelson JE, Cannon RO, Bacharach SL, Rumble TF, Bonow RO. Beta-adrenergic stimulation with isoproterenol enhances left ventricular performance in hypertrophic cardiomyopathy despite potentiation of myocardial ischemia: comparison with rapid atrial pacing. *Circulation* 1989;79:371–382.

139. Mazzotta G, Bonow RO, Pace L, Brittain E, Epstein SE. Relation between exertional ischemia and prognosis in mildly symptomatic patients with single or double vessel coronary artery disease and left ventricular dysfunction at rest. *J Am Coll Cardiol* 1989;13:567–573.

141. Bonow RO. Left ventricular structure and function in aortic valve disease. *Circulation* 1989;79:966–969.

142. Bonow RO. Left ventricular ejection dynamics and outflow obstruction in hypertrophic cardiomyopathy. *J Am Coll Cardiol* 1989;13:1280–1282.

144. Udelson JE, Bonow RO, O'Gara PT, Maron BJ, Van Lingen A, Bacharach SL, Epstein SE. Verapamil prevents silent myocardial perfusion abnormalities during exercise in asymptomatic patients with hypertrophic cardiomyopathy. *Circulation* 1989;79:1052–1060.

145. Dilsizian V, Cannon RO, Tracy CM, McIntosh CL, Clark RE, Bonow RO. Enhanced regional left ventricular function after distant coronary bypass via improved collateral flow. *J A, • Coll Cardiol* 1989;14:312–318.

146. Brush JE, Udelson JE, Bacharach SL, Cannon RO, Leon MB, Rumble TF, Bonow RO. Comparative effects of verapamil and nitroprusside on left ventricular function in patients with hypertension. *J Am Coll Cardiol* 1989;14:515–522.

149. Epstein SE, Quyyumi AA, Bonow RO. Sudden cardiac death without warning: possible mechanisms and implications for screening asymptomatic populations. *N Engl J Med* 1989;321:320–324.

154. Cuocolo A, Sax FL, Brush JE, Maron BJ, Bacharach SL, Bonow RO. Left ventricular hypertrophy and impaired diastolic filling in essential hypertension: diastolic mechanisms for systolic dysfunction during exercise. *Circulation* 1990;81:978–986.

155. Bonow RO. Regional left ventricular nonuniformity: effects on left ventricular diastolic function in ischemic heart disease, in hypertrophic cardiomyopathy, and in the normal heart. *Circulation* 1990;81(suppl III):III-54–65.

157. Hennein HA, Swain JA, McIntosh CL, Bonow RO, Stone CD, Clark RE. Comparative assessment of chordal preservation versus chordal resection during mitral valve replacement. *J Thorac Cardiovasc Surg* 1990;99:828–837.

158. Dilsizian V, Rocco TP, Freedman NMT, Leon MB, Bonow RO. Enhanced detection of ischemic but viable myocardium by the reinjection of thallium after stress-redistribution imaging. *N Engl J Med* 1990;323:141–146.

159. Udelson JE, Bacharach SL, Cannon RO, Bonow RO. Minimum left ventricular pressure during beta-adrenergic stimulation in human subjects: evidence for elastic recoil and diastolic "suction" in the normal heart. *Circulation* 1990;82:1174–1182.

164. Bonow RO, Dilsizian V, Cuocolo A, Bacharach SL. Identification of viable myocardium in patients with coronary artery disease and left ventricular dysfunction: comparison of thallium scintigraphy with reinjection and PET imaging with ^{18}F-fluorodeoxyglucose. *Circulation* 1991;83:26–37.

169. Perrone-Filardi P, Bacharach SL, Dilsizian V, Bonow RO. Impaired left ventricular filling and regional diastolic asynchrony at rest in coronary artery disease and relation to exercise-induced myocardial ischemia. *Am J Cardiol* 1991;67:356–360.

170. Dilsizian V, Smeltzer WR, Freedman NMT, Dextras R, Bonow RO. Thallium reinjection after stress-redistribution imaging: does 24 hour delayed imaging following thallium reinjection enhance detection of viable myocardium? *Circulation* 1991;83:1247–1255.

171. Cannon RO, Dilsizian V, O'Gara PT, Udelson JE, Bonow RO. Myocardial metabolic and hemodynamic significance of reversible thallium-201 perfusion defects in hypertrophic cardiomyopathy. *Circulation* 1991;83:1660–1667.

173. Dilsizian V, Perrone-Filardi P, Cannon RO, Freedman NMT, Bacharach SL, Bonow RO. Comparison of exercise radionuclide angiography with thallium SPECT imaging for detection of significant narrowing of the left circumflex coronary artery. *Am J Cardiol* 1991;68:320–328.

175. Bonow RO, Lakatos E, Maron BJ, Epstein SE. Serial long-term assessment of the natural history of asymptomatic patients with chronic aortic regurgitation and normal left ventricular systolic function. *Circulation* 1991;84:1625–1635.

176. Perrone-Filardi P, Bacharach SL, Bonow RO. Identification of viable myocardium in patients with chronic ischemic heart disease and left ventricular dysfunction: correlation of flow, metabolic activity, and regional function. *Cardiologia* 1991;36:299–307.

177. Clyne CA, Arrighi JA, Maron BJ, Bonow RO, Cannon RO. Systemic and left ventricular hemodynamic responses to exercise stress of asymptomatic patients with significant aortic stenosis. *Am J Cardiol* 1991;68:1469–1476.

184. Bonow RO. Prognostic applications of exercise testing. *N Engl J Med* 1991;325:887–888.

186. Bonow RO. Radionuclide angiographic evaluation of left ventricular diastolic function. *Circulation* 1991;84 (suppl I):I-208–I-215.

187. Bonow RO. Radionuclide angiography in the management of aortic regurgitation. *Circulation* 1991;84 (suppl I):I-296–I-302.

189. Dilsizian V, Freedman NMT, Bacharach SL, Perrone-Filardi P, Bonow RO. Regional thallium uptake in irreversible defects: magnitude of change in thallium activity after reinjection distinguishes viable from nonviable myocardium. *Circulation* 1992;85:627–634.

191. Dilsizian V, Bonow RO. Differential uptake and apparent thallium-201 "washout" after thallium reinjection: options regarding early redistribution imaging before reinjection or late redistribution imaging after reinjection. *Circulation* 1992;85:1032–1038.

194. Bonow RO. Determinants of exercise capacity in hypertrophic cardiomyopathy. *J Am Coll Cardiol* 1992;19:513–515.

195. Cannon RO, Dilsizian V, O'Gara PT, Udelson JE, Tucker E, Panza J, Fananapazir L, McIntosh CL, Wallace RB, Bonow RO. Impact of operative relief of outflow obstruction on thallium perfusion abnormalities in hypertrophic cardiomyopathy. *Circulation* 1992;85:1039–1045.

197. Perrone-Filardi P, Bacharach SL, Bonow RO. Effects of regional systolic asynchrony on left ventricular global diastolic function in patients with coronary artery disease. *J Am Coll Cardiol* 1992;19:739–744.

198. Quyyumi AA, Panza JA, Diodati JG, Callahan TS, Epstein SE, Bonow RO. Relation between left ventricular function at rest and with exercise and silent myocardial ischemia. *J Am Coll Cardiol* 1992;19:962–967.

200. Perrone-Filardi P, Bacharach SL, Dilsizian V, Maurea S, Marin-Neto JA, Arrighi JA, Frank JA, Bonow RO. Metabolic evidence of viable myocardium in regions with reduced wall thickening and absent wall thickening in patients with chronic ischemic left ventricular dysfunction. *J Am Coll Cardiol* 1992;20:161–168.

201. Bonow RO, Udelson JE. Left ventricular diastolic dysfunction as a cause of congestive heart failure: mechanisms and management. *Ann Intern Med* 1992;117:502–510.

202. Perrone-Filardi P, Bacharach SL, Dilsizian V, Maurea S, Frank JA, Bonow RO. Regional left ventricular wall thickening: relation to regional uptake of ^{18}F-fluorodeoxyglucose and ^{201}Tl in patients with chronic coronary artery disease and left ventricular dysfunction. *Circulation* 1992;86:1125–1137.

209. Dilsizian V, Bonow RO. Current diagnostic techniques of assessing myocardial viability in hibernating and stunned myocardium. *Circulation* 1993;87:1–20.

210. Quyyumi AA, Panza JA, Diodati JG, Callahan TS, Bonow RO, Epstein SE. Prognostic implications of myocardial ischemia during daily life in low risk patients with coronary artery disease. *J Am Coll Cardiol* 1993;21:700–708.

211. Perrone-Filardi P, Bacharach SL, Dilsizian V, Panza JA, Maurea S, Bonow RO. Regional systolic function, myocardial blood flow, and glucose uptake at rest in hypertrophic cardiomyopathy. *Am J Cardiol* 1993;72:199–204.

212. Quyyumi AA, Diodati JG, Lakatos E, Bonow RO, Epstein SE. Angiogenic effects of low molecular weight heparin in patients with stable coronary artery disease. *J Am Coll Cardiol* 1993;22:635–641.

214. Dilsizian V, Perrone-Filardi P, Arrighi JA, Bacharach SL, Quyyumi AA, Freedman NMT, Bonow RO. Concordance and discordance between stress-redistribution-reinjection and rest-redistribution thallium imaging for assessing viable myocardium. *Circulation* 1993;88:941–952.

215. Marin-Neto JA, Dilsizian V, Arrighi JA, Freedman NMT, Perrone-Filardi P, Bacharach SL, Bonow RO. Thallium reinjection demonstrates viable myocardium in regions with reverse redistribution. *Circulation* 1993;88:1736–1745.

216. Dilsizian V, Arrighi JA, Diodati JG, Quyyumi AA, Bacharach SL, Marin-Neto JA, Uddin S, Bonow RO. Myocardial viability in patients with chronic ischemic left ventricular dysfunction: comparison of ^{99m}Tc-sestamibi, ^{201}thallium, and ^{18}F-fluorodeoxyglucose. *Circulation* 1994;89:578–587.

217. Perrone-Filardi P, Bacharach SL, Marin-Neto JA, Dilsizian V, Maurea S, Arrighi JA, Bonow RO: Clinical significance of reduced regional myocardial glucose uptake in regions with normal blood flow in patients with chronic coronary artery disease. *J Am Coll Cardiol* 1994;23:608–616.

219. Arrighi JA, Dilsizian V, Perrone-Filardi P, Diodati JG, Bacharach SL, Bonow RO. Improvement of the age-related impairment in left ventricular diastolic filling with verapamil in the normal human heart. *Circulation* 1994;90:213–219.

220. Mazzotta G, Pace L, Bonow RO. Risk stratification of patients with coronary artery disease and left ventricular dysfunction by exercise radionuclide angiography and exercise electrocardiography. *J Nucl Cardiol* 1994;1:529–536.

221. Bonow RO. Asymptomatic aortic regurgitation: indications for operation. *J Card Surg* 1994;(suppl)9:170–173.

223. Bonow RO. Management of chronic aortic regurgitation. *N Engl J Med* 1994;331:736–737.

232. Bonow RO. The hibernating myocardium: Implications for the management of congestive heart failure. *Am J Cardiol* 1995;75:17A–25A.

233. Ritchie JL, Bateman TM, Bonow RO, Crawford MH, Gibbons RJ, Hall RJ, O'Rourke RA, Parisi AF, Verani MS. Guidelines for clinical use of cardiac radionuclide imaging. Report of the American Heart Association/American College of Cardiology Task Force on Assessment of Diagnostic and Therapeutic Cardiovascular Procedures (Committee on Radionuclide Imaging). *Circulation* 1995;91:1278–1303, *J Am Coll Cardiol* 1995;25:521–547.

235. Bonow RO, Nikas D, Elefteriades JA. Valve replacement for regurgitant lesions of the aortic or mitral valve and advanced left ventricular dysfunction. *Cardiol Clin* 1995;13:73–83.

240. Hendel RC, Chaudhry FA, Bonow RO. Myocardial viability. *Curr Prob Cardiol* 1996;21:145–224.

245. Bonow RO. New insights into the cardiac natriuretic peptides. *Circulation* 1996;93:1946–1950.

248. Bonow RO. Identification of viable myocardium. *Circulation* 1996;94:2674–2680.

249. Davidson CJ, Fishman RF, Bonow RO. Cardiac catheterization. In: Braunwald E, ed. *Heart Disease: A Textbook of Cardiovascular Medicine* 5th Edition. Philadelphia: W.B. Saunders Company, 1996:177–203.

251. Gheorghiade M, Bonow RO. Coronary Artery Disease. In: Kelley W, ed. *Textbook of Medicine* 3rd Edition. Philadelphia: J.B. Lippincott Company, 1996:371–385.

252. Kong TQ, Davidson CJ, Meyers SN, Tauke JT, Parker MA, Bonow RO. Prognostic significance of creatine kinase elevation following elective coronary artery interventions. *JAMA* 1997;277:461–466.

256. Bonow RO. Need more research on heart disease. *Chicago Tribune* Feb 19,1997;1:14.

260. Gheorghiade M, Bonow RO. Chronic heart failure in the United States: a manifestation of coronary artery disease. *Circulation* 1998;97:282–289.

261. Bonow RO, Carabelló B, de Leon AC, Edmunds LH Jr, Fedderly BJ, Freed MD, Gaasch WH, McKay CR, Nishimura RA, O'Gara PT, O'Rourke RA, Rahimtoola SH. ACC/AHA guidelines for the management of patients with valvular heart disease. A report of the American College of Cardiology/American Heart Association Task Force on Practice Guidelines (Committee on Management of Patients with Valvular Heart Disease). (submitted for publication).

DAVID COSTON SABISTON, Jr., MD:
A Conversation With the Editor*

Dr. David Sabiston is one of the most recognized names in surgery worldwide. He was born in Onslow County, North Carolina, on October 4, 1924. He graduated from the University of North Carolina at Chapel Hill at age 19 in 1944 and was a member of Phi Beta Kappa. He graduated from the Johns Hopkins University School of Medicine in 1947 at age 22 and he was a member of Alpha Omega Alpha. His internship and residency in surgery was at The Johns Hopkins Hospital under Dr. Alfred Blalock. After completion of his surgical training in 1953, he went into the U. S. Army Medical Corps for 2 years, spending that time with Dr. Donald Gregg in Washington, DC, in the Army Medical Service Graduate School. Dr. Sabiston returned to Hopkins in 1955, and except for a year at Oxford and London, United Kingdom, he remained there until 1964 when he became Professor and Chairman of the Department of Surgery at Duke University Medical Center in Durham, North Carolina. Shortly before leaving Hopkins, where he had already become a full professor of surgery, he did the first aortocoronary bypass operation ever performed. From 1964 until 1994 Dr. Sabiston was Chairman of the Department of Surgery at Duke. He built one of the finest departments of surgery ever created at any medical school. His Department of Surgery included not only general and cardiothoracic surgery but also neurosurgery, orthopedic surgery, plastic surgery, otolaryngology, and urology. His trainees who finished the general surgical program also were qualified in cardiothoracic surgery. Many of them went on to become division chiefs and chairmen of various departments of surgery around the country.

Despite his large administrative, operative, organizational and teaching activities, his own research work has continued throughout his career. He focused primarily on disorders of the coronary and pulmonary circulations. His investigative endeavors resulted in nearly 300 publications in medical journals.

In addition to his own writings and investigations, Dr. Sabiston has been the most prolific editor of surgical books during the latter half of this century. He is the long-time sole editor of *Textbook of Surgery* and coeditor (with Frank Spencer) of *Surgery of the Chest*. The former was begun in 1972 and the latter in 1976 and each was revised about every 4 years. Additionally, he has authored *Pulmonary Embolism* (1980), *Essentials of Surgery* (1987, 1994), *The Southern Surgical Association* (with Dr. Robert Sparkman), *Atlas of General Surgery* (1994) among others. In addition, he is the editor of *Atlas of Operations in General Surgery: Including Laparoscopic Procedures* and also the editor of *Atlas of Cardiothoracic Surgery*. And as

if these accomplishments were not enough, he has served as Editor in Chief of the *Annals of Surgery* for the last 31 years, and it is one of the most highly regarded surgical journals.

Dr. Sabiston has spent a great deal of time teaching housestaff and medical students. I doubt if any surgeon in the last half of this century was as good a teacher as he. He got to know his students well. He received the Golden Apple Award as Best Clinical Teacher by Duke Medical Students on 4 occasions (1966, 1977, 1982, and 1993), and the Thomas D. Kinney Award for Outstanding Teacher of the Year (presented at graduation exercises at Duke University Medical School) on 4 occasions (1976, 1981, 1982, 1983). In 1992, he received the Alpha Omega Alpha Distinguished Teacher Award presented at the Annual Meeting of the Association of American Medical Colleges. The latter award is given to only 1 physician yearly in the USA.

Because of his personal qualities and many professional accomplishments, Dr. Sabiston has been elected by his peers to the highest positions of leadership in American surgery. He has served as president of the American Surgical Association, the American College of Surgeons, the American Association for Thoracic Surgery, the Society of University Surgeons, the Southern Surgical Association, the Whipple Society, and the Society of Surgical Chairmen. He has served as Chairman of the American Board of Surgery, the Board of Regents of the American College of Surgeons, the Board of Governors of the American College of Surgeons, the Surgical Forum Committee, the American College of Surgeons, the Accreditation Council for Graduate Medical Education, and the Surgery Study Section of the National Institutes of Health.

And he has been an active lecturer and teacher outside his own medical center. He has given 164 named lectures in a similar number of cities in the USA and 61 lectures at various meetings abroad; he has been a visiting professor at 166 university medical centers in the USA.

For his accomplishments he has received many honors. He was elected to the Institute of Medicine of the National Academy of Sciences. He is an honorary fellow in 22 surgical societies around the world. He has received the Michael E. DeBakey Award for Outstanding Achievement; the American Heart Association Scientific Council's Distinguished Achievement Award; Distinguished Alumnus Awards from the University of North Carolina and the Johns Hopkins University, and an Honorary Alumnus Award from the Duke Medical Alumni Association; the Bigelow Medal from the Boston Surgical Society, and an honorary degree from the University of Madrid.

And he is a gracious, friendly, true Southern gen-

*This series of interviews are underwritten by an unrestricted grant from Bristol-Myers Squibb.

0002-9149/98/$19.00
PII S0002-9149(98)00324-5

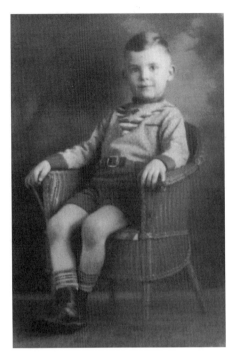

FIGURE 1. DCS at age 4.

tleman, who has always received the strong support of Aggie, his lovely wife of 43 years, and of their 3 lovely daughters.

William Clifford Roberts, MD[†] (hereafter, WCR): *Dr. Sabiston, it is a treat to be here in your home in Durham, North Carolina, today (February 15, 1998), and I appreciate very much your willingness to talk with me and share your illustrious career with the readers of* The American Journal of Cardiology. *Let me start by asking where were you born? Could you talk about your early upbringing?*

David Coston Sabiston, Jr., MD[‡] (hereafter, DCS): Thank you Bill. It is a real pleasure having you in our home. Your being a friend of long standing I have looked forward to this discussion with you. In answer to your first question, I was born in North Carolina in 1924 on my grandfather's farm. He showed me early the value of knowing the land and what it would produce. Later, my parents and I moved from there into town (Jacksonville), which is where I grew up and had my education through high school. I then went to Chapel Hill to college.

WCR: *Dr. Sabiston, where is Jacksonville, North Carolina?*

DCS: It is on the coast of the Atlantic Ocean. It is the county seat of Onslow County. Onslow is named for an English Lord, Darwin Onslow.

[†]Baylor Cardiovascular Institute, Baylor University Medical Center, Dallas, Texas 75246

[‡]James Buchanan Duke Professor of Surgery and Director of International Programs, Department of Surgery, Duke University Medical Center, Durham, North Carolina 27710.

WCR: *Who were your parents?*

DCS: My father was the son of the grandparents I just mentioned. My mother was Marie Jackson from Morehead City, North Carolina, which also is on the Atlantic Coast. She was a school teacher, very interested in education, both learning and teaching. She was a great stimulus to me to be an academic faculty member.

WCR: *What about your daddy?*

DCS: He was a businessman, a salesman for a grocery company.

WCR: *Did he travel a lot or was he home most of the time?*

DCS: He traveled but was also home a lot.

WCR: *What was Jacksonville like?*

DCS: Jacksonville was a small town. In the 1940 census, the population numbered 739.

WCR: *So you went to grammar school, junior high school, and high school in Jacksonville, North Carolina. What was grammar school like? Was it a one-room school?*

DCS: No. It was a good school for the times. There was a nice building and big classrooms. There were about 30 students in every class. I was very fortunate to have a good background before I went to Chapel Hill.

WCR: *How was early school divided; into grammar school and then high school?*

DCS: The first 7 grades were all preparatory to high school. Eighth through 11th are what we called high school.

WCR: *How many students were in your graduating high school class?*

DCS: About 30.

WCR: *You were the valedictorian of your class?*

DCS: That is correct.

WCR: *So that meant you were the first in your class from a scholastic standpoint? Did you have sports in high school? Did you participate in those activities?*

DCS: Yes. I ran track. In those days sports were not organized like they are today. They were very informal without real teams.

WCR: *What did you do in track?*

DCS: I ran the 100 and 220 yard dashes.

WCR: *What did you do in the summer time when school was not going on?*

DCS: When I was with my grandparents, I used to work on the farm a lot. I was very close to the soil and I have had a great respect for it ever since then. My paternal grandfather grew corn and tobacco. My grandmother also had a vegetable garden and I also worked in it.

WCR: *Did you know your mother's parents?*

DCS: Yes. They lived in Morehead City and I saw them from time to time, but not on a daily basis like I saw my other grandparents.

WCR: *You finished high school at age 16?*

DCS: Yes.

WCR: *That was younger than most of your classmates?*

DCS: Yes. I started early.

WCR: *Your mother, I presume, being a teacher herself, and scholastically oriented, taught you how to read pretty quickly?*

DCS: She stayed right on me academically all the time.

WCR: *Do you have brothers and sisters?*

DCS: I have 1 sister.

WCR: *Is she older or younger than you?*

DCS: She is younger.

WCR: *Is your sister living?*

DCS: Yes. She lives in Wilmington, North Carolina, near where we grew up.

WCR: *Were you and your sister close when growing up?*

DCS: Yes.

WCR: *How did you decide to go to the University of North Carolina to college?*

DCS: In North Carolina at the time that was the usual thing that happened. Of course students went elsewhere too, but for some reason North Carolina has been very singular in the fact that most of the high school graduates who go to college go to Chapel Hill and have since the University opened in the 1700s.

WCR: *You were 16 and it was 1941 when you entered Chapel Hill? What did you study in college?*

DCS: I majored in chemistry and zoology.

WCR: *Did you know you wanted to be a physician?*

DCS: Quite early. I had an uncle, my father's brother, who was a physician and I used to spend time in the summers with him. He would take me on rounds and let me sit in his office. So quite early I became intrigued with the idea of medicine. I held to it all through high school and college.

WCR: *Your uncle, the physician, was in Jacksonville?*

DCS: No, Kinston, a nearby town.

WCR: *Your parents, I presume, encouraged you to do that as well?*

DCS: They supported me the whole time.

WCR: *Did you enjoy college?*

DCS: Yes. Chapel Hill is a wonderful place to be. Great place to have fun. Great place to work. I had very good professors and we in North Carolina were very lucky to have a state institution as good as it was. I thoroughly enjoyed the time in Chapel Hill because it was such a good school. It is the oldest state university in the nation. The institution just recently celebrated it's 200th anniversary.

WCR: *Did any teachers in high school or college have a particular impact on you?*

DCS: Yes. There was one Professor of Chemistry, Dr. Edwin Carlyle Markham, who was very much a teacher and scholar, Dr. James Talmage Dobbins, also a Professor of Chemistry, and Dr. John N. Couch, a well-known botanist throughout the country.

WCR: *Were you a member of a fraternity in college?*

DCS: Yes, I was a member of Sigma Chi.

WCR: *Did you participate actively in the social activities at college?*

DCS: Yes.

WCR: *How far is Jacksonville from Chapel Hill?*

DCS: About 150 miles.

WCR: *You finished college in 3 years?*

DCS: Yes.

WCR: *Did you go in the summers or did you just take a lot of courses each semester?*

DCS: Yes. I went every summer. The war was going on and that is why I went into the Naval V12 program which was a part of the whole training.

WCR: *When it came time to pick a medical school, how did you select Hopkins?*

DCS: My roommate, Dotson Palmer, in college at the time asked me where I was going to apply. I had already put in my applications. I thought I was going to Chapel Hill. He said, "Why don't you try Hopkins?" I said I would never be able to get in there. He said, "You never know until you try." Out of the blue, I sent an application to Hopkins, frankly not expecting to be accepted, and I went to my mailbox one day and there was a letter from the committee saying I could be a member of the class of 1947.

WCR: *So you applied to only 2 medical schools, the University of North Carolina and The Johns Hopkins, and it was just by chance that you applied to Hopkins.*

DCS: It was by chance. I was not going to apply to Hopkins at all, although a number of boys in the South used to apply there before World War II. It had a good reputation, but known to be very hard to get into. I did not think I needed to put that stumbling block in front of me. I have always been thankful to my roommate for pressing me to apply to Hopkins.

WCR: *In college you were Phi Beta Kappa. You must have made all A's or virtually all A's.*

DCS: I did all right I think.

WCR: *Here you grew up in a small town in North Carolina, came to college to a larger but still small town, and now at age 20, big Baltimore. How did that strike you?*

DCS: It was quite different because I had never spent any significant time in a large city and, of course, Baltimore was just that. It took a little bit of time but I was so busy in medical school that I did not have much time to think about it. I was deeply engrossed in my studies and I had to work very hard. I tried to do everything I was supposed to do and that took about every minute of the day.

WCR: *You obviously did extremely well in medical school. Did learning come easy for you or did you have to work hard at it?*

DCS: I had to work hard at it. There were students in my class, for example, who could go to a lecture, learn everything, and repeat it to you in 2 or 3 days, but I had to work hard. I think I had to work harder than some other students.

WCR: *Do you think the fact that you had to work hard for your superb grades became an advantage to you later when you began doing a lot of teaching? Did it make your teaching better that everything had not always come easy for you?*

DCS: That is a very good question. I think that is right. I tried to plan teaching exercises in a way that I hoped the students would remember. I have always said for the students to remember that it did not make so much difference what you said, but it was the way you said it. You could talk to them all day and not make an impression and then you have lost a day.

WCR: *Who influenced you in medical school?*

DCS: Two people, Dr. Alfred Blalock, who caught my imagination and desire to be like him, and second, Dr. Arnold R. Rich, who I got to know pretty well. Dr. Rich was a very accomplished scholar. He was Professor of Pathology at Hopkins for many years. He succeeded William Welch and William McCallum in the Chair of Pathology there. Rich was the third Professor of Pathology at Hopkins and he was a very good professor. I was taught very well. I used to go to a weekly conference where he taught. I remember to this day how he would go around the class and ask each of us, by our names, what the answer was to this or that question. He would go over things informally, but it was a session we all enjoyed because he was such a complete scholar.

WCR: *He knew the names of medical students? That must have meant something to you? I understand that you knew the names of most medical students who rotated through your service?*

DCS: He was a good teacher and had quite an influence on me because he was a real scholar.

WCR: *How many medical students were in your class?*

DCS: Seventy-five.

WCR: *You entered medical school in 1943 and finished in 1947?*

DCS: Yes.

WCR: *You mentioned Dr. Blalock. What influence did he have on you when you were a medical student?*

DCS: He had done the first blue baby operation in 1944. Almost overnight, he became a household name. These children would pass in a wheelchair or be carried in the hallway panting for breath, nail tips and lips blue, very cyanotic, and often with oxygen tanks, and then they would walk out the front door of the hospital 2 weeks later pink and running around. It was almost like a miracle. This came about when I was a second-year medical student. When I was first introduced to surgery I knew that that was what I wanted to do. I was impressed with what he had been able to accomplish, first by his research on animals, and then by doing the same procedure in children. He was a great teacher and a great role model, an example to all of us.

WCR: *How did Dr. Blalock teach? Did he teach medical students a lot or just his housestaff?*

DCS: He pitched the tenor of his remarks differently to medical students than to housestaff because he realized there was a difference. He tried to present things that would get their attention and they would remember. At the end of every 1 hour session with him you went away with 2 or 3 major points. That was what he tried to do. He did not try to be encyclopedic and give a total review of the whole field but just the high points.

WCR: *How did he instill such loyalty in those of you who trained under him?*

DCS: That is a very perceptive question and it really is the basis of his whole being. He was always so loyal to us that naturally we would feel that way about him. He stood by everyone of his residents. We soon understood that so it was a 2-way equation. We owed our allegiance to him.

WCR: *You interned at The Johns Hopkins Hospital beginning in 1947. Did Dr. Blalock ask you to intern in surgery there? Did you apply elsewhere? How did it come about that you stayed at Hopkins?*

DCS: Actually, I had gotten to know Dr. Blalock as a medical student pretty well. He had just done the first blue baby operation as mentioned. He had filmed his very early operations on the blue babies. He needed to show these films to foreign visitors and he did not have anyone on the housestaff at that time who knew how to operate a motion picture machine. He found out that I knew how to use a motion picture machine. He would call me when someone was there from England or France and ask if I would mind showing the film for him that afternoon. He would always ask what time would be convenient for me. Actually, I wanted to be convenient for him. He got accustomed to me because previously he had had several of his films chewed up in the machine when it was run by people who did not know how to use it. That was very annoying to him. Every time I ran a film for him I would put it back just like it came. He got to know me by my first name when I was a third-year medical student. That is how we got close. I have often thought how smart it was that I knew how to run a motion picture machine, because I probably would not have had that relationship with him.

WCR: *How did you learn about films? Was that a hobby earlier on?*

DCS: Yes. I had taken some motion picture films when I was growing up. I could always thread one of those Bell and Howell Projectors. The main thing was that I did not chew up the film in the projector.

WCR: *Did you take a lot of still pictures also when you were young?*

DCS: Not so many. I really was not much of a photographer, but I did know how to run the projector.

WCR: *How did Dr. Blalock learn that you were an expert in this arena?*

DCS: That is a good question. I have often tried to solve that. I do not know exactly how he came to know that. I believe he went to one of the conferences when I was showing a film and he liked what he saw and asked me if I would do it. I told him to call me anytime. He would call me out of class. Naturally, admiring him like I did I was always there 5 minutes early. He was a great man for punctuality. He did not hold anyone up because he did not expect to be held up himself. He would often say that I was there early and he appreciated it. Those things made an impression on me.

WCR: *He knew he could count on you. Did you apply for a surgical internship anywhere other than Hopkins?*

DCS: I don't think I did. I did go around and visit a lot of programs. I have forgotten exactly if he told me I could stay on, but I was pretty confident. He asked me to apply and I figured knowing him like I did he would not have asked me to apply if he were not going to take me on.

WCR: *When you started your surgical internship in 1947 how many surgical interns were there in your group?*

DCS: Twelve.

WCR: *After the first year of residency that came down to what?*

DCS: Two. Two chief residents.

WCR: *Then for the rest of your 5 years you were one of those 2. Who was the other one with you?*

DCS: Jack Grayhack from Chicago. He later became Professor of Urology at Northwestern.

WCR: *During your training as an intern and as a houseofficer under Dr. Blalock from 1947 to 1953, I gather the program was set up so that you got to do an awful lot of operating.*

DCS: That was characteristic of the program. It was very thorough and you got a tremendous amount of experience. When we finished we had confidence in ourselves and the people knew that.

WCR: *Who were some of the other surgical trainees with you during that 6-year period?*

DCS: There was William P. Longmire, who became a faculty member while I was an intern. Later, he became the Professor and Chairman of Surgery at the University of California at Los Angeles. William Harry Muller was another; he became Professor and Chairman of Surgery at the University of Virginia. Another was Henry Bahnson who became Professor and Chairman of Surgery at the University of Pittsburgh. There were a whole group of surgeons like that at that time who took academic posts.

WCR: *The people that Dr. Blalock selected to be these special 2 each year all essentially turned out extremely well and became leaders in 1 medical center after another around the country. What was Dr. Blalock's ability to pick talent?*

DCS: That is a very good question and I have thought about it many times. He seemed to have had the ability to put the whole thing together and look at all facets of a person's life, their being and their productivity. He had uncanny ways of doing this. I don't think I have ever fully understood this because he was so much on target every time. He made very few mistakes in selecting his people. They were all hard workers and devoted to people. He put a lot of emphasis on character. He did not have any place for people who were not gentlemen. He was an exemplary Southern gentleman himself with high standards and honesty. He put a lot of emphasis on that. I think that is a very key thing. You can choose 5 people who are all very honest, straight forward, and of high character, and you are not going to lose on that. He had the ability to pick people who were really scholars and gentlemen.

WCR: *You obviously have picked a lot of people in your career during your 30-year period as Chairman*

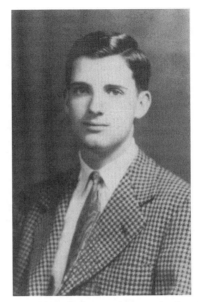

FIGURE 2. DCS when a freshman at the University of North Carolina.

of the Department of Surgery here at Duke. I gather your experience with Dr. Blalock was useful in that regard? You obviously have an ability to smell out those who were going to do well. You are obviously good at selecting talent. What are you looking for more than anything else?

DCS: You know I always tried to think how he would do it, because he was so sure fire in his choices. He always seemed to pick the right ones. I know he thought a lot about it. I certainly used everything that I learned from him in coming to that conclusion and selecting who I would have stay on. I had the wisdom to follow up on those people he chose and did well. Naturally, you want to check out the person's productivity to see if he can be a valuable member of the scientific community. I think one can do that by looking at their past performance. You have to have something to go on that is objective, and that usually is something you can find out from a person by asking the right questions. Usually you know some of that beforehand—what they have done, why they have done it, and how they are apt to do it in the future. Of course, it is a matter of pot luck. You don't always pick the right ones, but you can come close to it.

WCR: *I noticed from your curriculum vitae that during your period as a surgical intern and resident at Hopkins that you published quite a few articles in medical journals? How did you get turned on? Once you started you have never stopped.*

DCS: I think it was due to Dr. Blalock. I had a hard time separating anything that I did from him. It always went back to him. He was very supportive of publications. He thought you should share your discoveries with other people very quickly. I recognized that and did well because I always had to submit the manu-

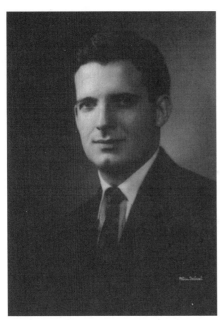

FIGURE 3. DCS in 1953 (age 28) when chief resident in surgery under Dr. Alfred Blalock.

script to him. He would go over it very carefully and make notes. Pretty soon I enjoyed handing him a paper and then getting it back and seeing his suggestions. That was extremely helpful in the formative years.

WCR: *Do you consider Dr. Blalock a scholar?*

DCS: Yes, no question. He could write extremely well, always in simple English. If you read his papers he expressed himself very well. He always used straightforward English. If a simple word would do he would use it in preference to a complicated word.

WCR: *After you finished your training at Hopkins you took your boards in both general surgery and thoracic surgery. Although you have always been in many aspects of surgery, I gather, you knew fairly early that you wanted to focus on cardiac and pulmonary surgery. That was before the cardiopulmonary machine came along.*

DCS: Extracorporeal circulation broke through about the time I was Chief Resident in Surgery. I finished the residency in 1953 and by 1955 the heart-lung machine was being used around the country. That was the heyday of cardiac surgery, as you know very well from your own interest in the field.

WCR: *When you finished your training, the only cardiovascular operations being done were closure of patent ductus arteriosus, production of a ductus (Blalock-Taussig), resection of coarctation of the aorta, pericardiectomy, and mitral valvulotomy. Dr. Sabiston, how did it come about that you went to Washington, DC, to work with Dr. Donald Gregg for 2 years?*

DCS: During the last 4 years of residency I had been a member of the Naval Reserve. I was required

to give the military 2 full years. I had been deferred until I finished my residency at Hopkins and then I had to go into the service. I went in 1953, the same year I finished the residency. I was supposed to go to Korea because we were in the Korean War at that time, but during the month of June or July, 1953, President Eisenhower ended the war in Korea. I was reassigned to Walter Reed.

WCR: *From looking over your bibliography it seems to me that you were interested in the coronary circulation before you went to work with Dr. Gregg. Is that right?*

DCS: Yes. Dr. Blalock said, "You know we have made advances in a lot of areas, but with the biggest problem, coronary artery disease, we have not made any advances at all." He said, "I want you to plan to be on the faculty and be in charge of that." So I worked with Donald Gregg on that because he was a coronary physiologist.

WCR: *What did you learn? You did 2 years of experimental work with non-human animals. That must have had quite an influence on you later on?*

DCS: That is right, Bill, because my association with Dr. Blalock was always learning things and he talked about some of the unknowns of the coronary circulation, how important they were, how it would be more important than all the other things we had done if we could find a way to help people with coronary disease. When I went to Walter Reed I had a chance to work with Don Gregg. I really took advantage of it. He was a great teacher, a competent constant investigator. He did everything multiple times to be sure. I can hear him say right now, "Doctor, you can never be too sure." He was so turned on by research that he worked many nights until after midnight in his laboratory. He never asked me to stay on after 5:00 P.M. because everyone else got off then, but I would stay. That was when I was dating my future wife. She was a student at Goucher College in Baltimore at that time. Often I would have planned a date and he would be working late in the lab. It would come time for me to go on my date and I would have to call her and tell her I am sorry but I have to work. I could not see leaving him in the laboratory by himself. He was so good about that. He always believed you should finish everything in 1 day and not put it off until the next. He worked many nights until midnight. He taught me the discipline of investigation.

WCR: *At that time, 1953 to 1955, Dr. Gregg was how old?*

DCS: He was probably 55 or 60.

WCR: *He was twice your age and he was still working pretty late hours.*

DCS: I knew that he was always very happy when I would stay on. I wanted to learn from him. Naturally, I wished he would not have worked at night but I did not want him to work without my being there.

WCR: *You got married in 1955 right after that period with Dr. Gregg, so you must have gotten out for a few dates here and there?*

DCS: Yes. I did all right, but I broke many dates. I must give Aggie credit. She was very understanding.

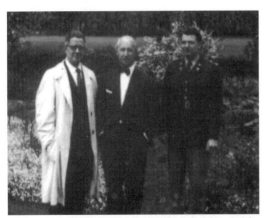

FIGURE 4. DCS *(right)* with Doctors Alfred Blalock *(left)* and Philip Allison *(center)* in 1960 (age 36).

That was not easy because she was still in college. She would make her plans to be off on a particular night and I would have to call her and tell her I could not come over that night. I was in Washington, DC, and she was in Baltimore. She had a good introduction to medicine. I met her when I was in Washington, DC. Her father was a United States Congressman who represented the Tidewater section of North Carolina for 26 years in the House of Representatives, so she lived in Washington when Congress was in session. She lived on campus while she was at Goucher, but the summer she would be with her parents in Washington.

WCR: *How did you 2 meet?*

DCS: It is a funny thing. I had an aunt who lived next door to me when I was growing up and she met Aggie at some function her father took her to. My aunt wrote me and said, "I met this very attractive lady who is in Baltimore right now. She is the daughter of Congressman Barden and I recommend her to you." I called Aggie for a blind date. First she was busy. She was dating a midshipman from Annapolis and she said, "No, I am sorry I am tied up." I said, "Well, may I call you some other time?" She said, "Yes, call me again." The next time we had a date.

WCR: *When you got married in 1955, you were 31 and Aggie was 22?*

DCS: Yes. She is almost 10 years younger than I am.

WCR: *Then in 1955 you both, I presume, moved back to Baltimore. You are now a member of the faculty and you remained in Baltimore, except for your year at Oxford and London, for the next 10 years, until 1964. How did that progress, particularly early on? You walked in and now you were no longer Chief Resident or resident, you were a real faculty person. How did it evolve?*

DCS: It evolved very well because Dr. Blalock always protected me. He had so many patients he could not see them all so he would channel some of them to me. They all had heart disease. That is how I really got my beginning. He never operated on a

patient with coronary artery disease. That was the way he would do with his former residents. He would do the same thing to Henry Bahnson, Frank Spencer, and all the rest. He helped us all get started.

WCR: *The young faculty members under Dr. Blalock at that time were yourself, Henry Bahnson, Frank Spencer, Jim Jude.*

DCS: Most Chief Residents under Dr. Blalock left Hopkins as soon as that last year was completed. They would get an appointment at another institution. Dr. Blalock would secure it for them.

WCR: *After you had been a faculty member for about 3 years you took a sabbatical to Oxford, United Kingdom. How did that come about?*

DCS: Although I had done coronary research with Dr. Gregg, Dr. Blalock told me, "You know a lot about the physiology of the coronary circulation, but you have not had any real activity in coronary atherosclerosis," and he said, "I want you to work with a person who has had a great deal of experience in experimental atherosclerosis." He sent me to Oxford to work with Howard W. Florey, the discoverer of penicillin. After he did his work on penicillin, Florey told me that he thought he had done about all he could do with penicillin and that he did not want to stay in that field anymore. He turned his attention to the biggest problem which was coronary atherosclerosis. We worked on that with Sir William Dunn in the Dunn School of Pathology at Oxford. I signed on to work with him and also with Dr. Phillip Allison, the Professor of Surgery there. Those 2 were my chief mentors while I was at Oxford as a Fulbright scholar. Dr. Blalock said, "You need some support while you are over there. I recommend that you apply for a Fulbright." That is why I did that. I was fortunate because research money was hard to come by in those days, particularly if you trained abroad. You might get an NIH scholarship in the United States but they were not honored if you went abroad. The scholarship, of course, allowed me to go to Oxford for a year.

WCR: *It sounds like Dr. Blalock had a pretty broad view of medicine and wanted you to be exposed, not only to other surgeons, but to people in other spheres.*

DCS: You are exactly right. He had had a year at Cambridge when he was a young man when he was at Vanderbilt and he knew the value of basic research. He had worked in the laboratories at Cambridge and was insistent that I spend some time in Cambridge, although he wanted me to work at Oxford with Florey and I did. I really enjoyed it. Blalock gave me a send off when leaving Baltimore. Florey said, "We must put our attention on the endothelium. I think it is more than just a plastic lining. A man cannot know too much about the endothelium, and how many enzymes it makes." I think how wise he was. Florey told me that the endothelium did a lot more than just line the vascular system. He did not know any facts but he knew how to get them. He was a brilliant man.

I knew why Florey was so interested in angina. He had it himself but he kept it a secret. People would not often let it be known that they had angina in those

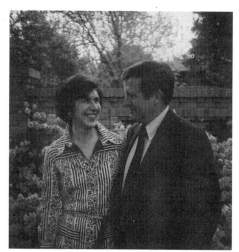

that period and that the experience expanded your horizons so to speak. Was that the first time you had been abroad?

DCS: I had been abroad one time before that when I was a resident under Dr. Blalock. He took me on a tour of England and France for 1 month and I thoroughly enjoyed that. That was in 1952. What I did then was carry his slides, projector, and all that kind of stuff. I was his handyman, but he introduced me to everybody and he knew them all. It was amazing. It was an honor for me for him to introduce me to those people. To be introduced by him might mean they would remember me. Dr. Blalock always gave everyone else more attention than he put on himself, and we all respected him for that. He knew it was so important to us and he was so genuine about it. He also would say, "This work was Dave's idea or Hank's idea." It made an impression on everyone. There were very few professors in those days who would say that such and such work was not all theirs.

WCR: *Dr. Blalock was relatively modest?*

DCS: Yes, very modest. He always gave his colleagues credit.

WCR: *During your sabbatical year, you did little operating? When returning to Baltimore in 1961, you rapidly were back into the swing of things? What were you looking forward to then? What were your goals?*

DCS: My goals were laid down by Dr. Blalock. He said, "I want you to come on the faculty and study coronary circulation and provide some means of revascularization. We have this problem of coronary disease and we have nothing for it." The Vineberg procedure was done but no one had any confidence in it. Blalock knew it would be a big thing and he said, "This would be bigger than all the congenital hearts we have put together." He started me off with that. He encouraged me to do the first bypass. It was the first time it was ever done. He was very instrumental in that and I would have never done it had it not been for his pressing me.

WCR: *So you did the first human bypass operation in 1962?*

DCS: Right.

WCR: *How did that come about? What exactly happened?*

DCS: The patient was referred to me after having had a heart attack and he was doing poorly. His cardiologist wanted something done, but something different than the Vineberg procedure. "I want you to do a direct operation," he said. He knew that Dr. Blalock had asked me to start that so I did. I did an aortocoronary anastomosis and the patient lived for about 24 hours and then suddenly died. We got our first real introduction to coronary bypass surgery in 1962!

WCR: *Did you use a saphenous vein?*

DCS: Yes.

WCR: *The conduit was inserted where?*

DCS: From the aorta to the coronary artery. I had a picture made of it at that time. Leon Schlossberg, as you know, worked in the hospital, and we called him into the operating room to sketch the operation be-

days because it had such a bad prognosis. He did not want that to be associated with him. When I got back to Baltimore he called me and said, "If I come over will you do a vascular operation on my heart. I have severe angina and I don't think I will live very long." I said "Let me do a little more on this, because it was not that certain in those days, and I will call you." Unfortunately, he had a heart attack before I got back to him. I don't know how long he had had it but it could not have been any worse.

WCR: *Dr. Florey was how old when you were working with him?*

DCS: I guess he was about 61 or 62 years old.

WCR: *What did you actually do when you worked there?*

DCS: I worked with him and some of his assistants on coronary atherosclerosis. We used to feed animals very high cholesterol diets and produce the atherosclerotic lesions. I made many photographs of histologic sections of atherosclerotic plaques.

WCR: *Did you enjoy working in the laboratory?*

DCS: Always. You could design experiments and see how they came out. The work produced a great sense of satisfaction. After producing the atherosclerosis, myocardial infarction often resulted. It was a positive academic endeavor.

WCR: *During your sabbatical you also spent some time in London?*

DCS: Yes. I went there and spent some time with some professors at the Great Ormond Street Hospital, the Children's Hospital for the British Isles. That was a very formative experience too. I thought a lot of Dr. Andrew Wilkinson who was Professor of Pediatric Surgery at the Great Ormond Street Hospital.

WCR: *You and Aggie must have had an enjoyable year?*

DCS: Yes. We had 2 of our 3 children with us then. They had a great time. We have always enjoyed England. We enjoy going back.

WCR: *I gather you met a number of people during*

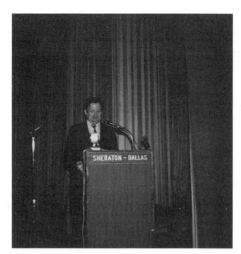

FIGURE 6. DCS presenting at the American Surgical Association meeting in Dallas, Texas, in 1978, the year he was President.

cause I knew it was the first time it had ever been done. So he did it and I later published the drawing. (Schlossberg was such a skilled artist. It was uncanny how well he could draw.)

WCR: *To which coronary artery?*

DCS: To the left anterior descending.

WCR: *Because you had done a lot of them in babies, this anastomosis must have been a piece of cake?*

DCS: It was a piece of cake as far as the technical aspects were concerned, but myocardial ischemia was always risky because the heart might fibrillate, although we did have a defibrillator available. Although the cardiopulmonary bypass machine was available, we did not use it because of its inherent risk.

WCR: *So you did the first coronary bypass operation without cardiopulmonary bypass? You just lifted the left anterior descending artery off the heart. Were you pleased with the result early on?*

DCS: Yes. I was. The patient got hypotensive early on, but, nevertheless, the result was encouraging and it gave us a greenlight to do it again. That was really important. At least the patient had not died on the operating table. In the early days, if you were not going to be successful, usually the patient died on the operating table. If they lived awhile afterwards, that was a very good sign. That is what happened to this first patient.

WCR: *Thus, this was not an operation carried out after an unsuccessful endarterectomy and you had no choice other than to put in a conduit. This operation was well planned beforehand. Both Dr. Blalock and certain cardiologists were behind it. You called the medical artist, Leon Schlossberg, in to record this event. You waited quite a period of time before you reported that patient. Why did you delay publication?*

DCS: Naturally, I wanted it to be successful long term and in this first patient it was not. I was not so impressed, but Dr. Blalock said I must report it, that it

was very important in the history of medicine. I later published it in an article on coronary surgery in general.

WCR: *In 1964, at age 39, you became a full Professor of Surgery at Hopkins. Dr. Blalock retired in 1964?*

DCS: Yes. He retired July 1964.

WCR: *That was the year you came to Duke?*

DCS: Yes, I stayed on just 1 month after he left the chairmanship. I am sure that he was very instrumental in getting the position for me at Duke.

WCR: *I gather that Dr. Blalock wanted you to be his successor at Hopkins?*

DCS: He told me that, but Hopkins rarely appoints a departmental chairman from its own faculty. They import somebody, and he said that is what they will probably do in his case. Although he told me that he would like for me to be his successor, and I appreciated that more than anything but Dr. Blalock was not permitted to pick his successor. The selection committee appointed someone from outside. Dr. Blalock recognized, however, that that was the way Hopkins did things.

Arnold Rich was holding the Department of Pathology together after McCallum had died, and not long afterwards the selection committee offered the Chairmanship of Pathology to somebody at Yale. That person came down to Hopkins and after several days said, "I appreciate very much your asking me to be Chairman, but that position belongs to Arnold Rich. You are passing over the greatest man in pathology because he is already here." Dr. Rich got the job because of the visitor from Yale's comment! Dr. Rich was a great person. Rich was the second best teacher I ever had.

WCR: *It was not long before Dr. Blalock's retirement that you were selected to be Chairman of Surgery here at Duke University. This was coming home, back to North Carolina. Were you very pleased to receive that opportunity?*

DCS: I was very pleased because, you have it right, it was coming back to North Carolina. Aggie appreciated that fact so much because she always wanted to come back. She liked Baltimore, since she had been there as a student at Goucher, but when she finished college she was ready to come home. We stayed in Baltimore for about 9 years. It was very good. Dr. Blalock had carcinoma and died in 1964. I was already in Durham. I used to go back on weekends to see him in Baltimore when he was in the hospital with cancer. He diagnosed his cancer himself. His physician believed that he had hepatitis, but Blalock felt his liver getting bigger and said he had cancer. I saw him on a Saturday before he died the following Tuesday. He told me he thought he had cancer. He had had an operation about 6 months before that for a slipped disc, but, in retrospect, that was due to a metastasis.

WCR: *Dr. Blalock was 65 when he died?*

DCS: Yes. He was born in 1899.

WCR: *At Duke you could run the show as you wanted to. You had been under Dr. Blalock for 17*

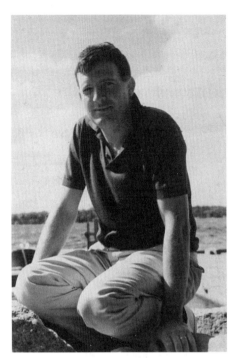

FIGURE 7. DCS while relaxing (about 1980).

years off and on. You obviously learned a good deal from him. You had spent time with Donald Gregg and Howard Florey. By that time you must have realized what kind of department of surgery you wanted and what kind of impact you could have on a medical center. When you came to Duke were you able to put your ideas into operation rapidly or how did it evolve?

DCS: You are very perceptive Bill. The early Chairman of the various departments at Duke had mainly come from Hopkins. Dr. William Welch was the one that dedicated the medical school and made the initial address here. He was very well liked at Duke. Welch was asked who they should appoint as Chairman of Pathology and he picked one of his own former residents, Wiley Forbus, who had trained at Hopkins under Welch. Forbus was a Hopkins graduate and Chief Resident under Welch. Then there were a series of physicians who came to Duke from Hopkins. They all had respect for Hopkins. I always thought that was the reason I got my position. Duke had a system of having strong Chairmen and turning things over to them, instead of letting the Dean make the decisions. The Chairman made them. Welch himself was the first Dean at Hopkins Medical School. He knew to pick good men and let them develop. All the people in the other departments were the same. Duke had a great history of that and that is how they chose their first Chairman. It was an environment where you were allowed to grow. That is what they did with me. I have always been very grateful because I could not have gone to a medical school that had as much

influence from Hopkins as they did. Not only that, they practiced it everyday.

WCR: *You must have had a bit of pride coming back to North Carolina. Did you say to yourself? "Well, I am going back home to my origins, and I am going to make Duke University the new Johns Hopkins. I am going to move Hopkins from Baltimore to Durham." You built your Department of Surgery and have produced the top leaders in surgery around this country during this last 30 years. They did not come out of Hopkins, they came out of Duke. How did you attract all these bright people that you surrounded yourself with in Durham, North Carolina. Durham is a pretty small place. A lot of the people you attracted did not grow up in Jacksonville, North Carolina, like you did. A lot of them, I suspect, grew up in Boston and New York City, and other large cities. How did you make this such an enticing department?*

DCS: You are very kind and generous to make those remarks and phrase them the way you did. It was a very simple thing for me. I set my sail as near to that as Dr. Blalock had done in trying to make Duke a place for young people to thrive, to give them opportunities, to make sure that they got credit for their accomplishments and rewards, such as being elected to a society. They then got their own appointments elsewhere very soon. They learned that they would be happier in academic work than in private practice. I did try to choose academic-type surgeons from the beginning. It was all a tremendously pleasant experience.

WCR: *Throughout most of your 30 years as Chairman, how many interns did you take on each year, more or less?*

DCS: When I first came here, Dr. Hart, the former Chairman of Surgery, had for good reason adopted his Hopkins system, starting off with 12 or 15 interns and then ending up with 2 Chief Residents. I soon figured out that that was very hard and, in a way, it made the program too competitive, and negatively so, because the housestaff fought against each other to rise to the top. I reduced the entering number down to the same number we finished with to cut out the competition. I had to do that by degrees. I could not do it overnight. If they were picked for an internship they would probably finish as Chief Resident. That was my goal.

WCR: *You must have taken a few more on as interns, since I gather, you finished 3 Chief Residents a year after a while? Some of those after internship, I presume, went into orthopedics or urology or something else. You felt comfortable that you were going to get your 3 through "Dave's decade" from the beginning? So you picked only people who had scholastically proven themselves and who, I presume, you felt comfortable with? You considered their character to be good and their manners gentlemanly?*

DCS: That is right. I always paid particular attention to what they said they wanted to do with their futures. I wanted it be crystal clear and unmistakably objective as possible. I listened to what they said and if they had the right message that would be the type of person I appointed.

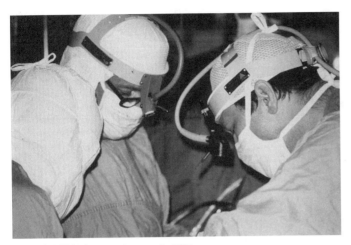

FIGURE 8. DCS in the operating room in 1984.

WCR: *Your Department of Surgery, I gather, included not only general surgery and cardiothoracic surgery, but also neurosurgery, orthopedic surgery, plastic surgery, otolaryngology, and urology. Despite heavy administrative responsibilities you also did quite a lot of operating yourself. You traveled a good bit, had many national and international societal and committee responsibilities, visiting professorships, wrote textbooks, and edited the* Annals of Surgery? *How did you put all this together?*

DCS: First, I have to tell you Aggie gets a lot of credit because she graciously never complained when I spent so much time working at home at night and on weekends. I had to do it that way, but she always provided a happy expression on her face and she was always good to me. Also, I had good people to work with on the faculty both at Hopkins and then at Duke. I shared a lot of things with them. I was always happiest when I was working. I did not like to waste time or do things that seemed to me not to be additive.

WCR: *You have spent a lot of time teaching, not only your housestaff that you carefully selected, but medical students who rotated through your service. Going through your curriculum vitae it looks like you were chosen the top teacher by the medical graduating classes 8 times! That is a tremendous honor. You were chosen as the one person in the country as best medical school teacher in 1992. That is an enormous honor. Have you enjoyed teaching through the years? You have obviously made that a major priority.*

DCS: Yes, you are right about that and again you are so perceptive. Without a doubt the single thing I enjoyed most was being a teacher. There is nothing like looking in a student's face and seeing it light up or observing a student's intense concentration while teaching, and have him tell you later something to that effect. It is a tremendous boost. It makes life worth living.

WCR: *How did you get into the textbooks?*

DCS: The Saunders Company came to me in the late 1950s and said they had been publishing for many years the most popular textbook of surgery by Christopher who was then Professor of Surgery at Northwestern. They wanted me to edit the next edition. That was a real bonanza. I took it on and was very fortunate to carry it through a number of editions. It was translated into 8 different foreign languages. Just the other day I got a notice from Russia that they wanted to translate some of our texts. I had a good publisher and a good book to start with and tried to build on that.

WCR: *How did you "capture"* Surgery of the Chest?

DCS: That was first written by Jack Gibbon who developed the heart/lung machine. He edited the first 3 editions. He turned it over to Frank Spencer and me. I was fortunate to be with it for a long time.

WCR: *Dr. Sabiston, how do you do your writing? Do you dictate? Do you write with pencil and paper?*

DCS: I wish I did use pencil and paper because I think some of the most productive authors are individuals who write it down. I dictate. My mind does not keep up with my handwriting. I get way behind when writing. I can talk much better. I have always dictated and had a secretary take it down. I go over it quite intensely afterwards and correct the dictation.

WCR: *Through the years have you done most of your writing (dictating) at home?*

DCS: Yes, on weekends and nights.

WCR: *When you were Chairman of the Department of Surgery here at Duke what were your daily activities like? What time would you get up in the morning?*

DCS: I have always gotten up early, had an early breakfast, and arrived at the hospital around 7:30 A.M. Usually, I would have a morning report with the Chief Residents, then make rounds, and then go to the operating room. That was my usual schedule for many years. When I got to be senior, I cut my own operating down to a more reasonable schedule.

WCR: *What time would you leave the hospital at night as a rule?*

DCS: I would usually be home by 8:00 P.M. with the family. I did not always make it in time for dinner, but I tried.

WCR: *After dinner you could work again?*

DCS: I would go back to my study. Aggie planned this house, Bill, and when she did she planned it so that I would have my study in the corner of the house, the quietest portion. I have 3 doors between my study and the children. They spent a lot of time in the family room, but there was a good distance between my study and the family room. Aggie took care of the children most of the time. That was the way it worked.

WCR: *You would have a full day, operate, teach, do administrative tasks, get home, eat dinner, and*

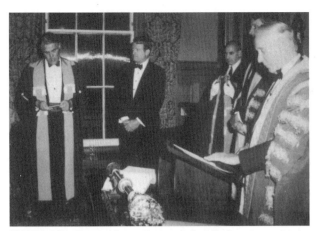
FIGURE 9. DCS when receiving an Honorary Fellowship from the Royal College of Surgeons of Edinburgh.

then you were back at your desk. How long were you good for? What time did you go to bed?

DCS: Usually about 10:00 or 10:30 P.M.

WCR: *You would wake up at 6:00 so you got a reasonable night's sleep most nights. When you were operating actively would you usually do 1 case a day, 2 cases, and how did you do that and also fulfill all of your other responsibilities?*

DCS: I thought it was very important to operate, so I always started off the day with at least an operation in the morning and sometimes 2. I would finish by noon. I would try to leave the afternoons open for appointments (faculty, residents, students and visitors) and my university and departmental responsibilities. I knew I could not be in the operating room in the afternoons when I should be attending committees because my people would not get treated right if I were not sitting at the table. I soon learned that there was nothing to be gained by being in the operating room in the afternoon.

WCR: *Through the years you have had a lot of responsibilities outside your Department of Surgery. In addition to other University responsibilities, you have been on numerous national and international committees; you have been an officer and/or board member of numerous professional societies. You have been president at one time or another of virtually every major surgical society in this country. How have you managed to fit in these additional responsibilities, not to mention your visiting professorships and your other travels, into your day-to-day local responsibilities?*

DCS: I suppose the first thing would be recognizing that these responsibilities that you refer to were very important to me and to my staff. I just needed to make room for them in the schedule and at the same time not let them take away from my local activities. Somehow, I had to put them all into the schedule. I think with proper attention it is possible to do that. It is hard sometimes but I think you should strive to do that.

WCR: *You have done so many different things. What are you most proud of in your career?*

DCS: There are a number of things. As you know yourself in your own experience, I am most proud of the trainees that have come out of the program and what they have accomplished in their own rights as they have gone off to other areas and sprouted new wings and new trees so to speak. The accomplishments of my faculty, residents, and students have brought me the greatest satisfaction.

WCR: *You have been Editor in Chief of the* Annals of Surgery *for 31 years. How did that come about? How much time do you spend a week editing that journal? Here is the premier surgery journal that you have had for over 3 decades!*

DCS: I have to spend a lot of time on it. You are exactly right. You know for a journal to be good, respected, and widely read it has to merit it. A journal cannot live on reputation for long. You have to have something there going for it. I always have given the journal prime time, each issue my best effort. It has been very valuable for me as a learning experience, and also hopefully for what I have been able to do for the authors. Again, it is just like so many things, it does not run by itself. It just takes hard work.

WCR: *How much time through the years would you estimate you spend a week on that journal.*

DCS: It is hard to tell because I did something on it almost every day. I would estimate probably a couple of hours a day.

WCR: *You have 3 daughters. Have you been a good daddy?*

DCS: I hope so. Fortunately, they say so. That is the biggest thing. I know I have not done as well as I might have because I spent a lot of time at the hospital, a lot of time on weekends working, but it has been a very satisfying experience. They know I have enjoyed them and they recognize that too.

WCR: *They have all done well. What do they do?*

DCS: One is an architect, one is a lawyer, and one has an interest in business.

WCR: *Do you have grandchildren?*

DCS: Five.

WCR: *Do they live in North Carolina?*

DCS: Yes, all of them do.

WCR: *Dr. Sabiston, when I was here at Duke one time you graciously invited me to speak to your house-staff. I remember coming into your office and speaking with you a few minutes and then each of your Chief Residents come into your office, and I met them. Then we went into your large conference room. All of your housestaff were seated, immaculately dressed in white, nobody came late, and they were quiet and respectful. It really was an eloquent way for me to see how you ran your department. I gather that you did not allow your surgical housestaff to run around the hospital in operating "pajamas." You encouraged*

INTERVIEW/DAVID COSTON SABISTON, JR. **369**

706

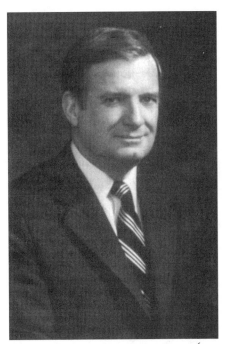

FIGURE 10. DCS in 1985 when President of the American College of Surgeons.

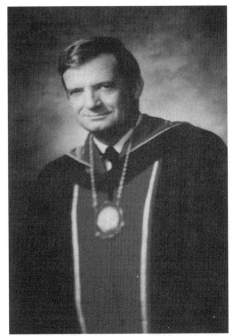

FIGURE 11. DCS in 1996 (copyright in 1996 held by the American College of Surgeons).

their keeping their shoes shined. In other words, I presume, you set a standard early on not just for your department but for other departments in the medical center to emulate. What kind of impact and what importance do you put on that?

DCS: That is a widely variable circumstance as you know so well. I have always thought surgeons ought not wear gowns outside the operating room, because of the unsterile environment. You should not be walking around in "pajamas" because that is just not the image I think we should be showing. You can carry that too far, of course, by making a scene out of every issue, but I think in the end it is the proper thing to do and my housestaff, I believe, usually kept the habit.

WCR: *You were Chairman at Duke for 30 years. Certainly you must have studied other contemporary departmental chairmen through the years. What other surgeons do you consider really led very enlightened departments?*

DCS: I've answered every question you have asked me but that gets down to so many personal features and so forth. I think I will use a well worn-out answer by saying "I think I will pass on that" if you will let me.

WCR: *What about surgeons for whom you have great admiration? There are a lot of surgeons who are, I gather, splendid surgeons, but don't spend a lot of time teaching medical students, teaching housestaff, and building their legacy so to speak in their trainees. You seem to have done all of that, but surely around*

the world there are a few other surgeons that you put on a pedestal above others.

DCS: I will answer that as carefully as I can, but I think I will mention only people who are senior to me. There are many. Francis Moore left behind a great legacy, Jonathan Rhoads is another one, and Robert Zollinger was a real power figure too, and he had a lot of trainees.

WCR: *You have enjoyed your influence in surgical societies, setting standards, I presume, for surgery all across this country and in other countries as well. Are there other surgeons in the National Academy of Sciences? I know you are a member of that?*

DCS: Yes. There are some that I know very well. They are usually individuals who have been investigators and done original work and who have been awarded for that by being elected to that group.

WCR: *Dr. Sabiston, you have done a lot of original work yourself. It seems that you have focused more on the coronary and pulmonary circulatory problems more than other things. What are you most proud of regarding your original contributions?*

DCS: I think probably the work on coronary circulation. I pursued that more than any other area.

WCR: *Are you disturbed about how medicine is going today?*

DCS: Yes. I am really worried about it. I am not a great supporter of the managed care system. I think we have the best medicine in the world in the United States. The economic burden we are asked to carry around our neck defeats many of the purposes of

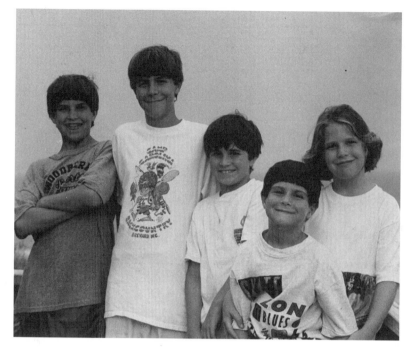

FIGURE 12. DCS's 5 grand-children: David Butler age 13, son of Agnes and Albert *(left)*; Carter Leggett age 13, son of Anne and Reid *(left center)*; Bill Butler age 10, son of Agnes and Albert *(center)*; Andrew Leggett age 7, son of Anne and Reid *(right center)*; Sarah Leggett age 10, daughter of Anne and Reid *(right)*.

medicine. They don't fit into the ideals of medicine or the objectives we ought to be following. The best medical care in every situation is getting increasingly hard to provide. Of course, the younger generation may come to live with it and enjoy it but it worries me.

WCR: *Through the years you have written quite a few pieces about other physicians, Dr. Blalock, for example. Who was Robert Kamish?*

DCS: He was an Administrator for the American College of Surgeons.

WCR: *Who was Theodore Drapanis?*

DCS: He was the Professor of Surgery at Tulane.

WCR: *You wrote on Trendelenburg?*

DCS: Trendelenburg was a very impressive German Professor at Leipzig. He did the first experimental work on pulmonary embolism and designed the procedure for pulmonary embelectomy which he did in calves in the early 1900s.

WCR: *You have always been interested in the lung it seems to me. In your books you have always written the chapter on cancer of the lung and mediastinum. That has always intrigued you it looks like?*

DCS: Yes. It has. I have been with them since the very beginning and some of it is associated with Dr. Blalock and some has been my own development of the medical interests through the years.

WCR: *When you were operating here at Duke, doing 1 or 2 cases a day, what operations were you primarily doing?*

DCS: Although I did some general surgery, I was primarily doing pulmonary and cardiac procedures. Dr. Blalock always did some general surgery. I think one of the last operations I did was a radical mastectomy.

WCR: *All of your Chief Residents when they finish take boards in both general surgery and thoracic surgery? That is pretty unusual in 1998. Is that going to survive?*

DCS: It probably will not. I don't know. It depends on many factors. Most of these trainees have gone out as cardiothoracic surgeons. I think they need to know as much about general surgery as they do about specialty surgery. That is one reason I have always held them to that.

WCR: *When you teach medical students, your array of topics appears to be nearly unlimited. I hear you give a great lecture on appendectomy, for example. Being Editor of the* Annals of Surgery *must have been useful to you in keeping up in areas other than cardiovascular and pulmonary?*

DCS: That is an easy way to keep up because you have to do that every day. No one knows that better than you. That keeps you alive in reviewing many different subjects. There is no way to avoid it. I think that is one of the great challenges and rewards of being an editor.

WCR: *A lot of manuscripts have passed over your desk. What do you particularly look for in a manuscript?*

DCS: It has to have a clear message, needs to be written well, and needs to show respect for the classics in medicine. If something has been done before, credit must be given for that and that is often missed by authors. They start out under the assumption that they are the first ones and sometimes I think they think they are. They have not investigated the subject enough to know about it.

WCR: *I bet there is hardly an appointment of Chairman of a Department of Surgery in this country without somebody's calling you and asking your opinion about it?*

DCS: You are kind to say that and it has been a pleasure of mine to be called in that situation. I can usually tell them the names of individuals who might be considered.

WCR: *Through the years have you taken time to develop one or more nonmedical hobbies?*

DCS: I have always been interested in general history. I certainly have had some role models such as Lincoln. I think he is a great figure. Studying the past greats has been a hobby of mine. I think it is very important that you know the people who have done a great deal for the country in one way or another and I try to do that.

WCR: *Was Dr. Blalock as historically oriented as you are?*

DCS: He was very historically oriented. He always referred to people who did things first and made great strides and I was very impressed with his ability to do that.

WCR: *Dr. Sabiston, I certainly appreciate your time and I am certain that the readers of* The American Journal of Cardiology *will as well. Is there any topic that you would like to discuss that we have not focused on?*

DCS: I would like to say that it has been a real honor to have been selected by you and *The American Journal of Cardiology* because it has such wide impact on the field and has for a number of years. I can only say I have been honored by your questions and your presence here in my home. I think very highly of what you and your colleagues have done in the same way as you have asked me about our group. Bill, thank you very much.

WCR: *Thank you, Dr. Sabiston. I sincerely appreciate your taking the time and also being so open in answering the questions.*

JOSEPH CHOLMONDELEY GREENFIELD, Jr., MD: A Conversation With the Editor*

Dr. Joseph C. Greenfield, Jr., was born in Atlanta, Georgia, on July 20, 1931. I first met him, I believe, in 1947 when he was a junior at Henry Grady High School in Atlanta, and I was a sophomore. Dr. Greenfield was in the class with my brother. Joe had a reputation of being a good guy, he was popular with his classmates, he was smart, he was on the rifle team, and he collected butterflies. He went to Emory University for 3 years, where he was elected to Phi Beta Kappa, and then he went to Emory University School of Medicine where he graduated in 1956 and was a member of Alpha Omega Alpha. His internship and residency in medicine were at Duke University in Durham, North Carolina. From there, he spent 3 years in the National Heart Institute in Bethesda, Maryland, working in the laboratory of Dr. Donald Fry. He returned to Duke in 1962. A year later he was appointed Chief of the Cardiology Section at the Durham Veteran's Administration Medical Center. In 1981, he became Chief of the Cardiology Division at Duke University Medical Center, and in 1983 he became Chairman of the Department of Medicine of Duke University Medical Center. He continued in that post until 1995. He also continued as Chief of Cardiology until 1989. Since 1970, he has been Professor of Medicine, and since 1981 he has been the James B. Duke Distinguished Professor of Duke University.

Until age 50 (1981), Dr. Greenfield spent about 80% of his time in his research laboratory working with animal models. He and his colleagues conducted a series of seminal studies focusing on the heart's response to ischemia and how the coronary arteries responded to a variety of stressors. His research, which generally asked fundamental physiologic questions, led to publication of nearly 150 scientific articles, appearing mainly in the *Journal of Clinical Investigation, Journal of Physiology, Circulation Research,* and *Circulation.*

Shortly after Dr. Greenfield's return to Durham in 1962, he began reading electrocardiograms in the heart stations at both the Veterans Administration and Duke University Hospitals. That endeavor has continued until the present, including during the period of his chairmanship. He often interprets 1,000 electrocardiograms a week.

During his 12 years as Chairman, the Department of Medicine underwent explosive growth. Total faculty grew from 152 MDs and 21 PhDs in 1983 to 290 MDs and 45 PhDs in 1995. Research funding from the National Institutes of Health grew from 13.6 to more than 34 million, boosting the department's NIH ranking from 14th in the nation in total funding to the top 6; clinical billings went from nearly $19 to $76 mil-

lion a year. Outpatient visits increased from 68,000 to 180,000; house staff grew from 95 to 145 physicians (US applicants for house staff positions grew from 600 to 1,200 a year); and fellowships went from 120 to 155. By the last of the Greenfield years, the department was recognized by *US News and World Report* as the third best internal medicine program in the United States. All of this growth occurred in the midst of difficult times for internal medicine in most parts of the country.

During his chairmanship, Greenfield made house staff and fellowship training a major priority not only for himself but for his entire department, with the goal of providing the best patient care anywhere. He considered the internship and residency years the most important part of the entire education, the time when one really learns to be a doctor. Greenfield created an exciting atmosphere for learning and achieving, and in doing so, this colorful and charismatic leader became almost a cult figure among those in the department. He both gave and received intense loyalty, and he was an extraordinary motivator and mentor.

Greenfield was always there for the house staff and faculty. He was gone no more than 10 days a year. He generally took morning reports 3 times a week; made general medicine attending rounds once or twice a week, and conducted "pizza rounds" every Friday night beginning at 11 P.M. or midnight. The latter was held in the departmental library; he would chat with the residents about patients, about their own families, and about what they needed to do better jobs. I doubt if any departmental chairman has been as much loved by his house staff and faculty as Joe Greenfield.

Greenfield is different from any other chairman I have met. His simple and small office is decorated by pictures of his hero, General Robert E. Lee, and an inspiring Civil War battle scene. Greenfield avoids social events, meetings ("Nothing was ever accomplished with more than 2 people in a room."), and trips. He rarely gives a talk. He has always driven to and from work in a truck. He is happy with his simple tastes, his unpretentiousness, his loyalties (to his family, colleagues, and institutions), his duties, his hobbies (Civil War, English-Pointer Birddogs, quail hunting, and butterflies), and his beliefs. We need more Joe Greenfields.

William C. Roberts, MD†(hereafter, WCR): *It is February 12, 1998, and I am in the office of Joseph C. Greenfield, Jr., in Durham, North Carolina. Joe, I appreciate your willingness to speak to me and the AJC readers. What I would like to do is start as early as you remember and try to learn where that spark to excel academically came from. Could you talk about*

---

*This series of interviews was underwritten by an unrestricted grant from Bristol-Myers Squibb.

†Baylor Cardiovascular Institute, Baylor University Medical Center, Dallas, Texas 75246.

0002-9149/98/$19.00 **219**
PII S0002-9149(98)00307-5

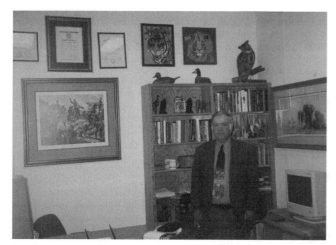
FIGURE 1. JCG in his office.

your growing up in Atlanta, your parents and siblings, and who had major influences on you during those early days?

Joseph C. Greenfield, Jr.,[†](hereafter, JCG): I was born in Atlanta in 1931, and lived there until 1956. (We lived in Richmond for about 1 year, when I was age 5 or 6, and then returned to Georgia.) My early years coincided with the depths of the Depression. I was, for better or worse, an only child. My earliest memories to excel came from my mother, who was academically inclined. Her father, my grandfather, who died in 1935, was a Methodist minister who received a PhD from Yale. He spent most of his life teaching ancient languages at what was then Florida State Women's College, now Florida State University. He instilled in my mother a love for academic endeavors. He was a Latin scholar, and, of course, when I went to high school I was made to take 4 or 5 years of Latin, which I promptly forgot, but which probably did help by making me do something I despised. After he died, I spent a fair amount of time in Tallahassee, Florida, with my grandmother who was originally from North Carolina. Her father was a surgeon in the Army of Northern Virginia during the Civil War. (I still have his surgeon's manual.) My father was a graduate of Georgia Tech. In the Depression, civil engineers were not in demand, and he went first into the insurance business, and finally into banking, working at First National Bank of Atlanta. His father, an Atlanta businessman, was involved in the development of the Crippled Children's Hospital. I remember his mother very well. She was born near Atlanta and the stories I remember from her were mainly those involving her family in and after the Civil War. She had 2 brothers killed, and the 1 surviving brother, a physician, lived with them. Because of her, I developed a life-long interest in the Civil War. When I grew

†James B. Duke Distinguished Professor, Duke University, Durham, North Carolina 27710.

up in Atlanta, many of the old Civil War trenches were still discernable, and I used to pick up "minie balls" on the school yard.

I had a very good education in the Atlanta public schools. The teachers that I remember in grammar school pushed us to excel. High school education for boys, at that time, in Atlanta consisted of 3 high schools: Boy's High, Tech High, and Commercial High. These were all public schools. The curriculum at Boy's High was designed to prepare for college. I had a wonderful education; the teachers really expected and demanded excellence. At that time, many of the classrooms were in old dilapidated wooden buildings heated with woodburning stoves. (We had a lot of fun putting firecrackers in them during class.) That experience made it clear to me that physical structure is not important in education. What we learned was dependent on the kind of people doing the teaching and what they demanded of us.

Another important factor in my growing up was World War II. I was 10 years old when Pearl Harbor was destroyed. The war affected our everyday life considerably with rationing, blackouts, and trying to help by collecting scrap, etc. My cousin was severely wounded in Germany and was hospitalized at Lawson Hospital near Atlanta. Weekly visits to him impressed on me the suffering associated with war.

During the summers while I was in high school and college, I worked in the pharmacology laboratory with Dr. Arthur Richardson, who was Chairman of Pharmacology at Emory University School of Medicine. I learned a lot and I enjoyed this research experience. At that time, Dr. C. Heymens from Belgium, who described the carotid sinus baroreceptors, was in the laboratory and I had a chance to interact with him. At Emory College, my primary mentor was Dr. Bell Wiley, a noted Civil War historian. At that time, you could enter medical school after 3 years, which I did, but during the summers while I was in medical school, I went back to college and got my AB degree in history. When I graduated from medical school, it became obvious to me that I was not going to be an historian, but my interest in history has continued.

I interned at Duke primarily because some of the house staff at Grady Hospital, who had graduated from Duke, told me that the training program was excellent. Obviously, Dr. Eugene Stead had a great influence on my life in demanding that the house staff enmesh ourselves in patient care. At that time, we worked 5 out of 7 nights sleeping in the hospital. It was not an ideal situation for family life, but we learned medicine.

As you remember, we were deferred from military service through medical school and house staff training. When I finished my training in internal medicine, I should have been placed on active duty under the

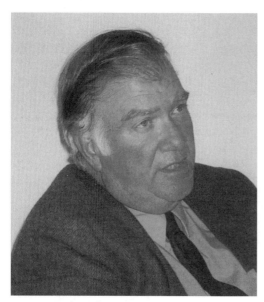

FIGURE 2. JCG during the interview

Berry Plan. I was very lucky in that I was accepted by the National Heart Institute at Bethesda, Maryland, to work with Dr. Bob Grant, an outstanding electrocardiographer. I joined the Public Health Service and went to work with Bob Grant. However, the day I arrived, Bob decided to become the Director of the National Heart Institute and left active research. I had to find a place to work and by sheer chance I found Dr. Donald Fry, who, I think, is one of the brightest and smartest people I have ever met. He had made a number of fundamental observations in both the mechanics of cardiac and pulmonary function. He was a superb individual and a very close friend. I was very lucky to have had the opportunity to work with him for 3 years. After completing my military obligations, I moved back to Duke and with Don's help and support developed my own research laboratory. We used a technique which we had developed to measure continuous cardiac output in patients. I became interested in studying the factors that regulate coronary blood flow and did most of my subsequent research work in this area.

WCR: *Let me go back a little bit. What was home life like for you when you were a youngster? You mentioned that your mother, in particular, was an intellectual person. What was it like sitting around the dinner table at night when you would come home from junior high school and high school?*

JCG: I grew up in what was the outskirts of Atlanta. (Now it's almost downtown.) I had the opportunity to do a lot of things outdoors, like hunting and fishing. A lot of our conversations were about these kinds of activities. We did not talk a lot about politics because my father hated Franklin Roosevelt so much that he would not talk about him. The kinds of conversations we had revolved mainly around day-to-day activities,

what was going on in the world, especially the World War.

WCR: *Where did you grow up in Atlanta? Where was your home located?*

JCG: It is about a mile from Emory University in Lennox Park.

WCR: *Were you close to your father? Did you hunt and fish with him?*

JCG: No. I did hunt with my great uncle, but my father was never a hunter or fisherman. He was a competitive pistol shooter and I went to a number of tournaments with him. Primarily because of his influence, I competed on the rifle team in high school.

WCR: *What about your mother?*

JCG: She was very much a stay-at-home person. Fortunately or unfortunately, raising me was almost her entire life.

WCR: *You were not a wealthy kid? How would you categorize yourself as far as opportunities that you had as a youngster versus some of your colleagues now?*

JCG: No, we were not wealthy, although we certainly were not destitute. We had a very difficult time financially in 1937 and had to live in Fayetteville, Georgia, with my grandmother. I went to a 1-room school and saw real poverty. I never will forget inviting a couple of my classmates to Sunday dinner; they ate so much they got sick. The lunch they brought to school each day was a cold potato. We did not have a lot when I grew up, but I did have an opportunity to go to college. I was expected to work, be it yard work or that type of thing, from an early age. My summers were spent working. I joined the Boy Scouts and got a lot out of that experience. I became an Eagle Scout, and again the drive to excel was very important. At that time Bert Adam's Boy Scout's Camp was right outside of Atlanta. I spent several weeks each summer there and got a lot out of the experience.

WCR: *Was your family religious?*

JCG: As I mentioned, my grandfather was a Methodist minister and my mother and I went to church every Sunday. My father was a Baptist. I am not sure he meant it to be particularly laudatory, but he described his mother as "an Admiral in the Lord's Navy." When he told her he was going to marry a Methodist she was absolutely convinced that "mixed marriages" would never work. When they baptized me but did not hold me under the water, she became so upset that she walked out. Although my father did not attend church regularly, my mother accompanied me to church weekly until I was perhaps 14 or 15 years old.

WCR: *Did you choose Emory to go to college because it was right there?*

JCG: It was near my house and at that time, cheap.

WCR: *You lived at home during college and medical school?*

JCG: Yes. I could walk, about a mile, to college. I was a member of Kappa Alpha (KA) social fraternity. That was a very important experience for me. When I entered college about half the class were returning World War II veterans. The other half were young smart alecs like me who had just graduated from high school. The older members of the fraternity put pressure on us to excel. I found the KA fraternity very important in that regard.

WCR: *You started college in 1949 when the GI bill was flourishing?*

JCG: Yes. College was filled with people that had been in World War II.

WCR: *They were anxious to do well?*

JCG: They were not there to play or to see how they could waste time in college. They made sure that we did the same thing.

WCR: *So they upped the standards for you folks coming right out of high school?*

JCG: My first semester I made all As and then dropped off and made a couple of Bs the second semester; I was dressed down by the president of the fraternity for making poor grades.

WCR: *In what way was being in the social fraternity important to you?*

JCG: It was very important to me. The members in the upper classes made sure that I excelled in school.

WCR: *Although it was a social fraternity, the members placed a lot of emphasis on doing well scholastically. Who influenced you in college? In college you majored in history?*

JCG: I majored in history as I mentioned. Dr. Bell Wiley was the main teacher I remember.

WCR: *What about sciences? Were you always turned on by biology and chemistry?*

JCG: I did well in them, but I never really liked them as much as I liked history. Some of the best courses I took in college were seminar courses where I read selected books and then discussed them with the professors.

WCR: *When you went to college had you already made up your mind that you wanted to go to medical school?*

JCG: Yes. I was in the accelerated 3-year program.

WCR: *You were put into the medical school track right out of high school? You knew you were going to medical school when you entered college?*

JCG: Yes, if I could get in. It was very competitive at that time to get into medical school.

WCR: *It was difficult at that time because the medical school classes were small, and because all those veterans were increasing the competition?*

JCG: That is exactly right.

WCR: *You went to Emory and finished college in 3 years? You went 12 years before that to school?*

JCG: Right. I did not skip any grades.

WCR: *When you finished college you were 20?*

JCG: Yes. I started medical school in 1952 at age 20 after 3 years in college. I had not finished college when I began medical school, but went back to college in the summers and that allowed me to get the (AB) degree in history.

WCR: *So you finished medical school at age 24? Did anybody turn you on in medical school?*

JCG: We had some very good basic science teachers. Probably the instructor I remember the best was the Chairman of Pathology, Dr. Walter Sheldon. He

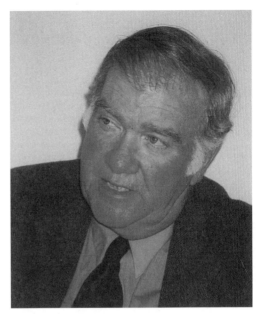

FIGURE 3. JCG during the interview.

was a superb teacher and demanded that we excel. In the clinical years, there were only a few full-time faculty. Thus, many of our clinical teachers were volunteers who were in private practice. Several of the major departments at the time did not have chairmen. Many of these volunteers and members of the·Emory Clinic were really superb role models. Dr. Bruce Logue, an outstanding cardiologist, was by far the best. Most of our clinical training occurred at Grady Hospital. There were not a lot of senior physicians in that hospital. It was mainly run by house staff. We learned by doing without much instruction. Actually, this training complimented what was available at Duke. At Grady Hospital, we had been able to do anything with patients, but there was no one to teach us what to do. When I got to Duke I saw the flip side in that there were a lot of staff physicians in the hospital and we were more constrained in making decisions about patients.

WCR: *When you were in medical school did you have a problem deciding what kind of physician you wanted to be or was that relatively easy for you?*

JCG: Primarily because of Dr. Logue, I wanted to be a cardiologist from the day I first went on the wards. Like most medical students, I went through a very transient period when I wanted to be a surgeon. However, I found out very quickly that I could not stand in the same place for a long period of time. This fact ended that potential career.

WCR: *When you came to Durham, Duke University Medical Center, in 1956, Dr. Stead had been here for 7 or 8 years? Except for the 3 years you were at NIH, you have not left Duke? What do you remember about medical internship and residency at Duke? You have* already mentioned that you lived at the hospital. You were essentially on call all the time?

JCG: We were totally enmeshed in medicine; we learned a lot. Primarily, I learned to enjoy delivering patient care. We ate, breathed, and lived medicine continually. In this respect, I think the things that I really enjoyed the most, which is so hard to get in training now, is to have personal relationships with so many patients. We had plenty of time to talk to them. It is hard to believe in 1998, but the first patient I took care of with a heart attack was a bank executive from Greensboro, North Carolina, who happened to be driving through Durham when he developed chest pain. At that time, there was no special place to put acute cardiac patients. The standard approach for patients with heart attacks was to put them in bed, relieve the chest pain, and have them on complete bed rest for 6 weeks. This meant they had to be fed by the nurses for at least 3 weeks. After that they could sit in a chair by the bedside. They were anticoagulated not to prevent cardiac clotting, but to try to prevent the complications of thromboembolism that so frequently occurred. In the acute patient, it was a maxim that if you could not make the patient pain free, he was going to die. I remember giving this patient large doses of morphine to no avail. After about 12 hours, he looked at me and said "Where do I go from here?" and died. I could do nothing except watch him die. On the other hand, we did know both the patients and families and we became physicians in the sense that we were involved with these people. They were not just a disease that you treated and discharged in 48 hours. This was a wonderful experience that physicians in training cannot get anymore. Of course, I had the opportunity to be involved in most of the changes that have taken place in cardiology from the beginning. When I began my internship the care of patients with heart attacks was not much different from the way patients with acute myocardial infarction had been treated for the preceding 100 years.

WCR: *You finished your house officer training and your 3 years at NIH in 1962. That was the year before Jack Kennedy was assassinated? So, in 1962, the therapy of acute myocardial infarction in actuality was about the same as it had been for the previous 100 years.*

JCG: I don't remember the exact date when defibrillators became available. We did have primitive pacemakers at that time. Actually, I was involved at the NIH in putting in one of the very early pacemakers. Also, I was at the NIH when the transeptal techniques to do left heart catheterizations were perfected. Cardiac care units became fairly widespread about 1965. The one at Duke was opened in 1964. The basic care of patients with acute myocardial infarction had not changed until we had the opportunity to put them in one place. The reason that cardiac care units were opened was to take care of patients who needed to be defibrillated or to have symptomatic bradycardia treated.

WCR: *You had an internship and 2 years as a resident in medicine and then you had 3 years at the National Heart Institute?*

JCG: The cardiology boards gave me credit for the 3 years at NIH. I had no other formal training in cardiology.

WCR: *When you returned to Duke in 1962, you were a cardiologist as it was defined at that time?*

JCG: That's right.

WCR: *How did things go when you came back to Durham? You set up your laboratory at the Veterans Administration Hospital. You started reading electrocardiograms daily?*

JCG: When I arrived at the NIH, Dr. Robert Berliner asked me to be responsible for the Heart Station at the Clinical Center (the NIH Hospital) and I read electrocardiograms for the next 3 years. When I returned to Duke, I became responsible for the ECG interpretation at the VA, and in 1969 I took over the Heart Station at Duke Medical Center, which I have continued until the present. I really enjoy reading ECGs and teaching electrocardiography to trainees.

In the beginning my research was helped immeasurably by Dr. George Tindall, a neurosurgeon, who let me use his laboratory until I could equip a laboratory of my own. We collaborated on a number of studies of cerebral blood flow. It was difficult at first to get money for research funding, but soon thereafter the NIH funds became readily available. Frankly, it was very easy to get grants beginning about 1964 and for the next 20 years. I obtained a Career Development Award, which funded my salary, and an RO1 and a VA Merit Review Award funded the research.

WCR: *How did you focus on coronary blood flow, coronary circulation, myocardial perfusion? Was that drawn out of your experience with Donald Fry?*

JCG: Not really. Don Fry taught me to think like a physiologist and to study the mechanics of the heart. I really became interested in coronary blood flow by visiting Donald Gregg at the Walter Reed Hospital. He was the "Father" of coronary flow physiology. He had developed an electromagnetic flow meter which allowed the continuous measurement of coronary flow. I had done similar blood flow work in the aorta at NIH and I brought this technique to Duke.

WCR: *You went over to see Donald Gregg in Washington, DC, on your own? You were already interested in it? How did you like working in the dog lab? I guess you used dogs primarily when you were working at the NIH?*

JCG: Most of the experimental work we did was with unsedated dogs. Because of Donald Gregg's influence, I tried to work on conscious, unsedated animals in an attempt to mimic the human pathophysiology as closely as possible. We developed a number of techniques to measure the factors which control coronary blood flow distribution in a number of different physiologic situations (e.g., exercise and pathologic conditions; e.g., cardiac hypertrophy). I was extremely lucky, in that 8 excellent graduate students completed their PhD thesis work with me. Two of these students, Judith Rembert and Philip McHale, remained in the

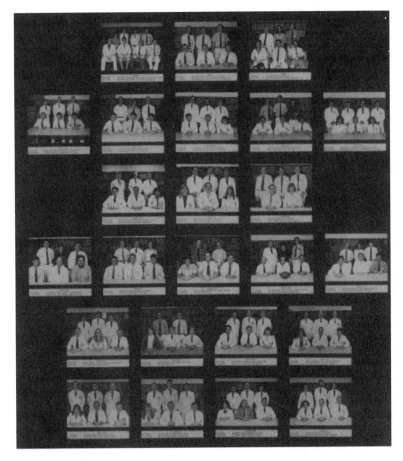

FIGURE 4 . Photographs of JCG with his chief residents and assistant chief residents at both Duke University Medical Center and the Veteran's Administration Medical Center during JCG's tenureship as Chairman.

laboratory and were largely responsible for our success in publishing high quality research.

WCR: *When you came back to Durham, North Carolina, from Bethesda, Maryland, you were entirely at the VA Hospital here?*

JCG: I had appointments at both Duke Hospital and at the VA Hospital, but I spent my day at the VA Hospital as Chief of Cardiology and doing research.

WCR: *When did you become Chief of Cardiology at the VA?*

JCG: 1963.

WCR: *How big was the division of cardiology in 1962, including your staff at the VA Hospital plus the staff at Duke University Medical Center?*

JCG: It would be a guess. There were no more than 15 senior staff physicians altogether.

WCR: *What is it today?*

JCG: About 52 full-time faculty.

WCR: *Just in cardiology?*

JCG: Yes.

WCR: *When you came back, I gather that you enjoyed teaching?*

JCG: Very much.

WCR: *You enjoyed taking care of sick people?*

JCG: Yes, but at the VA Hospital I was not the primary physician. The house staff actually took care of the patients and I functioned as a mentor or attending physician. I did not spend a lot of time in clinics seeing patients; I never did, as a matter of fact.

WCR: *You spent a lot of time in the laboratory at that time. That was the thing that was really turning you on then, I gather? You were enjoying this research and you were quite productive. When did it occur to you that maybe you would also like to be Head of Cardiology at Duke University Hospital? When is the first time that the idea of Chairmanship of the Department of Medicine was ever entertained by you?*

JCG: Very early on, I got a number of offers to look at academic positions, both as Chief of Cardiology and Chief of Medicine. The more I looked, the more I was happy with what I was doing. I primarily spent my day doing research and teaching. Thus, for a 20-year period, research in cardiovascular physiology and pathophysiology occupied more than 90% of my endeavors—I thought about research and little else. I really did not take a serious administrative job until 1981, when I became Chief of Cardiology at Duke.

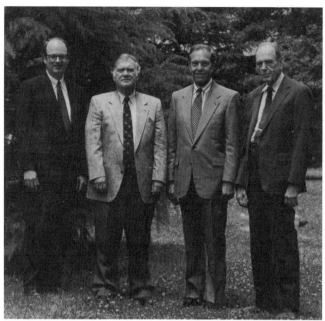

FIGURE 5. JCG (second from left) with the 2 previous chairman (Drs. James B. Wyngaarden [center right] and Eugene A. Stead [far right]) and the present chairman (Dr. Barton F. Haynes [far left]).

that we could make a major impact on the health care of patients with coronary disease in this state. At the time, we certainly were doing bypass surgery, but really not large numbers. We were not doing angioplasty, although angioplasty was being done in a number of other institutions. Thrombolytic therapy was not available at that time. However, it was very clear to me that interventional techniques were going to be the future and we could help the institution grow as well as make a major impact on health care in this state.

I had an experience in 1982 with a neighbor, a lady in her early 60s, who came to the hospital with mild chest pain. When she arrived in the emergency room, she developed complete heart block, cardiogenic shock, and for all intents and purposes, would have died. One of our cardiologists, Dr. Jess Peter, took her immediately to the cardiac catheterization laboratory and did an emergency coronary angioplasty. She walked out of the hospital a few days later a well person. As a matter of fact, she lived another 14 years. Based on my experiences with the first patient I had as an intern (who died with an acute myocardial infarction and I could not do anything for him), and the experience with this lady (who for all intents and purposes was "dead," but walked out of the hospital 5 days later a well person), I knew that we needed to dramatically alter our approach to the treatment of patients with acute myocardial infarction. Since Durham is a small community, we needed to develop a mechanism of rapidly transporting patients to the hospital. Helicopters at that time were primarily used for patients with trauma. We had a major knock-down war with the hospital administration in making them understand that we knew we could get the acute cardiac patients referred. I don't know the actual data, but the first year 75% of the transports by helicopter were cardiology patients. The program was so successful that we dramatically increased the number of patients admitted for cardiac disease, increasing the number of cardiac catheterizations and patients undergoing bypass surgery. In so doing, we improved the health care of the people in this state. At this point, I need to recognize the work of several of my colleagues who were primarily responsible for this growth: Dr. Rob Califf, Director the Cardiac Care Unit, initiated many of the clinical trials of thrombolytic therapy; Dr. Richard Stack, Director of the Interventional Laboratory, developed a number of successful devices; and most importantly, Dr. Harry Phillips, who was largely responsible for the enormous increase in the number of cardiac patients referred to this institution.

WCR: *At the same time, as a byproduct, it also improved the image of this medical center across the*

Thus, I spent nearly 2 decades without any major administrative responsibilities. It could not have worked out better. When I did take an administrative position, I cut the scope of my research effort significantly so that a limited amount of high quality work could be maintained. This afforded me time for my duties. Many of my colleagues have tried to manage academic administrative positions and run a large research program—to the detriment of both.

WCR: *In actuality you were 50 years old when you became Chief of Cardiology, not only at the VA Hospital but also at Duke University Medical Center. What was it that turned you on to the potential usefulness of invasive cardiology? It is my understanding, for example, that you were the one that really made Duke Cardiology shift gears. You got all these patients, not only in this area, but all over the state, and set up the helicopter service. It seems to me you were quite a visionary. You were ahead of other people by a long shot in getting that done. As you reflect on it, what did you forsee that others did not at that time?*

JCG: We need to answer this question from a couple of directions. First, the primary mandate of this institution, Duke University Medical Center, as defined by Mr. Duke was to deliver health care to the patients of North and South Carolina. Duke Medical Center was not developed as a primary research institution. It was built to take care of patients, and to this day plays a major role in caring for indigent patients without compensation. We had been very successful in setting up referral patterns from an area within a 100-mile radius of Durham. It was very clear to me

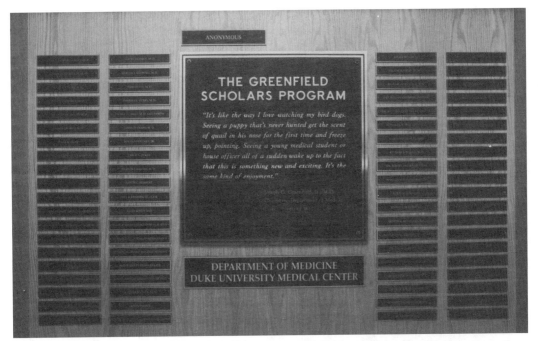

FIGURE 6. Photograph of the donors to The Greenfield Scholars Program, provided by JCG's colleagues in his honor. The program was initiated to provide salary support for the training of physician-scientists at Duke University Medical Center.

state, I suspect, enormously. You were paid for those procedures, so your Division of Cardiology must have been extremely well appreciated at that time by the medical center.

JCG: I'm not sure "appreciated" is the right word, but results were certainly recognized.

WCR: You became Chief of Cardiology at Duke Medical Center in 1981 when you were 50 years of age. Then, low and behold, the next year you were offered the Chairmanship of Medicine here. How did that come about?

JCG: Jim Wyngaarden, as you know, became the Director of the National Institutes of Health. There was a year's search, and basically it did not seem to be going anywhere. They had asked me to look at the job earlier and I really was not interested. The longer the search went it looked like things were going to deteriorate, so I talked to Dr. William Anlyan and was offered and accepted the position. It was kind of a defensive action. I did not think this place could keep going without a Chairman of Medicine; we were not making any headway without one.

WCR: So you became Chairman of Medicine in 1983. You stayed Chairman until 1995. That is a 12-year period. What were your goals when you took that Chairmanship?

JCG: To try to make absolutely certain that in every one of the medical subspecialties we excelled in patient care, in research, and in training. I have always viewed the Duke Medical Center as primarily a place to train specialists. Certainly, we have trained good general internists, but during my time, 90% of the

house staff that finished their internal medicine training went into a subspeciality. I think the thing I concentrated on as much as anything else was our house staff program, trying to get the best students we could, and to train them to be physicians. About half of those trainees also did their fellowships at Duke. The bulk of the people that we kept on the senior staff as clinicians came through our training program. From the outside we recruited primarily research-trained physicians. We did recruit a number of physician-scientists and the department became well funded from external sources such as the NIH. However, the main thing I concentrated on was making sure that the house staff program was the best it could be and that we delivered the best possible care we could.

WCR: I understand, Joe, that you spent an incredible time with your medical house staff. You knew each one of them very well. Your door was always opened to them or to anyone else, I gather, on your staff, and, furthermore, you were always here. You were not traveling on the circuit.

JCG: I tried to do 2 Visiting Professorships a year at the maximum. I went to the American Society for Clinical Investigation about every other year and I served on the American Board of Internal Medicine. That was it. I did not take any other jobs or anything else. I never was significantly involved in the committee work of American Heart Association, the American College of Cardiology, or other academic organizations.

WCR: So you took a maximum of 3 or 4 trips a year. Therefore, you were here, you were accessible, and

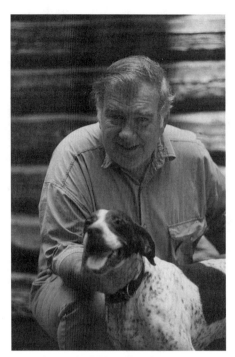

FIGURE 7. Photograph of JCG with one of his beloved bird dogs (Photography by Will & Denni McIntyre, McIntyre Photography, Inc., 3746 Yadkinville Road, Winston-Salem, North Carolina 27106.)

you were part of the house staff team in a way. You took morning reports?

JCG: I took morning reports every Monday and Wednesday and gave a clinical conference on Friday. Grand Rounds were held on Friday; I came in every Friday night to eat pizza with the house staff and to do 11:00 P.M. sign-out rounds with them. Many times these sessions went on to 2:00 in the morning.

WCR: *These 11:00 Friday night rounds, that was something you initiated. That had not gone on here before? What gave your that idea? What was your purpose?*

JCG: To try to get to know the house staff and also to make them understand that I was very interested in the quality of care they were delivering.

WCR: *That meant your whole medical house staff was here from 11:00 P.M. Friday night to whatever time you left Saturday morning?*

JCG: Just the ones rotating on the general medicine service at that time.

WCR: *So you had a relatively small group you could get to know?*

JCG: They usually would come from the VA Hospital also, at least those that were on call that night. I would say that on the average we would have 20 people there.

WCR: *You would bring the pizza?*

JCG: No. The department furnished the money and the house staff had a good time trying to get pizza as cheaply as possible.

WCR: *Would you actually make rounds or would you discuss patients?*

JCG: I initially started out doing the sign-out rounds with them. At Duke, we have a policy that the Chief Resident in medicine sees the new admissions every night. I initially did that and later on it became more of a social gathering.

WCR: *I understand you had a cardiology conference with the cardiology fellows and staff on Saturday morning.*

JCG: We did for a long time.

WCR: *You did at the time you were making these midnight rounds, and the cardiology conference started at 8:00 A.M.?*

JCG: Yes, that is right.

WCR: *Do you need much sleep?*

JCG: I am not a Napoleon. I can't get by on 3 hours, but I probably can get by on 5 without any real trouble.

WCR: *What do you usually do? What time did you wake up in the morning when you were Chairman of Medicine, Head of Cardiology, etc.?*

JCG: Six o'clock.

WCR: *What time do you go to bed?*

JCG: Midnight.

WCR: *What time do you come to the hospital?*

JCG: I had to be at the hospital at 8:00 A.M.

WCR: *You live on a farm?*

JCG: I have about 25 acres which is surrounded by a large tract of land, the Duke forest. A friend of mine built a log cabin and it is an ideal retreat. It is only a 5-minute drive from the hospital. I have a home in town, but I spend a lot of time at this place.

WCR: *I understand that your house staff had an incredible degree of loyalty to you and you instilled in them a tremendous loyalty to the Duke institution? What in you, as you examine yourself, gave you those characteristics to be such a mentor to all these young house officers?*

JCG: I think that I thoroughly enjoyed doing it. If you don't, you can't do it at all. I did enjoy trying to solve their problems and help them. The other thing is that I put myself in a position to have enough time to do it properly. I was not away from the institution very much, I was at Duke. I thoroughly enjoy hunting, quail hunting particularly. I have trained bird dogs all my life. There is nothing any more fun than seeing a young bird dog for the first time smell quail and really start doing what he was put on this earth to do. House staff and students are similar. The first time that you see them really get excited about medicine is a very rewarding situation.

WCR: *Once you took a house officer you sort of treated them as your kid in a way. You brought them along, made sure they got the fellowship they wanted, and they knew you would take care of them, but, at the same time, you apparently instilled in them to give their best. How did you do that? Everyone wants to get the best out of people who are under them, but apparently you did it?*

JCG: I think it was the obvious combination of carrot and stick, putting them where they could excel and making damn sure that they did. A major factor is peer pressure. The house staff did extremely well because they did not want their peers to see them not perform.

WCR: *You gave up cardiology after awhile? 1989?*

JCG: Yes.

WCR: *You were Head of the Division of Cardiology and the Department of Medicine simultaneously for about 6 years? Why did you keep cardiology?*

JCG: This sounds a little bit self-serving, but at that time, I really enjoyed cardiology more than medicine. Also, if you looked around the country, at that particular time, there was a lot of unrest among various cardiology divisions because they were supporting departments of medicine financially. There were a lot of arguments back and forth about cardiology's breaking off and being their own department. I just did not want to fight about finances with the Chief of Cardiology, because basically cardiology underwrote everything.

WCR: *What did you enjoy most about being Chairman?*

JCG: Developing people, be it house staff or young faculty.

WCR: *You enjoy being the mentor?*

JCG: Yes. Giving people opportunities and watching them to see how they do.

WCR: *Did anybody take care of you when you were coming along? Do you owe your career, in other words, to somebody who kept supporting you, or do you think primarily you are a self-made person professionally?*

JCG: I think Dr. Stead was that person. He mentored me in my early formative career and really tried to help me develop.

WCR: *You seem to be very loyal to your institution. Is that just the way you were put together or did you develop a love for Duke and instill that in others with time?*

JCG: Probably the latter is the way I was put together; I felt and still do feel, this institution did an enormous amount for me, gave me opportunities I could not have dreamed of having anywhere else. I owe back to them the kind of loyalty we talked about.

WCR: *I gather that while you were chairman you really upgraded the gastrointestinal, neurology, hematology-oncology, and cardiology divisions. Did you find that difficult in these arenas that you had not been in for 20 years essentially?*

JCG: I was lucky to pick very good people and I left them alone. I have always felt that the way you excel is to find the best person and then get the hell out of their way. That is what I did.

WCR: *It sounds like you have a good sense for talent. You sense it. What are you looking for in people that you want to surround yourself with?*

JCG: Bright people. I have always said that everyone around you should be smarter than you are. (In my case, that is pretty easy.) Above all, they need to be interested in developing other people's careers, not building everything for their own self-satisfaction. Any person, no matter how good they are professionally, but who are extremely self-centered and only interested in themselves will never build anything. I think the key thing is to try to find people who get a certain amount of enjoyment out of watching other people do well. I look for these characteristics more than anything else. Most of us get to where we are in medicine by being extraordinarily self-centered and looking after ourselves. That is one of the real failings in academic medicine. Not many people are interested in anybody else.

WCR: *What would be an example you would see in a house officer, somebody who is not trying to get credit for being clever or giving credit to others?*

JCG: Somebody who does extra work and does not complain about it or just covers for people and nobody even knows about it. That is the kind of person you are looking for.

WCR: *When you came on as Chairman of Medicine in 1983, how many faculty did you have at that time?*

JCG: Around 175: 152 MDs and 21 PhDs.

WCR: *When you stepped down in 1995, 12 years later, how many faculty did you have?*

JCG: It got up to about 250 MDs and 45 PhDs.

WCR: *How many house officers did you have in medicine most of the years?*

JCG: We usually had 45 to 50 interns, and about 35 or 40 junior and senior residents.

WCR: *And the total house staff?*

JCG: Somewhere in the neighborhood of 100 or 110. We also had an equal number of subspeciality fellows.

WCR: *One hundred to 110 house staff, 100 to 110 fellows in the various divisions, and then 250 or so faculty. You knew all those people?*

JCG: I would say I knew the faculty fairly well, knew the house staff well, about half the fellows came from the house staff, so I knew them, but it was very hard to know the fellows who had come from other places.

WCR: *If you traveled around a lot, there is no way you could remember the names of 500 people.*

JCG: No.

WCR: *If you add technicians in the Department of Medicine, secretaries, and financial people, you are talking about 1,000 folks?*

JCG: About 1,000.

WCR: *It has always amazed me how you seemed to have managed a huge department of medicine, a very large division of cardiology. Your office was always small. Your desk was always clean. Your door was always open. You must be very decisive and make these decisions, at least they have the appearance of being made quickly. I presume you have thought a lot about them before the decision was made.*

JCG: Several things enter into that. One of them is that I have never been impressed that any important decision was made with more than 2 people in the room. I think large meetings are a complete waste of time. The only reason to have such meetings is to convey what has already been decided. The reason for the small office is obvious. We don't have a lot of space at Duke, so I made sure I had an office that was

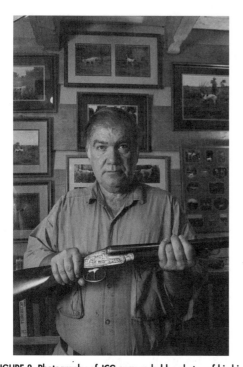

FIGURE 8. Photography of JCG surrounded by photos of his bird dogs, past and present. Dr. Greenfield displays the most recent addition to his collection of shotguns. Shortly before Greenfield stepped down from his chairmanship, he received a phone call late one afternoon from one of his faculty members, who had called to let him know that he and other departmental faculty would be meeting that night at a Durham restaurant to discuss a plan to begin charging the house staff for a statistics course that they would soon be required to take. Irate, incensed, absolutely livid that the faculty would even consider levying a fee on the house staff, Greenfield stormed off to the restaurant and barged into the meeting room. He was stopped short by the sight of about 40 or so grinning departmental faculty who had tricked him into a surprise dinner in his honor. They presented Greenfield with a rare, one of a kind, Purdy shotgun, that he had admired a few months earlier in a national hunting magazine. It is this gun that JCG displays in this photograph. The gun was made entirely by hand, with intricate carvings in both the stock and the metal. The shotgun is as much a work of art as it is a firearm. (Photography by Will & Denni McIntyre, McIntyre Photography, Inc., 3746 Yadkinville Road, Winston-Salem, North Carolina 27106.)

small and I had the cheapest desk available. When people would walk in and tell how cramped they were for space I would tell them to look at my office. If they wanted an expensive desk I would say "Fine, you write a check for the difference between my desk and yours and we will get you a bigger desk." It seemed to work very well. As far as keeping my desk clean, I have always had a big waste paper basket. I don't look at a lot of this stuff that comes through. I just throw it away.

WCR: *Joe, I understand you don't pay the best salaries in the country? What is your view on how much it takes to retain a good staff financially?*

JCG: I followed Dr. Stead's approach; try to balance the salary level and the unscheduled time. Thus,

a faculty member who works in a situation where patient responsibilities define their day completely made a higher salary. Faculty who are primarily doing research and can, to a large extent, dictate their own schedule, make less. Promotions come faster when faculty have the time to do more academic things. Many of my colleagues don't believe that is a fair approach. However, one thing is certain. The money generated by patient care activities underwrites a portion of the cost of doing research and allows some of the faculty the freedom to function as physician-scientists. That is how I arrived at faculty members' salary. A private institution like Duke simply can't compete salary wise with state institutions because our only sources of money are grants and what we get from patient care revenues. Endownments provide a trivial portion of the overall budget.

WCR: *When did you get married?*

JCG: I got married in 1955.

WCR: *That was immediately before you came to Duke? You married a lady from Atlanta?*

JCG: Yes. She was a technician I met at Grady Hospital. She was from Cochran, Georgia.

WCR: *You have 3 girls?*

JCG: Yes.

WCR: *Have you been a good daddy all these years?*

JCG: At least reasonably good. My oldest daughter has been severely retarded from birth. She lives with us and works everyday at a sheltered workshop and does extremely well. The second is a cardiologist in electrophysiology at Duke. The other is involved in developing the outreach programs at Duke.

WCR: *So they are all right here?*

JCG: Yes.

WCR: *Do you have grandchildren?*

JCG: No.

WCR: *Joe, what do you do in your spare time? I hear you like quail hunting?*

JCG: Right. I hunt and train bird dogs.

WCR: *How many dogs do you have now?*

JCG: Currently, I have probably 15.

WCR: *What kind of dogs are they?*

JCG: English pointers. At the present, all of my dogs are in Florida. They, like rich Yankees, winter in Florida and summer with me in North Carolina.

WCR: *Your quail hunting started when you were in Atlanta?*

JCG: It was very early, about age ten.

WCR: *I hear that you have gone to Africa to do some big game hunting. What was that like?*

JCG: Until recently, I had no interest in big game hunting. I hunted deer and turkeys a few times, but I did not enjoy it at all. The man I have hunted quail with in Florida since 1984 became a professional guide in Africa and he enticed me into going there for the first time in the summer of 1996. I went cape buffalo hunting in Tanzania. The mystique of this country captures you like nothing else; it is very hard to explain. I really enjoyed buffalo hunting. I got into a situation where we nearly got killed by a cape buffalo. Last year, I went to South Africa near Kruger Park where elephants have not been hunted in about 5 years. I had the opportunity to hunt bull elephant with a man whose father was a professional ivory hunter and who had spent the first 30 years of his life hunting elephants. This was by far the most emotional and rewarding experience I've had hunting.

WCR: *These adventures are new in your life?*

JCG: Brand new, like everything else, I seem to do things late.

WCR: *You were gone a little longer than usual for these trips?*

JCG: Sixteen days.

WCR: *Before 1995, you never did that.*

JCG: The longest I ever was gone was to Florida to hunt for 4 days at a time and then come back.

WCR: *During your major period of your Chairmanship you were gone 2 to 3 weeks a year at most?*

JCG: I did not take summer vacations at all, so the only time away was just when I hunted or went to an occasional meeting.

WCR: *You got interventional cardiology, acute care cardiology, going at this institution and expanded it over the state. How do you think angioplasty and stents and atherectomies and these invasive procedures are going to pan out with time?*

JCG: The initial clinical presentation of coronary disease, particularly acute myocardial infarction and unstable angina, has been dramatically improved by these techniques. Now we are able to really take care of people extraordinarily well, assuming you can intervene early enough after the onset of acute myocardial infarction. These procedures must be viewed as palliative, which may add an extra 10 years to life, but should never be considered, as many people do unfortunately, as curative. It is a mystery to me why coronary disease may progress very rapidly for reasons totally unknown, then not change for a long period of time, and then progress again. I still think there is a tremendous opportunity to do more positive things to improve the status of patients with coronary disease. What we are running up against, as always, is money. The initial manifestations of coronary disease have been moved primarily to the age group of 60 and 70 years of age. Who will pay for new treatment modalities? Certainly not Medicare. Does it cost less to die of cardiovascular disease or something else? This is a major issue as far as the cost of health care is concerned and there is no ready answer.

WCR: *Coronary bypass should be viewed the same way.*

JCG: Absolutely. It, too, is a palliative procedure.

WCR: *Joe, you seem to have a pretty good business mind. Your department during your chairmanship did quite well financially?*

JCG: We made a lot of money from clinical endeavors. For the last 3 years, we had problems with reimbursements going down, but we still did well.

WCR: *Where did your financial savvy come from?*

JCG: I was lucky to pick one of the best business managers in academic medicine, Paul Thacker. He is superb and he saved us all kinds of money.

WCR: *What is your advice for young doctors today? Managed care, how do you sense it now?*

JCG: There is one thing I always tell them, "Look, when you get your MD degree, no matter what happens you are going to eat, i.e., you are going to make enough money to live on, you don't have to worry about that. What you want to do is enjoy taking care of patients, get up in the mornings and be a physician. If you allow all the problems associated with health care reimbursements, managed care, etc., to become dominate in your thinking, it will destroy your effectiveness as a physician." Where I have a problem, is to try to honestly advise students who are interested in a basic research career as an MD, or even doing a lot of clinical research as an MD, and tell them that they are going to do well. This is very difficult because I am not sure myself. The physician-scientist, and I really believe in the concept of physician-scientist, is having a very difficult time. It is hard to talk people into going into a career where they are concerned about whether they can make a living.

WCR: *Joe, I gather there are 125 chairmen of medicine around the country. I suspect you are the only one who drives an old Chevy truck to work.*

JCG: 1991 is not too old.

WCR: *How did that come about?*

JCG: I started driving a pickup truck before pickup trucks were the in thing. I got my first one in 1964 as a hunting vehicle. To be candid, I needed to be able to haul dogs without having to smell them—thus, a truck's ideal.

WCR: *There are other chairmen across the country and I suspect you know most or at least many of them pretty well. Who have you respected enormously as a departmental chairman in medicine and why?*

JCG: Clearly, Dr. Stead was by far the best. However, chairmen such as Drs. Don Seldin, David Kipnis, Eugene Braunwald, Holly Smith, Frank Abboud, and Claude Bennett had that extra something special and were able to put together and maintain superb departments.

WCR: *It sounds to me like being a departmental chairman with so many people, the less selfish you are, as you have already mentioned, the better your department. It sounds to me like you can't think of yourself at all during this period of time.*

JCG: That is correct. You need to sublimate all of your own particular goals and enjoy watching your people excel.

WCR: *But at the same time, you were able to keep your lab going while chairman?*

JCG: From 1981 until the present, although funded reasonably well, we gradually decreased the scope of our work. I was able to continue to produce high quality research but at a much lower volume. I still have a Merit Review from the VA which will end in October 1998. It is very difficult to be competitive in research unless you concentrate almost entirely on research. I do most of my best work after waking in the morning by thinking about what I am going to do during the day. When you are chairman you are thinking about the department rather than what you are going to do in research.

WCR: *I understand that you have read hundreds of electrocardiograms every week at Duke University ever since you came back here in 1962. You must get to know a lot about people by reading electrocardiograms with them. Why have you done that? Is it because this is just a professional hobby for you?*

JCG: For a number of reasons: (1) it is the best way to know about every sick patient in the hospital automatically because they are going to have an electrocardiogram, and you can keep up with the clinical service; (2) I thoroughly enjoy it; and (3) the financial situation is such that nobody could accuse me of not pulling my weight because the professional fees more than pay my salary and always have.

WCR: *Although you have probably read more electrocardiograms than about anybody now, have you ever written a paper on electrocardiography?*

JCG: A few.

WCR: *That's it?*

JCG: I worked with Ray Bonner of IBM to develop a program for reading electrocardiograms. I thoroughly enjoyed this work and we wrote a couple of papers.

WCR: *Joe, you are 66 years old now? As you look back over your career, you have been a terrific scientist. You have been a loved teacher. You have been a mentor to numerous young physicians. You are responsible for a large number of their careers. You have lead one of the world's great departments of medicine, one of the world's best cardiology divisions. Your research has always been thought of to be on the highest level. What are you most proud of among all your endeavors?*

JCG: Probably the people I have interacted with and helped to develop their careers.

WCR: *When you get home at night do you do much medical work?*

JCG: No.

WCR: *You do it in the morning or at the hospital?*

JCG: Yes.

WCR: *Joe, does anything bother you about cardiology today?*

JCG: The thing that has distressed me the most has been the failure of the cardiology community to grasp the fact that they needed to develop criteria for the training of invasive cardiologists and to certify them. There are a significant number of inadequately trained invasive cardiologists (e.g., a large number of angioplasties in this country are done by physicians who do <30 a year.)

WCR: *Do you think we need all these cardiologists? Why at a center like this do you keep pouring out so many cardiologists?*

JCG: We are pouring out a few less, but I think it is an interesting question. I believe that when I get sick I want to see the best specialists possible to take care of me who understand my disease. It is very hard to prove that cardiovascular specialists are worthwhile, but we are beginning to get data now which shows what you knew to be true. If you have a heart attack and you are taken care of by a cardiologist, you are going to do better in terms of all the parameters than

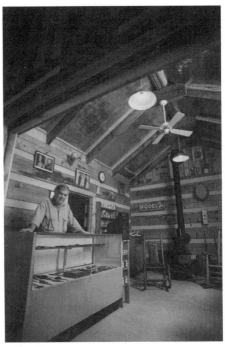

FIGURE 9. Photograph of JCG behind the counter in the old-fashioned country store he has recreated on his farm in rural Durham County. The farm has long been a favorite retreat for Greenfield, who built this cabin a few years ago with the help of friends. (Photography by Will & Denni McIntyre, McIntyre Photography, Inc., 3746 Yadkinville Road, Winston-Salem, North Carolina 27106.)

if cared for by a noncardiologist. I don't subscribe to the notion that health care costs are going to be lowered by getting rid of specialists. Currently, a large portion of the health care dollar is going to support the administrative aspects of medicine, such as advertising, highly paid corporate executives, and a gaggle of administrators, but not to physicians. I have not seen that this new approach actually reduces overall health care costs. I am concerned that we are at a point where the ability to deliver first class care health care has been severely curtailed. Maybe the nation can tolerate this situation, but I think it is a shame. The other answer to your question is that Duke Medical Center is in a position to train excellent subspecialists better than most other institutions. It strikes me as ridiculous that we should reduce the number we train while others don't.

WCR: *What is your view on preventive cardiology in general? Cholesterol lowering, blood pressure lowering?*

JCG: It depends on what we are going to prevent. I am certain that if the general population were willing to comply and all the known risk factors for the development of cardiovascular disease were eliminated, the disease on the average would occur some-

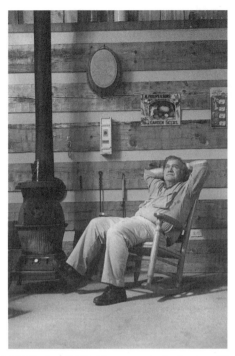

FIGURE 10. Greenfield in his country store by the stove. (Photography by Will & Denni McIntyre, McIntyre Photography, Inc., 3746 Yadkinville Road, Winston-Salem, North Carolina 27106.)

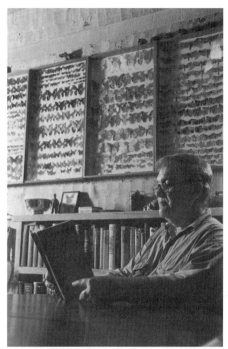

FIGURE 11. Photograph of Greenfield showing his butterfly collection in his farm cabin. Greenfield began the butterfly collection as a young boy. He is still an occasional collector. He once caught a rare natural hybrid that he gave to the American Museum of Natural History. (Photography by Will & Denni McIntyre, McIntyre Photography, Inc., 3746 Yadkinville Road, Winston-Salem, North Carolina 27106.)

what later in life. Whether or not the number of people actually developing cardiovascular disease would be reduced is a moot question. Certainly people will live longer. On the other hand, it is axiomatic that in the long run death will not be prevented. Thus, preventative strategies are unlikely to lower health care costs. If anything, living after the age when Social Security and Medicare take over will drain the national coffers. One thing is certain, we are all going to die. It is not clear to me that dying of something other than cardiovascular disease is cheaper.

WCR: *Talk a bit about your research. From age 30 to 50 you were straight ahead. As you look back over your own work, the training of others in your laboratory, the standards you set, the demand for accurate reproducible data, how does it hit you now?*

JCG: I cannot really say that anything we ever did was of major importance, but we published a body of excellent, solid research which will stand the test of time. I am very proud of it.

WCR: *The research made you a better doctor, a better teacher?*

JCG: A better doctor and a better teacher, because of the necessity to understand what the scientific method is all about and what it takes to prove an hypothesis.

WCR: *I suspect that you could not have been a chairman of a department which is as research based as yours without having gained an enormous amount*

of confidence from the success of your own research work.

JCG: There are 2 parts to this issue: (1) you have to be able to talk about research to people doing research in order to gain their respect if they are going to work for you. You have to produce research on your own to really make them comfortable, and (2) I think it also enables you to pick out people that are likely to be productive in the research arena.

WCR: *A lot of people talk about how much they have learned on travels, but I gather that as you reflect on your basic lack of travel, you are very pleased that you did it your way rather than the other way.*

JCG: Yes.

WCR: *That would be your advice to any young physician?*

JCG: What you learn primarily from traveling is that you have a very good situation at home—you better get back to it.

WCR: *You have mentioned your hobbies (Civil War, hunting). I gather you have been a student of butterflies all your life? Do you have other hobbies?*

JCG: No. I still collect butterflies. I am not a lepidopterist, but I have a reasonable collection and have had some fun with it.

WCR: *How many do you have?*

JCG: I have no idea.

WCR: *Do you have a butterfly list like bird watchers have a bird list?*

JCG: Yes. I was able several years ago to catch a couple of hybrids which are not supposed to occur in the wild. They're in the American Museum of Natural History.

WCR: *I understand, Joe, that you are a student of the Civil War.*

JCG: I got this interest from both my grandmothers.

WCR: *Are you a collector of Civil War books?*

JCG: Yes.

WCR: *Are you a first edition collector?*

JCG: No. I am more interested in what's in the book than what it looks like.

WCR: *So you still do a lot of reading on that topic?*

JCG: Yes. Also, I have recently gone on a number of walking tours of Civil War battlefield sites.

WCR: *I noticed that when you were in college you were a history major. Did you focus in any particular area during that time?*

JCG: Primarily in American History.

WCR: *Do you think these hobbies, the ability to get away by hunting, the ability to engross yourself in a Civil War tale, to find a beautiful butterfly has made you a better doctor and a better person? Do they help you communicate much better with people you talk to? Do you think your being a straight-shooter, which is what you are, trying to be enormously fair with everyone, were major assets in making your 12 years as departmental chairman so successful?*

JCG: I don't think there is any question about it. Sure. People will work for you for a variety of reasons. If you can pay them well, most people will work for you no matter what kind of person you are. If you can't do that, you have to substitute a number of things and the things you mentioned are the things you substitute. Try to develop a milieu where they want to work and promote the feeling that you are really going to try to do the best you can to meet their needs.

WCR: *Joe, thank you. I think that was terrific. I appreciate your willingness to do this.*

JCG: Bill, I am very delighted. I feel honored.

JCG's BEST PUBLICATIONS AS SELECTED BY JCG

5. Greenfield JC Jr., Patel DJ. Relation between pressure and diameter in ascending aorta of man. *Circulation Res* 1962;10:778–781.

12. Fry DL, Griggs DM Jr., Greenfield JC Jr. Myocardial mechanics; tension-velocity-length relationships of heart muscle. *Circulation Res* 1964;14:73–85.

13. Hernandez RR, Greenfield JC Jr., McCall BW. Pressure-flow studies in hypertrophic subaortic stenosis. *J Clin Invest* 1964;43:401–407.

25. Greenfield JC Jr., Tindall GT. Effect of acute increase in intracranial pressure on blood flow in the internal carotid artery of man. *J Clin Invest* 1965;44:1343–1351.

27. Greenfield JC Jr., Fry DL. Relationship between instantaneous aortic flow and the pressure gradient. *Circulation Res* 1965;17:340–348.

40. Greenfield JC Jr., Tindall GT. Effect of norephrinerine, epinephrine, and angiotensin on blood flow in the internal carotid artery of man. *J Clin Invest* 1968;47:1672–1684.

43. Greenfield JC Jr., Harley A, Thompsson HK, Wallace AG. Pressure-flow studies in man during atrial fibrillation. *J Clin Invest* 1968;47:2411–2421.

47. Harley A, Starmer CF, Greenfield JC Jr. Pressure flow studies in man: an evaluation of the duration of the phases of systole. *J Clin Invest* 1969;48:895–905.

52. Ruskin J, McHale PA, Harley A, Greenfield JC Jr. Pressure-flow studies in man: effect of atrial systole on left ventricular function. *J Clin Invest* 1970;49:472–478.

62. Greenfield JC Jr., Rembert JC, Young WG Jr., Oldham HN Jr., Alexander J, Sabiston DC Jr. Studies of blood flow in aorta-to-coronary venous bypass grafts in man. *J Clin Invest* 1972;51:2724–2735.

63. Bonner RE, Crevasse L, Ferrer MI, Greenfield JC Jr. A new computer program for analysis of scalar electrocardiograms. *Comp Biomed Res* 1972;5:629–653.

70. Ruskin J, Bache RJ, Rembert JC, Greenfield JC Jr. Pressure-flow studies in man: effect of respiration on left ventricular stroke volume. *Circulation Res* 1973;48:79–85.

71. Starmer CF, McHale PA, Cobb FR, Greenfield JC Jr. Evaluation of several methods for computing stroke volume from central aortic pressure. *Circulation Res* 1973;33:139–148.

77. Bache RJ, Cobb FR, Greenfield JC Jr. Effects of increased myocardial oxygen consumption on coronary reactive hyperemia in the awake dog. *Circulation Res* 1973;33:588–596.

81. Bache RJ, Cobb FR, Greenfield JC Jr. Myocardial blood flow distribution during ischemia-induced coronary vasodilatation in the unanesthetized dog. *J Clin Invest* 1974;54:1462–1472.

86. Bache RJ, Ball RM, Cobb FR, Rembert JC, Greenfield JC Jr. Effects of nitroglycerin on transmural myocardial blood flow in the unanesthetized dog. *J Clin Invest* 1975;55:1219–1228.

88. Wesly RLR, Vaishnav RN, Fuchs JCA, Patel DJ, Greenfield JC Jr. Static linear and nonlinear elastic properties of normal and arterialized venous tissue in dog and man. *Circulation Res* 1975;37:509–520.

102. Rembert JC, Kleinman LH, Fedor JM, Wechsler AS, Greenfield JC Jr. Myocardial blood flow distribution in concentric left ventricular hypertrophy. *J Clin Invest* 1978;62:379–386.

105. Swain JL, Parker JP, McHale PA, Greenfield JC Jr. Effects of nitroglycerin and propranolol on the distribution of transmural myocardial blood flow during ischemia in the absence of hemodynamic changes in the unanesthetized dog. *J Clin Invest* 1979;63:947–953.

109. Fedor JM, Rembert JC, McIntosh DM, Greenfield JC Jr. Effects of exercise- and pacing-induced tachycardia on coronary collateral flow in the awake dog. *Circulation Res* 1980;46:214–220.

114. Schwartz GG, McHale PA, Greenfield JC Jr. Hyperemic response of the coronary circulation to brief diastolic occlusion in the conscious dog. *Circulation Res* 1982;50:28–37.

115. Schwartz GG, McHale PA, Greenfield JC Jr. Coronary vasodilatation after a single ventricular extra-activation in the conscious dog. *Circulation Res* 1982;50:38–46.

123. Stack RS, Phillips HR III, Grierson DS, Behar VS, Kong Y, Peter RH, Swain JL, Greenfield JC Jr. Functional improvement of jeopardized myocardium following intracoronary streptokinase infusion in acute myocardial infarction. *J Clin Invest* 1983;72:84–95.

136. Sadick N, Dubé GP, McHale PA, Greenfield JC Jr. Metabolic mediation of single brief diastolic occlusion reactive hyperemic responses. *Am J Physiol* 1987;253:H25–H30.

141. Bauman RP, Rembert JC, Greenfield JC Jr. Regional atrial blood flow in dogs: effect of hypertrophy on coronary flow reserve. *J Clin Invest* 1989;83:1563–1569.

147. Dubé GP, Bemis KG, Greenfield JC Jr. Distinction between metabolic and myogenic mechanisms of coronary hyperemic response to brief diastolic occlusion. *Circulation Res* 1991;68:1313–1321.

148. Bauman RP, Rembert JC, Greenfield JC Jr. Regional blood flow in the canine atria during exercise. *Am J Physiol* 1993;265:H629–H632.

151. Bauman RP, Rembert JC, Greenfield JC Jr. Uniform vascular reserve in canine atria and ventricles during rest and exercise. *Am J Physiol* 1995:H1578–H1582.

CASE REPORTS, EDITORIALS, AND CLINICAL REVIEWS

6. Platt AP, Greenfield JC Jr. Inter-specific hybridization between Limenitis Arthemis Astyanax and Archippus (nymphalidae). *J Lepid Soc* 1971;25:278–284.

21. Rozear MP, Massey EW, Horner J, Foley E, Greenfield JC Jr. R. E. Lee's Stroke. *The Virginia Magazine of History and Biography.* 1990;98:291–308.

28. Rozear MP, Greenfield JC Jr. "Let us cross over the river": The final illness of Stonewall Jackson. *The Virginia Magazine of History and Biography.* 1995; 103:29–46.

NORMAN MAYER KAPLAN, MD: A
Conversation With the Editor*

Dr. Norman M. Kaplan was born on January 2, 1931, in Dallas, Texas, where he grew up. He went to public high school and then to the University of Texas where he graduated from the pharmacy school in 1950 at age 19 and from the University of Texas Southwestern Medical School in Dallas in 1954. His internship and residency in medicine were at Parkland Memorial Hospital in Dallas. From there he served as Chief of the Endocrinology Service at Lackland Air Force Base in San Antonio, Texas, and from there he went to Bethesda, Maryland, where he was a research fellow in the Clinical Endocrinology Branch in the National Heart Institute. He returned to Dallas in 1961 as a faculty member at Southwestern Medical School where he became full professor in the Department of Medicine 9 years later. He headed the Division of Hypertension from 1977 until 1997. His research endeavors have focused primarily on therapy of systemic hypertension. He is an extremely popular lecturer who has spoken at numerous meetings all over the world. His book, *Clinical Hypertension*, first appeared in 1973, and the seventh edition appeared in 1998. That book is the most popular one on clinical aspects of hypertension ever produced.

William Clifford Roberts, MD[†] **(hereafter, WCR):** I am speaking with Dr. Norman Kaplan in his apartment complex in Dallas, Texas, on January 14, 1998. Dr. Kaplan, I would like to try to get to know you better as a person. I wonder if you might start by telling about your growing-up period. What was it like growing up in south Dallas? What were your parents like? I gather that they had a grocery store. Did they go to college? What about your siblings? When you were home at night after school, did you have some meaningful conversations around the table? I gather the synagogue played a major role in your growing-up period?

Norman M Kaplan, MD[‡] **(hereafter, NMK):** I was "a mistake." My mother and father had had 3 children and they thought they were finished. In the middle of the depression, when things were really bad, I came along. My mother rather jokingly commented to me that she tried to end the pregnancy by jumping off the flour barrel in the grocery store but it did not work. Despite that questionable beginning, I grew up in a very supportive family. My parents both came over in the early 1900s from the "old country": my father,

from white Russia and my mother, from Poland. They married in 1918 right after my father came back from being in the Army in World War I. They started a small grocery store close to the black ghetto area in south Dallas. I grew up in this small ramshackle grocery store with the attached living quarters. We were really poor, but never wanted. By having a grocery store we always had enough to eat. I never felt deprived. I was always carefully looked after by my father and mother. My father died suddenly, I assume from coronary artery disease, when I was 17. My mother was by far the matriarch of the family. She was the daughter of a Rabbi who was brought over here because many of the congregation that he had ministered to in a small community in Poland, about 80 miles from Warsaw, had come to Dallas. They decided they wanted their Rabbi from the old country to come over and they brought him with my mother and one of her siblings. Eventually, 6 other siblings, the whole family, came over. I think it happened to a lot of immigrants in those days that the first member or 2 who could afford the passage came over, and then as they made a little money they sent for the rest of them. They settled in Dallas in the early 1900s.

I was 7 years younger than my next sibling, my sister, and, therefore, I spent a lot of time by myself. My 2 older brothers are 9 and 11 years older than I am. I was sort of an independent but well-behaved little kid. I went to regular school and after hours to Hebrew school. The Hebrew school was every day, Monday to Thursday, and then, of course, synagogue on Friday night and Saturday, and Sunday school on Sunday morning. I spent a lot of time at our Orthodox synagogue.

Growing up, I was pretty much a loner. I had a few friends but pretty much took care of myself. I did very well in school. I basically made straight A's without any real effort and I was the salutatorian of my high school class. I was upset that I was not the valedictorian, but that was because I made a bad grade in typing. I never could type. I was doubly promoted and graduated from high school at age 16. I was socially a very backward kid. I did not date a lot or have a lot of friends, but I did begin to date the classmate who later became my first wife. When I went away to Austin to the University of Texas to undergraduate school at age 16, this was the first time I had ever really interacted with a lot of other young people my age. Becoming a member of a fraternity was a lifesaver for me and helped me form close friends, many of whom I still have. They have been very meaningful to me. It was an important formative time. I continued to date my first wife at the University and we married my freshman year in medical school, when I was only 19. I was in a big hurry. I am not sure why.

I got accepted at Southwestern Medical School

*This series of interviews are underwritten by an unrestricted grant from Bristol-Myers Squibb.
†Baylor Cardiovascular Institute, Baylor University Medical Center, Dallas, Texas 75246.
‡Department of Internal Medicine, University of Texas Southwestern Medical School, Dallas, Texas.

0002-9149/98/$19.00
PII S0002-9149(98)00366-X

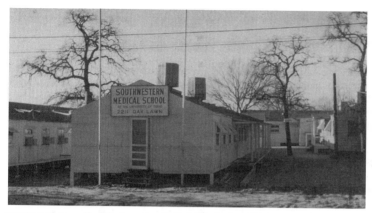

FIGURE 1. Photograph of Southwestern Medical School when NMK was a student, 1950-1954.

western but came here as a house officer, and subsequently became a leader of gastroenterology; *Dan Foster* who is now the Chairman of our department and a leading diabetologist; and *Jean Wilson* who became an outstanding endocrinologist; and *Charles Baxter* who became an outstanding burn surgeon. There were another 5 or 6 students who Seldin identified and he sent them all to the NIH. We are now talking about the late 1950s. For a young person who wanted to go into academic medicine, NIH was a necessity at the time. Seldin arranged with *Fred Bartter* to have me train as an endocrinologist at the NIH.

when I was 19. The decision to go into medicine was something I sort of fell into. My 2 older brothers had become pharmacists and they opened two drug stores. I thought that if I did not get into medical school I would become a pharmacist, so I took pharmacy as an undergraduate. I worked like a demon. I took 21 hours of courses each semester and went to school each summer. In 3 years I accumulated 144 hours of credit. If I had it to do it over I would never have gone into pharmacy, but would have taken liberal arts courses and gotten a good basic education.

Southwestern was a new and floundering medical school at the time. It had started during World War II after Baylor University College of Medicine moved from Dallas to Houston. Several Dallas physicians then started Southwestern Medical School, which initially was private. They built a little facility next to Parkland Hospital. By the time I got to medical school in 1950, it was about to go under. They almost lost their accreditation because *Tinsley Harrison*, who had been one of the primary strengths at the medical school, decided he had had enough of it and went back to Alabama, and *Carl Moyer*, a famous surgeon at that time, also left. In the late 1940s, the school did not have any significant financial support and was just about to go under when some people in Dallas exerted some influence on the state legislature and the University of Texas took it over in 1953 as its second medical branch, the first being the medical school in Galveston. At that same time, *Donald Seldin* who had just finished his fellowship in nephrology at Yale under *John Peters* and who was responsible for the future development of the school and who was my major mentor, became the Chairman of the Department of Internal Medicine. There were about 7 or 8 of us in the 1954 and 1955 classes of 100 students whom Seldin recognized as people he wanted to develop into his faculty. These included *Floyd Rector*, who subsequently went to San Francisco and was Chairman of the Department of Medicine there for the last few years; *John Fordtran*, who was not a student at South-

The medical school experience was a lot of fun. I never felt particularly threatened by what went on in medical school and I graduated tops in my class. I became Chief Resident at Parkland Hospital in 1957. I went into the Air Force for 2 years thereafter and spent 2 lovely years in San Antonio, having for the first time a little money to spend. We ended up with 4 daughters. I was a young Captain with a little money and a very easy job in the Air Force.

I then spent a year with *Fred Bartter* at NIH doing just bench laboratory research, studying the synthesis of aldosterone. I learned how to do the rather complex chromatographic isotopic assays for aldosterone and the rat bioassay for plasma renin activity. I got interested in aldosterone and renin as part of endocrinology. It was many years later that I really developed my primary interest in hypertension.

I came back to Southwestern in 1961 as an instructor, working as part of the endocrine group, which included *Leonard Madison, Roger Unger*, and *Don Seldin*, although he was primarily interested in the kidney. Gradually, as more younger investigators arrived, such as *Dan Foster, Jean Wilson*, and *Marvin Siperstein*, I got more interested in hypertension. When I came back from the NIH, Dr. Siperstein had joined the faculty and he worked with me for over a day in developing my first NIH grant. I had never put together a grant proposal and he had no interest in what I was doing. I was not planning to work with Dr. Siperstein, but Dr. Seldin asked him to help me put this together.

In those days, we had a rather small, probably 25-member, Department of Medicine, so all of us were close and collegial. Seldin, as the Chairman, went over every manuscript that any member of his department wrote and edited them extensively. He never put his name on them but he did spent a lot of time on manuscripts emanating from his faculty. We also had a fabulous series of sessions before any major society meeting where the research work was presented. As the faculty increased, the numbers of accepted abstracts also increased. We would spend 3 to 5 hours about 2 weeks before a meeting going over everyone's presentation. Seldin invariably detected flaws in the way the presentations had been put together or the slides composed. It was amazing; he would do this time after time. We were the people doing the work, we thought we knew everything on the subject, and had put it together logically. Yet, when we would present our work to the whole group, Seldin would stand up and say, "Look, this does not produce a logical sequence. You have to put it together this way, go from here to there instead of from there to here."

Southwestern Medical School was fortunate in having Seldin as the Head of Medicine. He began accumulating a faculty of young, bright, and imaginative people. You could go in and discuss problems with people who really were not working in your area because we were such a close group. It was a heady time for a young faculty person to be able to have those types of interactions, not only with the Chief, but also with other faculty. Today, the Department has over 200 members and it is very difficult to feel the same way. There are people here in our department now, where I have been for 38 years, who I don't even know. The close interrelationships made the foundation for my career.

I consider myself today mainly a communicator. I have done some good original work but most of what I have done and take most pride in is being able to take the work of others and put it together in a rational way that makes sense. I am not an elegant writer, but I try to keep it clear and simple. My major accomplishment is probably being able to look at a developing area, and, after much reading and listening, put together the information in a way that others can utilize meaningfully and apply to the care of patients. Maybe my rabbinical background, not only from my grandfather but from 5 generations of rabbis in my family before my grandfather, rubbed off a bit on me.

I have taken on through the years 3 major areas that have been contentious. The first was *primary aldosteronism*. *Jerome Conn*, at the University of Michigan, had put together the concept of the syndrome of aldosteronism due to a tumor of the adrenal gland in 1954. In the next 10 years, his group published a large amount of data on their experience with this syndrome. In 1964, Dr. Conn wrote in the *JAMA* that 20% of all hypertension was due to primary aldosteronism. I questioned this high frequency from the very beginning and began to accumulate data from patients in Dallas with hypertension and hypokalemia, the usual hallmarks of the syndrome. We measured aldosterone, we took tumors at autopsy (what we refer to now as "incidentilomas" but in those days were thought to be benign tumors of the adrenal gland) and measured the steroid synthesis in those tumors as well as in the tumors in patients who had the syndrome. We measured a whole variety of patients who had hypokalemia. Instead of finding a 20% frequency, we found <1% frequency of the syndrome among our hypertensive patients.

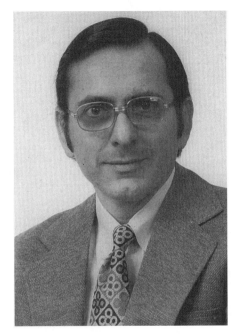

FIGURE 2. NMK in 1970.

My first national exposure was at the meeting of the Central Society for Clinical Research in Chicago in 1964 at the height of Dr. Conn's prominence from primary aldosteronism. When presenting for the first time before a major group (maybe 1,000 people) in Chicago with Jerome Conn sitting on the front row, I indicated that primary aldosteronism was not as common as he had claimed. He said it was simply a matter that we weren't looking at the right place and in the right manner. It turned out that I was closer to the truth than he was. Because Dr. Conn had become the world's authority in this area at the University of Michigan in those days, it is very possible that 20% of all their hypertensives did have the syndrome because the patients were being drawn there from all over the world. This is a phenomenon that happens in every disease that has been initially described by a new investigator. When physicians recognize new syndromes they accumulate such patients, funneling them into their own investigative area.

The same thing happened with renovascular hypertension and a number of forms of secondary hypetension. We must be cautious about the claims that come from investigators who describe a new syndrome. Because of the referral patterns they oftentimes recognize their problem much more frequently than is true in the general population. In those days, maybe less so today, there would be few laboratories that could study a described disease. These patients would come from far away places to be studied by a particular investigator. That is what happened with Dr.

Conn. At that time Ann Arbor was literally one of the few places in the world where the assays for aldosterone and renin could be done. I think Conn's mistake was that he interpreted his own experience to be applicable to the rest of the world.

The second thing I got involved with was *renin* and what it meant. *John Laragh*, who has been one of the original thinkers in the field of hypertension for the last 30 years, started in the early 1970s to look at the relation of plasma renin to hypertension. All the work that he and his group have done on the renin assay, on how to perform the assay, and what it means for diagnosis, prognosis, and treatment were all important contributions. But again I think John had blinders on. His experience, wherein renin was very important in diagnosis and in assessment of therapeutic responses, he felt applied to everyone where it obviously did not. Back in the early 1970s, I began to publish papers on the relation of renin measurements and other aspects of the renin-aldosterone system to the prevalence, prognosis, and therapy of hypertension. The years since that time have shown that John overstated his evidence although he still believes that renin plays a very important role in the diagnosis of hypertension, in the decision as to what its prognostic indications are, and in making therapeutic choices. The plasma renin level is important; it does add a great deal in the diagnosis of some low renin states, like primary aldosteronism, and in high renin states, like renovascular disease, but in most (>90%) hypertensive patients, renin assays do not give much additional information. It is now done relatively infrequently.

The third area concerns the *relation of calcium to blood pressure*. Dr. *David McCarron* of the University of Oregon was the strong advocate for calcium supplements to lower elevated blood pressure, claiming that calcium had a major impact on blood pressure. We found that calcium supplements lowered blood pressure only minimally, and we were one of the first to question this whole relation. Today, it is generally recognized that calcium supplements play a minimal role in lowering blood pressure.

I have been one who has questioned the implications of other people's work, but I have also made a few original observations, including some of the original work on mechanisms of the control of aldosterone synthesis (This was work I started at the NIH and continued here in Dallas for a few years.), on ways of assessing renin status via various clinical tests, and the mechanisms of oral contraceptive-induced hypertension. We described the "angiotension infusion test" which was an indirect way of assessing renin status. It was not a difficult procedure, but it was quickly supplanted by the ability to measure renin in a peripheral blood sample. The angiotensin-infusion test has been used, however, by obstetricians to detect early manifestations of preeclampsia.

In 1973, I published a book on hypertension. At that time, there was only one book on hypertension and it was by Sir George Pickering from Oxford, England. There were no journals devoted to hypertension. Pickering's book was wonderful, but his latest

(second) edition was 8 years earlier (1964). I decided it was time for another book and I decided to do it by myself. At that time, single-authored books were not rare. The first edition was published by MEDCOM, a company in New York started by 2 young entrepreneurs. The book had a lot more illustrations and a lot more fancy layout than most books that were being published in those days. This first edition was reasonably successful. The latest edition, the 7th, appeared in 1998, 25 years after the first. The first printing of this latest edition by Williams & Wilkins was for 50,000 copies. The 6th edition was translated into 7 languages (Japanese, Chinese, Spanish, French, Italian, Russian, and Greek) and I was just informed that the 7th will be translated into Turkish and Polish. It makes me very proud that the book has been so well accepted. The Japanese particularly seem to love my book and I have become sort of a "guru" of hypertension in Japan. All 7 editions are single-authored except for the 1 chapter on childhood hypertension which has been written by my friend, *Dr. Ellen Lieberman*. A third or more of my time is occupied with keeping up with the literature for the next edition of this book. I would not maintain as much of an interest, for instance, in pregnancy hypertension if I did not need to include that area in the next edition. I am 67 years old and fortunately in good health so I hope to continue the book by doing all this reading and synthesizing. I hope there will be an 8th edition, but I am not so sure after that.

WCR: Let me go back a little bit. You have talked about mentors during your training, Donald Seldin, for example. Could you go back to your early childhood? You mentioned that your home or living quarters were next to the grocery store. Your next oldest sibling sister was 7 years older than you were. I presume you worked in the grocery store a good bit. What was life like on a day-to-day basis then?

WMK: In looking back, it was a lonely experience. I remember every afternoon after coming home from grammar school that I would throw a tennis ball up against the wall as my primary extracurricular activity. I also went to Hebrew school every afternoon. We did not have television. There was not much else to do. I was a fairly avid reader. I went to the library, located about 6 blocks from home, often. I did not have a lot of close relatives or friends that I was growing up with. We also tended to be very separate, being a member of the Jewish community. My mother, who was very Orthodox, wanted my older brothers and me to become rabbis. None of us did. She was very protective of us in a very gentile world, and she wanted and insisted that we practice our Orthodox/Jewish beliefs. We were a reasonably close family and as long as my mother was alive and well the family got together for all of the Jewish holidays and festivals. At Hebrew School, I did relate to other young Jewish kids in the community, but I don't remember any of them living anywhere near where I was. Most of them came from more affluent areas. Although south Dallas in those days was not a wealthy area, most people had established small stores and began to move up in the world. Most Jews lived in an

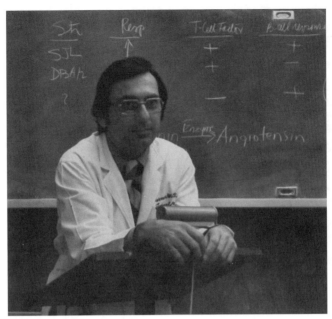

FIGURE 3. NMK teaching in 1982.

area of south Dallas which is today a very affluent area for African-Americans.

When I was around 12 or so there was a group called Young Judea, young Jewish kids who were looking to support Israel, which, of course, was not yet in existence. I remember as a kid collecting money, usually nickels and dimes, every Sunday morning at the delicatessen on Forest Avenue. They would let us out of Sunday School an hour early so we take a little blue box for the Jewish National Fund.

Maybe the fact that I have stayed pretty much a single investigator, written a single authored book, does reflect on the fact that when growing up I was pretty much by myself and did not have a lot of these nurturing relationships with a lot of other people.

WCR: I gather neither your mother nor father went to college?

NMK: Correct. I felt my mother was knowledgeable in the Jewish religion and in Jewish affairs. She was smart, but she was not an educated woman. She came to the USA and Dallas at about age 8 and did go to the public schools, but not beyond high school. My father came over at about age 14 years from "White Russia" near Kiev. He was an uneducated man, but he could read. Although he practiced as an Orthodox Jew he did not have the knowledge and the background that my mother did, having grown up with her father as a rabbi. My mother was educated in Jewish religious beliefs and prayer and such, but not in the outer world. I was 16 when I went to a symphony for the first time. It was my first exposure to anything outside of movies. But I never felt deprived. I thought we had every-

thing we needed and I did. I went to school with good clothes on, but I used to walk or hitch rides. We did not have an automobile. My father never did have a car. He drove a wagon with a horse until about 1940, and after that items were delivered to the grocery store. The first few years when I was at the University of Texas I had a bicycle. That was my way of getting around Austin. It was only when I was a senior in college and planning to come back to Dallas to enter medical school that I convinced by mother that I needed a car, and she, I think, went and borrowed some money to help me buy my first automobile. Coming out of that I guess has made me a little bit more aggressive about money than I would have been otherwise. Maybe that is one of the reasons I do so much lecturing and writing for the honoraria, although my faculty salary is obviously enough to keep me in good shape.

WCR: Your living quarters, being adjacent to the grocery store, must have been relatively small? Did you have a room of your own? Did you always room with your sister or one of your older brothers? Did you work in the grocery store there?

NMK: I slept with my mother and father in a bed next to theirs when I was a little kid. I remember that we had a black woman who was sort of a nanny to me during the daytime. She raised me as much as anybody because my mother and father were working in the grocery store. Apparently, I kept drinking out of a bottle until I was about 3 years old. I remember dropping the bottle and getting a real bawling out and

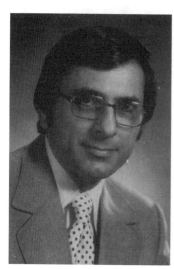
FIGURE 4. NMK in 1985.

then I decided that it was time to quit. I did work in the grocery store, mainly straightening out the shelves.

The second World War was a traumatic time because my mother had a lot of family left back in Poland. I remember vividly listening to the radio about what was going on in Europe and my mother's being very disturbed by the fact that Poland had been overrun quickly.

WCR: It sounds like school, whether grammar school, high school, college, or medical school, flowed very easily for you. Did your mother or father encourage you in school? Did they support your academic endeavors vigorously? Were your brothers and sisters similarly good students as you were?

NMK: I never had a lot of pressure put on me. When growing up, it seemed natural to excel in school. My strict Jewish Orthodox background encouraged me to learn all I could about Judism and religious practices. I don't remember ever being told that I should go to medical school. It just seemed something that sort of happened without any particular outside motivation. It must have been part of an ingrained attitude that being a good student and accomplishing something was expected. I don't ever recall being told that I didn't do well and should have made an A instead of a B. My academic achievements seemed to be self motivated or it came from sources that I never really identified. That whole attitude about reading and studying was just a natural assumption that my mother made and her children followed.

WCR: Were there any teachers in high school that had an impact on you?

NMK: A Mrs. Melson. She taught English literature. She motivated me to really work and go beyond what was expected. I remember having gone to the library and picking up books to read because of her

encouragement. She was about as tough a teacher as I remember having.

Forest High School, in those days, had about one third Jewish kids. The remainder were non-Jewish Caucasian since it was a segregated school. I encountered little overt anti-Semitism. I was nurtured by having a very strong Jewish family and my friends were almost entirely Jewish.

At the University of Texas as a student in the school of pharmacy, there was little special motivation provided. Although I did very well and came out with whatever honors you get from the University, it was not a place where I was stimulated. If I were able to go back, and, as I did with my children, I would have taken many liberal arts courses. In those days the University of Texas was very inexpensive. All 6 of my children, 4 by my first marriage and 2 stepchildren, went to the University of Texas. Two of my daughters, who subsequently became physicians, went through what was called Plan B at the University which was a group of 600 students considered special and brought into an intense liberal arts education. I wish that I had had that exposure.

WCR: It was expected that you would go to college. Your 2 brothers had gone off to pharmacy school. I gather your sister did?

NMK: In those days girls were not expected to do what the boys did. My sister went for only about 2 semesters to SMU, then quit, and got married. She was working as a secretary.

WCR: Do all 3 of your siblings now live in Dallas?

NMK: Yes. My father passed away early at about age 55 when I was 17. None of us knew of his having any medical problems. He died suddenly after having had chest pain. My mother lived 84 years. She was active until she was 80, serving as a cashier at my brother's drug store.

WCR: I gather that not only were you receiving your education at public high school but the Hebrew education you were receiving at the synagogue was a very important aspect of your education. I gather you learned to speak Hebrew fluently and your siblings as well. Could you discuss that briefly?

NMK: The speaking of Hebrew is something I never really picked up. I could read it and I could understand it pretty well, but in Dallas it is difficult to maintain your fluency. It did, however, play an important role in my life. When I was a junior medical student in Dallas in 1952, a friend of my family had a son who was going to have his Bar Mitzvah, and to do that the child has to stand up and read a part of the Bible in Hebrew. This kid did not know how to read Hebrew and he wanted to have the ceremony so they asked me if I would teach their kid how. I did and for about 5 years I supported myself and my family by teaching Jewish kids how to do their Bar Mitzvah. I would go out to their homes and charge $4.00 per hour to give these lessons. Four dollars an hour in 1954 or 1955 was a lot of money. I would make probably at the end of the week $25 to $30 from these lessons. That was a sizable part of our income.

I have always tried to maintain a reasonably close

Jewish identity. We have become, as has been true for a lot of Jewish people in the USA, less and less Orthodox. My wife and I now attend a conservative and occasionally one of the reform temples in Dallas. We have always tried to maintain a pretty close identity to the Jewish community. I have served, for example, on the board of the Dallas Jewish Federation. I was the first President of the Dallas Memorial Center for the Holocaust.

About 1964 I got involved in some Dallas Public School politics. This was right after the Kennedy assassination and Dallas was going through a major search of its own consciousness because many of us felt that Dallas had become somewhat reactionary in its attitude about a lot of things. About 6 weeks before the Kennedy assassination, Adlai Stevenson had come to Dallas and was spat on when speaking at SMU. There was a lot of antigovernment feelings in Dallas, which was sort of a "redneck haven." The public schools were woefully inadequate and underfunded. We had no kindergartens, no vocational education, no bilingual education. The teachers were paid at the very bottom of the level of teacher pay. Our tax base was very low. The whole system was run by what we referred to in those days as "the Dallas oligarchy," a small group of downtown businessmen, mainly bankers and insurance executives. They did things in Dallas because they were good for business. For instance, the integration of the schools, which had to be done because the courts were pressing all the school systems, was done without any agitation whatsoever. The reason was because the business community did not want to have Dallas look like Little Rock. Therefore, they passed an ordinance that prohibited 3 or more people getting together without the police being able to disperse them. Public protests consequently were prevented.

In early 1964, I happened to go to a meeting called by a few people to do something about our public schools. At the meeting, I spoke up and said, "We have to get organized. If we are going to change anything, we have to take over the school board." The school board was elected by the whole city in 1 at-large election. We decided that we would start a group of citizens trying to influence the vote for the Dallas School Board. We started an organization called the League for Educational Advancement in Dallas. Dr. Richard Crout (who later ran the FDA) and I were among those who started this organization and I was president for the first 4 years. In the next 5 to 7 years we really took over the Dallas school system by electing a group of outstanding citizens to the Dallas School Board, including Dan Foster who is now Chairman of our Department of Medicine. We got rid of the superintendent, who had been there for 24 years, and had been running it as a tight oligarchy. We brought in a young man, who, would you believe, came from the federal government, a native Texan named Nolan Estes, and he took over the Dallas School System. Subsequent to that a lot of changes came and a lot of improvements were made. Then we were forced by the courts to integrate the Dallas School System and that resulted in busing. Virtually all the improvements we made in the Dallas School System were destroyed by the public antagonism to the idea of busing. Busing, though it accomplished integration, polarized the community. Even people who wanted to work to improve the public school system took their kids out of public schools and put them in private schools. This happened over much of the country. It unfortunately was a major detriment to the attempts that good citizens were making to try to upgrade the public schools. Eventually in Dallas, the minority populations (Hispanics and African-Americans) became the majority in the Dallas public schools. The white citizens fled to the suburbs. I was involved with the school system for about 10 years (1965-1975). Because of the integration of the school system much of the support that we had engendered from the general community was dissipated. Unfortunately, busing destroyed this amalgam that we had of citizens wanting to do what we had to do to improve the public school system.

I have considered myself a good liberal Democrat all these years. That has become a rare bird in Dallas, which is a very Republican community.

WCR: Dr. Kaplan, let me go back a little bit. I am intrigued by your growing up. When you were in high school, did you participate very much in extracurricular activities? Were you in the band? Did you play an instrument? Did you participate in sports?

NMK: I did play some tennis. I had begun to play tennis when I was in my young teens and I got to be fairly good. I lettered in tennis at Forest High School my senior year. I got involved in the debate team. That may have had a considerable influence on my latter public speaking abilities because we did have that same woman, Mrs. Melson, as the sponsor of the debating team. We debated once a week after school. I think that may have also helped sharpen my communicative skills. I was asked to run for the presidency of the senior class. I came up against a tall handsome WASP who promised that if he were elected that he would allow people to chew gum and get out of school an hour early, both of which obviously were totally irrelevant, but he got elected by a landslide. I was gangly and not very outgoing.

WCR: How did you get back and forth to the University of Texas?

NMK: Hitchhiking. In those days it was safe. Every 6 to 8 weeks when I came home or returned to college I made a sign and went out on the highway. The sign said, "Ride to Dallas or Ride to Austin." I had no problem. I probably was able to get back and forth as fast as you could drive. I was an ordinary looking kid with a little suitcase. I don't think I ever paid and I never flew on an airplane. I did get into a fraternity in Austin, likely because my older brother was a founding member. I think that played a major role in my social development, getting in with a group of somewhat more mature and socially advanced young men, and also some veterans. We did have some of the older guys who had come back from the Army under the GI Bill of Rights.

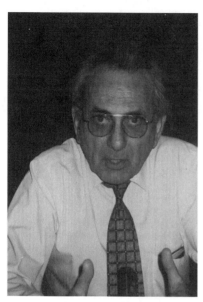

FIGURE 5. NMK at the time of the interview.

My mother sent me $100 a month to live on, for room, board, and books. Occasionally, I ran out of money and sent postcards (that my mother saved) that said, "Mom, please send me $7.50 so I can get a haircut and get my bicycle tire fixed." I waited tables at one the women's dorms to add to my income, and also to be able to get free meals. I worked all through college as a waiter at the LittleField Dorm. I was entranced by a lot of the young women and I certainly had not seen so many women up close in one place in all my life.

WCR: You and your high school girlfriend went to the University of Texas at about the same time?

NMK: Yes.

WCR: You got married at age 19?

NMK: We got married about 4 or 5 months after I came back to Dallas, after entering medical school.

WCR: Did you work during medical school? Was that a financial burden for you?

NMK: Fortunately, my wife worked as the secretary for the Rabbi at Temple Emmanuel, Levi Olin, who later became a member of the Board of Regents at the University of Texas. She supported me during medical school. I added to our income by teaching Hebrew to the Bar Mitzvah kids. During the first 2 summers, when we were out of school, I worked as a pharmacist in my brother's drug store.

WCR: When you finished medical school in 1954, you were debt free?

NMK: Yes. I then started internship at Parkland Hospital and it paid $25.00 a month, plus meals and laundry. My wife again supported me when I was a

house officer. We had our first child delivered the day before I graduated. I gave the Regent a cigar as he handed me my diploma. We had 4 daughters between 1954 and 1960. Two of them have become doctors, the other 2 are married to businessmen. Each of the 4 have children, and they have provided me with 9 grandchildren. I went into a second marriage 22 years ago and took on 2 stepsons who are out in California. My wife on her side has 4 grandchildren so between us we have 13 grandchildren. We are planning a large Passover together in April in Santa Fe, where we have a little house, with 12 adults and 13 grandchildren. We don't get together as a single family very often. I see the kids mainly when I travel to give talks. One daughter is an infertility obstetrician at Emory (Atlanta), and one daughter is a psychiatrist at the University of Cincinnati Medical School. Both of them married physicians who are on the same faculties. One daughter is in real estate in Austin with her husband, and 1 is in Detroit, Michigan, married to a real estate developer.

WCR: Other than Dr. Seldin, who mentored you in medical school and during your house officer period?

NMK: There was *Abraham Braude*, who came here as one of the very first appointees that Dr. Seldin made as Head of Infectious Disease. Abe Braude was a very gentle but tough investigator and teacher. As a second year resident, he took me under his wing and I did a little research project with him, and it resulted in my first publication. Abe had a strong influence; he encouraged me to become an academic physician. Beyond that, I think I got a lot of encouragement from my fellow residents, because as Seldin took over the department and developed it, we had a good group of bright young people. When I was at the NIH, 4 or 5 of these fellow house officers were also there. He was sending them up to NIH and to other places. He sent John Fortran to Boston to work with Franz Ingelfinger in gastroenterology. At the time there were only 12 to 18 interns and residents in Medicine. Today there are about 40 each year.

Parkland was and still is a great teaching hospital. I am very proud of the way Parkland has developed through the years and has become one of the premier teaching hospitals in the country. Dallas has continued to support Parkland in a very outstanding way. *Dr. Ron Anderson*, who has been our Chief Executive Officer, I think is an outstanding person. As is common now in a lot of places, we have opened up about 12 community outpatient facilities where people are now able to get their primary care and only come to Parkland when they get sick and need to be hospitalized or need to be seen by a specialist.

WCR: When you left your chief residency in 1958 and went into the military (San Antonio), you had actually not had any subspecialty training? I gather when you went to Lackland Air Force Base you were Head of Endocrinology and Metabolism there? Was that something you sought or how did that come about? You wrote several papers during your military experience?

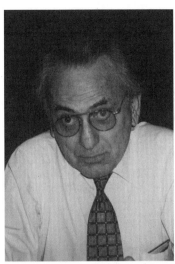

FIGURE 6. NMK at the time of the interview.

NMK: That was almost luck. *Dr. Arthur Grollman* was Head of Experimental Pharmacology at the medical school. He was one of the outstanding people in experimental medicine. He had developed the process of measuring cardiac output by using the Fick principle about 1920. He also developed peritoneal dialysis as an experimental tool to keep dogs alive after he had excised their kidneys. Arthur was a true loner, very critical, and a very tough investigator. He wrote the standard textbook on pharmacology that was used countrywide for a long time. Arthur was also a Brigadier General in the Air Force Reserves and at that time he was the major consultant to the Air Force for endocrinology. When I was a third year resident I started some projects with Dr. Leonard Madison and Dr. Seldin as my mentors on diabetic nephropathy on rats. I had also done a couple of studies on insulin passing through the liver under the direction of *Dr. Leonard Madison*. So as a third year resident I got involved in some research projects that related to endocrinology, mainly to diabetes. I was deferred by the Berry Plan until completion of my residency.

In 1958 when I completed my residency, I went into the Air Force. I was assigned to the SAC Headquarters in Omaha, Nebraska. I looked on the map and saw where Omaha was and I realized I did not want to go there. I had never really worked with Dr. Grollman but I had been told that he was somebody that the Air Force respected. I went to Arthur: "Dr. Grollman, can you help me get a better assignment in the Air Force?," and he said "No problem." He picked up the phone, talked to somebody in Washington, and I was reassigned to Lackland Air Force Base and appointed

the Head of Endocrinology there. They were looking for a young doctor who was trained in endocrinology. This was a consultant hospital for the entire Air Force and patients were referred there from all over the world. I had not had a lot of formal training in endocrinology. Once I wrote down that my interest was endocrinology, even though I had no Boards or fellowship specific to that field; when I arrived there they appointed me head of Endocrinology. We took care of all the diabetic and the thyroid patients. There were many young outstanding physicians who came into the Air Force at that time. There was *Roscoe Robinson* who became the Dean at Vanderbilt, retiring just last year, *Bill Ord*, a cardiologist who helped develop the program for space medicine, and *Steve Boehring* who became the Dean of Indiana Medical School. We saw literally 100s of patients with pituitary problems, because this was the primary neurosurgery hospital where they did most of the neurosurgery for the entire Air Force. Even though I was the Chief I really was not that well trained, but I was able to manage, and learned a lot.

WCR: How did it come about that you went to the National Heart Institute at the National Institutes of Health in Bethesda, Maryland? I gather you were there just one year under Fred Bartter?

NMK: That arrangement was made by Dr. Seldin.

WCR: That was the first experience you had, I gather, doing basic laboratory research. Did you enjoy that? How did it impact you in later years?

NMK: I learned the techniques. I did not particularly appreciate or enjoy the laboratory bench type of work. I did it and I think we did some good work which was published in the *Journal of Clinical Investigation*, but it was not the sort of thing I felt I really wanted to do long term. I was much more interested in the clinical aspects from the beginning. At the Clinical Center (the NIH Hospital) there were lots of patients under Dr. Bartter's supervision with Addison's disease, postural edema, calcium abnormalities, hypertension and, of course, Bartter's syndrome of juxtaglomerular hyperplasia. Bartter was a very eclectic endocrine investigator, interested in a lot of different problems. Once or twice a week we would make rounds on the patients that were in the Clinical Center under his direction, and it was a very eye-opening experience for a young clinical investigator. Bartter was an excellent researcher. He was very quiet and soft spoken, and when making rounds with him you had to bend over and try to catch what he was saying. Bartter was not a good teacher but he was a wonderful investigator. He was very tough and very critical about his work. I certainly accepted that as a necessary requirement to become an academic physician.

When I came back to Dallas I immediately set up the steroid assays that I had learned at the NIH and got involved in aldosterone. That led very quickly into looking for primary aldosteronism clinically. We continued some studies on the basic mechanisms of steroid production of aldosterone synthesis, but then that became less and less of my interest. I became more and more clinically oriented.

WCR: So although you sort of got started as an endocrinologist, you evolved into a systemic hypertension expert. How did that come about? When did you realize that this is the thing you wanted to focus on?

NMK: I was interested in aldosterone and renin and was asked to see patients who had problems with endocrine hypertension. Then one day I said to myself, "I don't need to be another one of the general endocrine people here because we have a lot of them around." *Charlie Pak* had come down here from the NIH where he had worked with Bartter and he took over the calcium area at the medical center. Siperstein, Unger, Madison, Foster, and Wilson were all there involved in diabetes. I decided to focus on hypertension and I opened the hypertension clinic. We started as a branch of endocrinology, and became a separate division of hypertension in the mid-1970s. Through the years we have had only 1 to 3 fellows and 1 or 2 faculty people. I never tried to develop a large group of people. That might be considered a fault because we were not able to attract big grants but I did maintain my NIH sponsorship through research grants for about 20 years. I did not get involved in large projects. Beginning in the 1970s and going on until now my interest has really been in the larger area of clinical hypertension. I focus more on the endocrine forms of hypertension, but I realize that is only 1% of the entire hypertension picture. I gradually looked at areas other than the endocrine one.

WCR: Could you describe what being an intern was like in 1954 or being a Chief resident in 1958 compared to the training schedules of today. Did you work every other night?

NMK: Those were the days when house officers were expected to work hard and not get paid very much. We always had good supervision. Dr. Seldin and the other members of the faculty made rounds with us every day. We had a lot of good conferences. Even in those days when there were relatively few house officers and few faculty, it was a fairly intense academic environment. We did a lot of work on our own. I recall some nights taking care of bad heart failure patients and various and sundry serious problems where I did not feel terribly adequate. Gradually, the house officers became a much more sophisticated group and we became a very strong academic department, but in those early times occasionally it got a little scary for having to deal with problems without a lot of ancillary help. You were expected to get help if you needed it and to go to the library. We did not have Medline searches then. I recall going to the library in the middle of the night to try to find out how to deal with a patient's problems.

It was a heady time here because things were just blossoming. New people were being brought in. *Carlton Chapman* was brought in as the Head of Cardiology. He later became President of the American Heart Association, President at Dartmouth. One of the things Dr. Seldin maintained for his 35 years as the Head of the Department of Medicine was that you had to do research. You could not just be a member of his

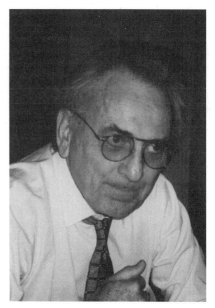

FIGURE 7. NMK at the time of the interview.

department unless you had a laboratory doing some kind of research. It was not required that it be bench research. Now, of course, the Department has changed. We now have a Department of General Medicine where the members are primarily taking care of patients, but that is a response to the managed care explosion to keep the medical school solvent. For many years, the medical faculty had very little contact with private patients. That was one of the reasons why we have a very good town-grown relationship. The members of the community of physicians in Dallas never looked upon the medical school faculty as competing with them. We are now competing with everyone else for patients.

WCR: When you were in medical school did you have a easy or difficult time deciding that you wanted to be an internist?

NMK: As a junior student, I thought I wanted to become either a pediatrician or a psychiatrist, but then Dr. Seldin grabbed me one day and said, "I'd like for you to go into internal medicine." His presence and what was happening in the Department of Medicine influenced me. Because I was still not absolutely secure about going into internal medicine, I decided to take a rotating rather than a straight medicine internship. By the time I started the internship, however, I was certain that I wanted to be an internist.

WCR: You became a full-time faculty member in 1961, and a full professor by age 41 in 1970. In the late 1960s, 1970s, and 1980s you started traveling a lot. You became recognized as a splendid teacher. I have participated in a few programs with you around the world and you are appreciated as the world's hypertension guru. You got your book going in 1973 and I gather you realized right away that this was a tremendous opportunity to have a worldwide impact. Let's say it's 1980. What were your daily activities like at that time? What time did you wake up in the mornings? What time did you get to work? When were you doing most of your writing? Do you do your writing with a pencil and paper or do you write on a computer? Do you dictate? Did you do most of that at home or did you do it at work? What time did you go to bed at night?

NMK: I have never been able to work in my office at the medical school. I have always done my writing and lecture preparing almost entirely at home where I've always had an office. I have done every bit of my writing with pencil and paper. I have the computers now, but I don't use them for this purpose. I still am not very good at it. If only I had passed typing in high school I think my whole future would have been different! I do work long and hard hours but likely no longer or harder than most academicians. We do a fair amount of traveling. Whenever I go to a nice place like Japan I take my wife and we do some vacationing at the same time. I don't recall taking a trip, maybe 1 or 2, through these years that was not medically related. Obviously, its very fortunate that somebody is paying for my travel. I have over the years accepted lectureships and professorships and have gone almost all over the world. I believe I am accepted here at our school as the hypertension person but I think I don't get the adoration and the acclaim that I get when I go elsewhere. I guess that is oftentimes true. You are probably more of a guru outside of your own home than you are at home.

It has been a very good life. I guess I am lucky that I picked hypertension because after all that is the most common disease that we all deal with; the most common indication for prescription drugs. I have enjoyed the travel very much. I obviously overdo it. I guess I am also lucky in having at the medical school the ability to take patients only as a consultant. I have not been the primary doctor for these patients so that I can get away without interfering with the care of the patients. I did not start it off purposely that way. I see 4 to 8 new consult patients a week on average. That is what I do in addition to the patients at Parkland that I deal with as a teacher. In the private realm, I see these patients sometimes for weeks or months, but follow them now mainly by phone and fax. They send me their home blood pressure readings and I give them advice. They don't have to come back frequently to have their blood pressures monitored. I see these patients and then send them back to their primary doctor which means I can go away to Japan for 10 days without the necessity of maintaining contact with a lot of sick people. I also find that the airplane is a wonderful place for me to write because there is nobody interfering.

WCR: I presume you never took summer vacations when you were growing up. When you went away to Austin to college was that the first time you had ever really been outside of Dallas, Texas? When was the first time you were outside of Texas, for example? Have you been given a hard time at the Medical School for traveling a lot? I put you in top rank among medical educators that I have witnessed personally. I have seen how hard you work at these places and how beneficial it is to Dallas, Texas, as well as to your medical school. Could you comment on that? Did your lack of travel in childhood make travel more exciting to you as an adult? Has your lack of money as a youngster made the seeking a dollar bill possibly a little more attractive as you have gotten older?

NMK: I think without question those influences must be playing a role. I remember the thrill of going to Galveston for a family vacation as a teenager. The first time I went out of Texas was for my fraternity's national convention when I was 18. Seeing the rest of the world has been enjoyable for me. I think my primary motivation has been the fact that I am being asked to do what I consider to be a legitimate part of an academic career, which is to lecture and participate in meetings and symposia. For me, lecturing and writing have become the primary purpose of my academic life. I don't have a lab anymore. Since I realized about 15 years ago that after having done that for 20 years, lab research was really not my primary interest.

Beyond the desire to teach, there is no question that getting the honoraria and the acclaim as you go to various and sundry places as a visitor has been a major influence on my willingness to do this. I also appreciate the fact that I must have a basic psychological insecurity when people ask me to do something, I have a hard time saying no, even if its not a matter of money or acclaim. I am asked to go down to San Antonio to the medical school and give a lecture to their class where I don't get anything but travel expense, and I would hardly ever say that I can't do it.

I don't think in looking back that my relationships with my kids and family were affected very much by it because I really did not get into this until the kids were grown and had left home. I attend on the inpatient medical services taking 1 or 2 rotations a year, which means about 3 months time when I don't go away, unless it is something like a major committee meeting of the Joint National Committee. When I am asked to have a conference with house staff or students I always make myself available. I do appreciate the fact that I would be doing a lot more in the way of patient contact if I were to stay in Dallas more rather than traveling.

The book has become quite successful and has also added significantly to my income, but even if I didn't make anything from that book I believe I would still work on it. I guess my bibliography has now gotten up close to 500 and most of those are things that people have invited me to do: to participate in supplements, symposia, etc. The ones that are on my basic investigative work probably are no more than 100. The rest have been invited in one way or another.

WCR: Dr. Kaplan, you have already mentioned how many people in the USA and around the world have systemic hypertension, an incredibly common occurrence. It is my understanding that possibly 60 million Americans have systemic blood pressures >140/90 mm Hg. You have already mentioned that you wrote the drug therapy section of the Joint National Committee Report. What you say about treatment of hypertension has an incredible impact, an effect not only on physicians but on profits to pharmaceutical companies. What you say can sway a lot of people whether or not, for example, to use calcium antagonists versus beta blockers versus ACE inhibitors. How do you handle this potential power? Do you think it is ethical for you in this power position to invest in pharmaceutical companies' stock, for example?

NMK: I recognize that what I say may have a goodly amount of influence upon the market at large and pharmaceutical sales of antihypertensives. It poses a challenge for me. I hope that I am not influenced by that sort of thing. In the Joint National Committee Report we did make a statement about the use of calcium antagonists that recommends broadening their use, but it was based upon a very good randomized controlled trial that was published in *Lancet* and had been presented earlier.

I know that there are people who have been very concerned about the calcium antagonist controversy. I have written favorable comments about calcium antagonists. I would believe, however, that has not been influenced by the fact that I have received honoraria from pharmaceutical companies that manufacture or market calcium antagonists, because I also receive honoraria from pharmaceutical companies that market every other class of antihypertensive drug. I don't have any particularly special relation with companies that market calcium antagonists. I try to be objective. I can't say that I have no bias, but, on the other hand, when I see the evidence that an α-blocker drug is good for lipids and insulin sensitivity, then I will write papers and talk about the usefulness of α blockers, whether they are being sponsored by one of the companies that make α blockers or not.

I am very careful when I present talks under the sponsorship of a pharmaceutical company. I also will not accept honoraria from pharmaceutical companies that market drugs that I do not approve or do not use. I have no problem in talking under the sponsorship of a β-blocker marketer, because as part of my talk, which is generally on all general aspects of treatment, I will say something nice about β blockers. Similarly, if I am talking under the auspices of an ACE inhibitor marketer, I will indicate that there are particular places where ACE inhibitors are useful drugs. I would not say only negative things about drugs marketed by a company that has asked me to give a talk under their auspices, but I do believe that my presentations are as unbiased as I can make them. I try to be very careful to maintain my integrity. I don't think I have given a talk on the treatment of hypertension in the last 10 years, where I have not emphasized the importance of non-drug therapy, lifestyle change, because I consider that to be a very important aspect of the treatment of hypertension. There is nobody marketing those lifestyle changes. I also recognize that I am there under

the sponsorship of a pharmaceutical company, and, therefore, I am going to say something about the products that this particular company makes, hopefully putting them in proper prospective which may include mention of adverse effects.

When I am asked to give a grand rounds at a medical school, and many of these are being sponsored by pharmaceutical companies, I rarely even do that much, because I assume that when I am asked to give a grand rounds it will be totally without any particular appreciation or attention to one pharmaceutical company's drugs. In those situations where I am presenting in an academic setting, my presentations are almost without any particular mention of one pharmaceutical company's products or another. Obviously, if I am talking about the drug treatment of hypertension I am talking about a variety of pharmaceutical companies' products and there is no way out of that.

WCR: You have been an advocate of non-drug treatment of hypertension for a long time. You seem to weigh less now than you did at one time in your life. You look quite healthy. What are you doing for your own health so that your blood pressure doesn't go up and your blood cholesterol levels don't get too high?

NMK: I try to live a life of moderation. I work out most every day, even when I am on the road. I believe that exercise is absolutely critical to good cardiovascular health and I practice what I preach. That is my way of keeping my weight under control, because part of travel is that you eat more than you do at home. I try to drink a little bit of alcohol on a regular daily basis. We keep a bottle of wine in our icebox and when I go out for a dinner I always have a glass or 2 of wine. I am a real believer in the protective effects of small amounts of alcohol. I eat a reasonably careful diet. I rarely have red meat or eggs. I think I follow the American Heart Association's guidelines of what is called the prudent diet, try to keep my weight under control, exercise regularly, drink a little bit, try to stay as unstressed as I can, although I admit I am a type A–but a happy type A. I am not one who is resentful or hostile. I taught Dean Ornish in Sunday School so he is someone I do relate to but I think his regimen is more than most patients will accept. I have not yet put myself on a statin drug because my cholesterol is only a little above 200 and since I don't have any other risk factors I figure I'm safe. But I recall some of your writings of a few years ago when you recommended that these drugs be much more widely advocated. I think time has actually proved you to be right. I thought you were a little bit wild at the time you were telling everybody to go on a statin, but I think we are all coming around to that because these drugs are so remarkably effective.

WCR: You talked about the "deadly quartet" and you popularized that syndrome: increased blood pressure, increased triglyceride levels, increased insulin, and increased upper body fat. That seems to put a lot of different things together. Could you comment on your analysis of that?

NMK: Actually other people, *Gerald Reaven* at Stanford and others, had talked about this syndrome, the insulin resistance syndrome, but in 1989 I gave a grand rounds here because of increasing awareness that hypertension was related to insulin resistance. I did extend the work of other people and I used that term first. I am not particularly proud of the "deadly quartet" as a term. Again, I don't think I made any original contributions to our understanding of this. I keep looking around America and we are so fat. You go to Japan and there is almost nobody overweight and they have one sixth as much coronary disease as we do. I clearly believe it has to be the lifestyle and the avoidance of obesity that makes the difference between our populations.

WCR: Dr. Kaplan, have you made any mistakes in your professional career? Is there anything you wish you had done that you did not do or certain things you did do that you wished you hadn't done?

NMK: I probably was a little bit too aggressive in attacking the aldosterone and the renin issues, but I have tried to be as objective and unbiased as I can be. I would have done more investigative work at our medical school, and been more actively involved in some projects with other associates in doing collaborative research. I headed the Hypertension Division at the medical school for about 18 years. *Ron Victor*, a bright young investigator, has recently replaced me. He is the prototype of the collaborative type of investigator. He has all kinds of people working with him. He is the kind of young man that I think if I were to go back I would try to emulate, doing collaborative work with other people to broaden the impact. The lecturing, writing, and teaching—I don't think I would want to change much of that. That is something I have enjoyed and I hope that I have been able to have a positive impact. I hope that I have been accepted as a relatively unbiased and objective person.

WCR: You talked about your being a loner as a child. In most of your publications you are usually the first author or the sole author. That can hardly be done today. When you started focusing on hypertension there was not anybody else to talk to. Now hypertension is being attacked by endocrinologists, cardiologists, nephrologists, etc. It has always bothered me that cardiologists as a group have ignored systemic hypertension. How do you get cardiologists interested in high blood pressure? They see oodles of patients with coronary disease, some of whom have hypertension.

NMK: I think part of it is because cardiologists have become so technologically oriented. There is nothing you really need to do that involves a catheter or an invasive procedure in the evaluation and management of patients with hypertension. Hypertension is a low technology area. For most patients all you have to do is take the blood pressure, take a good history and physical, get a little lab work, and start treating. I would hope that things are changing with cardiologists because of the recognition that heart failure, the most common indication for admission to general hospitals, is in large part the result of hypertension. The aging population with this tremendously high frequency of heart failure is forcing cardiologists to take a more active role in the earlier aspects of the disease so that they can treat the hypertension to prevent future heart failure.

Preventative cardiology has really never been a very popular aspect of medical care. Prevention is something that managed care operations might aggressively promote and pay for, and yet, when you spend an hour talking to a patient about the need for exercise and diet and all the other things, they don't pay any more than if you spend 5 minutes doing your regular office visit. I don't think it is true just of cardiologists. I think the same thing could be said of most areas. As specialists, we tend to deal primarily with the end results of problems that occur in patients.

WCR: What are your plans from here on? What do you want to accomplish now?

NMK: I have not thought about that seriously, although I did decide that now that I have gotten beyond age 65, I don't need the administrative hassling, so I voluntarily dropped the divisional Chiefship, although it was never a big responsibility of my life. I also wanted to make room for a younger person who I felt would be much better in expanding research on hypertension at our school. I am very pleased and satisfied with my current life situation. I would love to be able to continue to write, lecture, and see patients. I am very happy with the prospect of continuing to deal with hypertensive patients. I won't ever quit that. But I never wanted to be a full-time practitioner just dealing with patients. I like the balance between patient responsibilities as a consultant physician, the ability to write and lecture, and travel that I am now doing. I think it is a very pleasant and very productive mix that I am very pleased to be able to continue, and as long as my health holds out, as long as people want to hear me and read what I write, I think I will keep doing what I am doing now.

WCR: You must have gotten some opportunities to join one pharmaceutical company or another through the years? You have obviously declined those offers. It seems to me that there are more and more physicians, however, who have moved into the pharmaceutical arena in recent years and they had pretty good academic careers going for them. Could you comment on that?

NMK: I have had opportunities. I would immediately lose the one thing I probably want more than anything else, which is the general respect as an unbiased objective commentator on the whole area of hypertension. I want to maintain my independence. My current situation keeps me as independent as I want to be, and, therefore, I have resisted all the temptations that have been made available to me to take on these higher paying but more limiting kinds of work.

WCR: Could you comment just a moment on your television show, "Here's to Your Health", which I gather you received an Emmy nomination. You did that for about 4 years, 1984-1988.

NMK: It was fun. Actually it was something that was started by our local PBS station in cooperation with the medical school. *Dan Foster* was the first commentator on this program. Subsequent to that *Al Roberts* took it on. Then they asked me do it and I did for 4 years. I did enjoy very much being a ham in front of the screen. I understand they were being shown on 300 different stations, all through the PBS system. The Emmy nomination for daytime television came as a surprise. That was the first time that PBS had ever been nominated. I was beat out that year by Phil Donahue. It was sort of an ego trip but I do believe in public communication and making people aware. We talked about all sorts of things: depression, epilepsy, osteoarthritis, hypertension, coronary disease, etc., and got some good people to come to Dallas and we did some traveling to interview people elsewhere. It became so expensive that after awhile they could not justify continuing. I think that television has not provided good health information to the public. I don't know why but perhaps the public just does not want to look at such programming, unless its ER. I know we have some commentators on national television that give little snips, like Tim Johnson on ABC. I really wonder why we can't do a better job of that, but obviously we can't and so far commercial television has never bought into it.

WCR: Dr. Kaplan, are you concerned about the changes in health care delivery in the USA?

NMK: We are all going through the major revolution of managed care. I am obviously concerned as I am sure every academician is about the continued support of medical education and indigent patient care. We do a good job of it in Dallas but it is a strain on the taxpayers. There are >40 million Americans without their own health insurance. We are the only industrialized country in the world without a national health scheme of some sort. I am enough of a realist to realize that the federal government oftentimes messes things up and we can't have a solitary national health scheme, but the idea of single payer of health care is appealing to me. Take Canada as a good example of the way we ought to look at the future of providing adequate health coverage for our population. I think they have recognized that there has to be tax based on income to provide health care and then let the government stand away and let practitioners take care of their patients without other interference. I wish the Clinton attempt 4 years ago had been better thought out because there were some very good aspects of it. I believe, however, that a monolithic federally controlled health care system would not be appropriate. A single payer to raise the funds to provide health care and insure the entire population seems to me to be a very rational thing.

WCR: Although we are a big country, Dr. Kaplan, with 268 million people, do we really need 125 medical schools? We have 8 in the state of Texas. Granted Texas is the second largest state in the country, but are we producing too many physicians? A hungry doctor it seems to me is one of the most dangerous humans walking around.

NMK: Yes. I have been a firm believer for a long time that any time you put a doctor out there, he or she is going to generate enough business to make a good living. I think that has been well shown. The more physicians, the more hospital beds you have, the more they are utilized. We have to cut down on the number of specialists and we have to increase the number of primary care physicians. The concept of managed care's providing a gatekeeper to bring people into appropriate medical care is absolutely correct. I have no inherent bias against managed care. As a consequence, we get swamped at Parkland Hospital in the emergency room everyday with people who don't have a primary care provider and don't have any insurance. The number of doctors clearly has to be controlled and we do have to try to ensure an adequate number of primary care physicians. Cutting back on the number of specialists makes good sense.

WCR: Dr. Kaplan, I have enjoyed our conversation, and I appreciate your sharing a bit of your life and your views with the AJC readers.

NMK: My pleasure, Bill.

BEST PUBLICATIONS OF NMK SELECTED BY NMK

10. Kaplan NM, Bartter FC. The effects of ACTH, renin, angiotensin II and various precursors on biosynthesis of aldosterone by adrenal slices. *J Clin Invest* 1962;41:715–724.

15. Kaplan NM, Silah JG. The angiotensin infusion test: a new approach to the differential diagnosis of renovascular hypertension. *N Engl J Med* 1964;271:536–541.

16. Kaplan NM, Silah JG. The effect of angiotensin II on the blood pressure in humans with hypertensive disease. *J Clin Invest* 1964;43:659–669.

19. Kaplan NM. The biosynthesis of adrenal steroids: effects of angiotensin II, ACTH and potassium. *J Clin Invest* 1965;44:2029–2039.

22. Kaplan NM. Hypokalemia in the hypertensive patient: with observations on the incidence of primary aldosteronism. *Ann Intern Med* 1967;66:1079–1090.

23. Kaplan NM. The steroid content of adrenal adenomas and measurements of aldosterone production in patients with essential hypertension and primary aldosteronism. *J Clin Invest* 1967;46:728–734.

25. Jose A, Kaplan NM. Plasma renin activity in the diagnosis of primary aldosteronism. *Arch Intern Med* 1969;123:141–146.

27. Jose A, Crout R, Kaplan NM. Suppressed plasma renin activity in essential hypertension: roles of plasma volume, blood pressure, and sympathetic nervous system. *Ann Intern Med* 1970;72:9–16.

32. Saruta T, Saade GA, Kaplan NM. A possible mechanism for hypertension induced by oral contraceptives: diminished feed-back suppression of renin release. *Arch Intern Med* 1970;126:621–626.

38. Saruta T, Cook R, Kaplan NM. Adrenocortical steroidogenesis: studies on the mechanism of action of angiotensin and electrolytes. *J Clin Invest* 1972;51:2239–2251.

46. Kaplan NM. The prognostic implications of plasma renin in essential hypertension. *JAMA* 1975;231:167–170.

51. Kaplan NM, Kem DC, Holland OB, Kramer NJ, Higgins J, Gomez-Sanchez C. The intravenous furosemide test: a simple way to evaluate renin responsiveness. *Ann Intern Med* 1976;84:639–645.

53. Kaplan NM. Renin profiles: the unfulfilled promises. *JAMA* 1977;238:611–613.

54. Kaplan NM, Kramer NJ, Holland OB, Sheps SG, Gomex-Sanchez C. Single-voided urine metanephrine assays in screening for pheochromocytoma. *Arch Intern Med* 1977;137:190–193.

73. Ram CVS, Garrett BN, Kaplan NM. Moderate sodium restriction and various diuretics in the treatment of hypertension: effects of potassium wastage and blood pressure control. *Arch Intern Med* 1981;141:1015–1019.

79. Kaplan NM, Simmons M, McPhee C, Carnegie A, Stafanu C, Cade S. Two techniques to improve adherence to dietary sodium restriction in the treatment of hypertension. *Arch Intern Med* 1982;142:1638–1641.

85. Kaplan NM. Mild hypertension—when & how to treat. *Arch Intern Med* 1983;143:255–259.

98. Kaplan NM. Dietary salt intake and blood pressure. *JAMA* 1984;251:1429–1430.

125. Kaplan NM, Carnegie A, Raskin P, Heller JA, Simmons M. Potassium supplementation in hypertensive patients with diuretic-induced hypokalemia. *N Engl J Med* 1985;312:746–749.

134. Kaplan NM, Meese RB. The calcium deficiency hypothesis of hypertension: a critique. *Ann Intern Med* 1986;105:947–955.

143. Meese RB, Gonzalez DG, Casparian JM, Ram CVS, Pak CM, Kaplan NM. The inconsistent effects of calcium supplements upon blood pressure in primary hypertension. *Am J Med Sci* 1987;294:219–224.

156. Kaplan NM. Maximally reducing cardiovascular risk in the treatment of hypertension. *Ann Intern Med* 1988;36–40.

161. Kaplan NM. Calcium entry blockers in the treatment of hypertension. Current status and future prospects. *JAMA* 1989;262:817–823.

171. Kaplan NM. The deadly quartet: upper body obesity, glucose intolerance, hypertriglyceridemia and hypertension. *Arch Intern Med* 1989;149:1514–1520.

214. Khoury AF, Kaplan NM. Alpha-blocker therapy of hypertension. An unfulfilled promise. *JAMA* 1991;266:397–398.

233. Kaplan NM. The appropriate goals of antihypertensive therapy: neither too much nor too little. *Ann Intern Med* 1992;116:686–690.

235. Khoury AF, Sunderajan P, Kaplan NM. The early morning rise in blood pressure is related mainly to ambulation. *Am J Hypertens* 1992;5 (6 Pt 1):339–344.

250. Kaplan NM. Management of hypertensive emergencies. *Lancet* 1994;344:1335–1338.

251. Kaplan NM. Alcohol and hypertension. *Lancet* 1995;345:1588–1589.

252. Kaplan NM. Difficult to treat hypertension. *Am J Med Sci* 1995;309:339–346.

270. Kaplan NM. Gifford R W JR. Choice of initial therapy for hypertension. *JAMA* 1996;275:1577–1580.

272. Kaplan NM. Anxiety-induced hypertension. *Arch Intern Med* 1997;157:945–948.

739

Author Index

Subject Index

Abciximab
  effects in diabetes, 265–266
  effects in unplanned coronary stent
    deployment, 307–308
  inhibiting cell adhesion, 269
  for platelet aggregation inhibition,
    253
  reducing ischemic complications in
    directional atherectomy,
    326–328
  and results of stenting with
    angioplasty, 293
  short-term therapy with, 324–325
  in treatment of narrowed saphenous
    vein grafts, 269
  in unstable angina, 190–191
  use after coronary stent placement,
    309
  and vascular access site
    complications, 264
Abdominal obesity in men, and
    hyperinsulinemia, 144
Adenosine
  effects on antegrade and retrograde
    fast pathway conduction,
    462–463
  intravenous, with lidocaine in acute
    infarction, 245
  perfusion imaging for left bundle
    branch block, 135
Adenosine triphosphate in diagnosis of
    dual AV nodal pathways, 462
Adhesion molecules
  estrogen affecting, 122–123
  expression in endothelial cells, 38
  in hypertriglyceridemia, 41–43
  intercellular, postangioplasty
    levels of, 258–259
  role in serine proteases, 37–38
  serum levels in atherosclerosis,
    25–26
β-Adrenergic blocking drugs. *See* Beta-
    blockers
Adrenomedullin predicting
    postinfarction left ventricular
    function, 239–230
African-American men, exercise effects
    in hypertension, 422–423
Age groups, cardiac findings at
    necropsy, 234–235

Aging
  and aortic valve replacement in older
    patients, 432
  and cardiovascular events in
    depressed elderly persons, 152
  and coronary stenting in patients 75
    years of age or older, 321
  and emotional support for elderly
    heart failure patients, 382–384
  and mortality in elderly patients after
    bypass grafting, 328
  and patterns of change in lipids,
    88–89
Albumin excretion rate predicting
    mortality, 225–226
Alcohol intake
  affecting lipoprotein levels, 52
  withdrawal from
    affecting LDL particle size, 56–57
    lipoprotein(a) levels in, 57
Alteplase compared to streptokinase in
    pulmonary embolism, 499
Amiodarone
  compared to sotalol in atrial
    fibrillation, 472
  effects in atrial flutter, 466
  for heart rate control in critically ill
    patients, 473
Amlodipine
  in angina, 181
    compared to diltiazem, 182
  in heart failure, 385
  safety of, 424–425
Amyloidosis, and sudden cardiac death,
    373
Anergy to skin tests, evaluation in heart
    failure, 370–371
Aneurysms
  abdominal aortic
    degradation of elastic tissue in,
      506–507
    in-hospital cost of repair, 508
    pathogenesis of, 509–511
  coronary, in Kawasaki disease,
    513–514
  thoracic aortic, inheritance of,
    508–509
Angina
  amlodipine in, 181
    compared to diltiazem, 182
  coronary calcium patterns in, 172

nonfenestrated, 566–567
protein-losing enteropathy after, 566
thromboembolism after, 567
Fosinopril compared to enalapril in
heart failure, 375

Gemfibrozil affecting endothelial
function, 39
Gender
and early outcome of myocardial
infarction, 215–216
and prevalence of intermittent
claudication, 487–488
and ventricular function in right
bundle branch block, 463
Gene transfer, intramuscular, for
angiogenesis in ischemic limbs,
496–497
Genetics
angiotensinogen gene variants and
insulin resistance in nondiabetic
men, 155–156
conotruncal defects with 22q11
deletions, 549–550
factor VII gene polymorphisms in
myocardial infarction, 224–225
β-fibrinogen polymorphisms in
carotid atherosclerosis, 488
gene mutations in long QT
syndrome, 445, 446–448
glycoprotein lbα polymorphism in
coronary artery disease, 214–215
inheritance of thoracic aortic
aneurysms, 508–509
methylenetetrahydrofolate reductase
gene polymorphism in strokes,
491
molecular diagnosis for
cardiovascular disease, 556–558
monocyte chemoattractant protein-1
gene expression in endothelial
cells, 35–36
myosin-binding protein C gene
mutations in hypertrophic
cardiomyopathy, 562
paroxonase gene polymorphism, 61
in coronary artery disease,
151–152
troponin T gene mutation in
hypertrophic cardiomyopathy,
393–394
tumor necrosis factor polymorphisms
in heart failure, 368–370
Genistein
affecting arterial compliance in
women, 90
and cholesterol production by basic
protein-2, 55–56
and oxidation of LDL, 17–18

Gla protein, matrix, role in vascular
calcification, 36
Glucose levels
hyperglycemia affecting
endothelium-dependent
vasodilation, 29–30
and lipoprotein(a) concentrations,
77–78
Glutathione affecting endothelial
vasomotor function, 26–27
Glycoprotein
1bα polymorphisms in coronary
artery disease, 214–215
platelet receptor blockade. *See*
Platelets, glycoprotein IIb/IIIa
receptor blockade

Hand grip
apexcardiographic test in
hypertrophic cardiomyopathy,
391–392
exercise with stress
echocardiography, 137–138
Heart block
duration after surgery, 563
left bundle branch, tomographic
perfusion imaging for, 135
neonatal, in maternal lupus, 552
right bundle branch
and gender difference in
ventricular function, 463
and ST segment changes in leads
V_1—V_3, 464
Heart failure, 363–414
advanced, low lymphocyte count in,
584–585
after aortic valve replacement,
431–432
amyloidosis in, 373
and anergy to skin tests, 370–371
brain natriuretic peptide levels in,
367
cardiac endothelin receptors in,
364–365
cellular expression of nitric oxide
synthase in, 367–368
circulating levels of C-C chemokines
in, 368
dopamine affecting ventilation in,
386
emotional support for elderly
patients in, 382–384
evaluation of pacing sites in, 384–385
exercise capacity in
with left ventricular assist device,
411–412
losartan or enalapril affecting, 377
medical therapy or
revascularization affecting,
388–389